Health Promotion

THROUGHOUT THE LIFE SPAN

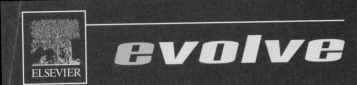

To access your *Student Resources*, visit:

http://evolve.elsevier.com/Edelman/

Evolve Student Resources for *Edelman/Mandle: Health Promotion Throughout the Life Span,* **sixth edition,** offer the following features:

Student Resources

- **WebLinks**
  An exciting resource that lets you link to numerous web sites carefully chosen to supplement the content of the textbook.

- **Web Site Resources**
  Resources such as forms, assessment tools, illustrations, and tables that supplement the chapter discussion.

- **Content Updates**
  The latest content updates to keep you current with recent developments in health promotion.

- **Glossary**
  Comprehensive list of all Key Terms and their definitions. Search capability allows searching by term, definition, or chapter.

Sixth Edition

Health Promotion

THROUGHOUT THE LIFE SPAN

Carole Lium Edelman, APRN, BC, CMC

Director of Outpatient Programs
Waveny Care Center
New Canaan, Connecticut;
Associate Faculty Member
Yale University School of Nursing
New Haven, Connecticut;
Fellow, Brookdale Center on Aging
Hunter College
New York, New York

Carol Lynn Mandle, PhD, RN, CS, FNP

Associate Professor
Boston College School of Nursing
Chestnut Hill, Massachusetts;
Co-Director, Medical Symptoms Reduction Programs
Mind-Body Medical Institute
Beth Israel Deaconess Medical Center
Harvard Medical School;
Kenneth B. Schwartz Fellow
Chaplaincy Department
Massachusetts General Hospital
Boston, Massachusetts

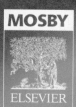

MOSBY

ELSEVIER

ELSEVIER
MOSBY

11830 Westline Industrial Drive
St. Louis, Missouri 63146

HEALTH PROMOTION THROUGHOUT THE LIFE SPAN

ISBN-13: 978-0-323-03128-8
ISBN-10: 0-323-03128-5

Notice

Knowledge and best practice in this field are constantly changing. As new research and experience broaden our knowledge, changes in practice, treatment and drug therapy may become necessary or appropriate. Readers are advised to check the most current information provided (i) on procedures featured or (ii) by the manufacturer of each product to be administered, to verify the recommended dose or formula, the method and duration of administration, and contraindications. It is the responsibility of the practitioner, relying on their own experience and knowledge of the patient, to make diagnoses, to determine dosages and the best treatment for each individual patient, and to take all appropriate safety precautions. To the fullest extent of the law, neither the Publisher nor the authors assumes any liability for any injury and/or damage to persons or property arising out or related to any use of the material contained in this book.

The Publisher

Previous editions copyrighted 2002, 1998, 1994, 1990, and 1986

ISBN-13: 978-0-323-03128-8
ISBN-10: 0-323-03128-5

Executive Editor: Darlene Como
Managing Editor: Linda Thomas
Publications Services Manager: John Rogers
Project Manager: Doug Turner
Senior Designer: Kathi Gosche

Printed in Canada
Last digit is the print number: 9 8 7 6 5 4 3

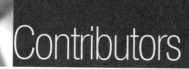

Contributors

Carolyn Spence Cagle, PhD, RNC
Associate Professor, Harris College of Nursing
College of Health and Human Services
Texas Christian University
Fort Worth, Texas
Chapter 16, The Prenatal Period
Chapter 20, School-Age Child

Martha Driessnack, PhDc, ARNP
Oregon Health & Science University
Portland, Oregon
*Chapter 15, Overview of Growth and Development
    Framework*
Chapter 18, Toddler
Chapter 21, Adolescent

Carole Lium Edelman, APRN, BC, CMC
Director of Outpatient Programs, Waveny Care Center
New Canaan, Connecticut;
Associate Faculty Member, Yale University School of
    Nursing
New Haven, Connecticut;
Fellow, Brookdale Center on Aging
Hunter College
New York, New York
*Chapter 1, Health Defined: Objectives for Promotion and
    Prevention*

Pamela Grace, PhD, ARNP
Assistant Professor, William F. Connell School of Nursing
Boston College
Chestnut Hill, Massachusetts
Chapter 5, Ethical Issues Relevant to Health Promotion

Philip A. Greiner, DNSc, RN
Associate Professor
Director, Undergraduate Program
Director, Health Promotion Center
School of Nursing
Fairfield University
Fairfield, Connecticut
*Chapter 1, Health Defined: Objectives for Promotion and
    Prevention*

Sheila Grossman, PhD, APRN-BC
Professor, FNP Specialty Director
School of Nursing
Fairfield University
Fairfield, Connecticut
Chapter 23, Middle-Age Adult

Susan A. Heady, RN, PhD
Associate Professor, Nursing Department
Webster University
St. Louis, Missouri
Chapter 10, Health Education

June Andrews Horowitz, PhD, APRN-C, FAAN
Associate Professor, William F. Connell School of Nursing
Boston College
Chestnut Hill, Massachusetts
Chapter 4, The Therapeutic Relationship
Chapter 13, Stress Management

Kathleen Huttlinger, PhD, FNP
Professor, College of Nursing
Kent State University
Kent, Ohio
*Chapter 25, Health Promotion in the Twenty-First Century:
    Throughout the Lifespan and Throughout the World*

Debora Elizabeth Kirsch, PhD(c), CNS, MS, RN
Assistant Professor, College of Nursing
SUNY Upstate Medical University
Syracuse, New York
Chapter 3, Health Policy and the Delivery System

Elizabeth C. Kudzma, DNSc, MPH, RNC
Professor, Division of Nursing and Health Studies
Curry College
Milton, Massachusetts
Chapter 22, Young Adult

Regina Lowry, RN, MSN, PhD(c)
Lecturer, College of Nursing
Energy Therapist, Markey Cancer Center
University of Kentucky
Lexington, Kentucky
Chapter 14, Holistic Health Strategies

Margaret K. Macali, MS, RN, CS
Director, Office of Public Health Nursing Services
Bergen County Department of Health Services
Paramus, New Jersey
Chapter 9, Screening

Carol Lynn Mandle, PhD, RN, CS, FNP
Associate Professor, Boston College School of Nursing
Chestnut Hill, Massachusetts;
Co-Director, Medical Symptoms Reduction Programs
Mind-Body Medical Institute
Beth Israel Deaconess Medical Center
Harvard Medical School;
Kenneth B. Schwartz Fellow, Chaplaincy Department
Massachusetts General Hospital
Boston, Massachusetts
Chapter 13, Stress Management
Chapter 23, Middle-Age Adult

Heather O'Brien Gillespie, MSPT
Senior Physical Therapist, Rusk Institute of Rehabilitative
    Medicine
New York University Medical Center
New York, New York
Chapter 12, Exercise

Anne Rath Rentfro, MSN, RN
Associate Professor, School of Health Sciences
University of Texas at Brownsville
Brownsville, Texas
Chapter 6, Health Promotion and the Individual
Chapter 7, Health Promotion and the Family
Chapter 8, Health Promotion and the Community
Chapter 19, Preschool Child

Susan Scott Ricci, ARNP, MSN, MEd
Nursing Program Director, Lake Sumter Community
    College
Leesburg, Florida;
Adjunct Instructor
University of Central Florida
Orlando, Florida
Chapter 17, Infant

Ratchneewan Ross, PhD, RN
Assistant Professor, College of Nursing
Kent State University
Kent, Ohio
Chapter 25, Health Promotion in the Twenty-First Century:
    Throughout the Life Span and Throughout the World

Linda Snetselaar, PhD, RD
Associate Professor, Department of Epidemiology
University of Iowa
Iowa City, Iowa
Chapter 11, Nutrition Counseling for Health Promotion

Marie Truglio-Londrigan, PhD, RN, GNPC
Associate Professor
Chair, Graduate Program
Lienhard School of Nursing
Pace University
Pleasantville, New York
Chapter 9, Screening

Geraldine Valencia-Go, PhD, MA, RN, CS
Associate Professor, School of Nursing
College of New Rochelle
New Rochelle, New York
Chapter 2, Changing Populations and Health

Meredith Wallace, PhD, APRN
Assistant Professor, School of Nursing
Fairfield University
Fairfield, Connecticut
Chapter 24, Older Adult

Study Questions

Darlene Nebel Cantu, MSN, RNC
Faculty, Department of Nursing Education
San Antonio College;
Director, Baptist Health System
San Antonio, Texas

Ancillary Contributors

Joyce Anderson, ND, cFNP
Assistant Professor, Nursing
Howard University College of Pharmacy, Nursing, and
    Allied Health
Washington, DC
Test Bank

Martha Driessnack, PhDc, ARNP
Oregon Health & Science University
    Portland, Oregon
Lecture Slides

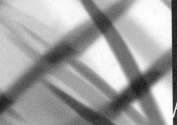

Mary E. Abrums, RN, MN

Marinda Allender, RN, MSN, CPN

Douglas Bloomquist, PhD

Philip Boyle, PhD

Jacqueline Clinton, PhD, RN, FAAN

Joni Cohen, RN, MN

Rebecca Cohen, RN, EdD

Katherine Smith Detherage, PhD, RN, CNAA

Lea Edwards, BSN, MEd

James A. Fain, PhD, RN, RAAN

Gail Park Fast, MN

Marilyn Frank-Stromberg, EdD, NP

Carol Scheel Gavan, EdD, RN

Qalvy Grainzvolt, BS

Krishan Gupta, MD

Lois Hancock, MSN, ARNP

Carolyn Hayes, PhD, RN

Janice Hooper, PhD, RN, CS

James S. Huddleston, MS, PT

Dennis T. Jaffe, PhD

Sally Stark Johnson, RN, MSN

Jeanette Lancaster, RN, PhD, FAAN

William Martimucci, MD

Ann Marie McCarthy, RN

Nancy Curro McCarthy, RN, EdD

Nancy Milio, PhD, FAAN, FAPHA

Katherine E. Murphy, MN, FNP

Lisa Newton, PhD

Jean M. O'Connor, MS, MPH, RNC, FNP

Reverend James O'Donahue, SJ, PhD

Ellen F. Olshansky, DNSc, RNC

Johanne Quinn, PhD, RN

Gurpal K. Sandhu, PhD

Jan Schurman, MN, FNP

Arlene Spark, EdD, RD

Carol L. Wells-Federman, MS, MEd, RN, CS

PURPOSE OF THE BOOK

The case for promoting and protecting health and preventing disease and injury has been established by many accomplishments throughout the twentieth century. Americans are taking better care of themselves as they enter the twenty-first century. Public concern about physical fitness, good nutrition, and avoidance of health hazards such as smoking has gone beyond a fad and has become ingrained in the American lifestyle.

Encouraging positive health changes has been a major effort of individuals, the government, health professionals, and society in general. In the United States, public and private attempts to improve the health status of individuals and groups traditionally have focused on reducing communicable diseases and health hazards. Now growing concerns exist to improve access to and reduce costs of health services and improve the overall quality of life for all people. Americans also recognize that the health of each individual is influenced by health environments of all individuals worldwide.

Personal lifestyles are known to influence health status in individuals and professionals who can use specific strategies to help families, communities, and groups maintain and adopt positive lifestyle behaviors. Indirect health information and informed decision or direct health education and resulting health-promotion, health-protection, and disease- and injury-prevention practices can all lead to the adoption of healthy lifestyles.

Health-promotion advances require a better understanding of health risks behaviors and intervention measures. Ten categories are identified as important determinants of health status:

1. Smoking
2. Nutrition
3. Alcohol use
4. Habituating drug use
5. Driving
6. Exercise
7. Sexual practices and contraceptive use
8. Family relationships
9. Risk management
10. Coping and adaptation

Outcome measures designed to assist individual efforts to change and improve behavior in these areas can lead to decreases in morbidity and mortality.

Professionals who undertake health-promotion strategies also need to understand the basics of health protection and disease and injury prevention. Health protection is directed at population groups of all ages and involves adherence to standards, infectious disease control, and governmental regulation and enforcement. The focus of these activities is on reducing exposure to various sources of hazards, including those related to air, water, foods, drugs, motor vehicles, and other physical agents.

Health care providers present the individual with disease- and injury-prevention services, which include immunizations, screenings, health education, and counseling. To implement prevention strategies effectively, it is essential to develop activities targeted to and tailored for all age groups in various settings, including schools, industries, the home, the health care delivery system, and the community.

Throughout the history of the United States, the public health community has assessed the health of Americans. In 1789 the Reverend Edward Wigglesworth developed the first American mortality tables through his study in New England. The *Report of a General Plan for the Promotion of Public and Personal Health* was completed by Lemuel Shattuck in 1880. *Healthy People, The Surgeon General's Report on Health Promotion and Disease Prevention* was first published in 1979 and followed by *Healthy People 2000: National Health Promotion and Disease Prevention Objectives*, which listed three goals to be achieved by the year 2000:

1. Increase the span of healthy life for Americans.
2. Reduce health disparities among Americans.
3. Achieve access to preventive services for all Americans.

This report presented many opportunities in the form of measurable targets, or objectives, which were organized into 22 priority areas within four broad categories: (1) health promotion, (2) health protection, (3) preventive services, and (4) surveillance and data systems.

Healthy People 2000 Mid-Course Review and 1995 Revisions and annual updates evaluated progress in selected areas of health promotion, health protection, preventive services, and surveillance data systems.

In this relatively short time, significant improvements have been made in the health behaviors and health of Americans. Examples of these improvements include reductions in infant mortality; teenage pregnancies; injuries; tobacco, alcohol, and illicit drug use; and death rates from coronary heart disease and cerebrovascular accidents. In addition, childhood vaccination rates are at the highest recorded.

Unfortunately, many more improvements are needed in the health of many Americans. Tobacco use by adolescents continues to increase. Nearly 40% of adults do not participate in leisure-time physical activity, and 40% of adults are obese. Violence and other abusive behaviors continue to destroy individuals, families, and communities across the United States. Chronic health problems, such as mental disorders and diabetes mellitus, continue to be undiagnosed and undertreated. Another example of this is the occurrence of HIV and AIDS disproportionately in black and Hispanic communities, especially in women.

Healthy People 2010 addresses these health problems by establishing goals and objectives for the first decade of the new millennium. The vision for *Healthy People 2010* is "Healthy People in Healthy Communities" because, as nursing has long recognized, the health of each individual is inseparable from the health of families, communities, the nation, and the universe. Health is significantly affected by the environments in which each individual lives, works, travels, and plays. Dimensions of the environment are not only physical, but also psychosocial and spiritual, including the behaviors, attitudes, and beliefs of each individual. Specific objectives in 28 focus areas support two major goals:

1. Increase quality and years of healthy life.
2. Eliminate health disparities.

These databases continue to provide assessments of health status and risk for evaluations and future planning, not only for health policy makers and health care providers, but for individuals, families, and communities (local, regional, national, and global).

The information in this edition of *Health Promotion Throughout the Life Span* includes these and other data and recommendations for health promotion, health protection, preventive services, and surveillance data systems, including those of the U.S. Preventive Services Task Force.

APPROACH AND ORGANIZATION

This edition presents health data and related theories and skills that are needed to understand and practice when providing care. This book focuses on primary prevention intervention, based on the Leavell and Clark model; its three main components are (1) health promotion, (2) specific health protection, and (3) prevention of specific diseases. Health promotion is the intervention designed to improve health, such as providing adequate nutrition, a healthy environment, and ongoing health education. Specific protection and prevention, such as massive immunizations, periodic examinations, and safety features in the workplace, are the interventions used to protect against illness.

In addition to primary prevention, this book discusses secondary prevention intervention, focusing specifically on screening. Such programs include blood pressure, glaucoma, and diabetes screening and referral. (The acute component of secondary prevention is not addressed in this book.)

This text is presented in five parts, each forming the basis for the next.

Unit One, *Foundations for Health Promotion*, describes the foundational concepts of promoting and protecting health and preventing diseases and injuries, including diagnostic, therapeutic, and ethical decision making based on the nursing emphasis of health patterns as described by Margaret Newman.

Unit Two, *Assessment for Health Promotion*, focuses on individuals, families, and communities and the factors affecting their health. The functional health pattern assessments developed by Gordon serve as the organizing framework for assessing the health of individuals, families, and communities.

Unit Three, *Interventions for Health Promotion*, discusses theories, methodologies, and case studies of nursing interventions, including screening, health education counseling, stress management, and crisis intervention.

Unit Four, *Application of Health Promotion*, also uses Gordon's functional health patterns, emphasizing developmental, cultural, ethnic, and environmental variables in assessing the developing person. The intent is to address the health concerns of all Americans regardless of gender, race, age, or sexual orientation. Although the human development theories discussed are primarily based on the research of male subjects, emerging theories based on female subjects have been included. The hope is to describe human development that more accurately reflects the complexity of human experiences throughout the life span.

Unit Five, *Challenges As We Enter the New Millennium*, presents a single chapter that discusses changing population groups and their health needs and related implications for research and practice in the twenty-first century. Throughout the text, research abstracts have been added to highlight state-of-the-art and the science of nursing practice and to demonstrate to the reader the relationship among research, practice, and outcomes.

Throughout these units, the evolving health care professions and the changing health care systems, including future challenges and initiatives for health promotion, are described. Emphasis is placed on the current concerns of reducing health care costs while increasing life expectancy and improving the quality of life for all Americans. This promotes the reader's immediate interest in and thoughts about the content of the chapters.

Key Features

- A **full-color design,** including color photos, has been implemented throughout for better accessibility of content and visual enhancement.
- Each chapter starts with a list of **objectives** to help focus the reader and emphasize the content the reader should acquire through reading the book. **Key Terms** are listed at the front to acquaint readers with the important terminology of the chapter.
- Each chapter's narrative begins with **Think About It,** the presentation of a clinical issue or scenario that relates to the topic of the chapter, followed by critical thinking questions. This promotes the reader's immediate interest in and thought about the chapter.
- **Research Highlights** boxes provide brief synopses on current health promotion research studies that demonstrate the links between research, theory, and practice.
- **Multicultural Awareness** boxes offer cultural perspectives on various aspects of health promotion.

- **Hot Topics** explores current issues, controversies, and ethical dilemmas with respect to health promotion, providing an opportunity for critical analysis of care issues.
- **Health Teaching** boxes present special tips and guidelines to use when educating people about health-promotion activities.
- The **Case Study** highlights a real-life clinical situation relevant to the chapter topic.
- The **Care Plan,** with the standardized sections of *Defining Characteristics, Related Factors, Expected Outcomes,* and *Interventions,* details nursing diagnoses relevant to health-promotion activities and the related interventions.
- **Innovative Practice** boxes highlight inventive and resourceful projects, programs, and research studies that draw upon new ways of implementing health promotion.
- A **Glossary** in the back of the book contains the Key Terms from each chapter and their definitions.
- **NEW! Healthy People 2010** boxes present a list of selected objectives that are relevant to the chapter's topic.
- **NEW! Web Site Resources** offer expanded chapter resources, such as assessment tools, developmental charts, and immunization schedules, on the book's website.
- **NEW!** Multiple choice **Study Questions,** in NCLEX-format, are located on perforated pages in the back of the book, to offer additional review and self-study practice.

ⓔⓥⓞⓛⓥⓔ ONLINE TEACHING/ LEARNING PACKAGE

New to this edition is an expanded website providing materials for both students and faculty, accessible at **http://evolve.elsevier.com/Edelman/.**

For Students

Web Site Resources: Resources that supplement the chapter discussion

WebLinks: Organized by chapter, these are direct links to numerous websites related to the chapter content.

Content Updates: Highlights of new information and findings that occur in health promotion after publica-

tion of the book, to stay current with trends and new developments.

Glossary: Comprehensive list of all Key Terms and their definitions. Search capability allows searching by term, definition, or chapter.

For Instructors

Chapter Outlines

Learning Objectives

Research Evaluation and Critique article

Sample Syllabi

Annotated Bibliography of teaching and education references

Image Collection, with approximately 40 images from the book

Lecture Slides, in PowerPoint

Test Bank, 250 questions in NCLEX format, including the new innovative item format

Glossary of Key Terms and their definitions, reproduced from the book

Many of the instructor resources are also available on CD-ROM. See your Elsevier sales representative for details.

The current trend to emphasize the developing health of people mandates that health care professionals understand the many issues that surround individuals, families, and communities in social, work, and family settings, including the biological, inherited, cognitive, psychological, environmental, and sociocultural factors that can put their health at risk. Most important is that they develop interventions to promote health by understanding the diverse roles these factors play in the person's beliefs and health practices, particularly in the areas of disease and injury prevention, protection, and health promotion. Achieving such effectiveness requires collaboration with other health care providers and the integration of practice and policy while developing interventions and considering the ethical issues within individual, family, and community responsibilities for health.

Carole Lium Edelman
Carol Lynn Mandle

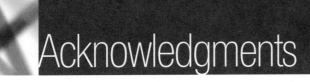

Acknowledgments

We had the good fortune of receiving much assistance and support from many friends, relatives, and associates. Our colleagues read chapters, gave valuable advice and criticism, helped clarify concepts, and provided case examples.

We also acknowledge the contributions of all the authors. In developing this text, they gave the project their total commitment and support. Their professional competence aided greatly in the development of the final draft of the manuscript. Special thanks go to Meghan Lynch for assistance with typing the manuscript and Barbara Abraham for her assistance in editing.

The editors worked and learned from each other during the planning and development of this book; throughout the entire process, close contact prevailed. They seemed to become the book and, in turn, the book now reflects them.

Both family and friends helped in the work and fulfilled the many responsibilities requested of them.

I am fortunate to have faith in the Lord, who gives courage and strength to face life's difficulties in a positive manner. My children, John and Megan Gillespie, Tom and Heather Gillespie, and Deirdre O'Brien, and my grandchildren, Ryan and Caroline, bring joy to me as an author and editor. Their patience and love are truly appreciated. Lenora and Rachel Pennacchia provide much encouragement and support. Fredric Edelman gives continued joy and happiness in our marriage.

Carole Lium Edelman

In the continued development of health, I acknowledge our faith in God and the strength of my mother, sister, and aunt; the joy of friends; the love of marriage and family with Robert, Jonathan, Stephanie, David, Dara, and Elizabeth; the commitments of nurses to social justice in the care of all people; and the knowledge we are just beginning.

Carol Lynn Mandle

To our wonderful families, friends, students, and colleagues—
that they promote health in themselves and others.

Contents

UNIT ONE   Foundations for Health Promotion, 1

1 Health Defined: Objectives for Promotion and Prevention, 3

Exploring Concepts of Health, 4
  Models of Health, 5
  Wellness–Illness Continuum, 5
  High-Level Wellness, 5
  Health Ecology, 6
  Functioning, 6
  Health, 6
Illness, Disease, and Health, 6
Planning for Health, 7
Healthy People 2010, 7
  Healthy People 2010 Goals, 7
  Healthy People 2010 Update, 10
Case Study, 10
  Problem Identification, 10
  Planning Interventions, 10
  What Was the Actual Cause of Frank's Problem?, 12
  Evaluation of the Situation, 13
Levels of Prevention, 13
  Primary Prevention, 13
  Secondary Prevention, 17
  Tertiary Prevention, 18
The Nurse's Role, 18
  Nursing Roles in Health Promotion and Protection, 18
Improving Prospects for Health, 20
  Population Effects, 20
Shifting Problems, 20
Moving Toward Solutions, 20

2 Emerging Populations and Health, 23

Emerging Populations in the United States, 24
Ethnicity, Ethnic Group, Minority Group, and Race, 25
Culture, Values, and Value Orientation, 26
  Health as a Value, 26
Folk Healing and Professional Care Systems, 27
Arab Americans, 27
  Health Care Issues of Arab Americans, 27
  Selected Health-Related Cultural Aspects, 28
Asian American–Pacific Islanders, 28
  Health Care Issues of Asian American–Pacific Islanders, 28

Selected Health-Related Cultural Aspects, 29
Latino/Hispanic Americans, 30
  Health Issues of Latino/Hispanic Americans, 30
  Selected Health-Related Cultural Aspects, 31
Black/African Americans, 32
  Health Care Issues of Black/African Americans, 32
  Selected Health-Related Cultural Aspects, 33
Native Americans, 34
  Health Care Issues of Native Americans, 34
  Selected Health-Related Cultural Aspects, 35
Emerging Rural and Urban Populations, 36
  Homelessness: A Continuing Saga, 36
  People Living With HIV-AIDS, 39
The Nation's Response to The Health Challenges, 42
  Healthy People 2010, 42
  Office of Minority Health, 43
Nursing's Response to Emerging Populations and Health, 43

3 Health Policy and the Delivery System, 50

History of Health Care, 52
  Early Influences, 52
  Industrial Influences, 53
  Socioeconomic Influences, 53
  Public Health Influences, 53
  Scientific Influences, 53
  Special Population Influences, 54
  Political and Economic Influences, 54
  Split Between Preventive and Curative Measures, 54
Organization of The Delivery System, 56
  Private Sector, 56
  Public Sector, 58
Financing Health Care, 61
  Costs, 61
  Sources, 63
  Mechanisms, 64
  Managed Care Issues, 65
  Health Insurance, 66
  Pharmaceutical Costs, 70
  The Uninsured: Who Are They?, 70
Health Care Systems of Other Countries, 71
  Canadian Health Care System, 71
  German Health Care System, 72
  United Kingdom's Health Care System, 72
Influencing Health Policy, 72

4 The Therapeutic Relationship, 77

Values Clarification, 78
Definition, 78
Values and Therapeutic Use of Self, 79
The Communication Process, 81
Function and Process, 82
Types of Communication, 83
Effectiveness of Communication, 84
Factors in Effective Communication, 85
The Helping or Therapeutic Relationship, 87
Characteristics of the Therapeutic
Relationship, 87
Ethics in Communicating and Relating, 89
Therapeutic Techniques, 89
Barriers to Effective Communication, 91
Setting, 93
Stages, 94
Brief Interactions, 95
Health Literacy, 95

5 Ethical Issues Relevant to Health Promotion, 100

Health Promotion as a Moral Endeavor, 101
Health Care Ethics, 101
Origins of Applied Ethics in Moral
Philosophy, 101
Types of Ethics, 102
Limitations of Moral Theory, 102
Feminist Ethics and Caring, 104
Professional Responsibility, 106
Accountability to Individuals and Society, 106
Codes of Ethics, 107
Advocacy, 108
Problem Solving: Issues, Dilemmas,
and Risks, 109
Preventive Ethics, 109
Ethical Principles in Health Promotion, 110
Autonomy as Civil Liberty, 110
Autonomy as Self-Determination, 112
Limits on Autonomy, 114
Confidentiality, 114
Veracity, 116
Nonmaleficence, 117
Beneficence, 117
Justice, 120
Strategies for Ethical Decision Making, 121
Locating the Source and Levels of Ethical
Problems, 121
Values Clarification and Reflection, 121
Decision-Making Considerations, 121
Ethics of Health Promotion: Cases, 122
CASE 1 Addressing Health Care System
Problems—Elissa Needs Help, 123
CASE 2 Assisted Suicide or Emotional
Support?—Ana and Victor, 123
CASE 3 How Much Money Can One Person
Spend?—Joe Does Not Like Taking Pills, 123
CASE 4 She's My Patient!—Lilly and "Jake"
(a.k.a. Paul), 123

UNIT TWO Assessment for Health Promotion, 127

6 Health Promotion and the Individual, 129

Functional Health Patterns: Assessment of the Individual, 131
Functional Health Pattern Framework, 131
The Patterns, 133
Individual Health Promotion Through the Nursing Process, 147
Collection and Analysis of Data, 147
Planning the Care, 148
Implementing the Plan, 149
Evaluating the Plan, 149

7 Health Promotion and the Family, 152

The Nursing Process and the Family, 153
The Nurse's Role, 154
The Family from a Systems Perspective, 154
The Family from a Developmental Perspective, 155
The Family from a Risk-Factor Perspective, 156
Functional Health Patterns: Assessment of the Family, 156
Health Perception–Health Management
Pattern, 158
Nutritional-Metabolic Pattern, 159
Elimination Pattern, 160
Activity-Exercise Pattern, 160
Sleep-Rest Pattern, 160
Cognitive-Perceptual Pattern, 161
Self-Perception–Self-Concept Pattern, 161
Roles-Relationships Pattern, 161
Sexuality-Reproductive Pattern, 165
Coping–Stress Tolerance Pattern, 166
Values-Beliefs Pattern, 166
Analysis and Nursing Diagnosis, 167
Analyzing Data, 167
Formulating Family Nursing Diagnoses, 171
Planning With the Family, 172
Goals, 172
Implementation With the Family, 172
Evaluation With the Family, 175

8 Health Promotion and the Community, 178

The Nursing Process and the Community, 179
The Nurse's Role, 179
Methods of Data Collection, 180
Sources of Community Information, 180
Community From a Systems Perspective, 181
 Structure, 181
 Function, 181
 Interaction, 182
Community from a Developmental Perspective, 182
Community from a Risk Factor Perspective, 182
Functional Health Patterns: Assessment of the Community, 183
 Health Perception–Health Management Pattern, 183
 Nutritional-Metabolic Pattern, 183
 Elimination Pattern, 183
 Activity-Exercise Pattern, 183
 Sleep-Rest Pattern, 183
 Cognitive-Perceptual Pattern, 184
 Self-Perception–Self-Concept Pattern, 184
 Roles-Relationships Pattern, 184
 Sexuality-Reproductive Pattern, 184
 Coping–Stress Tolerance Pattern, 185
 Values-Beliefs Pattern, 185
Analysis and Diagnosis With the Community, 185
 Organization of Data, 185
 Guidelines for Data Analysis, 186
 Community Diagnosis, 188
Planning With the Community, 188
 Purposes, 188
 Planned Change, 191
Implementation With the Community, 193
Evaluation With the Community, 193

UNIT THREE **Interventions for Health Promotion, 197**

9 Screening, 199

Advantages and Disadvantages of Screening, 200
Selection of a Screenable Disease, 201
 Significance, 201
 Can the Disease Be Detected by Screening?, 201
 Should Screening for the Disease Be Done?, 203
Ethical Considerations, 205
 Health Care Ethics, 205
 Economic Ethics, 205
Selection of a Screenable Population, 206
 Person-Dependent Factors, 206
 Environment-Dependent Factors, 210
Commonly Screened Conditions, 211
 Phenylketonuria, 211

 Breast Cancer, 212
 Cervical Cancer, 212
 Colorectal Cancer, 212
 Prostate Cancer, 212
 Cholesterol, 213
 Hypertension, 213
 Glaucoma, 213
 Human Immunodeficiency Virus, 214
 Lead, 214
 Diabetes Mellitus, 214
The Nurse's Role, 215

10 Health Education, 217

Nursing and Health Education, 218
 Definition, 219
 Goals, 220
 Learning Assumptions, 221
 Family Health Teaching, 221
 Health Behavior Change, 222
 Ethics, 223
 Cultural Considerations in Health Teaching, 223
Social Marketing and Health Education, 224
Teaching Plan, 224
 Assessment, 224
 Determining Expected Learning Outcomes, 225
 Selecting Content, 226
 Designing Learning Strategies, 226
 Evaluating the Teaching-Learning Process, 227
 Referring Individuals to Other Resources, 228
Teaching and Organizing Skills, 228

11 Nutrition Counseling for Health Promotion, 231

Nutrition in the United States: Looking Forward From The Past, 232
 Classic Vitamin-Deficiency Diseases, 232
 Dietary Excess and Imbalance, 232
Healthy People 2010: Nutrition Objectives, 232
 Nutrition-Related Health Status, 233
 Nutrition Objectives for the United States, 234
Food and Nutrition Recommendations, 234
 Dietary Reference Intakes, 234
 Dietary Guidelines for Americans, 236
MyPyramid: A New Food Guidance System, 236
 Food Guide Pyramid, 236
 MyPyramid, 236
Dietary Supplements and Herbal Medicines, 236
 Circumstances When Nutrient Supplementation Is Indicated, 239
 Vitamin Toxicity, 239
Food Safety, 241
 Causes of Food-Borne Illness, 241
 Food Safety Practices, 241
Food, Nutrition, and Poverty, 242
 Poverty and Income Distribution, 242

Food Assistance for the Poor, 242
Nutrition Screening, 245
Nutrition and Disease, 245
Cardiovascular Diseases, 245
Heart Disease, 245
Hypertension, 247
Cancer, 250
Osteoporosis, 251
Obesity, 253
Diabetes, 255
Human Immunodeficiency Virus and Acquired
Immunodeficiency Syndrome, 258

12   Exercise, 261
Defining Physical Activity in Health, 262
Healthy People 2010 **Objectives, 262**
Physical Activity Objectives: Making
Progress, 262
Aging, 264
Effects of Exercise on the Aging Process, 265
Coronary Heart Disease, 265
High-Density Lipoprotein and Serum
Triglyceride Levels, 266
Hypertension, 266
Hyperinsulinemia and Glucose Intolerance, 267
Obesity, 268
Osteoporosis, 269
Arthritis, 270
Low Back Pain, 270
Immune Function, 271
Mental Health, 272
How Much Exercise Is Enough?, 272
Aerobic Exercise, 273
Warm-Up and Cool-Down Periods, 275
Flexibility, 276
Resistance Training, 276
Exercise the Spirit: Relaxation Response, 276
**Monitoring the Inner and Outer
Environment, 279**
Fluid News, 279
Special Considerations, 279
Coronary Heart Disease, 280
Diabetes, 281
Building a Rhythm of Physical Activity, 282
Adherence and Compliance, 283
Creating a Climate That Supports Exercise, 284

13   Stress Management, 289
Sources of Stress, 290
**Physical, Psychological, Sociobehavioral, and
Spiritual Consequences of Stress, 291**
Physiological Effects of Stress, 291
Psychological Effects of Stress, 292
Sociobehavioral Effects of Stress, 293
Spiritual Effects of Stress, 293

Health Benefits of Managing Stress, 293
Assessment of Stress, 294
Stress Management Interventions, 296
Developing Self-Awareness, 296
Healthy Diet, 299
Physical Activity, 299
Sleep Hygiene, 300
Cognitive Restructuring, 300
Affirmations, 301
Social Support, 302
Assertive Communication, 302
Empathy, 303
Healthy Pleasures, 304
Spiritual Practice, 304
Clarifying Values and Beliefs, 305
Setting Realistic Goals, 305
Humor, 305
Effective Coping, 306

14   Holistic Health Strategies, 310
Holism, 311
Interventions, 312
Energy Work, 312
Movement Arts, 316
Meditation, 318
Prayer and Distant Healing, 319
Guided Imagery, 320
Music Therapy, 320
Bodywork, 320
Aromatherapy, 321
Presence, 322
Self-Knowledge, 322

UNIT FOUR   **Application of Health
Promotion, 327**

**15   Overview of Growth and
Development Framework, 329**
Overview of Growth and Development, 330
Concept of Growth, 330
Concept of Development, 339
Theories of Development, 340
Psychosocial Development: Erikson's
Theory, 340
Cognitive Development: Piaget's Theory, 340
Moral Development: Kohlberg's Theory, 341
Moral Development: Gilligan's Theory, 341

16   The Prenatal Period, 344
**Physical Changes in Maternal and Fetal
Systems, 345**
Duration of Pregnancy, 345
Fertilization, 345
Implantation, 345

Fetal Growth and Development, 345
Placental Development and Function, 346
Maternal Changes, 346
Changes During Transition From Fetus to Newborn, 352
Nursing Interventions, 352
Mucus, 352
Apgar Score, 353
Gender, 353
Race and Culture, 353
Genetics, 353
Gordon's Functional Health Patterns, 354
Health Perception–Health Management Pattern, 354
Nutritional-Metabolic Pattern, 356
Elimination Pattern, 357
Activity-Exercise Pattern, 357
Sleep-Rest Pattern, 358
Cognitive-Perceptual Pattern, 358
Self-Perception–Self-Concept Pattern, 360
Roles-Relationships Pattern, 361
Sexuality-Reproductive Pattern, 363
Coping–Stress Tolerance Pattern, 363
Values-Beliefs Pattern, 363
Pathological Processes, 364
Physical Factors and Diagnostic Tools, 364
Biological Agents, 365
Chemical Agents, 367
Mechanical Forces, 370
Radiation, 370
Social Processes, 370
Community and Work, 370
Culture and Ethnicity, 371
Legislation, 371
Economics, 372
Health Care Delivery System, 372
Nursing Interventions, 372

17   Infant, 376
Age and Physical Changes, 378
Developmental Tasks, 378
Concepts of Infant Development, 378
Denver Developmental Screening Test, 382
Gender, 382
Race, 383
Genetics, 383
Gordon's Functional Health Patterns, 384
Health Perception–Health Management Pattern, 384
Nutritional-Metabolic Pattern, 384
Elimination Pattern, 388
Activity-Exercise Pattern, 389
Sleep-Rest Pattern, 390
Cognitive-Perceptual Pattern, 392
Self-Perception–Self-Concept Pattern, 393
Roles-Relationships Pattern, 394

Sexuality-Reproductive Pattern, 397
Coping–Stress Tolerance Pattern, 397
Values-Beliefs Pattern, 399
Pathological Processes, 399
Unintentional Injuries, 400
Biological Agents, 401
Chemical Agents, 403
Motor Vehicles, 406
Radiation, 406
Cancer, 407
Social Processes, 407
Community and Work, 407
Culture and Ethnicity, 408
Legislation, 410
Economics, 411
Health Care Delivery System, 412
Nursing Interventions, 412

18   Toddler, 416
Age and Physical Changes, 417
Gordon's Functional Health Patterns, 419
Health Perception–Health Management Pattern, 419
Nutritional-Metabolic Pattern, 419
Elimination Pattern, 421
Activity-Exercise Pattern, 421
Sleep-Rest Pattern, 423
Cognitive-Perceptual Pattern, 423
Self-Perception–Self-Concept Pattern, 426
Roles-Relationships Pattern, 427
Sexuality-Reproductive Pattern, 429
Coping–Stress Tolerance Pattern, 429
Values-Beliefs Pattern, 429
Pathological Processes, 430
Accidents, 430
Motor Vehicles, 431
Biological Agents, 432
Poisoning, 432
Social Processes, 433
Day Care, 433
Culture and Ethnicity, 433
Legislation, 433
Economics, 434
Health Care Delivery System, 434

19   Preschool Child, 436
Age and Physical Changes, 437
Gender, 438
Race, 438
Genetics, 440
Gordon's Functional Health Patterns, 440
Health Perception–Health Management Pattern, 440
Nutritional-Metabolic Pattern, 440
Elimination Pattern, 442

Activity-Exercise Pattern, 442
Sleep-Rest Pattern, 443
Cognitive-Perceptual Pattern, 444
Self-Perception–Self-Concept Pattern, 449
Roles-Relationships Pattern, 449
Sexuality-Reproductive Pattern, 451
Coping–Stress Tolerance Pattern, 452
Values-Beliefs Pattern, 453
Pathological Processes, 454
Injuries, 455
Mechanical Forces, 457
Biological and Bacterial Agents, 457
Chemical Agents, 458
Cancer, 458
Asthma, 460
Social Processes, 460
Community and Work, 460
Culture and Ethnicity, 460
Legislation, 461
Economics, 461
Health Care Delivery System, 461
Nursing Interventions, 461

20 School-Age Child, 466
Age and Physical Changes, 467
Gender, 469
Race, 470
Genetics, 470
Gordon's Functional Health Patterns, 471
Health Perception–Health Management
Pattern, 471
Nutritional-Metabolic Pattern, 471
Elimination Pattern, 474
Activity-Exercise Pattern, 475
Sleep-Rest Pattern, 476
Cognitive-Perceptual Pattern, 476
Self-Perception–Self-Concept Pattern, 480
Roles-Relationships Pattern, 482
Sexuality-Reproductive Pattern, 483
Coping–Stress Tolerance Pattern, 484
Values-Beliefs Pattern, 486
Pathological Processes, 486
Accidents, 486
Mechanical Forces, 489
Biological Agents, 490
Chemical Agents, 491
Radiological Agents, 492
Social Processes, 492
Community and Work, 492
Culture and Ethnicity, 493
Legislation, 495
Economics, 495
Health Care Delivery System, 496
Nursing Interventions, 497
School and the Nurse, 498

21 Adolescent, 502
Age and Physical Changes, 503
Scoliosis, 504
Acne, 504
Gender, 505
Genetics, 506
Gordon's Functional Health Patterns, 506
Health Perception–Health Management
Pattern, 506
Nutritional-Metabolic Pattern, 508
Elimination Pattern, 509
Activity-Exercise Pattern, 510
Sleep-Rest Pattern, 510
Cognitive-Perceptual Pattern, 510
Self-Perception–Self-Concept Pattern, 511
Roles-Relationships Pattern, 512
Sexuality-Reproductive Pattern, 513
Coping–Stress Tolerance Pattern, 515
Values-Beliefs Pattern, 516
Pathological Processes, 516
Accidents, 516
Sports, 516
Violence, 517
Mechanical Forces, 517
Biological and Bacterial Agents, 518
Chemical Agents, 518
Cancer, 519
Social Processes, 519
School, 519
Culture and Ethnicity, 519
Legislation, 520
Economics, 520
Health Care Delivery System, 520

22 Young Adult, 523
Age and Physical Changes, 524
Gordon's Functional Health Patterns, 525
Health Perception–Health Management
Pattern, 525
Nutritional-Metabolic Pattern, 529
Elimination Pattern, 531
Activity-Exercise Pattern, 531
Sleep-Rest Pattern, 532
Cognitive-Perceptual Pattern, 532
Self-Perception–Self-Concept Pattern, 533
Roles-Relationships Pattern, 533
Sexuality-Reproductive Pattern, 535
Coping–Stress Tolerance Pattern, 538
Values-Beliefs Pattern, 540
Pathological Processes, 542
Accidents, 542
Pollution, 542
Occupational Hazards and Stressors, 542
Chemical Agents, 542
Cancer, 544

Social Processes, 544
  Community and Work, 544
  Culture and Ethnicity, 545
  Legislation, 545
  Economics, 545

23 Middle-Age Adult, 548
Age and Physical Changes, 549
  Mortality Rates, 549
  Gender and Marital Status, 550
  Genetics, 550
Gordon's Functional Health Patterns, 552
  Health Perception–Health Management
    Pattern, 552
  Nutritional-Metabolic Pattern, 552
  Elimination Pattern, 555
  Activity-Exercise Pattern, 555
  Sleep-Rest Pattern, 556
  Cognitive-Perceptual Pattern, 556
  Self-Perception–Self-Concept Pattern, 557
  Roles-Relationships Pattern, 558
  Sexuality-Reproductive Pattern, 561
  Coping–Stress Tolerance Pattern, 562
  Values-Beliefs Pattern, 564
Environmental Factors, 565
  Physical Agents, 565
  Biological Agents, 565
  Chemical Agents, 565
Social Processes, 566
  Culture and Ethnicity, 566
  Economics, 567
  Health Care Delivery System, 567
Nursing Interventions, 567

24 Older Adult, 571
Age and Physical Changes, 573
Goals of Health Promotion, 573
Theories of Aging, 574
Gordon's Functional Health Patterns, 575
  Health Perception–Health Management
    Pattern, 575
  Nutritional-Metabolic Pattern, 575
  Elimination Pattern, 576
  Activity-Exercise Pattern, 577
  Sleep-Rest Pattern, 579
  Cognitive-Perceptual Pattern, 579
  Self-Perception–Self-Concept Pattern, 582
  Roles-Relationships Pattern, 583
  Sexuality-Reproductive Pattern, 584
  Coping–Stress Tolerance Pattern, 585
  Values-Beliefs Pattern, 586
Pathological Processes, 586
  Accidents, 586

Biological Agents, 588
Drug Use, 588
Alcohol Use, 589
Tobacco Use, 589
Cancer, 590
Social Processes, 590
  Environments of Care, 590
  Cultural Diversity, 594
  Health Care Delivery System, 594

UNIT FIVE   Challenges in the Twenty-
             First Century, 599

25 Health Promotion in the Twenty-
   First Century: Throughout the Life
   Span and Throughout the
   World, 601
Health Promotion: Past Developments and
  Future Directions, 604
Global Strategy of Health for All, 604
  Health for All, 604
  Health Care Systems, 605
  New Public Health Movement, 606
  Socioecological Foundations of Health
    Promotion, 606
  Goals and Targets for Health Promotion, 606
  Health Rather than Health Care as a Starting
    Point, 607
Reform of Health Promotion and Health
  Care, 608
  Clinical Effectiveness of Preventive Health
    Care, 608
  Cost Effectiveness of Preventive Health
    Care, 608
  Health Promotion and Vulnerable
    Populations, 610
Implications for Nursing Leadership in Health
  Promotion, 611
  Implications for Policy Development, 611
  Implications for Practice, 612
  Implications for Education, 612
  Implications for Research, 613

Glossary, 618

Index, 630

Study Questions, 663

Answer Key, 678

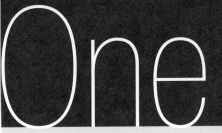

Unit One

Foundations for Health Promotion

1 Health Defined: Objectives for Promotion and Prevention

2 Emerging Populations and Health

3 Health Policy and the Delivery System

4 The Therapeutic Relationship

5 Ethical Issues Relevant to Health Promotion

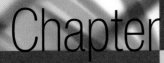

Chapter 1

PHILIP A. GREINER
CAROLE LIUM EDELMAN

Health Defined: Objectives for Promotion and Prevention

objectives

After completing this chapter, the reader will be able to:

- Analyze the term *health* as it has been used historically and as it is used in this textbook.

- Evaluate the consistency of *Healthy People 2010* goals with definitions of health.

- Analyze the progress made in this nation from the original *Healthy People* document to the foci in *Healthy People 2010.*

- Differentiate among health, illness, disease, disability, and premature death.

- Compare the three levels of prevention (primary, secondary, and tertiary) with the levels of service provision available across the life span.

- Critique the role of research and the nurse's role in the research process for the promotion of health for individuals and populations.

key terms

Applied research
Asset planning
Community-based care
Disease
Epidemiology
Evidence-based practice
Functional health

Health
Health disparities
Health promotion
Healthy People 2010
High-level wellness
Illness
Levels of prevention

Qualitative studies
Quality of life
Quantitative studies
Well-being
Wellness
Wellness–illness continuum

THINK About It

Use of Complementary and Alternative Therapies

One of the biggest challenges to health care providers is the blending of Western medicine and health practices with those from other cultures and ethnic groups. The federal government formed the National Center for Complementary and Alternative Medicine (http://nccam.nih. gov/) to conduct and support basic and applied research and training and to disseminate information on complementary and alternative medicine to practitioners and the public. As demographics of the United States shift, more people use a combination of therapies in self-care and for the treatment of illnesses.

1 What questions should the student ask to obtain information from people about their use of nontraditional therapies?

2 What should the student know about the benefits or drawbacks of using complementary therapies, such as acupuncture, spiritual healing, herbal remedies, or chiropractic methods?

3 What resources should the student trust for information on the efficacy and use of herbal remedies and relative to prescription medications?

Continued

THINK About It

Use of Complementary and Alternative Therapies *cont'd*

4 Which ideas of health would be most compatible with alternative therapies?

5 How can alternative therapies be integrated into *Healthy People 2010* objectives, given that the emphasis of these objectives is the use of available community resources and the development of partnerships?

Health is a core concept in society. This concept is modified with qualifiers such as *excellent, good, fair,* or *poor,* based on a variety of factors. These factors may include age, gender, race or ethnic heritage, comparison group, current health or physical condition, past conditions, social or economic situation, or the demands of various roles in society. This chapter will discuss health as a concept and related concepts such as illness, disease, disability, and functioning. Some motivating factors behind the move toward disease prevention and health promotion in society will be examined with an introduction to *Healthy People 2010.* Implementation of these concepts as nursing actions will also be addressed from ideal and pragmatic standpoints. Research supporting these concepts and recommendations for further research will be presented. Nurses need to understand the pivotal role they play in health promotion and disease prevention, the important role of research in the knowledge of what is healthy, the central role of **epidemiology** (the study of health and disease in society), and public health theory use in the everyday practice of nursing.

EXPLORING CONCEPTS OF HEALTH

Newman (1987b, 1995, 2003) states that nursing literature can be classified broadly within two major paradigms. The first is the **wellness–illness continuum,** a dichotomized portrayal of health and illness with many configurations, ranging from **high-level wellness** to depletion of health (death). High-level wellness is conceptualized further as a sense of **well-being,** life satisfaction, and **quality of life.** Movement toward the negative end of the continuum includes adaptation to disease and disability through various levels of functional ability. The wellness–illness conceptualization was the focus of early research and is consistent with the some of categories Smith (1983) identified in her philosophical analysis of health. Research based on the paradigm conforms primarily to scientific methods that seek to control contextual effects, provide the basis for causal explanations, and predict outcomes (Newman, 1987b, 1995).

The second paradigm characterizes health as a unidirectional development phenomenon of unitary patterning of the person-environment. The development perspective of health has been present in the nursing literature since 1970, but it was not identified clearly with health until the late 1970s and early 1980s. It has been conceptualized as ex-

panding consciousness, pattern or meaning recognition, personal transformation and, tentatively, self-actualization. This shift toward a developmental perspective has had clear implications for the way in which health is conceptualized (Newman, 2003). Although not endorsing the development perspective to the extent of Rogers (1970) and Reed (1983), Pender, Murdaugh, and Parsons (2002), Kaplan, Everson, and Lynch (2000), and Grzywacz and Fuqua (2000) state that health is an outcome of ongoing patterns of person-environment interaction throughout the life span. Research within this paradigm seeks to address the dynamic whole of the health experience through behavioral and social mechanisms. Health can be better understood if each person is seen as a part of a complex, interconnected, biological, and social system. This ecological view is useful to those who promote health.

People involved in health promotion should consider the meaning of health for themselves and for others, because a focused definition clarifies their work and enhances the quality of the health care system. Because the term *health* is used to describe a number of entities, such as a philosophy of care (health promotion and health maintenance), a system (health care delivery system), practices (good health practices), behaviors (health behaviors), costs (health care costs), and insurance, the reason that confusion continues regarding its use becomes clear. People's experiences with health in all of its entities have also changed over time.

Americans born before 1940 have experienced the greatest changes in how health is defined. Infectious diseases claimed the lives of many children and young adults; therefore, health was viewed as the absence of disease. The physician was the primary provider of health care services in independent practice, with services provided in the private office. The federal government was just establishing a federal role in working with states to address public health and welfare issues (Barr, Lee, & Benjamin, 2003).

As the national economy expanded during and after World War II in the 1940s and 1950s, the idea of role performance became a focus in industrial research and entered the health care lexicon. Health became linked to people's abilities to fulfill their roles in society. Increasingly, the physician was asked to complete physical examination forms for school, work, military, and insurance purposes as physician practice became linked more directly to hospital-based services. The federal government expanded its role through funding for hospital expansion and establishment of a new U.S. Department of Health, Education, and Welfare (USDHEW), currently the U.S. Department of Health and Human Services (USDHHS) (Barr, Lee, & Benjamin, 2003). There was recognition that a person might recover from a disease, yet might not be able to fulfill family or work roles because of residual changes from the illness episode. The work or school environment was viewed as a possible contributor to health or illness.

From the 1960s to the present, there have been incredible changes in the health care delivery system as federal and state governments have attempted to control spending and health care costs have escalated (Barr, Lee, & Benjamin, 2003). The growing number of primary care providers, including nurse practitioners and other advanced practice nurses, now attempt to involve individuals and their families in the delivery of care as individual responsibilities and lifestyle choices have become an important part of care. Health care has become an interdisciplinary endeavor, even as managed care companies limit the health-promotion options available under insurance plans. During this time, the idea of adaptation has had an important influence on the way Americans view health. Health has become linked to the changing environment to which individuals could react and change rather than becoming a fixed state. Adaptation fit well with the self-help movement during the 1970s and with the progressive growth in knowledge from research about disease prevention and health promotion.

There has been a more recent emphasis on the quality of a person's life as a component of health. Research on self-rated health (Cano et al., 2003; Idler & Benyamini, 1997; Johnson & Wolinsky, 1993) and self-rated function (Greiner, Snowdon, & Greiner, 1996, 1999) indicates that numerous factors contribute to a person's perception of health. In addition to the ability to function cognitively and physically (that is, **functional health**), fulfill social roles, and obtain health services, health is related to environment, socioeconomic level, race, and geographical location. Health is also directly linked to how providers perceive the recipients of services and to the options that providers offer.

Models of Health

Throughout history, society has entertained a variety of concepts of health (David, 2000). Smith (1983) describes four distinct models of health.

Clinical Model

In the clinical model, the absence of signs and symptoms of disease indicates health. Illness would be the presence of conspicuous signs and symptoms of disease. People who use this model of health to guide their use of health care services may not seek preventive health services, or they may wait until they are very ill to seek care. The clinical model is the conventional model of the discipline of medicine.

Role Performance Model

In the role performance model, health is indicated by the ability to perform social roles. Role performance includes work, family, and social roles, with performance based on societal expectations. Illness would be the failure to perform a person's roles at the level of others in society. This model is the basis for work and school physical examinations and physician-excused absences. The sick role, in which people can be excused from performing their social roles while they are ill, is a vital component of the role performance model.

Adaptive Model

In the adaptive model, the ability to adapt positively to social, mental, and physiological change is indicative of health. Illness occurs when the person fails to adapt or becomes maladaptive toward these changes. As the concept of adaptation has entered other aspects of American culture, this model of health has become more widely accepted.

Eudaimonistic Model

In the eudaimonistic model, health is indicated by exuberant well-being. Derived from Greek terminology, this term indicates a model that embodies the interaction and interrelationships among the physical, social, psychological, and spiritual aspects of life and the environment. Illness is reflected by a denervation or languishing, a wasting away, or lack of involvement with life. Although these ideas may appear to be new when compared with the clinical model of health, aspects of the eudaimonistic model predate the clinical model of health. This model is also more congruent with integrative modes of therapy, which are used increasingly by people in the United States and the rest of world.

These ideas of health provide a basis for how people view health and disease and how they view the roles of nurses, physicians, and other health care providers. For example, in the clinical model of health, a person may expect to visit a health care provider only when there are obvious signs of illness. Personal responsibility for health may not be a motivating factor for this individual, because the provider is responsible for dealing with the health problem and returning the person to health. Therefore attempts to teach health-promoting activities may not be effective.

Wellness–Illness Continuum

The wellness–illness continuum, as stated earlier, is a dichotomous depiction of the relationship between the concepts of health and illness. In this paradigm **wellness** is a positive state in which incremental increases in health can be made beyond the midpoint (Figure 1-1). These increases represent improved physical and mental health states. The opposite end of the continuum is illness, with the possibility of incremental decreases in health beyond the midpoint. This depiction of the relationship of wellness and illness fits well with the clinical model of health.

High-Level Wellness

From a dichotomous representation of health and illness as opposites, Dunn (1961) developed a health–illness continuum that would assess a client based on his or her relative health compared with others and the environment (Figure 1-1). A second dimension, high-level wellness, was added to the health–illness continuum, in which a matrix of a favorable environment allows high-level wellness to occur and an unfavorable environment allows low-level wellness to exist.

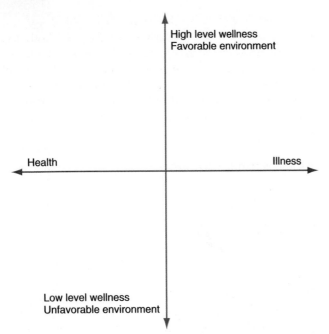

Figure 1-1 Wellness–illness continuum with high-level wellness added. Moving from the center to the right demonstrates movement toward illness. Moving from the center to the left demonstrates movement toward health. Moving above the line demonstrates movement toward increasing wellness. Moving below the line demonstrates movement toward decreasing wellness. (Modified from U.S. Department of Health and Human Services, Public Health Service, 1982.)

With this addition, it became possible to characterize a person's health status based on the clinical model of health and other social and environmental parameters. The concept demonstrates that a person can have a terminal disease and be emotionally prepared for death, while acting as a support for other people and achieving high-level wellness. High-level wellness involves progression toward a higher level of functioning, an open-ended and ever-expanding future with its challenge of fuller potential, and the integration of the whole being (Ardell, 2004). This definition of high-level wellness contains ideas similar to those in the eudaimonistic model of health. Additionally, high-level wellness emphasizes the interrelationship between the environment and the ability of achieving health on both a personal and a societal level.

Health Ecology

An evolving view of health recognizes the interconnection among people and their physical and social environments. Newman (2003) expressed this interconnection within a developmental framework, and the work of Gordon (1994) applies this interconnection to functional health patterns as presented in subsequent chapters. Health from an ecological perspective is multidimensional, extending from the individual into the surrounding community and including the context within which the person functions. It incorporates a systems approach within which the actions of one

portion of the system affect the functioning of the system as a whole. This view of health expands on high-level wellness by recognizing that social and environmental factors can enhance or limit health and healthy behaviors. For example, most people can benefit from physical activity such as walking. People are more likely to walk in areas where there are sidewalks or pathways and where they feel safe. Nurses can work to encourage people to walk, but they may also need to advocate for safe walking areas and work with others to plan for people-friendly community development.

Functioning

One of the defining characteristics of life is the ability to function. Similar to the concept of health, functional health can be characterized as being present or absent, at high level, or at low level. Functioning is integral to health. Physical, mental, and social levels of function are reflected in terms of performance and social expectations. Function can also be viewed from an ecological perspective, as in the example of walking used previously. Loss of function may be a sign or symptom of a disease. For example, sudden loss of the ability to move an arm or leg may indicate a stroke. The inability to leave the house may indicate overwhelming fear. In both cases the loss of function is a sign of disease, a state of ill health. Loss of function is an indication that the person may need nursing intervention. Research in older adults indicates that decline in physical function may predict loss of physical function and death (Greiner, Snowdon, & Greiner, 1996).

Health

Health, as defined in this text, is a state of physical, mental, and social functioning that realizes a person's potential. Health is an individual's responsibility, but it requires collective action to ensure a society and an environment in which people can act responsibly. The culture and beliefs of the people can also influence health. This definition is consistent with the World Health Organization (2004) definition of health as the state of complete physical, mental, and social well-being and not merely the absence of disease and infirmity. In addition to being measurable in process and outcomes, this definition is applicable across the life span, particularly for older adults whose functional abilities may determine needed services.

ILLNESS, DISEASE, AND HEALTH

It is easy to think of health or wellness as the lack of disease and to consider *illness* and *disease* interchangeable terms. However, *health* and *disease* are not simply antonyms, and *disease* and *illness* are not synonyms. **Disease** may be defined as the failure of a person's adaptive mechanisms to counteract stimuli and stresses adequately, resulting in functional or structural disturbances. This definition is an ecological concept of disease, which uses a multifactorial perspective rather than a search for a single cause. This approach increases the chances of discovering the various factors that may be susceptible to intervention. Health and disease must be viewed as inseparable, as variations of development over time. If disease does not exist, then there is no need to discuss health. **Illness** is a social construct in which people are in an imbalanced, unsustainable relationship with their environment and are failing in their ability to survive and create a higher quality of life. Illness is a response characterized by a mismatch between a person's needs and the resources available to meet those needs. Additionally, illness signals to individuals and populations that the present balance is not working. Disease is a biomedical term indicating the presence of a recognizable health deviation, whereas illness is a state of being. Illness has social, psychological, and biomedical components. A person can have a disease without feeling ill (e.g., asymptomatic hypertension). The theory that health and illness are dynamic patterns that change with time and social circumstances leads to the conclusion that health assessments must be made frequently during the life cycle. Most health evaluations are relative and based on a series of perceptions and observations rather than a limited standard of measurement. Health arises from a finely graded continuum of functional ability and disability, not from mutually exclusive categories. Health, illness, and disease are neither static nor stationary. Behind every condition is the phenomenon of almost constant alteration.

PLANNING FOR HEALTH

Prevention of disease in society has always been the focus of public health. However, over the past 30 years, health promotion has moved to the forefront within the public health sector and has become a driving force in health care.

A key milestone in promoting health was the advent of *Healthy People* (USDHEW, Public Health Service [PHS], 1979), the surgeon general's first report on health promotion and disease prevention issued during the waning years of the Carter administration. This document identified five national health goals addressing the reduction of death rates in adults and children and the reduction of sick days in older adults. Further, the document identified three causes of the major health issues in the United States as careless habits, pollution of the environment, and permitting harmful social conditions that destroy health to persist (hunger, poverty, and ignorance), especially for infants and children.

Healthy People was a call to action and an attempt to set health goals for the United States for the next 10 years by issuing 226 health objectives. Unfortunately, a change in political leadership and the spiraling costs of hospital-based health care caused this document to be placed on the back burner for 7 years. The need to report on progress toward the national objectives led a larger, renewed effort in the form of *The 1990 Health Objectives for the Nation: A Midcourse Review* (USDHHS, PHS, 1986). This midcourse review noted that although many goals were achievable, the unachieved goals were hindered by current health status, limited progress on risk reduction, difficulties in data collection, and a lack of public awareness.

Healthy People 2000 (USDHHS, PHS, 1990) and its *Mid-Course Review and 1995 Revisions* (USDHHS, PHS, 1996) were landmark documents in that a consortium of people representing national organizations worked with U.S. Public Health Service officials to create a more global approach to health. Additionally, a management-by-objectives approach was used to address each problem area. These two documents became the blueprints for each state as funding for federal programs became linked to meeting these national health objectives. As the objectives became more widely implemented, methods for collecting data became formalized, and the data flowed back into the system to form the revisions set in 1995. The core of these health objectives remained; that is, prevention of illness and disease was the foundation for health. *Healthy People 2000* set out three broad goals: increase the span of healthy life, reduce **health disparities,** and provide access to preventive services for all.

Additionally, the work included 22 specific areas for achievement, with objectives in each area based on age, health disparities, and health needs. By 1995, progress was made on 70% of these objectives. However, on 30% of the objectives, movement on goals was either in the wrong direction, had not changed, or could not be determined because the data were insufficient.

HEALTHY PEOPLE 2010

Healthy People 2010 (USDHHS, PHS, 2000) is the latest of the *Healthy People* documents. This document sets out 28 specific areas for health improvement in 467 objectives.

Healthy People 2010 Goals

Two goals of *Healthy People 2010* are to:
1. Increase quality and years of healthy life
2. Eliminate health disparities

Each goal is important. The first goal addresses the issues of longevity and quality of life. Increasing the number of years of healthy life addresses the concern that people are living longer but with chronic health problems that interfere with the quality of their lives. However, quality of life is also an issue for people who are unable to achieve long lives. Combining these two ideas places an emphasis on both longevity and quality of life as areas that need improvement. The second goal, eliminating health disparities, addresses the growing problems of access to care; differences in treatment based on race, gender, and ability to pay; and related issues such as urban versus rural health, insurance coverage, Medicare and Medicaid reimbursement, and satisfaction with service delivery.

These two goals set out the territory in which health promotion and disease prevention efforts take place. Research in a variety of areas has indicated clearly that health disparities are linked directly and indirectly to longevity and quality of life issues. For example, it is known that black men and women live fewer years than do white men and women, respectively. Research from the Agency for Health Care Research and Quality demonstrates that

Healthy People 2010
Selected National Health Promotion and Disease Prevention Objectives for Nutrition and Overweight

- 19-1. Increase the proportion of adults who are at a healthy weight.
- 19-2. Reduce the proportion of adults who are obese.
- 19-3. Reduce the proportion of children and adolescents who are overweight or obese.
- 19-5. Increase the proportion of people aged 2 years and older who consume at least two daily servings of fruit.
- 19-6. Increase the proportion of people aged 2 years and older who consume at least three daily servings of vegetables, with at least one third being dark green or deep yellow vegetables.
- 19-7. Increase the proportion of people aged 2 years and older who consume at least six daily servings of grain products, with at least three being whole grains.
- 19-8. Increase the proportion of people aged 2 years and older who consume less than 10% of calories from saturated fat.
- 19-9. Increase the proportion of people aged 2 years and older who consume no more than 30% of calories from fat.
- 19-10. Increase the proportion of people aged 2 years and older who consume 2400 mg or less of sodium daily.

From U.S. Department of Health and Human Services, Public Health Service. (2000). *Healthy People 2010* (conference edition, in two volumes). Washington, DC: U.S. Government Printing Office.

black men and women are provided with less invasive and less expensive interventions for cardiac disease than are white men and women (Canto, Allison, & Kiefe, 2000). By choosing not to offer reperfusion therapy to one racial group when it is warranted and offering the same therapy to another group contributes to the racial disparity in health care in this country and to the shorter life spans of blacks as compared with that of whites (Multicultural Awareness box).

The *Healthy People 2010* focus areas and objectives are the road map for this territory and a guide for health care research, practice, and communications in a way that should allow the health care community to measure progress on the broader goals.

The detailed objectives can be found on the Internet at *http://www.healthypeople.gov*. The 28 specific focus areas are listed alphabetically in Box 1-1. A quick look through these focus areas provides an indication of the scope of the *Healthy People 2010* areas compared with earlier *Healthy People* documents. These focus areas span age categories from conception to death and incorporate prevention, access, treatment, and follow-up at the individual, family, provider, work site, and community levels. *Healthy People 2010* is centered on 10 leading health indicators that

MULTICULTURAL AWARENESS

Influence of Personal Cultural Values on Health Care Delivery

Culture influences every aspect of human life, including beliefs, values, and customs regarding health care. As health care providers, nurses need to be aware of their beliefs, values, and customs and how these ideas translate into behavior. It is easy to assume that an individual's own perspective is correct and shared by others. This is especially true when working with other health care providers of the same culture. This concept is referred to as *ethnocentrism* and can lead to a devaluing of the beliefs, values, and customs of others, known as *racism*. Although it is impossible for any person to ignore the cultural influences on their lives, nurses and other health care providers have a special obligation to be aware of their own cultural biases and to focus more on the cultural influences in the lives of their clients by developing *cultural competence*. This ability to view others' situations from their perspectives is known as *empathy*. Multicultural health issues will continue to challenge providers to pursue lifelong learning about those for whom they provide care as the racial and ethnic mix in society changes.

Box 1-1 The 28 Focus Areas in *Healthy People 2010*

- Access to quality health services
- Arthritis, osteoporosis, and chronic back conditions
- Cancer
- Chronic kidney disease
- Diabetes
- Disability and secondary conditions
- Educational and community-based programs
- Environmental health
- Family planning
- Food safety
- Health communication
- Heart disease and stroke
- Human immunodeficiency virus
- Immunization and infectious diseases
- Injury and violence prevention
- Maternal, infant, and child health
- Medical product safety
- Mental health and mental disorders
- Nutrition and overweight
- Occupational safety and health
- Oral health
- Physical activity and fitness
- Public health infrastructure
- Respiratory diseases
- Sexually transmitted diseases
- Substance abuse
- Tobacco use
- Vision and hearing

From U.S. Department of Health and Human Services, Public Health Service. (2000). *Healthy People 2010* (conference edition, in two volumes). Washington, DC: U.S. Government Printing Office.

Box 1-2 **The 10 Leading Health Indicators in**
Healthy People 2010

- Physical activity
- Overweight and obesity
- Tobacco use
- Substance abuse
- Responsible sexual behavior
- Mental health
- Injury and violence
- Environmental quality
- Immunization
- Access to health care

Data from U.S. Department of Health and Human Services, Public Health Service. (2000). *Healthy People 2010* (conference edition, in two volumes). Washington, DC: U.S. Government Printing Office.

"reflect the major public health concerns in the United States and were chosen based on their ability to motivate action, the availability of data to measure their progress, and their relevance as broad public health issues" (USDHHS, PHS, 2000, p. 11) (Box 1-2). One example of an objective is presented here for illustration of the scope of this project.

Objective 22-2. Increase the proportion of adults who engage regularly, preferably daily, in moderate physical activity for at least 30 minutes per day. This objective directly addresses the first two leading health indicators, physical activity and weight (obesity). Arguably, other indicators such as tobacco and substance abuse and mental health are related indirectly to this objective. A person who smokes or uses drugs regularly has a limited ability to meet this objective. Nevertheless, physical activity can contribute to mental health through stress reduction and physical fitness. Access to health care to obtain a complete physical examination before starting to exercise and the quality of the work or neighborhood environment available for exercise can contribute to success or failure of this objective. This objective is related to other objectives such as nutrition and control of high blood pressure.

Current knowledge about physical activity and specific populations was considered when creating the *Healthy People 2010* objectives. Women, low-income populations, black and Hispanic peoples, those with disabilities, and those over the age of 75 exercise less than do white men with moderate to high incomes. These health disparities can influence the number of people in these groups who develop high cholesterol levels or high blood pressure, which further increases their risk of heart disease and stroke. Although this objective addresses adults, other objectives address the need to begin exercise activities at an early age and to encourage young adults to be actively engaged in exercise. How might this objective be adjusted to the needs of an older adult population?

Another important feature of *Healthy People 2010* is its emphasis on responsibility for intervention. Individuals need to accept responsibility for their lifestyle choices and behaviors. This emphasis on personal responsibility gives each individual a role in the quality of life and the length of healthy life each may have.

Health care providers need to be responsible for offering preventive health services and monitoring behaviors. Unfortunately, many of the incentives for providers are to do tasks and procedures rather than to counsel and help individuals choose among various behaviors. Providers need to take the time to discuss behaviors that may improve the quality of life and add years of life. For example, the addictive nature of tobacco and its effect on the development and course of a variety of chronic health conditions is now well recognized. Providers should ask every person about tobacco use and should provide ways to quit smoking, including economic and social incentives.

Providers also need to look for partnership in the community through which they can better serve the needs of individuals. *Healthy People 2010* emphasizes the efforts of partnerships and partnership building as essential to health promotion. One approach is to develop and use community nursing centers (*http://www.rncc.org*). The Health Promotion Center (HPC) operated by Fairfield University School of Nursing in Fairfield, Connecticut, is one example. The nurses and student nurses who provide health education, screening, and referral services at the HPC work with community organizations to better meet the health care needs of underserved people. The HPC staff works with senior housing organizations and senior centers to provide comprehensive cardiovascular screening and medication review. As an extension of this work, funding was secured for a program called Step Up to Health, a project to increase physical activity in this population through interactive planning and consumer ownership of the activities. The project is part of the National Blueprint Project supported by the Robert Wood Johnson Foundation (*http://www.agingblueprint.org*). The project is engaging older adults in walking programs, line dancing, gardening, and low-impact exercise programs, including the People with Arthritis Can Exercise (PACE) program from the National Arthritis Foundation (*http://www.arthritis.org/events/getinvolved/ProgramsServices/PACE.asp*). Another approach to partnerships is to have providers serve as active participants on community boards and advisory committees, which enables them to become more aware of the service needs in the community and the resources available to help meet those needs.

Work sites and communities need to become partners in providing opportunities for people to lead healthy lives through flexible work schedules, work site wellness programs, safe parks, and exercise facilities. Converting empty lots into community gardens provides beautification of the area, an opportunity for exercise in caring for the garden, and a source of fresh vegetables.

The faith community is a vital partner in meeting *Healthy People 2010* objectives. Faith communities can cut across economic, social, racial, and gender barriers, making them an excellent source for sharing information on health promotion and disease prevention. Parish nurses are becoming increasingly prevalent and they incorporate *Healthy People 2010* objectives into their activities (Berry, 2004).

Public health officials at all levels are necessary partners in meeting *Healthy People 2010* objectives. As part of the core public health functions of assessment, policy development, and assurance, the U.S. Public Health Service and all state, county, and local health departments need to collect data, make information available to the public, create policies that support *Healthy People 2010* objectives, and ensure that needed services are available from a competent workforce.

Healthy People 2010 can form the basis for planning, service delivery, evaluation, and research in every aspect of the health care system. Nurses need to be familiar with this document and its intent. They should compare their practices with the objectives in *Healthy People 2010*. Additionally, nurses need to be aware of the research and practice changes that occur as a result of the work toward these objectives.

Healthy People 2010 Update

In the years following publication of the *Healthy People 2010* document, the USDHHS, Public Health Service, has conducted a series of progress reviews on many of the 28 focus areas. The up-to-date listing of these reviews can be found at the *Healthy People 2010* Web site (*http://www.healthy people.gov/data/PROGRVW/default.htm*). The midcourse review of these objectives is due in 2005.

Progress in many of the focus areas is limited at this time. For example, in the area of access to quality health services, only small increases were noted in the number of people under 65 with health insurance. Although the 2010 goal is to have 100% coverage, that of this population in 2001 was 84%, leaving 16% of the under-65 population without insurance. Health disparities continue in that most health insurance coverage in the United States is linked to employment, with black and Hispanic populations less likely to have the education and opportunity to work in jobs with health benefits. There was improvement in the area of difficulty or delay in receiving needed health care for those without health insurance, and the federal initiative to increase the number and availability of services through federally qualified health centers should contribute to reductions in this area. A second example is the area of heart disease and stroke, where substantial progress was made by 2000. Both heart disease and stroke prevention will require significant effort to move from the mortality rate of 196 per 100,000 to the 2010 goal of 166 per 100,000 people for heart disease, and from 61 per 100,000 to the 2010 goal of 48 per 100,000 people for stroke. Health disparities remain for blacks, whose rate of mortality due to heart disease and stroke was 46% and 39% higher, respectively, than the national average in 2000. Progress in this area may be offset by the increasing age of the U.S. population and the number of people living with existing disease and risk factors.

CASE STUDY

Refer to the Case Study about Frank Thompson and his family. Read carefully, because some of the concepts covered thus far are applied in the following sections.

Problem Identification

How many problems does Frank's situation present? The answer depends on who is asked and the person's relationship to Frank. Each point of view focuses on different aspects of Frank's life. His physician, using a clinical model of health, might say that Frank had coronary heart disease with an acute myocardial infarction, hypertension, hyperlipidemia, chronic bronchitis, and obesity. Frank's problems represent a failure to meet several of the *Healthy People 2010* objectives on a personal level. His nurse might add that he paid little attention to his lifestyle, even after changes were recommended. He continued to overeat, drink too much, smoke, not exercise, and to live a stressful life. Frank's employer saw a man who had potential, but who was now too disabled to take on new responsibilities and perhaps unable to continue performing his previous duties. Frank's children might feel that he could no longer take them on jaunts or play with them. His wife, Sada, knew that their plans for educating their children and for travel and enjoyment might suffer. The human resource personnel who managed Frank's health insurance and pension programs would say that he had an expensive disease, and the state health planner would point out that Frank's problem was only one of a growing number of disabling illnesses that result from preventable causes.

To Frank, the health problems were multidimensional. His initial fear of dying, pain, dependence, and frustration decreased as he began to feel better, but his realization that he might never be able to achieve his dreams for himself and his family haunted him. Although theoretically in his prime, Frank suddenly saw himself as far older than his years, both in body and in social achievement. He believed he had reached his limit and that he would never again have the freedom to choose his future. He and his family needed to evaluate their situation and make alternative plans based on **asset planning.** A care plan has been developed for them (Care Plan box).

Planning Interventions

Rather than emphasizing chronic health issues and related problems, the nurse can begin with asset planning within the family. Asset planning is an approach that, given the realities of the present, helps the family and their providers focus on the building blocks for the future. It focuses on the assets or strengths of the individual, the family, and the community, applying those assets to improve or maintain the level of functioning.

Frank's physician and nurse can begin with Frank's survival of his first myocardial infarction. The coronary damage resulting from this event becomes the baseline for determining change in the lives of Frank and his family.

CASE STUDY

Assessment of Frank Thompson and Family

Frank Thompson's large brick home is located off a sparsely traveled country road. A few yards away stands the uninhabited shack where Frank was born during World War II.

Frank was raised knowing the odds that he faced as a poor tenant farmer. He helped his father, Ben, with their small tobacco and corn crops. They were unaware that the hazardous chemicals in the pesticides they used would later affect Ben's life. As his father often reminded him, Frank had to do better than others in school so he would not be doomed to the tenant farmer's life. However, Frank's school attendance was erratic because it was interrupted by the frequent demand of tending field crops. Thin and often tired, he had recurrent infections. The school nurse helped the Thompson family obtain medication for Frank's initial infection, but the family was never able to afford the penicillin that was necessary to prevent recurrent infections.

Inspired by the early work of Martin Luther King, Jr., Frank was intent on helping at home and building something better for his future. Frank managed to more than make up for his lost time at school. He passed his college entrance examinations and was awarded one of the new equal opportunity grants, which offered him a choice of attending any of the Ivy League schools in the Northeast. Instead, he chose the prestigious Southern University and eventually earned a master's degree in business administration. He married Sada, his long-time girlfriend, and the two planned their future.

With a good job in a large local sales firm, Frank built his house and started a family. He was promoted from a salesman to a division head and often traveled to regional meetings, sometimes accompanied by Sada and their three children. Frank's dream of sharing his success with his family included using part of his earnings to help his brothers and sisters with their education.

This new way of life meant little time for relaxation and frequent attendance at business luncheons and career-promoting social occasions. Frank kept late hours and worked long weekends. Good food, drinks, and cigarettes helped him relax before and after important business and social encounters; these softened the edges of hard bargaining and were status symbols.

Not surprisingly, Frank gained weight. He had a persistent cough, which was probably a result of the smoking habit he developed during the early years of his career. Frank's physician, with whom Frank visited regularly at the corporation's health maintenance organization, said Frank's blood pressure and serum lipid levels were both higher than normal and that he had chronic bronchitis. The physician urged Frank to do what he already knew he should: cut down on smoking, drinking, saturated fats, and calories; get more exercise; and find ways to relax. However, Frank's schedule was too busy for exercise. He had to work harder as he moved up in his company, but he also had to appear relaxed, which was an essential characteristic for a prospective vice president. To meet these goals, he tended to drink and smoke more. He also refused to take medication for problems he could not see. Lacking outward signs of disease, Frank believed he was out of shape but generally healthy. Then Sada pointed out that his chance for promotion might actually improve if he lost some weight; therefore, he registered for a physical fitness program for executives that he could attend on Sunday mornings and before work during the week. During his first workout, the classic sharp pain gripped his chest and Frank had a massive heart attack.

Weeks later, Frank was convalescing at home after being released from a university hospital coronary care facility. He was lucky to have survived the heart attack, but he was also lucky because most of the services were covered by his medical insurance plan and because 80% of his earnings were protected by the company's disability pension. Most people in the United States do not have this protection.

However, Frank's dreams of promotion were shattered. For many months he could go to the office only 2 or 3 times a week at most, simply to deal with routine matters. He could not travel, for business or otherwise, for a long time. He was also skeptical about his cardiac rehabilitation program because his heart attack happened during exercise.

Reflective Questions
1. As a nurse, how would you explain to Frank that his heart attack was not caused by exercise?
2. How might a family approach to diet and exercise work with this family, given its structure and background?
3. Are there negative behaviors in your life that you see as status symbols?

Earlier, Frank's physician had taken a broader time perspective when he advised Frank to cut down on smoking, which was contributing to both his bronchitis and his hypertension, and to change his high-fat diet and sedentary habits, which contributed to his weight problem and aggravated his high blood pressure. These lifestyle changes now become tools for Frank's recovery and for change within his family. His cardiac event becomes a risk factor for heart disease in the lives of his children.

Looking at the immediate future, Frank's employer saw the effect of the event on Frank's position within the company. Frank would have a long recovery that could be successful if he adhered to his cardiac rehabilitation program. Asset planning at this level meant examining how to move Frank back into his work role without further jeopardizing his health. Frank and Sada also needed to examine if he could continue in this position, given its potential effect on his health.

Frank and his family used a broader perspective than the medical personnel or the corporation. They knew that to achieve the family's economic and educational goals and still spend time together, they made decisions that ultimately affected Frank's health. Similar to many Americans, they had been willing to live with Frank's job pressures and stressful lifestyle. The family members were aware of their impoverished roots and had no wish to go back to them. However, they also recognized that the strength of their family, their ability to work together to achieve goals, and

CARE PLAN

Frank Thompson and Family

Nursing Diagnosis Risk for Ineffective Coping Due to Change in Role Performance and Self-Esteem

DEFINING CHARACTERISTICS

- Inability to complete tasks
- Lack of focus on needs
- Feelings of inadequacy
- Inability to make decisions
- Sense of being overwhelmed
- Rest and sleep disturbance
- Frequent stress-related headaches
- Emotional fragility
- Assessment of situations does not match assessments by others

RELATED FACTORS

- Unexpected life changes
- Chronic disease
- Stressful life events
- Uncertainty of family supports
- Unrealistic expectations of self
- Unpredictable future
- Need to reassess abilities
- Insecure job status

EXPECTED OUTCOMES

- The person will develop realistic expectations of capabilities based on rehabilitation potential.
- The nurse and person will set mutually agreeable milestones for resuming functions.
- The person will develop a revitalized sense of self.
- The person and family will use available resources to examine social and role shifts that affect the family.
- The person and spouse will express to each other their hopes and fears about the future.

INTERVENTIONS

- Listen to the concerns of the person and spouse regarding job, social, family, and medical concerns.
- Counsel the individual and spouse about realistic goals and expectations of cardiac rehabilitation.
- Assist the individual in setting realistic and attainable short-term goals.
- Assist the individual in developing more effective problem-solving skills.
- Provide support and positive feedback as short-term goals are met.
- Explore community services that match the goals of the family.
- Facilitate family access to needed services through advocacy and supportive guidance.
- Supervise and teach about prescribed and other medications.
- Coordinate communications between providers, employers, and other organizations to meet coping needs of the individual and his or her family.

their faith were assets that were missing in other families they knew.

Frank's social network of friends, relatives, and church members became an additional asset. They helped the family through the difficult initial weeks at home by providing meals, taking care of the yard work and laundry, and providing companionship so that Sada could shop and have time alone. As Frank recovered, they provided support for the social and lifestyle changes that Frank and his family needed to make.

The visiting nurse played a vital role in Frank's recovery. As the physician continued to monitor Frank's cardiac status, the visiting nurse began the long process of helping Frank change his habits. He had stopped smoking while in the hospital, but with more free time than usual, he was craving cigarettes again. Using an asset planning approach and Gordon's functional health patterns (1994), the visiting nurse identified the changes that Frank needed to make to decrease the risk of a second heart attack. A plan was developed to help him begin to take control of his life through behavior changes. These changes included relaxation techniques, diet modification, smoking cessation, and mild chair exercises. The support of the family was enlisted to reinforce the changes Frank was willing to make. His employer was contacted and agreed to a plan enabling Frank to work from home using a computer as the office became a nonsmoking workplace. Frank became an asset to the workplace, serving as a spokesperson for the benefits of lifestyle change. He was enlisted to talk with other employees about stress management and smoking cessation based on his personal experiences.

Health planners and public health officials used the broadest perspective in asset planning by viewing Frank as an example of a person whose potential shifted as a result of a preventable, disabling illness. The planners looked to public and private community patterns and policies that increase healthful habits and living conditions. Work schedules and work load; stress and safety in work environments; affirmative action programs for jobs and wages; availability of public transportation systems, recreational facilities, and economically accessible housing; farm price subsidies for food and tobacco crops that affect buying patterns; and excise taxes and regulation of health-damaging drugs such as alcohol and nicotine are all taken into consideration (Grzywacz & Fuqua, 2000). The asset planning approach emphasizes the positive actions that can be made to minimize the effects of Frank's illness and related diseases.

What Was the Actual Cause of Frank's Problem?

It is not possible to separate one cause from another, because causes are not single factors. In Frank's case the sources of illness were found in the many interrelationships in his life. Attempting to treat or change each factor as a separate entity can have a limited effect on the improvement of overall health. Frank's health problems were numerous. In addition to a poor diet, weight gain, lack of exercise, and smoking, his hyperlipidemia, an adaptive biological response to the pressures in his life, could not sustain him indefinitely. It eventually clogged his coronary vessels, becoming maladaptive. His hypertension, resulting from his diet and time-constrained lifestyle, was also a biological attempt to adjust to a situation that contributed to an imbalance between his personal resources and the demands of his family and the economic world. Frank's smoking was a psychosocial means to help him relieve some of the emotional pressures. It may have served this short-term purpose, but only at a silently rising cost to his health. Cigarette use by people who have hypertension or high serum cholesterol levels multiplies their risk of coronary heart disease (Izzo & Black, 2003).

Evaluation of the Situation

The health status of an individual or population depends on a sustainable balance of the complex responses between internal (physiological and psychological) and external (social and environmental) factors. Health was conceived initially as a biological state, with genetic endowment as the starting point. However, health involves psychological and social aspects and is interpreted within the context of the immediate environment.

The interconnections between biophysical, psychological, and environmental causes and consequences did not end with Frank's heart attack. His heart attack was only the most dramatic sign that health-damaging responses outweighed health-promoting ones. The "tip of the iceberg" analogy is used frequently to illustrate the importance of identifying individuals with subclinical symptoms. High blood lipid levels, high blood pressure, obesity, smoking, and persistent worrying were no less important than the infarction in shaping the status of Frank's health. To repair the damage to Frank's heart without changing his lifestyle, habits, and work environment would buy only a brief amount of time before further damage would occur.

The infarction and resulting disability also permanently reshaped Frank's environment. After a few months of working full time, Frank realized that he needed to find a less stressful job. He recognized that his sales administration skills were an asset and began interviewing in the nonprofit sector. Ultimately, he landed a job at half his previous salary, but with excellent benefits and a flexible work environment. His reduced income meant that his children's educational opportunities were more limited than they were before his heart attack, but his family responded by asking for tuition support from community organizations. Frank found that his contacts in both the corporate and the nonprofit sectors increased his value to his new employer. Frank's entire life, internal and external, had changed. He had learned to adapt to his health problems and had developed a more eudaimonistic approach to health and life.

Frank's situation illustrates how causes and effects in life and health tend to merge into constant, inseparable interconnections between individuals and their worlds. A person's health status is a reflection of a web of relationships that characterize that person's life. Health is not an achievement or a prize, but a high-quality interaction between a person's inner and outer worlds that provides the capacity to respond to the demands of the biological, psychological, and environmental systems of these worlds.

After reviewing the list of *Healthy People 2010* focus areas listed in Box 1-1, which ones apply to the promotion of Frank's health? Clearly, the area of heart disease and stroke is most applicable. The *Healthy People 2010* Web site lists a number of objectives that relate directly to prevention of heart disease, hypertension, and hyperlipidemia, including objectives that relate to treatment options and training the public to recognize and respond to heart attacks and stroke. Based on the information about Frank and his experience, determine what his children should be taught based on the *Healthy People 2010* objectives in this focus area.

LEVELS OF PREVENTION

Prevention, in a narrow sense, means averting the development of disease that will manifest in the future. In a broad sense prevention consists of all measures, including definitive therapy, that limit disease progression. Leavell and Clark (1965) defined three **levels of prevention**: primary, secondary, and tertiary (Figure 1-2). Although the levels of prevention are related to the natural history of disease, they can be used to prevent disease and provide nurses with starting points in making effective, positive changes in the health status of their clients. Within the three levels of prevention, there are five steps. These steps include:

1. Health promotion (primary prevention)
2. Specific protection (primary prevention)
3. Early diagnosis and prompt treatment (secondary prevention)
4. Disability limitation (secondary prevention)
5. Restoration and rehabilitation (tertiary prevention)

Some confusion exists in the interpretation of these concepts; therefore, a consistent understanding of primary, secondary, and tertiary prevention is essential. The levels of prevention operate on a continuum but may overlap in practice. The nurse must clearly understand the goals of each level to intervene effectively in keeping people healthy.

Primary Prevention

Primary prevention precedes disease or dysfunction. However, primary prevention is therapeutic in that it includes health as beneficial to well-being, it uses therapeutic treatments and, as a process or behavior toward enhancing health, it involves symptom identification when teaching stress-reduction techniques. Primary prevention intervention includes health promotion, such as health education about risk factors for heart disease, and specific protection, such as immunization against hepatitis B. Its purpose is to decrease the vulnerability of the individual or population to disease or dysfunction. Interventions at this level encourage individuals and groups to become more aware of the means of improving health and the things they

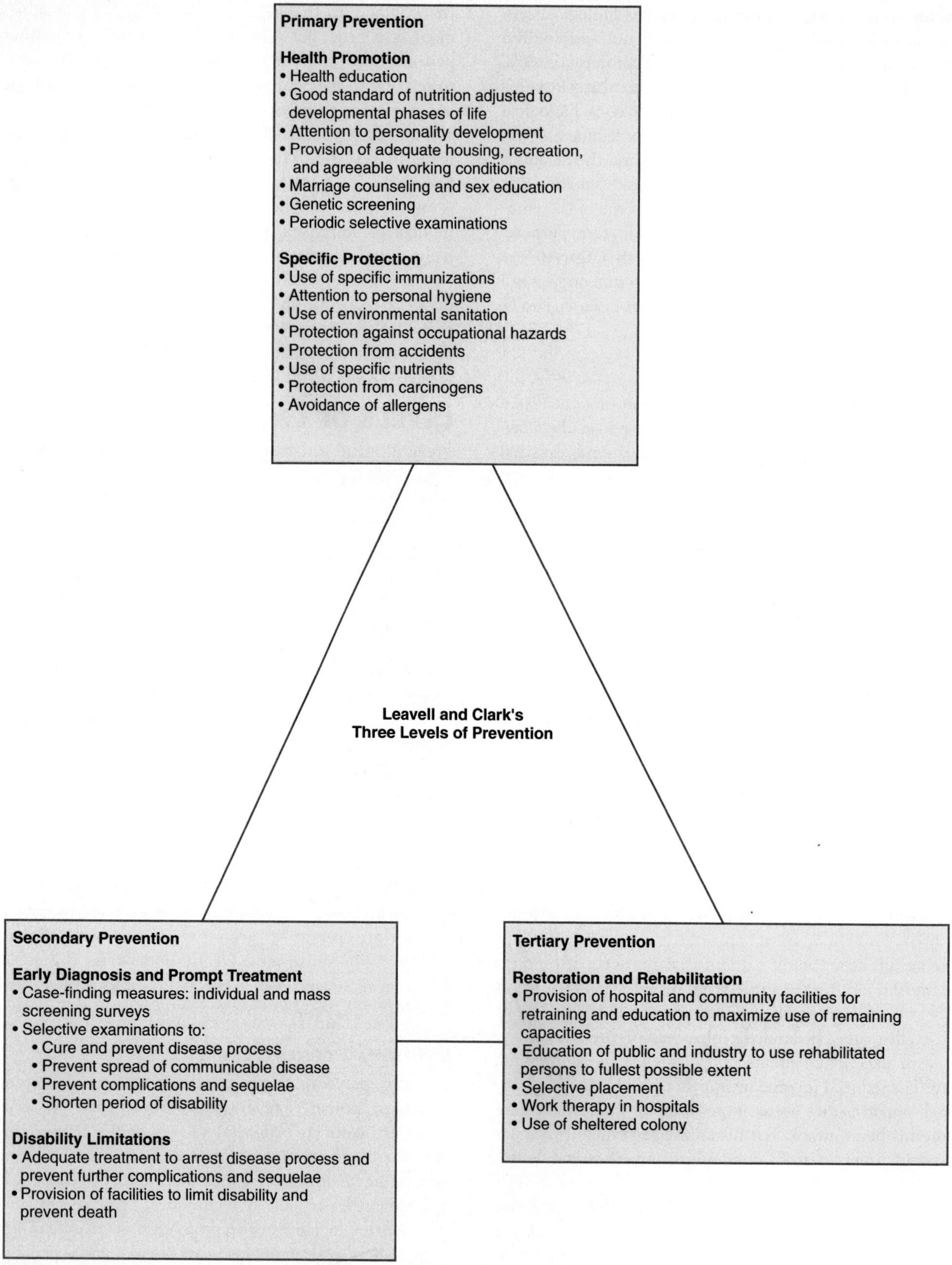

Primary Prevention

Health Promotion
• Health education
• Good standard of nutrition adjusted to developmental phases of life
• Attention to personality development
• Provision of adequate housing, recreation, and agreeable working conditions
• Marriage counseling and sex education
• Genetic screening
• Periodic selective examinations

Specific Protection
• Use of specific immunizations
• Attention to personal hygiene
• Use of environmental sanitation
• Protection against occupational hazards
• Protection from accidents
• Use of specific nutrients
• Protection from carcinogens
• Avoidance of allergens

Leavell and Clark's Three Levels of Prevention

Secondary Prevention

Early Diagnosis and Prompt Treatment
• Case-finding measures: individual and mass screening surveys
• Selective examinations to:
  • Cure and prevent disease process
  • Prevent spread of communicable disease
  • Prevent complications and sequelae
  • Shorten period of disability

Disability Limitations
• Adequate treatment to arrest disease process and prevent further complications and sequelae
• Provision of facilities to limit disability and prevent death

Tertiary Prevention

Restoration and Rehabilitation
• Provision of hospital and community facilities for retraining and education to maximize use of remaining capacities
• Education of public and industry to use rehabilitated persons to fullest possible extent
• Selective placement
• Work therapy in hospitals
• Use of sheltered colony

Figure 1-2 The three levels of prevention developed by Leavell and Clark. (Data from Leavell, H., & Clark, A. E. [1965]. *Preventive medicine for doctors in the community.* New York: McGraw-Hill.)

can do at the primary preventive health level and the optimal health level.

People are taught to use appropriate primary preventive measures. However, primary prevention can also be viewed as advocating for health policies that promote the health of the community and electing public officials who will enact legislation that protects the health of the public—a social and ecological role.

Health Promotion

Health promotion is a relatively new field; therefore, its definitions vary. O'Donnell (1987) has defined health promotion as "the science and art of helping people change their lifestyle to move toward a state of optimal health" (p. 4). Kreuter and Devore propose a more complex definition in a paper commissioned by the U.S. Public Health Service. They state that health promotion is "the process of advocating health in order to enhance the probability that personal (individual, family, and community), private (professional and business), and public (federal, state, and local government) support of positive health practices will become a societal norm" (Kreuter & Devore, 1980, p. 26).

The theoretical underpinnings for health promotion have evolved since the early 1980s. Most of these theories are derived from the social sciences and have been researched extensively. These theories include the theory of reasoned action by Ajzen and Fishbein (1980), theories of behavior by Bandura (1976, 1999), stages of change theories by Prochaska (Nigg et al., 1999), the health belief model by Rosenstock (Janz, Champion, & Strecher, 2002), and Pender's health promotion model (Pender, Murdaugh, & Parsons, 2002). Internet searches on each of these theories will provide numerous sites where more detailed information is available. Of particular interest to nurses are the most recent works by Bandura (1999) on self-efficacy and Pender, Murdaugh, and Parsons (2002) on the health promotion model.

Health promotion goes beyond providing information. It is also proactive decision making at all levels of society. A few of the strategies that have been identified within this decision-making process are screening, self-care of minor illness, readiness for emergencies, successful management of chronic disease, environmental changes to enhance positive behaviors, and health-enhancing policies within an organizational setting (Folding, 1988). These ideals are reflected in the *Healthy People 2010* objectives. Health promotion holds the best promise for lower-cost methods of limiting the constant increase in health care costs and for empowering people to be responsible for the aspects of their lives that can enhance well-being. Based on the significance of health-promotion activities within the health care system, efforts must be made to identify the determinants of health, identify relevant health-promotion strategies, and delineate issues relevant to social justice and access to care. Individuals, families, and communities must be active participants in this process so that the actions taken are socially relevant and economically feasible.

Health-promotion efforts, unlike those specific efforts directed toward protection from certain diseases, focus on maintaining or improving the general health of individuals, families, and communities (Health Teaching box). These activities are carried out at the public level (e.g., government programs promoting adequate housing), at the community level (e.g., Habitat for Humanity), and at the personal level (e.g., voting for improved low-income housing). Nursing interventions are directed toward developing people's resources to maintain or enhance their well-being, a form of asset-based planning.

HEALTH TEACHING   Process for Assessing, Evaluating, and Treating Overweight and Obesity in Adults

Overweight and obesity are major concerns in public health, because they contribute to other health problems such as high cholesterol, high blood pressure, diabetes mellitus, heart disease, functional limitations, and disability. As part of the National Heart, Lung, and Blood Institute's (NHLBI) Obesity Education Initiative, nurses have an important role to play in health education related to obesity prevention and control. The complete guide can be retrieved from *http://www.nhl bi.nih.gov/guidelines/obesity/prctgd_b.pdf*.

Assessment:

Nurses need to be able to explain body mass index and why it is the preferred method of determining overweight and obesity in adults. They need to understand the methods of data collection and measurement of height and weight, as well as waist circumference, risk factors, and co-morbidities. Nurses need to develop skill in determining weight loss readiness and motivation in their clients.

Management of Care:

Nurses should know best practices in weight management and weight loss. Fad diets, dietary supplements, and weight loss pills may be inappropriate for most people, and formal weight loss programs may be too expensive for low-income and moderate-income families. Use recommended diets that restrict caloric intake, set activity goals with your clients, encourage clients to keep a weekly food and activity diary and review with the client, and provide the client with information on diet and activity. Be sure to record client goals and the treatment plan, including a health education plan.

Be Prepared to Explain Therapies:

Nurses should become knowledgeable about current treatment options and their success rates. Holistic approaches are needed, because food behaviors are influenced by many factors. Listen to the clients' stories about food and its role in their lives. Therapies should fit the individuals' goals and should lead to lifestyle change.

Data from the National Heart, Lung, and Blood Institute. (2000). *The practical guide: Identification, evaluation, and treatment of overweight and obesity in adults* (NIH Publication No. 00-4084). Bethesda, MD: National Institutes of Health.

Two strategies of health promotion involve the individual and may be either passive or active. In passive strategies the individual is an inactive participant or recipient. Examples of passive strategies include: (1) public health efforts to maintain clean water and sanitary sewage systems to decrease infectious disease rates and improve health and (2) efforts to introduce vitamin D into all milk to ensure that children will not be at high risk for rickets when there is little sunlight. These passive strategies must be used to promote the health of the public when individual compliance is low.

Active strategies depend on the individual becoming personally involved in adopting a program of health promotion. Two examples of lifestyle change are daily exercise as part of a physical fitness plan and a stress-management program as part of daily living. A combination of active and passive strategies is best for making an individual healthier. Reexamine the Case Study to determine when Frank could have incorporated some of these strategies to decrease his risk of heart disease.

This text is concerned almost entirely with active strategies and the nurse's role in these strategies. Some passive strategies are included, but they are presented with the implicit belief that each individual must take responsibility for improving health. It is undeniable that passive strategies also have a valuable role, but they must be used within a context of encouraging and teaching individuals to assume more responsibility for their health.

Although health promotion would seem to be a practical and effective mode of health care, the major portion of health care delivery is geared toward responding to acute and chronic disease. Preventing or delaying the onset of chronic disease and adding new dimensions to the quality of life are not as easy to implement, because they take time to implement and evaluate and require personal action. These actions are more closely associated with everyday living and the lifestyles adopted by individuals, families, communities, and nations. Habits such as eating, resting, exercising, and handling anxieties appear to be transmitted from parent to child and from social group to social group as part of a cultural, not a genetic, heritage. These activities may be taught in subtle ways, but they influence behavior and have as much of an influence on health as does genetic inheritance. Although the public may not appreciate the causal relationships between behavior and health, it should be apparent to health professionals. Arguably, the concept of risk is the most basic of all health concepts, because health promotion and disease protection are based on this concept.

Health-promotion strategies have the potential of enhancing the quality of life from birth to death. For example, good nutrition is adjusted to various developmental phases in life to account for rapid growth and development during infancy and early childhood, physiological changes associated with adolescence, extra demands during pregnancy, and the many changes occurring in older adults. Good nutrition is known to enhance immune system function, enabling individuals to fight off infections that could lead to disabling illnesses. Other individual activities are adapted to the person's needs for optimal personality development at all ages. As seen in Unit Four, much can be done on a personal or group basis, through counseling and properly directed parent education, to provide the environmental requirements for the proper personality development of children. Community participation is also an important factor in promoting individual, family, and group health (see Chapters 7 and 8).

Personal health promotion is usually provided through health education (see Chapter 10). As an important function of nurses, physicians, and allied health professionals, health education is principally concerned with eliciting useful changes in human behavior. The goal is the inculcation of a sense of responsibility for an individual's own health and a shared sense of responsibility for avoiding injury to the health of others. This objective implies the encouragement of child-rearing practices that foster normal growth and development (personal, social, and physical). Health education nurtures health-promoting habits, values, and attitudes that must be learned through practice. These must be reinforced through systematic instruction in hygiene, bodily function, physical fitness, and use of leisure time. Another goal is to understand the appropriate use of health services. For example, a semiannual visit to a dentist may teach a child better oral health habits and to visit the dentist regularly, although this is not the primary purpose of the visit. Parents, teachers, and caregivers play a vital role in health education. In addition to teaching individuals, nurses need to develop skills in group teaching and in working within community organizations.

Research clearly shows an increase in longevity, a decrease in early mortality and morbidity, and an improvement in the quality of life for individuals who have been involved in health-promotion activities such as physical activity and avoidance of smoking. It must be emphasized that health promotion requires lifestyle change (Nigg, et al, 1999). Once a lifestyle change has been adopted, vigilance is needed to ensure that it is maintained and modified to fit developmental and environmental changes.

Empirical data linking risk factors, health-promotion activities, and outcomes are sufficient to drive the development of the *Healthy People 2010* objectives and to be incorporated into quality improvement measures in managed care. One of the challenges posed in *Healthy People 2010* is the development of measurable outcome objectives that are based on more realistic economic models.

Health promotion is an important concept for nursing, because it embodies many other concepts that nursing is concerned with today. As stated earlier, much of the nursing role is involved with health teaching. Standard 5B of the *Nursing: Scope and Standards of Practice* document (American Nurses Association [ANA], 2004) requires nurses "to promote health and a safe environment" (p. 28) through health teaching and evaluation of teaching effectiveness in clinical practice (Hot Topics box).

HEALTH-PROMOTION PROGRAM INCENTIVES

The concept of health-promotion program incentives is multidimensional. Incentives are best defined relative to their purpose, type, and form for either groups or individuals.

An incentive is a reward designed to influence an individual to make a desired change that might otherwise not be made based solely on the intrinsic benefit of the changed behavior. For example, a person may not choose to stop smoking because of the cost of the smoking cessation materials. If the person is given the smoking cessation materials for free and provided with a $10 incentive each week for using them, that person might decide to make the change. The benefits of not smoking are not enough of an incentive to stop smoking, but the incentives help to make the behavior change possible.

One example of an integrated incentive program in an employee wellness program is the HEALTH Plus program at Vanderbilt University (2004). Full-time employees and faculty can participate in an incentive program that rewards them for participation and achievement of specific health and wellness goals. Participants receive monetary incentives for completing a health risk assessment on-line. They can then select a level of behavior change based on increasing levels of commitment (bronze, silver, or gold). For each level, participants choose wellness categories and actions they are willing to take within each category. They then work on those actions over the following year and complete another health risk assessment at the end of the year to note achievement. Information is available on each category and action, and wellness staff can assist participants in reaching desired goals. The incentive for the participants is an additional $10 to $15 in each paycheck, participation in groups working on specific actions, and recognition of achievement of each level. The university benefits from healthier employees, which is recognized to increase productivity, limit health care costs, and improve quality of life.

Based on data from Vanderbilt University, Human Resources Department. HEALTH Plus Vanderbilt Faculty and Status Fitness Program. Retrieved March, 20, 2005, from: *http://www.vanderbilt.edu/HRS/wellness/hpgftg.htm*.

Specific Protection

This aspect of primary prevention focuses on protecting people from disease by providing immunizations and reducing exposure to occupational hazards, carcinogens, and other environmental health risks. Primary prevention intervention is considered health protection, because it emphasizes shielding or defending the body (or the public) from injury. Implementing nursing interventions that prevent a specific health problem may seem easier than promoting well-being among individuals, groups, or communities, because the variables are delineated more clearly in prevention than in promotion and the potential influences are less diverse. Two examples may help demonstrate these differences.

• Immunization for influenza is quite popular and has become a regular activity for older adults each autumn. Nurses participate in this specific protection role by giving the influenza injections in clinics and offices.

• Creating nut-free schools to protect hypersensitive children from life-threatening allergic reactions to peanut products have largely been the result of grassroots parent organizations working with formal community organizations to adopt policies that protect the health of these children. Nurses may be involved in the parent organizations or the school or public health boards that review the proposed policies. Additionally, nurses must be able to address the need to protect portions of the population at risk.

Secondary Prevention

Although primary prevention measures have decreased the hazards of chronic diseases such as cardiovascular disease, conditions that preclude a healthy quality of life are still prevalent. Secondary prevention ranges from providing screening activities and treating early stages of disease to limiting disability by averting or delaying the consequences of advanced disease.

Screening is secondary prevention, because the principal goal is to identify individuals in an early, detectable stage of the disease process. However, screening provides an excellent opportunity to offer health teaching as a primary preventive measure. Screening activities have become an important aspect in the control of chronic diseases such as heart disease, stroke, and colorectal cancer. Additionally, screening activities provide early diagnosis and treatment of nutritional, behavioral, and other related problems. Nurses play an important role in screening activities, because they can provide clinical skills and educationally sound health information during the process.

Delayed recognition of disease results in the need to limit future disability in late secondary prevention. Limiting disability is a vital role for nursing, because preventive measures are primarily therapeutic and are aimed at arresting the disease and preventing further complications. The paradox here is that health education and disease prevention activities are similar to those used in primary prevention, but applied to a person or population with existing disease. Modifications to the teaching plan must be made based on the individual's current health status and ability to modify behavior. In the Case Study, Frank needed secondary prevention after his heart attack. The lifestyle changes needed to prevent a second heart attack were similar to the steps he could have taken to prevent his initial heart attack, but with a recognition that his coronary status was now compromised. As a result, exercise had to be increased gradually as part of a cardiac rehabilitation program, and diet modifications had to be made with support from a registered dietitian to ensure adequate nutrition and weight loss.

Tertiary Prevention

Tertiary prevention occurs when a defect or disability is permanent and irreversible. The process involves minimizing the effects of disease and disability by surveillance and maintenance activities aimed at preventing complications and deterioration. Tertiary prevention focuses on rehabilitation to help people attain and retain an optimal level of functioning regardless of the disabling condition. The objective is to return the affected individual to a useful place in society, maximize remaining capacities, or both. The responsibility of the nurse is to ensure that people with disabilities receive services that enable them to live and work according to the resources that are still available to them. When a person has a stroke, rehabilitating this individual to the highest level of functioning and teaching lifestyle change to prevent future strokes are examples of tertiary prevention.

THE NURSE'S ROLE

Evolving demands are placed on the nurse and the nursing profession as a result of changes in society. Emphasis is shifting from acute, hospital-based care to preventive, **community-based care,** which is provided in nontraditional health care settings in the community. This demand for community-based services, with the home as a key community setting for care, is closely related to the changing demographics of the United States. As the home and community become the sites for care, nurses must assume more blended roles, with a knowledge base that prepares them to practice across settings using **evidence-based practice.** Within these roles, nurses assume a more active involvement in the prevention of disease and the promotion of health. Nurses can be more independent in their practices, can place a greater emphasis on promoting and maximizing health and, more than ever, are accountable morally and legally for their professional behavior.

Nursing Roles in Health Promotion and Protection

Although nurses often work with people on a one-to-one basis, they seldom work in isolation. Within today's health care system, nurses collaborate with other nurses, physicians, social workers, nutritionists, psychologists, therapists, individuals, and community groups. Nurses fill the roles of advocate, care manager, consultant, deliverer of services, educator, healer, and researcher.

Advocate

In the advocacy role the nurse helps individuals obtain what they are entitled to receive from the health care system, tries to make the system more responsive to client and community needs, and assists clients in developing the skills to advocate for themselves. The nurse strives to ensure that all people receive quality, appropriate, and cost-effective care and may spend a great deal of time identifying and coordinating resources for complex cases. Other examples of advocacy will be seen in subsequent chapters.

Care Manager

The nurse acts as a care manager to prevent duplication of services and reduce costs. The basis for care management is data. Information gathered from reliable sources enables the care manager to help individuals avoid care that is unproven, ineffective, or unsafe. Reliable sources of information on best practices, evidence-based practices, and standard protocols are available from Internet sites sponsored by the federal government (e.g., *http://www.nih. gov, http://www.cdc.gov*), specialty organizations (e.g., *http://www.arthritis.org, http://www.nursingworld.org*), and private foundations (e.g., *http://www.rwjf.org, http:// www.jhartfound.org*). Successful care management depends on a collaborative relationship among the care manager, other nurses and physicians, the individual and his or her family, the payer, and other care providers who work with the person. The wishes of the individual and family need to be clear to the care manager. Facilitating communication among parties is one of the care manager's most important functions.

Consultant

Nurses may act as consultants to provide knowledge about health promotion and disease prevention to individuals and groups. Some nurses have specialized areas of expertise or advanced practice standing, such as in gerontology, women's health, or community and public health, and they are equipped to provide information as consultants in these areas of specialization (ANA, 2004). For example, a gerontological nurse specialist might serve on a community planning board, offering advice about what type of health-promotion activities should be considered in planning a new senior housing development. In contrast to those doing independent consultation, all nurses need to develop consultation skills that can be integrated into practice and allow the individual nurse to take advantage of opportunities to provide support on an individual client level or for future development at the organizational level (Berragan, 1998).

Deliverer of Services

The core role of the nurse is as deliverer of direct services such as health education, flu shots, and counseling in health promotion. Visible, direct delivery of nursing care is the foundation for the public image of nursing. The public demands that nurses be knowledgeable and competent in their delivery of services. This role is clearly expressed in the Nursing's Social Policy Statement (ANA, 2003) and in the ANA Code of Ethics (ANA, 2001).

Educator

Health practices in the United States are derived from the theory that health components such as good nutrition, industrial and highway safety, immunization, and drug therapy should be within the grasp of the total population. Even with its rich resources, society falls far short of attaining the goal of maximal health for all. The problem is not a lack of knowledge, but rather the lack of application; therefore, it is incumbent on nurses to be excellent health educators. To teach effectively, the nurse must know essential things about the learner and the teaching-learning process (see Chapter 10).

In addition to their storehouse of scientific knowledge, nurses who are committed to their teaching role know that individuals are unique in their response to efforts to change their behavior. To expand their options in teaching methods, nurses explore the literature to find various ways to present health information. Teaching may range from a chance remark by the nurse, based on a perception of desirable client behavior, to structurally planned teaching according to client needs. Selection of the methods most likely to succeed involves establishing teacher-learner goals. Health promotion and protection rely heavily on the individual's ability to use appropriate knowledge. Health education is one of the primary prevention techniques available to avoid the major causes of disability and death today and is a critical task for nurses.

Healer

The role of healer requires the nurse to help the client return to the natural state of that individual through the integration and balance of various parts (McKivergin, 2005). Healing resides in the ability to glimpse or intuit the "interior" of an individual's care, to sense and identify what everyone else has missed or underappreciated, and to incorporate the specific insight into a care plan that assists that person to develop the capacity to heal. Nurses are "artists" who have a special ability to help people heal. The art of nursing is the extraordinary ability to manage a broad array of clinical, financial, and psychosocial issues—analogous to the way a sculptor might use a wide array of materials—to create something meaningful, sensible, and whole (see Chapter 14.)

Researcher

In today's health care environment, nurses are constantly striving to understand and interpret research findings that will enhance the quality and value of client care. To provide optimal health care, nurses need to use research findings as their foundation for clinical decision making. When nurses or other clinicians use research findings and the best evidence possible to make decisions, the outcome is termed *evidence-based practice*. Evidence-based practice is defined as the conscientious, explicit, and judicious use of current best evidence in making decisions about the care of individual clients. The practice of evidence-based medicine means integrating individual clinical expertise with the best available external clinical evidence from systematic research (ANA, 2004).

The National Institute of Nursing Research (NINR) serves as the focal point in developing research themes for the future of the profession. The NINR supports research to establish a scientific base for the care of individuals through-

out the life span, from management of illness and recovery to the reduction of risks for disease and disability. The five themes NINR has identified are: (1) changing lifestyle behaviors for better health, (2) managing the effects of chronic illness to improve health and quality of life, (3) identifying effective strategies to reduce health disparities, (4) harnessing advanced technologies to serve human needs, and (5) enhancing the end-of-life experience for clients and their families. Notice that health promotion is the basis for four of these themes. See the Research Highlights box for information related to studies of health promotion and disease prevention.

Evidence-based practice results from tracking down the best external evidence with which to answer clinical research questions. Evidence can be gathered from

---

research highlights

Behavioral Interventions in Health Care

The fields of health education, health promotion, and disease prevention have become more widely accepted, and the role of the nurse in primary, secondary, and tertiary disease prevention has expanded. Research studies initiated to evaluate the health effects and cost effectiveness of these programs use both public health and medical models. According to Dr. David Sobel, director of Health Promotion and Patient Education at Kaiser Permanente, Northern California Region, the influence of behavioral interventions in health care may be measured through (1) health improvement, (2) behavioral change, (3) increased satisfaction, and (4) cost savings and cost-effectiveness. A review of controlled studies indicates that behavioral and educational interventions significantly decreased the use of more expensive medical treatment, as follows:

- 17% reduction in total ambulatory visits
- 35% reduction in visits for minor illnesses
- 25% reduction in pediatric acute illness visits
- 149% reduction in office visits for acute asthma
- 140% reduction in office visits for arthritis
- 156% reduction in rate of cesarean sections
- 185% reduction in use of epidural anesthesia in labor and delivery
- 11.5-day reduction in length of hospital stay for clients requiring surgery

The literature addressing chronic disease indicates that almost one third of people visit a physician for bodily symptoms that are a manifestation of psychological distress; another one third have medical conditions resulting from poor lifestyle choices, such as smoking, unhealthy diets, and substance abuse. Therefore the other one third who have disorders such as arthritis, heart disease, diabetes, and asthma should demonstrate significant improvement through educational-behavioral interventions (stress management and relaxation techniques, nutrition education, pain management strategies).

Data from Connecticut Hospital Association. (1996). *Guidelines for the practice of health promotion.* Wallingford, CT: The Association; Sobel, D. (1993). Cost effectiveness of health and patient education. *Eighth Annual Interregional Health Education Conference.* Berkeley, CA: Kaiser Permanente.

quantitative studies that describe situations, correlate variables related to care, or test causal relationships between those variables. Results of these studies become incorporated into screening and treatment standards such as those from the U.S. Preventive Services Task Force (2002). Evidence can also be gathered from qualitative studies that describe phenomena or define the historical nature, cultural relevance, or philosophical basis of aspects of nursing care. Applied research is done to directly affect clinical practice (Burns & Grove, 2003). Sackett, Rosenberg, Gray, Haynes, and Richardson (1996) stressed the use of the best external evidence available to answer clinical questions and explore the next best evidence when appropriate. The next best evidence may include the individual clinical judgment that nurses acquire through clinical experience and clinical practice and other qualitative approaches to research.

Nurses need to recognize the importance of research as a basis for their practice and that they often participate in the research process by collecting data. For example, both home health nurses and nurses in long-term care facilities are required to collect extensive data on the cognitive and physical functioning of their clients using the Outcome and Assessment Information Set (OASIS) and Minimum Data Set (MDS) assessment tools. These data are used as part of the quality improvement process to indicate areas for improvement in care, thereby contributing to nursing protocols.

Chapters 16 to 24 highlight health-promotion research studies in specific age groups. Time should be taken to review this material and explore the relationship between behavior and disease, to identify which populations are at risk, and to discover what types of health-promotion programs work and why they work. Through knowledge of research, nurses can strengthen their confidence in making daily decisions about quality care.

IMPROVING PROSPECTS FOR HEALTH
Population Effects

Cultural and socioeconomic changes within the population unequivocally influence lay concepts of health and health promotion. In some areas of the United States the Hispanic population is larger than any other group. By the year 2050, it is predicted that most Americans will not be of white European descent. Taken as a portent for future health-promotion strategies, these predictions about the population indicate that current knowledge about and approaches to health promotion may not meet the needs of the future American population (see Chapter 2).

In addition to changes in the ethnic and racial distribution within the population, the projected changes in age distribution will affect health-promotion practice. Considerable growth is expected in the proportion of the population that is 25 years and older. For example, the post World War II baby boom will increase the number of people in the 65-and-older age group between the years 2010 and 2030. Although there was a drop in the birth rate after 1960, this decrease has been offset by an increase in immigration, both legal and illegal. More restrictive immigration rules related to the Bush administration Homeland Security Act have begun to limit legal immigration since 2002 (U.S. Department of Homeland Security, 2003). Analysis of these population trends and projections helps health professionals determine changing needs. Additionally, analysis of the social environment is necessary for social policy concerning health.

SHIFTING PROBLEMS

Provision of personal health services must be informed by environmental health. Environmental pollution is a complex and increasingly hazardous problem. Diseases related to industry and technologies, including asthma and trauma, have become important threats to health.

The physical and psychological stresses of a rapidly changing and fast-paced society present daily problems, such as economic pressures and poor health habits. Obesity, partly attributed to a lack of exercise and increasing food portion size, is a growing health issue. Ingestion of potentially toxic, nonnutritious, high-fat foods is another factor contributing to poor health (see Chapter 11). Abuse of tobacco, drugs, and alcohol also negatively affects health.

The emphasis on treating disease by applying complex technology is not only costly, but it also contributes minimally to the improvement of health. An orientation toward illness clearly focuses on the effects rather than the causes of disease.

A substantial change in wellness patterns is occurring. Infectious and acute diseases were the major causes of death in the early part of the twentieth century, whereas chronic conditions, heart disease, cerebrovascular accident (stroke), and cancer are the major causes today. Diagnosis and treatment of disease, which were highly successful in the past, are not the answer for today's needs, which are closely related to and affected by biochemical make-up, environment, and lifestyle.

MOVING TOWARD SOLUTIONS

Solutions are neither simple nor easy, but they can be focused in two major directions: individual involvement and government involvement. The first direction concentrates on actions of the individual, especially actions related to lifestyle across the life span. The learning and the inherent changes that are involved require the adoption of a new set of skills by people who will need the assistance of nurses to make those changes. Approximately one fifth of the population is faced with the problem of getting the basic necessities of food and shelter. The other four fifths, whose basic necessities have been met, must overcome problems that result from affluence.

Motivational factors play a large role in influencing attitudinal change. As discussed in Chapter 10, programs for health promotion and health education are only part of the answer. Financial incentives for prevention may be another motivating factor, and health advocacy by professionals in the health field is critical. Additionally, private and public action at all levels is needed to reduce social and environmental health hazards. Toxic agents in the environment such as particles from diesel emissions and social conditions such as school overcrowding can present health hazards that may not be detected for years; therefore, it is necessary for individuals and government to play a role.

Legislation and financing that relate to primary prevention are discussed in Chapter 3. Government activity, in the form of legislation, is increasing in this area. For example, bicycle safety, seat belts, and a graduated tax on cigarettes are areas for governmental intervention. Health ecology and planning are important areas for government involvement in the future. Redirection of the existing health care delivery system, putting more emphasis on primary prevention, is probably the most difficult and the most far-reaching goal; however, an emphasis on a wellness system is necessary to improve the health of the U.S. population.

SUMMARY

The way individuals define health and health problems is important, because definitions influence attempts to improve health and care delivery. In the Case Study, Frank Thompson's health was affected by obvious, immediate, and personal factors, such as his diet and employment pressures. Nevertheless, his problems had their roots in the social and economic conditions of his parents; in his own early history of illness, education, and work; and in his and his family's hopes and aspirations. His physician, who defined Frank's problem in immediate biomedical terms, used the tools of personal services to help repair the short-term effects of his heart attack. Public health planners, who saw Frank's problem on a longer-term population basis, sought policy solutions to the problem of cardiovascular disease.

The view taken in this text is such that a broad and longer-term perspective of health can guide toward promoting health more effectively, even as nurses deal with individual problems on a day-to-day basis. Health is a sustainable balance between internal and external forces. Health allows people to move through life free from the constraints of illness and allows healing to take place.

Illness represents an imbalance that human choices (intertwined social, political, spiritual, professional, and personal) create. In the United States, communities may yet have time to slow the onslaught of chronic disability and shift the direction, slow the pace, and humanize the scope of economic and social life.

To shift directions in today's health care patterns may be possible only when nurses and other health professionals do what is expected of them as leaders in the care of health: to work with others through open processes; to provide leadership in finding the vision and the path; and to inform, educate, and reeducate themselves, their colleagues, the media, and the general public using research findings and evidence-based practice methods. **Web Site Resource 1A** presents 21 competencies for health professionals in the twenty-first century developed by the Pew Health Professions Commission.

The responsibility of nurses as health professionals today calls for seeing the health problem in new ways and helping others to do the same. Responsibility means developing new roles and looking at the problem through others' eyes, including the eyes of individuals, the public, other professionals, and other nations. Responsibility also means evaluating the social and individual consequences, the long-term and short-term effects, and the public and private interests that are involved when deciding on the set of tools to use in the care of health.

ADDITIONAL STUDY MATERIAL

Study Questions in the back of the book, see page 663.

evolve WEB SITE MATERIALS

These materials are located on the book's Web site at http://evolve.elsevier.com/Edelman/.

- WebLinks
- Content Updates
- Web Site Resources

1A   Twenty-One Competencies for the Twenty-First Century

REFERENCES

Ajzen, A., & Fishbein, M. (1980). *Understanding attitudes and predicting social behavior.* Upper Saddle River, NJ: Prentice Hall.

American Nurses Association. (2001). *Code of ethics for nurses with interpretive statements.* Washington, DC: American Nurses Association.

American Nurses Association. (2003). *Nursing's social policy statement.* Washington, DC: American Nurses Association.

American Nurses Association. (2004). *Nursing: Scope and standards of practice.* Washington, DC.: American Nurses Association.

Ardell, D. B. (2004). *What is wellness.* Retrieved June 18, 2004, from: http://www.seekwellness.com/wellness/articles/what_is_wellness.htm.

Bandura, A. (1976). *Social learning theory.* Upper Saddle River, NJ: Prentice Hall.

Bandura, A. (1999). *Self-efficacy: The exercise of control.* New York: W. H. Freeman.

Barr, D., Lee, P., & Benjamin, A. (2003). Health care and health policy in a changing world. In Wallace, H. (Ed.), *Health welfare for families in the 21st century* (2nd ed.). Boston: Jones and Bartlett.

Berragan, L. (1998). Consultancy in nursing: Roles and opportunities. *Journal of Clinical Nursing, 7*(2), 139-143.

Berry, R. (2004). Community-oriented nurse as parish nurse. In M. Stanhope & J. Lancaster (Eds.), *Community & public health nursing* (6th ed., pp. 1092-1113). St. Louis: Mosby.

Burns, N., & Grove, S. K. (2003). *Understanding nursing research* (3rd ed.). Philadelphia: Saunders.

Cano, A., Scaturo, D., Sprafkin, R., Lantinga, L., Fiese, B., and Brand, F. (2003). Family support, self-rated health, and psychological distress. *Primary Care Companion Journal of Clinical Psychiatry, 5,* 111-117.

Canto, J. G., Allison, J. J., & Kiefe, C. I. (2000). Relation of race and sex to the use of reperfusion therapy in Medicare beneficiaries with acute myocardial infarction. *New England Journal of Medicine, 342*(15), 1094-1100.

Connecticut Hospital Association. (1996). *Guidelines for the practice of health promotion.* Wallingford, CT: The Association.

David, R. (2000, June). Keynote address: Leadership for innovation in health care. In *Ford Foundation, John F. Kennedy School of Government, Summary of Proceedings, Local Innovations in Health Care Conference.* Cambridge, MA.

Dunn, H. (1961). *High-level wellness.* Arlington, VA: R. W. Beatty.

Folding, J. (1988). The proof of the health promotion pudding. *Journal of Occupational Medicine: Official Publication of the Industrial Medical Association, 30*(2), 113.

Gordon, M. (1994). *Nursing diagnosis: Process and application* (3rd ed.). St. Louis: Mosby.

Greiner, P., Snowdon, D., & Greiner, L. (1996). The relationship of self-rated function and self-rated health to concurrent functional ability, functional decline, and mortality: Findings from the nun study. *The Journal of Gerontology. Series B, Psychological Sciences and Social Sciences, S51B*(5), S234-S241.

Greiner, P., Snowdon, D., & Greiner, L. (1999). Self-rated function, self-rated health, and postmortem evidence of brain infarcts: Findings from the nun study. *The Journal of Gerontology. Series B, Psychological Sciences and Social Sciences, 54B*(4), S219-S222.

Grzywacz, J., & Fuqua, J. (2000). The social ecology of health: Leverage points and linkages. *Behavioral Medicine, 26*(3), 101-115.

Idler, E., & Benyamini, Y. (1997). Self-rated health and mortality: A review of twenty-seven community studies. *Journal of Health and Social Behavior, 38*(1), 21-37.

Izzo, J., & Black, H. (2003). *Hypertension primer* (3rd ed.). Philadelphia: Lippincott Williams & Wilkins.

Janz, N., Champion, V., & Strecher, V. (2002). The health belief model. In K. Glanz, B. Rimer, & F. Lewis (Eds.), *Health behavior and health education: Theory, research and practice* (3rd ed.). San Francisco: Jossey-Bass.

Johnson, R., & Wolinsky, F. (1993). The structure of health status among older adults: Disease disability, functional limitation, and perceived health. *Journal of Health and Social Behavior, 34,* 105-121.

Kaplan, G. A., Everson, S. A., & Lynch, J. W. (2000). The contribution of social and behavioral research to an understanding of the distribution of disease: A multilevel approach. In B. Smedley & S. Syme (Eds.), *Promoting health: Intervention strategies from social and behavioral research* (pp. 37-80). Washington, DC: National Academy Press.

Kreuter, M., & Devore, R. (1980). Update: Reinforcing the case for health promotion. *Family & Community Health, 10,* 106.

Leavell, H., & Clark, A. E. (1965). *Preventive medicine for doctors in the community.* New York: McGraw-Hill.

McKivergin, M. (2005). The nurse as an instrument of healing. In B. Dossey, L. Keegan, & C. Guzzetta (Eds.), *Holistic nursing: A handbook for practice* (pp. 233-254). Sudbury, MA: Jones and Bartlett.

National Heart, Lung, and Blood Institute. (2000). *The practical guide: Identification, evaluation, and treatment of overweight and obesity in adults* (NIH Publication No. 00-4084). Bethesda, MD: U.S. Government Printing Office.

Newman, M. (1987a). *Health as expanding consciousness.* St. Louis: Mosby.

Newman, M. (1987b). Health conceptualizations: Nursing's emerging paradigm—the diagnosis of pattern. In V. A. McLean (Ed.), *Classification of Nursing Diagnosis* (proceedings of the 7th conference). St. Louis: Mosby.

Newman, M. (1995). *A developing discipline. Selected works of Margaret Newman.* New York: National League for Nursing Press.

Newman, M. (2003). A world of no boundaries. *ANS Advances in Nursing Science, 26*(4), 240-246.

Nigg, C. R., Burbank, P., Padula, C., Dufresne, R., Rossi, J. S., Velicer, et al. (1999). Stages of change across ten health risk behaviors for older adults. *The Gerontologist, 39,* 473-482.

O'Donnell, M. (1987). Definition of health promotion. *American Journal of Health Promotion, 1*(1), 4.

Pender, N. J., Murdaugh, C. L., & Parsons, M. A. (2002). *Health promotion in nursing practice* (4th ed.). Upper Saddle River, NJ: Prentice Hall.

Reed, P. G. (1983). Implications of the life-span development framework for well-being in adulthood and aging. *ANS Advances in Nursing Science, 6*(1), 18-25.

Rogers, M. (1970). *An introduction to the theoretical basis of nursing.* Philadelphia: F. A. Davis.

Sackett, D. L., Rosenberg, W. M. C., Gray, J., Haynes, R. B., & Richardson, W. S. (1996). Evidence of bad medicine: What it is and what it isn't. *British Medical Journal, 312,* 71-72.

Smith, J. A. (1983). *The idea of health: Implications for the nursing profession.* New York: Columbia University Teachers College Press.

Sobel, D. (1993). Cost effectiveness of health and patient education. *Eighth Annual Interregional Health Education Conference.* Berkeley, CA: Kaiser Permanente.

U.S. Department of Health and Human Services, Public Health Service. (1986). *The 1990 health objectives for the nation: A midcourse review.* Washington, DC: U.S. Government Printing Office.

U.S. Department of Health and Human Services, Public Health Service. (1990). *Healthy People 2000: The Surgeon General's report on health promotion and disease prevention* (Publication No. 7955071). Washington, DC: U.S. Government Printing Office.

U.S. Department of Health and Human Services, Public Health Service. (1996). *Healthy People 2000 mid-course review and 1995 revisions.* Boston: Jones and Bartlett.

U.S. Department of Health and Human Services, Public Health Service. (2000). *Healthy People 2010* (conference edition, in two volumes). Washington, DC: U.S. Government Printing Office.

U.S. Department of Health, Education, and Welfare, Public Health Service. (1979). *Healthy People.* Washington, DC: U.S. Government Printing Office.

U.S. Department of Homeland Security. (2003). *Yearbook of immigration statistics, 2002.* Washington, DC: U.S. Government Printing Office.

U.S. Preventive Services Task Force. (2002). *A guide to delivering clinical preventive services: A systems approach* (AHRQ Publication No. APPIP01-0001). Washington, DC: U.S. Government Printing Office.

World Health Organization. (2004). *About the World Health Organization.* Accessed July 18, 2004, from: *http://www.who.int/about/en/.*

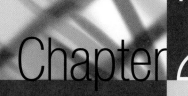

Chapter 2

GERALDINE VALENCIA-GO

Emerging Populations and Health

objectives

After completing the chapter, the reader will be able to:

- Distinguish voluntary from involuntary migration.
- Differentiate among ethnicity, ethnic group, race, and minority group.
- Describe demographic data relative to emerging populations:
  - Arab Americans
  - Black/African Americans
  - Native Americans
  - People afflicted with human immunodeficiency virus–acquired immunodeficiency syndrome (HIV-AIDS)
  - Asian Americans and Pacific Islanders
  - Latino/Hispanic Americans
  - Homeless people
- Discuss selected cultural factors that may have an impact on the health and well-being of emerging populations.
- Describe health concerns and issues of emerging populations.
- Contrast the folk caring system with the professional care system.
- Explain strategies of the nursing profession to meet the needs of emerging populations.
- Describe initiatives to address the health care concerns of emerging populations.

key terms

Culture	Gentrification	Skid row
Ethnic group	Involuntary migration	Taoism
Ethnicity	Minority group	Value orientation
Ethnocentric perspective	Professional care system	Values
Folk healing system	Race	Voluntary migration

THINK About It

Working With Ethnic Groups Made Easy

Establishing a knowledge base about a particular group can pose many challenges, including gaining entrée and earning the acceptance and respect of members.

In her research with Arab Americans, Jaber identified general fear, suspicion, and distrust of large institutions and governmental agencies as major barriers that were resolved by eliciting the collaboration of an important community-based organization that provides advice on awareness and acceptance. In addition, "attending major public events and programs involving the community by the principal investigator of the same ethnicity served to increase visibility and promote the study" (Jaber, 2003, p. 514). Other barriers such as misconceptions about the characteristics of the ethnic group are resolved easily by having adequate knowledge of the culture and, when possible, by using study personnel of the same ethnic background. Resources and materials should be in the language of the ethnic group and should be linguistically and culturally accurate. Protocols for recruitment and follow-up should be laid out carefully.

Similarly, African Americans "are sometimes reluctant to participate in studies" (Plowden & Wenger, 2001, p. 34). Feelings of mistrust of researchers stem partly from the Tuskegee Syphilis Study, contributing to a general perception that African Americans are used to collect data without getting benefits from the results. These barriers need to be addressed in working with these individuals. Therefore, a caring approach is recommended in which the researcher, initially identified as a stranger, becomes a friend and research enabler. "Unknowing," a way of knowing, entails an openness that is free from bias, prejudices, and stereotypes. Reflection facilitates awareness of the research informant's experience and all aspects of it. Being available and attentive to someone's needs, identified as presence and knowing, facilitates understanding the individual's feelings, thoughts, and ways of being. From a stranger to a trusted friend, the researcher can then formulate culturally appropriate strategies to resolve health issues.

An example of this process follows. Boesch (2002) described "The Native American Primer: A Partnership in Wisdom" as a resource to introduce Native American women to the topic of breast cancer and to the Study of Tamoxifen and Raloxifene (STAR). This resource includes a traditional story. The exchange of stories is a major component of the sharing in a social gathering where food is served. This is consistent with the cultural norm of extending hospitality through the sharing of food. The use of storytelling and community groups as partners in the research ensures increased participation in clinical trials.

Data from Boesch, M. (2002). Developing cancer clinical trial resources for Native Americans. *Cancer Practice, 10*(5), 263-264; Jaber, L. (2003). Barriers and strategies for research in Arab Americans. *Diabetes Care, 26*(2), 2003-2004; and Plowden, K. O., & Wenger, A. F. (2001). Stranger to friend enabler: Creating a community of caring in African American research using ethnonursing methods. *Journal of Transcultural Nursing, 12*(1), 34-39.

The United States and other countries became a family of countries during the event considered to be one of the worst transgressions against humanity: the September 11, 2001, attack on the World Trade Center in New York City. The impact of the event and the threats that may lie ahead in the near and distant future were envisioned. The sharing of concerns and people caring about each other transcended the usual barriers that divide a nation. People from diverse backgrounds bonded to deal with the trauma of this horrific event.

Fortunately, people bond not only during crises but also during celebratory events such as the New Year's Eve celebration in New York City. As the television cameras roam around Times Square, one can view every conceivable diversity. What becomes clear is that the United States is a country of diverse populations, unique in their cultural customs and traditions. Yet as this century progresses with advances and discoveries, there are shared concerns, hopes, and issues, such as good health, peace, and an acceptable standard of living, things that ensure a quality of life but continue to be elusive for many people. Perhaps an awareness and understanding of different populations that are emerging in this century will provide the basis for strategic planning to ensure quality of life.

EMERGING POPULATIONS IN THE UNITED STATES

Emerging populations include ethnic minorities, the homeless, and those afflicted with HIV-AIDS. Ethnic minority populations include Asian American–Pacific Islanders (AAPIs), black/African Americans (BAAs), Latino/Hispanic Americans (LHAs), Native Americans, and Arab Americans (included for the first time in this edition). Statistical data on each of these groups do not include data that are under the category of two or more races as reported in the U.S. Census Bureau.

The presence in the United States of the major **ethnic groups** that are the foci of this chapter can be attributed to a number of factors. One major factor is **voluntary migration,** large-scale immigration generally motivated by the quest of the individual or group for one or more goals including: (1) educational opportunities, (2) economic benefits, (3) social improvements, and (4) political or religious freedom (Fox, Burns, Popovich, & Ilg, 2001). Those who come to the United States for more positive experience are identified as immigrants and those who "leave their homeland under threat of injury or loss of life due to political or religious persecution" (Fox et al., 2001, p. 778) as refugees.

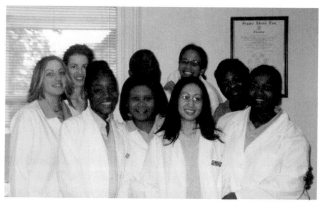

An ethnically diverse group of future nurses.

Orozco (2001) classifies immigrants on the basis of permanence in the new country; there are the immigrants whose move is permanent and "sojourners" (p. 7212) who stay for a specified length of time and then return to their homelands. Contract workers such as farm workers fall into this category, as do those who travel back and forth from the adopted country and their homeland to see remaining family members, check on business enterprises, or escape the winter months.

Another type of migration is **involuntary migration.** Meilaender (2001) identified flight from a hostile army, civil war, and political anarchy as reasons that cause involuntary movement of people to other lands. Natural disasters such as fires, floods, famines, earthquakes, and volcanic eruptions cause people to search for safer, more secure places to live. An even more severe situation occurs when people are literally forced out of their countries as in the slave trade of Africans, who were considered an abundant source of cheap labor (Bookman, 2002). More recently, there is "indentured servitude" (Bookman, 2002, p. 140) that entails deceitful movement of people who are lured by attractive job opportunities in another country and then find themselves trapped in low-paying menial jobs or prostitution.

Involuntary and voluntary migratory movements result in ethnic diversity that presents both problems and advantages. "Advantages might include a wide array of cultural activities such as festivals and restaurants. Problems include widespread uneven political representation, inequities in housing and employment, language instruction difficulties in schools, and interethnic tensions" (Vigil & Roseman, 2001, p. 410). As this nation of diverse peoples faces the challenges of the twenty-first century, will there be a unified quest to address the basic needs of every individual? Awareness and understanding are key elements of this goal.

ETHNICITY, ETHNIC GROUP, MINORITY GROUP, AND RACE

The U.S. Census Bureau, in its official reports, uses a system of classification that groups people into ethnic, racial, or **minority groups** (Holmes, 2003; Williams, 2000). How-

ever, the U.S. Office of Management and Budget issued a policy directive that established four races and two ethnicity categories. "The racial categories include white, black, American Indian/Alaska Native, and Asian Pacific Islander. The ethnicity categories, Hispanic origin and not of Hispanic origin" (Holmes, 2003, p. 1) are used by the U.S. Census Bureau in presenting data about individuals and families. There are, however, differences in these terms as proposed in numerous anthropological and sociological resources. It is reassuring to note that the U.S. Census Bureau is continuing its work in refining the categories. This work is difficult and challenging given that many people in the United States are "multiracial and multiethnic in ancestry" (Williams, 2001, p. 1436).

Race emphasizes "physical properties and biological heredity" (Bookman, 2002, p. 4). Early in the eighteenth century, race was used as a designation for "the descendants of a common ancestor, emphasizing kinship rather skin color or other physical characteristics" (Feagin, 2001, p. 12711). Later in the century, race evolved as a categorical system to designate people with distinctive physical characteristics such as skin color, physique, hair texture, and facial features. Leading intellectuals of the late eighteenth and early nineteenth centuries "increasingly proclaimed the virtues and privileges of whiteness" (Feagin, 2001, p. 12712). Crystallization of the distinction between white race and inferior race became widespread as "Europeans expanded their colonial adventures overseas. Colonizers developed racist rationalizations for their destruction of indigenous societies, enslavement of Africans, and other colonial pursuits" (Feagin, 2001, p. 12712).

The use of race to categorize people is losing ground as research data indicates that "there is more variation within races than between them and although there are patterns to the distribution of genetic characteristics, our racial categories do not capture biological distinctiveness. Racial taxonomies are arbitrary, and race is more of a social category than a biological one" (Williams, 2001, p. 4831). In American society, race is socially constructed (Yancey, 2003). "Americans attach social meanings to the perceived biological differences associated with racial differences. This definition leads to the construction of a racial identity that has profound sociological implications" (Yancey, 2003, pp. 10-11). Further, "race is only a rough proxy for socioeconomic status, culture, genes, but it precisely captures the social classification of people in a race-conscious society such as the United States" (Jones, 2000, p. 1212).

Ethnicity is a reference to a collective identity, a sense of uniqueness within the larger society, and a distinction from nonmembers. Ethnicity denotes a sharing of customs, food, dress, music, religion, and of symbols, such as language, among those who see themselves as fellow members of the group (Ben-Rafael, 2001; Gabaccia, 2002; Greene, 2000; Henslin, 2001). An ethnic group may have "common geographic origins, family patterns, language, religion, values, traditions, and symbols, music, dietary preferences, and employment patterns" (Williams, 2000, p. 210). The ethnic group includes those members with the sense of belonging to the collective identity. An "ethnic group is a group that is set apart by insiders or outsiders primarily on the basis of cultural or national origin characteristics subjectively selected" (Feagin, 2001, p. 12712). Although ethnic groups can share a range of phenotypic characteristics due to shared ancestry, the term *ethnicity* typically is used to highlight cultural and social characteristics instead of biological ones (Bookman, 2002; Williams, 2001). "Ethnic groups are socially organized groups with salient differences with respect to other groups in society" (Winkelman, 2001, p. 283). Ethnic groups provide some common identification with members. They are reference groups from which a member "acquires personal characteristics, social and psychological attachments, definitions of self, and a sense of common membership or group belonging" (Winkelman, 2001, p. 286).

Values and perceptions about health and illness evolve from the socialization process within a person's ethnic group. A sense of ethnicity also inspires the person to form a network of individual and group relationships that are maintained and nurtured by frequent interactions. The importance that individuals place on their families and other relatives as sources of formal and informal support during illness and crisis is a significant aspect of ethnic culture. Ethnicity plays an important role in relationships between people (Winkelman, 2001). Specific roles and expectations regarding different life situations facilitate optimal functioning of individuals. For example, "children learn basic facts of their family history and origins and the cultural content and practices associated with their ethnicity in their households" (Waters, 2001). Finally, ethnicity provides a basis for assessing the value systems of other groups (Winkelman, 2001).

The misuse of racial and ethnic group identity created another group category, the minority group. "Racial categories reflected a hierarchy of racial preferences: whites at the top, blacks at the bottom, and other groups in the middle" (Williams, 2000, p. 210). Therefore, "racial categories capture some of the inequalities that emerged as attitudes and beliefs about racial groups that became policies and societal arrangements to limit the opportunities and life chances of stigmatized groups" (Williams, 2000, p. 210). A minority group may be perceived as consisting of people who receive less than their share of wealth, power, or social status (Greene, 2000). "Minority status reflects the convergence of ethnic origin and socioeconomic disadvantage" (Williams, 2000, p. 211). In addition, minority group members "are subjected to unequal treatment through prejudice and discrimination by a dominant group" (Williams 2000, p. 211). The intertwining of race, ethnicity, and minority issues was noted in the fraud and larceny trial of a Polish worker and Jewish Tyco executives. An ex-school teacher serving as a juror hypothesized that the ethnicity of the two defendants was at issue and that they were "scapegoats for blueblood corporate directors" (Saul, 2004, p. A7).

CULTURE, VALUES, AND VALUE ORIENTATION

Ethnicity is evidenced in customs that reflect the socialization and cultural patterns of the group. **Culture,** as an element of ethnicity, consists of shared patterns of values and behaviors that characterize a particular group (Winkelman, 2001). It is "shaped by values, beliefs, norms, and practices that are shared by members of the same cultural group" (Giger & Davidhizar, 2001, p. 113).

Values are beliefs about the worth of something and serve as standards that influence behavior and thinking. "The value that an individual holds reflects cultural and social influences, relationships, and personal needs" (Ecker, 2001, p. 406). Cultural values "are unique, individual expressions of a particular culture that have been accepted as appropriate over time. They guide actions and decision making that facilitate self-worth and self-esteem" (Giger & Davidhizar, 2001, p. 113). Relative to health, cultural values "shape human behaviors and determine what individuals will do to maintain their health status, how they will care for themselves, and others who become ill, and where and from whom they will seek health care" (Boyle, 2003, p. 321).

A **value orientation,** learned and shared through the socialization process, reflects the personality type of a particular society. The dominant value orientations are shared by the majority of the group. Kluckhohn's model (1953) of value orientations incorporates themes regarding basic human nature, the relationship of human beings to nature, human beings' time orientation, valued personality type, and relationships between human beings. **Web Site Resource 2A** presents some solutions to the questions proposed by Kluckhohn.

Health as a Value

Fifty years ago, transcultural nursing was founded "as a formal area of legitimate study and practice" (Leininger, 2000, p. 69), intended to transform health care and help people of diverse cultures. Underlying this initiative is the belief that optimal health for all is an essential cultural value. Additionally, society generally believes that all people have a right to health care (Potter, 2001). "Educational programs, research projects, and clinical practices in transcultural nursing continue to be established and implemented to provide culturally sensitive, safe, competent, and meaningful care to people of diverse and similar cultures" (Leininger, 2000, p. 69). An analysis of Leininger's vision for the work of transcultural nurses indicates that there are many barriers and issues in health care, particularly for people from diverse cultures. For instance, health care for poor Americans and ethnic minorities is less than optimal, because they are unable to pay for services because of lack of insurance (Holmes, 2003). Health care insurance is not affordable for many poor Americans, whose priorities are the basic needs of life including food, clothing, and shelter rather than health care. Availability of health care facilities and resources does not mean accessibility because of difficulties traveling to a facility, long waiting periods in clinics, the unattractive and impersonal surroundings of health care facilities, and lack of consumer understanding of the process of obtaining care. Fragmentation of care and ethnocentric and impersonal attitudes of some health care providers place individuals in uncomfortable situations when intimate personal information is sought from them. For ethnic groups, health as a value may have different definitions and their behavior may reflect this.

Incongruent beliefs and attitudes about health and health care services among ethnic groups, the rest of the population, and particularly health care providers are major barriers to improving the health status of ethnic group members. Leininger (2001) believes that "our rapidly growing multicultural world makes it imperative that nurses understand different cultures to work and function effectively with people having different values, beliefs, and ideas about nursing, health, caring, wellness, illness, death, and disabilities" (pp. 6-7). Health care providers need to become responsive to the cultural values of different peoples and how these could augment effective and humanistic care delivery.

FOLK HEALING AND PROFESSIONAL CARE SYSTEMS

A group has within its cultural or ethnic customs and traditions a healing system that incorporates the beliefs and practices deemed essential in maintaining and restoring health. Andrews (2003) identified three components of the healing systems of people, including self-care, **professional care systems**, and folk healing systems. Self-care is seen in 70% to 90% of the general population, and this is used when one experiences a minor illness. "Professional care is characterized by specialized education and knowledge, responsibility for care, and expectation of remuneration of services rendered" (Andrews, 2003, p. 81). A **folk healing system** embodies the beliefs, values, and treatment approaches of a particular cultural group that are products of cultural development. Folk health practices are seen in a variety of settings, including community groups, kinship groups, private homes, and healers' shrines. Folk healers range from priests and medicine men and women to fortune-tellers, astrologers, and geomancers. Unlicensed practitioners such as lay midwives, bone setters, some dentists, and herbalists are part of the folk sector, as are religious practitioners such as spiritualists, Christian Scientists, and scientologists. Other areas of differences between folk and professional care systems are summarized in **Web Site Resource 2B.**

The choice of health care system varies among ethnic groups and among individuals within a group. Individuals' preferences for their folk healing systems is motivated by their familiarity with the folk healer, who usually speaks the same language and is knowledgeable of the beliefs, customs, and traditions of the ethnic group. Easy access and the individual's ability to pay for the healer's services are real advantages when compared with the difficulty of getting

appointments, the long waits, and the unfamiliar institutional settings in the professional care system. When folk healing practices are not effective, the individual may turn to the professional care system. Through a culturally sensitive assessment process, nurses can determine what folk remedies individuals are using and whether their continued use would interfere with the prescribed medical regimen. Andrews and Boyle (2003) have developed a transcultural assessment guide that nurses and other health care providers can use when working with ethnically diverse populations. Health care professionals must avoid an ethnocentric perspective when working with ethnic groups. An **ethnocentric perspective,** which views other ways as inferior, unnatural, or even barbaric, can serve as a major obstacle to establishing and maintaining good working relationships with consumers of health care services.

Ethnic groups will continue to use folk remedies and healing. Therefore, health care professionals need to take a look at the many positive aspects of folk systems. A caring, holistic approach, that incorporates family and support systems and considers the individual's viewpoint, is one of the more positive aspects of folk systems. This approach is getting recognition by the professional care system. A blend of both systems would optimize health care for ethnic Americans.

ARAB AMERICANS

Arab Americans come from several countries; Lebanon is the home of most. Other countries include Syria, Palestine, Iraq, Egypt, Yemen, and Jordan. The term *Arab* is a "cultural, linguistic, and to some extent, political designation" (Abraham, 1995, p. 84). Politically, the Arab world is usually said to include 18 countries. In the linguistic sense, the term *Arab* "refers to those areas where most people speak Arabic as their native language" (Donner, 2001, p. 584). Arab Americans came to the United States in three immigration waves. The first, who came between the late 1800s and World War I, were mostly from Greater Syria. The second wave came after the close of World War II and included many Muslims and refugees displaced by the 1948 Palestine War. The last wave occurred during the 1960s and consisted of many professionals, entrepreneurs, and skilled and semi-skilled laborers (Abraham, 1995; Stussy, 2000). In 2000, 1.2 million people reported Arab ancestry. The three largest groups are the Lebanese, Syrians, and Egyptians. About 48% of the Arab population lives in California, Florida, Michigan, New York, and New Jersey. Arab Americans accounted for 1.2% of the total population of Michigan in 2000 (U.S. Department of Commerce, 2003). Three major religions are represented among Arab Americans, including Christianity, Judaism, and Islam (Chelala, 2002).

Health Care Issues of Arab Americans

There is scarcity of health-related information (Kulwicki, Miller, & Schim, 2000) and a paucity of scholarship about Arab Americans (Sayed, 2003). Resources indicate that the most prevalent health problem is adult-onset diabetes, and coronary artery disease is on the rise (Hatahet, Khosla, & Fungwe, 2002). One of the largest groups of Arab Americans lives in Dearborn, Michigan (Jaber, Brown, Hammad, Zhu, and Herman, 2003b). A study on diabetes among 542 participants revealed a 15.5% prevalence rate in women and 20.1% in men. Further, the prevalence of undiagnosed diabetes was 10%.

Risk factors for diabetes among Arab Americans include obesity, age, gender, low employment rates for both males and females, and lack of a high school education in women. The last two factors were examined in relation to the process of acculturation. Jaber et al. (2003a) suggested that acculturation issues play an important role in the development of diabetes. The phenomenon called *postwesternization* has been suggested to "explain the lower rates of diabetes associated with acculturation." "Acculturation is associated with the adoption of healthy western habits (such as isocaloric low-fat diets and regular physical activity) rather than detrimental western habits (such as hypercaloric high-fat diets and sedentary lifestyles)" (Jaber et al., 2003b, p. 2013).

Another health concern is mental health, where work has just begun. Sayed (2003) looked at the concept of mental illness and mental health in Arab Americans. Analyses of several case studies indicate that therapists need to be fully aware of cultural meanings and significance of therapeutic approaches, such as psychotherapy, in order to bring about a comfortable therapist-client relationship. Similarly, Nassar-McMillan and Hakim-Larson (2003) looked at counseling considerations among Arab Americans. They suggested integrating Arab Americans' receptivity to counseling, cultural and religious backgrounds, and self-perceptions of identity in counseling approaches. The last one is important as it relates to how an individual perceives the United States and thereby a non-Arab therapist.

Many barriers prevent Arab Americans from using professional care services. These include religious beliefs and practices, cultural norms relating to modesty, family values of upholding the family's reputation, gender issues such as preference for same-sex health provider, use of folk remedies, and stresses of assimilation and acculturation such as lack of English skills. Other barriers related to health care providers include lack of culturally competent services and attitudes such as stereotyping and discrimination (Kulwicki, Miller, & Schim, 2000; Nassar-McMillan & Hakim-Larson, 2003). Additional barriers extend to other areas such as research. (See Think About It box at the beginning of the chapter.)

Selected Health-Related Cultural Aspects

Arabs value the family and the ties it maintains. Therefore, the extended family, clan, and tribe are common kinship groups. Customs center on hospitality around food, family, and friends (Abraham, 1995; Donner, 2001). Religion plays an important part in Arab culture, and there are dietary rules and prescribed rituals for praying and washing (Kavanaugh, 2003; Nassar-McMillan & Hakim-Larson, 2003). The male role is dominant and women are expected to play a submissive role (Adib & Mikkey, 2003; Mikkey, 2003; Nagaty, 2003). The emphasis on preservation of female chastity and fidelity prohibits adult males from being alone with women, except for spouses. Some women do not shake hands with men, and touching is done only within the marital relationship (Kavanaugh, 2003). Arab Americans are present oriented and view the future as uncertain.

ASIAN AMERICAN–PACIFIC ISLANDERS

The AAPI population grew tremendously with two streams of immigration (Kim, 2001). Chinese, Koreans, and Filipinos came during the first stream and their numbers, 46.2% of all immigrants, added to the already large numbers in the United States. Currently, these are the largest groups of Asians. They were mostly highly educated and many came to join families and seek employment (Holmes, 2003). Current demographic data for AAPIs can be found in **Web Site Resource 2C.** Native Hawaiians or Pacific Islanders include Hawaiians, Guamanians, Samoans, and other Pacific Islanders. The categories for Asian include Asian Indians, Chinese, Filipinos, Japanese, Koreans, Vietnamese, and others such as Cambodians, Laotians, Thais, Hmongs, and Malaysians (Qiu & Ni, 2003). AAPIs are most likely to live in Hawaii, California, and New York.

A look at the status of AAPIs reveals that they are doing relatively well in the United States. In spite of their short history, Asian Americans "distinguished themselves in many areas of American culture" (Kim, 2001, pp. 812b-812c). The importance of education from their perspective is evident at all levels. Among first-time kindergartners, Asians surpassed all groups in persistence at tasks, eagerness to learn, and paying attention. Dropout rates for Asians ages 16 to 24 were the lowest among all ethnic groups and whites (Holmes, 2003). A greater percentage earned bachelor's and master's degrees in 2000 than did Hispanics and Native Americans. See **Web Site Resource 2D** for a comparison of higher education among the major ethnic groups. Additionally, AAPIs surpassed all ethnic groups in the number of earned doctoral degrees (U.S. Census Bureau, 2001).

Health Care Issues of Asian American–Pacific Islanders

Variations in the health status of AAPIs are a result primarily of subcultures within the larger group. AAPIs have "indicators of being one of the healthiest population groups in the United States" (U.S. Department of Health and Human Services [USDHHS], 2000, p. 12). AAPIs have lower morbidity and better health status than other ethnic groups, probably because of lifestyle and other sociocultural factors (Chin, Takeuchi, & Suh, 2000). AAPIs have health problems similar to those of the U.S. population as a whole. However, "there is great diversity within this population group, and health disparities for some specific segments are quite marked" (USDHHS, 2000, p. 12). Heart disease, cancers, and cerebrovascular problems are the leading causes of death. AAPI women are less likely to die from breast cancer and resultant mortality rates are lower compared with the other ethnic groups. However, AAPIs have the highest rates of tuberculosis, 36.6 cases per 100,000 people. The infant mortality rate of 5.5 deaths per 1000 live births is lower than for any other race. Only 16.9% of AAPI women did not receive prenatal care, lower than all other ethnic groups (Holmes, 2003).

Health care issues of AAPIs are relative to their status as immigrants and an ethnic group. Some Asian American immigrants have brought diseases from the home countries, and they may subsequently experience new diseases because of their new lifestyles and living conditions. Others develop mental health issues such as depression relative to their inability to cope in a new culture (Fox et al., 2001). Others exhibit a level of cultural rigidity that hinders their adjustment and, thus, access to the health care system that is wrought with barriers. Important social problems that serve as barriers to health include (1) living in poverty, (2) socioeconomic conditions that stress intergenerational relationships when adult children cannot support and provide for elderly parents, (3) cultural norms that prevent people from seeking help outside the family, (4) incongruence between role expectations and fulfillment that strain spousal relationships, (5) change in child-rearing practices that challenge family harmony, and (6) loss of important social networks, which could lead to depression and anxiety (Dhooper, 2003).These factors combined with poor access and underutilization of health services increase the risks and produce negative health outcomes in this group.

Mental health problems among Asian Americans can be attributed to the stresses of adjustment to a new culture including "pressure to succeed (model minority myth), immigration and acculturation stressors, shame and denial, discrimination and racism" (Kuramoto & Nakashima, 2000, p. 58). Leong and Lau (2001) looked at cognitive, affective, value orientation, and physical barriers to providing effective mental health services to Asian Americans. Cognitive barriers include cognitions that "encompass traditional Asian notions of the nature, causes, and cures of mental illness and of well-being" (Leong & Lau, 2001, p. 203). Thus, Asian Americans may not readily seek help for mental illness unless the behaviors are "upsetting to the social group" (Leong & Lau, 2001, p. 203). Further, most would first rely on folk healers. Affective barriers include "culturally-based affective responses" (Leong & Lau, 2001, p. 303) such as shame and stigma that are avoided at all costs to protect the reputation of the family.

Closely related to the cognitive barriers are those that relate to value orientation. Asian Americans put emphasis on the family as a group rather than the individual. Hence when "many traditional psychotherapy orientations place high value on open communication, exploration of intrapsychic conflicts, and a focus on the individual" (Leong

| Box 2-1 | Selected Cultural Values of Asian American–Pacific Islanders |

- The family is extended, with grandparents, uncles, aunts, and cousins as part of the household.
- Within the family, there is differential treatment based on age and gender. The oldest adult male usually is considered the head of the family.
- The family's interests and honor supersede those of the individual; therefore, every member strives to avoid situations that may bring shame on the family.
- Older individuals are respected and their authority is unquestioned. Filial piety ensures loyalty and devotion from children.
- Maintenance of harmony is a priority; therefore, there is a strong emphasis on the avoidance of conflict and direct confrontation.
- Strong values conflict with mainstream cultural values, such as passivity to avoid conflict versus assertiveness.
- Emphasis on respect for authority figures is strong; therefore, disagreements are avoided.

& Lau, 2001, p. 204), Asian Americans perceive these to be in conflict with their value of collectivism versus individualism. Physical barriers, not necessarily unique to Asian Americans, include "lack of awareness of available services due to economic and geographic realities" (Leong & Lau, 2001, p. 204).

Selected Health-Related Cultural Aspects

AAPIs share many traditional values. A comprehensive description of traditional values in several Asian groups indicates commonalities and differences (Andrews & Boyle, 2003; D'Avanzo & Geissler, 2003). A list of some of the most important values of AAPIs is presented in Box 2-1.

The family is the most important social institution for AAPIs (Dhooper, 2003; Kim, 2001; Kuramoto & Nakashima, 2000). The family is often the source of functional and psychological support and there is "extensive family involvement in help-seeking" (Leong & Lau, 2001, p. 204). AAPIs try to inculcate cultural values in their children. Children and their well-being are the main concerns of mothers. Children become more cherished when mothers lose their spouses and they look to children as their main resource (Valencia-Go, 1999). However, many people find the task of parenthood in a new country difficult, because some of their cultural values conflict with the mainstream cultural values, such as passivity to avoid conflict versus assertiveness. Exposure of children to different cultures in schools and in their neighborhood facilitates their adoption of other cultural beliefs and attitudes in their socialization. Additionally, the employment of immigrant women outside the home has exposed their children to other caretakers. The absence of a parent in the home for a large portion of

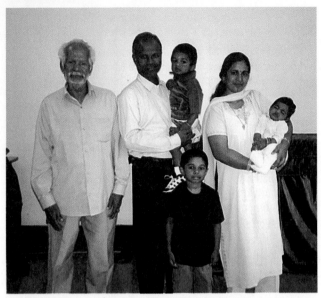

A three-generation Asian American–Pacific Islander family of Indian origin. The mother wears a sari, traditional Indian women's clothing.

the day forces children to assume adult responsibilities, a cultural inconsistency that parents have to tolerate. An environment in which children are deprived of parental guidance often results in negative behaviors that correlate with alcohol, tobacco, and other drug use (Kuramoto & Nakashima, 2000). The common absence of grandparents, who are important transmitters of culture, contributes to children's identification with the dominant host culture.

Asian folk medicine and philosophies have a strong Chinese influence as a result of early Chinese migration throughout Asia. Therefore, the folk medicines of Filipinos, Japanese, Koreans, and Southeast Asians are all imbued with Chinese principles. **Taoism** was the philosophical and theoretical foundation of Chinese medicine. According to Tao doctrine, humans are microcosms within the universe. Achieving harmony between the two is essential because the energies of both intertwine. Two forces, Yin and Yang, keep innate energy, called Chi, and sexual energy, called Jing, in balance. Yin is feminine, negative, dark, and cold; Yang is masculine, positive, light, and warm. An imbalance in energy can be caused, for instance, by yielding to strong emotions or eating an improper diet. In their interactions, humans and the universe are both susceptible to the elements of earth, fire, water, metal, and wood (Andrews, 2003; Kavanaugh, 2003; Yue, Lee, & Wong, 2003).

Asian folk medicine uses a wide variety of herbs for healing purposes including roots, leaves, seeds, tree bark, and parts of flowers. Some aspects of Asian folk medicine have gained popularity within the professional care system. Of these, the best known is acupuncture (Andrews, 2003). Other alternative treatment modalities that are slowly gaining wide acceptance are meditation, therapeutic touch, massage, imagery, relaxation, and bipolarity.

LATINO/HISPANIC AMERICANS

The LHA population makes up the largest ethnic group in the United States. See **Web Site Resource 2C** for selected demographic data about LHAs. "A high rate of immigration and high birth rate have combined to make Hispanic Americans one of the fastest-growing groups in the United States" (Garcia, 2001, p. 258). The 2005 and 2010 population projections indicate that they will continue to be the largest ethnic group. LHAs are relatively young. For the U.S. population, 25.7% of members are under 18 years of age, while for the Latino/Hispanic population this number is 35% (U.S. Census Bureau, 2001).

Hispanic Americans are also called *Latinos* because of their Latin American origins (Garcia, 2001). The census bureau revisited the term *Hispanic* and in 1996 redefined it, and in 1997 "the Office of Management and Budget issued a standard by which the terms Latino and Hispanic were to be used interchangeably" (Chong, 2002, p. 5). The largest Hispanic American subgroups are Mexicans, Puerto Ricans, and Cubans. Most Hispanics live in New York, Florida, and California (U.S. Census Bureau, 2001). Overall, LHAs tend to be urban dwellers (Benson, 2003; Garcia, 2001).

Hispanic Americans are making educational strides in spite of many barriers. "Discrimination continues to plague many Hispanic American students. Studies have shown that Hispanic students have often been assigned to classes for low achievers, forced to repeat grades, or classified as mentally handicapped because they do not speak English well or because of other cultural differences" (Garcia, 2001, p. 258). In 2001 among those 25 years and older, 57% completed high school, up 1.5% from 1999. Associate, baccalaureate, master's, and doctoral graduates all have increased in number since 1999 (Benson, 2003).

Health Issues of Latino/Hispanic Americans

Although cardiovascular disease and cancer are the first and second causes of morbidity and mortality among LHAs, their incidence in the general population is higher. Diabetes is twice as prevalent in Latino/Hispanics than non-Latino white Americans (D'Arrigo & Keegan, 2000; "Uninsurance among Latinos," 2000; West et al., 2001). A discussion of issues revolving around socioeconomic conditions and the health profile of this group has led to two explanatory models, the epidemiological paradox and the healthy migrant effect (Chong, 2002). Some possible reasons for the paradox include diet, family structure, mind-body connections, and genetics ("The Latino Paradox," 2003, p. 3). However, LHAs have higher rates of diabetes (Carter-Porkas & Zambrana, 2001; D'Arrigo & Keegan, 2000; Holmes, 2003; "New Campaign," 2002). Among adults 25 to 44 years of age in the Hispanic American population, HIV infection was ranked as the leading cause of death (Holmes, 2003). Among Hispanic American subgroups, socioeconomic status has been linked to health status. Cubans have a higher percentage (35%) of people whose families earn $35,000 or more. Additionally, fewer families live below the poverty level. Overall, Puerto Ricans and Mexicans have the lowest incomes and have higher rates of living below the poverty level. Cubans report better health status than the other two subgroups. Health care contact and restricted activity days were lowest for Cubans (Hayat, Lucas, & Kington, 2000).

LHAs use and receive less preventive health care. They are at a "greater risk for reduced access to regular medical care, delays in getting necessary diagnosis and treatment, poorer health outcomes, increased suffering, and even death" ("Uninsurance among Latinos," 2000, p. 4). Most LHAs are employed in occupations that do not provide health insurance (Carter-Porkas & Zambrana, 2001; Holmes, 2003). Only 49.9% of Hispanics have private insurance coverage, lower than the percentage among other ethnic groups and the white population. Several factors are offered as barriers. LHAs might not have acquired citizenship; therefore, they have lower odds of being insured by employers. In addition, lack of a high school diploma diminishes the opportunities to work in places that offer health insurance. Many Latinos are employed in agricultural, mining, service, domestic, and construction industries that are not as likely to provide health coverage (Carrillo, Trevino, Betancourt, & Coustasse, 2001).

The difficulties experienced by LHAs in receiving appropriate health care services are identical to those of the poor and other ethnic minorities. Additional barriers include the lack of racial and ethnic diversity in the leadership and workforce of the health care system. Lack of interpreter services for Spanish-speaking clients and lack of or inadequate culturally appropriate health care resources serve as barriers in the delivery of care. Guendelman and Wagner's (2001) study on Hispanic experience within the health care system indicates the importance of emphasizing culturally appropriate personal interactions. Guendelman and Wagner propose that "culturally appropriate personal interactions may serve as the basis for monitoring satisfaction with health care plans in the future" (p. 44). Poor access to health care providers and health care facilities also serve as deterrents to obtaining care (Carrillo et al., 2001).

Many Hispanic Americans may not readily seek care because they have continued reliance on their folk system of healing. Their preference for this is logical given their lack of health insurance and perceived difficulties negotiating the health care system because of language and other sociocultural barriers.

One must note that underlying all the statistical data about the health status of LHAs is a major issue in classification of ethnic groups in the United States. "Racial and ethnic identification—and its public reporting—among Hispanic-Latinos in the United States is embedded in dynamic social factors. Ignoring these factors leads to significant problems in interpreting data and understanding the relationship of race, ethnicity, and health among Hispanic-Latinos" (Amaro & Zambrana, 2000, p. 1724). Furthermore, a careful study of the diversity of Latino and Hispanic cultures and more accurate reporting of demographic data based on a more effective system of surveying are essential in creating policies for the health and well-being of the largest ethnic group in the United States.

Selected Health-Related Cultural Aspects

Each subgroup of the LHA population has distinct cultural beliefs and customs. However, a common heritage determines similar values and beliefs. For instance, the emphasis on family and religion are the two most important aspects of all Hispanic cultures. For older Hispanic Americans, the family is an important component of good health. The family is the most important source of support; therefore, the needs of the family as a whole supersede the needs of the individual. During times of illness and crisis, the family is there for the individual. Older family members and other relatives are accorded courtesy and respect and are often consulted on important matters (Andrews, 2003; Carbonell, 2003; Chong, 2002; Dumonteil & Gamboa-Leon, 2003).

LHAs' dependence on spiritual strength to aid them in illness and dying is evident in their use of prayer. They have "profound reverence for God and for other powerful forces they believe exist" (Chong, 2002, pp. 26-27). Furthermore, "health and disease are believed to be consequences of God's approval or disapproval of a person's behavior" (Chong, 2002, pp. 26-27). LHAs attribute the origins of disease and illness to spiritual or natural punishments, hot and cold imbalances, magic, dislocation of internal organs, natural diseases, and emotional and mental issues. The hot and cold concept of disease was derived from the Hippocratic theory of pathology. Illness occurs when there is an imbalance. This concept of hot and cold guides Hispanic people when they categorize illnesses and select appropriate treatments. For example, an elevated body temperature is managed by giving the person a cool drink to lower the fever. For a person who has a cold, drinking warm fluids is considered therapeutic (Chong, 2002).

LHAs attribute illness and disease to many supernatural and psychological causes. The evil eye, or the *mal de ojo*, is an example. Fright, or *susto*, and hysteria, or *ataque de nervios*, are caused by strong emotions, crises, and traumatic experiences (Chong, 2002). LHAs still resort to many home remedies and consult folk healers, including the *curandero*, spiritualist, *yerbero*, and the *sabador*. *Curanderos* use a variety of folk remedies, including prayers, rituals, herbs, and the laying on of hands. Spiritualists use medals, amulets, and prayers to effect a cure. The *yerbero* is knowledgeable in the use of herbs, while the *sabador* is an expert in massage and manipulation of bones and muscles (Andrews, 2003). Other Hispanic Americans such as Cubans practice *Santeria*. People who are ill may seek the advice of a "godfather" who is a member of the *Santeria*. Wearing white clothes for a year, performing rituals, and following dietary restrictions are involved in bringing forth a cure for an illness (Carbonell, 2003).

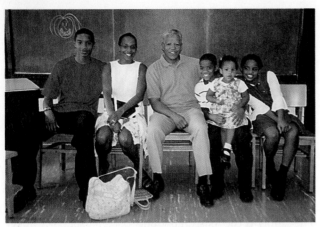

This father is a Latino/Hispanic American from Puerto Rico and this mother is a black African American. Religion is important to both of these cultures. The family is photographed in a classroom of their church.

Folk remedies are used in combination with professional care approaches. The individual's belief in the folk remedy can have positive effects on well-being. Therefore, professional care personnel need to find ways to blend the two systems to the optimal benefit of LHAs and their families.

BLACK/AFRICAN AMERICANS

The 2000 census indicates that there were 36,247,000 BAAs, or 12.7% of the total population, in 2001 (U.S. Census Bureau, 2002). They have been surpassed as the largest ethnic minority group by LHAs. More demographic data on BAAs can be found in **Web Site Resource 2C**.

The immigration history of blacks to America is significantly different from that of Europeans, Asians, and Hispanics. Most BAAs identify their ancestral heritage from the western part of Africa that was controlled by three great and wealthy empires, Ghana, Mali, and Songhai. "Africans had practiced slavery during the ancient period. Slaves captured in warfare were sold to Arab traders of northern Africa" (Hornsby, 2001, pp. 136c-136d). Portugal and Spain, as leaders in exploration and colonization, were involved in slave trade. Some believe that the first blacks in America came with Christopher Columbus in 1492. Black slaves also traveled with other expeditions. The migration of BAAs can be identified as involuntary, because this was forced, impelled, or imposed by explorers of the New World from Spain and Portugal. In the New World, many thriving industries had high demands for labor that the Native Americans could not fill; therefore, Africans were captured and sold as slaves.

The beginning of black America is recorded as the time when "the first laborers were brought to Virginia from the Caribbean in 1619" (Gabaccia, 2002, p. 25). When these laborers completed their service, they were free to buy property. "But racial prejudice among white colonists forced most free blacks to remain in the lowest level of colonial society" (Hornsby, 2001, p. 136d). Yancey (2003) contends

that the "overarching feature of African American history is slavery, and the American slave system set the tone for future racism and alienation towards African Americans" (p. 44). Further, African Americans were not given the same treatment extended to other migrant groups who had the opportunity to assimilate into the dominant majority culture. "Slavery made it necessary for majority group members to maintain a caste system for African Americans that deprived them of any possible social acceptance, and despite the adoption by African slaves of many European American cultural aspects, such as Christianity, they were unable to engage in the process of assimilation that other racial and ethnic groups experienced" (Yancey, 2003, p. 45). As one of the largest ethnic groups in the United States, BAAs are considered a minority group, a label originating from their slavery roots. Therefore, they continue, in many ways, to experience extreme segregation and exclusion from mainstream society, and discrimination by the majority group.

BAAs have made substantial progress in many areas during the past century. However, there are still inequities in many areas such as business, education, political participation, and leadership. Educationally, BAAs have made substantial gains. More blacks earned high school diplomas compared with Hispanics and Native Americans. Nevertheless, black Americans still lag behind whites in all levels of education (U.S. Census Bureau, 2002).

Health Care Issues of Black/African Americans

A complex set of social, economic, and environmental factors can be identified as contributors to the current health status of BAAs. However, poverty may be the most profound and pervasive determinant of health status. In the United States, health care is a commodity that can be purchased according to an individual's ability to pay (Keith, 2000), and health care is expensive. Individuals and families who are below the poverty level or lack adequate resources are obviously the most affected. Poor people cannot afford health insurance, which limits their access to health care services such as prenatal and maternal care, childhood immunizations, dental checkups, well-child care, and a wide range of other preventive services. Decreased resources for preventive care may necessitate more expensive services, such as emergency room care and intensive care in times of severe illness (Mays, Cochran, & Sullivan, 2000). In 2000, only 35.6% of BAAs had private insurance coverage compared with 63.1% of the total population. Private insurance through the workplace was 25% compared with 35.6% for the total population (Black Americans: A Statistical Source Book, 2003).

Two indices of the effects of poverty can be seen in the high rates of infant and maternal mortality. Despite changes in living conditions, advances in infection control, and improved standards in neonatal care, BAAs still experience high infant and maternal mortality rates. In 2000, the rate of low birth weight for BAA babies decreased slightly;

however, infant mortality rate has remained high at 13.9 deaths per 1000 live births, double that of whites. BAAs have the second highest percentage of women who lack prenatal care during the first trimester of pregnancy. Life expectancy for males is 68.3 years compared with 74.8 in white males. For black African females, life expectancy is 75 years compared with 80 in white females (Holmes, 2003).

Black American children living below the poverty level experience numerous health problems, including malnutrition, anemia, and lead poisoning. These problems and illness resulting from lack of immunizations combine to inhibit normal growth and development and affect school performance.

Poverty-stricken families usually live in depressed socioeconomic areas where housing conditions are unsafe and unhygienic. Unsafe buildings and other environmental structures cause accidents and injuries among young children. Young children have fallen to their deaths from windows that were unprotected by metal railings. Older people have suffered falls and other injuries from poorly lit stairways and hallways. Other hazards include uncollected garbage and abandoned buildings that are used as dump sites or as meeting places for a variety of illegal activities.

The incidence of cancer and mortality rates for BAAs is higher than for white Americans. The 5-year survival rate for cancer for those diagnosed from 1992 to 1998 was 52.6% compared with 63.8% in whites. BAAs have significantly higher incidence and mortality rates from many types of cancers. The mortality rate for breast cancer was 26.1% compared with 18.7 % among whites in 1998. In the same year, the incidence rate for prostate cancer was approximately twice for BAA males (Holmes, 2003).

The death rates from cardiovascular disease and cancer are about the same as in the general population. However, BAAs have a 45% higher incidence of lung cancer. A higher rate of death for black Americans occurs after a diagnosis of cancer. There were 51.6 deaths per 100,000 people compared with 22 from the white population. Severe high blood pressure is more common for black Americans in both men and women. In 1999, there were 46.8 deaths per 100,000 BAAs compared with 12.8 deaths among whites (Holmes, 2003).

Health issues of BAAs are receiving more attention. Currently, a number of excellent publications address health issues and problems. Selected ones are listed in **Web Site Resource 2E.** In addition, studies on how to overcome barriers to research are also being addressed. (See Think About It box at the beginning of the chapter.)

Selected Health-Related Cultural Aspects

Differences in cultural beliefs, attitudes, and practices exist between rural and urban black Americans; however, they share some basic cultural beliefs. Black American culture is centered on the family and religion. The family, the strongest institution for them, provides strong extended kinship bonds with grandparents, aunts, uncles, and cousins. The family is considered the strongest source of support, especially in times of crisis and illness. Family members and relatives are consulted before BAAs seek care elsewhere. There is a "need to be involved in the family's caring, nurturing, and healing process" (Bailey, 2000).

Religion and religious behavior are an integral part of the BAA community. BAAs are said to be "the most religious group in the world" (McGadney-Douglass, 2000, p. 202). The church, as the second most important institution for BAAs, has many purposes including (1) serving as a place to meet where members can pass news, take care of business, and find strength of purpose, (2) providing direct social welfare services, (3) acting as a stabilizing force in the community, (4) facilitating citizenship training and community social action, (5) serving as a transmitter of cultural history, and (6) providing the means for coping and surviving in a hostile world (McGadney-Douglass, 2000).

The BAA church and spirituality also play an important role in health issues. For instance, prostate education for older men is received more favorably when done within the parish nursing approach than elsewhere (Lambert, Fearing, Bell, & Newton, 2002). African American churches were used as the sites for an earlier study that looked at the perceived health needs of urban African American church congregants. This study was an important milestone in establishing parish nursing where nurses, as members of the congregation, "may be uniquely positioned to work within the culture of the congregation and establish trusting, effective relationships" (Baldwin, Humbles, Armmer, & Cramer, 2001, p. 301). A study that looked at screening behaviors and beliefs in God indicated that higher levels of belief in God were negatively associated with breast cancer screening. This is consistent with findings of earlier studies that indicated BAA beliefs that the disease is God's will (Kinney, Emery, Dudley, & Croyle, 2002). Samaan (2000) looked at the influence of race, ethnicity, and poverty on the mental health of children. Although the views of black children and white children regarding the importance of religion are not that different, Samaan found that black children's attendance of religious services is "more pronounced" (p. 108). The researcher indicated that this factor could account for the lower rates of psychiatric illness attributed to the "communal buffering factor in attending church" (p. 108).

Black Americans define *health* as a feeling of well-being and the ability to fulfill role expectations. They hold beliefs that diseases can be caused by natural or spiritual forces (Bailey 2000; Kavanaugh, 2003), and their approach to health care is guided by these beliefs. Readers are referred to Bailey (2000) for an enlightening historical overview of African American alternative medicine. BAAs continue to use their own traditional health system, especially when they lack access to the professional care system (Fletcher, 2000). Family members, such as grandmothers, and other community members are often consulted for traditional home remedies. Traditionally, roots, herbs, potions, oils, powders, rituals, and ceremonies are still used in many Southern communities. The use of healers is also common, including the old lady, who is knowledgeable about folk remedies and child care; the spiritualist, who assists with financial, personal, spiritual or physical problems; and the voodoo priest or priestess, who is knowledgeable about herbs, signs, and omens (Andrews, 2003).

As noted with the folk health practices of Asian and Hispanic Americans, BAAs' folk healing beliefs and practices can augment the professional care system. Black Americans often find comfort in the support that their religious leader or traditional healer can give them. Health care providers must find an appropriate place for these nontraditional modalities when caring for BAAs.

NATIVE AMERICANS

Native Americans lived in America for thousands of years before the arrival of Europeans. Most scientists believe that Native American people came to Alaska via land bridges now known as the Bering Strait (Campbell, 2000; Fixico, Kolata, & Neely, 2001), although Native Americans say they have always been here. Native Americans came to be known as Indians, a label given by Columbus when he encountered the native people in the West Indies, which he mistook for the East Indies. This label was then extended to all the native peoples of North and South America, from the Arctic to Tierra del Fuego.

Before 1492 there were an estimated 5 million Native Americans. Columbus' discovery brought colonization and settlement by various European groups (Snipp, 2000). Thus, the ancestral lands of the Native Americans were usurped, and the people were forced to labor on farms and in mines. Thousands died from disease and hard labor or were killed in attempts to escape from slavery. Other events, such as the removal of the Southeastern tribes in 1830, the Navajos' Long March to Fort Sumner in 1864, and the massacre at Wounded Knee in 1890, caused the Native American population to dwindle to 250,000 by 1890 (Fixico et al., 2001).

The 1950 census, the first to obtain a complete count of Native Americans, reported an increase from 237,000 in 1900 to 357,000 in 1950. The period from 1950 to 1980 was a time of rapid growth. However, "conquest, subjugation, corruption, genocide, and ethnocide brought considerable transformations in the lives and governments of Native Americans from coast to coast" (Grinde, 2002, p. xiii). Current Native American–Alaskan Native demographic data is presented in **Web Site Resource 2C**. Native Americans are concentrated in Oklahoma, California, Arizona, New Mexico, Alaska, Washington, North Carolina, Texas, New York, and Michigan. Of the total Native American population of almost 2 million, 62.3% live off reservations and 37.7% live on Native American lands. There are 314 reservations and 542 tribes, most of which have fewer than 1000 members. The Navajo reservation is the most populous (Snipp, 2000). The Cherokees make up the largest tribe (Holmes, 2003).

Native Americans also experience minority group status. In important aspects of life, such as educational attainment and income levels, Native Americans lag behind whites and other major ethnic groups. Native American percentages for higher education degrees are low in proportion to their total number. For example, in 2000 Native Americans ranked last in the numbers of associate, baccalaureate, and master's degrees compared with the other ethnic groups. Only 159 Native Americans earned doctoral degrees, an increase of 1 over the number earned in 1999. Among registered nurses, Native Americans have the lowest percentage, 0.5%, of the more than 2 million in the total population (USDHHS, 2001). Native Americans are making some progress in all levels of college education. However, low educational attainment and income levels combined with high rates of poverty are socioeconomic issues that affect health and the quality of life. Native Americans experience the many negative situations that confront poor people, both on the reservations and in the larger society.

Health Care Issues of Native Americans

Many of the health problems of Native Americans can be linked directly to the social and economic conditions described here. These conditions predispose Native Americans to illnesses and health problems that afflict the poor. Some of these problems have been discussed in the section on BAAs. Although Native Americans have responded well to prevention and treatment of infectious diseases, other health problems are closely linked to poverty and harmful lifestyle practices (Brenneman, Handler, Kaufman, & Rhoades, 2000). For instance, Native Americans have the highest percentage of smoking of all groups in the United States (Kegler, Cleaver, & Yazzie-Valencia, 2000).

Many Native American deaths can be attributed to unintentional injuries, cirrhosis, homicide, suicide, pneumonia, and complications of diabetes (USDHHS, 2000). Among Native American men 15 to 44 years old, unintentional deaths from accidents and intentional deaths from suicide and homicide account for 80% of all deaths each year. Cirrhosis afflicts Native Americans more frequently than other groups. It is the fourth major cause of death in Native Americans ages 45 to 54 and the fifth major cause for those 55 to 64 years old (Brenneman et al., 2000). Alcohol-related deaths are 62.7% higher than all races in the United States (Bohn, 2003). Alcohol use has been implicated as major factor in the abuse of Native American women (Bohn, 2003; Lauderdale, 2003). "Living with abuse and becoming dependent on alcohol and other drugs are intertwined problems for many women, especially Native American women. The use and abuse of alcohol or drugs is one way of coping with an abusive relationship, but also places the women and developing fetus at considerable health risk" (Lauderdale, 2003, p. 124). Although based on a sample of 30 Native American women, Bohn (2003) found that one half of study participants reported a history of substance abuse, including alcohol.

There is a high incidence of non–insulin-dependent diabetes (type 2), in Native Americans (USDHHS, 2000). Harmful lifestyle practices, including nutritional intake and activity levels, are implicated in the development of diabetes. Hence, health researchers focus on lifestyle interventions to forestall complications (Gilliland, Azen, Perez, & Carter, 2002). Boyle (2003) outlined the beliefs and practices related to diabetes. These beliefs include one's image and control of the body and illness as an unpleasant topic that needs to be avoided. Between 1990 and 1997, the number of Native Americans and Alaskan Natives with diagnosed diabetes increased from 43,262 to 64,474 individuals, indicating a 29% increase (Burrows, Geiss, Engelau, & Acton, 2000). Wittig (2004) showed that "diabetes was cited most frequently by students as a disease that nurses should be knowledgeable about when caring for Native Americans because of the high incidence of this condition among the population" (p. 58).

Many mental health problems confront Native Americans. Difficult life situations and stresses of daily life contribute to an array of problems, including feelings of hopelessness, desperation, family dissolution, and substance abuse, specifically alcohol. In 1998, there were 13.4 suicides per 100,00 Native Americans (Holmes, 2003).

The health problems of Native Americans are complicated by difficult access to health care. Of all ethnic groups discussed here, Native Americans have the second highest percentage of people who have not visited a doctor during the previous 12 months. For instance, a survey of oral health care showed that nearly two thirds of Native Americans have unmet dental needs. Only 1% of Medicaid-eligible babies get a dental examination before 1 year of age (Benn, 2003). People who live on reservations and are served by the Indian Health Service may find that this federally funded agency does not provide the services they need. Those who live in rural areas are underserved, with inadequate facilities and a lack of qualified personnel.

Selected Health-Related Cultural Aspects

Native Americans are generally present oriented; therefore, they emphasize events that are occurring now rather than events that will happen later. They take one day at a time, and in times of illness their way to cope is through hoping for improvement the following day (Kavanaugh, 2003; Reid & Rhoades, 2000). Native Americans value cooperation rather than competition. Sharing of resources, even among the poor, is an important component of this cultural value. Native Americans place great importance on their families and relatives. Three or more generations form an extended kinship system, which is enlarged by the membership of nonrelatives who are included through various religious ceremonies (Boyle, 2003). Faith and prayer are also integrated in Native American healing practices (Research Highlights box).

research highlights

Faith, Prayer, and Health Outcomes in Elderly Native Americans

The purpose of this correlational study was to examine the relation of faith and prayer to overall health status in elderly Native Americans. The researchers considered important cultural factors and used a conceptual framework that incorporated prayer, faith, and health.

Faith was conceptualized as "the individual's strength of belief in a Higher Power; faith represents the centrality or importance of this belief to the individual" (Meisenhelder & Chandler, 2000, p. 193). Individual, rather than group, prayer was conceptualized as "communicating with a perceived Higher Power" (Meisenhelder & Chandler, 2000, p. 193).

The study's hypothesis was that people with higher scores in faith and prayer would experience a more positive health status. The sample consisted of 36 men and 35 women, with 9% of them identifying themselves with an organized Christian religion. The researchers found that (1) the sample's "self report of health indicated a high level of functioning overall" (Meisenhelder & Chandler, 2000, p. 191), (2) age and social support had the strongest correlation with health, (3) "importance of faith, frequency of prayer, and extent to which people relied on their religion for coping were all significantly related to social functioning and, most strongly, mental health" (Meisenhelder & Chandler, 2000, p. 197), and (4) the importance of faith was a significant contributor to mental health.

The researchers concluded that age and social support were related to health outcomes, but did not influence mental health. Further, importance of the individual's faith in her or his life was strongly associated with mental health and that a "belief in a Higher Power appears to be associated with a positive mental outlook" (Meisenhelder & Chandler, 2000, p. 199).

Meisenhelder, J. B., & Chandler, E. N. (2000). Faith, prayer, and health outcomes in elderly Native Americans. *Clinical Nursing Research, 9*(2), 191-203.

Despite the great diversity in Native American groups in their beliefs and practices concerning health, illness, and healing, they share a common philosophical base. Native Americans believe that a state of health exists when a person lives in total harmony with nature (Rhoades & Rhoades, 2000). The earth is seen as a living entity that should be treated with respect; failure to do so harms the body. Illness is viewed not as an alteration in a person's physiological state, but rather as an imbalance between the ill person and natural or supernatural forces (Boyle, 2003). Native Americans believe that a person's sickness can be traced directly to having committed a violation against natural and spiritual laws; an individual can also inherit such a violation. The violation causes the person to get out of balance, and imbalance causes illness mentally, physically, emotionally, and spiritually. A framework for looking at Native American culture is described in the Hot Topics box.

A NEW EYE ON NATIVE AMERICAN CULTURE

HOTtopics

Each Native American tribe is distinct and unique in its culture, traditions, way of life, and beliefs. Similarities among tribes facilitate cohesiveness and bonding, a sense of "ethnicity or shared collectivity." A health culture exists in every group and it defines health, wellness, illness, and death. Native American nurses, as members of their tribes, view the world within their health culture and hence are guided by this in their work. Researchers looked at the essence of Native American nursing (Lowe & Struthers, 2001).

Using a qualitative research approach, the researchers identified "seven themes that describe the core principles of Native American nursing. These themes resulted in the development of a conceptual framework comprised of the following dimensions: (a) caring, (b) traditions, (c) respect, (d) connection, (e) holism, (f) trust, and (g) spirituality" (Lowe & Struthers, 2001, p. 280).

A schematic diagram of the model shows a circle that represents the holistic view of Native American culture. The roundness for the circle depicts "the interrelatedness, intertwining, and interlacing of all seven dimensions of the phenomenon of nursing in the Native American culture" (Lowe & Struthers, 2001, p. 282). Other parts of the circle denote symbols of the culture. The seven dimensions are written in the feathers of the great thunderbird that wrap around the circle of the medicine wheel. Thus, "the thunderbird, a sacred bird in Native American culture, is the frame for the circle" (Lowe & Struthers, 2001, p. 282).

Although the diagram uses Native American symbols, the framework can be used in working with any culture, because the core dimensions underlie the basic values of any ethnic group.

From Lowe, J., & Struthers, R. (2001). A conceptual framework of nursing in Native American culture. *Image: The Journal of Nursing Scholarship,* 33(3), 279-293.

Traditional health practices are an important part of the Native American way of life. Rituals and healing ceremonies that are believed to restore balance when illness occurs may be carried out by the medicine man or woman, who is believed to have hypnotic powers, the gift of mind reading, and expertise in concocting drugs, medicine, and poisons. More recently, the terms *traditional, shaman,* and *medicine person* are considered imprecise. The term "traditional medicine is generally used to describe the healing and beliefs of the Indian population" (Rhoades & Rhoades 2000, p. 402). The crystal gazer hand trembler identifies the cause of an illness and the shaman is called to induce a cure. The shaman is usually a powerful individual in the tribe. Although the power and reverence given to shamans may vary among tribes, they are treated with respect for their role in inculcating religious beliefs and promoting spirituality, good health, and good living for the people (Andrews, 2003; Boyle, 2003).

EMERGING RURAL AND URBAN POPULATIONS
Homelessness: A Continuing Saga

Homelessness is a complex social and economic problem that continues to persist and grow. It has been on the "American policy agenda for close to two decades" (Burt, Aron, Lee, & Valente, 2001, p. 1). Many services and programs have been put in place, yet homelessness has not been resolved. In the fifth edition of this book, Chapter 2 provided an overview of the causes of homelessness and earlier strategies to approach it. Perhaps a return to some basic information about it would shed light on its persistence as a societal problem.

The universal definition of homelessness has been quite elusive; therefore, who is considered homeless is difficult to define. Burt and colleagues (2001) proposed three elements that characterize homelessness, "transience or instability of place, the instability or absence of connections to family, and the instability or absence of housing" (p. 2).

Transience or instability of place characterize people who have no fixed place to live, such as nomadic tribes, people who work in a circus, carnival workers, and many migrant farm workers, peddlers, or tinkers. In the modern world, single people hired for construction or industries may have a place to stay, but not a fixed one. The instability or absence of connections can be seen in people without family such as the skid row population. **Skid row** is "a general term for an impoverished urban area where cheap housing, day labor, and marginal businesses can be found" (Hombs, 2001, p. 280). The Bowery in lower Manhattan, New York, is the most well-known domain for the skid row population. "The skid-row Bowery grew out of the Civil War which created homelessness on a vast scale" (Isay & Abramson, 2000, p. xiv). The men in the Bowery had flophouses that offered the "shabbiest accommodations" (Isay & Abramson, 2000, p. xiii). They had no connections with family. Some of the residents in these flophouses included recovering substance abusers, ex-prisoners, poor immigrants, and people discharged from mental institutions, just to name a few. Finally, people whose housing is unstable or absent include those who have experienced fire, flood, or natural disasters. Loss of one's dwelling characterizes this third type of homeless person. Additionally, when a person's family is no longer able to provide accommodation or when a community cannot provide housing, then this person is considered houseless, and this type is considered homeless in the United States.

The Stewart B. McKinney Homeless Assistance Act (PL 100-77) defines *homelessness* as the lack of a fixed, regular, and adequate nighttime residence. A homeless person's nighttime residence may be a supervised or publicly operated shelter designed as temporary living quarters, an institution serving as a temporary residence for people who require institutionalization, or any public or private place not intended for regular sleeping accommodations (Hombs, 2001). This definition is extremely limited and presents multiple issues and problems in resolving the homeless situation.

Burt et al. (2001) maintain that inclusive definitions of homelessness become useless, because entire populations who are poor or poorly housed will be eligible for services and benefits. On the other hand, these researchers say that "if the definitions are too specific, they focus too exclusively on the homelessness of the moment" (p. 6). With these perspectives in mind, it is suggested that a look at the causes of homelessness would facilitate the formulation of a definition that would address all related issues.

Why Families and Individuals Become Homeless

A look at homeless people over the last 2 decades reveals that they are individuals who were affected by changes in the (1) housing markets for low-income families and single people, (2) opportunities for people with only a secondary education or less, and (3) institutional supports for people with severe mental illness. In addition, persistent poverty and racial inequalities were added to what were identified as structural causes. There are also individual causes: (1) child and adult victimization, (2) mental illness, (3) substance abuse, (4) low levels of education, (5) poor or no work history, and (6) too early childbearing (Burt et al., 2001). Structural and personal factors alone or in combination lead to lack of resources to secure or maintain housing. Burt and colleagues (2001) propose that "housing affordability was and still is assumed to be the immediate cause of homelessness" (p. 8).

Depastino (2003) described the events in the 1980s when many federal programs for social welfare and housing lost funding in the face of soaring poverty. There were also changes in long-term economic and labor markets that had an impact on employment of men and women. The contraction of the government "safety net" resulted in many cuts in funding for programs such as the Aid to Families with Dependent Children. Women caring for dependent children were affected severely by this. There is also **gentrification,** a process of "transformation of a neighborhood to a higher income area, through the displacement of lower-end tenants, renovation of buildings, and the opening of higher-priced business" (Hombs, 2001, p. 278). Further, the release of mentally ill into the community starting in the 1950s swelled the numbers of people without affordable housing. Thus, the era of the new homeless came to being. "Old skid row refugees, displaced by urban renewal and gentrification, suddenly found themselves outnumbered by legions of newcomers: men, women, and even children pushed to the streets by the lack of affordable housing" (Depastino, 2003, p. 247). The new homeless consisted of "unprecedented proportions of women, children, and non-whites living in shelters and on the street" (Depastino, 2003, p. 256). "The homelessness of the late 20th century involved not only an economic crisis of shelter and housing, but also a cultural crisis of race, family, and gender" (Depastino, 2003, p. 249).

A striking feature of the new homeless is the large number of adolescents, estimated to be between 1 and 2 million. "Adolescents who are homeless in the United States come from every socioeconomic stratum in urban, suburban, and rural areas. Homeless youth are both males and females of every racial/ethnic identity" (Rew, 2002, p. 423). Rew (2002), in a descriptive study of homeless adolescents, found that nearly one half of her sample reported a history of sexual abuse. "Over half (51%) were thrown out of their homes by their parents; 37% left home because their parents disapproved of their alcohol or drug use, and nearly one third left home because parents sexually abused them" (Rew, Taylor-Seehafer, Thomas, & Yockey, 2001, p. 33). In another study, Rew, Fouladi, and Yockey (2002) reported that 35% of a convenient sample of 425 homeless adolescents left home because of homosexual or bisexual orientation.

Selected characteristics from the profile of homeless people includes more than 50% with less than a high school education, no health insurance, and reported substance abuse. History of victimization, incomes below the poverty level, many days without eating, and only a few days of temporary work add to the grim life of homeless people (Hombs, 2001).

The multidimensionality of homelessness serves as a negative consideration, because contraction or expansion of the definition would depend on availability of resources to alleviate the situation.

Estimates of Numbers of Homeless People

Given the multiple definitions of homelessness and the lack of a universal system for counting this population, estimates vary from resource to resource. "Substantial problems of methodology exist in trying to count homeless people. Street counts have always been the Achilles heel of homeless studies" (Hombs, 2001, p. 8). Additionally, "the kinds of living arrangements defining one as [homeless] can vary considerably from one investigator to another, adding a further note of uncertainty and making historical or regional comparisons risky" (Hopper, 2003, pp. 60-61). Estimates for the number of homeless people range from as low as 250,000 to as high as several million. These cannot be taken as accurate without considering some basic issues of estimating or counting. Homeless people "work very hard to obscure their homelessness by dress, appearance, and daily schedule. They try to make their homelessness invisible to those who might not otherwise recognize it" (Hopper, 2003, p. 8). For instance, those who do not use shelters, where counts are done, sleep in abandoned buildings, in their cars, in depots on the streets, or in tents in the woods. Recently a group of homeless people was found in a shanty area "tucked among tall ferns, twisted tree branches, and a thicket of overgrown grass and weeds behind the Supreme Industrial Equipment Co." (Schienberg, 2004, p. A32).

The homeless situation is a problem not only of individuals, but also of families, communities, and societies. This problem needs to be addressed as a dynamic and not a static phenomenon, for as societies change, evolve, and even move forward, there will always be those who are excluded and suffer consequences. These risks must be actively anticipated so that strategic planning can forestall any devastating and long-lasting effects.

Health Care Issues of Homeless Individuals and Families

The lives of homeless individuals and families are constant battles for daily survival. Homeless people experience exposure to extremes in temperatures, unsanitary living conditions, crowded shelters, poor nutrition, and unsafe situations, wherever they live. They experience the same situations relative to health care: poor access because of lack of health insurance and lack of resources to get to health facilities. A survey of health care access by homeless people identified the predominant physical and psychological health problems. Homeless people report respiratory ailments such as asthma and infections, ulcers, sexually transmitted diseases, dental caries, and vision difficulties. Psychological problems include alcohol and drug abuse, behavior disorders, depression, and posttraumatic stress disorder. Pregnancy rates are higher than comparable cohorts in the general population (Hatton, Kleffel, Bennett, & Gaffrey, 2001).

Homeless people lack preventive care and fail to return for follow-up care or comply with prescribed treatment (McCabe, Macnee, & Anderson, 2001). Exceptions are veterans who comprise almost 40% of the homeless population. Homeless veterans have better health care benefits but do not utilize them (Nyamathi et al., 2004). Lack or nonuse of preventive care among the homeless population often leads to expensive emergency room care.

Han and Wells (2003) looked at whether the use of the Health Care for the Homeless Program services by homeless adults was associated with a reduced risk for inappropriate use of emergency care services. Data indicate that misuse was not from lack of insurance but from inadequate access to primary care.

Homeless people suffer from mental health problems, often the primary cause of their homelessness. Homelessness also creates mental problems. Stresses of living in shelters and on the streets, physical problems, lack of resources, psychosocial issues such as shame and stigma, and feelings of hopelessness and despair often tax the homeless person's ability to cope.

Substance and drug abuse accompany their mental health problems (North, Egrich, Pollio, & Spitznagel, 2004). Nyamathi and colleagues (2004) examined perception of health status by homeless U.S. veterans. The researchers used a nonveteran comparison group. Both groups reported alcohol dependency and use of crack cocaine. Perceptions of fair to poor health were associated with injection drug use, and perceptions of worse health status were associated with symptoms of depression. Veterans' treatment for mental illness is often fraught with difficulties, because the illness is complicated by substance abuse, lack of insurance, and poverty, which serve as barriers to receiving care from providers who may harbor negative attitudes toward them (Lafuente, 2003; Sochalski & Mark, 2001).

The large numbers of homeless youth and the problems and issues they face have caught the attention of nurse researchers such as Rew, who has established a track record of research on this population. Homeless youth suffer the health problems of the general population of homeless people. "Homeless adolescents must learn to survive in environments that are highly stressful and filled with greater health risks than those encountered by household youths. Although many have fled from homes that were chaotic, all of them find that having no permanent place for food, shelter, or social support creates a formidable challenge to healthy growth and development" (Rew, 2002, p. 425). Homeless youth have increased rates of respiratory infections and other communicable diseases, including tuberculosis. They are at high risk for sexually transmitted diseases, including HIV-AIDS (Rew et al., 2002). Substance abuse is also commonly seen, as are mental problems including depression, self-harm, and suicide (Rew, 2002).

A Mosaic of Strategies to Address Homelessness

Homelessness has long been recognized as a multidimensional problem of modern society. A review of past strategies would reveal that approaches must go beyond the shelter approach. In addition to shelters, traditional approaches currently in use in varying degrees include (1) community-based residence programs, (2) residential services for the mentally ill, (3) foster family care, (4) halfway houses, (5) community lodges, and (6) satellite housing. Readers are encouraged to seek resources that these programs offer. A discussion of shelters as the predominant temporary residences for homeless people was presented in the fifth edition of this book.

Hombs (2001) provides an extensive resource and services list on homelessness. Other professionals who have done extensive work on the topic provide a variety of solutions and strategies to resolve this situation. One approach addresses mainstream social programs like "welfare, health care, mental health care, substance abuse treatment, veterans assistance and so on. These programs, however, are oversubscribed" (Hombs, 2001, p. 142). These social programs have been shifting their responsibility to the homeless assistance system that "ends homelessness for thousands of people everyday, but are quickly replaced by others" (Hombs, 2001, p. 143). Chronically homeless people and those who are chronically ill should be given housing that comes with supportive services. These two concurrent approaches that "close the front door" and "open the back door" are believed to reduce the costs of "expensive public systems such as jails and hospitals" (Hombs, 2001, p. 143).

Community health nurses who are at the forefront of homelessness advocate for changes and strategies to deal with the problems of the homeless. Strategies include assisting homeless people to gain access to the health care system and benefits, working with the community to obtain services and resources, educating the homeless about their health, and educating health care personnel about homeless people. Nurses are also encouraged to advocate for adequate transportation, day care, "one-stop shopping" for services, elimination of stigma, and policies that promote a healthy community (Hatton et al., 2001).

The problem of homelessness centers on the person who is part of a family, a community, and society. How much data and information are needed to solve a problem? In the case of homelessness, there is a critical need to know more about these men and women. It is the author's belief that the solutions to this problem are at the basic level of the homeless individual. A few selected works that support this view are worthy of mention. Rew's work, mentioned earlier, on homeless youth sheds light on how to address their health issues. One study on resilience showed that homeless youths who perceived themselves as resilient "reported feeling less lonely, less hopeless, and less engaged in life-threatening behaviors than those who perceived themselves as not being resilient" (Rew et al., 2001, p. 39). They hypothesized that "in the banding together to form living arrangements, they interacted more with each other than they would have in the mainstream world from which they may feel alienated" (Rew et al., 2001, p. 39). In another study, Rew, Fouladi, and Yockey (2002) looked at sexual health practices and recommended the use of "brief culturally-relevant interventions" (p. 144) for safe sexual behaviors.

Communities also need to continue their in-kind work with homeless people. Many schools and houses of religious worship have worked with local governments in extending support to the homeless. Food, clothing, night shelter, and short-term socializing have been provided. Parishioners may donate their time cooking meals, preparing the shelter, and serving as chaperones during the night. Much work is still needed to reduce rates of homelessness. The needs of the recently identified rural homeless must be addressed. Every citizen must be educated so that each person can serve as an advocate. Neighborhood coalitions must be established to prevent the increase in numbers of homeless and to support the return of the homeless person as a dignified, contributing member of society. Health care providers must continue to seek effective ways to coordinate their efforts through the creation of comprehensive resource materials. Technology must be put to its maximal capability to facilitate assessment and monitoring. Preparation for nursing and health care for the homeless in both rural and urban settings should be strengthened as an essential part of the curricula of the health care disciplines. Finally, more research regarding health care outcomes should be supported and data should be disseminated in a timely manner.

There is an increasing degree of optimism today in dealing with the problem of homelessness. Individuals and communities are showing concern through increased involvement. Homelessness is everyone's problem, and people can ultimately affect the establishment of priorities to facilitate an improved quality of life. Increasing awareness and knowledge of the current status of homeless people will aid in understanding the problem and its ramifications. This understanding will serve as an excellent guide in providing input, taking necessary action, and making the final decision as to what will make a healthy nation.

People Living With HIV-AIDS

Soon the HIV-AIDS epidemic will make its twenty-fifth year of known devastation to the lives of people, families, countries, and the world. Through 2002, a total of 859,000 people had been reported as having AIDS in the United States, dependencies, and associated nations. The diagnosis of HIV-AIDS decreased among children and in the 25 to 34 age group, but increased in all other age groups. BAAs accounted for 54% of new cases. From 1999 through 2002, increases were seen each year in men who have sex with men, among injection drug users, and in people exposed through heterosexual contact (Centers for Disease Control and Prevention [CDC], 2002b). "The majority of HIV infectees in the United States are minorities, and the vast majority of young and bisexual men in the United States who turned up HIV positive in a new study were unaware of their infection" (United States HIV, 2003, p. 34). Other statistics on people with HIV-AIDS are presented in Boxes 2-2 and 2-3.

Much has changed since the identification of HIV-AIDS over 20 years ago. Once it was considered a disease of gay, white people. Currently this disease affects people of all ages, both genders, and different populations in the United States. Through December 2001, BAAs accounted for 35%

Box 2-2 HIV and AIDS Statistics for 2002

Total number reported: 384,906
 Age group with highest incidence: 30 to 44 years old (43%)
 Females: 82,764 (61% through heterosexual contact, 36% through injection drug use)
 Males: 298,248
 Highest is in men who have sex with men (MSM): 58%
 Injection drug use (IDU): 23%
 Heterosexual contact: 10%
 MSM and IDU: 8%
 States with largest numbers of cases: New York, Florida, and California

Selected data from the U.S. Department of Health and Human Services. (2002). Cases of HIV infection and AIDS in the United States 2002. *HIV/AIDS Surveillance Report, 14*. Atlanta, GA: Centers for Disease Control and Prevention.

Selected HIV and AIDS Data on Ethnic Minorities

**People Living With AIDS:
Cumulative Through 2002**

Black, not Hispanic: 347,491
Hispanic: 163,940
Asian–Pacific Islander: 6924
American Indian–Alaska Native: 2875

NUMBER AND RATES OF AIDS DIAGNOSIS IN 2002

Non-Hispanic black: 21,049 or 76.4%
Hispanic: 6979 or 26%
Asian–Pacific Islander: 471 or 4.9%
American Indian–Alaska Native: 205 or 11.2%

EXPOSURE CATEGORIES

1. Male-to-male contact (highest)
2. Injection drug use
3. Heterosexual contact

Selected data from U.S. Department of Health and Human Services. (2002). Cases of HIV infection and AIDS in the United States, 2002. *HIV-AIDS Surveillance Report, 14.* Atlanta, GA: Centers for Disease Control and Prevention.

of total AIDS cases. Of the estimated 40,000 new HIV infections each year, more than 50% occur among African Americans (CDC, 2002b). The LHA population has the second largest number of members affected by HIV-AIDS. The AIDS incidence rate per 100,000 of the population in 2000 was 22.5, more than 3 times that of the white population rate of 6.6%. Cumulatively, in the Latino/Hispanic population, men accounted for 81% of cases reported; females represented 19% (23% in 2000 alone); 60% were born in the United States. The three modes of transmission yielding the highest numbers of infected are men having sex with men, injection drug use, and heterosexual contact, the latter accounting for the major mode for adult and adolescent Hispanic women (CDC, 2002a). In 2000, HIV-AIDS was the second leading cause of death for Hispanic men ages 35 to 44 and the fourth leading cause of death for Hispanic women in the same age group (CDC, 2002a).

AAPIs accounted for less than 1% of all AIDS cases in the United States but represented 27% of those found in Hawaii. At the end of December 2001, 6157 infected AAPIs had been reported and an additional 639 people with HIV were reported from areas with confidential reporting. Men accounted for 87% and women 13% of these cases. Although the numbers of infected people and those having the disease are low compared with the other groups, there is concern about this population because of rapid growth, high teen pregnancy and sexually transmitted disease rates, and increased mobility, immigration, and tourism (CDC, 2002b).

Like all the other ethnic groups, the Native American population has been witnessing increases in numbers of members afflicted with HIV-AIDS. At the close of 2001, a

total of 2537 Native Americans were reported to have the disease. These were men ages 25 to 34 and women ages 20 to 39 years. Fifty-two percent of HIV cases reported were attributed to men having sex with men. Forty percent were attributed to heterosexual contact (CDC, 2002b).

Issues in HIV-AIDS Prevention and Management

The most effective approach to HIV-AIDS is prevention, rapid diagnosis, symptom management (Coyne, Lyne, & Watson, 2002), and highly active antiretroviral chemotherapy (HAART) (Comulada, Swendeman, Rotheram-Borus, Mattes, & Weiss, 2003; Harris & Brown, 2001). Implementation of these approaches has been met with insurmountable multidimensional barriers. There are the stigma, poverty, lifestyles, behaviors, culture, beliefs, and values. Then there are the socioeconomic factors and political machinery of a nation. However, in the absence of a vaccine, there must be continued and sustained efforts to deal with the increase in numbers of infected people and deaths from this disease. Because prevention is the most important goal to contain the HIV-AIDS epidemic, the author's strong belief is that any strategy should have as its focal point individuals who are both the carriers and victims and their relationship in their families and communities. The discussion of HIV-AIDS prevention is, at best, only cursory in this chapter because of space limitations. An advance apology is extended to those who work tirelessly in continuing the mission of prevention. The material presented here is not sufficient recognition of their commitment and dedication. Further, the material will emphasize the situation of BAAs, who are most severely affected. The critical elements of preventive strategies, although identified in African Americans, could be applicable to other ethnic groups.

During the late 1990s, a sense of diminished priority for HIV-AIDS was considered to be the reason for the escalation of this problem among BAAs. A look at the factors that contribute to the AIDS epidemic in this group indicates that these are applicable to the other ethnic groups discussed here. First, BAAs have low educational attainment **(Web Site Resource 2D)**. They are underrepresented in the health care professions. For instance, BAAs comprise only 133,041, or 4.9%, of all registered nurses in the United States (USDHHS, Bureau of Health Professions, 2001). The insufficient number of health care professionals from minority groups has implications for culturally appropriate preventive care and management of HIV-AIDS in ethnic minority populations. Second, there are communication gaps between health care professionals and BAAs. "Cultural differences, lack of access to available services, racism, and misconceptions are some of the barriers to effective HIV-AIDS education and health promotion services" (Williams, 2003, p. 297). Third, there are myths, misconceptions, apathy, and lack of awareness of the consequences of the disease and other related social problems within the affected population. BAAs have many health issues, as discussed previously. They also have high poverty levels that contribute to their lack of access to resources about the disease and its consequences. Further, they have a lingering mistrust of the health care system that exploited them without benefits for the population (e.g., the Tuskegee Syphilis Study). Compounding factors include "high levels of stress, street violence and crime, homelessness, as well as heavy alcohol and illicit drug use" (Williams, 2003, p. 298). Fourth, there is evident sustained health disparity and the problem of drug abuse. "Sharing of hypodermic needles and trading sex for drugs are two ways that substance abuse can lead to HIV and other STD [sexually transmitted diseases] transmission" (Williams, 2003, p. 299).

Those who monitor the HIV-AIDS epidemic can attest to the important role that culture plays in prevention and management of the disease. When the value orientation relative to man's relationship to nature is fatalism, members perceive no control over their lives. African Americans (Plowden, Miller, & James, 2000) and Asian Americans (Chng & Collins, 2000) have fatalistic orientations. *Fatalism* is defined as a "surrendering of power to external forces of life which destroy personality, potential, hope, and life" (Powe & Johnson, 1995, p. 123). Research studies indicate that "in communities where the fatalism was high, participation in primary and secondary screening programs was low" (Plowden et al., p. 89). Additionally, the importance of the family could serve as a deterrent in seeking early diagnosis. Fear of shame and stigmatization of the family (Yoshioka & Schustack, 2001) prevent the individual from disclosing the diagnosis. On the other hand, loyalty and commitment to the family as a cultural norm could serve as strong motivators for providing assistance and support for an afflicted family member (Miner, 2000).

Since the early 1990s, the Jemmotts and their colleagues have conducted intervention studies that emphasize preventive outcomes. Their research has incorporated what they know about preventive measures and approaches that are culturally appropriate and have sound theoretical bases. Further, they study the most vulnerable groups that could exert the most significant impact on prevention of the disease. A synthesis of these studies is found in an excellent resource in which HIV-AIDS is discussed under lifestyle behaviors (Jemmott, Jemmott, & Hutchinson, 2001). These researchers' important contributions to the research on HIV-AIDS include not just the positive outcomes, but also the lessons that have been learned and the sharing of these lessons with the research community. "Racism, distrust of researchers, religious beliefs, homophobia, economic variables and diversity within the community" (Jemmott et al., 2001, p. 329) must be addressed, because these could serve as barriers. Additionally, substance abuse, women's issues, and adolescents' issues within the context of family and other relationships must also be considered in designing prevention strategies. The bases for interventions must be those theoretical models that "suggest new ways of thinking about program elements and provide a framework for organizing program content" (Jemmott et al., 2001, p. 334).

Knowledge taught should be complemented by skill-building content. "Several studies have suggested that interventions that address safer sex skills and perceived self-efficacy are more likely to be effective than information-only programs" (Jemmott et al., 2001, p. 335). Culturally sensitive approaches that consider social norms and values of the African American community should also be integrated into intervention programs. Culture plays an important role in HIV-AIDS, because it "strongly affects values, beliefs about health, disease, pain and suffering, expectations regarding health care professionals, religious doctrine, and world views, in general" (Brown, 2001, p. 61). Relative to religious beliefs, faith communities remain strong cultural influences in the lives of African Americans. Therefore, "It is important that any work in the African American population takes into consideration the impact of religion and the faith community on behavior because faith communities serve as means of social support for many African Americans" (Plowden et al., 2000, p. 91). Finally, researchers should build a relationship with the community. (See Think About It at beginning of the chapter.) Communities could provide "input in the design, planning, and implementation of risk-reduction studies" (Jemmott et al., 2001, p. 337).

Two other aspects of prevention must be addressed to limit the transmission of HIV. One aspect is early detection and the other is prevention of infection in women. "Unrecognized HIV infection is a major problem with important individual and public health implications" (Johnson et al., 2003, p. 277). "Failed early detection of HIV infection prevents any possible early educational interventions or behavior modification and precludes pre-AIDS treatment with highly active antiretroviral therapy (HAART)" (Johnson et al., 2003, p. 278). "Failed early detection is also failed secondary prevention. Persons with HIV infection who are unaware of their status may continue to engage in high-risk practices which promote transmission of the virus" (Johnson et al., 2003, p. 280). "For some AIDS cases, delays have been long as several years. About 52% of AIDS cases were reported to CDC within 3 months of diagnosis and about 88% were reported within 1 year" (USDHHS, 2002a, p. 37). Weinstock, Dale, Linley, and Gwinn (2002) surveyed clients who attended sexually transmitted disease clinics. Of the 52,260 clients, 14,750, or 28%, of the clinic clients reported not having had an HIV test. Similarly, Johnson and others (2003) conducted a survey of adults recently diagnosed with AIDS. The date of first HIV-positive test result was one of the questions asked. Researchers found early HIV detection less likely for women and ethnic minorities. An important recommendation from this research is the expansion of "behavioral intervention programs to reduce HIV risk behaviors" (Johnson et al., 2003, p. 281).

HIV prevention in women, particularly those of childbearing age, is a priority because of the potential devastation to future generations. Heterosexual contact among adult or adolescent females is the mode of transmission.

Cumulative data from 1998 indicate that 56,492 women have been infected. Additionally, since 1998, "of the 3374 children living with HIV-AIDS, 92% had been exposed perinatally" (USDHHS, 2002a, p. 7).

There are many issues in HIV-AIDS prevention, particularly among women from ethnic minority populations. Amaro, Vega, and Valencia (2001) describe the cultural, economic, educational, and social influences on HIV prevention among Latinas (Hispanic women). Cultural factors include beliefs that nothing can be done to prevent HIV. Hispanic culture is identified as having a fatalistic concept of man's relationship to nature (**Web Site Resource 2A**). Additionally, Latinas tend to assume submissive roles in the marital relationship. Therefore, their negotiation skills with regard to condom use might be ineffective. Moreover, Latino men are more likely to view condom use as interfering with sexual pleasure. Latinas suffer from poverty, low educational attainment, and poor English-language skills that hinder opportunities for health education and knowledge crucial in prevention. Others are involved in abusive relationships that hamper their abilities to control their lives and heighten their risks for HIV. Illegal status among many Latinas makes them vulnerable to victimization and exploitation. Given the complex set of factors that exert a strong influence in HIV prevention in Latinas, it is recommended that prevention efforts be concentrated on empowerment strategies that incorporate all the contextual factors and socioeconomic circumstances.

HIV-AIDS prevention is beyond assessment. There is now a core body of knowledge that could guide the design and implementation of preventive programs and strategies. Continued and increased support from the government for research, collaboration of health care disciplines, and involvement of individuals and families through community initiatives and political activism and advocacy could bring a rapid halt to transmission, with hope for a vaccine in the near future.

Other HIV-AIDS Prevention Initiatives

Selected initiatives for prevention that consider the issues discussed in the previous section can be found in many communities in the United States. The Alternative Co-Therapies Project in New York City serves HIV-positive African women and their families. Its services include child care, transportation support, comprehensive health care services, alternative co-therapies, increased accessibility of family members to health care services, and culturally competent clinicians (Miner, 2000). Another initiative is the Racial and Ethnic Approaches to Community Health (REACH), "a two-phased 5-year demonstration project to support community coalitions in the design and implementation of unique community-driven strategies to eliminate health disparities" (Ma'at et al., 2001, p. 94). One of the health problems addressed is HIV-AIDS. The U.S. Department of Health and Human Services in collaboration with the Congressional Black Caucus created Rapid Assessment, Response, and Evaluation (RARE), a community-based

technical assistance strategy. "RARE methodologies can provide a means through which municipalities can augment the role played by public health research in curtailing the HIV-AIDS epidemic" (Needle et al., 2003, p. 978).

THE NATION'S RESPONSE TO THE HEALTH CHALLENGES
Healthy People 2010

Healthy People 2010 outlines a comprehensive, nationwide health promotion and disease-prevention agenda. This initiative is designed to serve as a "road map" for addressing and improving the health of all people in the United States. *Healthy People 2010* is its foundation. With its 28 identified focus areas, the central goals are to increase quality of life and eliminate health disparities (USDHHS, 2000). The anticipated success of *Healthy People 2010* would include significant decreases in infant mortality, declines of death rates for coronary heart disease and stroke, and advances in cancer management. The complex and dynamic interplay of economic, political, social, and technological factors will require active participation in advocating for health, home, community, business, state, and the nation. Selected objectives relevant to the foci of this chapter are found in the *Healthy People 2010* box.

Healthy People 2010
Selected National Health Promotion and Disease Prevention Objectives for Emerging Populations

- Increase the number of people with health insurance to 100% (baseline: 83% [lower in ethnic minorities] of people under 65 years covered by health insurance in 1997).
- Increase the proportion of people who have a specific source of ongoing care to 96% (baseline: 87% in 1998).
- Reduce the overall cancer death rate. The target is 159.9 deaths per 100,000 of the population (baseline: 202.4 deaths per 100,000 of the population in 1998).
- Prevent diabetes. The target is 2.5 new cases per 1000 per year (baseline: 3.5 new cases, 3-year average, 1994 to 1996).
- Increase the proportion of people with diabetes who receive formal diabetes education. The target is 60% (baseline: 45% of people with diabetes received formal education in 1998).
- Reduce coronary heart disease deaths. The target is 166 deaths per 100,000 (baseline: 208 coronary artery disease deaths per 100,000 in 1998).
- Reduce AIDS among adolescents and adults. The target is 1 new case per 100,000 (baseline: 19.5 cases of AIDS per 100,000, aged 13 and older in 1998).

From U.S. Department of Health and Human Services. (2000). *Healthy people 2010* (Vol. 1). Washington, DC: U.S. Government Printing Office.

Office of Minority Health

The U.S. Department of Health and Human Services has an Office of Minority Health. "On July 10, 2002, it convened the National Leadership Summit on Eliminating Racial and Ethnic Disparities in Health" (USDHHS, 2002b). To eliminate health disparities, several strategies have been proposed including: "(a) broadening scientific research and data on racial and health disparities, (b) increasing awareness of the challenges facing minorities, (c) establishing partnerships to mobilize the larger community and stakeholders, (d) developing and enforcing policies, laws, and regulations to support the needs of racial and ethnic minorities and (e) ensuring access to critical health and human services" (USDHHS, 2002b, p. 1).

Many initiatives have been created to protect the health of minority communities. They address common health problems such as diabetes, substance abuse, and AIDS. There are also minority health research studies sponsored by the National Institutes of Health, Centers for Disease Control, and the Agency for Healthcare Research and Quality. Support for these initiatives and future ones must continue at all levels.

NURSING'S RESPONSE TO EMERGING POPULATIONS AND HEALTH

The American Nurses Association's (ANA) Code of Ethics explicitly states the profession's commitment to provide service to people regardless of background or situation (American Nurses Association, 1985). The ANA's Council on Cultural Diversity supports the work of nurses in their development of culturally competent care. The organization and its leadership, through the Ethnic-Minority Fellowship Program, has had an essential role in supporting the work and efforts of AAPIs, BAAs, LHAs, and Native Americans with master's and doctoral work. Nurses continue to make many positive moves toward understanding culturally diverse populations. See the Case Study about an elderly immigrant woman and the Care Plan that addresses interventions for her care.

Worthy of mention is the research focusing on health concerns and issues of ethnic populations. In addition, wide dissemination of research findings has been made possible through the *Journal of Transcultural Nursing* and through annual conferences and other workshops. Additionally, nurses with advanced preparation have committed their time and energy to developing approaches and models for transcultural nursing. These models are in Box 2-4.

Several other nursing journals focus on cultural diversity, such as the *Journal of Cultural Diversity* and the *Journal of Multicultural Nursing and Health*. These journals and a variety of other publications are constantly helping professionals increase their knowledge of health-related cultural issues. In addition, the *Minority Nurse Newsletter* provides excellent summaries of research studies, legislative updates affecting ethnic minorities, and relevant topics in education and practice. Ethnic nursing organizations are having an effect on greater cultural understanding through their dissemination of important works by clinicians, educators, and

CASE STUDY

Mrs. Denuval and Her Life in the United States

Mrs. Denuval came to the United States with her daughter, her daughter's husband, and their four children. All settled on the West Coast upon arrival. The daughter and her daughter's husband immediately got full-time employment befitting their educational credentials. Full-time employment was necessary to raise and support four children. In addition, they needed all the basic necessities including a place to live, warm clothing for the winter, and a means of transportation.

Mrs. Denuval assumed responsibility for caring for the kids and preparing their meals, which she enjoyed immensely. During her free time, she walked to the community library, the church, and the grocery store. On weekends, the entire family would go to parties and browse in the shopping mall. Soon, Mrs. Denuval met other older women and developed a social network. She had her own friends, who took her to movies, shopping, dances, and other activities. As her grandchildren got older and more involved with their friends, Mrs. Denuval found a great deal of free time.

When senior citizen housing became available in the metropolitan area, Mrs. Denuval's children suggested she move so that she could participate fully in all the senior citizen activities that the city had to offer. After a brief adjustment period, she volunteered her time teaching (she was a teacher in her native country) and participated actively in a senior citizen center that had many members from her country. She participated in dance presentations, outings, parties, and religious activities.

After living independently for almost 5 years, Mrs. Denuval's mobility became limited because of arthritic knees. She agreed to have one knee surgically replaced. Following the surgery and rehabilitation, she was diagnosed with Parkinson's disease. Living with her daughter was eliminated as an option because of the suburban location and difficult access to important resources.

Mrs. Denuval's health status would eventually be compromised with a degenerative disease like Parkinson's. Because she is a naturalized citizen, she is eligible for health programs such as Medicare. At the time of diagnosis, Mrs. Denuval was still functioning independently and living in senior housing. To ensure quality of life for her, short-term and long-term interventions must be considered. All her children and grandchildren would need to make a commitment to assist, encourage, and support her to maintain an optimal level of health and well-being. Involvement of all members of her immediate family would be consistent with cultural traditions and would facilitate informed decision making.

Reflective Questions

1. Describe culturally appropriate strategies and resources to assist the family in dealing with an aging parent with a chronic degenerative illness.
2. Suggest health care approaches or modalities for ensuring quality of life for Mrs. Denuval and her family.

CARE PLAN

Elderly Immigrant Woman

(Related to Mrs. Denuval Case Study)

Nursing Diagnosis Potential for Enhanced Family Coping

DEFINING CHARACTERISTICS

- Positive relationships among members of the family
- Extensive social support network
- Knowledge of wide range of resources by children
- High level of initiative and resourcefulness for problem solving
- Appropriate economic resources of children

RELATED FACTORS

- Socioeconomic status of children stable and supportive of standard of living
- High level of motivation of family

EXPECTED OUTCOMES

Mrs. Denuval and her family will:
- Utilize available and culturally appropriate resources
- Develop an effective communication system and shared caregiving
- Formulate a realistic plan for visiting and spending quality time together
- Discuss alternatives and strategies for future living arrangements

INTERVENTIONS

- Facilitate active participation of all members in decision making
- Keep family informed of available resources, services, and new health care information
- Provide referrals and consultation for counseling, support groups, and respite care
- Consult with members of the multidisciplinary team to address all aspects of care including physical therapy, speech therapy, nutritional support, and social services
- Discuss long-term strategies and end-of-life issues in the care of a person with Parkinson's disease, including alternative living arrangements

The role of professional nurses and other health care providers is a critical one in ensuring positive coping by the family and the client. Advocacy, counseling, health teaching, and referrals facilitate informed decision making. Sharing information about resources that can be tapped to meet the needs of the client in maintaining independence and quality of life are important functions of health care professionals. Respite care and support groups help to alleviate the stress of caregiving. Culturally appropriate approaches such as those that make use of family strength must be considered.

Box 2-4 Selected Models for Transcultural Nursing

- Process of cultural competence in the delivery of health care services (Campinha-Bacote)
- Transcultural assessment model (Giger and Davidhizar)
- Transdisciplinary, transcultural model for health care (Glittenberg)
- Culture care theory (Leininger)
- Purnell model for cultural competence (Purnell)
- Health traditions model (Spector, Rachel)

From Douglas, M. (2002). *Journal of Transcultural Nursing, 13*(3).

---

bodies for nursing education, such as the National League for Nursing and the Commission on Collegiate Nursing Education, create standards for including diversity in the academic preparation of students in baccalaureate and master's programs. Additionally, a cadre of nurses conduct research on the cultural practices and beliefs of individuals and families, which gives professionals a sound base for improving practice and designing cost-effective and humanistic health care strategies. The quest to deliver culturally competent care has provided the impetus for nursing faculty to require transcultural courses in the nursing curriculum to facilitate awareness and understanding of cultural diversity (Multicultural Awareness and Health Teaching boxes). Some widely used textbooks focusing on specific clinical areas of practice devote material to health care issues of ethnic minorities. Other resources include a chapter or two on cultural diversity. In addition, discussion of specific health care problems and nursing care always includes cultural aspects. In the clinical setting, health care workers, through staff development and in-service programs, are provided opportunities to learn and develop culturally sensitive care approaches.

The U.S. Department of Health and Human Services has funded programs for students from ethnic minority backgrounds and who also have economic issues as they pursue their basic nursing programs. The author's academic institution received a 3-year (1997 to 2000) grant for an initiative known as Growth and Access Increase for Nursing Students (GAINS). The author served as project director and, with the help of two full-time personnel, college and school administration and faculty, and external consultants, the student retention rate rose from 50% to 77% (Valencia-Go, 2000). A recent follow-up survey of GAINS participants indicates that only one participant had to retake the licensing examination; all others were successful on the first attempt. In addition, over 85% of the graduates are practicing in areas considered medically underserved. To this extent, the GAINS project achieved its goal of preparing ethnic minority people to return to and serve their communities (Valencia-Go, 2005).

SUMMARY

This century will be a time of great challenges as the United States continues to be a nation of diverse peoples. Emerging populations share similar concerns including health, an

---

researchers. A list of suggested readings can be found in **Web Site Resource 2E**.

Major organizations such as the ANA, the National League for Nursing, and the American Association of Colleges of Nursing publish culturally relevant materials to guide students, clinicians, and educators. Accrediting

MULTICULTURAL AWARENESS

Facilitating Transcultural Education

Nursing, as a health care discipline, has taken great strides in addressing the issue of multiculturalism. Credit is given to nurse educators who prepare students to care for multicultural populations. Many excellent resources produced by nurses address cultural concepts and strategies to facilitate multicultural awareness. Textbooks focusing on clinical areas of practice have integrated cultural diversity into nursing care strategies. However, how can students move above and beyond awareness to provide culturally competent care?

A transcultural course can open a world of knowledge on cultures. Students can get excited knowing about differences and similarities. They can participate in creative projects such as dress and food presentations. However, do these ensure culturally competent caring?

Clinical courses in nursing must build on the learned transcultural concepts. It is imperative that clinical faculty support students who are caring for people who are culturally different. Students should implement care modalities that meet the unique needs of each person. For instance, students might want to learn to braid the hair of a black individual. This aspect of nursing care would also facilitate the establishment of an effective working relationship. Are students able to recognize the hygienic practices of a Filipino person? Faculty should allow students time to think about their care modifications and consider cultural practices and how these fit within standards of care. Faculty should recognize their efforts informally through positive comments and formally through clinical performance evaluations.

As students progress in the curriculum, they will acquire other knowledge and skills essential to the role of a future professional. Courses in research, politics, and leadership may provide other perspectives to advocate for culturally competent care. In each of these courses, faculty can design action projects that will integrate learned transcultural concepts. For instance, students can be directed to assess the health needs of an ethnic community and then design a project with the members of the community to meet a specified need. Strategies should be selected that involve reviewing the research literature and getting the support of a legislator. Students should be encouraged to build on learned communication skills and to collaborate with a community leader. An example of a community-based project is the transformation of a garbage dump into a small park with benches. People in the neighborhood take care of the annual flowers and plants donated by local garden shops. This park became the collective effort of students, residents, and legislators.

Students need to see that their efforts to provide culturally competent care is the responsibility of the professional whose mission is to improve health, quality of life, and well-being of ethnic minorities.

HEALTH TEACHING   Facilitating Culturally Appropriate Teaching-Learning Projects

A culturally diverse academic institution provides many opportunities to facilitate students' abilities to communicate with each other and their clients in a health care setting. One project is a teaching initiative at a senior citizen nutrition site. Students work with peers who are ethnically diverse.

When students assess the needs of the senior site participants, they become aware that older adults are also ethnically diverse and that there is an inherent "culture" in the center that all the participants are aware of. This culture includes a mutual respect for each other regardless of personal or professional attributes. Students see that older people are able to transcend ethnic, economic, social, and other barriers for a positive experience in the center. Students assess the characteristics of the older adults and take these into consideration in the development of the teaching plan. Student diversity is reflected in the mosaic of ideas brought forth from each student's background and experiences. Culturally competent strategies learned from a transcultural course are adopted. If a student belongs to the same ethnic group as some of the elders, that student demonstrates specific ways to interact effectively with seniors of the same ethnicity. The students make visits to local neighborhood facilities and resources. They survey grocery stores and pharmacies to determine whether these meet the needs of the elders. For instance, the teaching project on nutrition considered ethnic foods that can be consumed when an individual is hypertensive or when there is a need to cut down on high-fat foods. When the teaching project focuses on mobility, students incorporate ethnic dancing as a form of exercise. Because gift giving is a way to acknowledge appreciation, students present ethnic minority elders with small gifts consisting of useful items, such as personal care products and problem solvers (e.g., reminder pads for medications, medication organizers, and bottle openers).

Students evaluate the learning of elders by using creative strategies such as games that are familiar to the elders. Further, they are asked to evaluate themselves as teachers. Did they incorporate the principles of teaching-learning? Did they integrate knowledge and experience into a culturally appropriate presentation? How did they grow as future professionals committed to working effectively with a culturally diverse client population?

---

acceptable standard of living, and quality of life for individuals, families, and communities. An array of cultural, economic, educational, social, and political barriers must be overcome at the local, national, and global levels to ensure the health and well-being of the people of the United States. The government, public and private industries, health care professions, and all individuals need to work together to ensure a healthy nation for future generations.

ADDITIONAL STUDY MATERIAL

Study Questions in the back of the book, see page 663.

evolve **WEB SITE MATERIAL**

These materials are located on the book's Web site at http://evolve.elsevier.com/Edelman/.

- WebLinks
- Content Updates
- Web Site Resources

2A Cultural Value Orientations
2B Comparison of Folk and Professional Care Systems
2C Demographic Data for Select Cultural Groups
2D Comparison of Major Ethnic Groups by Higher Education Degrees Conferred
2E Suggested Additional Readings About Select Ethnic Groups

REFERENCES

Abraham, N. (1995). Arab Americans. In R. J. Vecoli, J. Galens, Sheets, A., & R. V. Young (Eds.), *Gale encyclopedia of multicultural America* (Vol. 1, pp. 84-98). New York: Gale Research.

Adib, S. M., & Mikkey, I. F. (2003). Lebanon. In C. E. D'Avanzo & E. M. Geissler (Eds.), *Cultural health assessment* (3rd ed., pp. 443-449). St. Louis: Mosby.

Amaro, H., Vega, R. R., & Valencia, D. (2001). Gender, context, and HIV prevention among Latinos. In M. Aguirre-Molina, C. W. Molina, & R. E. Zambrana (Eds.), *Health issues in the Latino community* (pp. 301-324). San Francisco: Jossey-Bass.

Amaro, H., & Zambrana, R. E. (2000). Criollo, mestizo, mulato, laitnegro, indigena, white, or black? The United States Hispanic/Latino population and multiple responses in the 2000 census. *American Journal of Public Health, 90*(11), 1724-1727.

American Nurses Association. (1985). *Code of ethics.* Kansas City, MO: American Nurses Association.

Andrews, M. M. (2003). The influence of cultural health belief systems on health care practices. In M. M. Andrews & J. S. Boyle (Eds.), *Transcultural concepts in nursing care* (4th ed., pp. 73-91). Philadelphia: Lippincott Williams & Wilkins.

Andrews, M. M., & Boyle, J. S. (2003). Andrews/Boyle transcultural nursing assessment guide. In M. M. Andrews & J. S. Boyle (Eds.), *Transcultural concepts in nursing care* (4th ed., pp. 533-539). Philadelphia: Lippincott Williams & Wilkins.

Bailey, E. (2000). *African-American alternative medicine: Using alternative medicine to prevent and control chronic diseases.* Westport: Bergin & Garvey.

Baldwin, K. A., Humbles, P. L., Armmer, F. A., & Cramer, M. (2001). Perceived health needs of urban African American church congregants. *Public Health Nursing, 18*(5), 295-303.

Benn, D. K. (2003). Professional monopoly, social covenant, and access to oral health care in the United States. *Journal of Dental Education, 67*(10), 1080-1090.

Ben-Rafael, E. (2001). Sociology of ethnicity. In N. J. Smelser & P. B. Baltes (Eds.), *International encyclopedia of the social and behavioral sciences* (Vol. 7, pp. 4838-4842). United Kingdom: Cambridge University Press.

Benson, S. G. (2003). *The Hispanic American almanac* (3rd ed.). Detroit: Thomson Gale.

Black Americans: A statistical source book (2003). Palo Alto, CA: Information Publications.

Bohn, D. K. (2003). Lifetime physical and sexual abuse, substance abuse, depression, and suicide attempts among Native American women. *Issues in Mental Health Nursing, 24*(3), 333-352.

Bookman, M. Z. (2002). *Ethnic groups in motion: Economic competition and migration in multiethnic states.* London: Frank Cass.

Boyle, J. S. (2003). Culture, family, and community. In M. M. Andrews & J. S. Boyle (Eds.), *Transcultural concepts in nursing care* (4th ed., pp. 315-360). Philadelphia: Lippincott Williams & Wilkins.

Brenneman, G. R., Handler, A. O., Kaufman, S. F., & Rhoades, E. R. (2000). Health status and clinical indicators. In E. R. Rhoades (Ed.), *American Indian health* (pp. 103-121). Baltimore: Johns Hopkins University Press.

Brown, G. (2001). The impact of HIV/AIDS on the African American woman and child: Epidemiology, cultural, and psychosocial issues and nursing management. *The ABNF Journal, 12*(3), 60-62.

Burrows, M. R., Geiss, L. S., Engelau, M. M., & Acton, K. J. (2000). Prevalence of diabetes among Native Americans and Alaskan natives. *Diabetes Care, 12,* 1786-1790.

Burt, M., Aron, L. Y., Lee, E., & Valente, J. (2001). *Helping America's homeless.* Washington, DC: The Urban Institute Press.

Campbell, G. R. (2000). American Indian demographics. In C. J. Moose & R. Wildin (Eds.), *Racial and ethnic relations in America* (Vol. 1, pp. 63-66). Pasadena, CA: Salem Press.

Carbonell, A. A. (2003). Cuba. In C. E. D'Avanzo & E. M. Geissler (Eds.), *Pocket guide to cultural health assessment* (3rd ed., pp. 218-233). St. Louis: Mosby.

Carrillo, J. E., Trevino, F. M., Betancourt, J. R., & Coustasse, A. (2001). Latino access to health care: The role of insurance, managed care, and institutional barriers. In M. Aguirre-Molina, C. W. Molina, & R. E. Zambrana (Eds.), *Health issues in the Latino community* (pp. 55-73). San Francisco: Jossey-Bass.

Carter-Porkas, O., & Zambrana, R. E. (2001). Latino health status. In M. Aguirre-Molina, C. W. Molina, & R. E. Zambrana (Eds.), *Health issues in the Latino community* (pp. 23-54). San Francisco: Jossey-Bass.

Centers for Disease Control and Prevention. (2002a). *HIV/AIDS among Hispanics in the United States.* Retrieved May 10, 2004, from Centers for Disease Control and Prevention online access http://www.cdc.gov/hiv/pubs/facts/hispanic.htm.

Centers for Disease Control and Prevention, U.S. Department of Health and Human Services. (2002b). Cases of HIV infection and AIDS in the United States, 2002. *HIV/AIDS surveillance report, 14.* Atlanta, GA: Centers for Disease Control and Prevention.

Chelala, C. (2002). A vibrant place: Arab Americans in New York. *Lancet, 360*(9330), 417-420.

Chin, D., Takeuchi, D. J., & Suh, D. (2000). Access to health care among Chinese, Korean, and Vietnamese Americans. In C. J. Hogue & M. A. Hargraves (Eds.), *Minority health in America* (pp. 77-96). Baltimore: Johns Hopkins University Press.

Chng, C. L., & Collins, J. R. (2000). Providing culturally competent HIV prevention programs. *American Journal of Health Studies, 16*(1), 24-33.

Chong, M. (2002). *The Latino patient: A cultural guide for health care providers.* Yarmouth, Maine: Intercultural Press.

Comulada, W. S., Swendeman, D. T., Rotheram-Borus, M. J., Mattes, K. M., & Weiss, R. E. (2003). Use of HAART among young people living with HIV. *American Journal of Health Behavior, 27*(4), 389-400.

Coyne, P. J., Lyne, M. E., & Watson, H. C. (2002). Symptom management in people with AIDS. *American Journal of Nursing, 102*(9), 48-56.

D'Arrigo, T., & Keegan, A. (2000). Diabetes & Latinos: A community at risk. *Diabetes Forecast, 53*(6), 42-47.

D'Avanzo, C. E., & Geissler, E. M. (2003). *Pocket guide to cultural health assessment* (3rd ed.). St. Louis: Mosby.

Depastino, T. (2003). *Citizen hobo: How a century of homelessness shaped America.* Chicago: University of Chicago Press.

Dhooper, S. S. (2003). Health care needs of foreign-born Asian Americans: An overview. *Health and Social Work, 28*(1), 63-73.

Donner, F. M. (2001). Arabs. In *The world book encyclopedia* (Vol. 1, pp. 584-590). Chicago: World Book.

Dumonteil, E., & Gamboa-Leon, M. R. (2003). Mexico (United Mexican States). In C. E. D'Avanzo & E. M. Geissler (Eds.), *Pocket guide to cultural health assessment* (3rd ed., pp. 520-525). St. Louis: Mosby.

Ecker, M. (2001). Ethnics and values. In P. A. Potter & A. G. Perry (Eds.), *Fundamentals of nursing* (5th ed., pp. 401-422). St. Louis: Mosby.

Feagin, J. R. (2001). Racial relations. *International encyclopedia of the social and behavioral Sciences* (Vol. 19, pp. 12711-12715). Kidlington, Oxford: Elsevier Science.

Fixico, D., Kolata, A. L., & Neely, S. (2001). American Indian. In *The world book encyclopedia* (Vol. 10, pp. 136-185). Chicago: World Book.

Fletcher, A. B. (2000). African American folk medicine: A form of alternative therapy. *The ABNF Journal, 11*(1), 18-20.

Fox, P. A., Burns, K. R., Popovich, J. M., & Ilg, M. (2001). Depression among immigrant Mexican women and Southeast Asian refugee women in the U.S. *The International Journal of Psychiatric Nursing Research, 7*(1), 778-791.

Gabaccia, D. R. (2002). *Immigration and American diversity.* Massachusetts: Blackwell.

Garcia, H. D. (2001). Hispanic Americans. In *The world book encyclopedia* (Vol. 9, pp. 244-259). Chicago: World Book.

Giger, J. M., & Davidhizar, R. (2001). Diversity in caring. In P. A. Potter & A. G. Perry (Eds.), *Fundamentals of nursing* (5th ed., pp. 113-137). St. Louis: Mosby.

Gilliland, S. S., Azen, P. P., Perez, G. E., & Carter, J. S. (2002). Strong in body and spirit: Lifestyle intervention for Native American adults with diabetes in New Mexico. *Diabetes Care, 25*(1), 78-83.

Greene, R. (2000). *Social work with the aged and their families.* New York: Aldine de Gruyter.

Grinde, D. A. (2002). *Native Americans.* Washington, DC: CQ Press.

Guendelman, S., & Wagner, T. (2001). Hispanics' experience within the health care system: Access, utilization, and satisfaction. In M. Aguirre-Molina, C. W. Molina, & R. E. Zambrana (Eds.), *Health issues in the Latino community* (pp. 15-46). San Francisco: Jossey-Bass.

Han, B., & Wells, B. L. (2003). Inappropriate emergency department visits and use of health care for the homeless program services by homeless adults in the northeastern United States. *Journal of Public Health Management Practice, 9*(6), 530-537.

Harris, W., & Brown, G. (2001). Antiretroviral agents used in the treatment of HIV infections. *The ABNF Journal, 12*(3), 67-69.

Hatahet, W., Khosla, P., & Fungwe, T. V. (2002). Prevalence of risk factors to coronary heart disease in an Arab-American population in southeast Michigan. *International Journal of Food Science and Nutrition, 53,* 325-335.

Hatton, D. C., Kleffel, D., Bennett, S., & Gaffrey, E. A. (2001). Homeless women and children's access to health care: A paradox. *Journal of Community Health Nursing, 18*(1), 25-34.

Hayat, A., Lucas, J. B., & Kington, R. (2000). *Health outcomes among Hispanic subgroups: Data from the National Interview Survey, 1992-1995. Advance data.* Hyattsville, MD: U.S. Department of Health and Human Services.

Henslin, J. M. (2001). Race and ethnic relations: Measuring inequality. In A. M. Garcia & R. A. Garcia (Eds.), *Race and ethnicity* (pp. 22-41). San Diego: Greenhaven Press.

Holmes, T. (2003). *Minorities: A changing role in American society.* Detroit: Thomson Gale.

Hombs, M. E. (2001). *American homelessness* (3rd ed.). Santa Barbara, CA: Contemporary World Issues.

Hopper, K. (2003). *Reckoning with homelessness.* Ithaca, NY: Cornell University Press.

Hornsby, A. (2001). African Americans. In *The world book encyclopedia* (Vol. 1, pp. 136b-136h). Chicago: World Book.

Isay, D., & Abramson, S. (2000). *Flophouse: Life on the Bowery.* New York: Random House.

Jaber, L. A., Brown, M. B., Hammad, A., Nowak, S. N., Zhu, Q., Ghafoor, A., et al. (2003a). Epidemiology of diabetes among Arab Americans. *Diabetes Care, 26*(2), 308-313.

Jaber, L. A., Brown, M. B., Hammad, A., Zhu, Q., & Herman, W. H. (2003b). Lack of acculturation is a risk for diabetes in Arab immigrants in the U.S. *Diabetes Care, 26*(7), 2010-2014.

Jemmott, L. S., Jemmott, J. B. III, & Hutchinson, K. M. (2001). HIV/AIDS. In R. L. Braithwaite & S. E. Taylor (Eds.), *Health issues in the black community* (2nd ed., pp. 309-346). San Francisco: Jossey-Bass.

Johnson, D. F., Sorvillo, F. J., Wohl, A. R., Bunch, G., Harawa, M. T., Carruth, A. (2003). Frequent failed HIV detection in a high prevalence area: Implications for prevention. *AIDS Patient Care and STDs, 17*(6), 277-282.

Jones, C. P. (2000). Levels of racism: A theoretic framework and a gardener's tale. *American Journal of Public Health, 90*(8), 1212-1215.

Kavanaugh, R. R. (2003). Transcultural perspectives in mental health nursing. In M. M. Andrews & J. S. Boyle (Eds.), *Transcultural concepts in nursing care* (4th ed., pp. 272-314). Philadelphia: Lippincott Williams & Wilkins.

Kegler, M. C., Cleaver, V. L., & Yazzie-Valencia, M. (2000). An exploration of the influence of family on cigarette smoking among American Indian adolescents. *Health Education Research, 15*(5), 547-557.

Keith, V. M. (2000). A profile of African Americans' health care. In C. J. Hogue, M. A. Hargraves, & K. S. Collins (Eds.), *Minority health in America* (pp. 47-76). Baltimore: Johns Hopkins University Press.

Kim, H. (2001). Asian-Americans. In *The world book encyclopedia* (Vol. 1, pp. 812-814). Chicago: World Book.

Kinney, A. Y., Emery, G., Dudley, W. M., & Croyle, R. (2002). Screening behaviors among African American women at high risk for breast cancer: Do beliefs about God matter? *Oncology Nursing Forum, 29*(5), 835-843.

Kluckhohn, C. (1953). Dominant and variant value orientations. In C. Kluckhohn, H. A. Murray, & D. A. Schneider (Eds.), *Personality in nature, society, and culture* (2nd ed.). New York: Alfred A. Knopf.

Kulwicki, A. D., Miller, J., & Schim, S. M. (2000). Collaborative partnership for culture care: Enhancing health services for the Arab community. *Journal of Transcultural Nursing, 11*(1), 31-39.

Kuramoto, F., & Nakashima, J. (2000). Developing an ATOD prevention campaign for Asian and Pacific Islanders: Some considerations. *Journal of Public Health Management Practice, 6*(3), 57-64.

Lafuente, C. (2003). Powerlessness and social disaffiliation in homeless men. *The Journal of Multicultural Nursing and Health, 9*(1), 46-54.

Lambert, S., Fearing, A., Bell, D., & Newton, M. (2002). A comparative study of prostate screening, health beliefs, and practices between African American men and Caucasian men. *The ABNF Journal, 13*(3), 61-63.

Lauderdale, J. (2003). Transcultural perspectives in childbearing. In M. M. Andrews & J. S. Boyle (Eds.), *Transcultural concepts in nursing care* (4th ed., pp. 95-131). Philadelphia: Lippincott Williams & Wilkins.

Leininger, M. (2000). Founder's focus: The third millennium and transcultural nursing. *Journal of Transcultural Nursing, 11*(1), 69.

Leininger, M. (2001). The theory of culture care diversity and universality. In M. M. Leininger (Ed.), *Culture care diversity and universality: A theory of nursing* (2nd ed., pp. 5-68). Boston: Jones and Bartlett.

Leong, F. T., & Lau, S. L. (2001). Barriers to providing effective mental health services to Asian Americans. *Mental Health Services Research, 3*(4), 201-214.

Ma'at, I., Fouad, M., Grigg-Saito, D., Liang, S. L., McLaren, K., Pichett, J. W., et al. (2001). REACH 2010: A unique opportunity to create strategies to eliminate health disparities among women of color (Special Issue). *American Journal of Health Studies, 17*(2), 93-101.

Mays, V. M., Cochran, S. D., & Sullivan, J. G. (2000). Healthcare for African American and Hispanic women. In C. J. Hogue, M. A. Hargraves, & K. S. Collins (Eds.), *Minority health in America* (pp. 97-123). Baltimore: Johns Hopkins University Press.

McCabe, A., Macnee, C. L., & Anderson, M. K. (2001). Homeless patients' experience of satisfaction with care. *Archives of Psychiatric Nursing, 15*(2), 78-85.

McGadney-Douglass, B. F. (2000). The Black Church response to the mental health needs of the elderly. In S. L. Logan & E. M. Freeman (Eds.), *Health care in the black community: Empowerment, knowledge, skills, and collectivism* (pp. 199-214). New York: Haworth Press.

Meilaender, P. C. (2001). *Toward a theory of immigration*. New York: Palgrave.

Mikkey, I. F. (2003). Syria. In C. E. D'Avanzo & E. M. Geissler (Eds.), *Cultural health assessment* (3rd ed., pp. 748-754). St. Louis: Mosby.

Miner, J. (2000). Black women and HIV/AIDS: Culturally sensitive family health care. In S. L. Logan & E. M. Freeman (Eds.), *Health Care in the black community* (pp. 185-197). New York: Haworth Press.

Nagaty, K. A. (2003). Egypt. In C. E. D'Avanzo & E. M. Geissler (Eds.), *Cultural health assessment* (3rd ed., pp. 748-754). St. Louis: Mosby.

Nassar-McMillan, S. C., & Hakim-Larson, J. (2003). Counseling considerations among Arab Americans. *Journal of Counseling and Developments, 81*, 150-159.

Needle, R., Trotter, R. T. II, Singer, M., Bates, C., Page, J. B., Metzger, D. (2003). Rapid assessment of the HIV/AIDS crisis in racial and ethnic minority communities: An approach for timely community interventions. *American Journal of Public Health, 93*(6), 970-979.

New Campaign says 'Cuide su corazon' to people with diabetes. (2002). *Diabetes Week,* (Aug 26), 9.

North, C. S., Egrich, K., Pollio, D. E., & Spitznagel, E. L. (2004). Are rates of psychiatric disorders in the homeless population changing? *American Journal of Public Health, 94*(1), 103-108.

Nyamathi, A., Sands, H., Pattatucci-Aragon, A., Berg, J., Leake, B., Hahn, J. E. (2004). Perception of health status by homeless United States veterans. *Family Community Health, 27*(1), 65-71.

Orozco, M. M. (2001). Immigration and migration: Cultural concerns. In M. J. Smelser & P. B Baltes (Eds.), *International encyclopedia of the social and behavioral sciences* (Vol. 11, pp. 7211-7217). Kidlington, Oxford: Elsevier Science.

Plowden, K O., Miller, J. L., & James, T. (2000). HIV health crisis and African Americans: A cultural perspective. *The ABNF Journal, 11*(4), 88-93.

Potter, P. A. (2001). The health care delivery system. In P. A. Potter & A. G. Griffin (Eds.), *Fundamentals of nursing* (5th ed., pp. 22-47). St. Louis: Mosby.

Powe, B. D., & Johnson, A. (1995). Fatalism as a barrier to cancer screening among African Americans: Philosophical perspectives. *Journal of Religion and Health, 135*(20), 119-124.

Qiu, Y., & Ni, H. (2003). Utilization of dental care services by Asians and Native Hawaiian or other Pacific Islanders: United States, 1997-2000. *Advance Data, #336.* Hyattsville, MD: United States Department of Health and Human Services.

Reid, R. R., & Rhoades, E. R. (2000). Cultural considerations in providing care to American Indians. In E. R. Rhoades (Ed.), *American Indian health* (pp. 418-425). Baltimore: Johns Hopkins University Press.

Rew, L. (2002). Characteristics and health care needs of homeless adolescents. *Nursing Clinics of North America, 37*, 423-431.

Rew, L., Fouladi, R. J., & Yockey, R. (2002). Sexual health practices of homeless youth. *Image: The Journal of Nursing Scholarship, 34*(2), 139-145.

Rew, L., Taylor-Seehafer, T., Thomas, N. Y., & Yockey, R. D. (2001). Correlates of resilience in homeless adolescents. *Image: The Journal of Nursing Scholarship, 33*(1), 33-40.

Rhoades, E. R., & Rhoades, D. A. (2000). Traditional Indian and modern Western medicine. In E. R. Rhoades (Ed.), *American Indian health* (pp. 401-417). Baltimore: Johns Hopkins University Press.

Samaan, R. A. (2000). The influences of race, ethnicity, and poverty on the mental health of children. *Journal of Health Care for the Poor and Underserved, 11*(1), 100-110.

Saul, S. (2004, April 6). Ethnicity became issue in jury room. *Newsday,* A7, A54.

Sayed, M. A. (2003). Psychotherapy of Arab patients in the West: Uniqueness, empathy, and "otherness." *American Journal of Psychotherapy, 57*(4), 445-460.

Schienberg, J. (2004, April 14). Day laborers on the outside. *Newsday,* A32.

Snipp, C. M. (2000). Selected demographic characteristics of Indians. In E. R. Rhoades (Ed.), *American Indian health* (pp. 41-57). Baltimore: Johns Hopkins University Press.

Sochalski, J., & Mark, H. D. (2001). Response to health service utilization patterns among homeless men in transition: Exploring the need for on-site shelter-based nursing care. *Scholarly Inquiry for Nursing Practice: An International Journal, 15*(4), 155-159.

Stussy, S. A. (2000). Arab Americans. In C. J. Moose & R. Wilder (Eds.), *Racial and ethnic relations in America* (Vol. 1, pp. 102-107). Pasadena, CA: Salem Press.

The Latino paradox. (2003). *Harvard Health Letter, 28*(3), 3.

Uninsurance among Latinos leads to health disparities. (2000, May). *The Nation's Health,* 4.

United States HIV: Majority are minorities says CDC. (2003, Spring). *AIDS Watch,* 34.

U.S. Census Bureau. (2001). *The Hispanic population: Census 2000 brief*. Washington, DC: U.S. Department of Commerce Economics and Statistics Administration.

U.S. Census Bureau. (2002). *Statistical abstract of the United States* (122nd ed.). Washington, DC: U.S. Government Printing Office.

U.S. Department of Commerce. (2003). *Census 2000 brief: The Arab population: 2000.* Retrieved from www.census.gov/population/www/ancestry.html.

U.S. Department of Health and Human Services. (2000). *Healthy People 2010. Understanding and improving health.* Washington, DC: U.S. Government Printing Office.

U.S. Department of Health and Human Services. (2002a). Cases of HIV infection and AIDS in the United States, 2002. *HIV/AIDS surveillance report (14).* Atlanta: Centers for Disease Control and Prevention.

U.S. Department of Health and Human Services. (2002b). HHS disparities initiative. Fact sheet. *Protecting the health of minority communities.* Retrieved April 29, 2004, from http://www.omhrc.gov/rah/indexnew.htm.

U.S. Department of Health and Human Services, Bureau of Health Professions. (2001). *The registered nurse population: National sample survey of registered nurses, March 2000.* Washington, DC: U.S. Government Printing Office.

Valencia-Go, G. N. (1999). Elderly Filipino women's adjustment to widowhood: Implications for health and well-being. In L. Zhan (Ed.), *Asian voices: Asian and Asian-American health educators speak out* (pp. 58-67). Boston: Jones and Bartlett.

Valencia-Go, G. N. (2000). *Uniform progress report for grants and cooperative agreements for FY 2000.* Arlington, VA: Health Resources and Services Administration Bureau of Health Professions.

Valencia-Go, G. N. (2005). Growth and access increase for nursing students: A retention and progression project. *Journal of Cultural Diversity, 12*(1), 18-25.

Vigil, J. D., & Roseman, C. C. (2001). Teaching ethnicity and peace in the United States. In I. Susser & T. C. Patterson (Eds.), *Cultural diversity in the United States* (pp. 405-413). Boston: Blackwell.

Waters, M. C. (2001). Personal identity and ethnicity. In A. M. Garcia & R. A. Garcia (Eds.), *Race and ethnicity* (pp. 66-71). San Diego, CA: Greenhaven Press.

Weinstock, H., Dale, M., Linley, L., & Gwinn, M. (2002). Unrecognized HIV infection among patients attending sexually transmitted disease clinics. *American Journal of Public Health, 92*, 280-283.

West, S. K., Munoz, B., Broman, A. T., Sanchez, R., Klein, K., Rodriguez, J., et al. (2001). Diabetes and diabetic retinopathy in a Mexican-American population. *Diabetes Care, 24*(7), 1204-1209.

Williams, D. R. (2000). Race, stress, and mental health. In C. J. Hogue, M. A. Hargraves, & K. S. Collins (Eds.), *Minority health in America* (pp. 209-243). Baltimore: Johns Hopkins University Press.

Williams, D. R. (2001). Ethnicity, race, and health. In *The world book encyclopedia* (Vol. 7, pp. 4831-4838). Chicago: World Book.

Williams, P. B. (2003). HIV/AIDS case profile of African Americans. Guidelines for ethnic-specific health promotion, education, and risk reduction activities for African Americans. *Family Community Health 26*(4), 289-306.

Winkelman, M. (2001). Ethnicity and psychocultural models. In I. Susser & T. C. Patterson (Eds.), *Cultural diversity in the United States: A critical reader* (pp. 281-301). Boston: Blackwell.

Wittig, D. R. (2004). Knowledge, skills and attitudes of nursing students regarding culturally congruent care of Native Americans. *Journal of Transcultural Nursing, 15*(1), 54-61.

Yancey, G. (2003). *Who is white? Latinos, Asians, and the new black/nonblack divide*. Boulder, London: Lynne Rienner.

Yoshioka, M. R., & Schustack, A. (2001). Disclosure of HIV status: Cultural issues of Asian patients. *AIDS Patient Care and STDs, 15*(2), 77-82.

Yue, Z., Lee, W., & Wong, F. (2003). China. In C. E. D'Avanzo & E. M. Geissler (Eds.), *Pocket guide to cultural health assessment* (3rd ed., pp. 180-186). St. Louis: Mosby.

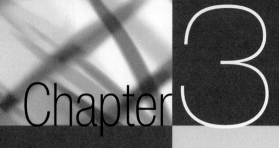

Chapter 3

DEBORA ELIZABETH KIRSCH

Health Policy and the Delivery System

objectives

After completing this chapter, the reader will be able to:

- Discuss key developments in the history of health care that influenced the philosophical basis of American health care and separated preventive from curative measures.

- Differentiate between private and public sector functions and responsibilities in the delivery of health care.

- Describe the mechanisms by which health care in the United States is financed in both private and public sectors.

- Discuss the influence of health legislation on health care delivery.

- Differentiate between the purposes, benefits, and limitations of Medicare and Medicaid programs.

- Describe the deficiencies of the health care system with regard to cost, access, and quality.

- Discuss the nurse's role in influencing health policy.

key terms

Advocate
Capitation system
Care management
Fee-for-service
Health maintenance organizations
Insurance

Lobbying
Lobbyist
Managed care
Nursing centers
Point-of-service
Policy decision making
Politics

Preferred provider organizations
Primary care
Primary care provider
Regulations
Self-insurance

THINK About It

Making Health Promotion a Reality

The inclusion of health-promotion activities and preventive measures in primary health care is supported by evidence-based practice. Combining clinical preventive services with population-based health-promotion activities, such as group smoking cessation programs, health education programs, and fitness programs in schools and on work sites makes sense. These combined measures are not only cost-effective, but they are essential to improve and maintain the health of present and future citizens.

The nurse is a key player in planning for a new health program based on recommendations from a community assessment. The nurse proposes a community fitness program be established by building a new recreational center in combination with the current athletic facilities at the local public high school. This primary preventive intervention would benefit students while in school and family and community members outside of school hours, thus promoting the fitness of the community. Individuals and

Continued

Making Health Promotion a Reality cont'd

THINK About It

families would join the center paying a reasonable membership.

1 How can the nurse "sell" the idea of the fitness health-promotion center to school board and other community members?

2 Why is the fitness program cost-effective?

The health care delivery system in the United States is a complex, multilayered entity that has the capacity to provide the newest technological treatments and implement the most advanced scientific interventions. Research findings have sparked the development of evidence-based practice, providing "gold standard" levels of medical and nursing care. The United States boasts a health care system equaled by no other country. Despite its impeccable reputation and breakthrough accomplishments, our health care system is plagued with escalating health care costs, limited access to care for some populations, workforce shortages, and quality of care issues. Health care is a big business, consuming more than 13% of the U.S. gross domestic product and exceeding $1.3 trillion (Sultz & Young, 2004). The salient issues of cost, quality, and access have been the focus of legislative agendas resulting in piecemeal reform efforts for decades. The dominant interest groups, government, employers, provider groups, pharmaceutical companies, medical personnel, and the public, are reluctant to make the necessary sweeping radical changes to correct the deficiencies of the system. Fear that individual interests of various stakeholders would be compromised and the level or quality of health care would decline has prevented bipartisan support for legislative reform to develop a system of universal health care. The market-driven American health care system has been unsuccessful in dealing with the issues of access, quality, and control of escalating costs.

The World Health Organization's (WHO) overriding objective is for all people to attain the highest possible level of health. WHO recognizes the importance of families and health promotion and has contributed to the family health policies of many nations by shaping global awareness for health promotion (WHO, 2004). WHO began the Health for All by the Year 2000 movement in 1977 by setting goals and targets for all member countries to attain a level of health that enables people to live socially and economically productive lives. Internationally, shrinking health care budgets have resulted in a variable level of achievement of these goals. In developing nations, such as those in Latin America and Africa, huge inequities in health care persist.

In 1990, the U.S. Department of Health and Human Services (USDHHS) published *Healthy People 2000*. Outlined were the core responsibilities of public health departments to protect the public from communicable diseases, exposure to toxic environmental pollutants, harmful

products, and poor quality health care. In addition, the document called for 90% of the population to be served by local health departments. Determinants were made in 1998 that of the 319 targets, only 15% had been met. Disparities among vulnerable populations, especially blacks and Native Americans, were increasing (Turnock, 2004). *Healthy People 2010*, the next set of 10-year targets, has even a more aggressive agenda of two broad goals:

1. Increase the number of years of healthy life
2. Eliminate health disparities among different populations

To meet these goals, improving the health of the population as a whole and reducing disparities will require different strategies.

Racial and Ethnic Approaches to Community Health (REACH) is a large-scale initiative of the Centers for Disease Control and Prevention (CDC) to eliminate racial and ethnic disparities in health. The groups targeted by REACH include African Americans, American Indians, Alaska Natives, Asian Pacificers, Hispanic Americans, and Pacific Islanders. Six priority health areas identified are cardiovascular disease, immunizations, breast and cervical cancer screening, diabetes, HIV-AIDS, and infant mortality. REACH 2010 supports community collaborations in designing, implementing, and evaluating community-driven strategies to eliminate health disparities, and 35 REACH 2010 projects were funded in 2003. Also in this initiative, the REACH Information Network (REACH IN), an Internet-based tool, will allow REACH coalitions to enter data and share information. The CDC and REACH 2010 will enter into partnership with local communities to plan and develop strategies for dissemination of lessons learned from earlier projects. It is expected the REACH IN databank will assist communities in not only collecting data but helping to evaluate community-specific strategies to reduce or eliminate health disparities. Education is a key factor in positive behavior changes in each of the REACH projects (CDC, 2004a). "Over the long term, public policies that narrow income disparities and increase access to education, jobs, and housing do far more to improve the health status of a population than do efforts to provide more health care services" (Turnock, 2004, p. 78). Nurses can be key agents of change in eliminating disparities with sound community education programs.

Public health nursing practice promotes and preserves the health of populations, looking at the community as a whole and its effect on the health of individuals, families, and groups. Community health nursing practice promotes, preserves, and maintains the health of populations through care provided to individuals, families, and groups and the effect of their health status on that of the community as a whole (Stanhope & Lancaster, 2004). *Healthy People 2010* emphasizes the relationship between individual health and community health, which is the health of the community and the environment in which individuals live, work, and play. Community health is affected by the collective behaviors, attitudes, and beliefs of all who live in it. The health of individuals is almost inseparable from that of the larger community, and the health of every community in every state determines that of the nation (USDHHS, 2000a).

In the first in a series of progress reviews on the 28 focus areas of *Healthy People 2010*, conclusions were drawn that only minimal progress has been made in meeting the population-based objectives. Considerations at this early review include: (1) increase efforts to provide access to care for those without health insurance and those with low income, (2) seek to improve the means of measuring health care access and disparities, (3) identify geographical areas and populations that are underserved, and (4) expand efforts to recruit minorities and people from disadvantaged backgrounds into health and allied health professions (Carmona, 2002). DATA2010 is a *Healthy People 2010* interactive database system accessible on the CDC Web site that tracks the most recent monitoring of the 28 focus areas.

"Following the terrorist assaults on September 11, 2001, lawmakers, prodded by the public, recognized a broader public health infrastructure was required to protect Americans against chemical or biological attacks" (Sultz & Young, 2004, p. 392). The Department of Homeland Security became effective on March 1, 2003, following months of debate. This massive federal government reorganization of 22 new and existing agencies seeks to restore an effective public health structure to strengthen the country's borders and comprehensive response and recovery operations should there be a terrorist attack with chemical or biological weapons. State and local health departments will serve an important role in maintaining the health and well-being of U.S. citizens (Sultz & Young, 2004). In addition, the public health system needs to address other equally important concerns. Chronic disease, the leading cause of death and disability in the United States, and the links between environment and health need to be primary considerations in building an effective public health system (Marmagus, King, Chuk, 2003). Strengthening this system should complement both goals of *Healthy People 2010*.

Nurses have a long tradition of involvement in health promotion, beginning with Florence Nightingale, the founder of modern nursing. While caring for wounded soldiers in the Crimean War, she fought for hospital reform in overcrowding, want of ventilation, and cleanliness. Her careful recordings of care outcomes quantified needed reform in health promotion (Neuhauser, 2003). Later, Lillian Wald, appalled by the lack of medical care, ignorance, and living conditions of the poor in 1893, developed a settlement program in New York City that trained nurses, provided care to families, and developed education programs for the community. Wald, a leader in political activism, spearheaded organized public health in the direction of health promotion for families and communities (Holder, 2004). These pioneers and others set the stage for nurses' unique role in health promotion.

The health care delivery system in the United States is experiencing significant changes. The Institute of Medicine (IOM), a nonprofit organization, conducts research from a systems approach to improve the health care of the nation. A 1999 IOM research study, To Err is Human: Building a Safer Health System, focused on prevention of medical errors, which account for approximately 98,000 deaths in hospitals each year. The startling findings concluded that the health care system, not bad practitioners, is the basic cause of medical errors. In November of 2003, the IOM released *Keeping Patients Safe: Transforming the Work Environment of Nurses* from the Work Environment for Nurses and Patient Safety Project. This report shows that work environments in hospitals and nursing homes contribute to nurses' errors. Four main problem areas in nurses' work environments are identified: (1) organizational management, (2) workforce management, (3) work design, and (4) organizational culture. Increased patient-to-nurse staffing ratios, fewer nurses, mandatory overtime, inadequate continuing education, and lack of nurse involvement in decisions about client care create an environment that contributes to error making. The data the IOM provided in this project support a direct link between nurse staffing and work environment to client outcomes (Institute of Medicine of the Academies, 2004; Kennedy, 2004). Nurses have a responsibility to understand the system in which they function, not only because of the influence the system has on their professional practice, but also the considerable impact on individuals and the public whom they serve (Maurer, 2000). Although health care often is equated with medical care, which focuses on the treatment of illness, this chapter presents the evolution and ongoing development of a broader concept of health based on the definition given in Chapter 1.

The complexities of the health care system necessitate an understanding of the system as a whole before focusing on the intermingled causative factors that have created a huge, fragmented enterprise. Many of today's problems have their roots in the decisions and directions of the past. It is not possible to identify and analyze current problems or to devise solutions without first exploring how the system developed. The relevance of the split between preventive and curative measures is apparent when the organization and financing of the delivery system is examined. The United States has established a system that uses two basic divisions of society to provide service: the public sector and the private sector. The merger of public health and welfare policies in the public sector is rooted in the Puritan ethic inherent in the historical development of the United States. The current focus on managed care as both an organizational strategy and a financing mechanism is highlighted in a discussion of how health care is delivered and financed. This discussion includes the role of the nurse as an **advocate** in the development of health policy.

HISTORY OF HEALTH CARE
Early Influences

Historical records of early civilizations (Egyptian, Indian, Chinese, Aztec, and Greek) show that ancient peoples were concerned with disease and practiced various methods of treatment. The earliest views of health can be seen as holistic in the sense of having a worldview. Primitive peoples understood illness in mystical terms; sickness and cure theories were tied to the cosmic view of life, with natural and supernatural forces often inseparable.

Most of the indigenous peoples of the world practice personal hygiene as part of their religious worldview. For thousands of years, epidemics were viewed as divine judgments on human wickedness, with a gradual awareness that pestilence has natural causes such as climate and other aspects of the physical environment.

During the Middle Ages, infectious diseases in epidemic proportions (leprosy, bubonic plague, smallpox, and tuberculosis [TB]) were the leading causes of death. Clearly, health was viewed in terms of survival and absence of disease.

Industrial Influences

The population of the Western world began to increase during the 1600s when America was first being explored. The New World had many things to offer explorers. An adequate food supply made it possible for the population to live longer, and advances in transportation made distribution of food supplies and other goods and services possible. Manufacturing advances during the eighteenth century, through the invention of the flush toilet and cast iron pipe, made sanitary engineering possible, saving many lives by preventing diseases such as typhoid, paratyphoid, and gastroenteritis.

Socioeconomic Influences

Although the Elizabethan poor laws (1601) in England provided a system of relief for the poor, which included infants, sick and elderly people, and laborers in the workhouses, a new poor law was enacted in 1834 based on the harsher philosophy that regarded pauperism among able-bodied workers as a moral failing. If the worker did not earn a subsistence-level income, then the attitude toward that worker was suspicious and punitive. These poor laws are the legal implementation of the Protestant work ethic that the Puritan forebears brought to the United States. People are held directly accountable for their state in life, and health maintenance is the responsibility of the individual. The far-reaching implications of this ethic can be seen today in the organization, financing, and delivery of health services.

Public Health Influences

Edwin Chadwick (1800-1890) is known as the father of British and American public health. Chadwick established an English Board of Health, which emphasized environmental sanitation but excluded physicians outside times of crisis. Additionally, he was secretary of the Poor Law Commission, which strove to improve the health of the masses for economic reasons. Chadwick's rationale was that disease among the poor was a major factor in their inability to support themselves. Therefore governmental health and welfare policies have been joined in England since the nineteenth century.

Lemuel Shattuck began the public health movement in the United States. He used the British system as the model, with public health services and welfare combined, despite the contradictory emphasis. Public health has focused on improving the health of the poor, whereas welfare has dictated subsistence at the minimal level. The influence of the Puritan ethic on the American health care system is apparent in the emphasis on the value of work and the attitude toward the poor. Today health and welfare departments continue their contradictory approach to the poor. (See the discussion of Medicaid later in this chapter.)

Scientific Influences

Until the twentieth century, epidemics of infectious disease (plague, cholera, typhoid, smallpox, and influenza) were the most critical health problems and major causes of death and disability for Americans. Scientific advances during the nineteenth century by Louis Pasteur (germ theory), Robert Koch (origin of bacterial infection), Joseph Lister (antisepsis), and Paul Ehrlich (chemotherapy) expanded public health from its earlier concentration on sanitation to control of communicable diseases through a broad biological base. Public health became an important force in decreasing death rates and increasing life expectancy through the application of bacteriology. Environmental conditions were improved by developing systems that safeguard water, milk, and food supplies, promote sanitary sewage disposal, and monitor the quality of urban housing.

Between 1936 and 1954, the discovery and use of sulfonamides and other antibiotics to treat bacterial infections reduced the death rate to its lowest point in history, with deaths caused by primary infections reduced to 4%, as compared with 33% only 50 years earlier (in 1886). The death rate did not change significantly between 1954 and the mid-1960s. Another decline in the death rate began after the mid-1960s. This decline has continued with the exception of a slight increase in 1995, with control of many infectious diseases. As the age of the population increases, chronic diseases such as heart disease, cancer, chronic lower respiratory disease, and diabetes are now among the leading or contributing causes of death as reported by the CDC for 2001 (Arias & Smith, 2003).

Despite the progress in conquering infectious diseases, for some age groups they are once again among the leading contributors to death in the United States. Diseases that were thought to be under control, such as measles and TB, are resurfacing and a new group of pathogens such as HIV and Ebola virus have emerged. Emerging infectious diseases are those in which the incidence (or number of new cases during a specified period) has increased significantly during the last 2 decades or is expected to increase. The incidence of AIDS in the United States rose alarmingly since general reports began in 1984, from an annual incidence of 1.88 new cases per 100,000 people in 1984 to 40.20 per 100,000 in 1993, and 15.0 per 100,000 in 2002. Combination antiviral therapy and primary prevention of opportunistic infections caused the number of deaths from AIDS to decrease

70% between 1995 and 1998. Despite a slowing decline in AIDS cases and deaths, it is estimated the number of new HIV infections per year has remained at 40,000 per year for the past decade, and 1 in 4 people are unaware that they are infected. Globally in 2003, 40 million people were estimated to be living with HIV-AIDS and 5 million people become infected with HIV annually (CDC, 2003). Since 1992, incidence rates for TB have been decreasing, following a resurgence over a 7-year period beginning in 1985. The national surveillance system at CDC reported a total of 14,871 new cases in 2003 (5.1 cases per 100,000 population), still not meeting the national interim goal set for 2000, which was 3.5 cases per 100,000 (CDC, 2004a). Drug-resistant strains of organisms (*Staphylococcus aureus*, *Streptococcus pneumoniae*, and *Salmonella typhimurium*) that cause communicable diseases are on the rise. For example, multiple drug–resistant TB is extremely difficult to treat and can be fatal, particularly among high-risk populations, including the homeless, drug abusers, and people with HIV. The most effective strategy for eliminating TB is to monitor this population and ensure completion of treatment by direct observed therapy. Resources are needed at local public health departments to provide follow-up in this typically elusive population. Elimination of public health appropriations that funded TB therapy and follow-up for nonadherent populations during the 1990s is a dramatic example of how legislative cuts in funding have cost the nation in both human and financial terms (Maurer, 2000). The national TB surveillance system at CDC reports elevated TB rates in both foreign-born persons residing in the United States and racial/ethnic minorities. Interventions to eliminate TB include not only adequate resources locally but a collaborative global effort as well (CDC, 2004b).

"For continued success in controlling infectious diseases, the U.S. public health system must prepare to address diverse challenges, including the reemergence of old diseases (sometimes in drug-resistant forms), large food borne outbreaks and acts of bioterrorism" (Lee & Estes, 2003, p. 35). Bioterrorism agents (anthrax, plague, smallpox) and chemical agents (ricin and sarin) pose potential threats to the public. Recent global outbreaks of the Hendra virus (1994), Nipah virus (1999), severe acute respiratory syndrome–associated coronavirus (2003), monkey pox, mad cow disease, and others (CDC, 2004) pose challenges to the global public health. An effective, comprehensive public health system in the United States is imperative.

Special Population Influences

The second goal of *Healthy People 2010* is to "eliminate health disparities among different segments of the population including differences that occur by gender, race or ethnicity, education or income, disability, geographical location, or sexual orientation" (USDHHS, 2000a, p. 11). For many of these disadvantaged people, the issues of preventing disease and promoting good health are often secondary to the problems associated with everyday survival. Determinants of health in a population are related strongly to socioeconomic status, with populations in the lower strata having worse outcomes. However, individual lifestyle behaviors including dietary choices, level of physical activity, use of alcohol and tobacco, substance abuse, and risky sexual behavior play a significant role in the health status of an individual. Access to health care for prevention, early detection, and treatment are paramount in diminishing health disparities, but programs promoting positive individual lifestyle behaviors are also needed (Lee & Estes, 2003). In addition, minority populations (even when access-related factors such as insurance status and income are controlled for) tend to receive lower quality health care than do nonminorities (Institute of Medicine, 2003) (Multicultural Awareness box).

Political and Economic Influences

Political and economic considerations are basic to the health care system. Politics determines which decision makers negotiate a desired outcome. Economics defines what resources are distributed and how they are distributed. The effect of economics and politics on the delivery of health care is illustrated by the situation in the United States following the Great Depression. Roosevelt's New Deal had an effect on health care, specifically in the passage of the Social Security Act (SSA) in 1935, which authorized grants-in-aid to individual states to improve state and local public health programs. Funds were available for "categorical assistance" programs, with cash grants first given to needy blind and elderly individuals and later to disabled people. Medical care was an allowable budget item, but payments often went for food, shelter, or other needs. Additionally, the SSA served as the basis for other assistance programs, such as Medicaid and Medicare, through subsequent amendments.

Split Between Preventive and Curative Measures

An orientation toward prevention has not been a part of the traditional medical education system, because physicians were excluded from early public health policies and because of the nature of medical education. Hospitals have had a monopoly on clinical medical education since the eighteenth century (Freyman, 1980). Hospitals were concerned with the treatment of overt disease, with a focus on activity and observable effects; people attracted to clinical medicine then, as now, were "activists."

The division between clinical medicine and public health is reinforced further by the custom of payment for a measurable act or, in this case, the treatment of visible illness. Monetary value cannot be placed on "intangibles" such as preventive services. Additionally, the Hippocratic oath, the basic philosophy of Western medicine, designates the physician's primary responsibility to the individual. This belief may prevent or inhibit the physician from seeing the broader needs of society, even when these needs coincide with those of the individual.

MULTICULTURAL AWARENESS

Transcultural Values and Beliefs About Health Care

WHY DO NURSES NEED TO BE CULTURALLY COMPETENT?

As the demographics of the United States continue to become more diverse, nurses need to be culturally competent or to practice transcultural nursing. The assumption that people are independently oriented and should assume responsibility for caring for themselves is based on Western values of autonomy, self-reliance, self-sufficiency and personal responsibility for health known as *individualism.* Some of these Western values are incongruent with non-Western cultural norms. In collectivist cultures, the need to maintain interpersonal harmony and group solidarity are valued (Andrews & Boyle, 2003). For example, cultures that are collectivist rather than individualist in orientation hold what Leininger (1997) calls "other-care values" (p. 342) such as interdependence, interconnectedness, and interrelatedness among group members. In some cultures, both group care and the inseparability of the environment and the individual are prominent values. Still other cultures value authoritarianism with specific rules about who has decision-making power or a deterministic view of the cause of illness with reliance on a higher power for matters of health and healing.

THE NURSE'S ROLE

Nurses need to support rather than interfere with family or group roles, challenge religious beliefs, or cause conflict with established lines of authority. For example, in many Mexican families, collective solidarity relies on the individuals in posi-tions of authority in the family to make decisions for other family members. The older males within the family may make the decisions for other members and hold responsibility and accountability for them. In Western society, competent adults are expected to be accountable and responsible for making decisions; autonomy is valued. Andrews and Boyle (2003) cite an example in which a competent adult Mexican widow was brought to the hospital by her daughter and required immediate surgery for gangrenous toes. The client and her daughter refused to sign the surgical consent form without consulting the client's oldest son who lived out of state. The son, in turn, contacted his uncle, still living in Mexico. The uncle finally consented to the surgery after several weeks when "He witnessed the client (his sister) suffering from much pain" (p. 516). The family in this example needed to make the decision based on their cultural norms and not on Western values. A nurse's attempt to promote the autonomy of the client in making her own informed decision to consent to surgery would not have been accepted in the collectivist social structure of this family (Andrews & Boyle, 2003).

For nurses to be culturally competent, they must assess cultural values that will enable them to provide culturally congruent nursing care. Unless nurses examine individuals' basic values and beliefs about health and health care, they might assume that all cultures share Western premises and values. Without meaning to impose their values, nurses may unwittingly encourage a behavior that is not culturally congruent for individuals from other-care cultures (see Chapter 2).

Data from Leininger, M. (1997). Transcultural nursing research to transform nursing education and practice. *Image: The Journal of Nursing Scholarship,* 29(4), 341-347; Andrews, M., & Boyle, J. (2003). *Transcultural concepts in nursing Care* (4th ed.). Philadelphia: Lippincott Williams & Wilkins.

The advances that conquered infectious disease involved a combination of social, educational, and medical efforts that integrated preventive and curative health care. Nevertheless, the shape of the current health care system stems from the 1850s, when separation of administration and staff for curative services (acute, chronic, and psychiatric illnesses) became the norm (Freyman, 1980).

The link between environmental health and personal medical care developed when sanitarians (people who work to maintain a clean environment) realized that their efforts alone were not sufficient to prevent and cure the diseases of the population as a whole; improvement of personal health was also necessary. Early preventive services directed toward individuals originated in medical practice rather than public health but were limited to welfare medicine (caring for individuals through state programs) or to salaried medical practice in factories. Community health centers that developed in the United States before World War I limited their scope to prevention and health education and, with the exception of some prenatal clinics, were generally located in poor neighborhoods. Delivery of preventive services developed separately from clinical medicine and became associated with public health. Most physicians, educated in hospitals, were interested in individuals for whom prevention had failed and whose illnesses brought them to the hospital ward.

Despite the separation of preventive and treatment services, the benefits of prevention eventually were incorporated into clinical medicine for individuals. Preventive and early detection measures became a part of pediatrics and obstetrics during the early part of the twentieth century, when vaccines and vaginal cytology examinations became available and accepted. Later in the twentieth century, internal medicine incorporated early detection of diseases such as diabetes, glaucoma, obesity, and hypertension. A shift to preventive medicine for the individual occurred, but the separate educational programs for public health and medicine still divided these areas. Not until the 1960s did the emphasis begin to turn from individual to societal values (Freyman, 1980). The U.S. focus on individual change toward better fitness, stress management, nutrition, and self-administered health care must follow the lead of many other countries' health-promotion efforts that call for changing the environment and health behaviors of individuals, families, and communities to promote health.

This new emphasis toward societal values parallels another evolution in the role of health in society. Increasingly, health care is regarded as a right rather than a privilege, with greater governmental involvement in and concern for the protection of that right. The future holds many more changes in the ongoing development of the role of health.

Individual health needs, financial resources, and the health care delivery system influence access to health care. Factors that limit a family's access to health care include the availability and location of health care facilities, geographical distance, transportation to these facilities, and the existence or type of health care insurance. Language barriers, hours missed from work or school, availability of child care, and excessively long waits for health care services all influence access to care (Spector, 2000). Each of these factors may be affected by the prevailing public policy of federal, state, and local governments. Technological developments, chronic illness, and the aging population each have an independent and interrelated influence on access to health care and the delivery of health services.

ORGANIZATION OF THE DELIVERY SYSTEM

The health care delivery system in the United States does not consist of a network of interrelated components, designed to work together like one might expect in a system. Instead "it is a kaleidoscope of financing, insurance, delivery, and payment mechanisms that remain unstandardized and loosely coordinated" (Shi & Singh, 2004, p. 4). This complex interrelationship involves providers, consumers, and settings, with both private and public sectors providing services. The public sector includes voluntary and nonprofit agencies and official or governmental agencies. Delivery of services is organized on three levels in both sectors: local, state, and national. Each of the three levels consists of private providers combined with official or voluntary public agencies. The nurse is often the professional who assists the health consumer throughout the complex delivery system; therefore, a basic understanding of the system's organization is essential.

Private Sector
Independent Practice

Traditionally, a person enters the health care delivery system by contracting directly with a health care provider for individual care based on **fee-for-service.** Free choice of provider has been the hallmark. However, more recently physicians and other health care providers are working within managed health care organizations. Although private practice traditionally has been disease oriented, the current emphasis on primary care necessitates a much broader perspective. **Primary care** involves continual and comprehensive care that includes efforts to keep people as healthy as possible and to prevent disease. It is delivered in settings close to where people live and work.

Private care may be delivered in numerous settings, from inpatient (hospital or extended care facility) to outpatient (ambulatory) settings. Outpatient care is defined as any health care services that are not provided on the basis of an overnight stay in which room and board costs are incurred. Ambulatory settings include two major categories: (1) care provided by owners and providers or (2) service settings (Shi & Singh, 2004, p. 239). These categories overlap, because many providers practice in their own offices and contract with one or more managed care organizations (see managed care discussion later in this chapter). Settings in the owner-provider category include independent physician practitioners, hospitals, community health agencies, managed care organizations, home health companies, and insurance companies. Settings in the second category include walk-in clinics, urgent care centers, outpatient surgery centers, chemotherapy and radiation settings, dialysis centers, neighborhood and community health centers, diagnostic and mobile imaging centers, occupational health centers, women's health clinics, wound care centers, fitness-wellness centers, health department clinics, and nursing centers (Shi & Singh, 2004).

Nursing centers, organizations that give the individual access to professional nursing services, are "strategically positioned to improve the health and well being of vulnerable populations" (Kinsey & Buchanan, 2004, p. 412). Nursing centers trace their origin to the Henry Street Settlements, founded by Lillian Wald in 1893 as discussed earlier (Holder, 2004). The modern movement to establish nursing centers began in 1965 when the nurse practitioner (NP) role was created, which allowed nurses to provide primary care to individuals. Nursing centers (ambulatory care centers and birthing centers) have provided high-quality nursing care from certified nurse midwives (CNMs), NPs, and other advanced practice nurses (APNs). During the 1970s, university-based centers and academic nursing centers were established to provide nursing services to communities, learning experiences for students, and settings for faculty practice and research. The key components of a community nursing center include (1) a nurse as chief manager, (2) nursing staff that are accountable and responsible for care and professional practice, and (3) nurses as the primary providers of care. Using a multidisciplinary collaboration framework, nurses have the opportunity to provide comprehensive primary care services, including a focus on wellness and health promotion, public health programs, and targeted interventions for populations with special needs. In recent years, more than one half have closed for financial reasons. The Council for Nursing Centers, established in 1988 within the National League for Nursing, promotes the mission and goals of nursing centers through educational programs, publications, research initiatives, and committee work. Members of the Council for Nursing Centers also provide mentoring and consultation to support colleagues in developing and advancing nursing centers. Nurses can continue to build community support, trust, and skills needed to make the nursing center model part of mainstream health care delivery in the twenty-first century (Kinsey & Buchanan, 2004; Vincent, Oakley, Pohl, & Walker, 2000) (Case Study).

A Nursing Center

A nursing student is completing her clinical experience in a nursing center. She follows a pregnant diabetic adolescent and her family in the home and for visits with a nurse midwife and dietitian in the center. She has the opportunity to participate in holistic nursing care and observe the delivery of a healthy infant during her clinical stay.

Reflective Questions
1. Compare the philosophy and subsequent care that individuals receive in a nursing center with the illness care they receive in a more traditional outpatient setting.
2. What kind of a role might the nurse pursue within a nursing center after graduation?

Managed Health Care Organizations

Managed health care organizations provide for both the delivery and the financing of health care for their members. "In 2002, 95 percent of all workers covered by employer health benefits were enrolled in some type of managed care plan" (Sultz & Young, 2004, p. 282). The principal force behind the growth of **managed care** is the belief that health care costs can be controlled by "managing" the way in which health care is delivered, controlling costs by controlling utilization (Sultz & Young, 2004).

The foundation of managed care organizations is the **primary care provider** (PCP), who may be a physician, physician's assistant, or nurse. Physician PCPs are usually general or family practitioners, but they may also be internists, pediatricians, or obstetrician-gynecologists. Physician's assistants are educated and prepared to work under the direct supervision of physicians. Nurses in advanced practice who provide primary care may be NPs or CNMs.

The PCP serves as a "gatekeeper" to coordinate and oversee individual care. The gatekeeper concept is designed to manage the individual's use of resources, to reduce self-referral to specialists, and to protect the individual from unnecessary procedures and overtreatment (Shi & Singh, 2004). Cost containment is achieved by decreasing hospital admissions and costly procedures and limiting referrals to specialists. An oversupply and abundance of specialists occur in some areas and a lack of primary care providers occurs in many rural areas. Specialist salaries typically exceed those of PCPs, and the number of specialists increased as technology developed. Box 3-1 provides a glossary of key terms used in managed care.

Health Maintenance Organizations

Health maintenance organizations (HMOs) deliver comprehensive health maintenance and treatment services for a group of enrolled individuals who prepay a fixed fee. The HMO accepts responsibility for the organization, financing, and delivery of health care services for its members. Several

Box 3-1 A Glossary of Managed Care

Capitation: a set amount or flat rate to cover an individual's medical care for a specified period

Care management: an organized approach to meet the needs of an individual, coordinating the delivery of all services in the most cost-effective manner

Gatekeeper: a primary care physician or APN who functions as the provider and who makes referrals for emergency services or specialty care

HMO: health maintenance organization; the type of managed care organization that provides comprehensive care for an enrollee through a predetermined annual fee structure

IPA: independent practice association; an organization that physicians in private practice can join so that the organization can represent them in the negotiation of managed care contracts

Managed competition: a health care reform proposal that would foster competition among integrated networks of insurance companies and health providers

Managed health care: a system that combines the functions of health insurance and the actual delivery of care. A gatekeeper controls costs and utilization of services

PCP: primary care provider; physician or APN who provides basic and routine health care services usually in an office or clinic

Per diem: reimbursement based on a flat rate per day for inpatient care

POS: point-of-service; a plan in which members decide where to receive services, either with a provider on the panel or to pay more and get services elsewhere

PPO: preferred provider organization; a plan that contracts with independent providers for services at a discount

Primary care: basic health care that emphasizes general health needs rather than specialized care

Reimbursement: the amount insurers pay to a provider, which may be a portion of the actual charge

Utilization review: a system used to monitor diagnosis, treatment, and billing practices, the purpose of which is to lower costs by discouraging unnecessary treatment

Modified from Shi, L., & Singh, D. (2003). *Delivering health care in America: A systems approach.* Sudbury, MA: Jones and Bartlett; Kongstvedt, P. (1996). *The managed health care handbook* (3rd ed.). Gaithersburg, MD: Aspen.
APN, advanced practice nurse.

models have evolved. The traditional HMO structure was a group or staff model, in which the fiscal agent employed a group of physicians and some specialty services to provide care to its members. Salaried providers generally spent all of their time serving members of the HMO. An example is Kaiser-Permanente Health Care System, which also has its own hospitals. The HMO through a prenegotiated contract, usually fee-for-service, purchased hospital care and other services for its members. Staff models were described as "closed panel," because employed physicians provided care only for members of the HMO. A community physician could not care for a member of the HMO without prearrangement or authorization by the HMO. As of 1999, less than 1% of individuals were enrolled in this type of HMO, partly due to the lack of flexibility, cost to expand facilities, and competition from independent practice associations (IPAs) (Sultz & Young, 2004).

Independent Practice Associations

IPAs are physician organizations composed of independent physicians in solo or group practices who provide health care services to members of an HMO in their private offices, eliminating the expense of the staff model HMO, which furnished and owned the facility in which care was provided. Hospital care and specialty services not within the IPA group can be purchased by the HMO for a fee-for-service or prepaid price. Physicians in an IPA contract may be restricted to caring only for members enrolled in the IPA, but some contracts may allow providers to care for nonmembers, as well. Other variations of the staff model and IPAs exist. In a group practice model, an HMO contracts with all physicians and specialists needed by the HMO enrollees, but physicians remain independent. Some contracts are exclusive, requiring physicians to restrict care to members of an individual HMO, and other variations allow physicians to care for members outside the HMO. In a network model, HMOs contract with individual physicians and with physician groups for both primary and specialty services. The HMO maintains control over fee arrangements. As of 2002, approximately 26% of individuals were enrolled in some sort of IPA (Sultz & Young, 2004).

Point-of-Service Plans

Point-of-service (POS) plans evolved in response to concern with lack of consumer choice in choosing providers and services. POS plans allow members, for an additional fee and higher co-payment, to use providers outside of the individual HMO network. Members can choose to pay for this enhanced POS or stay within the HMO network for reduced co-payments, allowing individual consumer choice. In 2002, 18% of HMO members were enrolled in various levels of POS plans (Sultz & Young, 2004).

Preferred Provider Organizations

Preferred provider organizations (PPOs), another delivery modeling the private sector, were formed by physicians and hospitals to serve the needs of private, third-party payer, and self-insured firms. Contracted providers in the PPO agree to deliver services to members for a fee-for-service negotiated discount price. To control costs, members must receive care exclusively from providers within the PPO or incur additional financial cost. "In 2002, PPOs were the most popular managed care plans, with a 52 percent market share" (Sultz & Young, 2004, p. 280). To control costs, the provider must receive preauthorization from the PPO for a member to be hospitalized, and second opinions are required before major procedures or surgery is performed. PPOs are beneficial to physicians and hospitals, because they are assured a certain volume of business (Sultz & Young, 2004).

Public Sector

The public sector contains official and voluntary public health agencies operating at the local, state, federal, and international levels. Health promotion and health protection or disease prevention receive greater emphasis in this sector than in the private sector.

Source of Power

The U.S. Constitution is based on the sharing of sovereign power between federal and state governments. The powers of the federal government in relation to health are not delineated specifically in the Constitution; they are derived from the financial authority to tax and to spend for the general welfare and from powers delegated to the government by the states, which reserve police power. Police power, the basis of the states' role in health, means that the states have the obligation and duty to protect the health, safety, and welfare of their citizens (Bonick, 2000). The state governor or legislature generally delegates police power to a specific health agency, usually the public health department. To protect citizens from the risk of contracting a disease, the public health officer can arrest an individual who has a communicable disease, such as TB, and refuses treatment. Police power also permits states to require licensing of professionals who deal in the public sector, such as nurses, physicians, and beauticians.

State health authority is based also on the Tenth Amendment, which reserves for the states, or for the people, those powers not delegated to the federal government by the Constitution. The states then use their powers to create local governments and delegate authority to them in health matters.

Influence of Political Philosophy

The prevailing political philosophy of societal health needs affects the relationship among federal, state, and local governments, as demonstrated by the 1930 New Deal philosophy. The trend toward increased federal government involvement continued during the Kennedy–Johnson era, when the government focused on societal needs and health care to an unprecedented degree. During the Nixon–Ford era, a New Federalism movement called for less federal encroachment into states' responsibilities and greater state and local responsibility related to the introduction of revenue sharing.

The Reagan-era version of New Federalism included pro-competition and deregulation policies as a means of dealing with limited finances (see the financing discussion later in this chapter). Clearly, the federal government's role varies according to political philosophy.

During the 1989-1993 Bush administration, little change occurred in moving new legislation toward health care reform. During his 4 years in the Oval Office, President George H. Bush worked toward two principal efforts, the Health Summit that convened in 1991 and the report issued by the Social Security Advisory Commission. These efforts provided no concrete solutions for the deep-set problems endemic to the health care system.

In 1993 the Clinton administration proposed the Health Security Act to achieve universal coverage in the United States, by mandating that all employers provide health insurance to their employees and by giving small businesses and unemployed Americans subsidies with which to purchase insurance. The plan met severe opposition from the insurance industry and the business community. Mass media advertisements by these stakeholders used a Harry and Louise–type media campaign to ask the public whether HMOs would provide choice and access to health care services. Large segments of the American public, especially the 80% who had employer-based private health insurance, began to fear being forced into HMOs, which would diminish their choice of, access to, and quality of health care. The financial cost of universal health care coverage was estimated to reach trillion-dollar levels. The act was defeated in Congress (Lee & Estes, 2003). A time of political caution followed in further movement toward a comprehensive system change. The portability of health care coverage bill was passed in 1996, and when Clinton was reelected the focus shifted to balancing the federal budget by 2002. Incremental legislation included the Balanced Budget Act (BBA) of 1997, which made significant reforms in Medicare. (See discussion about Medicare later in this chapter.) In 2000, despite a budget surplus, neither Al Gore nor George W. Bush offered plans for universal coverage in the 2000 presidential election campaign. The closest opportunity to enact universal health care for all citizens had passed.

The current administration has expressed a belief that all Americans should have access to affordable, high-quality health care. To achieve this goal, President George W. Bush has (1) requested the creation of new health savings accounts, (2) signed legislation for a prescription drug benefit under Medicare, (3) recommended an increased access to care with a 5-year plan to fund 1200 new or expanded community health centers, (4) strengthened Medicaid and the State Children's Health Insurance Program (SCHIP), (5) and committed to medical liability reform (*Bush's agenda*, 2005).

Managed Competition

Although the Clinton health reform plan did not become reality, many changes in the health care marketplace occurred in response to or in preparation for it. Managed competition, the basis of the Clinton proposal, not only incorporated the coordinated delivery system of managed care, but also encompassed large purchasing groups of businesses, government employees, and individuals. The health care market, not the government, was the driving force behind these networks that were formed in major metropolitan areas. Providers and insurers positioned themselves for success under increasing competition and decreasing financial resources in the health care marketplace. The rising cost of health care is not slowing. "The average annual premium of a health insurance policy is now more than $6000 (Canada $8910) for a family and more than $3000 for an individual" (Lee & Estes, 2003, p. 363).

Future Health Policy

Historical evolution of health policy in the United States clearly has revealed the problems facing the health care system. There remains a lack of consensus among the major stakeholders regarding the solutions to the problems. Deadlocks in the policy process of the 1993-1994 health system reform shifted the focus away from comprehensive reform. Instead, incrementalism as the principal means of health policy reform in a free-market system would prevail. Cost, access, and quality will continue to be major factors in policy development by all levels of government: local, state, and federal (Lee & Estes, 2003). A new health insurance paradigm surfaced in 2000, consumer-driven health plans. These employer-supplied insurance plans are an alternative to managed care health plans and may allow businesses, especially small businesses, an avenue to provide health care coverage to their employees. A health care reimbursement account, a medical savings account (MSA), or a health savings account is established for the employee. Individual members receive approximately $1000 annually to cover general health care expenditures, and unused monies are rolled over for the next year. Screening and preventive care are generally covered 100%, but higher cost care (catastrophic, surgery or hospitalization) has high deductibles. Policy considerations include making health savings accounts tax exempt, which would increase the appeal to both employees and employers. These plans are expected to grow in number as an alternative to managed care (Herrick, 2004).

Nursing's Role in the Search for Health Care Reform

The last decade of the twentieth century was one of great unrest for nurses. Major issues of rising costs, access to care, and accountability for the health care system were addressed in the American Nurses Association (ANA) proposal, "Nursing's Agenda for Health Care Reform," which emphasizes universal access to care under an expanded Medicare system focusing on health promotion and disease prevention. The first point in nursing's agenda is to provide primary care in convenient, familiar, community settings where individuals live and work, such as schools, work sites, and the home (Research Highlights box). A new proposal in 2000, Achieving Access for All Americans, recommitted to the principle that all Americans are entitled to ready access, affordable, quality health care services. The ANA proposes the Medicare program be expanded to a seamless, universal Medicare program that serves the broader American population. Discussed in this proposal are the growing numbers of uninsured, gaps in coverage, rising insurance premiums costs, and failure of comprehensive federal health care reform (American Nurses Association [ANA], 2000).

research highlights

Community-Based Program for Spanish-Speaking Hispanics With Chronic Disease in Northern California: Taking Control of Your Health

A growing health disparity between Hispanics and non-Hispanics, as well as the increase in the prevalence of chronic disease in the Hispanic population, sparked investigators to study participant outcomes of a 6-week peer-led community-based program for Spanish-speaking Hispanics with known chronic disease. The program, Tomando Control de su Salud (Taking Control of Your Health), was similar to a previously successful English Chronic Disease Self-Management Program. The participants of the study were recruited via community outreach to churches, community centers, and clinics in 4-month cohorts over a 3.5-year period. Participants were eligible for inclusion if they had heart disease, lung disease, or type 2 diabetes. Two and one-half hour class segments focused on exercise, positive thinking, nutrition, relaxation techniques, and problem solving. Disease specific content was not taught.

Participants were randomized into two groups, intervention and usual care participants. Intervention participants took Tomando immediately, whereas the usual care participants were put on a wait-list for 4 months. Treatment participants in this study numbered 327 and were compared with those placed on the wait-list (224 participants). After 4 months participants were compared with usual care subjects and demonstrated improved health status, health behavior, and self-efficacy, as well as fewer emergency room visits. After 1 year the improvements were maintained and remained significantly different from the baseline condition. In conclusion, this community-based program has the potential to improve the lives of Hispanics with chronic illness while reducing emergency room use.

Lorig, K., Ritter, P., Gonzalez, V. (2003). Hispanic chronic disease self-management: A randomized community-based outcome trial. *Nursing Research, 52*(6), 361-369.

Official Agencies

Official agencies are tax supported and therefore accountable to the citizens through elected or appointed officials or boards. The purpose and duties of official agencies are prescribed or mandated by law. This discussion is from the perspective of the individual gaining knowledge of or access to the health care system.

Local Level. The health department of a town, city, county, township, or district is the local health unit and is usually the first line of access and health responsibility for the population that it serves. The chief administrator, the health officer, is appointed by the mayor, the board of health, or some other executive governing body. The local health department's role and functions usually center on providing direct services to the public and depend on the state mandate and community resources. Local governments, but usually not health departments, have the responsibility to provide general health care services for the poor. (See the Medicaid section later in this chapter.)

State Level. Public health services are organized by each state, with wide variation from one state to another. The chief administrator is usually a state health officer or commissioner appointed by the governor. One agency, typically the state health department, carries out the primary responsibilities in policy, planning, and coordination of programs and services for local units under its jurisdiction.

Federal Level. The federal government assumes overall responsibility for the health protection of its citizens. Although all three branches of the government make health-related decisions, the major policy decisions are made by the president and his staff (executive branch) and Congress (legislative branch). These two branches determine health policy. Once policy is determined, other government agencies are responsible for oversight to ensure implementation.

The USDHHS is the main federal body concerned with the health of the nation and consists of a number of separate individual agencies. USDHHS agencies that relate directly to nursing include the Health Resources and Services Administration and the National Institutes of Health (NIH). The Bureau of Health Professions, within the Health Resources and Services Administration, contains a division of nursing, which is a source for nursing education and training grants. The National Center for Nursing Research, established in 1986, became the National Institute of Nursing Research within the NIH in 1993. The NIH funds nursing research, including health-promotion and illness-prevention studies. With a budget that has increased from an initial $16 million in 1993 to nearly $90 million in 2000, nurses have increased opportunities to make significant research contributions, particularly related to health promotion (NIH, National Institute of Nursing Research, 2000). **Web Site Resource 3A** describes the various agencies within the USDHHS and their major functions.

Other departments that are involved in health care at the federal level include (1) the Veterans Administration, an independent agency directly under the president that provides health care services for four categories of veterans, and (2) the Department of Defense, which sponsors health care for military personnel on active duty. For military dependents and retirees, care is covered through the former Civilian Health and Medical Program for the Uniformed Services (CHAMPUS) insurance program, renamed TRICARE.

Departments engaged in health-related activities include the following:

1. U.S. Department of Agriculture, which provides inspection of and research on crops and animals and also provides food stamps
2. U.S. Department of Housing and Urban Development, which constructs facilities such as rural hospitals and neighborhood clinics
3. U.S. Department of Labor, which provides preventive services in the workplace through the Occupational Safety and Health Administration

The federal agency that has major accountability for control of the environment is the Environmental Protection Agency. Established in 1970 as an independent (nondepartmental) government agency, its responsibilities include quality and pollution control of air and water; control of solid waste disposal, radiation hazards, and toxic substances; and pesticide regulation. Functions of the Environmental Protection Agency include conducting research on pollution control and the effects of pollution on humans, developing criteria and promulgating national standards for pollutants, and enforcing compliance with these standards.

Starting in 1992 health care providers, both as employers and as providers of public services, were required to comply with requirements of the Americans With Disabilities Act of 1990. The act is considered the most sweeping civil rights legislation since the Civil Rights Act of 1964. The two parts that apply most directly to health care providers are the prohibitions of employment discrimination and the requirements for provision of services to people with disabilities. An example of health care provider accommodation is to install wheelchair lifts in their shuttle bus systems. Despite their need for health promotion and disease prevention, individuals with disabilities face numerous problems gaining access to health-promotion programs and preventive services. The barriers are financial, social, physical, and logistical.

In 1990 President George H. Bush signed the Patient Self-Determination Act, which took effect in December 1991. This law was designed to increase individual involvement in decisions about life-sustaining treatment, ensuring that advance directives for health care are available to physicians at the time that medical decisions are being made and ensuring that individuals who have not prepared such documents are aware of their legal rights. As a condition of Medicare and Medicaid payment, the Patient Self-Determination Act requires health care facilities to comply with the law.

International Level. WHO, the United Nations' specialized agency for health, was established in 1948. Comprised of membership of more than 190 countries, the core functions of WHO include (1) giving worldwide guidance in the field of health, (2) setting global standards for health, (3) cooperating with governments in strengthening national health programs, and (4) developing and transferring appropriate technology, information, and standards (WHO, 2004). WHO also encourages and coordinates international scientific research.

Voluntary Agencies

The voluntary (not-for-profit) health movement, which began in 1882, stems from the goodwill and humanitarian concerns that are part of the nongovernmental, free enterprise heritage of the people of the United States. Powerful forces in the health field, voluntary agencies, foundations, and professional associations are nonprofit entities that maintain a tax-free status. Voluntary agencies are influential in promoting health affairs at the national policy level and often have significant influence on health legislation. Their prominent role in public influence was demonstrated by the American Cancer Society's early mass media announcements about the health hazards of smoking.

Philanthropic foundations provide valuable stimulation to the health field and operate under fewer constraints than do other sources in supporting research or training projects. Nurses interested in research or advanced clinical study that relates to the special interests of voluntary agencies or foundations may find grant monies available to support their work. Most libraries, available on-line, contain references detailing specific grant interests and available monies.

Professional associations, organized at the national level with state and local branches, are powerful political forces. For example, the American Medical Association's role in legislation for comprehensive health insurance was in opposition to that endorsed by the ANA. Nurses can support their professional organizations (the ANA and the National League for Nursing) in influencing the direction of health policy through membership and active participation.

FINANCING HEALTH CARE
Costs

The health care industry is the largest service industry in the United States today (Levit, Smith, Cowan, Lazenby, & Martin, 2003) and the most powerful employer in the nation, employing 3% of the total labor force (Shi & Singh, 2004). National health expenditures in the United States were projected to be $1.8 trillion in 2004 and $3.4 trillion by 2013, growing at an annual average rate of 7.3% from 2002 to 2013. In 2002 health spending was 14.9% of the gross domestic product and projected to be 18.4% by 2013. These projections do not include the impacts of the Medicare Prescription Drug Act of 2003. In 2000, the U.S. population was 280.2 million and per capita expenditure for health care was $4637. By 2006, per capita cost is estimated to be $6937 (Centers for Medicare & Medicaid Services, 2003). The United States spends far more on health care than any other industrialized country (Table 3-1).

Health care analysts predict the accelerations in health care cost will continue, putting pressure on public and private payers to finance them. Factors driving costs include 6 consecutive years of double-digit growth of prescription drugs costs (17.3% in 2000) and medical and scientific advances. Introduction of new therapies for chronic conditions and the aging population contributes to the rising number of prescription drugs used per capita. In 2000, the number of retail prescriptions per capita was 10.5, compared with 8.3 in 1995 (Levit, et al., 2003). Newer policies created in SCHIP to benefit uninsured children and teens cost $2.8 billion in 2000, and Medicaid spending increased 8.3% in 2000. Medicare spending rose 5.6% in 2000. Health care premiums rose 8.4% in 2000, costing $443.9 billion, in part due to rising prescription drug costs.

| Table **3-1** International Comparisons of Gross Domestic Product and Per Capita Health Expenditures |

	1980		1990		1998		2000	
Country	GDP	Per Capita	GDP	Per Capita	GDP	Per Capita	GDP	Per Capita
Canada	7.1%	$710	9.0%	$1676	9.3%	$2250	9.2%	$2535
Germany*	8.7%	$824	9.9%	$1600	10.6%	$2400	10.6%	$2748
United Kingdom	5.6%	$444	6.0%	$972	6.9%	$1450	7.3%	$1763
United States	8.7%	$1067	11.9%	$2738	14.0%	$4270	13.1%	$4672

Data from the Organization for Economic Cooperation and Development. *Health, United States* (p. 305). Retrieved March 15, 2005, from: *http://www.cdc.gov/nchs/data/hus/tables/2003/03huslle.pdf*
*For years prior to 1990, Germany refers to West Germany.

| Table **3-2** Total Personal Health Care Expenditures: Projections for 2004 |

Type of Service	Total Dollars in Billions	Percentage of Total
Personal health care	1540.7	100
Hospital care	551.7	35.8
Physician and clinical services	386.8	25.1
Dental care	78.0	5.1
Other professional services	51.0	3.3
Other personal health care	56.2	3.7
Home health care	40.6	2.6
Nursing home care	111.7	8.2
Prescription drugs	207.9	13.5
Durable medical equipment	20.6	1.3
Other nondurable medical products	36.4	2.4

Based on data from Centers for Medicare & Medicaid Services, Office of the Actuary. Table 2: Selected Calendar Years 1990–2013: National Health Expenditures Amounts. Retrieved February 2, 2005, from: *http://www.cms.hhs.gov/statistics/nhe/projections-2003*.
NOTE: Numbers are rounded; may not add to totals.

The growth in health expenditures, particularly since the onset of Medicare and Medicaid in 1965, is attributed quantitatively to four factors: (1) general inflation, (2) health care cost inflation, (3) application of more advanced and more types of technology, and (4) new pharmaceutical agents to treat acute and chronic conditions. Some of the qualitative factors that have influenced the increase in care costs include (1) growth in the proportion of the elderly, (2) rising expectations about the value of health care services, (3) government financing of health care services, (4) the nature of third-party reimbursement, (5) lack of competition which would promote efficiency in the delivery of services, (6) misdistribution of health care providers and services, (7) expansion of medical technology and specialty medicine, and (8) the growing number of uninsured and underinsured people (Chang, Price, & Pfoutz, 2001; Lee & Estes, 2003; Shi & Singh, 2004). For example, diagnostic and therapeutic techniques, including computer-aided technology and noninvasive imaging (such as magnetic resonance imaging), cardiac surgery, organ transplantation, and operations on joints (particularly hips and knees), enhance the capabilities of medicine while increasing costs.

Changes in hospital care—more outpatient services, shorter inpatient stays, and more care of chronic illness than

acute illness—mean that hospitals have less time to offer prevention or health-promotion education to individuals. Moreover, workforce shortages, especially in nursing, increased the use of nonprofessional caregivers. Inadequate resources, reimbursement, and numbers of nurses may prevent health care professionals from offering the range of health-promotion educational efforts called for in the *Healthy People 2010* objectives.

Although most industrial countries have adopted some version of a national health care system, the United States has relied on a free-market approach, with the private sector providing insurance coverage and the system providing for some individuals who are unable to pay. Since the 1980s the nation's employers, who are generally large payers of health care costs, have experimented with various payment mechanisms, such as employee cost sharing, self-insurance, and alternative delivery systems. The effects of this influx of business into health care and the subsequent emphasis on competition to resolve the financial problems are still being realized.

Projected national health expenditures for 2004 are shown in Table 3-2. The largest component is hospital care (35.8%), which experienced declining growth between 1990 (41.7%) and 1999 (36.9%). Spending for professional services (physician, clinical. and other) totaled 33.5%, with physicians and clinical services accounting for 25.1%, dental services 5.1%, and other professionals almost 3.3%. Another 2.6% went for home health care, 13.5% for prescription drugs, and 1.3% for durable medical products such as eyeglasses, wheelchairs, and hearing aids. Of the nondurable products, two thirds of the expenditures were for drugs and one third for over-the-counter medicines and medical sundries. Spending for nursing home care accounted for nearly 8.2% (Levit et al., 2003). In 2002, 14% of all health care costs were paid out-of-pocket, a total of $231.3 billion (Healthcare Spending, 2004).

Sources

Ultimately, the American people pay for all U.S. health care costs. Money is transferred from consumer to provider by various mechanisms. The major sources are government (federal, state and local), third-party payment (private insurance), independent plans, and out-of-pocket support (Sultz & Young, 2004).

Figure 3-1 shows funding sources for health care in 2002 and where the money went. The largest percentage went to hospital care (31%) and physician and clinical services (22%). The cost of private health insurance accounted for 35% of all expenditures. Consumers paid out-of-pocket for 14% of health care costs. The federal government paid one third (33%) of health care expenses, and state and local governments accounted for almost 12%.

Since 1989 the private share of health care expenditures has increased at a faster pace than the public share. Although employees covered by managed care plans accounted for 86% of all insured workers in 1998, premiums and benefits paid have increased (Levit et al., 2000). Enrollees choose from a preapproved list of providers in return for smaller premiums, co-payments, and deductibles. The trend is away from HMOs to less restrictive plans, such as POS plans and PPOs (Levit et al., 2000). As the number of consumers enrolled in managed care plans has grown, the breadth of insurance coverage has increased to more fully cover preventive services.

Although the public sector's share of health care spending increased from the 1960s through the 1980s, primarily because Medicare and Medicaid costs rose, it has stabilized at approximately 42% of the total costs of health care. Medicare experienced rapid benefit-payment increases (at average annual rates of 13.7%) between 1969 and 1993, with some slowing in growth since that time (down to 2.5% in 1998). Despite the aging of frail older enrollees, Medicare spending in 1998 has experienced "the slowest growth on record" (Levit et al., 2000, p. 130). Medicare costs escalate during the last year of a person's life. This decline between 1994 and 1998 reflects three interacting factors: (1) limits legislated to restrain growth in Medicare payments to providers, including the BBA of 1997 (see further discussion under Medicare later in this chapter), (2) continuing government detection activities for fraud and abuse of Medicare, and (3) a slight slowing of growth in the

Where It Came From

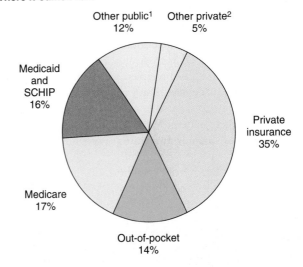

Where It Went

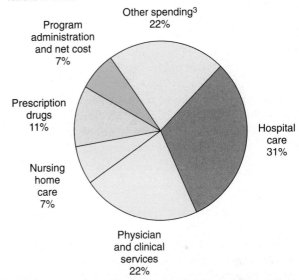

Figure 3-1   The Nation's Health Dollar in 2002. From Centers for Medicare & Medicaid Services, Office of the Actuary, National Health Statistics Group, 2002.
[1]"Other public" includes programs such as Worker's Compensation, public health activity, Department of Defense, Department of Veteran's Affairs, Indian Health Services, state and local hospital subsidies, and school health.
[2]"Other private" includes industrial in-plant, privately funded construction, and nonpatient revenues, including philanthropy.
[3]"Other spending" includes dentist services, other professional services, home health care, durable medical products, over-the-counter medicines and sundries, public health, research, and construction.

Medicare population, which is predicted to rise again. Almost 16% of Medicare recipients were enrolled in managed care plans in 1998 (Levit et al., 2000).

Federal and state Medicaid spending showed an increasing pattern similar to that discussed earlier in this chapter with Medicare (300% growth from 1980 to 1990), until recent years when spending growth rates have become more stable. Welfare-to-work requirements for people covered under Temporary Assistance for Needy Families (TANF) (1997) was combined with strong job growth to decrease the number of Medicaid recipients. (See further discussion of TANF under Medicaid later in this chapter.) By 2000, 55.8% of recipients were in enrolled some form of managed care. The largest share of Medicaid monies goes for institutional services. Namely, two thirds of program expenditures were for services providing care to elderly or disabled people. Less than 25% of expenditures went to nondisabled working age adults and children (Lee & Estes, 2003). In 2001, Medicaid provided health and long-term care coverage for almost 44 million individuals. The total cost of the Medicaid program in 2000 was $202.7 billion, an 8.3% increase from 1999. Each state receives from the federal government a different percentage of revenue to run a Medicaid program, leaving state budgets responsible for the remaining cost. For instance, New York state receives only 50% of its revenue from the federal level. The New York state budget contributes 25%, and the individual counties must pick up the additional 25%. In 2004, residents saw rising state and county taxes, as well as double-digit increases in property taxes to meet the needs of the Medicaid population in New York state. Medicaid is the largest third-party payer of nursing home care, paying about one half of the total expenditures for nursing facilities.

Mechanisms

Payment

Although some health care providers and other professionals in the private sector are paid on a fee-for-service basis, by third-party private insurance, or by public-supported insurance, most health workers, including nurses in institutional or community agencies and in the military, receive salaries. Most nurses are salaried; therefore, the separation of nursing costs from all other health-related costs is difficult. The cost of nursing care typically is incorporated in the room and board charge in the acute care setting. Without documentation of specific nursing costs, validating the need for skilled nursing services is difficult.

In recent years, nurses—especially APNs, NPs, clinical nurse specialists (CNSs), certified registered nurse anesthetists (CRNAs), and CNMs—have entered independent practice to provide direct services. Nurses who are academically prepared for advanced practice represent about 6% of all registered nurses. In 1998, there were approximately 78,000 NPs, 54,000 CNSs, 34,000 CRNAs, and 8000 CNMs in the United States (Kovner & Salsberg, 1999; Pearson, 2000).

A landmark study in an ambulatory care setting that randomly assigned clients to either NPs (part of Columbia Advanced Practice Nurse Associates) or physicians confirmed what NPs and their clients have known for a long time: NPs provide effective, quality primary care. NPs had the same authority, responsibilities, productivity, adminis-

trative requirements, and client populations as physicians and, more importantly, client outcomes were comparable (Mundinger et al., 2000).

Independent nursing practice may be viewed as a logical outgrowth of seeking higher levels of professionalism. The nurse practice acts of some states encourage nurses to use their knowledge more comprehensively than many agencies sanction. In independent practice, the nurse is directly accountable to individuals and is paid either directly or by third parties. The philosophical and realistic issues of private nursing practice range from questions about the equity of fee-for-service to the practical problems of setting up this type of practice. Independent practice's chance to become commonplace in nursing's future depends on decisions about reimbursement by third parties in both private and public sectors, because reimbursement continues to be a restriction on practice. Although legislation in 1997 included the reimbursement of APNs by Medicare, not all plans and provider groups include these nurses as primary care practitioners. Maine passed legislation in 1999 that requires managed care organizations to permit NPs to become credentialed PCPs. In 2003 NPs were granted primary care status in the state's Medicaid program. Maryland also has a new law allowing managed care consumers to choose an NP as a PCP. At the federal level, NPs are encouraging and lobbying lawmakers to allow them to order hospice and home health care (Rollet, 2003). Clearly the nursing practice roles and prescriptive authority of APNs varies state to state. Incremental steps have been taken to advance the APN role at both the federal and state levels.

Alternative forms of payment are salary and capitation. The salary system involves a set amount for services provided in a specified time frame. This system provides the employer with a fixed nursing income that is protected from changes in supply and demand, includes fringe benefits, and obviates fee collection problems. The salary system's flexibility makes it easier to fill unpopular jobs or jobs in underserved areas. Disadvantages of this system include a limit on income and constraints on schedules, vacations, and peer review. The nurse may have to meet goals other than personal ones.

In the **capitation system,** such as in an HMO, each provider receives a flat annual fee for each participant regardless of how often services are used. Individuals who enroll in an HMO pay a fixed amount on a monthly basis whether they use the services or not; prepayment provides an incentive to provide efficient care. The objective is to keep people healthy to prevent costly services. Cost consciousness dictates that illness be treated as early as possible and in the most cost-effective setting. Capitation is simple to administer; no third-party insurance payments are present and the HMO bears the risk of illness. Preventive primary care that avoids costly hospitalization keeps costs down, and the savings revert to the organization. On the negative side, individuals may make unnecessary visits, the increased number of people necessary to provide more monies may decrease comprehensive care, and there may be limits to quality of care, services, and access to all types of providers.

Cost Containment

The government's interest in hospital treatment cost containment is exemplified by the passage of the Social Security Amendments of 1983 (Public Law 98-21), which mandate the establishment by the Health Care Financing Administration of a prospective payment system for Medicare. This system means that providers are paid at preset rates based on 470 diagnosis-related group categories that are used to classify the illness of each Medicare-insured person. Rates for each diagnosis are established according to regional and national amounts based on each hospital's urban and rural cost experience. Average hospital occupancy rates declined by nearly 11% between 1980 and 1990; since the mid-1990s hospital use has stabilized (Levit, et al., 2000).

The revolutionary prospective payment system cost-containment mechanism was the first in a series of changes for the health care industry. The development of managed care plans provided a realignment of the nation's health care system. This variety of forms of prepaid and managed fee-for-service health care is designed to control the use and cost of health care. The intended effects of managed care are more comprehensive care for more people while containing both the use and costs of services. During the 1990s restrictions on managed care programs have been lifted to allow conversion to for-profit plans. For-profit status allows these plans to contain their costs (Thorpe & Knickman, 1999). The effect on quality and access to care remains to be determined.

Another recent piece of legislation that targets cost containment is the BBA of 1997, which also affected Medicare. This act reduced Medicare spending by limiting provider payments, increased options in the choice of managed care plans, and made MSAs an option (Lee & Benjamin, 1999). (See further discussion with Medicare later in this chapter.)

In **care management,** an experienced health care professional, such as an NP or CNM, determines what care is necessary, monitors that care, and arranges for clients to receive it for the most appropriate cost and in the most effective setting. Essential to the promotion of the health of individuals is an integration of financing, management, and delivery of health care in a continuously changing delivery system (Cary, 2000). Care managers are especially effective in meeting the needs of the elderly, high-risk pregnancy clients, those with spinal cord injuries, clients with AIDS, and other complex cases requiring multiple levels of care (Shi & Singh, 2004, pp. 394-395). Emphasis must be on health management across the continuum of health care delivery. As Medicaid and Medicare managed care systems continue to develop, demand for nurses to fill the care management role will continue.

Care management began through public programs with nurses in public health departments, social workers in

---

Box **3-2**   Care Management Services
Assessment: evaluating a person's physical, social, functional, psychological, and financial needs, including family situation
Care planning: setting goals, identifying specific services to meet individual needs, including how to allocate resources
Service coordination and referral: facilitating and coordinating access to needed providers
Care monitoring and periodic reassessments: evaluating progress, access to and use of services, and changes in needs

---

public welfare systems, and caseworkers in mental health departments. Managed care organizations rely on care management as one method to control costs, reduce inappropriate use of services, and improve quality of care. Care management takes numerous forms, but basic elements involve an individual who coordinates and monitors needed services in a supportive, effective, efficient, and cost-effective way (Cary, 2000). Basic care management services are described in Box 3-2.

Depending on the model used, care management services can be implemented in a broad or a narrow manner. Assessment broadly defined might include health needs and social and family needs; narrowly defined, assessment might focus solely on individual health concerns. Care managers are particularly important for people with catastrophic or complex acute or chronic illnesses, disabilities, or injuries, or for members who may experience high risk, volume, cost, or use. The care manager must achieve a balance between cost and quality and must collaborate effectively with all providers involved, both inside and outside the health plan and with the person's family, to ensure appropriate quality care. Pervasive problems faced by care managers include ethical and liability concerns, such as underservice and barriers to access and practice constraints, emanating from the labor-intensive, time-consuming, and costly nature of care management (Cary, 2000).

An individual with complex chronic health problems requires multiple services from providers in a variety of settings. For example, under managed care, hospitalizations are reserved for individuals who are acutely ill and require complex technological care. Americans are admitted to hospitals later and sicker, with discharges earlier than ever before. This delayed entry and accelerated community reentry, whether to the home or to a rehabilitative or extended care facility, requires complex coordination of services and providers. The care manager nurse is the key to efficient allocation of resources, coordinated care planning, and documentation of outcomes (Shi & Singh, 2004).

Managed Care Issues

Ninety-two percent of people with employer-based health insurance coverage are in a managed care program. Low co-payments and less paperwork are welcomed by individuals, but concerns about the quality of care provided when the overall emphasis is cost control is an issue. Gatekeeping is not seen by some clients as a way to maintain or improve quality of care; rather the PCP may be seen as the way managed care attempts to limit health care costs by decreasing the amount of care provided, especially by limiting referrals. Health care analysts describe several issues for managed care programs and the services they provide to their enrollees. Among these issues are consolidation of health plans, the effect on providers, conflicts of interest, and protection of the public (Torrens & Williams, 1999). As more and more health insurers merge, the tendency is for large organizations to exert more influence in controlling purchasers and payers and providers, with subsequent lack of variation and choice in plans in addition to potential monopoly issues. Managed care has created new systems, with groups of providers delivering care in more efficient ways. However, with an emphasis on providing fewer services, there may be less humane and compassionate personal care, the opposite of which has been a hallmark of the nation's health care system. Conflicts of interest among and between the many players in a managed care system in reducing the use of various services may affect clients who are unable to get needed services.

Clients' bill of rights proposals have in common efforts to restore control over health care decision making to clients and their providers (Angell, 2000). Some versions include language that would allow clients to sue their managed care companies. The argument against this stipulation is that lawsuits would tend to increase costs for the managed care companies, which will be passed along to employers; employers may then decide to reduce or drop health care coverage and increase indirectly the number of uninsured. These bills also provide for appeal mechanisms when services are denied, for treatment in hospital emergency departments when clients believe it is essential, and for referral decisions to be made by providers and clients rather than health plans and employers.

Nurses must be advocates to ensure that people receive quality care. An information resource for consumers is the National Committee for Quality Assurance's Quality Compass, a national database of comparative information about the quality of managed care. Through this database, consumers and employers can compare information such as accreditation status, regional and national averages, and other report card measures. The Internet is a tool nurses can use for their own continuing education needs, as well as to enhance client education within a facility, public library, or home. Nurses can steer clients toward appropriate Web sites for health-promotion and disease-oriented information (Health Teaching box).

Health Insurance

Positive elements of the health care system in America were mentioned in the introduction to this chapter—excellent

---

HEALTH TEACHING Access Health Care Information From the Internet

Mary Jones, age 38, and her family are new to a primary care clinic. Mary asks the nurse for advice in choosing a health plan that will best meet the needs of her growing family. Mary is 4 months pregnant with her third child. She and her husband, Joe, work for a state agency that provides multiple health plan choices. Joe, age 48, has many of the symptoms of coronary artery disease. Their son Billy, age 8, has asthma, and their daughter Laurel, age 4, has Down syndrome.

The nurse discusses Mary's family's general health-promotion and protection needs and the special needs presented by the diseases that have been identified. She provides some resources for Mary to learn more about the plans available in her area. The Joneses have a computer at home and are eager to access the Web sites suggested to them.

- From the Agency for Healthcare Research and Quality (AHRQ), a federal government agency with health information for consumers on guidelines to consumers in choosing a health plan: *http://www.ahrq.gov/consumer/hlthpln1.htm*
- From the U.S. Department of Labor, a federal agency that provides information on health plans, benefits, and has many links: *http://www.dol.gov/dol/topic/health%2Dplans/*
- For information and links on pregnancy and childbirth with many links: *http://www.childbirth.org*
- For additional information on pregnancy topics, birth, and tests, with many graphics and links: *http://pregnancy.about.com*

- For information on childhood asthma, care and treatment, news and research with many professional references and links, Ask NOAH About: Asthma, New York Online Access to Health: *http://noah-health.org/en/lung/conditions/asthma/issues/children/index.htm*
- For information about Genetic Diseases: Down Syndrome, care and treatment, news and research with many professional references and links, Ask NOAH About Genetic Diseases: Down Syndrome, New York Online Access to Health: *http://www.noah-health.org/genetics/conditions/downs/what/index.html*
- The National Down Syndrome Society Web site has information and resources on Down syndrome, advocacy, support groups, education, and links: *http://www.ndss.org/content.cfm*
- The American Heart Association Web site contains information on heart disease, diet, exercise, treatment, news, and links: http://www.americanheart.org
- For information about heart disease, symptoms, cholesterol, prevention, exercise, diet, and links, Ask NOAH About Heart Disease, New York Online Access to Health: *http:www.noah-health.org/en/blood/disease/causes/index.html*

clinicians, health care facilities, and equipment—all of which are available to people with good health insurance or adequate finances. The U.S. system exhibits a high degree of technological change and innovation and excellent information, quality, and cost-accounting systems. Financial outlays for education of health care workers; products such as drugs, medical equipment, and supplies; and research are second to those of no other country (Shi & Singh, 2004). In 2000, 72.4% of Americans had private health insurance; 64.1% had an employer-based plan, 24.7% a government plan, 3% a military plan, 13.4% a Medicare program, and 10.4% of Americans were on Medicaid. More than 41.2 million people, or 14.6% of the population, did not have health insurance in 2002. The uninsured or underinsured typically delay seeking health care until an urgent problem arises and then utilize the emergency department, an expensive and inefficient means. If the United States could find a way to offer affordable primary care to all Americans, better client outcomes would occur and less utilization of expensive services might ensue. (See the discussion of the uninsured later in this chapter.)

Health care forecasters and strategists predict that the Internet will change the health system. From its beginnings as an "experimental, Defense Department funded, secure data network," the Internet has become a new "social institution" (Goldsmith, 2000, p. 148). Predictions are that the Internet will accelerate the "virtualization" of health care plans and systems and help with the clerical aspects of caregiving and insurance. Consumer access to information, as described previously, is an ongoing benefit. Privacy concerns and professional resistance are two problems that remain to be solved (Goldsmith, 2000).

Insurance refers to individual payment to a fund to provide protection for each contributor against financial losses resulting from an unlikely but possible occurrence. Medical insurance began in this tradition in 1847, with payments made to offset income lost as a result of an accident. Sickness benefits began as an extra benefit and again emphasized the loss of income. Blue Cross and Blue Shield originated the reimbursement of general health care costs in the 1930s.

The term *insurance* is a misnomer, because health care is often required and is not a rare occurrence. *Assurance* is the term used in England to mean coverage for expected happenings (life assurance), whereas insurance covers unexpected happenings, such as fire and theft.

Private Health Insurance

The private health insurance industry in the United States has changed dramatically since the growth of managed care and the consolidation of health plans (see earlier discussion). Conventional indemnity fee-for-service insurance covered less than 15% of employees, and 86% of all insured workers were participants in some kind of managed care plan in 1998 (Levit, et al., 2000). Managed care approaches to cost control range from measures such as second surgical opinion, preadmission certification review, and length of stay reviews to measures to transfer some of the cost to the enrollee through deductibles and coinsurance costs (Thorpe & Knickman, 1999).

In the private sector, the following five types of organizations provide health care insurance:

1. Traditional insurance companies (including the earliest insurer, Blue Cross and Blue Shield, a nonprofit charitable organization) and for-profit commercial insurance companies
2. PPOs acting as "brokers" between insurers and health care providers
3. HMOs, which are independent prepayment plans
4. POS plans, which combine features of classic HMOs with client choice characteristics of PPOs
5. Self-insurance and self-funded plans, in which either the employer takes on the role of insurer or the enrollee sets up a trust account with tax savings

Traditionally, private insurers charged employers or individuals annual premiums and provided services on a fee-for-service basis. Organized at the state and local level, Blue Cross and Blue Shield generally complement each other, with Blue Cross reimbursing hospitals and Blue Shield covering physicians and other providers. After World War II, insurance companies began to provide health insurance plans in competition with Blue Cross and Blue Shield. Today, more than 800 commercial, profit-making insurance companies, such as Metropolitan Life and Aetna, offer policies that cover hospitalization and in-hospital or office-based physician care, major medical expenses directed primarily at catastrophic illness, or cash payments as a flat sum of money per day of hospitalization. Fewer insurers every year offer insurance coverage for individuals, which is extremely expensive. They contract with employers to offer group plans (Whitted, 1999). Much of the individual insurance sold today is supplementary, such as that designed to supplement Medicare, known as *Medigap*. These plans reimburse only deductibles and coinsurance payments associated with Medicare.

HMOs attempt to lower health care costs by emphasizing preventive rather than curative care, possibly decreasing the severity of some illnesses. Outpatient care is the focus, with lower hospitalization rates than in the fee-for-service area, almost entirely a result of lower admission rates. HMOs tend to use fewer services, with emphasis on the least costly means of providing a service.

POS plans enable enrollees to choose, at the point of service, whether to use the plan's provider network or seek care from nonnetwork providers. Typically, network providers are paid on a capitated or discounted fee basis, and nonnetwork providers are paid on a fee-for-service basis. Coinsurance (about 30%) and deductibles (about $300 per year) for nonnetwork providers are higher, to dissuade enrollees from choosing this option (Thorpe, 1999).

Another change in the structure of the insurance industry is the growth of self-insured or self-funded plans. **Self-insurance** means that an employer (or union) assumes the claims risk of its insured employees, whereas self-funding refers to paying insurance claims from an established fund, such as a bank account or trust fund. Self-insurance gives employers a financial advantage, including an Employee Retirement and Income Security Act (ERISA) exemption from state taxes on health insurance premiums and interest earnings on reserves before claims payment (Sultz & Young, 2004). Between 1993 and 1997, the promotion to use self-insured employers dropped from 19% to 13% (Shi & Singh, 2004).

Public Health Insurance and Assistance

Medicare. Medicare is a federal program which finances medical care for people over 65, disabled individuals who are entitled to Social Security benefits, and people with end-stage renal disease requiring dialysis or a kidney transplant. The Medicare program, also known as Title XVIII of the SSA, went into effect in 1966 after decades of debate and is currently operated under the administrative oversight of the Centers for Medicare and Medicaid Services. Medicare is an entitlement program. "People have contributed to Medicare through taxes, they are 'entitled' to the benefits regardless of the amount of income and assets they have" (Shi & Singh, 2004, p. 205). The intent of Medicare was to protect older adults against the catastrophic financial debts often incurred in managing chronic illness and to assist in the payment of health care. This was the first time that federal legislation was enacted to remove financial barriers to medical care for the elderly. In 1983 Medicare added hospice benefits for the last 6 months of life to cover services for the terminally ill. Hospice is based on a philosophy that views death as a normal part of the life cycle and emphasizes living the remainder of life as fully and comfortably as possible. Hospice care is only 1% of the total Medicare expenditures, covering about two thirds of cost, or $2.8 billion per year (Sultz & Young, 2004). See **Web Site Resource 3B,** which presents Medicare insurance–covered services for 2004.

Medicare, Part A, is financed by mandatory taxes paid by employers and all working people, including the self-employed, into the Hospital Insurance Trust Fund. Part A covers inpatient services, care in a skilled nursing facility, home health visits, and hospice care. Medicare, Part B, is supplementary voluntary medical insurance financed partly by general tax revenues and partly by required premium contributions. In 2001, 94% of all Medicare enrollees in Part A also had Part B coverage, because the premium is far less than the cost of private insurance (Shi & Singh, 2004). Part B covers physician services, hospital outpatient services (outpatient surgery, diagnostic tests, radiology and pathology services, emergency services, ambulance services, outpatient rehabilitation services, renal dialysis), medical equipment, supplies, and some preventive services (Papanicolaou smears, mammography, screening for colorectal and prostate cancer, glaucoma screening, flu and pneumonia vaccines).

Neither Part A nor Part B of Medicare offers comprehensive coverage. Inherent in the program are deductibles, set amounts that the individual must pay for each type of service before Medicare begins to pay, and coinsurance, a percentage of charges paid by the individual. There are also limitations on the amount of coverage provided. For example, hospital benefits end after 90 days (with a lifetime reserve of an additional 60 days) and extended care facility benefits last a maximum of 100 days.

Except for end-stage renal disease and some diabetes monitoring (discussed later in this chapter), Medicare does not provide for catastrophic chronic illness. Nor does it cover continual health needs such as routine physical examinations, vision care (including eyeglasses), dental care (including dentures), or hearing aids. Furthermore, custodial care (routine assistance with activities of daily living not requiring medical or nursing care) is not covered. Custodial care can be the most costly and financially catastrophic service.

The limits in Medicare coverage mean that older adults pay a substantial portion of their health care costs beyond the expected 20%, especially when they have a chronic illness. Unlike most private insurance, Medicare does not include an annual limit on out-of-pocket spending. The main population at risk, the elderly, may have limited financial access to preventive health services not covered.

Quality and cost of care have been issues for Medicare for more than 25 years. Numerous pieces of legislation and Medicare amendments have attempted to solve various aspects of the cost and quality concerns.

The Tax Equity and Fiscal Responsibility Act of 1982 established a case-based reimbursement system, namely diagnosis-related groups, which were designed to provide cost-containment incentives. Subsequently, in 1983, Title VI of Public Law 98-21 established a prospective payment system for inpatient services for Medicare clients. This legislation also encouraged growth in the number of HMOs and other comprehensive plans enrolling Medicare beneficiaries. Although the prospective payment system has slowed the growth of inpatient hospital Medicare spending, that of outpatient spending continues to rise (Thorpe, 1999).

In 1988, Congress passed the Medicare Catastrophic Act, designed to expand Medicare to shield beneficiaries from catastrophic hospital and physician costs related to acute illnesses. Although new benefits for long-term care were not provided, the bill included coverage for outpatient prescription drugs. In 1989, before it could be implemented, this bill was repealed as a result of pressure from older adults who objected to the legislation's financial approach. Costs of the program were passed on to the elderly as new premiums and income-related surcharges connected to their federal income tax.

In the Omnibus Reconciliation Act of 1989, Medicare revised its payment scheme for physicians. First, a new payment system that went into effect in 1992 assigned relative values to services based on the time, skill, and intensity required to provide them. Second, a limit was set on the amount that physicians could charge individuals above the amount that Medicare pays. This restriction was designed to limit growth of Medicare costs for physician payments.

The BBA of 1997 included Medicare+ Choice, which offers the option of managed care plans such as HMOs, POS plans, PPOs, or private fee-for-service plans in which the enrollee pays extra when costs for care are higher than Medicare rates. Additionally, MSA plans are available whereby Medicare pays a health insurance policy, putting money into an MSA. Enrollees use the MSA and their own money for care (up to a certain amount per year); when that amount is reached, the insurance covers all Medicare-approved expenses for the rest of the year. If an enrollee has money in the MSA at the end of the year, that amount is rolled over for the next year (USDHHS, 2000b).

The BBA of 1997, the Balanced Budget Refinement Act of 1999, and the Benefits Improvement and Protection Act of 2000 have added services to the Medicare benefits package. These services include coverage for screening tests for breast, cervical, vaginal, prostate, and colorectal cancer; bone mass measurements; diabetes monitoring and diabetes self-management; and influenza, pneumonia, and hepatitis B vaccinations.

The missing Medicare benefit causing great concern was the rising cost and lack of coverage for outpatient prescription drugs. Americans age 65 and over account for over one third of all drug spending, but they represent only about one eighth of the population (Deets, 2000). Although some HMO plans provided this benefit for seniors, less than 16% of seniors were enrolled in managed care plans in 1998 (Levit, et al., 2000). Of the average 19% of older adults' out-of-pocket income ($2430) spent on health care in 1999, 17% of that amount was for prescription drugs (Deets, 2000). On December 9, 2003, President George W. Bush signed into law the Medicare Prescription Drug, Improvement and Modernization Act of 2003, Public Law 108-173. This lengthy piece of legislation amends Title XVIII of the SSA to provide for a voluntary program for prescription drug coverage and modernize the Medicare program, including a provision to provide teaching hospitals with increased indirect medical education payments. The new Medicare prescription drug benefit will start on January 1, 2006. All people with Medicare will be able to enroll in plans that cover prescription drugs. According to the consumer government site for Medicare information:

1. Individuals will choose a prescription drug plan and pay a premium of about $35 a month.
2. The first $250 (called a deductible) will be paid by the individual.
3. Medicare will pay 75% of drug costs up to $2250, with individuals paying 25% of these costs.
4. Individuals will pay 100% of drug costs between $2250 and $3600.
5. Medicare will pay 95% of drug costs after an individual has spent $3600.

The revision to the Medicare program is expected to cost $400 billion over the next 10-year period (Altman, 2004).

Prior to the full enactment, incremental steps will begin in May 2004, starting with the ability to purchase a prescription drug card. Much skepticism and debate occurred at the time of enactment of the new law. Some advocates saw the act as a step in the right direction to assist the elderly with prescription drug costs. Others felt the law did not go far enough in controlling prescription drug prices, thus further filling the coffers of pharmaceutical companies. For others, the failure to enact universal health coverage in 1994 was also a failure to assist elders in the rising cost of prescription drugs. Although not a comprehensive plan, any help was welcomed. Because health care policy typically is enacted in increments, this first step may pave the way for added coverage in the future. The full effect of the new law is yet unknown.

Medicaid. Medicaid is a health insurance program available only to certain low-income individuals and families who fit into an eligibility group that is recognized by federal and state law. Medicaid pays health care providers if they participate in the Medicaid program.

Medicaid is an assistance program, commonly referred to as *welfare*, managed jointly by the federal and state governments to provide partial or full payment of medical costs for individuals and families of any age who are too poor to pay for the care. Medicaid legislation, Title XIX of the amendments to the SSA, went into effect in 1967. The federal government provides funds to states on a cost-sharing basis, with 50% to over 80% from the federal government and the remainder from the state, according to the per capita income of each state, to guarantee medical services to eligible Medicaid recipients. **Web Site Resource 3C** presents a comparison of Medicare and Medicaid.

People eligible for Medicaid are those who receive Supplemental Security Income (SSI) and TANF (see discussion of welfare reform). Additionally, Medicaid pays the Medicare premiums, deductibles, and coinsurance for certain low-income Medicare recipients (Koch, 1999). Medicaid eligibility varies state to state, as do the program benefits. In 2000 Medicaid consumed 50% of total state health care expenditures. Medicaid plans are open-ended, meaning a state must admit into the program at any time all individuals who meet the criteria. A state is not allowed to cap the Medicaid budget for a particular fiscal year, thus making it difficult to determine exactly how much money needs to be appropriated. The program encourages its own growth and expansion (Lee & Estes, 2003).

States administer Medicaid under broad federal requirements and guidelines. Each state establishes its own eligibility standards; determines the scope, type, duration, and amount of services to be provided; sets the rate of payment; and administers its own program. Programs vary widely from state to state in terms of services covered.

For a list of basic health services mandated, refer to **Web Site Resource 3C**. Included are inpatient and outpatient care; laboratory and radiology services; prenatal care; family planning services and supplies; rural health clinic services; federally qualified ambulatory and health center services;

physician services; nurse midwife, and pediatric and family NP services; home health care for people eligible for skilled nursing services; skilled nursing facility services for people 21 years of age and older; and early and periodic screening, diagnosis, and treatment (EPSDT) of people under 21 years of age. Other services, such as dental care, eyeglasses, or intermediate care facility services, may be added at the state's option.

The EPSDT provision signified the federal government's recognition of the need for primary prevention and health promotion. The emphasis on prevention rather than treatment—the focus of this text—was a positive approach toward health and required development and implementation of new methods of health care delivery. The EPSDT program has five phases: (1) outreach and case findings, (2) screening, (3) testing, (4) compiling and reporting of results, and (5) follow-up and treatment.

State Medicaid programs must cover all pregnant women and children up to 6 years of age with family incomes less than 133% of the federal poverty level; children age 12 or younger in families with incomes below 100% of the poverty level (all poor children under age 19 were covered in 2002); poor families who lose cash assistance resulting from work earnings (for a transition period); for a 12-month period, two-parent families whose principal wage earner is unemployed; and disabled people losing eligibility due to work pay (Thorpe & Knickman, 1999).

States have looked to managed care to lower their Medicaid costs. In 1998 more than one half of all Medicaid recipients used some type of managed care plan, most using the HMO model (Levit, et al., 2000). As the number of Medicaid beneficiaries in managed care increases, the effect of these changes must be monitored to determine access to and quality of care for low-income individuals.

Several states are participating in the Robert Wood Johnson model program of purchasing long-term care insurance to protect a specific amount of money. Once the insurance monies are paid out up to that amount, the insured individual qualifies for Medicaid. This program is considered an attempt to cut Medicaid costs for long-term care of individuals over the age of 65.

Traditionally, states determine Medicaid eligibility, covered benefits, and provider-payment mechanisms; therefore, Medicaid programs vary widely from one state to another and may be inadequate to meet the health care needs of covered individuals. The previously discussed legislation that separated Medicaid from the receipt of cash assistance, such as covering low-income pregnant women and children, is meant to produce greater uniformity in Medicaid. However, each state still determines its Medicaid budget and optional services based on its financial status. Despite the program expansions and that Medicaid is the largest program that provides health care services to the poor, it covers only 40% of individuals with income below the poverty level (Thorpe & Knickman, 1999).

Passage of the welfare reform bill in 1996 (Personal Responsibility and Work Opportunity Reconciliation Act of 1996, Public Law 104-193) reveals a significant philosophical shift in federal thinking about welfare assistance in the United States. For the first time, Medicaid is not linked directly to welfare programs. Ending a 61-year guarantee of federal aid, the TANF program (formerly Aid to Families With Dependent Children), established by this legislation, provides temporary financial aid with a 5-year lifetime limit. Legal immigrants who arrive in the United States after the passage of this bill must wait 5 years to become eligible for programs. The aim is to help parents become self-sufficient through welfare-to-work programs. Some states have changed the name of their official department of social services (Family Independence Agency) to reflect the change in philosophy from dependency to temporary assistance (Clemen-Stone, McGuire, & Eigsti, 2002). As welfare changes dramatically, there is concern about an increase in health disparities among Americans and restriction of resources for children, especially in states with high rates of immigration such as California and Texas. Changes in Medicaid eligibility resulted in an increased number of uninsured (O'Grady, 2000).

Pharmaceutical Costs

The spiraling cost of prescription drugs continues to add to the complexity of providing adequate health care. Newer drugs cost more than the drugs they replace and contribute 50% of the increased cost. Increased utilization of prescription drugs adds to an increased cost per day of medications. Consumer demand sparked by drug advertisements, new indications for use, and increased consumer knowledge of available drugs have placed an increase in the demand for the prescription medications. Increased drug cost is attributed to inflation, more days of therapy per user, greater number of drugs per user, cost of research and drug development, and advertising. (See previous discussion on prescription medications.)

The Uninsured: Who Are They?

The United States has the highest proportion of population with no health insurance of all developed countries. In 2002, 41.2 million Americans (14.6% of the population) had no health insurance, an increase of 1.4 million people since 2000. The lack of health insurance is greatest for Hispanics and blacks, younger Americans (18 to 34 years of age), people with low educational attainment, men more than women, and particularly people living in the South and the West (Koch, 1999). Most of the uninsured have at least one family member who is working full time; over one half have family incomes of less than 200% of the federal poverty level (about $33,000 for a family of four) (O'Grady, 2000). Even among the 20% of uninsured who have access to employer-sponsored health insurance, they are unable or unwilling to obtain coverage because the cost of premiums is high (O'Grady, 2000). The largest numbers of the uninsured work in part-time jobs, minimum wage jobs, or are employed by small firms. Children are typically not covered on their families' health insurance plan when turning 19 unless they are full-time college students. Consolidated Omnibus Budget Reconciliation Act (COBRA) plans are available for a fee to cover the gap between reaching age 19 and securing a job with employer-based benefits. Some uninsured adults do not have jobs in which health care is provided, and the cost of individual private health insurance is usually high. Some young adults have employer-based plans but choose not to utilize them due to cost. Other young adults, typically a healthy group, choose not to spend money on a plan due to necessity or personal choice. Instead they seek health care only when necessary and pay out-of-pocket. For those with acute or chronic health care needs, the price of being uninsured is detrimental to financial solvency. Solutions to providing health care to the uninsured vary, with some success in offering tax breaks or other financial incentives for businesses to offer health insurance plans and in expanding eligibility requirements for Medicaid. Programs that facilitate an individual's pursuit of education can move a person into a better paying job, which increases the likelihood of employment-based insurance being available and affordable. Unlike in some other countries, individuals cannot be mandated to carry health insurance at this time. Without solutions, the projection is for the number of uninsured to increase to 55 million by 2010 (O'Grady, 2000).

The uninsured incur increased health risks because they delay care more than 3 times as often as do people with coverage. They more often need hospital treatment that could have been avoided, more often are diagnosed with cancer in a later stage, and increase their likelihood of dying in a hospital more than 3 times the rate of people with health insurance (O'Grady, 2000). Without health insurance, low-income families frequently must rely on a fragmented and difficult-to-use public system of health care. Regular preventive care, including prenatal care, immunization, and well-child care, is sometimes difficult to obtain, and its availability may not be adequately understood.

A plan that targets poor, uninsured children who are not eligible for Medicaid is included as a provision of the BBA of 1997, which established SCHIP. Implemented at the state level, these programs have experienced problems with lower-than-expected enrollments, which may be a result of a lack of awareness of the program, eligibility requirements, or other unknown factors (ANA, 2000).

Another step toward addressing part of the problem for the uninsured and underinsured was the Health Insurance Portability and Accountability Act (HIPAA) (Public Law 104-191) in 1996, which took effect in 1997. The portability provision means that individuals with health insurance who lose or leave their jobs can maintain coverage even when they are sick. However, cost may be a prohibitive factor, because it does not regulate premium costs. Insurers are also prohibited from refusing coverage based on an individual's health status, although limited waiting periods may apply. Additionally, the bill allows individuals in small firms, uninsured individuals, or self-insured individuals with high-deductible plans to set up a tax-exempt MSA. This MSA allows tax deductions for long-term care insurance premiums and for qualified, unreimbursed home health and long-term care services; it allows the terminally ill earlier access to earnings built up in life insurance policies without tax penalties; it establishes fraud and abuse guidelines; it provides liability coverage for medical volunteers who provide free medical care to low-income individuals in medically underserved areas; and it mandates that USDHHS develop regulations and standards for the electronic transfer of medical information, confidentiality, and a unique health identifier. One of the most costly and complicated changes mandated by HIPAA is that health care companies must design interactive data systems that allow the transfer of health data while maintaining client confidentiality (Goedert, 2000).

HEALTH CARE SYSTEMS OF OTHER COUNTRIES

Interest in universal health care makes for a reasonable discussion. By examining the international health care continuum, perspectives on reform of the U.S. system may prove worthwhile. The United States spends the highest proportion of gross domestic product on health care of all industrialized countries, and has the highest cost per capita, as well. Canada, Germany, and the United Kingdom represent a select sampling of international countries, each having some form of universal health care plan, and these are compared with that of the United States in Table 3-1. Of the countries examined, the United Kingdom spends the least amount on health care and the least per capita.

Canadian Health Care System

The Canadian universal coverage social insurance plan is similar to the Social Security and Medicare programs for older people in the United States. Physicians practicing in Canada do not work on salary for the government, but are private practitioners paid on a fee-for-service basis as in the United States. Every Canadian, regardless of income or job status, has the same basic health insurance. Many Canadians have supplemental insurance through their employers to help pay for uncovered services like dental care.

Canadians pay for health care through a variety of federal and provincial taxes, just as Americans pay for Social Security and Medicare through payroll taxes. The federal government appropriates funds to the provinces and territories. Because the government is the primary payer of medical bills, Canada's health care system is referred to as a *single-payer arrangement*. Benefits vary among the provinces, but most cover hospital care, medical care, long-term care, and mental health services, as well as prescription drugs for people over age 65. Younger Canadians pay for prescriptions out-of-pocket on an income-based sliding scale. Canadians with supplemental insurance may have prescription drug coverage. Although each province runs its own insurance program as it sees fit, all are guided by the five principles of the Canada Health Act, as shown in Box 3-3. If an individual moves from one province to another, the provincial policy will continue. At one time, the Canadian system

Box **3-3** **Five Principles of the Canada Health Act**

Universality: everyone in the nation is covered
Portability: people can move from province to province and from job to job or onto the unemployment roles and retain their health coverage
Accessibility: everyone has access to the system's health care providers
Comprehensiveness: provincial plans cover all medically necessary treatment
Public administration: the system is publicly run and publicly accountable

seemed to be an ideal model that the United States should adopt; however, increasing health care costs and access issues are unresolved. In 1998 a report indicated that 212,990 Canadians were on hospital waiting lists for surgical procedures, with an average wait time of 13.3 weeks, and four out of five Canadians are unhappy with their socialized health care system. This report came from Manitoba, a predominately rural province (Reed, 2000).

Over the years, the federal government has decreased contributions to the provinces and territories due to large budget deficits and limited fee increases to physicians for services. Regionalization of hospitals has caused access to care issues for those outside of major cities. Canadians tend to have longer waiting times than do U.S. citizens for health care services, diagnostic testing, and surgery. Expansion to offer better access to home care and community-based services are emerging issues. A greater percentage of physicians are PCPs, not specialists like in the United States. The Canadian system in 2000 spent $2535 per capita, compared with $4672 in the United States (Bodenheimer & Grumbach, 2002; Chang et al., 2001; Shi & Singh, 2004). Would the American public tolerate waiting for health care services?

German Health Care System

Germany provides near universal access to health care through sickness funds. Over 600 sickness funds provide health coverage for approximately 90% of the population. Approximately 8% of people have private insurers. Private insurers pay physicians higher fees than do sickness funds, allowing preferential treatment to the wealthier. About 0.2% of the population (which is wealthy) has no insurance. If a person retires, changes jobs, or stops working for any reason, that person and the family maintain membership in the sickness fund (Geyman, 2002, p. 392). Employers and workers pay a percentage into the sickness fund. Employees pay about 12% of their annual income into the sickness fund. The funds are nonprofit and are required to cover hospital costs, physician services, prescription drugs, dental care, prevention, and maternity care with modest co-payments (Bodenheimer & Grumbach, 2002, p. 160). Germans are free to see any "ambulatory" (general) practi-

tioner they choose. If hospitalization is needed, usually a referral is needed and care is received from a hospital-based physician. Ambulatory physicians are required to join their regional physician's associations, which are paid a fee each year from the sickness fund. Ambulatory physicians are paid according to a detailed fee schedule. "Since 1986, physician's associations, in an attempt to stay within their global budgets, have reduced fees on a quarterly basis if the volume of services delivered by their physicians was too high" (Bodenheimer & Grumbach, 2002, p. 162). Hospital physicians are salaried. Problems include a two-tiered system, with some people who can afford private care bypassing and weakening the public system, friction between ambulatory and hospital physicians, and low reimbursement of physicians resulting in more clients being seen in a shorter period of time.

United Kingdom's Health Care System

The British health system is named the National Health Service, which is founded on the mission of primary care and community health services. Each person living in a geographical area is assigned to a primary care group, of which general practitioners (GPs) are members. A typical primary care group has 100,000 clients and 50 GPs and is responsible for population-based care. The system is financed over 80% from taxes, 13% from employer-employee contributions, and 4% user charges. About 11% of the British population holds private health care insurance, allowing preferential treatment. GPs do not care for clients in the hospital. The acute care and specialist physicians are salaried employees of the United Kingdom. Health care costs are strictly controlled by the supply of personnel, facilities, medical resources, and salaries. Primary care is readily available, but wait time for consultants and elective surgery (e.g., a hip replacement or cataract surgery) may be 3 months or more. Renal dialysis is performed less in the United Kingdom, especially for those over the age of 60. In the United Kingdom, physicians perform fewer surgeries and fewer diagnostic tests, and fewer medications are prescribed. (Bodenheimer & Grumbach, 2002; Chang et al., 2001; Shi & Singh, 2004).

INFLUENCING HEALTH POLICY

The primary responsibility of the nurse is to the individual, family, group, or community served. A major portion of the nurse's role is to **advocate** not only for the individual, but also for justice in health care delivery. Nurses need to be aware of issues that have an effect on the health of the American people and to know how to work for needed change.

Health cannot be separated from its environment; therefore, it is essential that nurses become involved in all aspects of planning to maximize the health potential of all Americans. This involvement needs to include attention to policy decisions and political action. Policy affects the broader aspects of environment, the biophysical and socioeconomic conditions of homes, schools, workplaces, communities, and the health care delivery environment. By virtue of their numbers, nurses, who make up the largest group of health care providers in the United States, have tremendous potential to influence decision making.

Participation in **policy decision making** requires the nurse take a proactive stance to determine needs before a problem arises. Policy development and change take place on many levels, from within the nurse's agency or work group to the community, state, and national levels. At the institutional level, clinical decisions influence policy, as do management issues. The nurse should examine the rationale behind an existing or planned policy and determine whether or not it is relevant now. Nurses are empowered by their education and experience to use their people skills and to apply change theory to influence policy development and change.

Much health-related decision making is the result of legislation at the local, state, or national level. Laws, rules enforced by a ruling authority by which society is governed, and **regulations,** agency or department rules developed for the implementation of laws, define what services are being offered to whom and who will pay how much. **Politics** influences change and is an arena for nursing's participation that is part of this nation's democratic heritage. The nurse can be politically involved in many ways. Voting, after becoming well informed on current issues and candidates, is an important way for nurses to be actively involved. The nurse should get to know the politically influential people in the community and disseminate to others what she learns from them.

The nurse can run for political office (many nurses now represent their local constituencies, and they have increasing visibility at the state and national levels) and support colleagues who represent nursing's interests. Financial contributions to Nurses for Political Action Coalition (N-PAC), ANA's political arm, increase the power base of nurses. Membership in professional and community groups provides the nurse with a collective voice to influence legislators. ANA's Nurses Strategic Action Team (N-STAT) network is an organized grassroots effort by nurses to help elect ANA-PAC–endorsed candidates and to inform members of Congress about policy issues of concern to nurses. When nurses join N-STAT, they receive *Action Alert and Legislative Update,* detailing specific legislative issues to enable them to be adequately informed and to respond to legislators in a timely manner.

Legislators are influenced by the information that they receive and by the sources of that information. Nurses have a wealth of knowledge about health care that legislators need to know. The process of trying to persuade legislators to vote for or against measures important to the interest group represented is called **lobbying.** A **lobbyist** is a registered representative of a special interest group. The ANA, located in Washington, DC, employs nurse lobbyists. Nurse lobbyists are active at the state level, also.

Communicating with a legislator is essential and can be done by phone, writing a letter, personal visits, or e-mail

Box **3-4**	Nursing's National Agenda for the Future: Ten Areas of Concern Demanding Action

Economic value*
Delivery system*
Education*
Work environment*
Leadership and planning
Legislation/regulation/policy
Professional/nursing culture
Recruitment/retention
Public relations/communication
Diversity

From American Nurses Association Web site. Accessed January 28, 2005, from: *http://www.nursingworld.org.* Report: Nursing's Agenda for the Future. Retrieved January 28, 2005, from: *http://www.nursingworld.org/naf/.*
*Top priorities of the December 2002 NAF's steering committee.

correspondence. Legislators have staffs of experts in various areas, and each legislator is assigned to committees. To understand the legislative process, the nurse needs to follow the progress of a bill. Thousands of bills are introduced at both the state and federal levels and must be passed within a 2-year time frame or die by default. "Nurses can influence the introduction of a bill as constituents and as members of professional nursing organizations" (Santa Anna, 2002, p. 452). Once a bill is introduced it is referred to committee, and the committee chairperson determines which bills will be considered. Hearings are then held on the considered bills. When finished in committee, a bill is "reported out" to the floor of the Senate or House of Representatives for a vote. Both the Senate and the House must pass identical versions of the bill and, once passed by both chambers, it is forwarded to the President for signing. If signed, it is enacted into law (Milstead, 1999). It is important for nurses to lobby, to inform legislators of new issues, and to give expert testimony on introduced bills. It is essential that nurses become politically aware and active to enable the collective voice of nursing to reach its full potential (Box 3-4).

Unfortunately, the collective voice of nurses is rarely heard. In 2002, of the 2.7 million registered nurses in the United States and the 2.2 million employed in nursing, only about 20% were members of the ANA or specialty nursing organizations. Networking and information used to be primary reasons to join an organization. The Internet has replaced this need by providing easy access to current information and networking via e-mail, listservs, and chat rooms for nominal or no cost. Membership dues in many organizations are high, and nurses may not see tangible benefits tied to membership. Younger nurses from generations X and Y as a group have little interest in politics and voting (Shinn, 2002). There are more than 100 professional nursing organizations. The few nurses who are members are divided among the many. In addition, nurses have not been unified on issues such as entry into practice. It is the responsibility of nurses to become and remain well informed. As

HOTtopics

NURSING'S AGENDA FOR THE FUTURE

The ANA held a summit in September of 2001 to determine what nursing should look like and where it should be by the year 2010. The summit brought together nurses from many other nursing associations in a collective effort to develop a strategic plan to address the growing nursing shortage and to move the profession forward while providing quality nursing care to consumers. The agenda developed by the steering committee focused on 10 areas of concern derived from an IOM study, Crossing the Quality Chasm: A New Health System for the 21st Century, and other evidence-based research (see Box 3-4). The ANA has a history of commitment to the idea that all Americans are entitled to accessible and affordable quality health care services. In

November 2003 nursing organizations submitted over 200 proposals to push forward the NAF agenda. As the nation's largest health care profession, nurses can bring about positive changes in both the nursing profession and health care delivery system.

Questions:

- How can nurses ensure safe, quality client care?
- What are the root causes of the growing nursing shortage?
- How can nurses work collectively to move the NAF agenda forward?

From ANA Web site 2004. Report: Nursing's Agenda for the Future and progress reports on NAF. Retrieved March 15, 2005, from: *http://www.nursingworld.org/naf/*.

well-informed, empowered professionals, nurses play a significant role in supporting legislative initiatives that promote and protect the health of the public (Hot Topics box).

SUMMARY

Nurses need to be proactive in shaping policy that affects the health care system. They need to understand the complexity of the system to be able to educate individuals and families about health care resources and to coordinate services. To accomplish this task, nurses need to become and remain well-informed citizens and health care consumer advocates.

A historical perspective and a description of the current health care delivery system in the United States provide a framework for the analysis of trends, values, and needs related to health. Comprehensive health services do exist, but they are fragmented, unequally distributed, and extremely expensive. Although there is more emphasis on health promotion, as evident by the broad goals of *Healthy People 2010,* the current system continues to concentrate on the delivery and financing of illness care. Promotion of health needs to be incorporated into a system that delivers health care to all Americans. The delivery system needs to move beyond a focus on short-term, episodic disease patterns that were predominant during the first half of the twentieth century and conquer the problems facing us today. Health problems that are chronic in nature require a system that supports long-term continual delivery and financing mechanisms. A change in emphasis and direction is needed.

The U.S. government provides the legal underpinnings for protecting and controlling the environment for health and delivery of health care services through the enactment of laws and the regulation of financing for the system. Social policy, as a reflection of society's values, has changed from a laissez-faire approach during the 1850s to one in which the federal government has had a prominent role in organizing and financing health care since the 1970s. Health care became a major political issue in 1991 and is likely to remain an issue until the problems of cost containment and universal access are solved. Other industrialized nations have managed to provide universal health care. The American public is becoming increasingly dissatisfied with the present system and the cost of care. Although cost containment was the primary concern during the 1990s, quality is paramount in this new century. Addressing quality, cost, and access to health care is the challenge for the future.

ADDITIONAL STUDY MATERIAL

Study Questions in the back of the book, see page 663.

evolve WEB SITE MATERIAL

These materials are located on the book's Web site at http://evolve.elsevier.com/Edelman/.

- WebLinks
- Content Updates
- Web Site Resources

3A Agencies Within the U.S. Department of Health and Human Services and Their Major Functions
3B Medicare Insurance–Covered Services for 2004
3C Comparison of Medicare and Medicaid

REFERENCES

Altman, D. (2004). The new Medicare prescription-drug legislation. *The New England Journal of Medicine, 350*(2), 9-10.

American Nurses Association. (2000). *Achieving access for all Americans: A proposal from the American Nurses Association for health coverage 2000.* Retrieved May 2, 2004, from: *http://www.nursingworld.org/readroom/rwjpaper.htm.*

Andrews, M., & Boyle, J. (2003). *Transcultural concepts in nursing care* (4th ed.). Philadelphia: Lippincott Williams & Wilkins.

Angell, M. (2000). Patients' rights bills and other futile gestures. *New England Journal of Medicine, 342*(22), 1663-1664.

Arias, E., & Smith, B. (2003). Deaths: Preliminary date for 2001 (On-line). *National Vital Statistics Report, 51*(5), 1-45. Retrieved May 1, 2004, from: *http://www.cdc.gov/nchs/data/nvsr/nvsr51/nvs51r_05.pdf.*

Bodenheimer, T., & Grumbach, K. (2002). *Understanding health policy: A clinical approach* (3rd ed.). New York: McGraw-Hill.

Bonick, J. (2000). Policy, politics, and the law. In M. Stanhope & J. Lancaster (Eds.), *Community and public health nursing* (5th ed., pp. 177-199). St. Louis: Mosby.

Bush's agenda for improving health care. Retrieved March 16, 2005, from: *http://gop.com/GOP Agenda/AgendaPage.aspx?id=4.*

Carmona, R. (2002). *Progress review: Access to quality health services. U.S. Department of Health & Human Services–Public Health Sector.* Retrieved April 30, 2004, from: *http://www.healthypeople.gov/data/2010prog/focus01/.*

Cary, A. H. (2000). Case management. In M. Stanhope & J. Lancaster (Eds.), *Community and public health nursing* (5th ed., pp. 380-399). St. Louis: Mosby.

Centers for Disease Control and Prevention. (2004a). *Racial and ethnic approaches to community health (REACH 2010): Addressing disparities in health at a glance 2004.* Retrieved April 30, 2004, from: *http://www.cdc.gov/nccdphp/aag/aag_reach.htm.*

Centers for Disease Control and Prevention. (2004b). Trends in tuberculosis—United States 1998-2001. *MMWR Weekly, 53*(10), 209-214. Retrieved March 15, 2005, from: *http://www.cdc.gov/mmwr/preview/mmwrhtml/mm531.*

Centers for Disease Control and Prevention, Department of Health and Human Services. (2004). *Health and safety topics A-Z.* Retrieved May 1, 2004, from: *http://www.cdc.gov/az.do.*

Centers for Disease Control and Prevention, National Center for HIV, STD and TB Prevention. (2003). *HIV/AIDS Update.* Retrieved May 1, 2004, from: *http://www.cdc.gov/hiv/stats.htm.*

Centers for Medicare & Medicaid Services, Office of the Actuary. (2003). *National health care expenditures projection: 2003-2013.* Retrieved March 15, 2005, from: *http://www.cms.hhs.gov/statistics/nhe/projections-2003/proj2003.pdf.*

Clemen-Stone, S., McGuire, S., & Eigsti, D. G. (2002). *Comprehensive community health nursing* (6th ed.). St. Louis: Mosby.

Deets, H. (2000, Feb.). Medicare drug coverage: It's smart medicine. *AARP Bulletin,* 28.

Freyman, J. G. (1980). *The American health care system: Its genesis and trajectory.* Huntington, NY: Krieger.

Geyman, J. (2002). *Healthcare in America: Can our ailing system be healed?* Boston: Butterworth-Heinemann.

Goedert, J. (2000). The dawn of HIPAA: What the Health Insurance Portability and Accountability Act means to you. *Health Data Management, 8*(4), 84-106.

Goldsmith, J. (2000). How will the Internet change our health system? *Health Affairs, 19*(1), 148-156.

Healthcare spending, 2002. (2004). *Family Practice News, 34*(3), 1.

Herrick, T. (2004). Consumer-driven health care. *Clinical News, 8*(7), 6-7.

Holder, V. (2004). From handmaiden to right hand—The infancy of nursing. *AORN Journal, 79*(2), 374-382, 385-390.

Institute of Medicine, Board on Health Science Policy. (2003). *Summary: Unequal treatment—Confronting racial and ethnic disparities in health care, 1-28.* Retrieved April 28, 2004, from: *http://books.nap.edu/books/030908265X/l.html#pagetop.*

Institute of Medicine of the Academies. (2004). A. Page (Ed.), *Keeping patients safe: Transforming the work environment of nurses.* Washington, DC: The National Academies Press.

Kennedy, M. (2004). Nurses' workplace must change. *American Journal of Nursing, 104*(1), 23-24.

Kinsey, K., & Buchanan, M. (2004). The nursing center: A model of community health nursing practice. In M. Stanhope & J. Lancaster (Eds.), *Community and public health nursing* (6th ed., pp. 412-416). St. Louis: Mosby.

Koch, A. L. (1999). Financing health services. In S. J. Williams & P. R. Torrens (Eds.), *Introduction to health services* (5th ed., pp. 113-150). Albany, NY: Delmar.

Kovner, C., & Salsberg, E. (1999). The health care work force. In A. Kovner & S. Jonas (Eds.), *Jonas and Kovner's health care delivery in the United States* (6th ed., pp. 64-115). New York: Springer.

Lee, P., & Benjamin, A. E. (1999). Health policy and the politics of health care. In S. J. Williams & P. R. Torrens (Eds.), *Introduction to health services* (5th ed., pp. 439-465). Albany, NY: Delmar.

Lee, P., & Estes, C. (2003). *The nation's health* (7th ed.). Sudbury, MA: Jones and Bartlett.

Leininger, M. (1997). Transcultural nursing research to transform nursing education and practice. *Image: The Journal of Nursing Scholarship, 29*(4), 341-347.

Levit, J., Cohen, S., Mason, D. (2002). Political analysis and strategies. In D. Mason, J. Leavitt, & M. Chaffee (Eds.), *Policy and politics in nursing and healthcare* (4th ed., pp. 71-91). St. Louis: Saunders.

Levit, K., Cowan, C., Lazngy, H., Sensenig, A., McDonnell, P., Stiller, J., et al. (2000). Health spending in 1998: Signals of change. *Health Affairs, 19*(1), 124-131.

Levit, K., Smith, C., Cowan, C., Lazenby, Martin, A. (2003). Inflation spurs health spending in 2000. In H. Wallace, G. Green, & K. Jaros (Eds.), *Health and welfare for families in the 21st century* (2nd ed., pp. 231-244). Sudbury, MA: Jones and Bartlett.

Marmagus, S., King, L., Chuk, M. (2003). Public health's response to a changed world: September 11, biological terrorism, and the development of an environmental health tracking network. *American Journal of Public Health, 93*(8), 1226-1230.

Maurer, F. A. (2000). The U.S. health care system. In C. M. Smith & F. A. Maurer (Eds.), *Community health nursing: Theory and practice* (2nd ed., pp. 53-90). Philadelphia: Saunders.

Milstead, J. (1999). *Health policy & politics: A nurse's guide.* Gaithersburg, MD: Aspen.

Mundinger, M., Lane, R., Lenz, E., Totten, A., Wei-Yann, T., Cleary, P., et al. (2000). Primary care outcomes in patients treated by nurse practitioners or physicians: A randomized trial. *Journal of the American Medical Association, 283*(1), 59-68.

Neuhauser, D. (2003). Florence Nightingale gets no respect: As a statistician that is. *Quality and Safety in Health Care, 12*(4), 317.

O'Grady, E. (2000). Access to health care: An issue central to nursing. *Nursing Economics, 18*(2), 88-90.

Pearson, L. (2000). Annual legislative update: How each state stands on legislative issues affecting advanced practice nurses. *Nurse Practitioner, 25*(1), 16-28.

Reed, L. (2000). *Socialized medicine leaves a bad taste in patients' mouths.* MAKINAC Center for Public Policy. Retrieved February 2, 2004, from: *http://www.mackinac.org/article.asp?ID=2748.*

Rollet, J. (2003). Annual legislative update. *Advance for Nurse Practitioners, 11*(12), 37, 40-42.

Santa Anna, Y. (2002). Legislative and regulatory processes. In D. Mason, J. Leavitt, & M. Chaffee (Eds.), *Policy and politics in nursing and healthcare* (4th ed., pp. 451-478). St. Louis: Saunders.

Shi, L., & Singh, D. (2004). *Delivering health care in America: A systems approach* (3rd ed.). Sudbury, MA: Jones and Bartlett.

Shinn, L. (2002). Contemporary issues in professional organizations. In D. Mason, J. Leavitt, & M. Chaffee (Eds.), *Policy and politics in nursing and healthcare* (4th ed., pp. 601-607). St. Louis: Saunders.

Spector, R. (2000). *Cultural diversity in health & illness* (5th ed.). Upper Saddle River, NJ: Prentice Hall.

Stanhope, M., & Lancaster, J. (2004). *Community & public health nursing* (6th ed). St. Louis: Mosby.

Sultz, H., & Young, K. (2004). *Health care USA: Understanding its organization and delivery* (4th ed.). Sudbury, MA: Jones and Bartlett.

Thorpe, K. (1999). Health care cost containment: Reflections and future directions. In A. Kovner & S. Jonas (Eds.), *Jonas and Kovner's health care delivery in the United States* (6th ed., pp. 439-473). New York: Springer.

Thorpe, K., & Knickman, J. (1999). Financing for health care. In A. Kovner & S. Jonas (Eds.), *Jonas and Kovner's health care delivery in the United States* (6th ed., pp. 32-63). New York: Springer.

Torrens, P. R., & Williams, S. J. (1999). Managed care: Restructuring the system. In S. J. Williams & P. R. Torrens (Eds.), *Introduction to health services* (5th ed., pp. 151-170). Albany, NY: Delmar.

Turnock, B. (2004). *Public health: What it is and how it works* (3rd ed.). Sudbury, MA: Jones and Bartlett.

U.S. Department of Health and Human Services. (2000a). *Healthy people 2010: Understanding and improving health*. Washington, DC: U.S. Government Printing Office.

U.S. Department of Health and Human Services, Health Care Financing Administration. (2000b). *Choices under Medicare, 2000*. Washington, DC: U.S. Government Printing Office.

Vincent, D., Oakley, D., Pohl, J., Walker, D. (2000). Survival of nurse-managed centers: The importance of cost analysis. *Outcomes Management for Nursing Practice, 4*(3), 124-128.

Whitted, G. (1999). Private health insurance and employee benefits. In S. J. Williams & P. R. Torrens (Eds.), *Introduction to health services* (5th ed., pp. 171-203). Albany, NY: Delmar.

World Health Organization. (2004). *Overview of WHO*. Retrieved May 1, 2004, from: *http://www.who.int/about/overview/en/*.

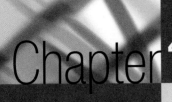

Chapter 4

JUNE ANDREWS HOROWITZ

The Therapeutic Relationship

objectives

After completing this chapter, the reader will be able to:

- Evaluate values clarification as a prerequisite to effective health promotion.

- Examine the elements and process of communication.

- Analyze differences between functional and dysfunctional communication.

- Develop strategies to promote therapeutic relationships with diverse populations across clinical settings, contexts, and nursing roles.

- Synthesize knowledge of the therapeutic relationship as an essential component of health promotion.

key terms

15–Minute interview	Input	Self-disclosure
Communication process	Metacommunication	Self-esteem
Empathy	Nonverbal communication	Telehealth
Feedback	Output	Therapeutic use of self
Health literacy	Reflection	Values clarification
Helping or therapeutic relationship	Relationship stages	Verbal communication
	Self-concept	

THINK About It

How Does a Nurse Respond When an Individual's Values Conflict With the Nurse's Values of Promoting Healthy Behaviors?

Samantha, a 17-year-old girl, comes into the health clinic at her school to ask the nurse practitioner to prescribe birth control pills for her and to check her for a vaginal discharge. The nurse begins the appointment by asking Samantha about her chief complaint of discharge. Samantha answers these questions until the nurse asks about her relationship with her boyfriend. Samantha comments, "Don't worry about me. We're in love and I just need birth control pills so I won't get pregnant." When the nurse introduces the topic of health risks associated with unprotected sex, Samantha says, "Look, I don't need a lecture. You sound like my mother. I know what I'm doing and I don't need condoms because he's not with anyone else."

1 How can this nurse bridge the apparent gap between the nurse's values and Samantha's values?

2 In this brief encounter, how can the nurse begin to establish a therapeutic relationship?

3 What responsibilities does the nurse need to weigh in responding to Samantha's request?

4 What health risks exist if the nurse does or does not do what Samantha wants at this visit?

5 What does the nurse need to know about policies and care decisions for individuals who are not legal adults?

6 What strategies could the nurse use to engage Samantha in a conversation about her sexual behaviors and related health issues?

The therapeutic relationship is the milieu in which nursing care occurs. Practice is shaped by the nurse's one-way interest in the individual that Peplau (1991) described as the nurse's ability to focus on the interests, concerns, and needs of the individual. The desired outcome is characterized as "knowing the patient": a process of understanding the individual as a unique person (Whittemore, 2000, p. 75).

Knowing the patient is the relational context for nursing interventions. Particularly in health promotion, this is essential. Health promotion requires sensitivity to each person's goals and values—the individual's and the nurse's. Assisting a person to adopt health promoting behaviors requires more than giving information; health promotion requires effective communication. Providing health communication is a focus area of *Healthy People 2010* (U.S. Department of Health and Human Services, 2000), making it a priority for nursing practice. Successful health promotion involves interpersonal skills, personal insight, accountability, mutual respect, and a supportive working milieu. Essential to this interactional process are values clarification, communication, and the helping relationship. See the *Healthy People 2010* box for the Leading Health Indicators and Priorities for Action.

Healthy People 2010

Leading Health Indicators

- Physical activity
- Overweight and obesity
- Tobacco use
- Substance abuse
- Responsible sexual behavior
- Mental health
- Injury and violence
- Environmental quality
- Immunization
- Access to health care

Priorities for Action

- Adopt the 10 Leading Health Indicators as personal and professional guides for choices about how to make health improvements.
- Encourage public health professionals and public officials to adopt the Leading Health Indicators as the basis for public health priority setting and decision making.
- Urge public and community health systems and our community leadership to use the Leading Health Indicators as measures of local success for investments in health improvements.

From Healthy People 2010: Leading Health Indicators. (n.d.). *Leading health indicators: Priorities for action.* Retrieved May 31, 2005, from *http://www.healthypeople.gov/thi/factsheet.htm.*

VALUES CLARIFICATION
Definition

Values are qualities, principles, attitudes, or beliefs about the inherent worth of an object, behavior, or idea. Values guide action by sanctioning certain behaviors and negating others. Values and beliefs are essential factors in design and implementation of nursing interventions (Guttman, 2000). Cognitive values are those that are ascribed to verbally and intellectually. Active values, in contrast, are those that are physically acted out. Judging the power of a given value by its ability to influence action is important. For example, a nurse may claim to value the worth of all people equally, but may treat individuals of various races differently and provide the most time and concern for those who are racially similar to the nurse. This cognitive value has little power to shape the nurse's behavior. If the nurse treated people of all races with equal respect, then the value would also be active and have great power to motivate behavior.

Many forces shape values. Passed down from one generation to another, values color an individual's identity, goals, and sense of personal meaning. Values are embedded in the culture and taught within a family and social context, giving meaning to the life events and happenings outside the family's boundaries (Wright & Leahey, 2000). Recognition that values are culture-bound is a critical step in exploring personal values and appreciating the values held by others (Guttman, 2000). To engage in health promotion, the nurse must explore how culture, traditions, and practices in a multiethnic and multicultural society influence health-related values. Without this understanding, the nurse is likely to relate to individuals with a limited awareness of assumptions and inadequate sensitivity to the uniqueness and perspective of the person, family, or community.

Values evolve; they are not static. Life events and social processes can spark a reappraisal of personal values. **Values clarification** is a method for discovering one's values and the importance of these values (Raths, Harmin, & Simon, 1978). Values clarification does not tell a person how to act, but it assists in recognizing what values are held to evaluate how they influence action.

Box 4-1 outlines seven steps in the valuing process. The first three steps of choosing involve a cognitive process, the next two steps involve the affective or emotional domain, and the final steps involve behavior (Raths, et al., 1978; Stuart & Laraia, 2001). The nurse uses values clarification to examine personal values and their potential influence on nursing care, and to assist people in identifying their values and reflecting on their connection to health-related behaviors. Box 4-2 lists suggestions for putting values clarification into action.

Values clarification becomes a clinical aim when individuals' values lead to behaviors that conflict with the nurse's value of promoting health. For example, a nurse tells a childbirth education class consisting of pregnant women and their coaches that alcohol use poses serious risks to the fetus. After the class, one woman comments, "Do you really think that having a drink once in a while is bad for the baby? I'm sick of being told that I can't do things because of the baby." In this example, an apparent conflict in values between the nurse and the patient exists. Intervention is needed to examine how this woman's wish for freedom from restrictions clashes with her desire to have a healthy child. Nurses must consider their own values related to health promotion for the individual and the fetus and must weigh the importance of respecting individuals' rights to make decisions about their own health behaviors. Such value conflicts result in ethical dilemmas. Resolution rests on the nurse's ability to examine conflicting values and available evidence

---

Box **4-1** The Valuing Process

CHOOSING
1. Choosing freely
2. Choosing from alternatives
3. Choosing after careful consideration of potential outcomes of each alternative

PRIZING
4. Cherishing and being happy with personal beliefs and actions
5. Affirming the choice in public, when appropriate

ACTING
6. Acting out the choice
7. Repeatedly acting in some type of pattern

Box **4-2** Techniques for Assisting Individuals to Clarify Values

IDENTIFY THE INDIVIDUAL'S VALUES

"What is important to you?"
"Which of the following statements sounds most like the way you think?"
"What do you value most in life?"

USE REFLECTION TO RESTATE THE VALUE AND MAKE IT EXPLICIT

"In what you've just told me, I hear that it is very important to you that . . ."
"I understand that you value . . ."

IDENTIFY VALUE CONFLICTS OR CONFLICTS BETWEEN VALUES AND ACTIONS

"What connection does this value have to your current health or illness and to the healthy behaviors, interventions, or treatments needed to maintain or restore your health?"
"How does this particular value affect your behavior and health?"
"What are some ways that you might put your values into action?"
"Are your actions consistent with your values? If not, then what might you change?"

---

about possible outcomes when fashioning health-promotion interventions.

Values and Therapeutic Use of Self

The self, the most precious and unique of all human endowments, is a personal concept of individuality as distinct from other people and objects. **Therapeutic use of self** is the application of one's cognitions, perceptions, and behaviors to create interpersonal encounters that promote health in another person, family, group, or community. Without self-awareness and clarification of values, therapeutic use of self is impaired. Self-concept and self-esteem are interrelated components of individuals' judgments and attitudes about themselves. **Self-concept** is a mental picture of the self, a composite view of personal characteristics, abilities, limitations, and aspirations. **Self-esteem,** the affective component of self-perception, refers to how individuals feel about the way that they see themselves. Internalized appraisals from others also influence self-concept and self-esteem.

Self-concept evolves throughout life. From birth, family experiences and parental identification mold the child's sense of identity. The classic research studies of Coopersmith (1967) and Sears (1970) demonstrated positive relationships between the self-reliance, self-esteem, and self-confidence of parents and children. Self-esteem is learned from experience (Schuster, 2000). To cultivate children's self-esteem and enable them to have a realistic perception of their strengths and weaknesses, parents should focus on positives, give feedback on abilities and limitations, and provide the child with a sense of belonging. Positive, rewarding, anxiety-free interactions contribute to security, esteem, and positive self-view. Positive but realistic appraisals from significant others, especially the parents, help the young child to develop this healthy self-view (Sullivan, 1953).

The self does not develop solely in response to the reflected appraisals of others. Genetic endowment, experiential opportunities, and the individual's action shape self-concept. People can accept or reject the appraisals of others and modify their behavior. The ability to control actions and evaluate outcomes of interactions allows individuals to modify and alter their views of self. As such, the self is dynamic, changing through interaction with the outside world and in response to the various maturational and situational crises of life.

The ability to examine, reflect on, and evaluate the self is a uniquely human talent. Self-awareness involves interactions between the self and the external world and the symbolic connections created by the individual. The self includes an unconscious component that is only partially accessible and influences behavior. Self-awareness is influenced by the degree to which an individual has an accurate concept of all dimensions of the self. The Johari window (Luft, 1984) provides a schema for understanding the various components of the self (Figure 4-1). Box 4-3 lists these four components of the self.

Together, these windowpanes represent the total self. Three principles guide an understanding of how the self functions in this representation: (1) change in one portion influences all other portions, (2) the smaller the first portion, the poorer communication will be, and (3) interpersonal learning enlarges the first portion and decreases the size of one or more other portions (Luft, 1969). The goal of self-awareness is to increase the size of the first windowpane while reducing the size of the other three areas (Figure 4-2) (Sundeen, Stuart, Rankin, & Cohen, 1998).

Consider the differences between windows A and B of Figure 4-2. Window A represents an individual with little self-awareness. Windowpane number 4 is large, suggesting that a good deal of the person's experiences, thoughts, and feelings are repressed or suppressed, probably a result of associated anxiety. Additionally, window A suggests a large "not me" portion of the self. In contrast, window B represents a person who is open to the world and is comfortable with his or her self-concept.

The goal of high self-awareness, as illustrated in window B of Figure 4-2, is reached through three steps. The first step is listening to oneself and paying attention to emotions, thoughts, memories, reactions, and impulses. Frequently, people tune out their feelings and thoughts because they are anxious or because they are in a hurry to accomplish some other task. Without self-reflection, people act automatically and lose some of the meaning of living. To improve the ability of self-reflection, ask questions such as the following:

- What am I feeling now?
- What emotions have I experienced today and in the past day or so? What were my thoughts?
- What events led up to these thoughts and feelings?
- What actions did I take? Did my behavior fit with my thoughts and feelings, or was there a lack of harmony?
- Was I aware of my reactions at the time that they took place?
- How have I responded in clinical situations lately? How did I react in response to a particularly happy, sad, or

1 Known to self and others	**2** Known only to others
3 Known only to self	**4** Known neither to self nor to others

Figure 4-1 Johari window. (From Luft, J. [1984]. *Group processes: an introduction to group dynamics* [3rd ed.]. Palo Alto, CA: Mayfield. Reprinted with permission from Mayfield.)

Box **4-3** Components of the Self

1. The public self, which is shown to others
2. The semipublic self, which is seen by others but may be outside the individual's awareness
3. The private self, which is known to the individual, but not revealed to others
4. The inner self, which is the unconscious portion not known even to the individual because it has anxiety-provoking content

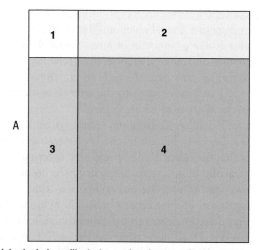
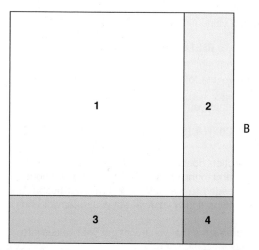

Figure 4-2 Johari windows illustrate varying degrees of self-awareness. **A,** Person has little self-awareness. **B,** Person has great amount of self-awareness. *1,* Public self. *2,* Semi-public self. *3,* Private self. *4,* Inner self. (From Sundeen, S. J., Stuart, G. W., Rankin, E. A. D., & Cohen, S. A. [1998]. *Nurse-client interaction: Implementing the nursing process* [6th ed.]. St. Louis: Mosby.)

difficult situation? In what way might I alter my actions now? What feelings and reactions did I experience while interacting with this individual?

The second step is listening to and learning from others. Feedback from others that conflicts with self-image can produce anxiety. In response, the feedback is ignored or translated incorrectly to preserve self-image and reduce anxiety. However, this pattern of responding limits knowledge of the self and inhibits the ability to examine the appraisals of others. Limited personal growth results. Asking reflective questions enables the nurse to use feedback effectively. Helpful questions include "What feedback have I received today?" and "What is the other person trying to tell me now?" A person also can ask others directly for feedback. For example, a student nurse might ask another student how he or she comes across. The feedback might be used to alter aspects of behavior that are ineffective or problematic before asking a faculty member for evaluative feedback. Using clinical supervision and consultation with colleagues provides needed opportunity for reflection on practice. "The intensity of interpersonal work necessitates that an arena be provided in which nurses can be helped to reflect on their practice" (DeMarco, Horowitz, & McLoed, 2000, p. 172). How the nurse comes across to the individual or family is crucial to successful health promotion, making self-awareness and sensitivity to feedback essential.

The third step is **self-disclosure;** sharing aspects of the self enriches interpersonal life. Through self-disclosure, people come to know themselves better because they have held thoughts, actions, and feelings up to the light for examination with others. Self-disclosure is an indicator of a healthy personality and a strategy for developing one (Jourard, 1971; Stuart & Laraia, 2001). Self-disclosure by one person tends to trigger self-disclosure by another in a reciprocal pattern of interaction. Therapeutic interactions characterized by reciprocity involve a mutual exchange—a pattern of communication between the nurse and an individual, not a one-way intervention from the nurse to the other person. Traditionally, clinicians have been wary of self-disclosure, because it may cross a boundary from a professional to a personal relationship. Additionally, the nurse's self-disclosure might burden the individual and shift the focus of attention from the individual to the nurse. Although these guidelines should be kept in mind to prevent excessive or inappropriate self-disclosure, appreciation that self-disclosure occurs within human interactions is needed. McCann and Baker (2001) found that revealing oneself was an effective clinical strategy to develop a helping relationship. Nurses are not blank screens, robots, or technicians delivering care; individuals value nurses who engage in interactions as real people and who are willing to share information about themselves.

Practical **reflection,** a thinking process described by Taylor (2004), involves bouncing back one's own thoughts and recollections of events to understand them and to take needed corrective action. The process of practical reflection dovetails with steps toward self-awareness previously described and offers complementary helpful tips. First, the nurse recalls an incident when something went wrong. Then the nurse experiences the incident again by remembering images and by privately retelling events, statements, outcomes, and associated emotions. Next, the nurse interprets the story of communication that failed by examining expectations, ideals, goals, influences, personal actions, and others' actions that occurred during the event. The last step involves honest inspection of the nurse's own role in the story. Insights gained then may be applied in new interactions to prevent things going wrong again in a similar way.

Why is it important for a nurse to clarify personal values and increase self-awareness? The things the nurse values and self-understanding influence behavior. The self is the nurse's greatest tool; to use the self effectively, the nurse must be fully aware of how it functions. Thus, reflection and self-awareness guide the nurse's practice framework. In addition, sensitivity to patients' perspectives is required to build a collaborative partnership, the cornerstone of the nurse-patient relationship (Gallant, Beaulieu, & Carnevale, 2002).

THE COMMUNICATION PROCESS

The **communication process** is the forum for all thought and relationships shared among people. In conjunction with the use of scientific and technological advances, communication is an essential tool for the nurse to engage in health-promotion interventions. "In the health promotion context, communication interventions aim to intervene by helping bring about desired changes in people's beliefs and behaviors or in their physical or social environments" (Guttman, 2000, p. 2). Communication is an information exchange between individuals through shared symbols and signs and commonly understood behavior (Ruesch & Bateson, 1987). This exchange involves all the modes of behavior that an individual uses, consciously or unconsciously, to affect another person. Communication includes the spoken and written word and nonverbal communication (gestures, facial expressions, movement, body messages or signals, and artistic symbols).

In nursing, communication is the cornerstone of a positive nurse-patient relationship (Attree, 2001; Thorsteinsson, 2002). Patient-centered, or person-centered, communication refers to a set of strategies and actions to enhance reciprocity, mutual understanding, and decision making. "Therapeutic communication involves use of carefully selected communication interventions to help patients and families overcome stress and adjust to the unalterable" (Schuster, 2000, p. 7). Focusing the clinical discussion around the person's story rather than a version reformulated by the provider is essential to person-centered communication. Box 4-4 highlights strategies associated with person-centered communication based on evidence from the research literature.

Box **4-4** Strategies Associated With Patient-Centered Communication

- Permitting people to tell their stories in their own words and chronology
- Using a conversational interviewing style
- Being friendly through humor and social conversation, and nonverbal cues such as smiling
- Eliciting people's views, perspectives, thoughts, wishes, goals, values, and expectations
- Inquiring about the nature of the person's life
- Attending to the person's needs
- Avoiding overemphasis on technical aspects of care and tasks
- Not being too busy to talk
- Responding to cues concerning emotional issues and problems
- Giving information about self-care and participation in decision making
- Developing mutual understanding
- Creating collaborative health care plans
- Showing empathy and concern for the individual's well being
- Connecting with individuals through humor, touch, and selective self-disclosure
- Tuning in to individuals' preferences and style
- Advocating for individuals' needs
- Maintaining confidentiality

Modified from Brown, S. J. (1999). Patient-centered communication. In J. J. Fitzpatrick (Ed.), *Annual review of nursing research: Vol. 17. Focus on complementary health and pain management* (pp. 85-104). New York: Springer; McCabe, C. (2004). Nurse-patient communication: An exploration of patients' experiences. *Journal of Clinical Nursing, 13,* 41-49; McCann, T. V., & Baker, H. (2001). Mutual relating: Developing interpersonal relationships in the community, *Journal of Advanced Nursing, 34,* 530-537; Moyle, W. (2003). Nurse-patient relationship: A dichotomy of expectations. *International Journal of Mental Health Nursing, 12,* 103-109.

Considerable evidence supports the effectiveness of these strategies. Research study results showed that nurses communicate effectively when they use a person-centered approach involving attending, empathy, being friendly (McCabe, 2004), being with the individual, and providing comfort (Moyle, 2003) (Research Highlights box). Although these strategies sound simple and basic, study participants have voiced that such appraisals are noticeably absent in many instances and that their presence makes the difference between good and not so good care (Attree, 2001).

Function and Process

Ruesch and Bateson (1987) have delineated the following functions of communication:

1. To obtain and send messages and to retain information
2. To use the information to arrive at new conclusions, to reconstruct the past, and to look forward to future events
3. To begin and to modify physiological processes
4. To influence others and outside events

research highlights

Exploration of Nurses' Communication

STUDY OVERVIEW

In a qualitative phenomenological study, McCabe (2004) explored patients' experiences of how nurses communicate with them. Using purposeful sampling, McCabe interviewed eight patients who had been hospitalized in a general teaching hospital in the Republic of Ireland. Hospitalization for a minimum of 4 days provided an opportunity for regular communication with nurses. Data were collected using unstructured tape-recorded interviews. Each participant provided informed consent. Interviews began with questioning about the participants' experiences of how nurses communicated. McCabe transcribed interview recordings and applied hermeneutic phenomenological techniques to examine the lived experience of the phenomenon under investigation. Data analysis revealed four themes: lack of communication, attending, empathy, and friendly nurses.

RESULTS

Lack of communication. Failure to provide adequate information and greater concern with tasks than talking with patients emerged as a major theme and impediment to effective nurse-patient communication. Task-centered communication, an aspect of lack of communication, indicated to participants that tasks were more important than they were. Participants also described being reassured when nurses used a patient-centered approach.

Attending. Attending comprised nurses' accessibility and willingness to listen to patients, indicated by nonverbal communication. Attending included subthemes of giving time and being there; open, honest communication; and genuineness. Helpful communications included verbal communication that responded directly to patients' concerns and nonverbal communication that indicated the nurse's self-awareness and genuineness.

Empathy. Empathy meant emotional engagement of the nurse with the patient. Empathy enhanced trust and understanding. Patient-focused interaction resulted from empathy and led to a sense of security and reassurance among participants.

Friendly nurses and humor. All participants noted that nurses were friendly and that they appreciated their use of humor. When nurses used humor to make participants laugh, nurses became more approachable. In addition, humor seemed to improve participants' self-esteem.

IMPLICATIONS

Findings indicated that nurses can communicate effectively when they use a patient-centered approach to interactions. A primarily task-centered approach, in contrast, interfered with effective nurse-patient communication. The researcher concluded that changes in health care organizations are needed to recognize the importance of a patient-centered communication approach to care delivery.

McCabe, C. (2004). Nurse-patient communication: An exploration of patients' experiences. *Journal of Clinical Nursing, 13,* 41-49.

Communication transmits information, both interpersonally and intrapersonally, and it provides the basis for action.

The process of communication consists of four components (Watzlawick, Beavin, & Jackson, 1967). Nurses must be able to diagnose communication difficulties in any of these components. **Input** involves taking in information from outside the individual or group. Once taken in, input must be transformed in some manner to be used. For example, symbols must be translated into words to transmit ideas. The flow and transformation of processed input refers to the way information is analyzed and stored within the individual, or the way it is transmitted from person to person within a human system (group or family) before communication with the external environment occurs. The outcome of information processing, **output,** involves further exchange with the environment or other person. A new information exchange is triggered at this point in the cycle by the response called **feedback,** a monitoring system through which the person or group controls the internal and external responses to behavior (output) and accommodates these responses appropriately. A feedback loop shows the dynamic nature of communication. Each piece of communication is both a stimulus designed to elicit a response and a response to a different stimulus (Figure 4-3).

When interpersonal communication is analyzed, two types of feedback can be identified: positive (encouraging change) and negative (encouraging homeostasis or no change). Parent's commands to a young child illustrate these types of feedback: (1) positive, "Try that again; you almost had it" and (2) negative, "Don't touch that; it's hot." The first statement shows the parent's attempt to encourage the child to continue new behavior; the second illustrates an effort to curtail undesired behavior. Rather than meaning "good" or "bad," positive and negative feedback refer to promotion of system change and stability, which is the process of balancing the direction and magnitude of change. Both types of feedback are needed, depending on the situation.

The situational context of communication is important. The context of communication is the setting's physical, psychosocial, and cultural dimensions. It includes the relationship between sender and receiver; their previous experiences, feelings, values, cultural norms, age and developmental stage, and the physical location (Kasch, 1986; Robinson, 2002; Stuart & Laraia, 2001).

Types of Communication

All human communication occurs in three forms: (1) verbal, (2) nonverbal, and (3) metacommunication. Each affects the meaning and influences the interpretation of the message.

Verbal Communication

Verbal communication is the transmission of messages using words, spoken or written. As symbols for ideas, words impart meaning defined by a specific language. The ability to communicate with language is a critical ability.

People who are deaf or hard of hearing often use sign language to communicate. Signs, similar to spoken or written words, are used consistently to represent a particular meaning. Words also may be spelled out through finger spelling in a manner parallel to written communication. Braille assists blind and visually challenged people to read. Touch is used to interpret markings that represent letters and words. Sign language and Braille blend aspects of verbal and nonverbal communication, but both forms of communication transmit meaning through a consistent language system.

Verbal communication with people who speak a different language poses a challenge. As societies become increasingly multicultural, assistance from specially trained interpreters is essential to providing culturally competent care (Robinson, 2002). Confidentiality issues, the complexity of health information, and the need to validate understandings and reach mutual decisions make it inappropriate to use untrained personnel or relatives to interpret simply because they are available.

The importance of language development is apparent in its three functions: (1) informing the person of others' thoughts and feelings, (2) stimulating the receiver of a message by triggering a response, and (3) serving a descriptive function by imparting information and sharing observations, ideas, inferences, and memories (Watzlawick, et al., 1967). The ability of verbal communication to fulfill these functions is influenced by many factors, including the communicator's social class, culture, age, milieu, and ability to receive and interpret messages.

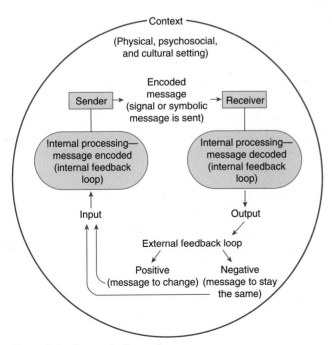

Figure 4-3 Communication system.

Nonverbal Communication

Nonverbal communication or language encompasses all messages that are not spoken or written. The channels of nonverbal communication are the five senses. Movement, facial and eye expressions, gestures, touch, appearance, and vocalization or paralanguage all constitute nonverbal modes of communication (Blondis & Jackson, 1982; Schuster, 2000). Although all communication has the potential of being misunderstood, nonverbal communication is particularly subject to misunderstanding because it does not always reflect the sender's conscious intent. Nonverbal messages also tend to be nebulous, without specific beginnings and endings.

Body motion or kinetic behavior includes facial expression (or facies), eye movements, body movements, gestures, and posture (Blondis & Jackson, 1982). When observing facial expression, the nurse notices the affect or emotion that is communicated. Does the person appear happy or sad; alert, distracted, or sleepy; or contented, agitated, or anxious? The degree of emotion expressed should also be noted. Does the person's face express what generally is considered an excessive degree of feeling for the situation, too little, or none at all? Eyes, in conjunction with the movement of other facial muscles, move in ways that convey affect. Eye contact conveys messages of interest or trust; lack of eye contact can imply lack of interest or anxiety; constant eye contact can send a message of hostility.

All of these nonverbal messages are culturally and situationally bound. Nonverbal behavior, particularly facial and eye expressions, is contextual. For example, in certain circumstances and cultures, avoidance of direct eye contact between some people can be a sign of respect. Yet, in other situations and cultures, it can be interpreted as indicative of disinterest, avoidance, or disrespect.

Sign language combines features of both nonverbal and verbal communication. Sign language involves nonverbal communication because, although it uses symbols that are communicated through specific signs, these are enhanced by facial expressions and body postures. However, sign language shares many aspects of verbal communication. It has syntax and grammar, words may be spelled out, and a standard meaning is assigned to specific signs to create symbolic language, just as words share common definitions.

Importance of Nonverbal Communication. Nonverbal communication has great power to transmit information about another's thoughts and feelings; therefore, careful observation is essential. Even silence can be very revealing. The significance of nonverbal communication is best captured by the axiom, "Actions speak louder than words." Nurses' nonverbal messages that communicate distance from the person, or signal an unfriendly or uncaring attitude, thwart development of a therapeutic relationship (McCabe, 2004; Moyle, 2003) and thereby render health-promotion efforts unproductive.

Metacommunication

Besides verbal and nonverbal communication, a phenomenon called **metacommunication** refers to a message about the message. Watzlawick, Beavin, and Jackson (1967) described metacommunication as the impossibility of not communicating; that is, "one cannot not communicate. Persons transmit a message about what is being communicated even when words are not spoken" (p. 49). Metacommunication is the relationship aspect of communication. In a sense, metacommunication involves reading between the lines or going past the surface content of the message to glean nuances of meaning. When the content and the relationship aspects, or metacommunication aspects, of a message are incongruent, interpreting the communication accurately may be difficult, leaving the receiver uncomfortable and confused.

Group Process

In group settings, a special type of metacommunication is called *process*. A basic principle of group theory states that all communication has content and process. Content is what is said; process is the relationship aspect of what is communicated. Group process occurs during every group encounter. Staff meetings and clinically oriented psycho-education, therapy, and counseling groups always involve group process. For example, consider two individuals in a smoking cessation group who always support each other by agreeing with each other and offering comments or criticism to any group member who disagrees. Although this pairing between the individuals offers them some protection from anxiety that may result from self-examination and feedback, it isolates them and curtails feedback from others. Examination of this group process is an essential task. The nurse leader and participants can transform this problematic situation into a learning opportunity by (1) identifying the pattern by pointing out the behavior after it has occurred frequently, (2) helping the pair and other group members to consider what needs are being met through this pattern, (3) looking at each person's role in fostering this process (e.g., why other group members have failed to confront the pair), and (4) discussing potential outcomes of changing the behavior. These steps can be applied in clinical situations when greater self-understanding is a goal.

Effectiveness of Communication

Understanding what makes communication effective improves the nurse's ability to assess needs and to intervene effectively to promote patients' health. Steps to functional communication include (1) firmly stating the case, (2) clarifying the message, (3) seeking feedback, and (4) being receptive to feedback when it is received.

To state the case firmly, the sender needs to make the content and the metacommunication congruent; when they conflict, the message is confusing. For example, a nurse is angry with a colleague for making statements to an administrator that undermined the nurse's plans for reconfiguring a health-promotion program in their agency. When the nurse had a chance to speak with this colleague, they exchanged pleasantries without mention of what the nurse thought about the colleague's statements to the administrator. When the colleague asked if something was bothering the nurse, the nurse responded that nothing was wrong. The colleague senses that the nurse's verbal and nonverbal communication did not match; in other words, the content of the message and the metacommunication were incongruent. The colleague was left feeling uneasy, and the nurse failed to express his or her thoughts or to take effective action to rectify the perceived problem with the colleague. To make the communication functional, the nurse needed to bring thoughts and feelings into awareness and reflect on the intended message. Once these steps are accomplished, the message's content and metacommunication can be adjusted to match, and the nurse's communication is likely to be effective.

To clarify the message, the sender must give a complete message. Important features should be emphasized and specifics of any request must be stated, not assumed. The message's importance also must be indicated. To illustrate, a woman mentions to her nurse that it is nearly June. The nurse responds that he has noticed how warm the weather is becoming. On the surface, this communication may seem functional until the intent of the woman's message is considered. She meant to imply that June is the 5-year anniversary of her remission from cancer, and she hoped that her nurse would somehow know that she wanted him to comment on the significance of this anniversary. To make this communication functional, the woman needed to expand the message (e.g., "My anniversary after cancer treatment is coming up") and then clarify her wish for a sensitive response from the nurse (e.g., "This anniversary marks the goal for you to be cancer-free"; "What will you do to celebrate?"). Additionally, she needed to show how important the message was (e.g., "I'd really like to do something special to mark this date"). If the nurse had been attuned to the metacommunication in this exchange, he could have clarified this woman's intent and met her need for recognition and dialogue.

One technique for clarifying and qualifying messages is called the *"I" statement*. Use of "I" statements assists the sender to state what he or she wants, feels, thinks, or plans (including likes and dislikes). For example, "I felt unimportant when you forgot to recognize this anniversary" is an "I" statement that the patient could have used to communicate effectively.

Questions can clarify and qualify, depending on the type of question asked. Open-ended questions tend to elicit descriptive responses rather than one-word answers. For example, the question, "Tell me what you did for exercise this week," is likely to yield a more elaborate description of a health behavior from a patient than the question, "Did everything go okay with your exercise plan?" However, direct questions that seek a one-word answer are useful

when a specific piece of information is sought. "Did you spend 15 minutes or more walking today?" may be a better approach than "What was your activity like today?" when it is important to discuss and promote minimum exercise requirements. Also, for individuals having trouble expressing more than the simplest thoughts, asking direct questions that call for brief replies can be helpful, such as, "Did you eat breakfast?" This approach is particularly useful with people who are depressed, regressed, cognitively impaired, or unable to handle complex information or communication at a particular time.

Seeking feedback is another element of functional communication. Consensual validation, confirming that both sender and receiver understand the same information, calls for the use of the clarification skills just described. In family communication, the parent, as the sender, should model this behavior for children by asking the child, as the receiver, to explain his or her sense of the message and how to ask the sender for further explanation. For example, "I want you to clean your room" (message from parent) can be followed by, "Tell me how you think you will do that" (validating that child and parent agree about what the task entails). This style of seeking validation can be adapted to nurse-nurse or nurse–other professional exchanges between colleagues and to therapeutic interactions. Such confirmation in communication is essential when providing health-promotion interventions. Without validating that the patient understands the information and its importance, and that the patient has a behavior plan to follow, health-promotion efforts are likely to fail.

Being open to feedback also is crucial. A "no questions" attitude blocks functional communication, whether in the home, classroom, or clinical setting. Children, students, individuals, and even other nurses may be afraid to question anyone in authority or may assume that the person should magically know what is intended or expected. For example, a person may avoid confronting a nurse who fails to explain the clinical plan and then communicates that the person should know how to follow through. Statements by the sender such as "Tell me what you think" and "What is your understanding of what I said?" are helpful.

Receiving and sending messages involves many of the same processes. Evaluation of the intent of the message, both the content and the metacommunication, is the first step. The receiver frequently needs to seek clarification and validate understanding of the message for communication to be effective. Clarification of expectations, active exchange of information, power sharing, and negotiation will enhance the quality of nurse-patient communication. The outcome is a nurse-patient relationship based on partnership (Gallant, et al., 2002).

Factors in Effective Communication
Listening

Effective listening, an important part of communication, is more than passively taking in information. Effective listening is actively focusing attention on the message. Asking questions to explore what is meant helps the listener reach an accurate assessment of the message's meaning.

Many forms of nonverbal communication have been identified that, from a Western or European perspective, commonly convey that the person is listening. These nonverbal communications include direct gazing and eye contact, head nodding, orienting one's body to maintain interpersonal closeness, leaning forward, facial expressions such as eyebrow animation and smiling, and brief verbal statements that indicate interest, such as "Please go on" or "Tell me more about that. . . ."

For behavior to communicate that the person is listening also depends on the context and intensity of the activities, and the cultural norms of each person. For example, leaning close to a person might be interpreted as intrusive. Yet, the same behavior could be seen as a sign of support, depending on the context and perspective of those involved. Sensitivity to nuances in communication and validation of meaning can be particularly helpful strategies when the nurse and patient come from different cultural backgrounds.

Reciprocity, the patterning of similar activities within the same interval by two people, can help the nurse communicate a listening stance in an effective way. When the nurse matches nuances of the individual's type and style of behavior, the chances that the person will interpret the nurse's behavior as an indication of active listening are increased, and the likelihood of misinterpretation is reduced. Nurses can enhance the quality of their communication, even when encounters are brief, by attending to reciprocity in their interactions and by validating whether or not reciprocity is associated with shared interpretations of meaning.

Poor listening blocks the nurse's understanding of the patient. The nurse's failure to listen may be caused by anxiety; lack of experience, which leads to excessive talking by the nurse; preoccupation with personal thoughts; or lack of practice (Stuart & Laraia, 2001). The importance of focusing on the individual's needs and concerns through effective listening is a recurrent theme in research concerning therapeutic interaction (Attree, 2001; Douglass, Sowell, & Phillips, 2003; McCabe, 2004; Moyle, 2003).

Flexibility

Flexibility is a balance between control and permissiveness. In overcontrol, every message is monitored. In exaggerated permissiveness, anything can be communicated in any way. For communication to be functional, rules are needed about what is appropriate, without rigid prescriptions that inhibit meaningful interchange. For example, the guideline that nurses will not answer questions concerning intimate details of their lives sets an appropriate limit; however, this does not mean that nurses should refuse to answer any question about themselves.

Silence

Silence between people is often uncomfortable for the nurse who is somewhat insecure about what should occur during a therapeutic encounter. However, silence can be beneficial when used carefully. When seeking a verbal response, silence can be perceived as a lack of interest. At other times, silence allows patients to reflect on what is being discussed or experienced, lets them know that the nurse is willing to wait until they are ready to say more, or simply provides them with comfort and support. Each situation needs evaluation and sensitivity. Rather than asking a flurry of questions to break the silence, the nurse should allow the person time to decide when to comment or should make brief comments that do not demand answers, such as "It can be helpful to take time to think about what we've been discussing." Also, comments such as "Try putting your thoughts or feelings into words" can help the person to share these thoughts or feelings when silence is blocking rather than improving the communication.

Humor

Humor is part of being human; it relieves tension, reduces aggression, and creates a climate of sharing. Humor can block communication when it is used to avoid subjects that might be uncomfortable or when it excludes other people. Humor can also inflict emotional pain and communicate negative views or stereotypes about particular individuals or groups through teasing and jokes concerning race, ethnicity, culture, country of origin, occupation, age, gender, sexual activity, or other traits that stand out or are devalued. A direct response to the latent content or message in this type of humor is an effective way to curtail its use and minimize its effect. For example, "That kind of joke makes me very uncomfortable. I don't find it funny to describe [the specific group in question] that way, and I would like you to stop." To be helpful, the meaning of the humor must be understood and its purpose supportive to the individual. Clarification of the meaning should be used when there is doubt or concern.

Touch

Touch is an interesting means of nonverbal communication for nurses, who often touch individuals while administering care. The nurse's concern can be expressed by a gentle or soothing application of touch. Nevertheless, in some instances touch is inappropriate. For example, in interactions with individuals who have trauma histories or acute psychiatric disturbances, touch might be misinterpreted. A woman who has been raped might interpret touch during an examination as an attack. Evaluation of the context and meaning of touch to the individual is based on knowledge of that person and interpretation of feedback. Figure 4-4 illustrates appropriate use of touch.

Space

Space between communicators varies according to the type of communication, the setting, and the culture. Hall (1973) researched proxemics, the use of space between communicators, and identified four zones of space commonly used

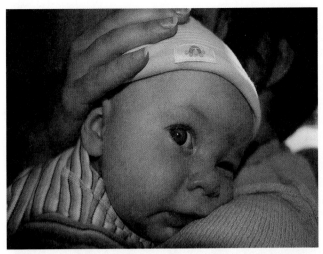

Figure 4-4   Touch is a powerful form of nonverbal communication. (Courtesy Boston College.)

Box **4-5**	Zones of Space Common to Interaction in North America

1. *Intimate space:* up to 18 inches (45.5 centimeters); used for high interpersonal sensory stimulation (Figure 4-5, *A*)
2. *Personal space:* 18 inches to 4 feet (45.5 centimeters to 1.2 meters); appropriate for close relationships in which touching may be involved and good visualization is desired (Figure 4-5, *B*)
3. *Social-consultative space:* 9 to 12 feet (2.7 to 3.6 meters); less intimate and personal, requiring louder verbal communication (Figure 4-5, *C*)
4. *Public space:* 12 feet (3.6 meters) and over; appropriately used for formal gatherings, such as giving speeches (Figure 4-5, *D*)

Based on data from Hall, E. (1973). *The silent language.* Garden City, NY: Doubleday/Anchor Press.

in interaction in North America that are presented in Box 4-5.

Understanding the appropriate distance for a given type of interaction helps the nurse to make nonverbal and verbal communication congruent and to avoid violating spatial norms (Schuster, 2000). Awareness of cultural customs concerning distance is important in shaping communication and interpreting the behavior of others. When people from different cultures or groups communicate, there may be discomfort about the acceptable distance between them when speaking. Recognition of differences helps the nurse adjust the distance and interpret the meaning of this nonverbal communication.

Many traits and components discussed in this chapter characterize functional communication. However, communication is a subtle and intricate process. Communication cannot be reduced to a set of parts and principles; its roles and nuances are far more complex and variable. To communicate by language and symbols is a special human ability. Healthy communication enables people to move from being alone to being together—clearly one of the crucial tasks of living. Effective communication is also the foundation for the helping relationship.

THE HELPING OR THERAPEUTIC RELATIONSHIP

A **helping or therapeutic relationship** is a process through which one person promotes the development of another person by fostering the latter's maturation, adaptation, integration, openness, and ability to find meaning in the present situation (Peplau, 1969). The therapeutic relationship emerges from purposeful encounters characterized by effective communication. In this relationship, the nurse respects the individual's values, attends to concerns, and promotes positive change by encouraging self-expression, exploring behavior patterns and outcomes, and promoting self-help (Moyle, 2003). This helping relationship is created by the

Box **4-6**	Characteristics Associated With Therapeutic Effectiveness

- Self-awareness and self-reflection
- Openness
- Self-confidence and strength
- Genuineness
- Concern for the individual
- Respect for the individual
- Knowledge
- Ability to empathize
- Sensitivity
- Acceptance
- Creativity
- Ability to focus and confront

nurse's application of scientific knowledge, his or her understanding of human behavior and communication, and his or her commitment to the individual. The therapeutic relationship is the foundation of clinical nursing practice—the essential element of care with every individual in every situation. Techniques, technology, interventions, and contexts vary, but the relational aspect of nursing practice produces a cohesive unity, allowing each nurse to see people holistically and as unique individuals.

No perfect profile or personality of a helping person exists. However, certain traits can be nurtured without thwarting the nurse's unique personality. These characteristics enable the nurse to be an agent of therapeutic care (Peplau, 1963; Stuart & Laraia, 2001). Box 4-6 lists characteristics associated with therapeutic effectiveness.

Characteristics of the Therapeutic Relationship

No recipe is available for a successful therapeutic relationship. Techniques and concepts serve only as tools. As a

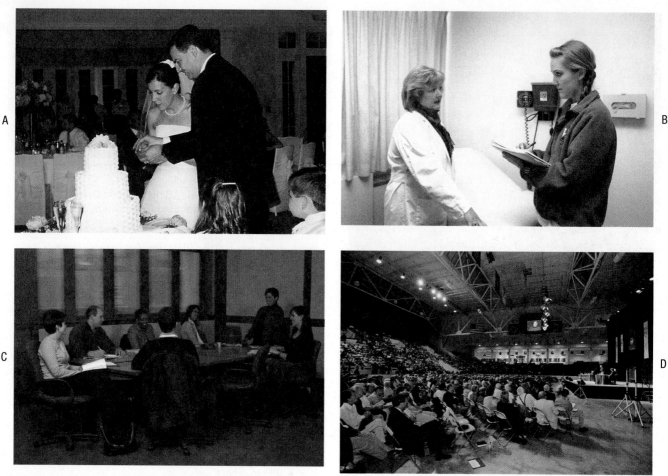

Figure 4-5 **A,** Intimate distance communication. **B,** Personal distance communication. **C,** Social-consultative distance communication. **D,** Public distance communication. (**B–D** courtesy Boston College.)

nurse develops and evaluates a helping relationship, the following guidelines may be useful.

Purposeful Communication

Purposeful communication means that the nurse focuses communication for a particular aim. Social chitchat, communication without a goal, should not make up the bulk of therapeutic interaction. This does not mean that the nurse should never discuss a social topic; nonetheless, there should be some purpose. For example, discussing the weather with a somewhat disoriented elderly individual serves the purpose of orienting that person to the environment. Goals guide the nurse in focusing communication.

Rapport

Rapport is a harmony and an affinity between people in a relationship (Rogers, 1965). The nurse is responsible for establishing an atmosphere in which rapport can develop, by using many of the traits listed for a helping person. To let the person know that his or her concerns interest the nurse and that working together may alleviate some of his or her difficulties and encourage growth, it is important to be genuine, open, and concerned.

Trust

Trust is a necessary component of any helping relationship. Trust is the reliance on a person to carry out responsibilities and promises, based on a sense of safety, honesty, and reliability. Trust is an important component of partnership (Gallant et al., 2002). The nurse promotes trust by modeling and structuring the relationship appropriately. Strategies that promote trust include:

- Trusting the individual to do as promised
- Clearly defining the relationship parameters and expectations, particularly the purpose and specifics of time, place, and anticipated behavior
- Being consistent
- Examining behaviors that interfere with trust

Empathy

Empathy is the ability to understand another's feelings without losing personal identity and perspective. Empathic nurses draw on emotions and experiences that enable them to place themselves in the other person's situation. As the person's sense that the nurse is understanding and accepting increases, the individual's distress decreases. Outcome from research studies are building knowledge about the role that empathic nursing care plays in outcomes. For example, Moyle (2003) conducted a phenomenological study to explore the experience of being nurtured while depressed. Interviews with hospitalized participants revealed the importance of nursing presence that included spending time listening and assisting participants to discuss problems, fears, and anxieties. Furthermore, participants described their disappointment when nurses distanced themselves by attending only to physical needs and by limiting contact.

Nurses can learn behavioral approaches that enhance empathic relations with people through supervised experiential learning. For example, nurses do not empathize by switching the focus of the interaction to themselves or by sympathizing (e.g., "I know exactly how you feel; that happened to me once"). Rather, they use clinical and personal experience to appreciate the individual's feelings and experiences. Using personal understanding while maintaining boundaries is the essence of empathy in the helping relationship. With empathic understanding, the nurse acknowledges the affective domain of personal experiences and uses this knowledge to appreciate the person's reactions. Empathy enables the listener to share human experiences as the basis for providing care.

Goal Direction

A helping relationship is special in its goal-directed nature. Although most human relationships focus on mutual benefit, a helping relationship exists solely to meet some need or to promote the growth of the recipient. Although the nurse may benefit from the interaction, the relationship is centered on the recipient.

Goals are formulated as desired individual behaviors. Short-term goals are likely to be achieved within 10 days to 2 weeks; all other goals are long term. All goals should be stated in measurable terms and should focus on a positive change or on the decrease of problematic behavior. Ideally, a person works with the nurse to establish goals. However, some individuals, such as those who are seriously ill, depressed, psychotic, or cognitively impaired, are unable to establish goals. When an individual is unable to negotiate appropriate goals, the nurse establishes realistic goals and shares them with the person, who is free to participate or to reject efforts to reach these goals.

Ethics in Communicating and Relating

Ethical decision making is closely linked with the goal-directed nature of helping relationships. Ethical issues are present in human interactions whenever behavior may affect others, whenever actions involve conscious choices of methods and ends, and whenever actions can be evaluated in reference to standards of right and wrong (Johannesen, 2002). Guidelines that may be adapted as ethical standards for interpersonal communication are highlighted in Box 4-7.

Frequently the nurse may wish to set goals that the individual does not want to reach; the nurse must remember

---

Box 4-7 Guidelines for Ethical Interpersonal Communication

Ethical interpersonal communication involves:
- Being aware and open to changing concepts of self and others
- Attending to role responsibilities; individual sacrifice, when it is required to make a "good" decision; and emotions, while guarding against letting emotions be the sole guide of our behavior
- Sharing personal views candidly and clearly
- Communicating information accurately, with minimal loss or distortion of intended meaning
- Communicating verbal and nonverbal messages with congruent meanings
- Sharing responsibility for the consequences among communicators
- Recognizing the multicultural context of all communication
- Respecting the dignity of every person
- Avoiding coercion and use of power in communicating
- Being sensitive to gender and cultural contexts of communication and interpretation
- Eliminating any elements of your communication that denigrate, stereotype, or devalue

Unethical communication involves:
- Purposefully deceiving
- Intentionally blocking communication, for example, changing subjects when the other person has not finished communicating, cutting a person off, or distracting others from the subject under discussion
- Scapegoating or unnecessarily condemning others
- Lying or deceiving that causes intentional or unintentional harm
- Verbally "hitting below the belt" by taking advantage of another's vulnerability

Modified from Bosek, M. S. D. (2002). Ethics in practice: Effective communication skills. *JONA's Healthcare Law, Ethics, and Regulation, 4*(4), 93-97; Johannesen, R. L. (2002). *Ethics in human communication* (5th ed.). Prospect Heights, IL: Waveland Press.

---

that the problem belongs to the person, as does the choice of care alternatives. The nurse assists the individual in decision making, with the decision based on the individual's value system. However, the nurse should not take a laissez-faire approach and avoid assisting the person. The nurse's responsibility is to help the individual to examine values, identify conflicts, and prioritize goals and desired health care outcomes. Action follows from understanding values and the best available information. Both the individual and the nurse must bring interpreted facts and personally clarified values to the interaction to establish goals. Recognizing this interplay, the nurse must clarify personal values, subsequently respect the individual's rights, and act to support and protect the integrity of the person and the family.

Therapeutic Techniques

Occasionally, clinicians who are novices in establishing helping relationships assume that they are bound to "say the wrong thing" and cause terrible damage to the person, or that they will learn some magical phrases and questions to create instant rapport. No nurse or other professional is so powerful that a "wrong word" will destroy the individual's self-concept or self-esteem. Even people with physical and emotional problems are resilient and have coped, at least to some degree, with a lifetime of stresses. Alternatively, no magical saying exists that the nurse can always plug into an interaction to communicate successfully. Although some techniques often are useful, they must be applied with purpose, skill, and attention to the individuality of each person and to the context of the interaction. The following techniques therefore should be viewed as guidelines, rather than prescriptions, for effective shaping of the therapeutic relationship.

Focus on the Individual

The first step to therapeutic communication is focusing on the individual and why the interaction is occurring. The nurse is not the focus; the person is. Although an overly businesslike style fails to communicate concern and support (Moyle, 2003), delving into one's own personal life to the extent that it diverts attention from the other person's concern also is problematic. Avoiding nurse-directed conversation can be difficult; a useful rule of thumb is to answer or respond to obvious questions and to switch the focus back to clinical concerns when other questions are asked. For example:

Individual (looks at female nurse's wedding ring): "Are you married?"

Nurse: "Yes, I am."

Individual: "What does your husband do for a living?"

Nurse: "Rather than get distracted by a discussion about me, let's get back to planning how you will manage at work."

Keeping focus on the person's concerns includes identifying the portion of the message that is clear and relevant to the purpose of the interaction, seeking validation, and helping the individual to clarify the rest of the message.

Help the Individual to Describe and Clarify Content and Meaning

Too often the nurse rushes to offer an interpretation of the nature of the problem and quickly follows up by suggesting a solution. Solving problems efficiently makes the nurse feel effective, important, and powerful; however, the person's needs may not be met. A crucial step in using the therapeutic relationship effectively is to assist the individual to describe a particular experience or concern. Description is enhanced when the nurse prompts the person to clarify the description and interpret its meaning.

Use of who, what, where, and when questions helps the person to clarify and expand the content and meaning of what is communicated. Phrases such as "tell me," "go on," "describe to me," "explain it to me," and "give me an example" also are likely to elicit description of important content and to diminish distracting generalizations and

abstractions. By seeking feedback, the nurse helps the individual to explain the meaning further. In clarifying, the nurse should avoid threatening, detective-like questions. Questions that begin with "why" often increase the person's anxiety because they demand reasons, conclusions, analysis, or causes (Peplau, 1964). Reformulating questions to obtain data first and then helping the individual to analyze links among events, thoughts, feelings, actions, and outcomes is generally a more helpful approach.

A problem-solving approach by the nurse assists the person to describe and clarify the content and meaning of experience. Sequential steps help the individual to explain events, to change circumstances and responses that interfere with health, and to solve problems (O'Toole & Welt, 1989; Peplau, 1963). This problem-solving approach can be adapted for use in health promotion to assist the person in problem solving by working through the steps outlined in the Health Teaching box. These steps are a useful guideline for keeping the focus of concern on the individual and his or her definition of the problem. Rather than telling the person what is wrong and how to fix it, the nurse's primary goal is helping the person to describe the problem and formulate solutions in partnership.

Use Reflection

Reflection is the restatement of what the individual has said in the same or different words. This technique can involve paraphrasing or summarizing the person's main point to indicate interest and to focus the discussion. Effective use of this approach does not include frequent, parrotlike repetition of the individual's statements. Instead, reflection is the selective paraphrasing or literal repetition of the person's words to underscore the importance of what has been said, to summarize a main concern or theme, or to elicit elaborated information.

Use Constructive Confrontation

Confronting an individual means that the nurse points out a specific behavior and then helps the person to examine meaning or consequences of the behavior. For example:

Nurse: "You missed your appointment for the consultation we had scheduled."

Individual: "Oh, I didn't notice the date."

Nurse: "You are usually very aware of time and appointments. What do you think was going on with you that you didn't notice the date this time?"

This type of confrontation is not an angry exchange, but a purposeful way of helping the person examine personal actions and their meaning.

Use Nouns and Pronouns Correctly

Some individuals have difficulty separating themselves from others or specifying the object or subject in their language. These individuals misuse pronouns by referring to we, us, they, she, he, him, and her, without clearly identifying the referent, and by making vague statements such as "They

HEALTH TEACHING   Steps in Promoting Problem Solving

Describe the experience or event of concern.

Helpful Verbal Nursing Strategies:

"Tell me what happened." "Describe the experience to me."

Analyze the parts of the experience and see relationships to other events.

Helpful Verbal Nursing Strategies:

"What meaning does this have for you?" "What pattern is there?"

Formulate the problem.

Helpful Verbal Nursing Strategies:

"In what way is this problematic?" "What do you want to see changed?"

Validate the formulation.

Helpful Verbal Nursing Strategies:

"Do you mean . . . ?" "Let me tell you what I understand you to be saying."

Use the formulation to identify ways to solve or manage the difficulty.

Helpful Verbal Nursing Strategies:

"What would you do the next time?" "In what way has your view changed?" "What actions are needed to solve the problem that you've identified?"

Try out the solutions, judge the outcomes, and adjust the plan accordingly.

Helpful Nursing Strategies:

Encourage application in new situations through role playing or through practice in appropriate settings; assist the individual to cycle through the above sequence as needed to evaluate the outcome and make adjustments to the plan.

Modified from Peplau, H. E. (1963). Process and concept of learning. In S. Burd & M. Marshall (Eds.), *Some clinical approaches to psychiatric nursing* (pp. 348-352). New York: Macmillan.

don't like me. They told me I was useless." Others may use general nouns, such as everyone, people, doctors, and nurses, to avoid clear communication about specific persons. The nurse can clarify by asking, "Who are they?" or "To whom are you referring?" Additionally, the nurse must be careful to use separate pronouns when speaking of herself or himself and the individual, particularly when the patient has disordered thinking. For example, when communicating with an individual who is confused or exhibits disordered thinking, the nurse should say you and I, rather than us or we, to promote clear thinking and communication and to assist the individual to maintain personal boundaries (Peplau, 1963).

Use Silence

Allowing a thoughtful silence at intervals helps the individual to talk at his or her own pace without pressure to perform for the nurse. Silence also permits time for reflection. Particularly helpful to the depressed or physically ill person, silence can reduce pressure and conserve energy. After several moments, the nurse can ask the person to share some thoughts. For example, "Try putting your thoughts into words," "Tell me what are you thinking or feeling now," or "I'll be here when you feel ready to talk."

Accept Communication

Acceptance of the person's mode of communication is an important ingredient in a helping relationship. Allowing the person to communicate verbally and nonverbally in a personal fashion promotes feelings of safety and respect. Nevertheless, acceptance of communication does not mean that the nurse always agrees with the individual or tolerates inappropriate behavior within the established limits of the setting, such as verbal or physical abuse. Rather, accepting

communication involves effective use of patient-centered communication, as described earlier in this chapter. Box 4-4 presents specific strategies associated with patient-centered communication.

Barriers to Effective Communication

Barriers to effective communication can originate with the nurse, the individual, or both. The most obvious barrier is the nurse's failure to use the types of therapeutic techniques just described. Lack of knowledge or experience can limit the nurse's ability to assess the individual's needs and repertoire of skills. Supervision and study can help the nurse apply the steps of the nursing process by using effective intervention approaches.

Communication is also ineffective when some part of the communication–feedback loop breaks down. Failure to send a clear message, receive and interpret the message correctly, or provide useful feedback can interfere with communication. Diagnosing the source of the communication breakdown, taking steps to correct it, and using knowledge of the communication process and appropriate therapeutic techniques are the nurse's responsibility.

Anxiety

When the nurse or individual is highly anxious during an interaction, perception is altered and the ability to communicate effectively is curtailed sharply. Defense mechanisms, such as denial, projection, and displacement, reduce anxiety at the expense of understanding the true meaning of an interaction. Severe anxiety and defense mechanisms distort reality and lead to disordered communication. To enhance interpersonal communication, the nurse identifies the feeling of anxiety and its source and uses anxiety-reducing interventions.

MULTICULTURAL AWARENESS

Multicultural Context of Communication

As health care providers, nurses might believe that they have expert knowledge about health promotion and the treatment of illness that will be beneficial to others. Therefore it seems logical that nurses would select appropriate information to share with individuals to help them maintain health and manage illness or alterations in health status. However, consider the possible influences of cultural differences between the nurse and individual.

Much of the knowledge generated from nursing-related disciplines and the sciences is rooted in a Western perspective. Particularly in the United States, knowledge is developed and interpreted from the perspective of the dominant cultural group, a white, Anglo-Saxon, Christian point of view. When this perspective remains unexamined, alternative perspectives are ignored and invisible. Nurses who are members of the dominant cultural group may be well-intentioned, but ineffective, when they attempt to engage a person of a different cultural group in a relationship without questioning how culture influences interactions, interpretations of events and information, and beliefs and values concerning health and health care practices. Preconceived ideas about people based on some characteristic or group affiliation, such as racial or ethnic identity, religion, country of origin, gender, or sexual orientation, can interfere with nurses' abilities to relate to people as individuals. At the same time, a lack of knowledge of other cultural groups hampers nurses' understanding of the individual's point of view.

Guidelines for recognizing the multicultural context of communication in therapeutic relationships include the following:
- Make ethnocultural assessment a critical component of every clinical evaluation.
- Allow other people to define themselves.
- Respect the language of others and do not assume superiority in language.
- Collaborate with trained translators and health promoters (people with the same ethnic or racial background as the individuals).
- Avoid use of racist, sexist, ageist, and other forms of denigrating language.
- Do not perpetuate stereotypes in communication.
- Adapt communication to the uniqueness of the individual.
- Reject humor that degrades members based on gender, race, ethnicity, religion, sexual orientation, country of origin, and so forth.

- Respect the rights of others to have different practices and customs.
- Do not allow injustice to continue through silence.
- Present information clearly to all people to help them make informed choices.
- Do not judge values, traditions, and practices based on their similarity or difference from personal values, traditions, and practices, but based on whether they facilitate human potential.

The following are some issues for the nurse to consider:
- When the nurse works with a person from a different cultural background, what are common barriers to establishing a therapeutic relationship?
- In learning about different cultural groups, is there a risk of creating new stereotypes that interfere with the ability to treat people as unique individuals?
- If the nurse has little or no knowledge about a person's culture, how can the nurse provide meaningful nursing care?
- Are the two previous questions contradictory? How can the nurse meet the different challenges that they imply?
- Research measurements typically are developed from the perspective of the dominant culture. If the nurse wishes to use a standardized instrument to measure clinical or research variables among members of different cultural groups, then what questions about the instrument should the nurse ask, and what problems might the nurse encounter? What would need to be done to determine whether or not an instrument truly measures the same phenomenon across different populations?
- Consider the possible influences of cultural differences between the nurse and the individual. Think of an example of two people from different cultural groups who developed a relationship. Examine how they got to know each other and what differences and similarities they uncovered. Did barriers to understanding each other exist? If so, how did they bridge these barriers? What did they learn about themselves? What did they learn about the ways that culture shapes perspective and interactions? Think about how a nurse can apply these insights to his or her relationships with people from cultural groups that differ from their own.
- How would a multicultural perspective change the practice?

Guidelines developed by the author and modified from information from Johannesen, R. L. (2002). *Ethics in human communication* (5th ed.). Prospect Heights, IL: Waveland Press; Robinson, M. (2002). *Communication and health in a multi-ethnic society.* Bristol, UK: Policy Press.

Attitudes

Biases and stereotypes can limit the nurse's and individual's ability to relate. When the difficulty is the individual's problem, the nurse can assist by examining those views that interfere with the person's relationships. When the problem is the nurse's, openness in the supervisory relationship to examination of personal behavior is crucial. When the nurse fails to examine his or her attitudes toward the person, negativity may be communicated and perceptions of the interaction may be distorted.

Gaps Between Nurse and Individual

Related to attitudinal barriers, differences in gender, age, socioeconomic background, ethnicity, race, religion, or language can block functional communication between the nurse and individual. These factors can cause differences in perception and block mutual understanding. Newly licensed nurses have attributed communication problems to differences in language proficiency among nurses, including English as a second language, as well as to problems in understanding non–English-speaking individuals (Smith

& Crawford, 2004). To reduce such gaps, nurses can question unclear verbal or written communications, seek clarification or assistance from translators, and explore how perceptions may be different and how to clarify meanings (Bosek, 2002). (See Multicultural Awareness box and Chapter 2).

Resistance

Resistance comprises all phenomena that inhibit the flow of thoughts, feelings, and memories in an interpersonal encounter and behaviors that interfere with therapeutic goals. Resistance arises from anxiety when a person feels threatened. To reduce this anxiety, the person implements resistant behavior, most often in the form of avoidance, such as being late, changing the subject, forgetting, blocking, or becoming angry.

Initially, the nurse should identify the behavior, whether it is the nurse's or the individual's behavior, and then attempt to interpret it in the context of the interaction. Exploration of possible threats in the relationship, goals, or a particular topic can lead to understanding the source of the resistance and finding the ability to handle these difficulties. Anxiety reduction is often a necessary step in dealing with resistant behavior.

Transference and Countertransference

Transference is reacting to another person in an exchange as though that person were someone from the past. Transference may involve a host of feelings that generally are classified as positive (love, affection, or regard) or negative (anger, dislike, or frustration). Typical transference reactions involve an important figure from the past such as a mother or father; however, at times transference may be more general to include all authority figures. Something about another person's characteristics, behavior, or position, in combination with individual dynamics, triggers this response. People in a therapeutic relationship often develop strong transference feelings toward the helping professional, arising from the interaction's intensity and the care provider's authoritative or nurturing role. To work with a patient's transference reactions effectively, the nurse first helps the person to examine feelings and thoughts about the nurse. Then the nurse assists the patient to compare and contrast the nurse with people from patient's past to remove distortions and comprehend the present reality.

Countertransference basically is the same phenomenon, but it is experienced by the health care professional rather than the patient. The nurse experiences many feelings toward the patient; these feelings are not problematic, unless they remain unanalyzed and block the nurse's ability to work effectively with the individual. For example, if a nurse has strong feelings for the patient and thinks that the person cannot possibly function after discharge without the nurse's aid, then the nurse is likely to distort the patient's abilities, encourage a childlike dependency, and interfere with the patient's progress. This nurse needs to examine such personal feelings to understand their source. Once understood, countertransference reactions generally cease to interfere with the relationship. Consultation with an advanced practice psychiatric nurse is recommended whenever transference or countertransference reactions are persistent and problematic.

Sensory Barriers

When the individual has sensory limitations, the nurse may need to use extra skill in communicating. Use of the other senses to send or receive messages should be attempted. Special help is often available from trained therapists and teachers; for example, many agencies have access to interpreters for deaf people, and visual aides may be useful. Nurses must be as creative as possible, learn from others who are skilled in alternative forms of communication, and make referrals as necessary.

Failure to Address Concerns or Needs

Failure to meet the individual's needs or to recognize the individual's concerns is the most serious barrier to effective interaction. This failure can arise from (1) inadequate assessment, (2) lack of knowledge, (3) inability to separate the nurse's needs from the individual's needs, and (4) confusion between friendship and a helping relationship, including unrecognized or unresolved sexual issues. To correct this problem, the nurse should recognize that a barrier to relating with the person exists. Using the supervisory process to determine the problem's source, the nurse should then take corrective action, such as obtaining more information or knowledge, performing a self-assessment with values clarification, and examining reactions, biases, and expectations.

Setting

The setting of a therapeutic interaction can affect the goals and the nature of the communication. The most important aspect of any setting is that the nurse and individual are able to attend to each other. The nurse's attention to the person helps create this atmosphere. The nurse should assess the influence of factors such as lighting, noise, temperature, comfort, physical distance, and privacy; potentially disturbing factors can be altered or controlled within the limits of the setting. Occasionally the nurse has only minimal control over the setting, as in a busy clinic, health center, inpatient unit, or the individual's home. Although far from the ideal of a quiet, pleasant, well-lit private office, these typical clinical settings can be used effectively by creating a sense of private space. Curtains can be drawn, doors shut, and two chairs pulled to a corner to shape an environment for interaction. When possible, however, nurses should seek offices or rooms to establish privacy during significant communication or when imparting important or complex health information. The nurse can also acknowledge verbally that some aspect of the environment, such as an interruption or noise, is bothersome. This strategy shows people that the nurse recognizes possible concentration difficulties and is sharing the environment with them.

| Box **4-8** | Key Topics of Discussion During the Orientation or Introductory Phase of the Therapeutic Relationship |

- What to call each other
- Purpose of meeting
- Location, time, and length of meetings
- Termination date or time for review of progress through follow-up
- Confidentiality (with whom clinical data will be shared)
- Any other limits related to the particular setting

Stages

Therapeutic relationships follow sequential phases, which may overlap, vary in length, or involve issues that appear over time rather than in a set sequence. Orientation (introductory), working, and termination phases have been identified by researchers and clinicians.

Originally these **relationship stages** were identified from clinical interactions that developed over a prolonged period of time. However, they can be observed in brief encounters that are effective; that is, interactions that meet individuals' needs rather than therapeutic interactions that have been reduced to little more than quick question-and-answer sessions. Whether the nurse is engaged in a long-term or short-term relationship with an individual, attention to the relationship stages is important. Brief therapeutic relationships will telescope the stages; therefore, it is particularly important that the nurse focus on meeting the key demands of each relationship phase. It is important to note that individuals may move in and out of direct care episodes while a therapeutic relationship is maintained over a longer period. A relationship exists even when the nurse and individual do not see each other for an extended period, and each encounter takes place within the trajectory of the relationship stages.

Orientation or Introductory Phase

The orientation or introductory phase begins when the nurse and individual meet. This meeting typically involves some feeling of anxiety; neither party knows what to expect. When the therapeutic relationship is primarily a counseling type of relationship, part of the nurse's role is to help structure the interaction by discussing several topics during the initial and sometimes during first few meetings. Box 4-8 lists topics appropriate to this phase. Discussion of these issues establishes a contract or pact and involves a mutual understanding of the parameters of the relationship and an agreement to work together.

The orientation stage is a critical juncture in any therapeutic relationship. Without successful transition through the orientation phase, no working alliance will exist and treatment goals will remain unmet. In a descriptive qualitative study of nurses' perceptions of their therapeutic relationships, Forchuck and colleagues (2000) identified helpful factors during the orientation phase: consistency, pacing, listening, positive initial impressions, and attention

to comfort and control. In contrast, factors that hamper relationships include inconsistency, unavailability, individual factors associated with trust, nurses' feelings about the other person, confrontation of delusions, and unrealistic expectations.

When the therapeutic relationship is not primarily structured as counseling with a specific number of sessions, the orientation phase may appear less distinct and the topics noted may seem irrelevant. In this case, the nurse can adapt the suggested topics to meet the specific situation. However, except in true emergencies, initial encounters should always include introductions by name, discussion of the purpose, and a plan for ongoing care or specific follow-up.

Working Phase

The working phase of the therapeutic relationship emerges when the nurse and the individual collaborate as partners in promoting the person's health. The working phase may last for an established number of sessions, as in brief psychotherapy, or it may extend over a longer period if the nurse is the primary care provider for an individual or family. During the working phase, the relationship is the context through which change takes place. Goals are set, and the nurse and individual work mutually toward their accomplishment. Interventions are tailored to the specific situation and health needs of the person and family. Solving problems, coping with stressors, and gaining insight are all part of the working phase. The nurse and individual recognize each other's uniqueness.

Resistant behaviors may be observed during this phase as the nurse and individual become closer and work on potentially anxiety-producing problems. The person may pull away through the use of defense mechanisms, because change can be difficult. Overcoming the resistance becomes an important nursing task.

Termination Phase

Termination marks the end of the relationship established in the therapeutic contract or negotiated in accordance with the limits of the contract. Ending a relationship can cause anxiety for both the individual and the nurse. Termination represents a loss; therefore, it can trigger feelings of sadness, frustration, and anger. Termination in this case is the loss of a relationship and the loss of future involvement, with its attendant realistic expectations or fantasies. Termination also reawakens feelings of previously unresolved losses, such as a death or divorce.

Working through any feelings related to termination is an important part of clinical care. Some individuals require the nurse's assistance to experience the feelings of loss and to connect present reactions to past real or symbolic losses. Box 4-9 lists additional interventions for use during the termination phase.

Both the nurse and the individual can learn much during termination; the process directs both participants to examine problems and progress in the relationship, feelings, and reactions. The experience also helps the nurse and individual

Box **4-9**	Interventions for Use During the Termination Phase of the Therapeutic Relationship

1. Let the patient know why the relationship is to be terminated.
2. Remind the patient of the date and how many meetings or appointments are left.
3. Collaborate with other staff so that they are aware of how the patient is reacting and any special needs that the patient may have.
4. Help the patient to identify sources of support and other people with whom a relationship is possible.
5. Review the gains and the remaining goals.
6. Discuss the pros and cons experienced during the relationship to help the patient to develop a realistic appraisal.
7. Make referrals for follow-up care as needed.

Box **4-10**	Key Ingredients for a 15-Minute Family Interview

1. Use manners to engage or reengage. Make an introduction by offering your name and role. Orient family members to the purpose of a brief family interview.
2. Assess significant areas of internal and external structure and function (obtain genogram-basic family composition information, and external support data).
3. Ask family members three key questions.
4. Commend the family on one or two strengths.
5. Evaluate usefulness and conclude.

gain practice in ending relationships and in exploring reactions, which can be most helpful when future losses occur.

Brief Interactions

Time constraints in practice are unavoidable. Although challenging, brief therapeutic encounters can be meaningful and useful. Limited time is not a valid reason to avoid interviewing or interacting with individuals. Rather, nurses purposefully can structure brief interactions to achieve specific clinical outcomes (Wright & Leahey, 2000). Box 4-10 delineates key ingredients for a **15-minute interview** with a family.

These guidelines for brief interactions with families can be adapted for interviews with individuals. An effective 15-minute interview is feasible if nurses plan to introduce themselves, state the purpose of meeting, validate understanding with the person or family, clarify parameters such as time, focus and listen, and elicit significant individual and family data. Most importantly, the goal of the interaction must be realistic and clearly defined. For example, the purpose may be to elicit a family's view of the problem for which the patient has sought care or to prioritize problems to be treated. Even when time is limited, the interview is structured to provide an opportunity for the person or family to engage in dialogue as an active participant in care, and the nurse's attention is completely focused on the individual.

Health Literacy

Clear communication improves the quality of health care encounters. **Health literacy,** the capacity to read, comprehend, and follow through on health information, is a critical component of health promotion. Yet, nearly half of American adults do not understand basic health information. This level of low health literacy costs an estimated $58 to $73 billion annually (Ask me 3. IOM report on health literacy, n.d.; Health care coalition promotes clear communication, 2004). To combat low health literacy, nurses can

encourage patients to ask three essential questions at every health visit:

"What is my main problem?"

"What do I need to do?"

"Why is it important for me to do this?" (Ask me 3. Tips for clear communication, n.d.).

Nurses also promote health literacy by creating a safe and comfortable environment, sitting down to establish eye contact rather than standing when communicating, using visual aids and models to illustrate conditions and procedures, and verifying understanding of care instructions by having patients teach the content back (Health care coalition promotes clear communication, 2004). The Case Study presents a detailed scenario of a home visit between a nurse and a patient and questions related to how the nurse can develop a therapeutic relationship with the patient. The Care Plan presents a plan of care for the patient, including communication interventions.

SUMMARY

Relating to patients offers many challenges and rewards for nurses. Although some aspects of this work are predictable, each person and family is unique and provides a chance for the nurse to learn, grow, and help in new ways. This chapter provides guidelines for developing therapeutic relationships, but these guidelines do not guarantee success or an easy job. The desire and skill of the individual nurse bring this information to life. The blend of the nurse's artistry, humanity, knowledge, skill, and ethics sparks concern and the ability to help another human being communicate effectively—essential components of the nurse-patient relationship.

The therapeutic relationship is the primary arena for health promotion. Values clarification, communication, and the helping relationship are its core components. Applying this knowledge to their varied nursing roles is essential to promoting health and providing quality care.

Rising use of technology and mounting pressures for cost-effective care are here to stay. In this climate, the importance of the therapeutic relationship is underscored (Hot Topics box). Without a relational context, the care

CASE STUDY

A Health-Promotion Visit

As part of a health-promotion visit for Maria Sanchez-Smith and Thomas, her 2-week-old infant, Jessica Mills, a registered nurse, planned to conduct an infant assessment, provide breast-feeding support, teach about normal infant development and care activities, and assess Mrs. Sanchez-Smith's adaptation to motherhood and her postpartum recovery status. Before the visit, Ms. Mills reviewed the clinical information she obtained during Mrs. Sanchez-Smith's hospitalization. Mrs. Sanchez-Smith is a 34-year-old Hispanic, primiparous woman who delivered a 7-pound, 10-ounce healthy boy after a 12-hour labor. The labor had progressed well without complication. Mrs. Sanchez-Smith received epidural anesthesia at 6-centimeters dilation and the baby was delivered vaginally. Her husband, Mark Smith, provided labor support and was present for the delivery. After a 2-day hospital stay, Mrs. Sanchez-Smith was discharged. At discharge, the infant was breast-feeding, had normal newborn examination findings, and weighed 7 pounds, 5 ounces. Ms. Mills had been impressed by both parents' preparation for the birth. They had attended childbirth classes and read several books about infant development and parenting. Mrs. Sanchez-Smith planned to take an 8-week maternity leave from her position as a lawyer in a large practice and had arranged for a childcare provider to come to the family's home to take care of the infant beginning 2 weeks before the end of her maternity leave. Mr. Smith had not planned to take time off from his job, because he had recently been promoted to a high-level managerial position in his company that required increased travel and time at work. He was able to postpone a business trip to be present at the delivery and had sent a plane ticket to his mother-in-law so she could come and stay at their home during the first week after Mrs. Sanchez-Smith and Thomas were discharged from the hospital.

During the visit, Ms. Mills first assessed the infant. She incorporated teaching concerning normal infant development and concluded that Thomas was a healthy 2-week-old infant who was feeding well. Jacob's circumcision was healing without complication and he had regained his birth weight.

When Ms. Mills asked how Mrs. Sanchez-Smith was doing, Mrs. Sanchez-Smith hesitated and then responded, "I'm not sure. I'm very glad that Thomas is doing well . . . but I worry sometimes that I'm not going to be able to do everything right for him. It's funny, but I've spent so many years getting an education and establishing my law career. It was hard work, but I managed to do well. Now a little infant overwhelms me. I don't know how I'll manage this." When Ms. Mills asked Mrs. Sanchez-Smith to talk more about her concerns, Mrs. Sanchez-Smith described how incompetent she felt while her mother was staying with her. "My mother could do everything so easily. I fumbled with every diaper. It felt like she criticized how I did things. When she told me about what she did when she had children, I felt pushed to do things 'her way' and not the way that I had planned. She even wanted to give him a bottle when I was trying so hard to get breast-feeding going. At least the doctor said Thomas had gained enough weight. Thomas' weight gain made me feel like I wasn't a total failure. I couldn't wait for her to go, but I fell apart after she left. I was alone. Mark is out of town until the weekend, and I couldn't get Thomas to stop crying yesterday. I thought I would scream so I put him down in his crib and I just sat there crying. What's wrong with me? I've never felt so out of control before. I want to be a good mother, but I feel like I can't give any more right now."

In response to Ms. Mills' follow-up questions about mental status, Mrs. Sanchez-Smith described frequently feeling irritated and sad, crying a few times over the last several days, difficulty sleeping even when the baby was asleep, feeling fatigued, and being worried about how she would be able to go back to work in only a few weeks. Ms. Mills also inquired about the family's cultural, ethnic, and religious backgrounds. Mrs. Sanchez-Smith responded, "Interesting that you should ask. That's actually another issue right now. I'm from New Mexico and my family is Hispanic and Catholic, but I'm not a practicing Catholic now. You might guess that I'm Latina from my hyphenated name. I added my maiden name to Smith when I got married to honor my family. Mark is Protestant, but not really religious. His family comes from New Jersey. They are very nice and were supportive when we got married. We were lucky that our families accepted us together. I have to admit, though, that we didn't really figure out what we would do about raising the baby. Mark thinks that we'd be hypocrites to have a Catholic christening. Plus my mother told me that I'd be selfish to go back to work so soon. Can you help me? I feel like I'm going out of my mind and I don't know what to do."

This case study raises a variety of clinical concerns. As the nurse in this encounter, Ms. Mills could begin by considering the following questions.

Reflective Questions

1. What are my feelings as I listen to her story and her distress? Am I aware of how my values and expectations affect my interaction with this person? How can I establish a therapeutic relationship to support Mrs. Sanchez-Smith during this stressful period?
2. What is the significance of the distress symptoms that Mrs. Sanchez-Smith reported? Given that the period during which many women experience postpartum blues has passed, what is the most appropriate action to obtain a thorough mental status examination for postpartum depression?
3. Who is the most appropriate health care provider to evaluate her for postpartum depression, and treat her if it is confirmed? How can I facilitate getting her the care she needs and can I remain available to her? How can I assist Mrs. Sanchez-Smith to meet the infant's developmental needs during this stressful period?
4. In what ways do family dynamics, values, and expectations related to differing cultural and religious heritages contribute to the problems described? What can I do to explore these issues further? What strengths can be harnessed? How can I engage support systems to ameliorate rather than exacerbate the difficulties? What can be done to engage both Mr. Smith and Mrs. Sanchez-Smith in a therapeutic relationship to focus on the couple and parenting concerns, and to involve both partners in treatment strategies?

CARE PLAN

Transition to Parenthood

(Related to Maria Sanchez-Smith Case Study)

Nursing Diagnosis Potential for Alteration in Parenting Related to Stress Involved in Transition to Parenthood

DEFINING CHARACTERISTICS

- Feeling overwhelmed with responsibilities of new parenthood
- Insecurity about tasks of infant care
- Crying
- Sadness
- Feeling out of control
- Difficulty sleeping even when the baby is asleep
- Worry about going back to work soon

RELATED FACTORS

- Transition from high career achievement to new role as mother
- Differing religious, ethnic, and cultural backgrounds of the two parents and extended families
- Confusion and lack of decisions about religious and cultural traditions to follow for their infant
- Conflicting expectations of extended families, particularly from Mrs. Sanchez-Smith's mother
- Job pressures on Mr. Smith to travel and be away from home
- Unanticipated social isolation for Mrs. Sanchez-Smith during this postpartum period
- Limited social support (particularly from husband due to work-associated travel)

INTERVENTIONS

- Health information is provided about normal newborn and postpartum adjustment.
- Infant care information is provided based on Mrs. Sanchez-Smith's needs.
- Expectations about postpartum adjustment and parenthood are elicited.
- Health information about postpartum depression is provided regarding prevalence and common symptoms.

- Personal and family history is conducted, with a focus on mental health.
- Postpartum depression is evaluated using interview questions and an assessment measure, such as the Edinburgh Postnatal Depression Scale (Cox, Holden, & Sagovsky, 1987), or the Postpartum Depression Screening Scale (Beck & Gable, 2001).
- If symptom levels suggest postpartum depression, a referral for mental health evaluation is made.
- Sources of social support are solicited and specific plans are made to use available support, such as husband, friends, and hired infant care providers.
- Conflicts and areas of shared values, plans, goals for raising the baby are explored.
- Pros and cons of options for raising the baby are examined in relation to religious, ethnic, and cultural considerations.
- A follow-up plan is made to reassess symptoms of postpartum depression and to discuss ongoing concerns about how to raise the baby with Mrs. Sanchez-Smith and Mr. Smith.
- Referral is made to local support and psychoeducational programs for interfaith couples.

EXPECTED OUTCOMES

- Competent mothering and infant care are displayed.
- Mrs. Sanchez-Smith describes her feelings, concerns, and needs.
- Indicators of postpartum depression are evaluated and referral for follow-up made for positive findings.
- Social supports are engaged.
- Mrs. Sanchez-Smith and Mr. Smith successfully negotiate immediate decisions about religious and cultural practice concerning their baby, and agree to use counseling services to work out decisions concerning their child's upbringing and involvement of extended family.

---

dimension in health care is lost, and health promotion is reduced to standardized, recipe-like prescriptions. Effective health promotion directed to the needs of individuals, families, and communities requires reflection on the value of caring, effective communication, and a helping relationship.

ADDITIONAL STUDY MATERIAL

Study Questions in the back of the book, see page 663.

evolve WEB SITE MATERIALS

These materials are located on the book's Web site at http://evolve.elsevier.com/Edelman/.

- WebLinks
- Content Updates

TELEHEALTH: THERAPEUTIC RELATIONSHIPS IN THE AGE OF THE INTERNET

Technological advances have produced rapid changes in communication. Automatic teller machines have replaced human tellers at banks for most routine transactions. Voicemail rather than a receptionist is likely to answer calls, and messages are recorded electronically. A response may come in the form of another voicemail message. E-mail and instant messaging are ubiquitous. Information in many areas is now available via access to a computer and an Internet connection. These technologies can speed up work and expand capabilities. Who would prefer to use a traditional typewriter to prepare papers and documents after mastering a word-processing program?

Telehealth, the use of telecommunications and data technologies to deliver health care services including diagnostic services, treatment, consultation, and health information (Jenkins & White, 2001; Office for the Advancement of Telehealth—Publications, 2004), is now omnipresent. Rather than replacing traditional care, telehealth is best understood as a complementary approach to long-distance care delivery. Telehealth has potential to expand access to care, particularly for patients in remote areas, and to contain costs.

Technological advances have produced benefits; however, technology also can reduce the need for direct interpersonal contact. Barriers to use include financial investment to establish networks, inadequate reimbursement mechanisms, risks to confidentiality with electronic transmission, and licensure issues when care is transmitted across state lines (Jenkins & White, 2001).

Consider the following questions about telehealth:
- What effects do technological changes have on the therapeutic relationship?
- Will face-to-face interaction become a rare occurrence? In the future might therapeutic interactions take place primarily via technology, such as voicemail, the Internet, and videotape transmission? What advantages and disadvantages will appear with the increasing use of technology in nursing practice?
- What creative approaches may evolve using technology in therapeutic relationships? Consider how to avoid making interactions impersonal when technology is used.

For additional information about telehealth, see Jenkins, R. L., & White, P. (2001). Telehealth advancing nursing practice. *Nursing Outlook, 49,* 100-105; Office for the Advancement of Telehealth—Publications. (2004, February). *Innovation, demand and investment in telehealth.* Retrieved May 9, 2004, from: *http://telehealth.hrsa.gov/pubs.htm.*

REFERENCES

Ask me 3. IOM report on health literacy. (n.d.). Retrieved May 7, 2004, from: *http://www.askme3.org/tips.asp.*

Ask me 3. Tips for clear communication. (n.d.). Retrieved May 7, 2004, from: *http://www.askme3.org/tips.asp.*

Attree, M. (2001). Patients' and relatives' experiences and perspectives of 'good' and 'not so good' quality care. *Journal of Advanced Nursing, 33,* 456-466.

Beck, C. T., & Gable, R. K. (2001). *Postpartum depression screening scale.* Los Angeles, CA: Western Psychological Services.

Blondis, M. N., & Jackson, B. E. (1982). *Nonverbal communication with patients: Back to the human touch* (2nd ed.). New York: John Wiley & Sons.

Bosek, M. S. D. (2002). Ethics in practice: Effective communication skills. *JONA's Healthcare Law, Ethics, and Regulation, 4*(4), 93-97.

Coopersmith, S. (1967). *The antecedents of self-esteem.* San Francisco: W. H. Freeman.

Cox, J. L., Holden, J. M., & Sagovsky, R. (1987). Detection of postnatal depression: Development of the 10-item Edinburgh Postnatal Depression Scale. *British Journal of Psychiatry, 150,* 782-786.

DeMarco, R. F., Horowitz, J. A., & McLoed, D. (2000). A call to intraprofessional alliances. *Nursing Outlook, 48,* 172-178.

Douglass, J. L., Sowell, R. L., & Phillips, K. D. (2003). Using Peplau's theory to examine the psychosocial factors associated with HIV-infected women's difficulty in taking their medications. *The Journal of Theory Construction & Testing, 7,* 10-17.

Forchuck, C., Westwell, J., Martin, M., Bamber-Azzapardi, W., Kosterewa-Tolman, D., & Hux, M. (2000). The developing nurse-client relationship: Nurses' perspectives. *Journal of the American Psychiatric Nurses Association, 6,* 3-10.

Gallant, M. H., Beaulieu, M. C., & Carnevale, F. A. (2002). Partnership: An analysis of the concept within the nurse-client relationship. *Journal of Advanced Nursing, 40,* 149-157.

Guttman, N. (2000). *Public health communication interventions: Values and ethical dilemmas.* Thousand Oaks, CA: Sage.

Hall, E. (1973). *The silent language.* Garden City, NY: Doubleday/Anchor Press.

Health care coalition promotes clear communication: Patients encouraged to ask "Ask me 3." (2004, July/Aug.). *Clinician News, 4.*

Jenkins, R. L., & White, P. (2001). Telehealth advancing nursing practice. *Nursing Outlook, 49,* 100-105

Johannesen, R. L. (2002). *Ethics in human communication* (5th ed.). Prospect Heights, IL: Waveland Press.

Jourard, S. (1971). *The transparent self* (Rev. ed.). New York: Van Nostrand Reinhold.

Kasch, C. R. (1986). Toward a theory of nursing action: Skills and competency in nurse-patient interactions. *Nursing Research, 35,* 226-230.

Luft, J. (1969). *Of human interaction.* Palo Alto, CA: National Press Books.

Luft, J. (1984). *Group processes: An introduction to group dynamics* (3rd ed.). Palo Alto, CA: Mayfield.

McCabe, C. (2004). Nurse-patient communication: An exploration of patients' experiences. *Journal of Clinical Nursing, 13,* 41-49.

McCann, T. V., & Baker, H. (2001). Mutual relating: Developing interpersonal relationships in the community, *Journal of Advanced Nursing, 34,* 530-537.

Moyle, W. (2003). Nurse-patient relationship: A dichotomy of expectations. *International Journal of Mental Health Nursing, 12,* 103-109.

Office for the Advancement of Telehealth—Publications. (2004, Feb.). *Innovation, demand and investment in telehealth.* Retrieved May 9, 2004, from: *http://telehealth.hrsa.gov/pubs.htm.*

O'Toole, A., & Welt S. R. (1989). *Interpersonal theory in nursing practice.* New York: Springer.

Peplau, H. E. (1963). Process and concept of learning. In S. Burd & M. Marshall (Eds.), *Some clinical approaches to psychiatric nursing* (pp. 348-352). New York: Macmillan.

Peplau, H. E. (1964). *Basic principles of patient counseling* (2nd ed.). Philadelphia: Smith Kline and French Laboratories.

Peplau, H. E. (1969). Professional closeness: As a special kind of involvement with a patient, client, or family group, *Nursing Forum, 8,* 342-360.

Peplau, H. E. (1991). *Interpersonal relations in nursing.* New York: Springer.

Raths, L., Harmin, M., & Simon, S. (1978). *Values and teaching.* Columbus, OH: Charles E. Merrill.

Robinson, M. (2002). *Communication and health in a multi-ethnic society.* Bristol, UK: Policy Press.

Rogers, C. (1965). *Client-centered therapy.* Boston: Houghton Mifflin.

Ruesch, J., & Bateson, G. (1987). *Communication: The social matrix of psychiatry.* New York: W. W. Norton.

Schuster, P. M. (2000). *Communication: The key to the therapeutic relationship.* Philadelphia: F. A. Davis.

Sears, R. R. (1970). Relation of early socialization experience to self-concepts and gender role in middle childhood. *Child Development, 41,* 267-289.

Smith, J., & Crawford, L. (2004). Issues in communication for newly licensed nurses. *JONA's Healthcare Law, Ethics, and Regulation, 6*(1), 15-16.

Stuart, G. W., & Laraia, M. T. (2001). *Stuart & Sundeen's principles and practice of psychiatric nursing* (7th ed.). St Louis: Mosby.

Sullivan, H. S. (1953). *The interpersonal theory of psychiatry.* New York: W. W. Norton.

Sundeen, S. J., Stuart, G. W., Rankin, E. A. D., & Cohen, S. A. (1998). *Nurse-client interaction: Implementing the nursing process* (6th ed.). St. Louis: Mosby.

Taylor, B. J. (2004). Improving communication through practical reflection. *Reflections on Nursing Leadership, 30*(2), 28-29, 38.

Thorsteinsson, L. S. C. H. (2002). The quality of nursing care as perceived by individuals with chronic illnesses: The magical touch of nursing. *Journal of Clinical Nursing, 11,* 32-44.

U.S. Department of Health and Human Services. (2000). *Healthy People 2010: Understanding and Improving Health* (2nd ed.). Washington, D.C.: U.S. Government Printing Office.

Watzlawick, P., Beavin, J. H., & Jackson, D. D. (1967). *Pragmatics of human communication: A study of interactional patterns, pathologies and paradoxes.* New York: W. W. Norton.

Whittemore, R. (2000). Consequences of not "knowing the patient." *Clinical Specialist, 14,* 75-81.

Wright, L. M., & Leahey, M. (2000). *Nurses and families: A guide to family assessment and intervention* (3rd ed.). Philadelphia: F. A. Davis.

Chapter 5

PAMELA GRACE

Ethical Issues Relevant to Health Promotion

objectives

After completing this chapter, the reader will be able to:

- Discuss the nature and purposes of health care ethics.
- Describe the responsibilities of health care professionals (the development and the role of professional codes of ethics, advocacy, political activity, preserving professional integrity).
- Relate the responsibilities of health care professionals to health promotion.
- Describe the tension between promoting the health of individuals and that of society.
- Evaluate salient theoretical approaches to ethical problem solving.
- Apply ethical perspectives and principles to health-promotion practice throughout the life span.
- Describe contemporary issues in health promotion (genetics, culture, end-of-life decision making).
- Analyze problems related to health promotion using an ethical decision-making framework.

key terms

Applied ethics
Codes of ethics
Descriptive theories
Dilemmas
Ethic of care

Ethics
Feminist ethics
Genetic counseling
Metaethics

Moral
Moral philosophy
Normative theories
Value theories

THINK About It

The Juvenile Interpreter

A recent Hastings Center Report by Levine, Glajchen, & Cournos (2004) presents the case of a middle-aged Chinese immigrant, Mr. C., who after an emergency admission for chest pain is diagnosed with end-stage heart disease. Neither Mr. C. nor his wife is very fluent in English and the couple's eldest daughter, a 15-year-old girl, is most often relied on to translate for them because an interpreter is not always readily available. Commenting on the case, Myra Glajchen notes that "the U.S. Office of Civil Rights has stated that every Medicare or Medicaid provider must provide language assistance" (p. 11) as needed. This, although a worthy ideal, is often difficult to accomplish because of the multicultural nature of our contemporary society and the diversity of languages spoken. With increasing frequency, health care providers are faced with the problem of assessing the degree to which an

Continued

THINK About It

The Juvenile Interpreter *cont'd*

interpreter has translated accurately (in either direction) information and thus the extent to which the patient is able to make informed decisions.

1 What are the ethical issues associated with asking a minor to translate and impart sensitive, complex, and serious information?
   • From the perspective of the child
   • From the patient's perspective
   • From the health care provider perspective
   • From society's perspective

2 What alternatives are possible?

3 What related health care policies should be formulated or supported by health-promotion professionals?

HEALTH PROMOTION AS A MORAL ENDEAVOR

Human health promotion is a moral endeavor. We can say that it is a moral endeavor, because it involves both a critique of arrangements that facilitate or obstruct the well-being of a society overall and of activities that promote, protect, and support health for the individual members of a society. Health is considered a human good, because it allows people to live well and achieve their goals. At the level of the individual, health promotion involves the provision of services that assist humans to function as well as possible given their particular circumstances. This necessitates consideration of a variety of influences on a person's health status such as mental, physical, spiritual, and environmental factors, as well as their relationships with others (social factors). In this way, understanding the contexts of people's lives is crucial to health-promotion endeavors. Viewing health promotion as a moral endeavor is consistent with the intent and goals of the U.S. government's prevention agenda for the nation as laid out in *Healthy People 2010* (2000). The two overarching goals of *Healthy People 2010* are:

1. Increase quality and years of healthy life
2. Eliminate health disparities

The purpose of health-promotion efforts, as discussed throughout this book, is to ensure that people have, or have access to, the tools and strategies to live at the highest level of well-being possible. Health-promotion efforts address environmental obstacles to human health, such as pollution, advertising campaigns for harmful products, and economic disparities. Thus health promotion is not the province of a single discipline but involves the collaboration of all professional groups that have the pertinent knowledge and skills to enable or protect health within a society.

This chapter is focused on understanding the health professional's moral responsibilities toward individuals and society with regard to facilitating health, well-being, or the relief of suffering. Professional responsibilities are those obligations incurred by disciplines that purport to provide a service to society. For example, the American Nurses Association's (ANA, 2001) code of ethics (see Box 5-3 later in the chapter) promises that "nursing encompasses the prevention of illness, the alleviation of suffering, and the protection, promotion, and restoration of health in the care of individuals, families, groups and communities" (p. 5). This document, along with the ANA's *Nursing's Social Policy Statement* (ANA, 2003), an excerpt of which is presented later in the chapter in Box 5-2, lays out the ethical responsibilities of U.S. nurses. The International Council of Nurses (2000) also has a code of ethics, which serves as a standard for nurses worldwide and is easily accessible via the Internet.

Health-promotion ethics is best viewed as a subset of health care ethics which, in turn, has its roots in moral philosophy and value theory. This section of the book, then, discusses the requirements of, as well as obstacles to, health promotion across the life span and in contemporary health care settings. To facilitate this, the development, scope, and limits of ethical theories and perspectives are explored in relation to problem recognition and resolution.

Included in this chapter's content is the position that just as illness prevention is a crucial aspect of health promotion, anticipation and prevention of ethical problems is a critical component of ethical professional action; thus preventive ethics is introduced (see Box 5-4 later in the chapter). To illustrate this exploration of ethical issues in health promotion, a variety of real and hypothetical cases are used. Strategies to aid the health care professional in identifying, anticipating, and addressing ethical issues are provided throughout.

The terms *ethical* and *moral* are used interchangeably throughout the chapter. Although some commentators have distinguished the two concepts from each other, they have the same root meanings. The term **ethics** is "derived from the Greek ethos . . . meaning customs . . . conduct and character" (Davis, Aroskar, Liaschenko, & Drought, 1997, p. 1). The term **moral** is derived from Latin *mores* and originally meant "to do with custom or habit" (Davis et al., 1997, p. 1).

HEALTH CARE ETHICS
Origins of Applied Ethics in Moral Philosophy

The discipline underlying practice, or **applied ethics,** is moral philosophy. **Moral philosophy** is concerned with discovering or proposing what is right or wrong, or good or bad, in human action toward other humans and other entities such as animals and the environment. Singer (1991) confirms that the crucial practical questions of moral philosophy are "What ought I to do? How ought I to live?" (p. vii). Among the tasks of moral philosophy is that of formulating theories or frameworks to guide action. Using a moral theory to propose and implement appropriate actions in troubling situations will most consistently result in good action or the avoidance of harmful actions.

The theories that emerge as a result of philosophical inquiry about good action are called **value theories,** because they are concerned either with discovering what humans seem to value (descriptive theories) or proposing what they ought to value (normative theories) given some presupposed philosophy about the nature, or purpose of being human, or in order to achieve predetermined goals. What is often called the *golden rule* is a classic example of a normative principle. The golden rule essentially commits us to treating other people in the manner that we, ourselves, would wish to be treated given similar circumstances. For example, if I were lost in a strange city I would expect that a knowledgeable person would give me directions if asked, because I would willingly assist someone who was lost in my city. Normative theories permit judgments about the value of actions based on the extent to which these actions are consistent with the assumptions of the theory.

Types of Ethics
Descriptive Value Theories

These theories are based on observations of human behavior over time and in a variety of settings. **Descriptive theories** do not tell us what actions we ought to take—they are not directive—they merely tell us how people act toward each other and their environments, what they seem to believe are good or moral actions.

Normative Theories

Normative theories, on the other hand, are concerned with ensuring good actions. They are either reasoned and logically explored explanations of the moral purpose of human interactions, or they are divinely "revealed" truths about good action (religious ethics). Actions that are in accord with the foundational principle or principles of the theory will be right or good actions; they are the types of actions we ought to take given that we believe the principles are valid.

Consequentialism. The foundational principle of John Stuart Mill's (1861) utilitarian theory proposes that actions are good insofar as they are aimed at yielding the greatest amount of happiness or pleasure or cause the least amount of harm or pain to people and overall within the society. It is often formulated as the greatest good for the greatest number. Pleasure for Mill was a complex concept; he did not mean unthinking pleasure. He defined pleasure in qualitative as well as quantitative terms. The utilitarian perspective is consequentialist. The consequences or intended consequences of actions matter. Therefore any decision making about intended actions or interventions from the consequentialist perspective must take into account all knowable potential consequences. Among the implications of this type of theory for health care professionals is the imperative that data gathering must be thorough and complete. Additionally, the professional is accountable for possessing the appropriate skills and knowledge to under-

take actions that will promote a good for people. The professional's decision can be evaluated as bad or good to the extent that actions are in accord with the theory, in this case "right actions" are those that are directed toward promoting the greatest good or causing the least harm. The propositions of the theory direct what is needed for moral action or, stated another way, for doing the right thing.

Duty-Based Theories. Other normative value theories are not as heavily weighted toward producing good consequences. For example, duty-based theories such as that of Immanuel Kant (1724-1804) and those of various religions (Judaism, Christianity, Islam) are more dependent upon adherence to duties than they are on good consequences. Individuals are viewed as having certain duties that cannot be circumvented, even if deliberately side-stepping the duty will result in good outcomes. For religions these rules are imparted, in some way, by a divine being.

For Kant, the use of our capacity to reason is what permits moral action. For example, Kant believed that lying is always wrong even if on some occasions it produces a good outcome. It is wrong because it is irrational to lie. If lying were widely practiced we would lose our ability to trust what others tell us, and this would make effective communication impossible. Kant based his theory on the idea that what separates us from other life forms is our ability to make rules for ourselves using our ability to reason. His main rule, whereby each of us can determine for ourselves a moral course of action, is the categorical imperative. The categorical imperative was framed several different ways by Kant; however, the easiest to understand for current purposes is the following conceptualization, "I ought never to act except in such a way that I can also will that my maxim should become a universal law" (Kant, 1967/1785, p. 318). This could be stated alternatively as a question to ask oneself prior to acting, "Could any other person in the same or similar circumstances also take this action or refrain from this action?" A variety of philosophical perspectives, including some contemporary ethical positions, is discussed in more detail later in the chapter in relation to individual cases.

Limitations of Moral Theory

It is important to keep in mind that moral theories arise out of a particular perspective or philosophy about the world. They are conceptualized as a result of this perspective and within a historical and political context. The philosophical approach that evaluates value theories or ethical perspectives for their congruence and usefulness in human decision making across environments is **metaethics.** Philosophers interested in metaethical questions investigate where our ethical principles come from and what they mean. Are they merely social inventions? Do they involve more than expressions of our individual emotions? Metaethics allows us to critique the adequacy of ethical approaches for application across a variety of practice settings and cultural environments. Other sorts of metaethical questions posed by moral philosophers include: Are there such things as absolute ethical truths? If so how do we go about discovering these, and if not what foundations should we use to guide our actions? What considerations are important? How do we know which actions are good? What is a valid moral theory? Should human values be congruent across settings and cultures?

For example, religiously based moral theories are dependent upon the idea that good actions are those that obey the laws of a supreme being. However, because the foundational tenets of religions do not mirror each other, what constitutes a moral action from a Jewish perspective may well be morally prohibited from a Catholic perspective (Clarfield, Gordon, Markwell, & Shabbir, 2003). Moreover, even within a religion, the tenets of its different sects or branches may not always lead to the same conclusions about good actions. For such reasons, there are equally strongly held but divergent views on what is the good for humans. Many contemporary philosophers have argued that there can be no singular approach that permits the identification or resolution of all moral problems (Rachels, 2003; Weston, 2001). Even the golden rule can be problematic from a cross-cultural perspective. For example, I might want to be treated as an autonomous being capable of making my own decisions, but a person from Thailand might be more used to family-centered decision making. Treating my Thai friend as I would wish to be treated would be a mistake. An understanding of cultural beliefs is necessary for good action in such cases (Multicultural Awareness box).

Additionally, utilitarian theories emerged out of a particular era and as a result of perceived injustices in societal arrangements in England during the turmoil of the industrial revolution. Utilitarians such as Jeremy Bentham (1748-1832) and John Stuart Mill (1806-1873) sought frameworks that would permit the rectification of unjust policy decisions and the vast economic inequities within their society. For this reason such theories have a tendency to privilege the good of the group over the needs of individuals viewed as individuals.

Therefore it is not prudent to adopt one theory to guide actions in every situation related to health promotion. All moral theories have flaws which when applied indiscriminately can lead to actions that are problematic, either for an individual or for a group or for a combination of both. Health-promotion activities mandate not only a general understanding of the nature of the problem or potential problem but also knowledge of the values, beliefs, needs, and desires of the person who is the recipient of the efforts in question.

Although it is true of ethical theories that they are not helpful in many health-related decision-making situations, certain principles, derived from a variety of ethical theories, have proved useful in exploring underlying assumptions; they permit the highlighting of salient aspects of complex problems. "Principles inherent in a variety of ethical theories do serve as useful tools with which to examine the implications of different proposed courses of action; they permit clarification of hidden issues or facets" (Grace, 2004, p. 299) of situations. However, selection of pertinent principles is dependent both upon the context of the problem and the beliefs and values of the individual or group for which action is needed. These tools (principles derived from a variety of ethical theories), although they

MULTICULTURAL AWARENESS
Self-Reflection and Other Skills

The increasingly multicultural nature of contemporary society and the diversity of languages spoken and values held presents health care providers with complex assessment and planning problems. Nurses and allied professionals are charged with facilitating optimal care for all, regardless of "personal attributes" and taking into account "the needs and values of all persons" (ANA, 2001, Provision 1 and interpretive statements). It is not possible to know details about every culture. However, there are strategies that a health provider or promoter can employ to ensure that an individual's unique values and particular needs are the focus of interventions. When a particular culture is part of your population base, opportunities exist and should be pursued for learning about that culture. Besides asking the patient or knowledgeable others generalities about the particular culture, it is important to discover individual differences in beliefs, values, and needs (as they are for any patient). To facilitate your assessment, perhaps the most important undertaking is self-reflection (group reflection can help introduce different "takes" on a situation and increase self-awareness). The following are self-reflection and other considerations for providing culturally sensitive care:

1. Commitment to increasing knowledge and skill in sensitivity to cultural differences
2. Self-awareness and awareness of one's own biases, beliefs, and values. Ask yourself:
   - What values and biases you bring to the relationship
   - How your background has influenced your beliefs
   - What knowledge and experience you have to draw on
   - What values you think you share with the patient—validate with the patient
   - How comfortable you are with who you are
   - What further information you need to facilitate culturally competent care
   - Who or what is the best resource for further information
3. Awareness of the validity of different beliefs and values
4. Attempts to understand the meaning behind patient behavior
5. Increased knowledge of the beliefs and values of other cultures
6. Developing cultural skills through encounters with people from other cultures

facilitate communication between professionals in the interests of people, cannot be used effectively in the absence of contextual considerations, because it is often just these contextual considerations that determine which principles are relevant. For example, a woman seeks assistance in deciding whether to undergo genetic testing for the breast cancer gene BRCA2, because several members of her immediate and antecedent family have been diagnosed with breast or associated cancers. She tells her nurse practitioner that she is not sure whether it would be beneficial to be tested. The nurse practitioner, in facilitating the woman's health-promotion efforts, understands that she must use clinical judgment to facilitate the woman's autonomous choice. Understanding the requirements of the principle of autonomy is important to the task of helping the woman with her decision making. However, it is not sufficient to understand the meaning of autonomy and its limits; we also have to know something about the woman's life, values, beliefs, and relationships in order to provide her with the information and resources necessary for her decision. People are contextual beings; therefore, the choices they make affect not only themselves but also others in their lives, sometimes in profound ways. If the woman is screened and the results found positive for the gene, she not only has to decide her next actions, but the results have implications for family members including any children she has. Box 5-1 presents information on **genetic counseling.** Individual principles of importance to decision making in health care

settings are explored in depth later in the chapter. They, along with associated ethical considerations such as professional, feminist, and virtue ethics, underpin a framework of moral decision making for health promotion that is offered shortly.

Feminist Ethics and Caring
Feminist Ethics

Feminist perspectives on ethics are derived from the concerns of the feminist movement to expose and rectify injustices to which women historically have been subjected. Nelson (1992) notes that "feminism raised the consciousness of a whole generation to the male-dominated power structures within American society" (p. 8). Feminist thought is not limited in its influence to the United States; it has also been influential on societal changes in other Western countries. The feminist movement perspectives have broadened to include problems common to all oppressed groups. **Feminist ethics,** emerging as it has out of feminist thought and feminist philosophy, is not another ethical theory as such; rather it presents a viewpoint on moral problems in health care, and other areas of life, that have been neglected historically.

Feminist scholars have noted the limitations of traditional moral theories, and the principles derived from them, when used in health care settings. These are viewed as unable to adequately capture the nature and origins of

---

Box **5-1** Genetic Counseling

Since the last edition of this book, the exciting announcement regarding the completion of the genome project was made by the International Human Genome Sequencing Consortium, led in the United States by the National Human Genome Research Institute and the Department of Energy, on April 14, 2003. This represents an important initial step in expanding our potential to understand the genetic contributors to disease and to formulate interventions. However, there are complex ethical issues associated with, and raised by, genetic advances. For health-promotion professionals, a crucial skill is the ability to refer individuals appropriately to specialized genetic counselors. Although many health care professionals have the skills to counsel patients about genetic testing issues, especially in their fields of expertise, genetic counselors are an increasingly important resource.

Genetic counselors are specially trained master's-prepared individuals. These professionals can obtain certification through the American Board of Genetic Counselors. Their professional society is the National Society of Genetic Counselors. Genetic counselors enter the field from a range of backgrounds including biology, genetics, nursing, psychology, public health, and social work.

The goals of the discipline are outlined in their Code of Ethics (National Society of Genetic Counselors, 2004). Genetic counselors provide counseling services that are nondirective (Andrews, Mehlman, & Rothstein, 2002), which means that they avoid coercion or persuasion. Although there is controversy about how directive or nondirective advice should be

used, and based on the ethical ideals of autonomy, counselors strive to be nondirective while at the same time tailoring information to fit the specific needs of patients. Andrews and colleagues (2002) note that nondirective methodology is a way for the genetic counseling community to avoid association with the eugenics movement. Because advances in embryo pre-implantation genetic testing, as well as in-utero fetal testing, permit screening for certain superior characteristics or the screening out of certain genetic diseases, the perceived need to distance the profession from this issue is understandable.

Ethical issues related to genetic counseling for screening purposes that apply both for genetic counselors and other health care providers include:
- Understanding the wider context of genetic testing implications (privacy, discrimination, economics, health insurance denials, implications for family members, anxiety and apprehension, and eugenics (striving for perfection) and its associated implications for individuals and society
- Assisting people to determine the risks and benefits of screening
- Assisting people to prepare for their future needs
- Assisting people with their procreative planning
- Understanding how cultural differences impact counseling needs

Societal issues related to genetic advances include determining research priorities, justice issues, and discrimination of the genetically disadvantaged.

health care problems. Feminist critics assert that moral decision making must include an investigation of both hidden and overt power relationships implicit in ethical problems. Additionally, the importance of understanding both the contexts of situations and the interrelationships of those involved should not be neglected, because human beings are not isolated individuals who may be viewed as totally independent of others. Thus moral decision making must include the illumination of hidden power imbalances in relationships and situations (Donchin & Purdy, 1999; Tong, 1997; Warren, 2001). This additional criterion for exploring the moral content of health care and health-promotion problems permits the underlying causes of complex problems to be uncovered. Feminist ethics, then, can be thought of as contributing a perspective that is mostly missing from traditional ethical approaches. This changes both the way problems are perceived and the way they are explored. Characteristics of feminist ethics include the following:

1. Understanding that human beings are inseparable from their relationships with others
2. A "focus on care and responsibility in relationships rather than on the application of abstract principles" (Davis et al., 1997, p. 58)
3. A concern with the development of character and attitudes that result in caring actions reflective of a person who is related to rather than detached from context
4. A concern for the rights of individuals and for equality that is not limited to the oppression of women

Feminist ethics, then, depending on perspective, allows both a critique of the treatment of individuals as contextual beings and of inequities in social arrangements that are problematic for marginalized groups (Thorne & Varcoe, 1998; Tong, 1997; Warren, 2001).

For health promotion the feminist ethic of care is an important concept, because it permits a focus on the nature of the health care professional–patient relationships and the nature of people as inseparable from their contexts. The concept of care has found increasing acceptance in nursing circles as both a virtue of the nurse and a responsibility of practice. Carol Gilligan's (1982) work, among that of others, has been instrumental in the acceptance of the concept of care as informing ethics in nursing practice.

The Ethic of Care

The **ethic of care** means a responsibility to attend to the individual as individual in all of his or her complexities. It requires certain characteristics and attitudes of the nurse or allied provider (in addition to the professional's knowledge and skills) that include a predisposition to engage with an individual in the interests of that individual. The focus is on the individual as unique and particular. The needs of particular unique individuals are uncovered as the result of a focused attention on that person. Benner, Tanner, and Chesla (1996) define care as "the alleviation of vulnerability; the promotion of growth and health; the facilitation of comfort, dignity or a good and peaceful death" (p. 233). For Benner and colleagues, an ethic of care requires knowledge

and experience and is not solely an emotion in the way that care or caring is understood in everyday life. Many of the current conceptualizations of care, viewed as a responsibility of practice, have their origins in the work of Carol Gilligan.

Carol Gilligan (1982) was a student and colleague of Lawrence Kohlberg, a developmental psychologist. The main focus of Kohlberg's (1981, 1984) body of work was the nature of moral character development. Kohlberg's developmental theory was informed by Piaget's work on the stages of cognitive development in children. Kohlberg's stages of moral development were derived from longitudinal studies of young men. These moral reasoning studies were designed around the idea that an ability to apply conceptions of justice, rules, and principles to difficult situations denoted the highest achievable level of moral development. Gilligan "challenged the male bias in his [Kohlberg's] work" (Liaschenko & Peter, 2003, p. 35). By studying women's experiences, Gilligan (1982) discovered that they had a moral orientation based in the caring and nurturing of others. In this framework interrelationships and contexts are important and must be included as particularities important to understanding the complexities of a given situation. One way to look at an ethic of care versus an ethic of justice is that justice demands that we treat people fairly and not to regard their incidental differences as important in determining what is required. So justice is impartial and nondiscriminatory. Care, however, does necessitate an understanding of situational particularities; it ensures that we understand a given individual's needs in the context of his or her life. Generally justice and care have been viewed as opposing concepts. Liaschenko (1999) presents a compelling argument for them to be viewed as interrelated concepts. Justice is in the interest of particular individuals. In other words, justice issues concern individuals within a society. What is important about people is that they have individual interests that are protected by just policies.

Fry (1990) has identified three models of caring in contemporary literature: cultural, feminist, and humanistic. She notes that the humanistic model best captures the essence of care viewed as an aspect of nursing practice. Care as a facet of nursing practice requires engagement on the part of the nurse with the person in a relationship that permits the meaning and context of the person's needs to be exposed. This requires an understanding of human relationships as complex webs of interdependencies and interrelationships. A person cannot be extricated successfully from this complex web and treated as an isolated entity for the purposes of decision making; to do so would be to miss the point of nursing judgment and the provision of a good for the person. For example, a focus on pathophysiology is liable to miss nonphysiologically based contributing aspects of illness or ill health (Grace, 2004). Effecting a physiological cure does not necessarily remove the factors that made the person vulnerable. It also requires that the nurse is willing to address those needs from the person's perspective where this is possible. Thus in nursing, *care* is best described as a concept that requires an engaged knowing of the person. Benner and colleagues (1996) note of care that it is "the dominant ethic found in [nurses'] stories of everyday practice" (p. 233).

Limits of the Ethic of Care

One problem with using care as an ethic of health-promotion practice has to do with the problem of moral predictability or certainty (Nelson, 1992). If the emphasis is on relationships and there are no criteria for right and wrong action, how can one be assured of the morally correct action in a given situation? An answer to this could be that a morally correct action is one that emerges as a result of nursing judgment that is based on prior knowledge, experience, and an engaged relationship with the person. Thus the process of the interaction, coupled with the character, knowledge, experience, and intent of the moral agent or carer, is the crucial factor that achieves the moral good for an individual person as individual. The action is right if the nurse possesses the right characteristics and the person's complex needs are met. However, when the solution to one person's problems affects others, the rightness of the action depends on more than the one-on-one caring relationship. The problem remains one of choosing between this person's needs and needs of related others who might be affected by the chosen actions. This problem is resistant to resolution via an ethic of care alone. The problem-analysis framework described later includes the ethic of care, among other considerations. Another criticism is that the care ethic does not permit a moral critique of such things as poor institutional practices or poor interprofessional relationships (Nelson, 1992). Both an ethic of care and principles derived from traditional moral theory may be needed for good health-promotion activities.

The purpose of ethical inquiry in health promotion is to gain clarity on actual or potential moral issues arising in the context of health-promotion endeavors and to understand what is expected of the health-promotion agent viewed as moral agent. Ethical inquiry will not permit the resolution of all problems, mainly because the environments in which health-promotion efforts are conceptualized are incredibly complex. It is impossible to foresee all possible consequences of action, but ethical reasoning can facilitate appropriate and in-depth data gathering, permit the uncovering of hidden agendas and interests, and focus us on the most salient aspects of a particular problem, thus enhancing professional judgment.

Professional judgment and ensuing actions have their impetus in the provision of a good for the population of concern. Thus health promotion is a moral endeavor requiring morally sensitive and knowledgeable agents, but what are the scope and limits of a health care professional's obligations to anticipate, identify, and address morally problematic issues related to the promotion and protection of health for individuals, groups, and society? How do health care professionals balance their duties to individuals with a duty to the society? The following section addresses these questions.

PROFESSIONAL RESPONSIBILITY
Accountability to Individuals and Society
Professions

Although this section focuses on the nursing discipline's mandate to promote health, this discussion can also be applied to the responsibilities of allied health professions who assume health-promotion responsibilities. Using the term *profession* to denote the status of nursing and other disciplines is controversial. Indeed, the term is ambiguous. I have explored this problem elsewhere (Grace, 1998, 2001). For the purposes of this chapter I will assume that nursing is a profession insofar as it provides a service to society, is self-governing, and its members are accountable for their actions. One important facet of professions, perhaps especially of those that provide crucial services to society such as "medicine or law" (Windt, 1989, p. 7) and in this case nursing, is that they have codes of ethics outlining what, in essence, are their promises of service to society. A significant consequence of professional status is that members can be held accountable for their practice formally by professional licensure boards. More importantly they are morally accountable for practicing according to their discipline's implicit or explicit code of ethics. Codes of ethics provide a normative framework for professional actions. There is implicit acceptance of these codes upon acquiring membership in the discipline. Professionals become members of their professions after completing a period of knowledge and skills acquisition and upon commencing practice in the professional role.

Trust

Service professions such as nursing, medicine, and law are exemplified by their relationships to those in need of services. This relationship is one of trust. The professional has the knowledge and skills to meet an individual's needs or the needs of a group. The potential recipient of services lacks the knowledge or ability to anticipate or meet his or her own needs or the needs of the group. Indeed, increasingly the individual or group may not have the option of choosing a health care provider. This is, in part, makes health care professional–citizen relationships fiduciary ones. An individual or group is in the position of having to trust that the professional will keep the given entity's best interests as the primary goal and will strive to meet those needs. For example, in the current health care environment in the United States, people may have trouble accessing a specialist provider because of their particular insurance coverage or the inability to afford health care insurance or to pay on their own. Newton (1988) argues that professionals' knowledge puts them in the best position to recognize and anticipate obstacles to optimal provision of service. This is an additional aspect of accountability. Newton

(1988) asserts that a profession's members are accountable for practices that are:

> . . . inadequate at any stage of the rendering of the service: if the client the ultimate consumer is unhappy; if he is happy but unknowing, badly served by shabby products or services; or if he is happy and well served by the best available product but the state of the art is not adequate to his real needs. (p. 49)

Recognizing Barriers

Therefore, health care professionals are responsible not only for promoting health and healing but for recognizing and addressing barriers to health-promotion activities. The ANA's (2003) recently revised *Nursing's Social Policy Statement* provides a detailed account of the nursing discipline's responsibilities and "expresses the social contract between society and the profession of nursing" (p. 1). An excerpt of this statement is presented in Box 5-2. The following definition of professional nursing includes a warrant to advocate for changes when health care services are threatened.

> Nursing is the protection, promotion, and optimization of health and abilities, prevention of illness and injury, alleviation of suffering through the diagnosis and treatment of human response, and advocacy in the care of individuals, families, communities and populations. (ANA, 2003, p. 6)

Codes of Ethics

Codes of ethics are examples of normative ethics in that they prescribe how members of a profession ought to act

given the goals and purposes of the profession related to individuals and society. In this sense the goals and purposes of the profession serve as foundational ethical principles. The provisions of the code provide direction and express "expectations of ethical behavior" (ANA, 2001, p. 5). They represent the profession's promises to society. "A code of ethics makes explicit the primary goals, values and obligations of the profession" (ANA, 2001, p. 5). The *Code of Ethics for Nurses* is presented in Box 5-3. Although the public is not directly involved in the formulation of such codes and, indeed, is for the most part not even aware of their existence, the profession is responsive to the evolving needs of a given society. It can be said that codes of ethics are the tentative end results of a discipline's political process in that they result from debate and discussion among the profession's scholars, leaders, and membership over time but they are not static.

For example, nursing's scholars and leaders, in light of a host of changes in the nurse's work settings, recognized the

---

Box 5-2 Social Policy Statement

Excerpt: Knowledge Base for Nursing Practice

The knowledge base for nursing practice includes nursing science, philosophy, and ethics.

Nurses partner with individuals, families, communities, and populations to address such issues as:

- Promotion of health and safety
- Care and self-care processes
- Physical, emotional, and spiritual comfort, discomfort, and pain
- Adaptation to physiological and pathophysiological processes
- Emotions related to experiences of birth, growth and development, health, illness, disease, and death
- Meanings ascribed to health and illness
- Decision making and ability to make choices
- Relationships, role performance, and change processes within relationships
- Social policies and their effects on the health of individuals, families, and communities
- Health care systems and their relationships with access to and quality of health care
- The environment and the prevention of disease

From American Nurses Association. (2003). *Nursing's social policy statement* (2nd ed.). Silver Spring, MD: nursesbooks.org.

Box 5-3 Code of Ethics for Nurses

1. The nurse, in all professional relationships, practices with compassion and respect for the inherent dignity, worth, and uniqueness of every individual, unrestricted by considerations of social or economic status, personal attributes, or the nature of health problems.
2. The nurse's primary commitment is to the person, whether an individual or part of a family, group, or community.
3. The nurse promotes, advocates for, and strives to protect the health, safety, and rights of the person.
4. The nurse is responsible and accountable for individual nursing practice and determines the appropriate delegation of tasks consistent with the nurse's obligation to provide optimal person care.
5. The nurse owes the same duties to self as to others, including the responsibility to preserve integrity and safety, to maintain competence, and to continue personal and professional growth.
6. The nurse participates in establishing, maintaining, and improving health care environments and conditions of employment conducive to the provision of quality health care and consistent with the values of the profession through individual and collective action.
7. The nurse participates in the advancement of the profession through contributions to practice, education, administration, and knowledge development.
8. The nurse collaborates with other health professionals and the public in promoting community, national, and international efforts to meet health needs.
9. The profession of nursing, as represented by associations and their members, is responsible for articulating nursing values, for maintaining the integrity of the profession and its practice, and for shaping social policy.

From American Nurses Association. (2001). *Code of ethics for nurses with interpretive statements*. Washington, DC: Author.

need for revisions to the 1985 *Code of Ethics for Nurses*. Input was solicited from nurses across the country and in a variety of settings, and the code was revised accordingly. Olson (2001) notes that the new code recognizes that problems associated with managed care and other health policy changes threaten the nurse's right to practice in settings that uphold safety and facilitate respect for patient rights. Further, the new code places more emphasis on the nurse's right to preserve his or her personal integrity defined as "an aspect of wholeness of character" (ANA, 2001, p. 19). When the nurse's strongly held values and beliefs or safety are challenged by a nursing care situation, the nurse has the right to decide whether to participate.

Decisions not to participate in a situation cannot be made trivially because of the trust relationship and a nurse's moral accountability for actions. The threat to the nurse's integrity must be serious and the risk to the person's well-being such that the person's safety is not jeopardized by the nurse's absence. Other arrangements must be made for care of the person in such circumstances. The nurse who encounters repeated threats to integrity has a responsibility to consider changing the situation in some way. Change efforts may be directed toward institutional policy or may require that an alternative work environment be considered. Some provisions of the ANA code of ethics (2001) are discussed in more depth later in the chapter in relation to health-promotion activities.

Codes of ethics tend to offer guidelines not only about responsibilities for ensuring good care, but also about responsibilities for recognizing and addressing barriers to service. The nursing profession in the United States, via the ANA code of ethics, proposes that "the nurse promotes, advocates for, and strives to protect the health, safety, and rights of the person" (ANA, 2001, Provision 3). This requires anticipation of future health needs and political activity when necessary to ensure health promotion. Codes of ethics represent the ideals of the profession and thus serve as general guides to action. The ANA code of ethics is nonnegotiable; that is, the goals and intent of the code may not be ignored, diluted, or downplayed by individuals or institutions employing nurses in the United States (ANA, 1994).

Advocacy

Advocacy, as an expectation of nurses, is strongly reinforced both in the code of ethics (ANA, 2001) and in innumerable scholarly articles. However, advocacy is also a controversial concept. The meaning of advocacy is hard to pin down and, consequently, there is no agreement about the boundaries of a nurse's responsibilities to advocate. The term *advocacy* is derived from its use in law. In legal jurisprudence, advocacy is aggressive action taken on behalf of an individual, or perhaps a group viewed as an individual entity, to protect or secure that individual's rights. The term *advocacy* can be traced to the fourteenth-century French *advocacie* which meant "the function of an advocate; the work of advocating; pleading for or supporting", while *advocate* is derived from the Latin *advocatus* meaning, "one sum-

moned or 'called to' another, esp. one called in to aid one's cause in a court of justice" (Brown, 1993, p. 194). "Therefore, a lawyer, while defending or representing a client, has this responsibility to the client as a foremost responsibility" (Grace, 2001, p. 154). Thus in law the individual lawyer does not have an opposing obligation to attend to social justice issues. This attention to broader questions of justice is the responsibility of other areas of the justice system.

Unlike advocacy within the justice system, advocacy in health care settings is not a simple concept (Grace, 1998). The adoption of the term *advocacy* to denote professional action in nonlegal settings gives rise to confusion. Nurses (and other health care professionals) have a responsibility to speak up on behalf of people whose rights have been interfered with or endangered in some way. However, that is not the end of their responsibilities. They must also consider that specific actions they undertake, in the name of advocacy (regardless of the prevailing definition of advocacy), may pose problems for other people who are relying on them for health care services.

For example, Sally Rimmer, a case manager, is assisting Jim Bailey to apply for services in a rehabilitation facility because he has residual hemiparesis secondary to a cerebrovascular accident. There is a waiting list at the facility, but Sally believes it is a priority for Jim to be treated there, because he lives with his elderly mother who is frail and will not be able to assist him with his activities of daily living. Because Sally represents other people who will also benefit from rehabilitation, her decision to advocate for Jim must be weighed against the needs of these other people. A moral responsibility associated with advocacy in health care settings is that the effect of actions on others is considered. When advocating extra attention or specialized care for a given person, an injustice may be rendered simultaneously to other people in the nurse's care. "Advocacy conceptualized as professional action stemming from the profession's purposes, and more properly termed 'professional advocacy' ... requires a balancing of the health needs of the individual with the health needs of the population" (Grace, 2001, p. 159).

Advocacy is an ideal of health care professions that requires attention to individuals and to broader societal concerns. Understanding the interdependent nature of individual and social needs facilitates preventive and health-promotion actions on the part of health care professionals both locally and more globally. Such actions may include political activity, in concert with others, on behalf of common populations of concern. Preemptive and sociopolitical advocacy permits the source of the ongoing problems to be accurately identified and challenged. Ballou (2000), among others, has strongly argued that nurses have moral obligations related to sociopolitical advocacy on behalf of their populations of concern. Sally Rimmer's obligations include recognizing the problems caused by a chronic shortage of rehabilitation services. Her concerns include discovering the source of this problem and joining with others in an attempt to address it at this level. Strategies for solving seemingly intractable problems of health care or the health care delivery system include collaboration with specialty nursing, medical or patient advocacy groups, and publication of the issues in the popular press.

Advocacy at the level of the care of individuals is related to trust. Trust is a necessary part of the health care professional–patient relationship. Davis and colleagues (1997) note that an ethical responsibility of the nurse's role is "to see that the person's rights and interests are protected" (p. 76). This is part of the role, because people may not recognize either what is needed to meet their needs or when the care they are receiving is substandard.

Advocacy for good health care including health promotion is a concept with broader implications. It necessarily includes those activities that are directed toward remedying socially based inequities or inadequacies in the health care delivery system. Gaylord and Grace (1995), among others, note that advocacy should be viewed as an ethic of practice that includes all activities directed toward the person's good. Further, it is proposed that advocacy may be required on an organizational or political level when obstacles to good care are recurrent (Ballou, 2000; Grace, 2001). "So advocacy is an obligation of professional role but not solely in the narrow sense of speaking up for, or acting on behalf of, individuals or groups in specific situations. This is because necessarily included in the nurse's moral decision making is consideration of which actions will be most supportive of the profession's goals overall" (Gaylord & Grace, 1995, p. 160). Advocacy is often a risky practice in that speaking up, or facilitating the good, for individuals or groups, may pit nurses against their peers or against other interested parties. Potential adversaries are those who do not share the same professional goals, or are not as reflective about what these goals entail, or have an economic or other interest in maintaining the status quo.

The health care professional role and its attendant responsibilities (advocacy) require that professional knowledge and judgment be brought to bear on a variety of situations, from the relatively simple to the complex. First, judgment permits the isolation, identification, and analysis of health problems or potential problems, often in collaboration with others. Second, appropriate actions are formulated and their likely consequences considered. Third, obstacles to action are recognized and addressed. Finally, actions are carried out and evaluated. These basic steps are evident whether the object of health care or health promotion is an individual, or a group, or society.

Problem Solving: Issues, Dilemmas, and Risks

The nature of health care settings and environments makes it inevitable that some extremely difficult decisions will have to be made. However, many of the ethical problems encountered in health-promotion settings are issues rather than dilemmas. As Chambliss (1996), a sociologist who studied nurses in acute care institutional settings, asserts, organizations such as hospitals often give rise to

"practical problems, not individual dilemmas" (p. 91). These are nonetheless moral problems, because they interfere with the goals of promoting health, or well-being, or the relief of suffering. In noninstitutional health care settings obstacles to good care are also caused by health care system arrangements, by interprofessional conflicts, and by the lack of resources. **Dilemmas** are ethical issues of a special sort. The term *dilemma* is a conjoining of *di*, meaning two, coupled with *lemma*, a Greek term meaning assumption or premises (Brown, 1993). In ethics, dilemmas are those situations in which a choice must be made between two (or among more) equally undesirable options. Weston (2001) claims that true dilemmas are actually quite rare and that options often can be found by changing the way the situation is scrutinized.

For the most part ethical problems in health promotion are not dilemmas. However, the goals of health promotion require that both issues and dilemmas be recognized and addressed. Neglected issues can become dilemmas. The situation that Graham Pink faced is an example of an ethical issue that became a dilemma. Mr. Pink was a charge nurse working on a geriatric ward in a British hospital. He had grave concerns about the treatment of people, especially during the night shift, which was chronically understaffed. First Mr. Pink went through the usual channels trying to get changes made. He notified his supervisors verbally and via written documentation but was unsuccessful in achieving change. Indeed, the situation deteriorated further. He went higher in the administrative chain of command with complaints that people were being neglected and endangered by the situation. He was unsuccessful at all levels. Finally, his moral concerns were such that he decided to report the situation to the local newspaper, even though he knew that he might lose his position as a result. He was fired in September 1991 but was eventually exonerated (Wilmot, 2000).

When a nurse is in danger of losing his or her position as a result of advocating for better conditions, one consideration is whether the people are liable to be better served overall by the action. This requires balancing the foreseeable risks of advocating with the likely benefits to the individual or group. A framework for making ethical decisions is offered and discussed later in the chapter. Included in this discussion are considerations for the health-promotion agent related to personal security along with preserving integrity.

Preventive Ethics

Preventive ethics, like preventive health care activities, aims to interrupt potential ethical problems before they develop. Preventive ethics is a requirement of health-promotion endeavors perhaps more specifically than it is of any other area of health-related activities. Preventive ethics requires the health promoter both to envision potential problems and to institute actions that halt their development. For example, it is possible to extend a dying person's life almost indefinitely using available technology, including vasoactive drugs and high-technology devices. It has become the norm (for a variety of reasons) for medical personnel to try to do so. Although a competent person has the right to refuse treatment and this right is legally recognized as a result of the Patient Self-Determination Act (PSDA) of 1991, many people become incapacitated quickly and before they are able to make their wishes known. Although all states recognize and honor advance directives, the legally recognized form varies from state to state (Box 5-4). Most people have not formulated advance directives. There are many reasons why this is true. Much more work needs to be done on engaging people in discussion and planning for such eventualities while they are still well (see the Research Highlights box). The work of communication with patients and families can begin before a problem arises. This is often missing both in institutional settings and primary care settings.

Preventive ethics using a feminist ethics perspective would permit addressing institutional practices that make it difficult for high-technology care to be more humanistic or addressing the underlying social issues that lead people to overeat, smoke, or be inclined toward violence. For example, preventive ethics would require investigating why as a society we have trouble discussing death and dying, and why we find it so hard to have a peaceful or good death. Weston (2001) notes that much of the energy used on the polarized abortion debate could be more profitably put to use in determining why people who don't want to be pregnant nevertheless become pregnant. Weston (2001) would reframe the question to ask "why pregnancy, or pregnancy at the wrong time, is so unacceptably burdensome for many women" (p. 43). We need to ask questions about lack of support, lack of education, poor or difficult-to-use birth control methods, resistance from spouses and lovers, lack of child care, and so on. Strategies for identifying potential ethical problems before they occur include examining problematic cases for their antecedents. We should ask fundamental questions about societal arrangements and influences on health trends.

On a local level, nurses and other health promoters need to bring to bear clinical judgment in anticipating and forecasting problems before they arise. For example, when a nurse observes that a person and family either do not understand information that has been given to them or the implications of following a given course of action, then the nurse engages in preventive ethics by supplying that information. The nurse acts to prevent negative consequences that can arise as a result of poorly understood information. Many problems in health care occur as a result of poor communication or because information has been provided too late for reasoned decision making.

Preventive ethics also includes social and political activism, in concert with other nurses or professional nursing organizations, to effect those changes in the health care environment needed to avert potential hazards. Some of these hazards result from inadequate access to health care. "*Nursing's Social Policy Statement*" is clear about the collective responsibility of nursing to influence . . . social and public policy to promote social justice" (ANA, 2003, p. 5).

So far the discussion has traced the origins of moral philosophy and applied ethics, along with providing a brief critique of the usefulness of these for guiding professional action. As noted, we cannot use a particular moral theory to exclusively guide health-promotion activities, because each theory has flaws that lead to further problems. The principles of duty-based theories can conflict with each other, as in the example, I must tell the truth but telling the truth might cause harm. Utilitarian or consequentialist approaches can lead us to neglect the needs of some individuals for the benefit of the larger group. An exclusive emphasis on care gives us no way to evaluate the good of our actual actions. This next section explores certain moral principles, derived from a variety of moral theories, which have proved useful to the project of clarifying problems in health care and permit us to locate the essential facets of a problem.

ETHICAL PRINCIPLES IN HEALTH PROMOTION

Although the tenets of nursing's codes of ethics and standards of practice provide some guidance about the nature of practice and the manner in which services will be provided, they tend to be vague and nonspecific, often leaving some ambiguity about the best course of action in morally troubling situations. The use of principles derived from a variety of ethical theories, along with feminist insights or an ethic of care, permits us to get a more nuanced and detailed picture of actual or potential morally problematic health situations. Beauchamp and Walters (1999) note "principles provide a starting point for moral judgment and policy evaluation, but, . . . more content is needed than that supplied by principles alone" (p. 19). In other words principles such as autonomy, beneficence, and justice often serve as helpful starting points in teasing out the tangled elements of complex issues, but taken alone they are usually insufficient to permit moral problem solving in health care environments. One must decide which principles are important to consider in a given case or situation, and this requires an exploration of the case as discussed in the decision-making framework provided later in the chapter.

Additionally, tenets of the code for nurses (ANA, 2001) and other ANA position statements provide guidance regarding what are a nurse's moral responsibilities in a particular type of situation. Certain tenets (see Box 5-3, provisions 6 to 9) also address the responsibilities of the nurse toward improving the larger health care environment. These obligations include facilitating "community, national, and international efforts to meet health needs" (ANA, 2001, p. 23).

Autonomy as Civil Liberty

In health-promotion settings and endeavors the concept of autonomy can be understood from two different perspectives. From the vantage point of public health, the extent

Box 5-4 Preventive Ethics: Patient Self-Determination Act and Advance Directives

One fact that all people face is the uncertainty and fragility of life. Health-promotion endeavors can increase individual capacities to withstand the vagaries of life and even permit humans to flourish while living with chronic illness. However, what often cannot be predicted is whether and when the ability to make our wishes for treatment and care known will be lost. Over the last 2 to 3 decades, great technological and therapeutic advances have been made, with the resulting ability to save the lives of people experiencing catastrophic illnesses and trauma. The side effect of these advances, unfortunately, is that sometimes we are successful only in prolonging the dying process. Although it is now recognized that people have a right to refuse treatment to prolong life, it is not uncommon that critically ill people lose the ability to articulate their wishes for treatment. Advance directives are a way for people to ensure that when they become incapacitated the care and treatment they receive matches their predetermined wishes. At their best, advance directives also have the potential to relieve the strain felt by loved ones as they strive to make the "right" treatment choices for a friend or relative. They also guide health professionals in their decision making regarding the person in question.

TYPES OF ADVANCE DIRECTIVES

All states have advance directive laws. However, they differ regarding what is the legal form of advance directive and what is required to validate it. For example, in Massachusetts the legal advance directive is a health care proxy. It requires the designation of a person to make one's health care decisions in the event of incapacity. Two people have to witness the signature, neither of whom can be the designee.

1. *Instructional.* A written document, this is also known as a *living will* or *terminal care document.* It can be very specific and tailored to order or may be a form document that can be downloaded from the Internet.
2. *Health care proxy.* This is also known as a *durable power of attorney for health care.* It allows a competent person to designate a decision maker in the event of incapacity.

   Fagerlin and Schneider (2004) found that living wills are the least effective advance directive in the absence of a health care proxy. The best advance directive is a combination of proxy and written directions.

   The PSDA of 1991, which was formulated in response to 2 decades of ambiguity and litigation involving right-to-die cases, represented an attempt to ensure that people's rights were honored. The PSDA required changes in public policy, public and professional education, institutional policy, and social awareness (Clarke, 1998). The PSDA was expected to improve communication related to end-of-life care issues and preferences among individuals, health care providers, and proxy decision makers. It requires institutions that receive Medicare and Medicaid funds to:

* Give written information on admission to all (not just the Medicare and Medicaid) patients about their rights under the law to make their own treatment decisions

* Inform people of their rights to complete state-allowed advance directives and provide written policies about those rights
* Document when a patient has an advance directive
* Not discriminate or make care conditional on the existence or absence of an advance directive
* Provide staff education about advance directives and personal rights

Although the PSDA has great potential, it serves its purpose only to the extent that it is taken seriously as a responsibility of a given institution. All too frequently institutions fail to ensure that a suitably qualified person is available to impart the information or to request personal preferences. It is important for those involved in health promotion to understand, and therefore address, why people may be reluctant to make an advance directive, why institutions are not diligent in providing information and education, and why even in the presence of the PSDA most people do not have advance directives (Miles, Koepp, & Weber, 1996).

RESERVATIONS ABOUT, AND IMPEDIMENTS TO THE USE OF, ADVANCE DIRECTIVES

* Discussions with health care providers about the implications of desired choices have been inadequate.
* People don't want to talk about future incapacity or death. They may have cultural prohibitions about discussing the possibility of serious illness or death.
* Past encounters with the health care system has led to distrust.
* People can't predict accurately their future preferences and they know too little about what constitutes life support.
* People may change their minds about what they will accept.
* Health care proxy may turn out to be a poor choice or may cause conflicts among other family members or loved ones. The patient or family may ask for something that is morally unacceptable.
* Treatments may be specified to which the provider has conscientious objections.
* Documentation may be lost, misplaced, or not accessible in an emergency.
* Written instructions are too vague, and open to divergent interpretation, to be useful guides.
* Even the most diligent proxy cannot always know what the person would have wanted in the absence of a detailed treatment directive.
* The proxy may make a treatment choice contrary to the person's directive.
* The proxy may make a decision with which the institution or physician disagrees.

Compiled from Fagerlin, A., & Schneider, C. E. (2004). Enough. The failure of the living will. *Hastings Center Report, 34*(2), 30-42; Miles, S. H, Koepp, R., & Weber, E. P. (1996). Advance end-of-life treatment planning: A research review. *Archives of Internal Medicine, 156,* 1062-1068; and Wolf, S. M. (2001). Sources of concern about the Patient Self-Determination Act. In W. Teays & L. M. Purdy (Eds.), *Bioethics, justice and health care* (pp. 411-419). Belmont, CA: Wadsworth/Thompson Learning.

of individual autonomy, or freedom of action, may be limited by the duty of protecting the health and safety of the society (Ovrebo, 2000). From this perspective there is an age-old struggle between civil rights and public safety. Moral questions center on the problem of how much liberty the society is justified in regulating in the interests of the health and safety of the society at large. Ovrebo (2000) reminds us that "controversies over coercive health measures" are at least "as old as the quarantining of ships carrying bubonic plague" (p. 23). The first outbreaks of shipborne bubonic plague were noted in ships that had sailed from the Orient to Italy in the 1300s (McGowan, 1995). Sailors on the ships were quarantined and not allowed to disembark; thus their freedom was restricted. There is an inevitable tension associated with curtailing civil liberties in the name of safety or health. This tension arises from perceptions that what is important about human life, in most Western contexts, is that some freedom of action is a prerequisite of human flourishing. Additionally, human rights' curtailment has permitted control of large populations by small, but powerful, minorities.

Currently there are many indirect threats to the health and safety of our society. Actions to resolve any of these have the potential to impinge on civil liberties including, but by no means limited to, bioterrorism, the spread of HIV-AIDS, drug-resistant tuberculosis, and advances in genetic knowledge. Advances in genetic knowledge present the possibility of discrimination from a variety of sources. It will be difficult to maintain individual privacy. Discrimination based on class or gene profile will be made easier. Genetic enhancement may be used by select individuals who can afford it (Bereano, 2000).

The current managed care environment, while having a stronger focus on inculcating healthy behaviors, can impinge on civil liberties. Prioritizing behavior change or modification in health-promotion endeavors over the need to address underlying social contributors, such as poverty and other forms of disadvantage, has been criticized by those who feel that a focus on the social determinants of health would permit more effective, less restrictive health promotion and protection (Cribb & Duncan, 2002; Marmot & Wilkinson, 1999; Ovrebo, 2000).

Autonomy as Self-Determination

The second, but related, sense of autonomy has to do with individual choice. In health care and health-promotion settings where individuals are the focus of concern, *autonomy* means the right to determine what treatments or interventions one will accept. It is perhaps the most powerful moral principle underlying the treatment of individuals, at least in Western societies. This principle asserts that people have the ability to reason, and a consequence of the ability to reason is the capacity to make choices. These choices concern both one's own behavior and how one should act toward others. Although the idea that the essence of being human is our ability to reason originated with Aristotle, Kant (1967/1785) developed this idea in meticulous detail

in his work, "Foundations of the Metaphysics of Morals." The human capacity for reason and thus for self-governance is also that which gives the individual moral worth. According to Kant, among all the animals only people are capable of conscious desires and goals. People are free agents capable of making decisions and setting their own goals as guided by their own reason. This principle is still a salient consideration in health care settings; it underpins the health provider and promoter–patient relationship and the issue of informed consent. However, there is limited agreement about the scope, limits, and strength of this principle (Beauchamp & Childress, 2001). When describing autonomy in the context of health or treatment choices, it is important to delineate what we mean by autonomy in the context of the problem under discussion. Feminist criticisms of an emphasis on autonomy highlight the problem that our choices necessarily affect others because we are contextual beings inseparable from our relationships with one another.

Generally, respecting autonomy requires that we permit individuals to make their own decisions, even when these decisions seem to others to be ill informed. There are exceptions to this rule. Exceptions include those situations in which there is a high risk of serious injury or death and when it cannot be determined whether the person's judgment is impaired (Box 5-5); that is, we make exceptions to the rule of autonomy when we suspect that an individual is not able to reason adequately, or to reason at the normal level (given that the normal level of functioning is self-sufficient). A person's reasoning ability may be impaired for several reasons. The difficulties may be psychological, physical, or a result of incorrect or incomplete information. Normally respect for people, which is another way of saying

---

Box **5-5** Proxy Decision Making

I. Autonomy based: person's previously articulated desires
  A. Written
    1. Living will, advance directive
    2. Document details to varying degrees what the person will or will not accept
  B. Substituted judgment
    1. Individual appoints a proxy who is expected to honor previously expressed preferences
    2. Informal (nonappointed significant other)
II. Best interests
  A. Surrogate chooses the actions that will give the highest overall benefit—may or may not be based on a person's previously expressed desires; a quality of life determination based when possible on knowledge about the person (Beauchamp & Childress, 2001)
  B. Best interests may trump the proxy's choice; doubt about the proxy's motives possible
III. Reasonable person standard
  A. Based on the answer to "What would a reasonable person want?"

respect for human dignity, or autonomy, permits individuals to make and learn from their own mistakes and holds them accountable for their actions.

In health care or health-promotion settings, respect for autonomy requires that individuals be given the information they need to make choices. Choices can be considered autonomous only if certain criteria are met. The criteria that determine whether or not a person is actually capable of autonomous (voluntary) choice include cognitive maturity, possession of appropriate information to permit decision making, intact mental capacities (the ability to reason logically), the absence of internal or external coercive influences, and the ability to appreciate the risks and benefits of alternative choices. This is quite a tall order. It is probably true that nobody acts totally autonomously at any given time because of the influences of entrenched beliefs and values which are derived, for the most part, from our cultural and environmental backgrounds. Some of these are under conscious control in the sense that we can recognize what values we hold and even revise them if they are dissonant with other values. However, some of these influences are not readily recognizable; they lie beneath the surface of consciousness and are hard to access even if we are willing to try. We all have blind spots; autonomy viewed as informed, uncoerced, and reasoned action is therefore an ideal. Many of us, and probably most of the time, fall short of the ideal. Autonomy is the moral principle that underlies the concept of informed consent to treatment, interventions, and health-promotion efforts.

Autonomy and Adolescents

Based on theoretical conceptions and findings from empirical studies related to development and decision making (Dickey & Deatrick, 2000; Ross, 1997; Weir & Peters, 1997; Weithorn & Campbell, 1982), adolescents 14 to 17 years of age are, generally, considered capable of meeting these criteria and making decisions as ably as adults. Involving adolescents fully in their own health care facilitates self-care agency (Research Highlights box). For nurse theorist Orem (1995), whose focus on self-care agency includes developmental considerations, there is a relationship between the deliberate self-care activities of mature and maturing people and ongoing optimal development and future functioning. Self-care is learned as a result of membership within family or other social groups. Although for the most part this includes some supervision by responsible adults, respect for an adolescent's developing autonomy facilitates health.

Informed Consent

Informed consent to research, treatments, or health-promotion endeavors is a process of ensuring that a person has all of the appropriate information necessary to come to a decision about participation that facilitates autonomous action. Beauchamp and Childress (2001) note that "informed consent occurs if and only if a person or subject, with substantial understanding and in the absence of substantial control by others, intentionally authorizes a professional to do something" (p. 78). The key phrase is "with substantial understanding." Informed consent may be seen as the (temporary) end result of a process. The consent is temporary, because new information may change the balance of risks and benefits of the proposed procedure. Thus even after a consent form is signed, a person has the right to rescind consent in light of changed consequences.

Components of the consent process include determining the person's competency to make the decision or to consent; that is, there must be no physical or mental impairments that hinder the person in question from understanding and processing information. For example, a person with pneumonia who is febrile and confused probably is not capable of making an informed decision until the fever is reduced and the confusion has cleared. To be substantially informed a person must be made aware of important details of the proposed intervention, including its nature, purpose, probability of success, and important risks, and must also understand what alternatives (if any) are available. This information must be tailored to meet the specific needs of an individual and thus requires that we know something about the person. In this way an ethic of care is important to our understanding of a person's unique needs. We can check understanding to a certain extent by asking the individual to

---

research highlights

Use of Advance Directives With Adolescents

Scholars of health care ethics have proposed that discussions related to advance directives for care should begin while people are healthy and should take place in an ongoing fashion as part of health maintenance activities (Grace, 2004; May, 2002; McCullough, 1998). McAliley, Hudson-Barr, Gunning, and Rowbottom (2000) took this idea one step further, noting that although "The American Academy of Pediatrics (AAP) supports giving children a voice in their health care decision-making, . . . how teens want to be involved in this is not known" (p. 471). To answer this question they conducted an interview study of 107 adolescents between the ages of 15 and 18 years related to having or making a living will.

Results of the study yielded a wide range of information about adolescents and advance directives. Participants were able to pass a test used for demonstrating decision-making competency. They were willing to answer questions related to their own health care treatments as they envisioned themselves in a coma, and those responses are similar to those reported for adults. The vast majority of participants felt it was "somewhat important" or "very important" for someone their age to have a living will. Most of the adolescent participants did not report feeling uncomfortable discussing these issues (McAliley et al., 2000, p. 471).

From McAliley, L. G., Hudson-Barr, D, C., Gunning, R. S., & Rowbottom, L.A. (2000). The use of advance directives with adolescents. *Pediatric Nursing, 26*(5), 471-482.

articulate how the proposed intervention will facilitate his or her own values and goals. There must be no subtle or overt coercion by professionals or others who are significant in the person's life or might otherwise have undue influence (e.g., employer). Finally, appropriate supports must be available to complete the proposed intervention.

Obtaining consent for any interventions, or for involvement in research, is best viewed as a process that entails ongoing assessment of the person's status and evaluation of needs for further information or support. People who are in stressful situations have limited abilities to process information; thus, we should assess for and validate understanding on an ongoing basis. It has been well documented that people do not grasp information well either when they are in stressful situations or when the information is complex.

Most health-promotion activities do not require formal informed consent. However, they do require us to understand both the philosophy behind, and the status and validity of, the supporting research before we assist people to be sure that we use health-promotion strategies that best fit their beliefs and values.

Exceptions to Autonomous Decision Making

Exceptions to the rule of permitting autonomous decision making exist. In some cases proxy decision making on behalf of the individual is required. Nevertheless proxy decision making must take into account what is known about the person and must follow a path of action that is most likely to respect that individual's previous goals and values when these are knowable. Certain populations are considered less than fully autonomous for a variety of reasons. People with Alzheimer's disease or other physical or psychological disruptions or deficits that prevent adequate comprehension may require proxy decision makers (see Box 5-5). Incarcerated people are restricted in their choices and may be subject to subtle or not-so-subtle coercion. Children are considered less than fully autonomous because they are not developmentally mature. Additionally, in people with certain mental illnesses, such as psychoses or bipolar disorders, their capacity for decision making that is in alignment with previous life goals may fluctuate. The President's commission (1982) formed to look at health care decision making has noted that the minimal capacities needed for competent decision making are: "1. Possession of a set of values and goals, 2. the ability to communicate and to understand information, and 3. the ability to reason and deliberate about one's choice" (p. 57). These criteria are generally accepted as a basic minimum (Beauchamp & Childress, 2001). It can be seen from these criteria that some children would be able to understand the implications of a given course of treatment, and others with cognitive impairments may nevertheless be deemed competent to make certain decisions. Buchanan and Brock (1989) have argued persuasively that competency to make autonomous choices is not an all-or-nothing capacity. They remind health care professionals that competency determinations are, as a rule, made for a given decision or task and thus

should be task relative. Moreover, they affirm that competency for decision making occurs along a continuum. Thus, a person may vacillate between competency and noncompetency, depending on either the task at hand (degree of difficulty or risk) or physical or psychological status during the period when a decision must be made.

When advocating decision making for a cognitively impaired person, it is important to consider the risks of permitting the decision compared with the benefit of allowing the individual to make his or own decision. The benefits in terms of self-esteem may well outweigh the risks of many choices. However, if the risk of injury is high and it is obvious that the person does not grasp this, decision making should not be allowed. In this case, either we are preserving the person's autonomy so that he or she may engage in decision making at a future time (and presumably death truncates autonomy) or because severe suffering is likely to occur and the person has not taken this into consideration.

Proxy Decision Making

When children are involved, it is often the parent or guardian to whom we turn for permission to treat. Nevertheless, in pediatric settings it is incumbent on people involved in health-promotion endeavors or in research with minors to gain assent from the child in addition to consent from the parent or guardian. For the child's assent to be meaningful, an assessment of level of maturity and comprehension is required, and information must be provided in language and terms that are appropriate for the developmental level. Conversely, when there is conflict between the decision of the parent and that of the child, the health care provider has a duty to ensure that the parental choice is in the child's best interest. Where there is serious doubt, it may be necessary to involve the courts.

Limits on Autonomy

Although autonomy remains an important principle for individual decision making related to interventions of various sorts, curtailments on autonomy are frequent in daily life. We are constrained by our work conditions, by access to information, by unconscious drives, by emotions, and by the impact of our behavior on others. For the sake of societal interests the autonomous actions of individuals may sometimes be curtailed. This is especially true when the health of other people are put at risk.

Confidentiality

Autonomy is also the principle underlying confidentiality. "The ability to maintain privacy in one's life is an expression of autonomy" (Burkhart & Nathaniel, 2002). People have the right to decide who shall have access to information about them, thus limiting the negative use of personal information by others. In certain situations the status of confidentiality between a person and others, such as clergy, is considered a privilege and as such is shielded from exposure by the legal system. In health care, confidentiality does not carry as strong a status as clergy-supplicant or lawyer-client privilege (Grace, 2004). There may be occasions when health care providers have a duty to warn others who are unknowingly endangered. This duty was highlighted by the landmark Tarasoff case. On October 27, 1969, Prosenjit Poddar killed Tatiana Tarasoff. Poddar was receiving psychiatric care during this period. He had informed his therapist 2 weeks earlier that he was going to kill a certain girl, easily identifiable as Tarasoff, on her return from Brazil. At the time his therapist tried to have him committed. The police detained Poddar briefly but decided he was rational, so they released him. No one warned Tatiana of the danger and Poddar killed her. The courts concluded that "once a therapist does in fact determine, or under applicable professional standards reasonably should have determined, that a person poses a serious danger of violence to others, he bears a duty to exercise reasonable care to protect the foreseeable victim of that danger" (Tarasoff v. Regents of University of California, 1976). The court recognized the difficulty of predicting dangerousness and the importance of maintaining confidentiality but determined that when the risk is high, confidentiality should be breached.

Health care professionals must strive to keep the person's personal information confidential so as to enhance trust within the health care professional–patient relationship. Therefore, in health care settings there are strong sanctions against breaching confidentiality. In theory the principle of confidentiality may be overridden only in situations in which extreme harm to self or others is imminent. In practice, confidentiality is breached frequently. In hospital settings many people have access to the person's information. Insurance companies demand access to information before payment for services is made. Additionally, there has recently been a push to institute a nationwide medical information bank. The ethical implications of this are many, and such implications are the subject of debates in the ethics literature (Etzioni, 1999; Goldberg, 2000; Gostin, 1997; Hodge, 2000).

In outpatient settings, barriers to privacy may occur when office or other personnel are personally acquainted with the patient. This is especially true in the types of settings where health promotion is the focus of practice. In such settings it is important that those supervising the health efforts address confidentiality issues with the staff they supervise. When health professionals are members of the community in which they practice, there may be confidentiality issues associated with the intimate nature of small communities. Nurses and other health-promotion professionals may find themselves being asked by friends and relatives of a patient for details about that person's health status. It can be very difficult to respond diplomatically while maintaining the person's privacy.

The Privacy Rule

The Privacy Rule (45 Code of Federal Regulations Part 160, 164 subparts A & E) was developed as a result of the Health Insurance Portability and Accountability Act (HIPAA). Its intent was to ensure that individuals' health information is

properly protected, while allowing the flow of information needed to provide and promote high-quality care (including using patient information for research) and to protect the public's health and well-being. HIPAA was meant to protect the privacy of individually identifiable health information in the face of advances in electronic technology and to limit the ways in which "health plans, pharmacies, hospitals, clinics, nursing homes and other covered entities (any provider that conducts or conveys information in electronic form, e.g., physicians, nurse practitioners)" can use medical information (U.S. Department of Health and Human Services [USDHHS], 2005). *Covered entities* basically means those covered by the privacy rule. The limitations on use of medical information extend to any identifiable information, written, oral, or computerized. Although there are some legal guidelines about disclosure, nurses and others are responsible for using clinical judgment in deciding what level of detail to share (USDHHS, 2004). It is important to understand that the purpose of the rule is protection of individual rights while still facilitating important public health and epidemiological research. Health-promotion activities include empowering people to exercise these rights when this is necessary. The Privacy Rule ensures that patients are given a copy of the privacy practices at a given institution. Additionally, under the rule individuals have the right:

- Of access to their own information
- To limit who may receive their information
- To request corrections for errors
- To receive an accounting of how their information has been used
- To request special confidential reporting of their information to them at a location of their choosing (e.g., this may be especially important for individuals at risk for intimate partner violence)
- To pursue complaints with the Department of Health and Human Services Office for Civil Rights

A rule of thumb for health professionals related to sharing information with others is to disclose only as much information as is necessary to permit optimal care and only information that is pertinent to the situation. A decision about disclosure of a person's information requires balancing of the risks of information sharing with the benefits of treatment. Although the privacy rule was meant to help safeguard people's rights, some commentators and researchers are finding the rule overly restrictive and worry that it might discourage important research, perhaps especially genetic research, with its far-reaching implications for individual privacy. As Kulynych and Korn (2002) write:

> Although the rule's drafters wisely opted not to create special standards for genetic information, the limits they have placed upon the use and disclosure of all "identifiable" health information will profoundly affect the conduct of genetic studies and many other forms of research. Research compliance efforts will become more costly and time consuming as institutions and individual providers who use or disclose health information for research confront new

procedural requirements and new liability for failures to meet the privacy rule's intricate compliance obligations. Investigators who use health information, as well as the institutional committees that must review human subjects research proposals, will need to familiarize themselves with a confusing array of new terminology, ambiguous standards and burdensome required paperwork. (p. 310)

Adolescents: Special Considerations of Confidentiality

Adolescents often provide health professionals with very tricky confidentiality issues. As Bandman and Bandman (2002) note, the adolescent is torn between wanting to challenge authority and to assert independence whilst still needing the "help and support of effective parents" (p. 195). The results of risk-taking behavior, such as drug and alcohol experimentation and risky sexual activity, and their normal developmental needs make teenagers a health-promotion challenge. The task of health promotion is to maintain and facilitate the adolescent's emerging autonomy and confidentiality needs, while mediating between the teenager and parental figures who feel that they have a right to information about the child. It is easy to become caught in the tension "between the anger and perceived duties of the parent and the defensiveness and vulnerability of the adolescent" (Bandman & Bandman, 2002, p. 200).

Although federal and state laws, in addition to (and as a result of) ethical considerations, generally serve to protect the privacy and autonomy of adolescents, health promotion involves more than mere protection. It involves facilitating the adolescent's health. Thus responsibilities include helping an adolescent to grasp his or her authentic options and rights, facilitating interaction between the adolescent and parents or guardians, maintaining trust, and conserving confidentiality.

On the other hand, clinical judgment (which includes ethical judgment) is important in determining risk. If the risk of preserving the adolescent's privacy is high, based on all pertinent and available evidence such as the presence of sexual or physical abuse, then it may be necessary to report this information to appropriate authorities. Mandatory reporting laws exist. Such laws are important for the general protection of a society's citizens. However, there may be rare occasions when a judgment must be made about whether upholding the legal obligation would cause more harm than good. In such circumstances there are two separate considerations. First, one must decide whether the risk to professional standing and licensure of not following the legally required path is something that the professional is willing to assume. The second consideration involves assessing the benefits and risks to the patient of not reporting. There is no easy resolution for these types of problems. If the situation is not an emergency, it is prudent to solicit appropriate advice from a peer, a counselor, or an ethics expert or resource. In any case, it remains the professional's ethical responsibility to handle the given situation in a manner that preserves trust and provides ongoing support.

Veracity

Veracity, or devotion to the truth, is another principle that supports health-promotion activities. Veracity is important in health care settings, because it involves trust, which is the basis of nurse or health care provider–patient relationships. People whose health is in question either do not have the knowledge or skills to address their vulnerability personally, or they are reliant upon the professional to supply this. In most cases they will not have the capacity to assess or access suggested remedies on their own. They are to varying degrees reliant upon the person who does possess the knowledge and skills to bring these to bear on their behalf. The contemporary bioethics literature favors characteristics of "veracity, . . . candor, honesty and truthfulness" (Beauchamp & Childress, 2001, p. 283) as virtues to be nurtured in the development of health professionals. This represents a change from the paternalistic (the physician knows what is best) attitudes that prevailed earlier in this century and up to the late 1960s.

Veracity in giving people information about their health care needs facilitates autonomous choice and enhances personal decision making. There are times, though, when health care professionals are tempted to withhold certain details from the person when this is seen as in the person's best interests or when family members demand it. In general it is difficult for health care providers to determine how much information and which types of information will best serve a person's needs. Knowledge of the person's beliefs, values, and lifestyle preferences are essential to the process of supplying adequate information to support autonomous decision making. One way to do this is to give the appropriate information while acknowledging that certain undesirable effects may occur and that these should be reported to the provider. Deliberately withholding information so that a person agrees to a treatment or interventions that the health-promoting agent considers important conflicts with veracity. It is tempting to avoid the longer route to resolving such problems (e.g., education, understanding people's motives, environmental challenges), but this eventually undermines trust and constitutes a moral problem. Veracity is compromised when the clinician withholds information that a person has a right to know or gives information that is misleading or incomprehensible. Veracity has some cross-cultural implications, in that some cultures have not traditionally valued truth telling in the case of terminal illness or cancer diagnosis. Decision making about whether to honor veracity in such cases must take into consideration what is known about the culture, the particular person, the strength of his or her personal and cultural beliefs, and whether there is evidence about what sorts of things the person would like to know (see the Multicultural Awareness box).

The absence of veracity may interfere with autonomous action. In the case of terminal illness it may deprive the person of the ability to plan the remainder of his or her life. It is rare, but may be possible, that a person does not want to know a certain diagnosis or a given trajectory. If this is known in advance it may prove an exception to the rule of veracity (e.g., a person may waive the right to certain information in advance).

Veracity can be a problem on a larger scale, for example, in health education endeavors aimed at changing patterns of behavior in social groups or in communities. Should nurses and others just present the facts or should they attempt to persuade? What are the limits of veracity? Is it permissible to exaggerate the dangers of certain behavior in the interests of the health of the society? These questions cannot be answered within the confines of this chapter but are important to keep in mind when assessing the merits of proposed population-based interventions.

Nonmaleficence

Related to autonomy is the principle of nonmaleficence, which enjoins people not to harm other people. In general society this principle constrains people from autonomous action when their actions are likely to harm others. In health care settings it prohibits clinicians from harming those for whom they provide services. For health promotion it means that in planning activities either on an individual level or the societal level, possible harms must be minimized. Some harms are acceptable if the overall benefits outweigh the risks of actions. Harms may be intentional or unintentional. It is often impossible to foresee all the risks of a given course of action. However, professionals who engage in health-promotion endeavors are responsible for foreseeing predictable adverse consequences and taking these into consideration. These responsibilities include addressing social or health care policies that are discovered to have unintended effects. Norton (1998) gives an example of a health policy that had unintended negative health effects. This concerned a government initiative in the United Kingdom designed to encourage nurses and midwives to facilitate breast-feeding over bottle feeding. At first this sounds like a worthy health-promotion strategy, because research has shown the advantages to the baby of breast-feeding. However, one health authority proposed that the nurses not discuss formula mixing unless the women themselves broached this subject. The problem is that many women, for a variety of reasons, either choose to or have to bottle feed their babies; therefore, there is "a responsibility for nurses and midwives to ensure that mothers are given accurate information about the safe preparation of these feeds" (Norton, 1998, p. 1273).

The possibility of unintentional harms is a hazard of most actions designed to promote health. Such risks can be minimized by well thought-out activities for which every effort has been directed toward trying to foresee possible negative effects and to avoid, or control for, these. Professionals are responsible for understanding the limits of their knowledge or the data to which they have access. A synthesis of the characteristics reflection, critical thinking, and knowledge, along with an understanding of the details and context of a situation, is required before embarking on a course of action aimed at facilitating a person's health or well-being. The overall discomfort encountered by the individual must be the minimum possible to achieve the primary good intended. In other words, the health care provider is accountable for his or her judgment and for providing interventions most likely to bring about the desired result. Thus more than just the intention not to do harm is required.

Nurses and allied professionals can do harm inadvertently through ignorance or incompetence, through referral to another provider who is incompetent or inappropriate, by inadequate supervision or training of those under one's supervision, and so on. A health care professional who genuinely attempts to minimize harms that are necessary to providing a greater good (beneficence) acts with nonmaleficence if what results is more beneficial than it is harmful. Alternatively, even if greater harm than good did actually ensue, if it could not have been anticipated based on available information and the clinician's competent judgment, then the action was not maleficent. For example, a course of exercise is designed for a person subsequent to a thorough physical. The person is educated about proper body mechanics, heart rate parameters, and appropriate exercise maneuvers but during an exercise session faints and fractures his arm. Further testing reveals a previously undetected cardiac anomaly that is subsequently surgically corrected. This is not maleficence; the main objective of the agent was therapeutic and the event was, if not totally unforeseeable, not identified upon routine preexercise testing. However, the duty of nonmaleficence does mean that health care professionals are accountable for foreseeing the consequences of their actions when this is possible. This places obligations on the practitioner to evaluate the problem thoroughly in its rich contextual facets. A meticulous and informed evaluation in turn requires professional competency. Thus harm caused through careless, indifferent, or expedient decision making violates the principle of nonmaleficence. Both deliberate harm and harm caused by indifferent or incompetent decision making should be considered maleficent and are morally problematic.

Beneficence

Beneficence is the quality or state of doing or producing good. As a moral principle, beneficence presents us with the duty to maximize the benefits of actions while minimizing harms. There are two related senses of the moral principle of beneficence in health-promotion settings. The principle of beneficence may govern actions taken to further the overall health or well-being of the society in general or it may govern actions taken to promote the good of a particular individual.

When society formulates rules that are designed to protect people against the negative effects of their own actions, these rules are considered beneficent. They are also sometimes described as paternalistic because they override a person's autonomy to disobey them. For example, seat belt laws are paternalistic, as are rules governing the use of therapeutic or so-called *recreational drugs*. "Paternalism is the interference of a state or an individual with another person, against their will, and justified by a claim that the person interfered with will be better off or protected from harm" (Dworkin, 2002). The term *paternalism* is derived from *parens patrie*, or the interest of the state in protecting the vulnerable in society.

The principle of beneficence, when used to justify overriding an individual's autonomous choice in order to serve that individual's interests, is sometimes justified when a person lacks the capacity to make personal or health care decisions. Thus any of the factors that interfere with autonomy, as discussed previously (coercion, cognitive impairment, lack of understanding), may require the health care provider to beneficently override the individual's decisions. Generally, though, beneficence permits interference only when the risks of the individual's proposed actions are high and we cannot determine how autonomous is the decision to act. This is because autonomy is such a powerful principle in Western societies that a decision to override is not taken lightly. I am justified in preventing a person from taking an overdose of sleeping pills or jumping off a cliff, because the risks of not doing so are high and if the person succeeds there is no possibility of future autonomous actions.

Beneficence, unlike nonmaleficence, is not necessarily a moral requirement of action on the part of societal members toward each other (Grace, 2004). Whether beneficence is viewed as a moral requirement of societal members to actively promote each other's good very much depends upon philosophical beliefs and the ethical theory or perspective ascribed to (if any); that is, as an ordinary citizen I am not necessarily morally required to go out of my way to help or benefit someone. The exception is when a person is endangered and my assistance would mitigate that danger, in which case failing to offer assistance, arguably, violates the principle of nonmaleficence. Exceptions to beneficence in everyday life include the actions of parents on behalf of their children and guardians on behalf of their wards. In other words, exceptions exist in which we have responsibility for vulnerable others.

In contrast to ordinary members of society, health care professionals have augmented duties of beneficence, because their professional goals involve meeting health care needs and thus are aimed at providing a good. For such reasons, beneficence is a moral expectation of health care professionals. "Beneficence is a requirement to produce net benefit for those on whose behalf health care workers undertake interventions" (Cribb & Duncan, 2002, p. 41).

Beneficence is a difficult principle in health-promotion settings because of the dual nature of health-promotion goals, health for individuals and healthy communities. There is often a tension between the two as noted earlier. Tones (1997) highlights this problem in a discussion of health educators aims. They "need on the one hand to prevent disease and safeguard the public health while, on the other hand, respecting individual freedom of choice—including the freedom to adopt an unhealthy lifestyle" (p. 33). Thus duties of beneficence may be at odds with facilitating autonomy viewed narrowly as freedom of action, even self-destructive action.

A paradox exists when we try to change unhealthy behaviors but don't address the underlying causes of those behaviors. For example, although smoking cessation programs do assist some people to stop smoking, and restricting areas where people may smoke tends to persuade some people that it is just becoming too inconvenient to continue, we ought also to be addressing the advertising campaigns that aim to gather new recruits from among adolescents. Popular press articles note the trend among adolescents to try flavored cigarettes. " . . . *bidis*, are flavored to taste like strawberry, chocolate, mandarin orange, vanilla, grape, lemon-lime, clove, mint, cinnamon, wild cherry, mango, cardamom, licorice, or raspberry. They are hand rolled into the leaves of an Indian plant, tied with string and attractively and exotically packaged. All in all, it looks like a product that was designed for teens. But these tobacco cigarettes are addictive, dangerous, and rapidly gaining in popularity" (Greater Dallas Council on Alcohol and Drug Abuse, 2002). Norton (1998) notes that a real problem with any education-based health-promotion endeavor is that in the absence of underlying societal changes it is ultimately doomed to fail. This supports the earlier argument about professional obligations to address deep-rooted social problems that jeopardize health or are associated with health disparities. See the Hot Topics and Health Teaching boxes for discussions of direct-to-consumer marketing (DTCM) of genetic testing for examples of this.

Beneficence: Conflict With Autonomy

From the previous discussion it can be seen that the principles of beneficence and autonomy sometimes conflict. For example, seat belt rules are ostensibly created to protect people from injury, but they take away autonomous choice. Beneficence may justify overriding the decision of a febrile confused patient who refuses to take her antibiotics for pneumonia. Permitting this patient to refuse may risk her life. What is the clinician's responsibility? Duties of beneficence seem to mandate medicating her against her will, ensuring that the good of health is facilitated although violating the principle of autonomy. The justification for this must include an assessment of her status related to capacity for autonomous decision making for this particular treatment. Preserving the person's life so he or she can make autonomous decisions in the future may be required by beneficence. However, it can be argued that beneficence takes precedence over autonomy only in those cases in which the choice cannot be considered autonomous. Thus we have to explore how autonomous the choice is. First, there has to be evidence that a choice has been made. In this case the choice was between accepting antibiotic treatment versus not accepting antibiotic treatment. Second, the

HOTtopics   DIRECT-TO-CONSUMER MARKETING: DRUGS AND TESTS

Commercial industries have discovered a novel way to increase profits. DTCM can occur via print, the Internet, or television. It impacts health-promotion efforts in a variety of ways and has serious ethical implications. DTCM of genetic testing, interventions for newly discovered diseases, or drugs shifts emphasis away from promoting healthy lifestyles or addressing environmental concerns to quick fixes that are more likely to benefit the commercial enterprise and its stakeholders than the individuals to whom the advertising campaigns are directed. Although similar problems apply to DTCM of drugs, genetic testing is used below as an exemplar of problems.

DTCM: Genetic Testing

In a workshop held in March 2003 sponsored by the National Human Genome Research Institute of the National Institutes of Health, various interested parties, including scientists, ethicists, company spokespersons, and consumers, discussed the pros and cons of this mode of promoting genetic testing. The workshop's summary report notes that "while this DTCM may increase public awareness about the availability of genetic tests, there may also be some risks in adopting this strategy." It was noted that, according to recent research, advertisements could increase consumers' awareness about diseases, but they often fail to accurately convey risk information including the implications of test results on the mental status of test takers and on related others. Additionally, the information may fail to reach those most at risk. Hull and Prasad (2001), reporting on her research, urges that more research be carried out to better understand consumer responses to advertisements.

Problems Associated With DTCM of Genetic Testing

Note: Some of these problems are also associated with genetic testing in general.

- Resource allocation (in terms of the implications of misdirected testing on consumer and provider time and counseling requirements)
- Lack of utility of available interventions
- Consumer inability to deal with the complexity of the information: confusion, false hope, false anxiety
- Economic harm to consumer
- Missed opportunities to pursue other health interventions
- Professionals with working knowledge of genetic testing not available to advise about testing
- Provider education (or lack thereof) with regard to genetics, nonhealth implications within families, and how to communicate genetic information
- Lack of regulatory oversight for tests, existing oversight is technology driven rather than public health oriented, lack of validated tests, lack of consensus on methods for validating genetic tests
- Scant data about harms or benefits of tests
- Questionable scientific accuracy and validity of the advertisements
- Misinformation in public sector about genetics

Modified from the summary report of the National Human Genome Research Institute, March 23, 2004.

HEALTH TEACHING   Helping Patients to Grasp the Health Implications of Direct-to-Consumer Marketing

1. Become educated about genetics, the scope and limits of genetic testing, and related marketing strategies, especially as this relates to your specific area of practice.
   - Thoroughly investigate the merits of any new marketing strategy that your patients bring to your attention.
   - Attend workshops.
   - Keep up to date on the related research and ethics literature (paper or electronic journals, articles, and forums).
   - Be aware of and use local resources for genetic advice (counseling services, ethics services at local hospitals, health care ethics or bioethics departments of local colleges and universities).
2. Assist patients to make a comprehensive assessment of their own needs and goals and to what extent the publicized testing or other offering is likely to help them meet these.

- Explore with them possible motivations for the particular marketing strategy.
- Formulate a list of pros and cons of using the test, drug, or device.
- Assess the extent to which the particular offering is likely to achieve patient goals.
- Explain the possible effects of the test, drug, or device on self, family, and others (psychological, physical, and economic).
- Provide ongoing advice, resources, and support as needed.
3. Refer patients to genetic counselors for further discussion (see Box 5-1 on genetic counseling).

---

reasonableness (or rationality) of the decision has to be discerned; that is, it must be ascertained whether the person really has grasped the implications of refusing treatment. The reasons given for the treatment refusal, then, should illuminate gaps in information delivery or processing.

Finally, it must be determined whether there are any external or internal coercion factors impinging on the decision. Perhaps the person feels she cannot afford the medicine (external) or perhaps she has a mistrust of antibiotics because of a previous experience (internal).

Agich (2003) has noted that competent decision making requires, among other things, that the person be in possession of adequate information, an understanding of benefits and costs of alternative treatments or plans, and knowledge of personal values and beliefs and the effects of these upon the decision. He is expressly discussing decision making in nursing home settings, but these ideas are applicable to decision making in all types of settings and perhaps especially in correctional facilities. These criteria can be used to permit clinicians to distinguish informed decisions from those that cannot be considered autonomous or when special measures must be taken to control coercive factors. When a decision cannot be said to be informed, the principle of beneficence directs us to decide treatment based on the person's best interests.

Justice

Justice is an ethical principle of major importance in health-promotion settings. There are various conceptions of justice, and the term is used in a variety of ways. For the purposes of this chapter the discussion is about social justice rather than criminal justice (also known as commutative justice). Social justice has to do with any formal or informal systems existing within a given society to determine what will be the distribution of goods such as health, education, food, and shelter. Buchanan (2000) notes that as a result of studying early records, we know "the concept of justice has been central to human understandings of socially significant values" (p. 155).

There are two broad socially oriented ideas regarding justice. One perspective views justice as being based on desert—those who are more worthy of merit, or who contribute more, are viewed as deserving of better social benefits. The other perspective views justice as equalizing benefits across society regardless of merit. This latter view is justice as fairness. The tendency when discussing the provision of health care for a society is to focus on justice viewed as fairness and as favoring equality. However, when the discussion turns to allocation of scarce resources, such as organs for transplant, one can detect in the discussion a justice standard that favors merit rather than equality. There are interesting and complex philosophical debates about the use of justice as merit, but they are beyond the scope of this chapter. Instead we will focus on the requirements of justice viewed as fairness, because we know that inequalities in health care exacerbate and are exacerbated by economic disadvantages stemming from a variety of causes.

The social justice arrangements in a society are indicative of what the society values. In democratic societies, the requirements of social justice generally include equitable distribution of the benefits and burdens of societal life. "Justice as fairness" reflects the ideas behind Rawls' (1971) *A Theory of Justice*. Rawls identifies two "rules of justice that he argues will enable humankind to resolve disputes fairly and justly" (Buchanan, 2000, p. 156). "First: each person is to have an equal right to the most extensive liberty compatible with a similar liberty for others. Second: social and economic inequalities are to be arranged such that they are both (a) reasonably expected to be to everyone's advantage, and (b) attached to positions and offices open to all" (Rawls, 1971, p. 60). Rawls formulates these rules as a result of his hypothetical method for deciding how a society's institutions should be arranged in order to provide for fairness. Rawls proposes that these rules of justice would emerge as a result of an average person's reasoning from behind a "veil of ignorance" (ignorant about their place in society, personal assets, or handicaps) about what social arrangements they would prefer if they did not know what their personal impediments or assets were going to be. Rawls theory, although respected by ethicists, is subject to criticism on a variety of fronts. The most significant criticism for present purposes is that justice as fairness does not provide a lot of guidance for some common social problems such as abortion, welfare, and the righting of previous wrongs (e.g., affirmative action, the rights of native people) and ignores the problems of those without legal rights such as undocumented workers (Buchanan, 2000; MacIntyre, 1984; Taylor, 1985). However, the standard of equality gives health-promotion professionals a ground to argue the need for just health care provisions and to criticize current conditions of inequity.

An emphasis on justice in health care settings is sometimes called the *impartialist perspective* in that it considers the needs of all who fall under its umbrella. For example, within the prison system, this view of justice would mandate access to care for prisoners in need. Thus it would not permit arbitrary obstacles to access (such as requiring good behavior or favors) that might be presented by prison officers or by other prisoners who wish to exert physical or psychological control. Justice would also require improved access to care for the poor and underprivileged, both in terms of receiving care and transportation or local availability of services.

Although justice might require consideration of the special needs of a disadvantaged group, it does so impartially; that is, it does not distinguish among the particulars of individuals. Each member within the group has an equal right to whatever is proposed. In an economically and profit-driven health care system injustices occur both at the local and societal levels. Because justice viewed as fairness is impartial about individual differences, that moral perspective taken alone is not a perfect tool with which to look at health care disparities and their causes. The combination of justice, feminist concerns about power and oppression, and the acknowledged responsibilities of health care professionals to promote health permit a comprehensive view of problems associated with health protection and promotion. This view incorporates problems both for a society and for individuals within the society. Buchanan (2000) captures this necessary synthesis of perspectives well, noting "the mutually reinforcing relationships among justice, caring and responsibility" which will help health care professionals to "enable people to live well" (p. 167).

STRATEGIES FOR ETHICAL DECISION MAKING

Locating the Source and Levels of Ethical Problems

Many problems associated with health promotion are not moral or ethical dilemmas in the sense described earlier. Although some dilemmas occur and must be addressed, most health-promotion problems are moral or ethical issues in the sense that obstacles exist to prevent an individual from living life well and flourishing, or obstacles exist to prevent or interfere with societal goals related to health. Throughout this chapter discussions of both the larger (societal) and narrower (individual) perspectives have been emphasized and their relationships highlighted. Sometimes tensions between the two require mediation and may force the health promoter to decide which problem must be addressed first. For example, a nurse at a family practice clinic cares for a teenager who is morbidly obese. At the level of the patient the nurse is charged with discovering underlying causes of the obesity (physical, psychological, contextual) and designing strategies in concert with the patient to help resolve the problem. However, as a professional who has, both anecdotally and on researching the issue, noted that this is an increasingly prevalent problem, the family practice nurse has responsibilities to address the issue at the more political level in concert with interested others. As Norton (1998) notes "health promotion . . . includes a variety of activities such as lobbying to bring about healthy public policy at both government and local levels" (p. 1270).

To address health-promotion issues effectively, professionals need not only possess their particular disciplinary expertise and an understanding of ethical language, principles, and perspectives, but also a willingness to understand their own values and preconceptions about health and people. Understanding personal philosophy, biases, and values permits one to control for these in the sense of being aware of the influences they have over our interactions with others.

Values Clarification and Reflection

Gaining confidence in moral decision making is a slow process. The following are suggestions that will permit development related to recognizing and addressing ethical issues.

Examine Beliefs and Values

Cultivate the habit of examining what are your personal values and beliefs related to the human condition, justice, and responsibility. Be willing to revise your beliefs in line with your professional knowledge base, experiences, or current research findings. For example, how do beliefs that "people get what they deserve" collate with what we know, that those of lower socioeconomic status have lower levels of health and that poor health interferes with functioning and is associated with depression? How do our attitudes change when we try to place ourselves in the context of the other person's life?

This is not to say that maintaining personal integrity is not important—it is. Maintaining both personal and professional integrity is essential to good practice. Integrity has to do with a sense of wholeness of the self and consistency of actions with truly examined beliefs and values. "Nurses have both personal and professional identities that are neither entirely separate nor entirely merged, but are integrated" (ANA, 2001, p. 19). Tenet 5 of the ANA (2001) *Code of Ethics for Nurses With Interpretive Statements* validates the nurse's preservation of integrity in those situations in which he or she feels that personal integrity is compromised. It notes that, "where a particular treatment, intervention, activity or practice is morally objectionable to the nurse . . . the nurse is justified in refusing to participate on moral grounds" (ANA, 2001, p. 20). When this involves risk to the patient, though, other arrangements must be made to safeguard patient care.

A true examination of beliefs and values requires a willingness to admit that these may not always be justifiable—they may be remnants from childhood indoctrinations of various sorts. For example, one might believe that certain ethnic groups are inferior in some way, or that one should not question authority. An honest and ongoing examination of one's values and biases permits one to control for these in situations in which personal values and biases are irrelevant to the care of patients.

The Influence of Personal Beliefs and Values

An understanding of how personal beliefs and values are either congruent, or are liable to interfere, with the task at hand is crucial to ethical problem solving. In any given situation, the nurse or allied health professional must ask him or herself, "What are my beliefs and biases in this situation? How are these likely to influence my actions?" For example, if the home health nurse believes her below-poverty-level, depressed, obese, diabetic patient who smokes is responsible for the poor healing of her own leg ulcer, she may be less inclined to work with the patient to discover and address the patient's goals.

Reflection on Practice

A third helpful strategy is to reflect on situations afterward to discover what worked, what didn't work, and what could be done differently in the future. It is often helpful to interact with peers or other experts after particularly difficult situations to discover alternative perspectives or resources for the purposes of future problem solving.

Decision-Making Considerations

Any decision making in health-promotion settings has inseparable moral components. This is true for the reasons outlined earlier, related to professional responsibility to further the good for individuals and society. Thus the careful exercise of experience, skill, and knowledge is warranted when trying to formulate the best course of action for a given individual or group, or in resolving particular as well as societal health-promotion problems. This framework is offered as a way of ensuring that clarity about a particular case or situation is gained. Because of the diverse nature of health-promotion activities, no straightforward models of decision making can realistically be applied in all situations. Additionally, it is often true of such issues that decision making is an ongoing process. Revisions to plans may be required in light of new information. The following are all important facets of decision making but do not necessarily occur in the order given.

Identify the Main Problem or Issue

What level of problem is this: social, group, or individual? If the location of the problem is societal, it will also impact individuals and groups and a decision has to be made about the order of interventions. Try to determine what is the main ethical principle involved or whether it is a problem of conflicting principles. For example, in order to provide benefit to the patient his autonomy must be overridden. Is this a social justice issue? An autonomy issue? What factors led to the problem? Is there coercion or are there other power imbalances? Who has an interest in maintaining the power imbalances and who gains the most from the imbalance? These are the questions feminist ethics would ask.

Determine Who or What Created the Problem

Who has a stake in the issue and in how it will be resolved? Answering this question will permit a determination of whose input is crucial to the decision-making process. Who or what are important considerations (institutions, individuals, businesses, social policy)? Does this issue result from a failure to predict the consequences of certain social policies?

Determine the Prevalent Values

What are the values held by all the different players? Are there value conflicts? The value conflicts might be individual versus social, for example, a patient with tuberculosis who refuses to take his medicines, thus putting at risk members of his family or of the community. Values conflicts might also be interpersonal among the health-promotion team or personal versus professional. As a general rule, more weight is assigned to the values of the individual who is most likely to be affected by a decision. It is important to consider the influence of culture upon values when the issue has to do with health promotion for culturally diverse groups. It is important to involve people who can help sort out the cultural beliefs, especially when language difficulties are present. A knowledgeable but neutral interpreter may be helpful when liaison between groups is needed.

Identify Information Gaps

This is a good place to reflect upon whether the decision maker(s) are confident about what they do and do not know. This is not always an easy task. Information may exist that has not yet reached our awareness, or we might fail to ask a question that would reveal important information. How can we be confident about the scope and limits of our

knowledge? Clinical judgment is a good tool but is not foolproof. When doubts exist or the decision is likely to have serious or risky consequences, we need to involve knowledgeable others or try to determine the best places to gain missing information.

Formulate Possible Courses of Action and Probable Consequences

Courses of action may involve further information gathering, brainstorming, and possibly collaboration with other experts or specialists. Although further data may be needed to resolve problems at the level of individuals or small groups, it is especially necessary to enlist additional help when the issue is one that requires political action to bring about policy changes. It may be necessary to bring in community members and leaders or to enlist the political power of specialty groups. Finally, a determination must be made about which proposed courses of action will be the least harmful and the most beneficial.

Initiate the Selected Course of Action and Evaluate the Outcome

Does the actual outcome match the anticipated outcome? If not, what happened that was unexpected? Would this have been foreseeable given more data? Would you do things differently in another similar situation given what you've learned? Does the problem need to be addressed at a different level (institutional or public policy)?

Engage in Self-Reflection and Peer or Expert Group Reflection

What could you have done differently? Would consulting with others have altered your conception of the problem or your course of action? What insights can you or your peers glean from this that could be appropriate for similar situations in the future? How might continuing education opportunities help you or your peers more appropriately address similar problems in the future? Would an ethics resource (committee or consultant) be helpful in such situations? Could you use this case as a focused learning experience for your peers and collaborators?

ETHICS OF HEALTH PROMOTION: CASES*

Some cases of especial relevance to health-promotion professionals are presented below. They are followed by questions that can be answered by individual readers, but they also provide a good starting point for group discussion. Try using the decision-making strategies suggested throughout the chapter as you explore these problems. It is anticipated that you will want more information than is provided. Deciding what extra information would be helpful is an important part of the exercise.

---

*The author would like to acknowledge the contributions of Carol Lynn Mandle and Carolyn Hayes. They contributed some of these cases.

CASE 1   Addressing Health Care System Problems—Elissa Needs Help

Elissa is 38 years old. She recently moved 200 miles from her home to a small town (population 6000) and separated from her abusive husband to escape his continuing threats and to be near her childhood friend. She suffers from chronic, sometimes incapacitating, depression for which she has in the past received antidepressant medications and counseling, with temporary relief. She has been unable to work and has no private health insurance. She is eligible for the state's Medicaid program, however, and has recently discovered that Medicaid will cover her health care needs. Her friend refers her to the only primary care center in the area, where she is seen by Jill, one of the two nurse practitioners. As part of her evaluation, Jill discovers that Elissa was also abused as a child and has very poor self-esteem, although Elissa affirms that her childhood friend is very supportive. Jill believes that longer term psychological counseling would benefit Elissa and facilitate her well-being, but she also knows that none of the counseling services within a 50-mile radius accepts Medicaid payment. Elissa has no transportation.

What are Jill's options? Responsibilities?

What actions might she pursue both on a local level and a political level?

What are her resources?

What is the responsibility of the health-promotion disciplines in cases like this?

CASE 2   Assisted Suicide or Emotional Support?—Ana and Victor

A nurse in a clinic is accountable for ongoing assessments of pain management in a population with chronic pain. One of the long-term patients, Ana, has been requiring increasing amounts of narcotics for her pain management over the last year. The nurse has known for over a year that Ana's husband, Victor, has amyotrophic lateral sclerosis, or Lou Gehrig's disease. Victor's disease adds a great deal of stress to both their lives, which has had a negative effect on Ana's physical health. The nurse assesses the emotional toll of Victor's illness as part of Ana's pain assessment. During one of these discussions, Ana asks the nurse how much of her narcotic medication her husband would need to take to end his life.

What does it mean to provide someone with the "means" to commit suicide?

What questions would you have for Ana at this point of the conversation?

What would you do with the answers?

Do you have any obligations to Victor?

Do you collaborate with Victor's physician?

What is in Ana's "best interests"?

Who or what are your resources?

What does nursing as a discipline say about assisted suicide?

What is the law in your state?

What should you do?

CASE 3   How Much Money Can One Person Spend?—Joe Does Not Like Taking Pills

A nurse practitioner is caring for people in an economically poor neighborhood. An older woman, Rose, frequently runs out of inhalers for her asthma. The insurance does not pay enough per month for her to be able to use the inhalers as directed. She struggles along as best she can but frequently cancels outings with loved ones because she "can't always catch her breath and it scares the little ones." The nurse practitioner has tried to advocate for more medication. Time and time again, the response of the insurance company is, "There is only so much money to spread around."

Across the street is Joe, who has been a patient for nearly 3 years. He needs to take diuretic medications to avoid frequent hospitalizations. He does not like to think of himself as a "man who needs pills." Consequently, he does not take the diuretic medication, resulting in preventable hospitalizations. If he changed his pattern of behavior, there would be money for Rose to receive more medication.

What are the ethical questions in this scenario?

Ethically, can the nurse practitioner tell Joe about Rose's situation to try to persuade him to take his pills?

Is there anything that the nurse practitioner should do individually to resolve this dilemma? Is there anything that nursing as a discipline should do?

What course of action would be in Rose's best interest?

CASE 4   She's My Patient!—Lilly and "Jake" (a.k.a. Paul)

A nurse practitioner is at a conference when a physician colleague discusses a difficult case. One of his patients, "Jake," is HIV positive but refuses any treatment. The physician explains that Jake fears that his wife will discover and recognize the names of the medications, because he knows "these drug names are discussed on television all the time." He has not told, nor does he ever intend to disclose to his wife, that he is HIV positive. Jake firmly believes his condition is his private information and, for now, the couple uses condoms for birth control. The physician is concerned that Jake will not tell his wife. The physician is presenting this case to colleagues to highlight the public awareness campaigns that, to some extent, have affected patient privacy. He argues, "Listen to how they call out your name and the drugs at the pharmacy counter."

The nurse practitioner recognizes bits and pieces of information and comes to the painful realization that Jake is really Paul, and Paul is the husband of one of her patients, Lilly. Lilly has begun to discuss with you that she wants to get pregnant soon. The town is too small for the nurse practitioner to be mistaken. Or is it?

Is it ethical for the nurse practitioner to ask the physician if Jake is Paul?

Is it ethical for her to tell Lilly she suspects Paul is HIV positive?

Should this information change how she counsels Lilly about a pregnancy?

What is in Lilly's best interests?

What resources are available?

SUMMARY

Health promotion is a vast and complex practice area; consequently, the associated ethical challenges are diverse and multileveled. This chapter has outlined the nature and purpose of health care ethics and related this to the responsibilities of nurses and allied health providers practicing in contemporary health and health-promotion settings. It has proposed that health promotion should be viewed as a moral undertaking of health care professionals. Health care professionals will have gained some of the tools and language needed to explore ethical issues, discuss these with others, and address problematic issues at both the individual and the societal levels. A selection of contemporary issues was used to illustrate points and provide examples. This selection represents a very small portion of potential contemporary problems; nevertheless, the tools and strategies provided are not specific to these problems but can be used to explore issues particular to their specialty settings. Perhaps the most important factor to keep in mind is that practice problems manifesting at the level of the individual almost always have their origins in the broader societal environment.

ADDITIONAL STUDY MATERIAL

Study Questions in the back of the book, see page 663.

evolve WEB SITE MATERIALS

These materials are located on the book's Web site at http://evolve.elsevier.com/Edelman/.

- WebLinks
- Content Updates

REFERENCES

Agich, G. A. (2003). *Dependence and autonomy in old age: An ethical framework for long term care.* Cambridge, UK: Cambridge University Press.

American Nurses Association. (1994). *Position statement: The nonnegotiable nature of the ANA code for nurses with interpretive statements.* Washington, DC: Author.

American Nurses Association. (2001). *Code of ethics for nurses with interpretive statements.* Washington, DC: Author.

American Nurses Association. (2003). *Nursing's social policy statement.* (2nd ed.). Silver Springs, MD: nursesbooks.org.

Andrews, L. B., Mehlman, M. J., & Rothstein, M. A. (2002). *Genetics: Ethics, law and policy.* St. Paul, MN: West Group/Thompson.

Ballou, K. A. (2000). A historical-philosophical analysis of the professional nurse obligation to participate in sociopolitical activities. *Policy, Politics & Nursing Practice, 1*(3), 172-184.

Bandman, E. L., & Bandman, B. (2002). *Nursing ethics through the lifespan* (4th ed). Upper Saddle River, NJ: Prentice Hall.

Beauchamp, T. L., & Childress, J. F. (2001). *Principles of biomedical ethics* (5th ed.). New York: Oxford University.

Beauchamp, T. L., & Walters, L. (1999). *Contemporary issues in bioethics* (5th ed.). Belmont, CA: Wadsworth.

Benner, P., Tanner, C. A., & Chesla, C. A. (1996). *Expertise in nursing practice: Caring, clinical judgment and ethics.* New York: Springer.

Bereano, P. (2000). Does genetic research threaten our civil liberties? Retrieved May 24, 2004, from: http://www.actionbioscience.org/genomic/bereano.html.

Brown, L. (1993). *The new Shorter Oxford English dictionary.* New York: Oxford Clarendon Press.

Buchanan, D. R. (2000). *An ethic for health promotion.* New York: Oxford University.

Buchanan, A. E., & Brock, D. W. (1989). *Deciding for others: The ethics of surrogate decision making.* New York: Cambridge University.

Burkhart, M. A., & Nathaniel, A. K. (2002). *Ethics and issues in contemporary nursing* (2nd ed.). Albany, NY: Delmar.

Chambliss, D. F. (1996). *Beyond caring: Hospitals, nurses and the social organization of ethics.* Chicago, IL: University of Chicago Press.

Clarfield, A. M., Gordon, M., Markwell, H., & Shabbir, M. H. A. (2003). Ethical issues in end-of-life geriatric care: The approach of three monotheistic religions—Judaism, Catholicism, and Islam. *Journal of the American Geriatrics Society, 51,* 1149-1154.

Clarke, D. B. (1998). The Patient Self-Determination Act. In J. F. Monagle & D. C. Thomasma (Eds.), *Health care ethics: Critical issues* (pp. 92-113). Gaithersburg, MD: Aspen.

Cribb, A., & Duncan, P. (2002). *Health promotion and professional ethics.* Malden, MA: Blackwell.

Davis, A., Aroskar, M. A., Liaschenko, J., & Drought, T. S. (1997). *Ethical dilemmas & nursing practice* (4th ed.). Stamford, CT: Appleton & Lange.

Dickey, S. B., & Deatrick, J. (2000). Autonomy and decision making for health promotion in adolescence. *Pediatric Nursing, 26*(5), 461-470.

Donchin, A., & Purdy, L. (1999). *Embodying bioethics: Recent feminist advances.* Lanham, MD: Rowman and Littlefield.

Dworkin, G. (2002). Paternalism. In E. N. Zalta (Ed.), The Stanford encyclopedia of philosophy. *Retrieved June 1, 2004, from:* http://plato.stanford.edu/archives/win2002/entries/paternalism/.

Etzioni, A. (1999). Medical records: enhancing privacy, preserving the common good *Hastings Center Report, 29*(2), 14-23.

Fagerlin, A., & Schneider, C. E. (2004). Enough. The failure of the living will. *Hastings Center Report, 34*(2), 30-42.

Fry, S. T. (1990). The philosophical foundations of caring. In M. Leininger (Ed.), Ethical and moral dimensions of care (pp. 13-24). Detroit Wayne State.

Gaylord, N., & Grace, P. (1995). Nursing advocacy: an ethic of practice. *Nursing Ethics, 2*(1), 11-18.

Genetic Counselors Code of Ethics (1992). *Journal of Genetics Counseling 1*(1), 41-43.

Gilligan, C. (1982). *In a different voice: Psychological theory and women's development.* Cambridge, MA: Harvard University Press.

Goldberg, A. I. (2000). Commentary. *Cambridge Quarterly of Healthcare Ethics, 9:*113-117.

Gostin, L. O. (1997). Personal Privacy in the Health Care System: Employer-Sponsored Insurance, Managed Care, and Integrated Delivery Systems. *Kennedy Institute of Ethics Journal, 7*(4), 361-376.

Grace, P. J. (1998). A philosophical analysis of the concept 'advocacy': Implications for professional-person relationships. (Doctoral dissertation, University of Tennessee, Knoxville, 1998). *Dissertation Abstracts, International,* UMI No 9923287.

Grace, P. J. (2001). Professional advocacy: Widening the scope of accountability. *Nursing Philosophy, 2*(2), 151-162.

Grace, P. J. (2004). Ethics in the clinical encounter. In S. Chase (Ed.), *Clinical judgment and communication in nurse practitioner practice* (pp. 295-333). Philadelphia: F. A. Davis.

Greater Dallas Council on Alcohol and Drug Abuse. (2002). *Candy flavored cigarettes gain popularity.* Dallas: Author. Retrieved May 28, 2004, from: http://www.gdcada.org/stories/bidi.htm.

Hodge Jr., J. G. (2000). National Health Information Privacy and New Federalism. *Notre Dame Journal of Law. Ethics and Public Policy, 14*(2), 791-820.

Hull, S. C., Prasad, K. (2001). Reading between the lines: Direct-to-consumer advertising of genetic testing in the USA. *Reproductive Health Matters, 9*(18), 44-48.

International Council of Nurses. (2000). *The ICN code of ethics for nurses.* Geneva, Switzerland: Author. Retrieved February 8, 2005, from: *http://www.icn.ch/icncode.pdf.*

Kant, I. (1967). Foundations of the metaphysics of morals (Trans. L. W. Beck). In A. I. Melden (Ed.), *Ethical theories: A book of readings* (2nd ed., pp. 317-366). Englewood Cliffs, NJ: Prentice Hall. (Original work published 1785.)

Kohlberg, L. (1981). *The philosophy of moral development: Moral stages and the idea of justice. Essays on moral development* (Vol. 1). San Francisco: Harper & Row.

Kohlberg, L. (1984). *The nature and validity of moral stages. Essays on moral development* (Vol. 2). San Francisco: Harper & Row.

Kulynych, J., & Korn, D. (2002). Use and disclosure of health information in genetic research: Weighing the impact of the new federal medical privacy rule. *American Journal of Law & Medicine, 28*(2-3), 309-324.

Levine, C., Glajchen, M., Cournos, F. (2004). A fifteen-year-old translator. *Hastings Center Report, 34*(3), 10-12.

Liaschenko, J. (1999). Can justice coexist with the supremacy of personal values in nursing practice? *Western Journal of Nursing Research, 21*(1), 35-50.

Liaschenko, J., & Peter, E. (2003). Feminist ethics. In V. Tschudin (Ed.), Approaches to ethics: nursing beyond boundaries (pp. 33-43). New York: Butterworth Heinnemann.

MacIntyre, A. (1984). *After virtue* (2nd ed.). Notre Dame, IN: Notre Dame University.

Marmot, M., & Wilkinson, R. G. (1999). *The social determinants of health.* Oxford, UK: Oxford University.

May, T. (2002). *Bioethics in a liberal society: The political framework of bioethics decision making.* Baltimore, MD: Johns Hopkins.

McCullough, L. B. (1998). Preventive ethics, managed practice, and the hospital ethics committee as a resource for physician executives. *HEC Forum, 10,* 127-135.

McGowan, T. (1995). *The black death.* New York: Watts Franklin.

Miles, S. H, Koepp, R., & Weber, E. P. (1996). Advance end-of-life treatment planning: A research review. *Archives of Internal Medicine, 156,* 1062-1068.

Mill, J. S. (1979). *Utilitarianism.* Indianapolis, IN: Hackett. (Originally published 1861.)

National Society of Genetic Counselors. (1992). *Code of ethics.* Retrieved June 3, 2004, from: *http://www.nsgc.org/newsroom/code_of_ethics.asp.*

National Society of Genetic Counselors. (1992). Retrieved February 8, 2005, from: *http://www.nsgc.org/.*

Nelson, H. L. (1992). Against caring. *The Journal of Clinical Ethics, 3*(1), 8-20.

Newton, L. H. (1988). Lawgiving for professional life: Reflections on the place of the professional code. In A. Flores (Ed.), *Professional ideals* (pp. 47-56). Belmont, CA: Wadsworth.

Norton, L. (1998). Health promotion and health education: What role should the nurse adopt? *Journal of Advanced Nursing, 28*(6), 1269-1275.

Olson, L. L. (2001). Nursing's new code of ethics: A collaborative process. *Chart, 98*(5), 8.

Orem, D. (1995). *Nursing: Concepts of practice* (5th ed.). St. Louis: Mosby.

Ovrebo, B. (2000). Health promotion and civil liberties: The price of freedom and the price of health. In D. Callahan (Ed.), *Promoting healthy behavior: How much freedom? How much responsibility* (pp. 23-36). Washington, DC: Georgetown University Press.

President's Commission for the Study of Ethical Problems in Medicine and Biomedical and Behavioral Research (President's Commission) (1982). *Compensating for Research Injuries: The Ethical and Legal Implications of Programs to Redress Injured Subjects.* Washington, DC: U.S. Government Printing Office.

Rachels, J. (2003). *The elements of moral philosophy* (2nd ed.). New York: McGraw-Hill.

Rawls, J. (1971). *A theory of justice.* Cambridge, MA: Harvard University.

Ross, L. F. (1997). Health care decision making by children—Is it in their best interest? *Hastings Center Report, 27*(6), 41-45.

Singer, P. (1991). *A companion to ethics.* Cambridge, MA: Blackwell.

Tarasoff v. Regents of University of California. (1976, July 1). California Supreme Court 131. *California Reporter,* 14.

Taylor, C. (1985). The nature and scope of justice. In C. Taylor, *Philosophy and the human sciences. Philosophical papers* (Vol. 2, pp. 289-317). Cambridge, UK: Cambridge University.

Thorne, S., & Varcoe, C. (1998). The tyranny of feminist methodology in women's health research. *Health Care for Women International, 19*(6), 481-493.

Tones, K. (1997). Health education as empowerment. In M. Siddell, L. Jones, J. Katz, & A. Peberdy (Eds.), *Debates and dilemmas in promoting health: A reader* (pp. 33-42). Buckingham, UK: Macmillan/Open University.

Tong, R. (1997). *Feminist approaches to bioethics: Theoretical reflections and practical applications.* Boulder, CO: Westview Press.

U.S. Department of Health and Human Services. (2003). *Fact sheet: Protecting the privacy of patients' health information.* Washington, DC: Author. Retrieved May 24, 2004, from: http://www.hhs.gov/news/facts/privacy.html.

U.S. Department of Health and Human Services. Office for Civil Rights. (2004). *HIPAA Privacy Rule.* Retrieved May 24, 2004, from: *http://www.hhs.gov/ocr/hipaa/.*

Warren, V. L. (2001). From autonomy to empowerment: Health care ethics from a feminist perspective. In W. Teays & L. Purdy (Eds.), *Bioethics, justice, & health care* (pp. 49-53). Belmont, CA: Wadsworth.

Weir, R. F., & Peters, C. (1997). Affirming the decisions adolescents make about life and death. *Hastings Center Report, 27*(6), 29-40.

Weithorn, L. A., & Campbell, S. B. (1982). The competency of children and adolescents to make informed treatment decisions. *Child Development, 53,* 1589-1598.

Weston, A. (2001). *A practical companion to ethics* (2nd ed.). New York: Oxford University.

Wilmot, S. (2000). Nurses and whistleblowing: The ethical issues. *Journal of Advanced Nursing, 32,* 1051-1057.

Windt, P. Y. (1989). Introductory essay. In P. Y. Windt, P. C. Appleby, M. P. Battin, L. P. Francis, & B. M. Landesman (Eds.), *Ethical issues in the professions* (pp. 1-24). Englewood Cliffs, NJ: Prentice Hall.

Unit Two

Assessment for Health Promotion

6 Health Promotion and the Individual

7 Health Promotion and the Family

8 Health Promotion and the Community

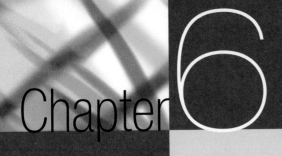

Chapter 6

ANNE RATH RENTFRO

Health Promotion and the Individual

objectives

After completing this chapter, the reader will be able to:

- Define the framework of functional health patterns as described by Gordon.

- Describe the use of the functional health pattern framework in assessing the individual throughout the life span.

- Give examples of the categories of behaviors within the health patterns: functional, potentially dysfunctional, and actually dysfunctional.

- Describe aspects to consider while diagnosing the risk factors or the etiological factors of actually or potentially dysfunctional health patterns.

- Discuss planning, implementing, and evaluating nursing interventions in health promotion with the individual.

- Develop a specific health-promotion plan based on an assessment of an individual.

key terms

Age-developmental focus
Cultural competence
Cultural focus
Expected outcomes
Functional focus

Functional health patterns
Health status
Individual-environmental focus
Nursing diagnosis

Nursing interventions
Pattern focus
Risk factors

THINK About It

Assessment of Alcohol Consumption

*Women have different patterns of alcohol consumption and different thresholds for problem drinking than men. Instruments such as the CAGE detect alcohol dependence and would not be a sensitive enough measure for some women, in particular pregnant women, who are less likely than men to be alcohol dependent. The T-ACE provides a much more sensitive measure of alcohol intake patterns than that derived from the CAGE test (considered **C**utting down on drinking, been **A**nnoyed by criticism of drinking, feeling **G**uilty about drinking, and using alcohol as an **E**ye*

opener). Instead, women are better assessed using the T-ACE test. This test, developed for use with women, was the first validated screening tool for assessing drinking risk in pregnant women. A pattern of drinking is established using the following questions:

- *How many drinks does it Take to make you feel high?*
- *Have you ever been Annoyed by people criticizing your drinking?*
- *Have you ever felt you ought to Cut down your drinking?*

Continued

Sections of this chapter are modified from the curriculum of the Adult Health Nursing, Master of Science Program, Boston College Graduate School of Nursing, Chestnut Hill, MA; Gordon, M. (1994). *Nursing diagnosis: Process and application* (3rd ed.). St. Louis: Mosby.

Assessment of Alcohol Consumption cont'd

- Have you ever had a drink first thing in the morning (eye opener) to steady your nerves or get rid of a hangover?
  Scores are calculated as follows:
- A reply of more than two drinks to question T is considered a positive response and scores 2 points, and an affirmative answer to question A, C, or E scores 1 point, respectively.
- A total score of 2 or more points on the T-ACE indicates evidence of problem drinking during pregnancy (Chang, 2001).

1 Why would a nurse tailor the assessments to individual characteristics of a population?

2 How effectively would this screening tool identify alcohol problems in women other than the pregnant women within the population? Why?

Healthy People 2010

Selected Examples of National Health-Promotion and Disease Prevention Objectives for Individuals

- 13-6a. Increase the proportion of sexually active people who use condoms.
- 22-2. Increase the proportion of adults who engage regularly, preferably daily, in moderate physical activity for at least 30 minutes per session.
- 22-7. Increase the proportion of adolescents who engage in vigorous physical activity that promotes cardiorespiratory fitness 3 or more days per week for 20 or more minutes per occasion.
- 25-11. Increase the proportion of adolescents who abstain from sexual intercourse or use condoms if sexually active.
- 27-1a. Reduce cigarette smoking by adults.

A central unifying theme has historically linked definitions, philosophies, and frameworks of nursing, known as holistic attention to pattern recognition during the examination of person-environment relationships throughout the life span. The purpose of nursing is to facilitate processes in these patterns that lead toward wellness. Health and illness within this context are seen as reflections of changing patterns of the life process. Disorganization or ineffective coping produce fluctuations in patterns and eventually result in illness. Patterns of strengths redirect the individual toward a more harmonious, free-flowing pattern (Newman, 2002). Long before the current focus on health promotion with the *Healthy People* initiatives in the United States, Florence Nightingale expressed the belief that the laws of both health and nursing are similar and pertinent to both the sick and the well individual (Nightingale, 1992).

The American Nurses Association (ANA) defines the practice of nursing as the performance of services using the nursing process in (1) promoting and maintaining health, (2) case finding and managing illness, injury, or infirmity, (3) restoring optimal functioning, or (4) helping the client achieve a dignified death (American Nurses Association [ANA], 2003). Although this definition was designed to provide a model for state nursing practice acts, the familiar terminology in the ANA social policy statement is more concise. "Nursing is the protection, promotion, and optimization of health and abilities, prevention of illness and injury, alleviation of suffering through the diagnosis and treatment of human response, and advocacy in the care of individuals, families, communities, and populations." (ANA, 2003b, p. 6). This is the definition of nursing used in most nurse practice acts in the United States. These responses are divided into health-restoring responses (reactions to health problems as illness) and health-supporting responses (concerns about potential health problems, such as susceptibility to illness) (ANA, 2003a, 2004). The

nursing process is the organized method of giving individualized nursing care to each person, family, and community, including assessment, diagnosis, outcome criteria, process criteria (including planned interventions), implementation, and evaluation. These components are explained comprehensively in the ANA (2004) publication called *Nursing: Scope and Standards of Practice*.

Based on this definition, primary prevention is a concept central to nursing and includes generalized health promotion and specific protection from disease. Health promotion connotes an active process involving protection (immunizations, occupational safety, and environmental control) along with a lifestyle, value and belief system, and set of behaviors that enhance health. Chapter 1 describes the health of any individual, family, or community as a sustainable balance involving complex responses among internal physiological and psychological systems and the external environment. Many reference materials describe the medical model of assessment of an individual's biophysical states, including the comprehensive review of systems and physical examination conducted by the nurse, physician, or physician's assistant (Bickley & Hoekelman, 2002; Jarvis, 2003). Within nursing theory, nursing knowledge development is a process of the whole. The patterns in the nursing contain parts. It is not a matter of merely adding to or summing up those parts. The nurse uses a framework to assess interactions among a person's biophysical, psychosocial, and spiritual states and the environment (Newman, 2002). Selected examples of the *Healthy People 2010* objectives that are related to individuals are presented in the *Healthy People 2010* box.

With health promotion serving as the underlying theme, this chapter addresses the nursing assessment of the individual. In most areas of nursing, tertiary care and prevention of further disease provides the focus of attention. This focus tends to limit reflection to problem solving rather than guidance for overall general health and wellness. Concentration on strengths provides the nurse in the health-promotion setting with a foundation to help individuals move toward improved health. When the person is not ill, support from the nurse enhances the ability to maintain or strengthen health. Most nursing diagnoses approved by the North American Nursing Diagnosis Association (NANDA) are problem oriented, and the framework is what nurses are most familiar with. The NANDA definition of **nursing diagnosis** includes life processes as well as actual or potential health problems. This inclusion of life processes provides a broad base for nursing diagnoses to depict healthy responses, although fewer than 10% of the approved nursing diagnoses reflect the concept of healthy response or the potential for healthy responses (Stolte, 1996). One function of a nursing diagnosis in the well individual is to focus on developmental or maturational tasks. An example of this kind of focus can be seen with well-child care or with anticipatory guidance in prenatal care.

Nevertheless, the accepted framework used for assessment in most areas of nursing is the functional health patterns assessment of the individual described by Gordon. This framework is the foundation for the underlying concepts that apply to most nursing diagnoses. As NANDA continues to develop wellness diagnoses for health promotion, Gordon's framework will most likely continue to provide the foundation for these diagnoses, as they have with the nursing diagnoses developed to date. This same framework is used throughout this unit to demonstrate assessment approaches with the family and community (see Chapters 7 and 8). This chapter also discusses components of the nursing process as they relate to health promotion of the individual (Gordon, 1994).

FUNCTIONAL HEALTH PATTERNS: ASSESSMENT OF THE INDIVIDUAL

Nursing assessment determines the **health status** of the individual. Table 6-1 demonstrates the aspects common to a complete nursing assessment. Assessment, in this case, refers only to collection of data that culminates in identifying a problem or stating a diagnosis. An artificial component separation—diagnosis or problem identification—is considered for clarity. This process of assessment follows guidelines used in the ANA's publications (ANA, 2004). Assessment of health status should consider not only physiological parameters, but also the entire human being interacting with the environment. Behavior patterns, beliefs, perceptions, and values are essential components of health (nursing) assessment when maximal health potential of the individual is considered. Pattern recognition supports our understanding the health of an individual (Newman, 2002; Rogers, 1970).

Historically, conceptual models in nursing have employed Gordon's (1994) health-related behaviors (van Achterberg, Frederiks, Thien, Coenen, & Persoon, 2002; Kozier, Erb, Berman, & Burke, 2003; Pryor & Smith, 2002). The framework has developed into an assessment model with 11 functional health patterns. Functional patterns interact to determine an individual's lifestyle. Using this framework, the nurse combines assessment skills with subjective and objective data to construct patterns reflective of this lifestyle.

Functional Health Pattern Framework

Holism and the totality of the person's interactions with the environment are the philosophical foundations of this text. Gordon's functional health patterns maintain these same philosophical foundations. This foundation provides a mechanism for data collection that encompasses the entire person and all life processes. By examining functional patterns and interactions among patterns, nurses accurately determine and diagnose actual or potential problems, intervene more effectively, and achieve outcomes that promote health and well-being (Gordon, 1994). In addition to providing a framework to assess individuals, families, and communities holistically, functional health patterns provide a strong focus for more effective **nursing interventions** and

Table 6-1 Aspects of a Nursing Assessment

Definition	Deliberate and Systematic Data Collection
Components	*Subjective data:* Health history, including subjective reports and individual perceptions *Objective data:* Observations of nurse Physical examination findings Information from health record Results of clinical testing
Function	Description of person's health status
Structure	Organization of interdependent parts describing health, function, or patterns of behavior that reflect the whole individual and environment
Process	Interview, observation, and examination
Format	Systematic but flexible; individualized to each person, nurse, and situation
Goal	Nursing diagnosis or problem identification Identification of areas of strengths, limitations, alterations, responses to alterations and therapies, and risks

outcomes. This stronger focus provides a solid position from which nurses participate as decision makers in health care systems at organizational, community, national, and international levels.

Definition

Functional health patterns are interrelated behavioral areas that provide a view of the whole individual. The typology of 11 patterns serves as a useful tool to collect and organize assessment data and to create a structure for validation and communication among the health care providers.

Each pattern, briefly described in Table 6-2, is a bio-psychosocial-spiritual expression of the whole person. Individual reports and nursing observations provide data to describe patterns. As a framework for assessment, functional health patterns provide an effective means for nurses to perceive and record complex interactions of the individual's biophysical state, psychological makeup, and their relationship to the environment.

Characteristics

Functional health patterns are characterized by their focus. Gordon (1994) identified five areas: (1) pattern, (2) individual-environmental, (3) age-developmental, (4) functional, and (5) cultural.

Pattern focus implies that the nurse explores patterns or sequences of behavior over time. Gordon's (1994) use of the term *behavior* encompasses biophysical, psychological, sociological, and any other classification of human behavior. The nurse's recognition of a pattern is a cognitive process that occurs during information collection. As information is collected, cues are identified and clustered. Then patterns emerge that represent historical and current behavior. Patterns are easiest to recognize when behavior or information is quantifiable, as with blood pressure, and pattern recognition is facilitated when baseline data are available. Patterns

within patterns are developed and assessed. Blood pressure, for example, is a pattern within the activity and exercise pattern. The individual baseline and subsequent readings may present a pattern within expected norms. Erratic blood pressure measurements indicate an absence of pattern. This lack of pattern forms a type of pattern in itself. The categories of functional health provide a structure for analyzing a factor within a category (blood pressure: activity pattern) and a structure to search for causal explanations, usually outside the category (excessive sodium intake: nutritional pattern) (Gordon, 1994).

Food intake examples can illustrate the **individual-environmental focus** of Gordon's framework. Although reference is made within many patterns to environmental influence, it often refers to the physical environments within and external to the individual. Common to each functional health pattern are environmental influences such as role relationships, family values, and societal mores. Personal preference, knowledge of food preparation, and ability to consume and retain food govern the individual's intake. Cultural and family habits, financial ability to secure the food, and crop availability also influence food intake. Additionally, the person who secures, prepares, and serves the food, such as the mother or father, controls nutritional intake for children.

Each pattern also reflects a human growth and **age-developmental focus** (Brown, 2002; Wong, Perry, & Hockenberry-Eaton, 2002). The previous discussion of health addresses the complexity of biopsychosocial-spiritual systems of the individual and their interaction with environment. Individual fulfillment of developmental tasks increases complexity. These tasks, however, provide learning opportunities for the individual to maintain and improve health. Over 25 years ago, Bruhn, Cordova, Williams, and Fuentes (1977) proposed a framework to organize specific health tasks for the individual to accomplish at each developmental phase of the life cycle, as iden-

---

Table **6-2** Typology of 11 Functional Health Patterns	
Pattern	**Description**
Health perception–health management pattern	Individual's perceived health and well-being and how health is managed
Nutritional-metabolic pattern	Food and fluid consumption relative to metabolic needs and indicators of local nutrient supply
Elimination pattern	Excretory function (bowel, bladder, and skin)
Activity-exercise pattern	Exercise, activity, leisure, and recreation
Sleep-rest pattern	Sleep, rest, and relaxation
Cognitive-perceptual pattern	Sensory, perceptual, and cognitive patterns
Self-perception–self-concept pattern	Self-concept pattern and perceptions of self (body comfort, body image, and feeling state); self-conception and self-esteem
Roles-relationships pattern	Role engagements and relationships
Sexuality-reproductive pattern	Person's satisfaction and dissatisfaction with sexuality and reproduction
Coping–stress tolerance pattern	General coping pattern and effectiveness in stress tolerance
Values-beliefs pattern	Values, beliefs (including spiritual), or goals that guide choices or decisions

Modified from Gordon, M. (1994). *Nursing diagnosis: Process and application* (3rd ed.). St. Louis: Mosby.

tified by Erikson (1994) and Havighurst (1972). This framework is presented in **Web Site Resource 6A.** Learning developmental tasks begins at birth and continues until death. By considering current epidemiological data and recommended health behaviors, this framework continues to be useful today for health promotion throughout the life span. Therefore, Unit 4 uses Gordon's framework to explore developmental tasks and their related health behaviors for health promotion.

Functional focus refers to the individual's performance level, a traditional area of concern in nursing models. Other disciplines examine functional patterns, but assessment data vary. Physical therapists and occupational therapists develop their plans with functional ability of the client at the core, but the central consideration is on the physical abilities of the individual (Nosek et al., 2004). For physicians, genitourinary functions refer to frequency or voiding patterns and characteristics of urine, such as color, odor, and laboratory analysis results. In addition to these factors of genitourinary function, nurses assess how the particular voiding pattern affects lifestyle, particularly how urinary frequency affects sleep patterns and the ability to perform activities such as shopping or socializing. Additional concerns might include the individual's ability to walk or climb stairs to the bathroom or to manage these activities safely at night (Brown, 2002).

Culturally based age, developmental, and gender norms influence the development of health patterns; therefore, **cultural focus** is another area to consider when assessing functional health patterns. Madeline Leininger defines *transcultural nursing* as a "theoretical and practice discipline focused on comparative cultural care, health, well-being, and illness patterns in different environmental contexts and under different living conditions" (Leininger & McFarland, 2002, p. 27). To demonstrate **cultural competence,** care is delivered with the knowledge of and sensitivity to the cultural factors that influence the health and illness behaviors of a client or family. The complexity of any culture reveals patterns of behavior, health practices, and activities that have been transmitted from former generations. Nurses who are sensitive to the underlying personal and cultural reality of an individual, identifying and using cultural norms, values, and communication and time patterns in collecting and interpreting assessment information, will provide more culturally competent care (Dossey, Keegan, & Guzzetta, 2000; Kozier et al., 2003).

Rationale for Use

These characteristics illustrate how the functional health pattern framework centers on the concept of health. Information collected for a functional pattern assessment is the foundation of most nursing assessments. Although various theoretical and conceptual frameworks of nursing collect holistic data about the person, variations exist in the interpretation of the data and the interventions used to achieve the desired outcomes. The assessment structure of the func-

tional health pattern framework is relevant to all conceptual models and is used by NANDA as the structure to support the nursing diagnosis nomenclature. Nursing classification and outcome nomenclature also use Gordon's functional patterns as a foundation (Carpenito-Moyet, 2003; Kozier et al., 2003).

Advantages of a functional health pattern framework specific to the practice of nursing include the following:

- The structure provides a consistent nursing focus through a means of collecting, organizing, presenting, and analyzing data to arrive at a nursing (not a medical) diagnosis.
- The format is flexible and can be tailored to the individual, the situation, or the nurse.
- The information collected is suitable to any arena of practice, whether in the home, clinic, or institution and whether assessing the individual (adult or child), family, or community.

Theoretical components of nursing (education and research) are also facilitated by functional health patterns. The student, educator, or researcher is able to do the following:

- Organize clinical knowledge in a way relevant to the nursing diagnoses, interventions, and outcomes
- Gain advanced knowledge of the individual's problems amenable to nursing care and of diagnosis-specific interventions and outcomes
- Identify areas in which knowledge in nursing requires expansion

Medical science data is incorporated into, but is not the focus for, organizing nursing knowledge.

The Patterns

Each pattern is a biopsychosocial spiritual expression of the individual and reflects lifestyle or life processes from the perspective of both the individual and the nurse. Additionally, this expression reflects (1) a pattern or sequencing of behaviors, (2) the role of the environment (physical environs and family, societal, and cultural influences), and (3) influences of a developmental nature.

The assessment of each pattern as functional (strengths), dysfunctional (nursing diagnosis), or potentially dysfunctional includes an indication of the individual's level of satisfaction with the pattern. Any problems reported should be assessed further to include the individual's explanation of the problem, remedial actions taken, and the perceived effect of these actions.

An important goal in assessing each pattern is to determine the individual's knowledge of health promotion, the ability to manage health-promoting activities, and the value that the individual ascribes to health promotion.

Each pattern is presented in this chapter, with details for the nurse to use when assessing the client using a functional health pattern framework and when making a diagnosis in clinical practice. Understanding the role each pattern plays in the individual's life and in the nurse's practice is also helpful; therefore, there will be a discussion of the individual significance and nursing implications of each.

Health Perception–Health Management Pattern

This pattern provides an overview of the individual's health status and the health practices that are used to reach the current level of health or wellness. The focus is on perceived health status and the meaning of health, along with the individual's level of commitment to maintaining health (Gordon, 1994). When eliciting information of this sort, the nurse will discover areas that may need further exploration under another functional health pattern. For example, when an individual can no longer mow the lawn without suffering shortness of breath or severe back pain, the nurse stores the information and retrieves it later when assessing the activity and exercise pattern or the cognitive-perceptual pattern.

The importance of the health perception–health management pattern to an individual is apparent. Lifestyle and ability to function are affected when people do not perceive that health problems are present, when they are unaware of necessary health promotion in the absence of problems, when they do not feel capable of managing their own health, or when they believe activity on their part is useless in promoting health. Health-promoting activities (adequate nutrition, activity and exercise, sleep and rest), routine professional examinations, self-examinations, immunizations, and safety precautions (auto safety restraints and locked medicine cabinets) are instrumental in improving or maintaining an optimal quality of life.

The objective in assessing the health perception–health management pattern is to obtain data about perceptions, management, and preventive health practices (Gordon, 1994). Exploring values may lead to identifying potential health hazards, such as noncompliance to a prescribed medical or nursing regimen or inability to manage health effectively.* In addition to these clues, the nurse may also identify unrealistic health and illness perceptions and expectations.

Assessment parameters to explore include the following:
- Health and safety practices of the individual
- Previous patterns of adherence or compliance
- Use of the health care system
- Knowledge of the availability of health services
- Patterns indicating at what point health care is sought
- Access to health care, including financial resources, health insurance, and transportation

In addition to methods of health management, the nurse explores health perception as the individual describes current health status, past problems, and anticipation of future problems associated with health or health care. Expectations are indicative of health beliefs, locus of

---

*The terms cues or clues to problems mentioned within this section refer to defining characteristics identified by NANDA (2003).

MULTICULTURAL AWARENESS

Self-Assessed Health Status of Hispanic Americans

	Excellent	Very Good	Good	Fair to Poor
Cuban	38%	22%	26%	14%
Mexican	28%	24%	31%	16%
Puerto Rican	28%	27%	28%	18%
Other (including Central and South American)	33%	28%	28%	12%

Data from Hajat, A., Lucas, J. B., & Kington, R. (2000). *Health outcomes among Hispanic subgroups* (Publication No. 310). Hyattsville, MD: National Center for Health Statistics.

control, and realistic understanding of health state and any health problems (Multicultural Awareness box).

The significance of this pattern to nursing cannot be overstressed. Health perceptions influence data collection and provide direction for all planning of care. Health beliefs, also discussed under the values-beliefs pattern, directly influence participation in care. Individuals are less apt to engage in self-care or preventive measures when they (1) believe it is the responsibility of health team members to keep them healthy, (2) do not recognize or acknowledge their susceptibility to an impending health problem, or (3) believe that they cannot influence their health status.

Past health management serves as a predictor of future health management. If there has been a lack of adherence to a prescribed regimen, a recurrence is likely unless the nurse is able to identify and remedy related causes. An illustration of this situation can be found in an individual with high blood pressure who fails to keep follow-up appointments, often "forgets" to take medication, and eats foods with high sodium content. An assessment must be made to determine whether this evident noncompliance is based on a conflict within the value system of the individual (health beliefs), inaccurate information, misunderstanding, inadequate ability to learn, retain, or retrieve information (knowledge deficit), or denial of illness (health perception). Variables such as financial resources, transportation difficulties, nutritional preferences, daily activities (individual and family patterns), and ability to read written instructions (literacy or visual acuity) may affect the individual's behaviors.

Nutritional-Metabolic Pattern

The nutritional-metabolic pattern describes nutrient intake relative to metabolic need (Gordon, 1994). This pattern includes not only the individual's description of food and fluid consumption (history), but also the nurse's observations and perceptions regarding adequate nutrition (physical examination). The nurse should elicit the individual's satisfaction with current eating and drinking patterns, including restrictions, and the individual's perception of problems associated with eating and drinking, growth and development, skin condition, and healing processes.

All bodily functions and the lifestyle of the individual are governed by intake and supply of nutrients to tissues and organs. Sufficient food and fluid intake is necessary to provide the energy needed for performance of all activities, which include both the internal physiological functioning of the organs and the external body movements. Interruption in the acquisition or retention of food or fluids offsets this balance and significantly alters the person's lifestyle. Nutrition and metabolism also govern the rate of an individual's growth and development.

The assessment objective in this pattern is to collect data about a typical pattern of food and fluid consumption, the adequacy of this pattern of consumption and, as with all patterns, perceived problems associated with nutritional intake. Clues may point to conditions of overweight, underweight, overhydration, dehydration, or difficulties in skin integrity, such as breakdown or delayed healing. Individuals may also be at risk for developing these problems.

Parameters for assessment fall into two broad categories: (1) parameters to evaluate nutrient intake and (2) parameters to evaluate metabolic demands. Intake may be assessed with a 24-hour recall of food and fluid consumption; a listing of dietary restrictions, food allergies, vitamin supplements, caffeine and alcohol ingestion (when not included in the medication history); and a schedule of eating and drinking patterns. Assessment includes screening for problems associated with swallowing or chewing.

When problems become apparent, a focused assessment might include patterns of food preference, feelings about present weight, and details of eating habits. Intake may be affected if the individual eats alone rather than with others. Frequent dining out may be indicative of problems in this or other functional patterns. When diets consist of fast foods, the consumption pattern may uncover deficits of essential vitamins or minerals. When appropriate, the nurse assesses areas pertinent to obtaining food. Who purchases food? Is shopping preplanned with a grocery list? Are financial resources and a food budget adequate? Is food stored properly? Who prepares the food? How are foods prepared (fried, broiled, steamed, boiled, or baked)?

Metabolic demands vary from individual to individual and within the same individual during times of illness, stress, growth, high or low activity levels, healing, or recovery. Developmental and environmental conditions may alter metabolic demands. Appetite and reported changes in weight, skin integrity, and general healing ability are explored during the interview or health history. The individual may also report a decreased tolerance for hot and cold weather.

Nurses' observations and perceptions play a vital role when assessing nutritional and metabolic pattern. Physical examination allows assessment of both nutrient supply to the tissues and metabolic needs of the individual. Objective findings serve as indicators to measure reliability of subjective reports concerning nutrient intake.

Gross metabolic indicators include temperature, height, and weight. The physical examination also focuses on the skin, bony prominences, dentition, hair, and mucous membranes. Skin and mucous membranes, in particular, use nutrients rapidly and provide excellent indices of adequacy of nutrient supply. Assessment of the skin includes color, temperature, turgor, and an evaluation of any skin lesions, areas of dryness or scaliness, rashes, pruritus, or edema. Mucous membranes are examined for color, integrity, moisture, and lesions. Dentition is evaluated for structure. Are teeth erupted at normal stages of development? Are teeth firmly implanted? Do dentures fit properly? Additionally, decay and evidence of oral hygiene are evaluated. Healing is assessed when there is evidence of injury.

Although problem identification occurs after assessment of all 11 functional health patterns, a problem in any one area serves as a clue to dysfunction in others. Assessment of one pattern is facilitated by synthesis and analysis of data collected in the other 10 functional health patterns. Nutrition and metabolism are particularly significant within the patterns of health management, elimination, activity, sleep, cognition, roles, and stress tolerance. The values-beliefs pattern may significantly alter all other functional patterns. Sociocultural values and ethnic backgrounds play a major role in determining an individual's pattern of eating.

Another area to consider is that eating habits, food preferences, and patterns of nutrient supply and demand vary over the life span. Raw fruits and vegetables may be fun "finger food" for the toddler, but the older adult, especially one with loose dentures or arthritis of the temporomandibular joint (jaw), may find it impossible to eat these foods.

Implications for practice using this pattern focus include emphasis on educational needs. Assessment aims to demonstrate strengths in functional patterns in addition to disclosing dysfunctional or potentially dysfunctional patterns. Good nutrition as part of health-promotion activities should be considered a strength. Health promotion in this pattern may provide a stepping stone for similar activities in the other patterns. For example, if balanced nutritional intake improves an individual's functional level, then that same individual may choose to learn relaxation techniques to decrease the stress response. Understanding food and fluid intake and balance of food and body requirements helps individuals adjust caloric intake as growth slows in order to prevent overweight problems during the adult years.

Elimination Pattern

The elimination pattern is designed to describe the function of the bowel, bladder, and skin. The nurse determines regularity, quality, and quantity of stool and urine, through the subjective reports of the individual about methods used to achieve regularity or control, and any pattern changes or perceived problems. Excretory function of the skin is evaluated by determining the amount of perspiration and associated odor control (Gordon, 1994).

The significance of the elimination pattern to the whole person varies from individual to individual. Many people view regularity of elimination as a measure of their health and as a sensitive indicator of proper nutrition and stress level. The individual's perceptions are important in determining whether the pattern is problematic or dysfunctional, and assessment is based on the individual's usual pattern. Many misconceptions about regularity exist, particularly of bowel function, an area in which self-treatment often is used to correct perceived problems. It is important to collect data about self-treatment methods used.

Difficulty with control of excreta has cultural implications. When lack of control exists, body image (self-perception) frequently is altered, and altered modes of elimination may affect perceptions of sexuality. Both lack of control and altered modes of elimination impinge on the activity level of the individual, adversely affect socialization, and even affect sleeping patterns.

Age and developmental levels direct the line of questioning. Assessment of children is geared to toilet training methods, whereas regularity is more often a concern of adults. In addition to constipation, older adults may begin to develop problems of urinary control. Women past the childbearing age are particularly prone to urinary stress incontinence.

The assessment objective is to collect data about regularity and control of excreta (Gordon, 1994). The nurse investigates clues suggesting constipation patterns, diarrhea, or any form of incontinence through focused assessment. Changes in elimination pattern, pain, discomfort, and any perceived problems are also assessed. Data collection includes an explanation of the problem, methods of self-treatment, and perceived results (Gordon, 1994).

Data such as quantity, quality (color, odor, and consistency), and frequency or regularity of stool, urine, and perspiration are determined. The nurse assesses excretory mode, time patterns, and control. Changes in pattern, perceived problems, and elimination habits are explored with the individual. Examination includes gross screening of specimens, noting amount, consistency, color, and odor. Any drainage from wounds or fistulas should be noted when skin is assessed.

The transition from nutrition to the elimination pattern often occurs naturally. Roughage level in the diet affects bowel elimination patterns, and urinary elimination problems are frequently linked to fluid intake. Even skin integrity may herald questioning about drainage and lead to discussion of additional elimination patterns.

Many individuals do not consider laxatives as medications. Therefore, the nurse must ask specific questions about any remedial actions taken when constipation is a problem. A perceptive nurse will note discrepancies between dietary intake and reported regularity of bowel movements. Assessment may disclose a dependency on laxatives, suppositories, or enemas and may indicate that the individual has a knowledge deficit regarding bowel elimi-

nation. Health education about normal bowel function, nutritional guidelines to assist the individual in elimination, or an exercise program may significantly improve elimination pattern dysfunction.

Urinary frequency also requires further health education. Research indicates that prolonged time between urinations is associated with increased incidence of urinary tract infections (Moore, Day, & Albers, 2002). Evidence-based practice guides the nurse in establishing a more suitable elimination routine for the individual.

Although any area perceived to be a problem by the individual is a problem, the nursing assessment is designed to evaluate patterns of dysfunction or potential dysfunction of which the individual is unaware. The nurse shares the analysis of the data with the individual, basing the care plan on shared goals.

Activity-Exercise Pattern

The activity-exercise pattern centers on activity level, exercise program, and leisure activities.

The following parameters are explored: movement capability, activity tolerance, self-care abilities, use of assistive devices, changes in pattern, satisfaction with activity and exercise patterns, and any perceived problems (Gordon, 1994).

Limitations of the individual's movement capabilities or ability to perform activities of daily living significantly alter the lifestyle and may affect every other functional health pattern. Movement and independent functioning in self-care is almost universally valued. Child-rearing practices demonstrate this value; parents boast about their infant who walks early, their toilet-trained toddler, and their preschooler who dresses without assistance.

The activity-exercise pattern provides an effective indicator of the individual's commitment to health promotion and preventive care (Figure 6-1). That exercise has an impact on health status has been documented thoroughly, and public awareness has grown tremendously in recent years. Problems associated with overweight and obesity are linked to sedentary lifestyle and lack of activity. Obesity is seen as an epidemic in some populations.

The number of people who jog or walk as a part of their regular fitness routine has certainly increased, and participants can be seen at nearly every public park in metropolitan areas. The growing number of health spas demonstrates increased membership, and companies involved in selling exercise programming to group consumers (businesses, church and social groups, and housing complexes) claim increasing participation. On the other hand there has been a rapid increase in obesity and overweight among children in the United States in recent years. From 1963 until 2000, the number of overweight children and adolescents in the United States rose from 4.2% to 15.3% of the population (Centers for Disease Control and Prevention, 2003). The Surgeon General has predicted that the prevention of obesity could have an effect on morbidity and mortality

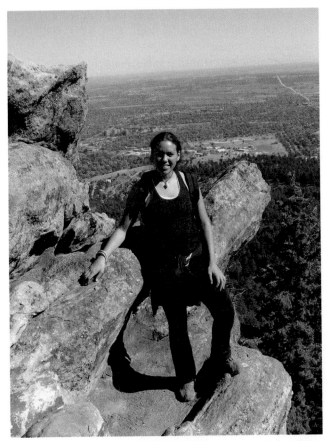

Figure 6-1 The activity of a young adult provides an indicator of the individual's commitment to health promotion.

exceeding that of cigarette smoking. With a $177 billion direct and indirect cost in 2001, obesity surely burdens the health care system immensely (U.S. Department of Health and Human Services, 2001). Assessment and planning to prevent obesity could have a major impact on the nation's health.

In addition to examining exercise and mobility levels, the activity-exercise pattern provides an indication of energy expenditure levels and activity tolerance levels. Leisure activities provide clues to the individual's value system. The American work ethic and competitive nature of many occupations often creates a void in leisure or recreational activities. Unless health promotion is brought to people's attention, they may be too preoccupied to recognize the loss of recreational activities.

The ability to move and perform activities of daily living directly affects control of the immediate environment; therefore, an obvious link exists between the activity-exercise pattern and the individual's health. Environment also affects mobility; individuals living alone in high-crime areas may limit their activity because they are afraid. Older individuals may live too far from public transportation to shop for groceries. In the past, a walk to the bus stop may have been the major mode of exercise. The number of stairs

the individual must negotiate with a cane may restrict activities. Weather may also play a role in altering exercise patterns. For individuals with any neuromuscular or perceptual disturbances, these environmental barriers may be a significant handicap. Only recently have legislators faced issues concerning wheelchair access to public buildings.

The objective of assessment within the activity-exercise pattern is to determine the pattern of activities that require energy expenditure. Components reviewed are daily activities, exercise, and leisure activities (Gordon, 1994). The nurse seeks clues to discover strengths and weaknesses within the pattern. Decreased energy levels, perceived problems, coping strategies, changes within the patterns, and associated explanations for these changes are all important clues that require further exploration. Generally, individuals with respiratory or cardiac disease warrant in-depth assessment, and focused assessment is indicated for individuals with neuromuscular, perceptual, or circulatory impairments.

Dimensions to be described and assessed include daily activities, leisure activities, and exercise. Daily activities include (1) occupation (position, hours of work or school, and amount of physical exercise versus cognitive or sedentary activities), (2) self-care abilities (feeding, bathing, grooming, dressing, and toileting), and (3) home-management routines (cooking, cleaning, shopping, laundry, and outdoor activities). Problems within any of these areas require explanation. Is it a problem of energy expenditure, mobility limitations, or decreased motivation caused by depression, grieving, or incongruent values?

Exercise parameters include type, frequency, duration, and intensity of the individual's regular exercise. The nurse should also assess the importance of exercise to the individual's feelings about it. A 24-hour recall of the previous day's activities provides an initial picture of the pattern; specifics are then addressed as described for each major component. A weekly log is particularly useful for follow-up visits and whenever a problem is suspected. In addition to the weekly log, a focused assessment includes details such as mode of transportation. Does the individual go everywhere in a car? Is public transportation used and, if so, how far away is the route? Are elevators used rather than stairs?

Factors interfering with exercise or mobility include dyspnea, fatigue, muscle cramping, neuromuscular or perceptual deficits, chest pain, and angina. As with other patterns, feelings of satisfaction and the individual's perception of problems always provide valuable indications of dysfunctional or potentially dysfunctional patterns.

The nurse carefully evaluates subjective reporting of complaints, such as dyspnea, by noting any difficulty for the individual during the interview and physical examination. Components of the examination assess circulatory, respiratory, and neuromuscular indicators. The nurse measures and records skin color and temperature, heart rate (apical and radial measurement), and blood pressure and notes respiratory rate, rhythm, depth of inspiration, and effort involved.

Ambulation is observed and gait, posture, and balance are recorded. Muscle tone, strength, coordination, and range of motion provide useful clues to validate reports of activity and exercise. Assistive devices or prostheses are evaluated for proper use, proper fit, and degree of assistance or support provided.

The history and examination are closely linked. Examination alone may not disclose early morning pain and stiffness of the joints, and this subjective reporting is invaluable. When appropriate, the nurse may ask the individual to climb stairs or perform self-care activities under observation, which is useful in assessing level of impairment. Direct observation is the best way to validate assessment findings. Various instruments have been designed to quantify level of ability or disability. For some individuals, a metabolic activity index, in which each activity is measured according to kilocalories of energy expended per minute, may be a helpful to quantify assessment results and plan care.

Developmental norms have been established for the infant and toddler. Childhood development is monitored carefully through milestones such as sitting, crawling, walking, running, and hopping. However, the nurse must remember that some degree of activity is needed regardless of age or health status. Careful assessment of ability, limitations, and interests helps to guide the nurse as improved patterns of activity and exercise are designed based on the holistic assessment. Problem identification is reserved for the conclusion of the assessment after all 11 patterns have been constructed. Useful clues within a pattern may guide the interview into other pattern areas, but premature closure is dangerous. At this point, only tentative diagnoses are possible. Often explanations to problems lie in another functional health pattern. For example, when the individual expresses an inability to perform exercise on a routine basis, barriers may be discovered in another pattern. The barriers may be associated with knowledge deficit, personal or family value system, overriding priorities, or that exercise is not valued. Is the inability to perform activities a result of general fatigue caused by inadequate or decreased sleep time associated with anxiety, nocturia, pain, or an infant waking every 3 hours for feeding? Are responsibilities associated with caring for several preschoolers and inadequate financial resources to secure a babysitter the cause? The assessment's purpose is to narrow the number of possible explanations.

Sleep-Rest Pattern

Perhaps the single most important factor that is assessed in the sleep-rest pattern is the perception of adequacy of sleep and relaxation. Subjective reports of fatigue or energy levels provide some indication of the individual's satisfaction.

People make assumptions about the roles that sleep and rest play in preparing the individual for required or desired daily activities. This pattern becomes extremely important when sleep and rest are perceived as insufficient. Although the exact function of sleep has not been identified clearly, it seems to serve a restorative function in most individuals.

Sleep-deprivation studies provide vivid demonstrations of the need for different types of sleep: light, deep, dream, and rapid eye movement sleep.

Again, problems within this pattern may cause problems in other patterns. A person who has difficulty with sleep may be tense and irritable, unable to tolerate stress, more prone to infectious processes, and incapable of making health-promoting relationships. Alterations in appetite, elimination difficulties, and activity intolerance will likely be experienced. Some degree of cognitive dysfunction generally occurs.

The objective when assessing the sleep-rest pattern is to describe the effectiveness of the pattern from the individual's perspective. Wide variation in sleep time (from 4 hours to more than 10 hours) does not necessarily affect functional performance; different individuals require different amounts of sleep. Pertinent information includes data suggestive of difficulties with sleep onset, sleep interruptions, and awakening. The nurse also evaluates disturbances such as dreaming and nightmares, sleepwalking, nocturnal enuresis, and penile tumescence. Counseling, institution of safety measures, or medical referral may be necessary.

In addition to sleep, the nurse assesses rest and relaxation according to the individual's perceptions. Activities of the sedentary isolate type, such as reading or crocheting, may be relaxing for some individuals. Passive involvement, as with television viewing, may provide the only source of relaxation for the individual. Daily naps or relaxation exercises (meditation, yoga, or breathing exercises) may also be a part of this pattern.

Assessment parameters of the sleep dimension are divided into two parts: (1) sleep quality and (2) sleep quantity. Sleep quality includes the individual's perception of sleep adequacy, performance level, and physical and psychological state on awakening.

Sleep quantity, in addition to the hours slept each day, is used to build a schedule of sleep times. The nurse assesses for regularity the time of retiring, time of awakening, and additional periods of sleep throughout the day. Sleep onset, the number of awakenings, and reasons for them provide clues to problems. The dimensions of rest and relaxation include the parameters of type, frequency or regularity, and duration. The perceived effectiveness of methods used to promote rest is also assessed.

When problems exist, focused assessment to evaluate efficiency of time spent in bed for sleep compared with actual sleeping time is warranted. The value attributed to sleep by the individual will largely affect both motivation to sleep and the ability to achieve sleep. Individuals are conditioned to sleep under certain circumstances, and maintaining bedtime rituals is a distinct advantage in sleep promotion. A person who expects to sleep usually will, provided that established patterns are maintained. The nurse should assess changes in schedule and routines associated with bedtime. When assessing bedtime routines, the nurse includes rituals along with other aids to sleep, such as natural aids (warm milk) or medications (prescription and nonprescription). Physical examination by the nurse includes general appearance, behavior, and performance changes.

As with pain, sleep is a subjective experience. Comprehensive examination may be performed (for example, with polysomnography), but discussion of this is beyond the scope of this text. Research indicates that subjective reporting of sleep quality and measures of sleep time closely approximate electroencephalographic findings. Most difficulties associated with sleep are amenable to nursing therapies.

Nursing implications focus on the need to be alert to evidence of sleep disturbances so that proper interventions can be instituted before sleep deprivation occurs. The nurse concentrates on subjective reports of difficulties or feelings of not being sufficiently rested. Care is taken not to interpret isolated findings; every person has experienced at least one poor night's sleep.

Frequent awakenings do not necessarily imply sleep interruption. Many individuals awaken numerous times during the night but return to sleep within seconds. This may be especially true of older adults who generally spend most of the night in stages of light sleep. Their normal developmental pattern does not include deep sleep; therefore, awakenings may not affect the sleep cycles and resultant feelings after awakening in the morning. More commonly, however, older individuals experience difficulty returning to sleep because they experience discomfort, fears, or other variables.

Gaining a sense of the individual's biological rhythm and peak performance time may be helpful to the nurse when planning health education and return visits. Individuals commonly refer to themselves as *morning people* or *night owls*; patterns of retiring and arising may provide clues. Patterns of sleep and rest in conjunction with subjective reports of physical and mental well-being help determine appropriate interventions.

Cognitive-Perceptual Pattern

Cognitive patterns include the ability of the individual to understand and follow directions, retain information, make decisions, solve problems, and use language appropriately. Auditory, visual, olfactory, gustatory, tactile, and kinesthetic sensations and perceptions determine perceptual and sensory patterns. Pain perception and tolerance are analyzed within this pattern area (Gordon, 1994).

Capacity for independent functioning is considered a major role of thinking and perceiving. Compensation for cognitive-perceptual difficulties ensures the individual's safety. Health requires a balance between the individual and the environment; decreasing levels of cognition or perception require increasing levels of environmental control. Sheltered work environments and group living arrangements for the mentally or sensory-impaired are examples of this process.

The developmental stage plays a significant role in cognitive and perceptual abilities. Vision and hearing do not reach full potential until school age; 20/30 vision is normal for the preschooler. The ability to problem solve and conceptualize is also marked by developmental stages proposed by the theorist Piaget (Wong et al., 2002). As the adult reaches maturity, declines in visual acuity, hearing, touch, and even taste begin and continue through the later years.

The interrelationships among the individual, the developmental stage, and the environment contribute to several patterns. For example, the behavior patterns of a 20-year-old high school dropout who works in a factory will differ from those of a 20-year-old second-year premedical student. Cognitive function must be evaluated within the context of the environment (Gordon, 1994). The complexity of the environment chosen by the individual results in different levels of functioning; the nurse's assessment should reflect this difference.

The objective in assessing the individual's cognitive-perceptual pattern is to describe the adequacy of language, cognitive skills, and perception relative to desired or required activities (Gordon, 1994). The nurse collects and assesses clues that may indicate potential problems, particularly sensory deficits, sensory deprivation or overload, and ineffective pain management. Cognitive dysfunction may cause impaired reasoning, knowledge deficits related to health practices, and memory deficits.

A number of assessment parameters are available. All individuals should be questioned regarding sensory-perceptual problems. Subjective reporting includes whether and when the individual has been tested recently for hearing and vision. Any changes in the sensation or perception of the individual should be noted. In addition to decreased ability or acuity in hearing, vision, smell, and taste, the nurse evaluates other perceptual disturbances, such as vertigo; increased or decreased sensitivity to heat, cold, or light touch; and visual or auditory hallucinations or illusions. The use and perceived effectiveness of assistive devices, such as hearing aids, glasses, and contact lenses, are noted.

Any discomfort or pain is evaluated further. Useful tools have been designed to record and quantify changes in pain perception (Aubrun, Paqueron, Langron, Coriant, & Riou, 2003; Clark, Gironda, & Young, 2003; Horgas, McLennon, & Floetke, 2003; Nicholson, 2003; Wentz, 2003). Location, type, degree, and duration of pain provide indicators of possible causes or sources. Relief measures used to control pain and their effectiveness provide data and a focus for health education. Medication, heat or cold applications, and relaxation are examples of relief measures that should be explored for their usefulness in a plan of care (McCaffery & Pasero, 1999; McCaffrey, Frock, & Garduilo, 2003). For all individuals, exploring tolerance to pain is appropriate, using questions such as "Do you feel you are particularly sensitive to pain?" and "What level of pain is associated with your (cut, sprain, broken bone, or labor contractions)?"

Other areas of cognitive patterning to be explored include educational level, recent memory changes, ease or difficulty in learning, and preferred method of learning. Even when no problems are apparent or suspected, the nurse may assess these areas in more detail to determine areas of strength for use with health-teaching plans.

Objective data are accumulated throughout the interview or assessment process. This data collection begins with the nurse's perception of the individual's general appearance: hygiene and grooming, proper use of clothing, neatness and appropriateness of dress, and indication that these are appropriate to the individual's developmental stage. Language and vocabulary use, the ability to convey an idea with words or with actions when speech is impaired or not yet developed, and grammatical correctness provide clues to cognitive functioning. Amplitude and quality of speech, affect and mood, as well as attention and concentration are all indicative of the individual's mental status. For many individuals, this information is sufficient to relay a sense of the level of understanding, memory, and mentation. Problem-solving abilities usually can be determined when the individual is asked to relate any perceived problems, explanation of the problems, actions taken to solve the problems, and results of the actions taken. Because this is a basic assessment in each functional health pattern, the nurse already has an idea of whether thought processes are logical, coherent, and relevant for this individual.

When problems within the cognitive realm do not surface, the information is recorded as part of the objective data or findings of the physical examination. Data to be noted include language, vocabulary, attention span, grasp of ideas, level of consciousness, orientation to person, place, and time, language spoken (whether primary or secondary), and behavior during the data collection process, including posture, facial expression, and general body movements.

When a problem is apparent or suspected based on age, hereditary factors, or inconsistencies in the assessment data, a focused assessment is essential. Coma scales or functional dementia scales may be appropriate. More commonly, a mental status examination is performed to assess orientation, attention, calculation, language (ability to name objects, repeat abstract ideas, and follow commands), and recall (immediate-term, short-term, and long-term memory). Abilities to read, write, and copy designs can also be assessed.

The examination of a sensory-perceptual pattern evaluates hearing, vision, and areas of pain at a screening level; comprehensive examinations are available and may be indicated. A full neurological assessment is warranted when specific sensory deficits are identified during the examination.

Although these assessment areas may seem overwhelming, the time required is generally less than in most other pattern areas, perhaps because more information relevant to the cognitive-perceptual patterns becomes available as each pattern is assessed. Transition into the cognitive-perceptual pattern from other patterns may be facilitated by referring to a problem already described, with a question such as "Do you generally find it easy to solve problems effectively?" The self-perception pattern follows the cognitive pattern particularly well, because mental status measures include feelings and perceptions of the individual regarding self. Mood, affect, and responses to the interviewer, such as eye contact, are indications of self-esteem. Cognitive-perceptual ability greatly influences the ability to function (self-care) or manipulate within the environment (activity and exercise).

The placement of each of the patterns in a sequence suitable to each nurse, individual, or situation has been discussed. When the cognitive-perceptual pattern is dysfunctional, however, the individual is most likely unreliable as the historian; therefore, it is wise to consider this pattern early in the assessment process. Approaching this pattern early saves valuable time and permits the identification of patterns that can be assessed more reliably.

Every person has experienced temporary memory lapses at one time or another. These events alone are not sufficient basis for judgments. Sequence of behaviors and clustering of appropriate signals (defining characteristics) are necessary to determine any nursing diagnosis. Equally important is the need to assess all pattern areas before data analysis and problem identification.

Cognitive data and sensory abilities guide the nurse in planning care, which is especially apparent in health teaching. Formulation of health teaching plans ideally reflects the individual's preferred method of learning. The effective plan considers the individual's demonstrated developmental level, the ability to store information, retrieve information, compensate for deficits, as well as the neuromuscular and sensory levels necessary for skills development. An individually tailored plan contains mutually developed goals and short-term objectives. Although self-care might be an outcome for any person newly diagnosed with diabetes mellitus, behaviors expected of an adult with diabetes will differ from those expected of a child.

Self-Perception–Self-Concept Pattern

The self-perception–self-concept pattern encompasses the sense of personal identity, goals, emotional patterns, and feelings about the self. Self-image and sense of worth stem from the individual's perception of personal appearance, competencies, and limitations, including the individual's self-perception and others' perceptions. The nurse assesses both verbal and nonverbal cues (Gordon, 1994).

The significance of the sense of self to the whole person is best exemplified by personal experiences. Individuals who feel good about themselves look and act differently from those who feel unable to accomplish anything worthwhile. Patterns of eating, sleeping, and activity usually change if self-concept changes.

The individual's developmental level affects and is affected by this pattern. Erikson (1994) identifies eight stages of human development, proposing that with each stage a central task or crisis must be resolved before healthy growth can continue. According to Erikson, in early childhood the individual develops a sense of autonomy and struggles with the sense of shame and doubt. When this developmental level is achieved or resolved, the child moves on to develop initiative during the next stage. One of the tasks Havighurst (1972) identifies during this later phase is building wholesome attitudes toward oneself (self-esteem), whereas the model proposed by Bruhn and colleagues (1977) refers specifically to self-concept development. In this model, delays in self-concept development affect progress toward subsequent tasks (see Table 6-3).

Family climate and relationships patterns provide the environmental impact that influences the self-concept pattern. The family's role in the individual's development is apparent when Erikson's developmental tasks and the appropriate stages of the family life cycle (see Chapter 7) are analyzed jointly. All people who are closely associated with the individual affect that person's self-esteem. Most people care about what others think of them; therefore, the support of significant others affects the self-perception–self-concept pattern (Faulkner & Davey, 2002; Schor, 2003).

Achieving a sense of "I" versus "we" is vital for the individual. A sense of "I" as a person, apart from the roles that the person may assume, is important. For example, the sense of "me" rather than roles such as mother, father, daughter, son, student, or nurse helps to establish self-perception.

The assessment objective in this pattern area is to describe the individual's patterns and beliefs about general self-worth and feeling states (Gordon, 1994). The nurse looks for clues that indicate identity confusion, altered body image, disturbances in self-esteem, and feelings of powerlessness. Anxiety, fear, and depression states can be identified and are responsive to nursing interventions (Barker, 2001; Farmer, 2002).

Erickson's framework describes sequential and healthy developmental patterns for the individual. Accomplishment of the wellness tasks may be apparent in other functional health patterns as well, providing additional indications of developmental level (see Unit 4) (Stolte, 1996). Feelings about self contribute additional information for this pattern. Knowledge of individual strengths and limitations along with attitudes toward these strengths and limitations becomes important data when planning care. To elicit this kind of information, questions are asked regarding personal appearance and capabilities in the cognitive, affective, and psychomotor domains. This portrayal provides evidence of a sense of identity and worth, self-image, and body image. A description of emotional patterns or a general feeling state concludes the history when no problems are indicated. A focused assessment may use specific tools, when necessary, to measure body image (Young, Polzin, Todd, & Simuncak, 2002).

The nurse notes general appearance and affect, which may have been assessed as part of a formal mental status examination. Low self-esteem may be indicated by head and shoulder flexion, lack of eye contact, and mumbled or slurred speech. Anxiety or nervousness might be revealed through extraneous body movements such as foot shuffling or tapping, facial tension or grimace, rapid speech, voice quivering, twitches or tremors, and general restlessness or shifts in body position. Any of these indicators demand further exploration to determine underlying problems.

Self-concept influences the individual's interaction with the nurse. Because the information in this pattern is personal, sharing the information may actually facilitate the process of goal setting and intervention planning when the nurse possesses strong communication skills and a caring attitude.

Roles-Relationships Pattern

The roles-relationships pattern describes the position assumed and the associations engaged in by the individual that are connected to that position. The individual's perception is a major component of the assessment, and exploration of this pattern should include the individual's level of satisfaction with roles and relationships.

The need for relationships with other people is universal. Dossey and colleagues (2000) have identified basic needs for communication, fellowship, and love in high-level wellness. Similarly, Maslow's hierarchy of needs includes a sense of love and belonging (Duvall & Miller, 1985).

The ability to communicate with other people in a meaningful way greatly affects the whole person (Figure 6-2). The concept of health as the harmonious balance between the individual and the environment indicates the major role that relationships with others play in health status (Dossey et al., 2000; Newman, 2002). The function development plays in health is apparent in Erikson's stages of ego development (Erikson, 1994). This series of hypotheses about readiness proposes that attainment of each stage is required to progress to the next stage. For example, a person can become immersed in a relationship of genuine intimacy only after self-identity has stabilized.

Certain tasks for family development have been identified similarly by Duvall and Miller (1985) (see Chapter 7). The emphasis within these models is on the individual's relationships within the family and within the larger context of society.

The objective of the roles-relationships pattern assessment is to describe an individual's pattern of family and shared circumstances, with the associated responsibilities. The individual's perception of satisfaction with the established relationship contributes to this assessment. Loss, change, and threat produce the major problems within this pattern. Clues indicative of impaired verbal communication, social isolation, alterations in parenting, independence-dependence conflicts, dysfunctional grieving, and potential for violence are pertinent.

Table 6-3 Relationship Between Selected Developmental Tasks and Wellness Tasks for Each Stage of the Life Cycle

Erikson's Eight Life Stages	Havighurst's Developmental Tasks	Examples of Minimal Wellness Tasks for Each Developmental Stage
1. Infancy (trust vs. basic mistrust)	Learning to walk Learning to take solid foods Learning to talk Learning to control elimination of body waste	Acquiring ability to perform psychomotor skills Learning functional definition of health Learning social and emotional responsiveness to others and to physical environment
2. Early childhood (autonomy vs. shame and doubt)	Learning gender difference and sexual modesty Achieving physiological stability Forming simple concepts of social-physical reality Learning to relate emotionally to parents, siblings, and others Learning to distinguish right from wrong and developing a conscience Learning physical skills necessary for ordinary games	Learning about proper foods, exercise, and sleep Learning dental hygiene Learning injury prevention (safety belts and helmets, sunscreen, smoke detectors, poisons, firearms, and swimming) Refining psychomotor and cognitive skills
3. Late childhood (initiative vs. guilt)	Building wholesome attitudes toward self as a growing organism Learning to get along with peers	Developing self-concept Learning attitudes of competition and cooperation with others Learning social, ethical, and moral differences and responsibilities
4. Early adolescence (industry vs. inferiority)	Learning appropriate gender identity: masculine or feminine role Developing fundamental skills in reading, writing, and calculating Developing concepts necessary for everyday living Developing conscience, morality, and scale of values Achieving personal independence Developing attitudes toward social groups and institutions	Learning that health is an important value Learning self-regulation of physiological needs—sleep, rest, food, drink, and exercise Learning risk taking and its consequences (injury prevention)
5. Adolescence (identity vs. role confusion)	Achieving new and more mature relations with peers and both sexes Achieving gender identity Accepting physique and using body effectively Achieving emotional independence of parents and other adults Achieving assurance of economic independence Selecting and preparing for occupation Preparing for marriage and family life Developing intellectual skills and concepts necessary for civic competence Desiring and achieving socially responsible behavior	Learning economic responsibility Learning social responsibility for self and others (preventing pregnancy and sexually transmitted diseases) Experiencing social, emotional, and ethical commitments to others Accepting self and physical development Reconciling discrepancies between personal health concepts and observed health behaviors of others (use of alcohol, drugs, tobacco, firearms, and violence) Learning to cope with life events and problems (suicide prevention) Considering life goals and career plans and acquiring necessary skills to reach goals Learning importance of time to self and world
6. Early adulthood (intimacy vs. isolation)	Selecting and learning to live with a mate Starting a family; managing a home Taking on civic responsibility	Committing to mate and family responsibilities Selecting a career Incorporating health habits into lifestyle
7. Middle adulthood (generativity vs. stagnation)	Accepting and adjusting to physiological changes Achieving adult social responsibility Maintaining economic standard of living Assisting adolescent children	Accepting aging of self and others Coping with societal pressures Recognizing importance of good health habits Reassessing life goals periodically

Table 6-3	Relationship Between Selected Developmental Tasks and Wellness Tasks for Each Stage of the Life Cycle *cont'd*	
Erikson's Eight Life Stages	**Havighurst's Developmental Tasks**	**Examples of Minimal Wellness Tasks for Each Developmental Stage**
8. Maturity (ego integrity vs. despair)	Adjusting to decreasing physical strength and health Adjusting to retirement and reduced income Adjusting to death of spouse Establishing an explicit affiliation with own age group Establishing satisfactory physical living arrangements	Becoming aware of risks to health and adjusting lifestyle and habits to cope with risks Adjusting to loss of job, income, and family and friends through death Redefining self-concept Adjusting to changes in personal time and new physical environment Adjusting previous health habits to current physical and mental capabilities

Modified from Bruhn, J., Cordova, F. D., Williams, J. A., Fuentes, R. G. (1977). The wellness process. *Journal of Community Health, 2,* 209-221; Erikson, E. (1986). *Childhood and society* (35th anniversary ed.). New York: Norton; Havighurst, R. (1973). *Developmental tasks and education* (3rd ed.). New York: David McKay; U.S. Department of Health and Human Services. (2000). *Healthy People 2010. National health promotion and disease prevention objectives* (Conference Edition). Washington, DC: Public Health Service; U.S. Preventive Services Task Force. (1996). *Guide to clinical preventive services: An assessment of the effectiveness of 169 interventions.* Baltimore: Williams & Wilkins.

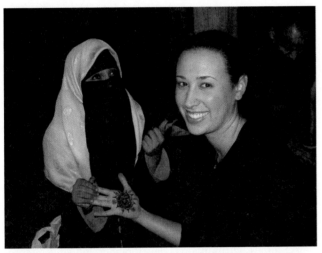

Figure 6-2 The ability to communicate with individuals of another culture greatly affects the development of an individual.

Assessment focuses on family, work, and community roles and relationships. Within the family, assessment parameters include the family structure, tasks performed, social support systems, and other dynamics, such as decision making, power, authority, division of labor, and communication patterns. Parenting or marital difficulties and family violence issues are explored. The roles of student and employee are explored to determine specific occupation or position, along with work responsibilities and work environment. Parameters such as stress, safety, and health factors should be included (Case Study and Care Plan). Financial concerns, job security, and retirement plans are elicited. Activity-rest patterns elicit information about time commitments, leisure activities, and physical exercise; therefore, the assessment at this point addresses the impact of these factors on the roles-relationships pattern. Community roles and relationships indicate involvement within the neigh-

CASE STUDY

Cindy

Cindy is a single 28-year-old woman. Cindy studies nursing and shares an apartment with two friends. She was having increasing difficulties with her course work and was placed on academic probation. Cindy became concerned about the effect of stress on her ability to finish her studies and on her future career. She grew increasingly nervous and began to ask, "Will I ever be okay?" and "Will I ever be able to finish school and function as a nurse?" Cindy expressed her fear of weakness and feelings of isolation, loneliness, helplessness, and loss of control. These feelings began to find expression in anger related to this major life disruption. She verbalized her anger at God for allowing this to happen to her. Her incapacity deprived her of her normal outlets for expressing and finding support for such concerns. Cindy was unable to participate in the practices of her faith, in which she previously had found strength in facing life's challenges. Her inability to concentrate and her growing feeling of lethargy added to her frustration. Expressing these fears and concerns was difficult for Cindy. The nurse, however, developed a trusting relationship with Cindy, permitting her to express her fears, anxieties, and concerns. Based on the nurse's assessment, the nursing diagnosis of spiritual distress was formulated.

Reflective Questions
1. What differential diagnoses should the nurse consider?
2. Describe other individuals you know who have experienced spiritual distress.

Modified from McFarland, G. K., & McFarland, E. A. (1993). *Nursing diagnosis and intervention: Planning for patient care.* St. Louis: Mosby.

borhood and other social groups, such as the level of socialization and amount of social support available. Within all three components (family, work or school, and community) the individual is asked to describe the level of satisfaction with the roles and relationships.

CARE PLAN

Spiritual Distress

(Related to Cindy Case Study)

Nursing Diagnosis Spiritual Distress Related to a Threat to Well-Being, Loss of Meaningful Role, and Separation From Religious and Family Ties

DEFINING CHARACTERISTICS

- Experiences a disturbance in belief system
- Demonstrates discouragement or despair
- Chooses not to practice religious rituals
- Shows emotional detachment from self and others
- Expresses concern, anger, resentment, and fear, related to a major life disruption

RELATED FACTORS

- Threat to well-being from change in role as a student and fear of failure
- Loss of meaningful role as a student
- Separation from religious and family ties

EXPECTED OUTCOMES

- Client will verbalize a greater sense of purpose, meaning, and hope.
- Client will express feelings of anger verbally and will discuss anger with another person.

INTERVENTIONS

- Take time to be present and available to listen to the client.
- Convey a nonjudgmental attitude.
- Encourage the client to verbalize feelings.
- Engage the client in values clarification.
- Encourage the client to acknowledge feelings of anger and to acknowledge and name any other feelings experienced.
- Reassure the client that it is acceptable to feel anger toward a supreme being.
- Encourage honest dialogue with a peer whom the client trusts.
- Offer consultation with an appropriate spiritual advisor.
- Inform the client of religious resources.
- Pray with the client as indicated.

Modified from Carpenito-Moyet, L. J. (2003). *Handbook of nursing diagnosis* (10th ed.). Philadelphia: Lippincott Williams & Wilkins.

Threat of change, actual change, and loss are areas to be explored further. In addition, family or work roles alone may not cause stress, but combining them may cause difficulties, as with the working mother or traveling husband and father.

Objective data for assessment within this pattern are usually unavailable unless the nurse makes a home visit or sees the individual in the company of significant others in some other capacity. Family interaction and communication patterns are noted whenever possible. Cognizant of meaningful relationships within the family, the nurse identifies potential problems, such as those that occur with the college student away from home, the individual who travels or moves frequently, and sole family survivors when older adults outlive their family members and friends (Kahana, Kahana, & Kercher, 2003; Kropf & Burnette, 2003; Peternelj-Taylor & Yonge, 2003).

The relationships among the functional health patterns are clearly apparent in light of the developmental stages. Difficulties within the self-concept pattern and difficulties with relationships often appear together (Erikson, 1994). Relationships affect the whole person; therefore, problems in the roles-relationships pattern may be exhibited in other areas such as sleep, appetite, and sexuality.

Sexuality-Reproductive Pattern

The sexuality-reproductive pattern describes the individual's sexual self-concept, sexual functioning, methods of intimacy, and reproductive areas. Data collection combines subjective information, nursing observations, and physical examination. Normal development and perceived satisfaction combine to provide the elements of this pattern (Gordon, 1994).

Sexuality is the behavioral expression of sexual identity. The importance of this pattern area to the individual's life and health are closely related to the self-perception and the relationships patterns. Body image, self-concept, and role and gender identity are linked to sexual identity. This concept of sexual self and the individual's relationships pattern indicate the level and the perceived satisfaction of sexual functioning. Sexual functioning involves, but is not limited to, sexual relations with a partner. Reproductive patterns are equally significant to this pattern assessment, the whole individual, and the family and community (see Chapters 7 and 8).

As discussed, individual development influences reproductive capacities; these include secondary sex characteristics, genital development, ego integrity, and the family life-cycle stage (Duvall & Miller, 1985; Erikson, 1994). Environment also plays a part in expression of the sexuality-reproductive pattern. Cultural and family norms may contribute to the expression of sexuality and combine with other factors, such as the family's financial stability, to influence reproductive patterns. Norms within society may create issues in expressions of sexuality.

One objective of assessment in this pattern is to describe behavioral problems or difficulties (Gordon, 1994). Equally important is assessing the individual's knowledge of sexual functioning and preventive health practices, such as breast and testicular self-examination, Papanicolaou smears, effective contraceptive use, and avoiding infection. Clues are evaluated for potential or actual sexual dysfunction.

Parameters assessed include (1) sexual self-concept, which may be derived from information collected in the self-perception–self-concept and the roles-relationships patterns, (2) sexual functioning, with the nurse noting evidence of some form of intimacy, the level of sexual activity or libido, and the effect of health or illness on sexual expression, and (3) reproductive patterns in which the nurse collects data pertinent to health-promotion factors, such as feelings related to aging, preventive practices, and knowledge of sexual functioning. For women, reproductive pattern assessment would also include information about menstruation, such as onset, duration, frequency, last menstrual period, discomfort, and menopause, as well as information about reproductive stage, such as pregnancy history and birth control methods.

Level of satisfaction with sexual self-concept, sexual functioning, and reproduction is also explored. Difficulties, such as ineffective or inappropriate sexual performance, discharges, infections, venereal disease, discomfort, and history of abuse, are evaluated. Focused assessment to collect additional information is warranted with sexual dysfunction or trauma. Physical examination evaluates genital development and secondary sex characteristics. Intimacy, such as holding hands and hugging, between partners is noted.

People may feel threatened by discussion of topics in this pattern; depth of exploration is governed in part by the individual's wishes. Dialogue is encouraged but may be postponed until a firm and trusting relationship is established.

A clear representation of the individual's knowledge and use of preventive practices facilitates planning for health promotion. Although sex education usually is associated with school programs, information and discussion about sexuality is just as important for adults. Sex education is a key element of parenthood classes. Improved understanding of sexuality and sexual function leads to discovery and increased satisfaction (Health Teaching box).

Coping–Stress Tolerance Pattern

Gordon (1994) describes the coping–stress tolerance pattern as a depiction of general coping and the individual's ability to effectively manage stress. This pattern includes the individual's ability to process life crises and to resist disruptive factors which will influence self-integrity of ego, mode of conflict resolution, stress management, and accessibility to necessary resources.

The ability to manage stress effectively in life is a learned behavior. Stress is a necessary part of life; without it there is no motivation to grow. Stress becomes a problem when tolerance is weak and daily activities are affected (Dossey et al., 2000; Peternelj-Taylor & Yonge, 2003).

Most stress comes not from great tragedies, but from an accumulation of minor irritations. Stress is not inherent in the event, but in the individual's perception of that event. Whereas one individual may experience stress from missing a bus and can think only of being 10 minutes late, another will consider the same event an opportunity to spend 10 minutes reading the newspaper. This difference in perception may represent the different values used to identify sources of stress or it may represent coping strategies.

For purposes of assessing this pattern, coping, which is considered the individual behavioral response to stress, includes both problem-solving ability and use of defense mechanisms. Coping is viewed not as a single act but as a process incorporating many behaviors. The function of coping is to deal with the threat or emotional distress of an event. Coping effectiveness is assessed from the individual's perspective and from the nurse's observation of the individual's ability to function in the presence of actual or potential stressors in the environment.

The perception of stress and the ability to manage it depends on personal development, amount of stress previously experienced, current level of stress within the environment, and sources of social support. For example, an elderly individual may have experienced many stresses during life and managed them effectively, but now coping may no longer be possible because too many stressors, such as physical incapacitation, fixed income, fear of illness or injury, and lack of transportation, exist or because a social support system is no longer available (Kahana et al., 2003; Kropf & Burnette, 2003).

HEALTH TEACHING   Sexuality and Aging Women: Common Myths

- Masturbation is an immature activity of youngsters and adolescents, not of older women.
- Sexual desire and prowess wane during the climacteric; therefore, menopause is the death of a woman's sexuality.
- Hysterectomy creates a physical disability that causes the inability to function sexually.
- Sex has no role in the lives of older adults except as perversion or remembrance of times past.

- Sexual expression in old age is taboo.
- Elderly adults are too old and frail to engage in sex.
- Sex is unimportant or over.
- Older women do not wish to discuss their sexuality with professionals.

Originally modified from Morrison-Beedy, D., & Robbin, L. (1989). Sexual assessment and the aging female. *Nursing Practice, 14,* 35; and Ebersole, P., & Hess, P. (1994) *Toward healthy aging: Human needs and nursing response* (4th ed.). St. Louis: Mosby. Updated with information from: *http://www.apa.org/pi/aging/sexuality.html.*

The objective in assessment is to determine the individual's stress tolerance and past coping patterns. The nurse evaluates clues to difficulties in managing past and current stressors and changes in the effectiveness of a coping pattern in order to determine personal coping capacity.

Assessment parameters include (1) the coping task, including the physical, psychological, and socioeconomic stimuli with which the individual must cope, (2) coping style, or the tendency to use a specific style, such as approach oriented, avoidance oriented, or nonspecific, (3) coping strategies, including specifics, and (4) coping effectiveness.

Coping strategy may be divided into information seeking, direct action (fight or flight), inhibition of action, or use of social support. Coping effectiveness is best assessed by eliciting the individual resources and the individual's functional level (Dossey et al., 2000). Individual resources include the variety of coping mechanisms used by the individual, flexibility of these mechanisms, and the health-promotion value associated with each.

Stress tolerance patterns elicit the amount of stress effectively processed in the past. Use of anticipatory coping is assessed along with whether the individual knows how to cope, but does not (production deficit), or simply does not know how to cope (skill deficit).

Other indicators of value within this pattern are discussed under the self-perception–self-concept pattern. Objective data of concern include physical signs of restlessness, irritability, and nervousness, such as increased heart rate and blood pressure and perspiration.

Evidence of coping ability and tolerance to stress are found in every other functional health pattern. Stress also affects the other patterns, thereby resulting in health problems such as insomnia, weight loss, and poor concentration (Dossey et al., 2000; Gordon, 1994; Jacobs, 2001).

Health can be promoted through early intervention. For example, Holmes and Rahe found a significant relationship between perceived stressful life events and subsequent illness (Cassidy, 2000). Coping patterns and stress tolerance in the past may uncover unhealthy behavior, such as smoking and drinking, that needs to be replaced by alternative coping strategies. Stress-reduction workshops would be helpful for most of the population, because the future undoubtedly holds stressful events, some of which may be overwhelming without coping strategies. See the Innovative Practice box for information about a unique company that offers stress management interventions.

Dossey and colleagues (2000) offer categories for stress management: (1) social engineering strategies, such as time management or planned change, (2) personality engineering strategies, such as assertiveness training or cognitive rehearsal, and (3) altered states of consciousness, such as meditation or relaxation. Planning based on the assessment of all functional health patterns to help determine a coping pattern should include these kinds of strategies.

innovative practice

The Humor Potential, Inc.

The Humor Potential, Inc., is a company that provides resources, products, and seminars for stress management with the use of humor. Company president Loretta LaRoche is an internationally recognized expert on stress management, emphasizing the importance of balancing daily living experiences with humor. The Humor Potential, Inc., offers seminars and lectures to health care professionals, schools, corporations, other organizations, and the general public. The corporation also produces television programs that have been shown on PBS, NBC, CNN, and HBO. The first PBS show, *The Joy of Stress,* was nominated for a regional Emmy Award.

Books, prints, audiotapes and videotapes, and other products dealing with humor can be purchased from her Web site. The collection consists of audiotapes and videotapes that have been developed for corporate meetings and training. An example is *Stressbusters!*, an audiotape and videotape and action guide that increases productivity by reducing stress. Two other tapes, *Not Another Meeting* and *Whoopee! Another Meeting*, are meeting openers for staff development programs given to employees to improve communication, productivity, and outcomes within an organization. A catalog is available for e-mail, fax, phone, and mail orders.

Contact information:
The Humor Potential, Inc.
Web site: *http://www.lorettalaroche.com*
Email: inquiries@lorettalaroche.com
Telephone: 800-99-TADAH (800-998-2324)

Values-Beliefs Pattern

The values-beliefs pattern describes values, including the individual's spiritual values, beliefs, and goals. This pattern also includes perceptions of what is right, what is good, and conflicts that beliefs or values impart.

Each of the 11 patterns addresses value systems of individuals and society. Individual beliefs or values develop over time and govern life through personal experiences and family and societal influences (Duvall & Miller, 1985; Wong et al., 2002).

The objective in assessing this pattern is to determine the basis for health-related decisions and actions (Gordon, 1994). Rosenstock (1974) suggests that an individual will engage in preventive health behavior when a threat to wellness or health status exists. Several other health belief models expand on this concept by including other motivations, such as personal values and environmental influences. Clues to conflict within the individual's value system or between the person's value system and that of the family or society are explored.

Dimensions of assessment include the individual's values, beliefs, or goals that guide choice or decisions that are related to health. The nurse collects information while exploring each pattern, while summarizing, clarifying, and securing additional information. Specifically, values and beliefs about self, relationships, and society are appraised. Individuals' beliefs, goals, and purposes of life are reviewed, along with any conflicts, perceived philosophies, and those of the family, culture, and society. Sources of strength, such as God or significant individual practices, are explored, including religious beliefs and preferences.

Past goals and expectations are assessed through the individual's satisfaction. The nurse must identify the individual's goals and expectations concerning health, clarifying to help the individual achieve them. To be effective, health-promotion interventions are based on the individual's value system and health beliefs (Dossey et al., 2000; Jarvis, 2003; Pender, Murdaugh, & Parsons, 2001).

The brevity of this discussion is no indication of the importance that the values-beliefs pattern plays in the assessment of the individual. Individual values play a role in all of the patterns.

INDIVIDUAL HEALTH PROMOTION THROUGH THE NURSING PROCESS

The nursing process—the systematic approach to reduce or eliminate the individual's health problem—is accomplished in several steps, first collecting the necessary data. With the individual, the nurse analyzes the data, identifies a nursing diagnosis, projects outcomes, prescribes interventions, and evaluates effectiveness. Reassessment, reordering of priorities, new goal setting, and revising the plan continues as part of the process toward outcome attainment (Carpenito-Moyet, 2003).

Collection and Analysis of Data

Assessment is a systematic technique for learning as much as possible about the individual. The main purpose in collecting data from a new individual is to see whether health problems exist and to identify the individual's health goals. An assessment of an adult based on the functional health patterns is presented in **Web Site Resource 6B.**

Data collection includes biographical data, such as age, sex, and the purpose of the visit. This process is followed by assessment of the previously outlined 11 functional health patterns. Subjective reporting, nursing observations and perceptions, and the physical examination are assessed and recorded. The remaining discussion focuses on nursing diagnosis.

Problem Identification

Although the concept of problem identification has been debated in the past, most nurses now have distinguished nursing diagnosis as the problem label. Diagnosis is a careful examination and analysis of the facts in an attempt to explain something. Nursing diagnosis is the naming of an individual's response to actual or potential health problems or life processes (Carpenito-Moyet, 2003; Gordon, 1994; NANDA, 2003).

Nursing diagnoses provide the basis for selection of nursing interventions to achieve outcomes for which the nurse is accountable (Gordon, 1994). NANDA has provided leadership in developing standardization of the descriptions of human responses that nurses manage. The most recent revision of this taxonomy has been approved for clinical testing and has been endorsed by the ANA (NANDA, 2003).

Gordon (1994) proposed the accepted format of nursing diagnosis that lists the problem, etiology, and signs and symptoms (PES), or defining characteristics, for each diagnosis accepted for clinical testing.

At the 1998 NANDA conference a multiaxial framework for nursing diagnoses was proposed but has yet to be completed and approved by the NANDA board. This proposed formation for nursing diagnoses is a more detailed clinical language and an improved structure for nursing diagnoses to be included in computerized databases. If approved in the future, nursing diagnoses will be expressed by six axes: (1) diagnostic concept (parenting), (2) acuity (altered), (3) unit of care (individual), (4) developmental stage (adolescent), (5) potentiality (at risk for), and (6) descriptor, creating the diagnostic statement (NANDA, 2003).

See Research Highlights for discussion of a study of a nursing versus nonnursing classification system.

In discussions of problems, the meaning of *problem* must be clearly defined and identified. The concept as used in this text refers to Gordon's (1994) proposition that a health problem is defined as a dysfunctional pattern and that nursing's major contribution to health care is in preventing

---

research highlights

Classification Systems

In a pilot study involving two classification systems, researchers explored the differences between a nonnursing classification system for function and disability (the International Classification of Impairments, Disabilities, and Handicaps-2 [ICIDH-2]) and the diagnostic classification system used by nursing. Experts were asked to identify and classify patient problems that were observed on a videotape of a clinical case or that appeared in patients' records as nursing problem statements from nursing diagnoses. Each problem statement was classified by a panel of three individuals. The findings suggest that the ICIDH-2 classification system is pertinent to the nursing discipline and permits classification of most nursing diagnoses. The classification system in its current form would be valuable for nurses, and the investigators recommended that nurses take an active role in further development of the ICIDH-2 system to improve its usefulness to nursing.

From van Achterberg, T. Frederiks, C., Thien, N., Coenen, C., & Persoon, A. (2002). Using ICIDH-2 in the classification of nursing diagnoses: Results from two pilot studies. *Journal of Advanced Nursing, 37*(2), 135-144.

and treating these patterns. A pattern is dysfunctional when it represents a deviation from established norms or from the individual's previous condition or goals. (Normative behavior is further discussed in Unit 4.) A dysfunctional pattern is a problem when it generates therapeutic concern on the part of the individual, others, or the nurse and when it is amenable to nursing therapies.

As patterns are assessed, the nurse proposes several hypotheses regarding functional or dysfunctional labeling. At the completion of the assessment, conclusions must be drawn. The possibility exists that all patterns are functional, that some are functional, and that others are dysfunctional or potentially dysfunctional.

Functional refers to wellness and optimal health. Dysfunctional patterns, indicating some health problems, may be present in the absence of disease; that is, nursing care may be needed for health promotion and health maintenance, not health restoration. The case history of Frank Thompson in Chapter 1 effectively illustrates the multiple nursing care needs of an individual who is not ill.

In potentially dysfunctional patterns, sufficient evidence exists or enough **risk factors** are present to indicate that a pattern dysfunction will likely occur if interventions are not made. Early identification of potential problems is possible through systematic data collection and analysis.

Contributing Etiological Factors

To plan care, the nurse must first determine what has caused the actual or potential health problem: its contributing etiological factors. The etiological factors of most dysfunctional patterns lie within another pattern or patterns. Although etiology is never an absolute within human sciences, the projection of outcomes or goals must be based on probable causes. Interventions then focus on mediating or resolving the probable causes. Most often, many factors are involved and problems are said to relate to rather than be a result of these factors.

Potential problems are not actual problems but risk states; therefore, they have no specific cause and are identified when risk factors are present. Nursing intervention is directed toward risk reduction through education (classes or brochures) to improve nutrition, prevent accidents, and so forth. Risk estimate theory and potential health problems are developed further in Chapters 7 and 8 and Unit 4 (Hot Topics box).

Diagnostic Variables

The ability to arrive at an accurate diagnosis, even when all the appropriate information is available, is governed primarily by the nurse's clinical skills. Experience improves the technique when nursing is performed as a scientific process. Nursing requires gathering information, interpreting it based on normative values, organizing and grouping inappropriate findings, identifying the problem, and then planning appropriate goals and interventions.

HOTtopics

HEART DISEASE IN WOMEN

Contrary to what many people think, heart disease is the leading cause of death in women. Approximately 370,000 American women of all races and ethnic groups die from heart disease each year. Black women have the highest death rate from heart disease (535 deaths per 100,000 population), followed by white women (388 deaths per 100,000 population), Hispanic women (265 deaths per 100,000 population), Native American women (259 deaths per 100,000 population), and Asian American and Pacific Islander women (221 deaths per 100,000 population). Nurses need to assess women for risk factors and symptoms of heart disease.

From Casper, M. L., et al. (2000). *Women and heart disease: An atlas of racial and ethnic disparities in mortality* (2nd ed.). Morgantown, WV: Office for Social Environment and Health Research, West Virginia University.

Difficulties are encountered when there are no available norms, which occurs frequently in the psychosocial assessment components. Using the 11 interdependent functional health patterns helps to solve these difficulties. By focusing on each of these areas, recognizing whether a problem does or does not exist is easier. Any change within the pattern may be a sign of dysfunction or an unhealthy but stabilized behavior. For example, a sign of dysfunction might be a 2-year-old child who is still not walking; developmental growth is a major factor in activity patterns of infants, toddlers, and children.

The use of physiological parameters clearly demonstrates the idea of a stabilized dysfunctional pattern, but equal attention must be given to psychological development. For instance, a 26-year-old man who lives with his mother and gives no indication of independent decision making should be evaluated.

It should be apparent that assessment information primarily comes from the initial contact with the individual and the database, which is generally the case in health-promotion activities. However, in any acute situation or emergency, quick assessment of the major problems is given high priority on a hierarchy-of-needs basis and the full nursing assessment is postponed temporarily.

For further understanding of the nursing diagnosis, the nurse is referred to books discussing the development of diagnoses, the diagnostic process, and specific details of each accepted diagnosis (Carpenito-Moyet, 2003; Gordon, 1994; NANDA, 2003).

Planning the Care

Planning, in the nursing process, is the proposal of diagnosis-specific treatment to assist the individual toward the goal, or expected outcome, of optimal health. The individual's goals and the determined nursing diagnosis provide the basis for planning. Clarity of the goals and diagnoses is critical to development of an effective plan of care.

Yura (1982) identifies the following purposes of the planning phase: (1) to assign priority to the problems diagnosed, (2) to specify the behavioral outcomes or goals with the individual, including the expected time of achievement, (3) to differentiate individual problems that can be resolved by nursing intervention, those that can be handled by the individual or family member, and those that should be handled with or referred to other members of the health team, (4) to designate specific actions, the frequency of these actions, and the short-term, intermediate-term, and long-term results, and (5) to list the individual's problems (nursing diagnosis) and nursing actions (frequency and **expected outcomes**, or goals) on the nursing care plan or blueprint for action. This plan provides the direction for individual and nursing activities and is the guide for the evaluation. There are many research studies involving outcomes from which nurses can draw to improve effectiveness of the care they provide.

Implementing the Plan

Implementation is the completion of the actions necessary to fulfill the goals for optimal health; it is the enactment of the nursing care plan toward the behaviors described in the proposed individual outcome.

The selection of a nursing intervention depends on several factors: (1) the desired client outcome, (2) the characteristics of the nursing diagnosis, (3) the research base associated with the intervention, (4) the feasibility of implementing the intervention, (5) the acceptability of the intervention to the individual, and (6) the capability of the nurse (Carpenito-Moyet, 2003).

A nursing interventions classification is being developed. As discussed in Unit 1, a critical component of effective communication is the accurate interpretation of the individual's information. This feedback process continues throughout all phases of the nursing process; the nurse continues to collect data to modify the plan as needed and does not blindly implement the care plan. As discussed in Unit 3, the most frequently used nursing interventions in health promotion are screening, education, counseling, and crisis intervention. All of these interventions require strong communication abilities from the nurse.

Evaluating the Plan

The process of analyzing changes experienced by the individual occurs in the evaluation phase of the nursing process, with the nurse examining the relationships between nursing actions and the individual's goal achievement. Nursing process emphasizes that evaluation is always considered in terms of how the individual responds to the plan of action

(Yura, 1982). As discussed, the nursing diagnosis, or health problems, and the goal, or expected outcome, guide the evaluation of the nursing care plan.

Many variables influence outcomes: the interventions prescribed by the health care providers, the health care providers themselves, the environment in which the care is received, the individual's motivation and genetic structure, and the individual's significant others. The task for nursing is to define which outcomes are sensitive to nursing care so as to identify the expected and attainable results of nursing care for each individual (Yura, 1982).

All of these components of the nursing process are documented by the nurse on the individual's health care record (Bickley & Hoekelman, 2002).

SUMMARY

Data relevant to the health-promotion activities of the individual focus primarily on the assessment of the current health status so that the nurse can identify problem areas, or areas of dysfunction, within the individual's health and lifestyle pattern. This process is a fundamental first step and precedes all other components of the nursing process. Without a clear picture of the problem, nursing activities are fruitless.

Gordon's functional health pattern framework provides guidance for the individual assessment. The focus of each pattern includes the age-developmental influences exerted, cultural and environmental roles played, functional ability displayed, and behavioral patterns specific to each individual. The interaction between internal mechanisms and the environment is assessed through these 11 functional health patterns.

When assessing each pattern, the nurse must understand the pattern definition, the significance of the pattern to the whole individual, the developmental influences, the environmental role, the assessment objectives, the assessment parameters and indicators, and the nursing implications. Assessment is essential to all components of the nursing process in health promotion for the individual.

ADDITIONAL STUDY MATERIAL

Study Questions in the back of the book, see page 663.

evolve WEB SITE MATERIALS

These materials are located on the book's Web site at http://evolve.elsevier.com/Edelman/.

- WebLinks
- Content Updates
- Web Site Resources

6A   Relationship Between Selected Developmental Tasks and Wellness Tasks for Each Life Cycle Stage

6B   Functional Health Patterns Assessment for an Adult

REFERENCES

American Nurses Association. (2003a). ANA's 'foundations of practice' revised. *American Nurse, 35*(5), 15.

American Nurses Association. (2003b). *Nursing's social policy statement* (2nd ed.). Washington, DC: American Nurses Association.

American Nurses Association. (2004). *Nursing: Scope and standards of practice.* Washington, DC: American Nurses Association.

Aubrun, F., Paqueron, X., Langron, O., Coriant, P., & Riou, B. (2003). What pain scales do nurses use in the postanaesthesia care unit? *European Journal of Anaesthesiology, 20*(9), 745.

Barker, P. (2001). The tidal model: Developing a person-centered approach to psychiatric and mental health nursing. *Perspectives in Psychiatric Care, 37*(3), 79.

Bickley, L., & Hoekelman, R. A. (2002). *Barbara Bates guide to physical examination and history taking* (9th ed.). Philadelphia: Lippincott Williams & Wilkins.

Brown, S. (2002). Systematic review of nursing management of urinary tract infections in the cognitively impaired elderly client in residential care: Is there a hole in holistic care? *International Journal of Nursing Practice, 8*(1), 2.

Bruhn, J., Cordova, F. D., Williams, J. A., & Fuentes, R. G. (1977). The wellness process. *Journal of Community Health, 2*(2), 209-222.

Carpenito-Moyet, L. J. (2003). *Handbook of nursing diagnosis* (10th ed.). Philadelphia: Lippincott Williams & Wilkins.

Casper, M. L., Barnett, E., Halverson, J. A., Elmes, G. A., Braham, V. E., & Majeed, Z. A., et al. (2000). *Women and heart disease: An atlas of racial and ethnic disparities in mortality* (2nd ed.). Morgantown, WV: Office for Social Environment and Health Research, West Virginia University.

Cassidy, T. (2000). Stress, healthiness and health behaviours: An exploration of the role of life events, daily hassles, cognitive appraisal and the coping process. *Counselling Psychology Quarterly, 13*(3), 293.

Centers for Disease Control and Prevention. (1997). Guidelines for school and community programs to promote lifelong physical activity among young people. *Morbidity and Mortality Weekly Report, 46*(No. RR-6), 1-36.

Centers for Disease Control and Prevention. (2003). *Prevalence of overweight among children and adolescents: United States, 1999.* Retrieved April 28, 2004, from: *http://www.cdc.gov/nchs/data/hus/tables/2002/02hus071.pdf.*

Chang, G. (2001). Alcohol-screening instruments for pregnant women. *Alcohol Research & Health, 25*(3), 204-209.

Clark, M. E., Gironda, R. J., & Young, R. W. (2003). Development and validation of the Pain Outcomes Questionnaire-VA. *Journal of Rehabilitation Research & Development, 40*(5), 381.

Dossey, B. M., Keegan, L., & Guzzetta, C. E. (2000). *Holistic nursing: a handbook for practice* (3rd ed.). Gaithersburg, MD: Aspen.

Duvall, E., & Miller, B. (1985). *Marriage and family development* (7th ed.). New York: Harper Collins.

Ebersole, P., & Hess, P. (1998). *Toward healthy aging: Human needs and nursing response* (6th ed.). St. Louis: Mosby.

Erikson, E. H. (1994). *Identity: Youth in crisis* (Austen Rigg Monograph, Reissue ed.). W. W. Norton.

Farmer, T. J. (2002). The experience of major depression: Adolescents' perspectives. *Issues in Mental Health Nursing, 23*(6), 567.

Faulkner, R. A., & Davey, M. (2002). Children and adolescents of cancer patients: The impact of cancer on the family. *The American Journal of Family Therapy, 30*(1), 63.

Gordon, M. (1994). *Nursing diagnosis: Process and application* (3rd ed.). St. Louis: Mosby.

Hajat, A., Lucas, J. B., & Kington, R. (2000). *Health outcomes among Hispanic subgroups* (Publication No. 310). Hyattsville, MD: National Center for Health Statistics.

Havighurst, R. J. (1972). *Developmental tasks and education* (3rd ed.). United Kingdom: Longman Group.

Horgas, A. L., McLennon, S. M., & Floetke, A. L. (2003). Pain management in persons with dementia. *Alzheimer's Care Quarterly, 4*(4), 297.

Jacobs, G. D. (2001). The physiology of mind-body interactions: The stress response and the relaxation response. *Journal of Alternative & Complementary Medicine, 7*(6), 83.

Jarvis, C. (2003). *Physical examination and health assessment* (4th ed.). Philadelphia: Saunders.

Kahana, E., Kahana, B., & Kercher, K. (2003). Emerging lifestyles and proactive options for successful ageing. *Ageing International, 28*(2), 155.

Kozier, B., Erb, G., Berman, A. J., & Burke, K. (2003). *Fundamentals of nursing: Concepts, process, and practice* (7th ed.). Upper Saddle River, NJ: Prentice Hall.

Kropf, N. P., & Burnette, D. (2003). Grandparents as family caregivers: Lessons for intergenerational education. *Educational Gerontology, 29*(4), 361.

Leininger, M., & McFarland, M. R. (2002). *Transcultural nursing: Concepts, theories, research and practice* (3rd ed.). New York: McGraw-Hill.

McCaffery, M., & Pasero, C. (1999). *Pain: Clinical manual* (2nd ed.). St. Louis: Mosby.

McCaffrey, R. L., Frock, T. L., & Garduilo, H. (2003). Understanding chronic pain and the mind-body connection. *Holistic Nursing Practice, 17*(6), 281.

Moore, K. N., Day, R. A., & Albers, M. (2002). Pathogenesis of urinary tract infections: A review. *Journal of Clinical Nursing, 11*(5), 568.

Morrison-Beedy, D., & Robbin, L. (1989). Sexual assessment and the aging female. *Nursing Practice, 14*(35).

Newman, M. A. (2002). The pattern that connects. *ANS Advances in Nursing Science, 24*(3), 1.

Nicholson, B. D. (2003). Diagnosis and management of neuropathic pain: A balanced approach to treatment. *Journal of the American Academy of Nurse Practitioners, 15*, 3.

Nightingale, F. (1992). *Notes on nursing; What it is, and what it is not* (Commemorative ed.). Philadelphia: Lippincott.

North American Nursing Diagnosis Association. (2003). *Nursing diagnosis 2003-2004: Definitions and classifications.* Chicago: North American Nursing Diagnosis Association.

Nosek, M. A., Hughes, R. B., Howland, C. A., Young, M. E., Mullen, P. D., & Shelton, M. L. (2004). The meaning of health for women with physical disabilities. *Family & Community Health, 27*(1), 6.

Pender, N. J., Murdaugh, C., & Parsons, M. A. (2001). *Health promotion in nursing practice* (4th ed.). Saddle River, NJ: Prentice Hall.

Peternelj-Taylor, C. A., & Yonge, O. (2003). Exploring boundaries in the nurse-client relationship: Professional roles and responsibilities. *Perspectives in Psychiatric Care, 39*(2), 55.

Pryor, J., & Smith, C. (2002). A framework for the role of registered nurses in the specialty practice of rehabilitation nursing in Australia. *Journal of Advanced Nursing, 39*(3), 249.

Rogers, M. (1970). *An introduction to the theoretical basis of nursing.* Philadelphia: F. A. Davis.

Rosenstock, I. (1974). *Health Education Monographs, 2,* 354.

Schor, E. L., American Academy of Pediatrics Task Force on the Family. (2003). Family pediatrics: Report of the Task Force on the Family. *Pediatrics, 111*(6), 1541-1571.

Stolte, K. (1996). *Wellness nursing diagnosis for health promotion* (1st ed.). Philadelphia, PA: Lippincott-Raven. Retrieved April 26, 2004.

U.S. Department of Health and Human Services. (2001). *The Surgeon General's call to action to prevent and decrease overweight and obesity* (Rep. No. 02NLM:WD 210 59593 2001). Washington, DC: U.S. Department of Health and Human Services, Public Health Service, Office of the Surgeon General.

van Achterberg, T. Frederiks, C., Thien, N., Coenen, C., & Persoon, A. (2002). Using ICIDH-2 in the classification of nursing diagnoses: Results from two pilot studies. *Journal of Advanced Nursing, 37*(2), 135-144.

Wentz, J. D. (2003). Assessing pain at the end of life. *Nursing, 33*(8), 22.

Wong, D. L., Perry, S. E., & Hockenberry-Eaton, M. J. (2002). *Maternal child nursing care* (2nd ed.). St. Louis: Mosby.

Young, L. K., Polzin, J., Todd, S., & Simuncak, S. L. (2002). Validation of the nursing diagnosis anxiety in adult patients undergoing bone marrow transplant. *International Journal of Nursing Terminologies & Classifications, 13*(3), 88.

Yura, H. (1982). *Human needs and the nursing process.* New York: McGraw-Hill Appleton Lange.

Zeiss, A. M., & Kasl-Godley, J. (2001). Sexuality in older adults' relationships. *Generations, 25*(2), 18.

Chapter 7

ANNE RATH RENTFRO

Health Promotion and the Family

objectives

After completing this chapter, the reader will be able to:

- Describe the use of the functional health pattern framework in assessing families throughout the life span.

- Describe examples of the clinical data to be collected in each health pattern during each of the family developmental phases.

- Give examples of the following behavioral changes within the health patterns of families: functional, potentially dysfunctional, and actually dysfunctional.

- Describe developmental and cultural characteristics of the family to consider while identifying risk factors or etiological factors of potentially or actually dysfunctional health patterns.

- Discuss planning, implementing, and evaluating nursing interventions in health promotion with families.

- Develop a specific health-promotion plan based on a family assessment, nursing diagnosis, and contributing risks or etiological factors.

key terms

Cultural competence
Developmental theory
Divergent family structures
Ecomap
Family developmental tasks
Family function

Family health status
Family nursing diagnosis
Family nursing interventions
Family pattern
Family resilience
Family risk factors

Family strengths
Family structure
Genogram
Risk factor theory
Systems theory

THINK About It

Caring for Older Adults

Adult family members, who may even have health problems of their own, find themselves caring for their elderly parents. This type of situation is expected to become more prevalent in the coming years.

1 What are the implications of this growing situation for individuals? Families? Communities? The nation?

2 How will this trend affect individual lives personally and professionally?

How family members relate to one another influences the understanding of behavior, which is demonstrated in the family's structural, functional, communicational, and developmental patterns (American Academy of Pediatrics [AAP], 2003; Brannigan, Gemmell, Pevalin, & Wade, 2002; Friedman, Bowden, & Jones, 2003). Therefore an important consideration in the appraisal of health promotion and disease prevention is the family assessment. Within families, children and adults are nurtured, provided for, and taught about health values by word and by example, and it is within families that members first learn to make choices to promote health.

Healthy People 2010 views families as means of providing an important opportunity for health promotion and disease prevention. This report asserts that beginning a family should be one of the joys of life. Through family planning, parents assume responsibility to care for and provide for their children. After the choice has been made, the mother has the responsibility to seek prenatal care during the first trimester of pregnancy. Breast-feeding also helps give infants a healthy start. Nutritious diets that support physical growth and development coupled with physical activity promote healthy habits. Within families, children first observe and learn behaviors. Patterns of nutrition, activity, oral hygiene, and coping develop at an early age, and family members support these patterns by example. Patterns of alcohol consumption and tobacco use are similarly established within families. For adolescents and young adults, learning about physical development can foster positive awareness of their sexuality. Promoting self-esteem and reinforcing positive behaviors also builds the mental health of children. Primary care providers support positive behaviors by providing family members with scientifically sound clinical preventive services, such as immunizations, screening for early detection, and appropriate counseling.

Pender believes that the family is a logical unit of assessment and intervention for health promotion, because families have primary responsibility for (1) developing self-care and dependent-care competencies within the family, (2) fostering resilience among family members, (3) providing resources, and (4) promoting healthy individuation while maintaining family cohesion. Furthermore, the task of fostering health and healthy behaviors should be an integral part of a functional family process (Pender, Murdaugh, & Parsons, 2001).

This chapter uses systems theory, developmental theory, and risk factor theory to guide the nursing process with families. The 11 functional health patterns described in the previous chapter are used to pose questions during data collection. The analysis phase of the nursing process categorizes these data within stages of family development and, from the analysis, a nursing diagnosis is formulated. **Family health status** is considered functional, potentially dysfunctional (potential problem), or dysfunctional (actual problem) (Gordon, 1994). The planning phase begins when family goals and objectives are stated. The family, the nurse, or another health professional facilitates implementation.

Four types of interventions are discussed for health promotion and disease prevention. Nurses assume various roles throughout the stages of family development, and these roles are also presented. Evaluation of a family plan considers outcomes that are specific, objective, and measurable and that rely on the family's subjective interpretation of concerns and probability of success (Friedman et al., 2003; North American Nursing Diagnosis Association, 2003).

THE NURSING PROCESS AND THE FAMILY

The goal of nursing is to facilitate the health of the family (Newman, 1995). Nursing process with families is a two-level process that includes the family as a group and the family member as an individual (Friedman et al., 2003). The home is the most natural environment for this encounter, although the process may occur in other settings, as well. Members of different age groups (infants, children, and older adults) are likely be available in the home. The nurse also observes the physical environment firsthand during a home visit. For example, household safety hazards are observed directly. The nurse can also monitor the family unit with their rituals, roles, and interpersonal interactions. Generally the nurse contacts the family and establishes an appointment time for the visit. Including each member of the family in the visit will provide the nurse with a broader perspective than interviewing a single member. During the visit, the nursing process takes place with the family, not for the family. The family joins with the nurse in all phases of the process. Guidelines for home visits are presented in Box 7-1.

Box **7-1** **Guidelines for Home Visit to Promote Health and Prevent Disease**

PLANNING THE VISIT

- Make arrangements with the family.
- Study information regarding the family from agency records, referral forms, and other sources.
- State the purpose of the visit.
- Obtain appropriate supplies and teaching aids for visits.

MAKING THE VISIT

- Offer an introduction and explain the purpose of the visit.
- Place the nurse's bag in an appropriate location.
- Include all family members in the discussion.
- Identify the family's request for assistance.
- Understand the situation from the family's perspective.
- Identify appropriate activities for health promotion and disease prevention.
- Identify how the home visit is to be financed.
- Make a contract with the family that states specific goals and objectives that the family wants to reach.
- Terminate the visit with specific instructions and information about the next visit: when it will occur, what will happen, who will be present, and what the family must accomplish before then.

Comprehensive family assessment provides the foundation to promote family health (Friedman et al., 2003). Several factors influence family assessment, such as the nurse's perception of what constitutes a family; knowledge of theories, norms, and standards; and an ability to put the family at ease during visits. In addition to factors that pertain to the nurse, familial factors also influence the assessment, such as cooperation from family members, mutual agreement to work toward a desired goal, and the family's ability to see the relevance of the implementation plans. A useful health-promotion family assessment involves listening to the family, engaging in participatory dialogue, recognizing patterns, and assessing the family's potential for active, positive change (Endo et al., 2000; Friedman et al., 2003).

The assessment phase of the nursing process seeks and identifies information from the family about health-promotion and disease prevention activities. To obtain this information, nurses follow the family's progress through developmental tasks and identify strengths in the family's ability to generate low risk–taking behaviors associated with disease prevention. The two approaches considered in this chapter are the developmental framework and the risk-factor estimate. Developmental norms as proposed by Duvall and Miller (1985) and risk-factor estimates as proposed in *Healthy People 2010* can be used to guide nurses through the steps of the nursing process when working with families.

The Nurse's Role

Working with families from a systems perspective helps the nurse understand ways in which family members interact, what the family norms and expectations are, how effectively members communicate, how families make decisions, and how families cope with needs and expectations. The nurse's role in health promotion and disease prevention includes the following tasks:

1. To become aware of family attitudes and behaviors toward health promotion and disease prevention
2. To serve as role model for the family
3. To collaborate with the family in assessing, improving, enhancing, and evaluating their current health practices
4. To assist the family in growth and development behaviors
5. To assist the family in identifying risk-taking behaviors
6. To assist the family in decision making about lifestyle choices
7. To provide reinforcement for positive health-behavior practices
8. To assist the family in learning behaviors to promote health and prevent disease
9. To serve as a liaison for referral or collaboration between community resources and the family
10. To provide health information to the family
11. To assist the family in problem solving and decision making about health promotion

How the nurse works with families will depend on the framework used to guide, observe, and classify the situation. Nursing roles for families in various stages of development are presented in **Web Site Resource 7A.**

THE FAMILY FROM A SYSTEMS PERSPECTIVE

The family can be defined as a set of interacting individuals who are related by blood, marriage, cohabitation, or adoption and who interdependently perform relevant functions through roles. Relevant functions of the family include values and practices placed on health. Health is viewed as any activity assumed by the family to promote health and prevent disease. Effective execution of health-related functions is based on how the family progresses through developmental tasks and how well the family generates low risk–producing behaviors associated with disease prevention. Choices regarding health-promotion and disease prevention behaviors determine the potential a family possesses to enhance health practices in its members.

Systems theory is used to explain patterns of living among the individuals who make up the family system. In systems theory, behaviors and family members' responses influence the family's pattern and life. Meanings and values are vital components of the family system and provide motivation and energy. Every family has a unique culture, value structure, and history. Values, which are described as the means of interpreting events and information, pass from one generation to the next. Values continually interact with the environment and change slowly over time. The family processes information and energy exchange with the environment through values; the values identify the meaning of the information for the family's use.

Systems have boundaries that separate the family system from the rest of the environment and control the flow of information, energy, and matter between the system and the surrounding environment to maintain the system. This characteristic becomes the family's psychic energy and internal manager, made up of interactions and relationships of members with one another and with those outside the family system. The family is considered a unified whole rather than the sum of its parts—an integrated system of interdependent functions, structures, and relationships that acts as a single whole.

Living systems are open systems. As a living system, the family must be open to a constant exchange of energy and information with the environment; the greater the openness of the family, the greater the changes can be. Change in one part or member of the family results in changes in the family as a whole. Change requires the adaptation of every member of the family as roles and functions take on new meanings. After the family has made the change, it does not revert to its former state; the change is incorporated into the system.

Families are composed of both structural and functional components. **Family structure** refers to the family's roles and relationships, whereas **family function** is the process of continual change in the system as information and energy are exchanged between the family and the environment.

THE FAMILY FROM A DEVELOPMENTAL PERSPECTIVE

Building on Erikson's (1994) theory of psychosocial development, Duvall and Miller (1985) identified stages of the family life cycle and critical **family developmental tasks.** Although Duvall's classification has been criticized for its middle class homogeneity and lack of diversity in family forms, this conceptual model helps to anticipate family events. Knowing family composition, interrelationships, and its particular life cycle helps nurses predict overall **family pattern.** Box 7-2 lists tasks essential to the family's survival and continuity. Duvall maintains that most families complete these basic family tasks. Each family performs these tasks in a unique expression of its personality. The nurse collects data to determine progress toward task attainment. In addition to general tasks of survival and continuity, stages of development exist in this model, with specific tasks related to each stage. Specific tasks are growth responsibilities that arise during the family's developmental stages. Failure in a task leads to societal consequences. For example, child abuse or neglect may result in intervention by police, welfare, health department, or other agencies (Health Teaching box). Life cycle tasks build upon one another. Success at one stage is dependent upon success at an earlier stage. Early failure may lead to developmental difficulties at a later stage of the family life cycle.

As families enter each new developmental stage, transition occurs. Events such as marriage, childbirth, releasing members as adolescents and young adults, and continuing as a couple or single person through the "empty nest" and aging years move families through new stages.

Each new developmental stage requires adaptation with new responsibilities. Concurrently, each developmental stage provides opportunities for families to realize their potential. The nurse anticipates change through analysis of the family's progress through each stage. Each new stage presents opportunities for health promotion and intervention.

Stages of family development, although reflective of traditional nuclear families and extended family networks, also apply to other family configurations. For example, when a couple marries and brings children from a previous marriage to the union, the blended family works toward achieving the developmental tasks of the couple stage along with the

| Box 7-2 | Tasks for Family Survival and Continuity |

- Providing shelter, food, clothing, health care, and similar needs for its members
- Meeting family costs and allocating resources, such as time, space, and facilities, according to each member's needs
- Determining who does what in the support, management, and care of the home and its members
- Ensuring each member's socialization through the internalization of increasingly mature roles in the family and in society
- Establishing ways of interacting, communicating, and expressing affection, aggression, sexuality, and similar interactions within limits acceptable to society
- Bearing (or adopting) and rearing children, then incorporating and releasing family members appropriately
- Relating to school, church, work, and community life and establishing policies for the inclusion of in-laws, relatives, guests, friends, mass media, and others
- Maintaining morale and motivation, rewarding achievement, meeting personal and family crises, setting attainable goals, and developing family loyalties and values

Modified from Duvall, E. M., & Miller, B. (1985). *Marriage and family development* (6th ed.). New York: Harper & Row.

HEALTH TEACHING   Domestic Violence

- Encourage all women to pursue education, employment, and other means of self-actualization to empower themselves and build self-esteem.
- Teach women to control their fertility with contraception and abortion services. This can have an empowering effect and help them avoid unwanted pregnancies that might lead to more abuse.
- Inform adolescents and young women that violence and abuse are not a normal part of intimate relationships. Help them avoid potential abusers, such as men who seem overly jealous, overprotective, or controlling; men who have a history of substance or alcohol abuse; or men who exhibit violent behavior toward animals, objects, or other people.
- Let the woman know that she is free to discuss this issue and encourage her to do so.
- Assure the woman that she is not alone and that many women share this problem. Explore the health conse-

quences of battering for her, her children, and other family-household members.
- Educate the woman about the cycle of violence and explain that without intervention, violent episodes will likely increase in both frequency and severity.
- Provide the woman with referral information for legal, law enforcement, shelter, financial, and counseling services.
- Help the woman develop an escape plan.

The National Coalition Against Domestic Violence provides information to health care providers, a network of shelters, and counseling programs and operates a national hotline: 800-799-SAFE (7233); telecommunications device for the deaf: 800-787-3224; Web site: http://www.ncadv.org/; address and telephone number: P.O. Box 18749, Denver, CO 80218, 303-839-1852.

From Star, W. L., Lommel, L. L., & Shannon, M. T. (1995). *Women's primary health care.* Washington, DC: American Nurses Publishing.

family stages for the children. Both the couple and their children bring values and beliefs from the past that must become integrated into the present union. Childless couples present developmental tasks that are different from those proposed for the couple with children.

Assessment of a family's developmental stage entails the use of guidelines for analyzing progress toward developmental tasks, family growth, and health-promotion needs. The family developmental tasks to use as guidelines during these stages are summarized in **Web Site Resource 7B.**

Family risk factors can be inferred from (1) lifestyle, (2) biological factors, (3) environmental factors, (4) social and psychological dimensions, and (5) the health care system. As outlined in the Frank Thompson case study in Chapter 1, lifestyle habits such as overeating, drug dependency, high sugar or cholesterol intake, and smoking can influence health outcomes. Biological risk factors would include the elements of genetic inheritance, congenital malformation, and mental retardation. To fully explore environmental risk factors that influence family function, the nurse would explore work pressures, stress, anxieties, tensions, and air, noise, or water pollution. Social and psychological dimensions such as crowding, isolation, or rapid and accelerated rates of change are areas to consider when assessing family risk factors. Finally, health care system factors such as overuse, underuse, or inappropriate use of accessibility should be considered in the family assessment of risk.

To reduce risk factors, families focus on influencing the health behaviors of their members. Society glamorizes many hazardous behaviors through advertising and mass media, and negative health consequences may not always be apparent. Families influence their members to weigh the consequences of risk-taking behavior. Awareness of risk factors may prompt families to strive to reduce modifiable risk factors. Healthy behavior, including use of preventive health care services, is a significant area of family responsibility.

THE FAMILY FROM A RISK-FACTOR PERSPECTIVE

Traditionally, epidemiology has used levels and trends of mortality and morbidity rates as indirect evidence of health. Data such as infant mortality rates, stillbirth rates, and leading causes of death have long been used as indicators of the collective health of a community. Healthy family functioning links the stages of the family life cycle and specific risk factors. Epidemiology often describes a disease association in terms of risk. Risks to health can be physiological or psychological. Physiological risks may arise when there is a genetic component, and psychological risks would include those related to low self-image. Risks also arise from the environment, including the physical environment and socioeconomic conditions (AAP, 2003; Becker, Hogue, & Liddle, 2002; Brannigan et al., 2002). **Risk factor theory** considers families a pivotal part of the environment and also an important support system used to decrease health risks for individuals.

To calculate risk estimates, a comparison is made between two groups: one with the risk factor and one without. Frequency of deaths, illnesses, or injuries from a specific cause in a group that has some specific trait or risk factor is compared with another group that does not have this trait, or in the population as a whole, to obtain a risk estimate. Some diseases may occur more frequently in certain families, such as sickle cell anemia in black families and Tay-Sachs disease in Ashkenazi (East European) Jewish families. These high-risk families are identified readily because of the hereditary component of the disease.

Other diseases not linked to heredity are more difficult to attribute to specific causes. The natural history of chronic disease may predispose individual members to greater risk, but the specific cause may be difficult to identify. Leppink (1982) identifies six progressive stages in the natural history of chronic diseases: (1) no-risk stage, (2) risk stage, (3) infiltration stage, (4) critical stage, (5) symptom stage, and (6) overt disease stage. These stages are defined in **Web Site Resource 7C.** These stages continue to hold meaning within the current nursing climate. Epidemiological strategies used to identify strategic points of control will often use similar concepts (Clark, Gironda, & Young, 2003).

Lung cancer follows the natural history of a chronic disease, because individuals may have no risk until they begin smoking tobacco. At some point the dysplasia of the epithelial cells of the bronchi indicates active disease. Intervention at stage three may prevent the disease, because anatomical changes reverse when smoking is discontinued.

Leppink's model applies to diseases such as cervical cancer, cerebrovascular accident, and heart disease. Changing behavior during the first three stages of the disease promotes prevention or reduction of morbidity.

Probabilities of risk change depending on the family's activities in health promotion and disease prevention. Stages of family development are used to classify risk factors. Age-specific developmental stages, along with their associated age-specific health problems, appear in Table 7-1. Periods during which the family is most sensitive to certain risk factors and the time during which health promotion and disease prevention can be enhanced are highlighted in Table 7-1. Many health problems listed correspond to risk behaviors, such as tobacco and alcohol use, faulty nutrition, overuse of medications, fast driving, and relentless pressure to achieve. Habits learned in the family setting help to develop an individual's lifestyle behaviors. At least 7 of the 10 leading causes of death listed in the *Healthy People 2010* report might be reduced substantially if the family improves only five habits: (1) diet, (2) smoking, (3) exercise, (4) alcohol use, and (5) stress. See the *Healthy People 2010* box for selected objectives related to families.

FUNCTIONAL HEALTH PATTERNS: ASSESSMENT OF THE FAMILY

Gordon's 11 functional health patterns (Gordon, 1994) help organize basic assessment information of the family (Denham, 2003; Friedman et al., 2003; Rossi, 2003;

Table 7-1 Family Stage: Specific Risk Factors and Related Health Problems

Stage	Risk Factors	Health Problems
Beginning childbearing	Lack of knowledge about family planning Adolescent marriage Lack of knowledge concerning sexual and marital roles and adjustments Low-birth-weight infant Lack of prenatal care Inadequate nutrition Poor eating habits Smoking, alcohol, and drug abuse Unmarried status First pregnancy before age 16 or after age 35 History of hypertension and infections during pregnancy Rubella, syphilis, gonorrhea, and AIDS Genetic factors Low socioeconomic and educational levels Lack of safety in the home	Premature baby in family Birth defects Birth injuries Accidents SIDS Respiratory distress syndrome Sterility Pelvic inflammatory disease Fetal alcohol syndrome Mental retardation Child abuse Injuries Birth defects Underweight or overweight
Family with school-aged children	Working parents with inappropriate use of resources for child care Poverty Abuse or neglect of children Generational pattern of using social agencies as a way of life Multiple, closely spaced children Low family self-esteem Children used as scapegoats for parental frustration Repeated infections, accidents, or hospitalizations Parents immature, dependent, and unable to handle responsibility Unrecognized or unattended health problems Strong beliefs about physical punishment Toxic substances unguarded in the home Poor nutrition	Behavior disturbances Speech and vision problems Communicable diseases Dental caries School problems Learning disabilities Cancer Injuries Chronic diseases Homicide Violence
Family with adolescents	Racial and ethnic family origin Lifestyle and behavior patterns leading to chronic disease Lack of problem-solving skills Family values of aggressiveness and competition Family values rigid and inflexible Daredevil risk-taking attitudes Denial behavior Conflicts between parents and children Pressure to live up to family expectations	Violent deaths and injuries Alcohol and drug abuse Unwanted pregnancies Sexually transmitted diseases Suicide Depression
Family with middle-aged adults	Hypertension Smoking High cholesterol levels Physical inactivity Genetic predisposition Use of oral contraceptives Sex, race, and other hereditary factors Geographical area, age, and occupational deficiencies Habits (i.e., diet with low fiber, pickling, charcoal use, and broiling) Alcohol abuse Social class Residence	Cardiovascular disease, principally coronary artery disease and cerebrovascular accident (stroke) Diabetes Overweight Cancer Accidents Homicide Suicide Abnormal fetus Mental illness Periodontal disease and loss of teeth Depression

Continued

Table 7-1 Family Stage: Specific Risk Factors and Related Health Problems *cont'd*

Stage	Risk Factors	Health Problems
Family with older adults	Age Drug interactions Metabolic disorders Pituitary malfunctions Cushing's syndrome Hypercalcemia Chronic illness Retirement Loss of spouse Reduced income Poor nutrition Lack of exercise Past environments and lifestyle Lack of preparation for death	Mental confusion Reduced vision Hearing impairment Hypertension Acute illness Infectious disease Influenza Pneumonia Injuries such as burns and falls Depression Chronic disease Elder abuse Death without dignity

Modified from U.S. Department of Health and Human Services. (2000). *Healthy people 2010*. Washington, DC: U.S. Government Printing Office. *AIDS*, acquired immunodeficiency syndrome; *SIDS*, sudden infant death syndrome.

Healthy People 2010
Selected Examples of National Health-Promotion and Disease Prevention Objectives for Families

- 1-4. Increase the proportion of people who have a specific source of ongoing care.
- 19-2. Reduce the proportion of adults who are obese.
- 19-3c. Reduce the proportion of children and adolescents who are overweight or obese.
- 26-10a. Increase the proportion of adolescents not using alcohol or any illicit drugs during the previous 30 days.
- 26-10c. Reduce the proportion of adults using any illicit drug during the previous 30 days.
- 26-11c. Reduce the proportion of adults engaging in binge drinking of alcoholic beverages during the previous month.

Wertlieb, 2003). The structure within the patterns represents a standardized format to use with a systems approach to family assessment of developmental stages and risk factor identification. Information obtained from the 11 functional patterns is judged against family developmental norms and age-specific risk factors. Dysfunctional patterns within a family are explored to determine causal factors and corresponding details in one or more of the other interdependent patterns (see Chapter 6).

Problems in functional patterns are identified as dysfunctional health patterns, not diseases. For example, a potential dysfunction is predicted when risk factors are present. Developmental risk and a risk of change toward a less functional health pattern are types of risk states. If risk factors are present, then a family is said to be susceptible to or at risk for a problem (see Table 7-1).

Gordon (1994) interprets a risk state as a potential problem, which indicates the presence of factors that predispose a family to a dysfunctional health pattern. To formulate a nursing diagnosis, the nurse names the problem and causative factor. Probable causes may be logically connected to the problem. Probable causes also may precede or occur concurrently with the problem. The nurse identifies causal factors to plan care. Intervention is directed toward causal factors that can be modified to influence a positive change. Risk factors indicate a potential problem, but the problem's origin may be nonspecific. Intervention in this case is directed toward reducing risk factors.

Family history is explored beginning with the health perception–health management pattern. Exploring issues within this pattern first provides an overview to help locate where problems exist in other patterns and to determine which ones may require more thorough assessment. Additionally, this pattern starts the history taking from the family's perspective and helps the family define the situation. The roles-relationships pattern defines the family structure and function. Lifestyle indicators are assessed through the remaining nine patterns.

Health Perception–Health Management Pattern

The health perception–health management pattern identifies characteristics of the family's general health perceptions and management and preventive practices. Pratt (1976) identified six characteristics of healthy families: (1) members facilitate an interaction process, (2) members enhance individual development, (3) role relationships are structured effectively, (4) members actively attempt to cope with problems, (5) members promote healthy home environments and lifestyles, and (6) members establish regular links with the broader community.

Health practices vary from family to family. Each family identifies and performs health-maintenance activities based on beliefs about health. What the family believes is feasible, as demonstrated in their lifestyle practices, also determines health practices. Nurses facilitate health within the family by assisting members to be conscious of their health beliefs, behaviors, and status. The nurse promotes the refinement of family responses to the individuals within the family, as well as to the world surrounding the family (Newman, 2002).

Exploration during the assessment includes the following areas:

- What is the family's philosophy of health? Does each family member hold similar beliefs? Do family members practice what they believe?
- In what behaviors or lifestyle practices, such as smoking, alcohol, and drug abuse, does the family engage?
- What chronic disease risk behaviors are exhibited within the family?
- Does the family engage in health-related behaviors, such as eating three meals a day at regular times, eating breakfast every day, exercising a minimum of 2 or 3 days a week, sleeping 7 to 8 hours each night, and abstaining from smoking?
- Are risk factors present for infections, such as lack of immunization, lack of knowledge of transmittable diseases, and poor personal hygiene?
- Are risk factors for bodily injury, accidents, or substance abuse present in the home?
- Are chemicals in the home within easy reach of children?
- Do elderly members know what medications they are taking and the reasons for using them?
- Are there medications in the home that are not being used and should be discarded?
- Is nutrition sufficient to maintain adequate energy levels?
- Are any unattended health problems present?
- Is there a history of repeated infections and hospitalization?
- Is safety lacking in the home?
- Is the home understimulating or overstimulating?
- Where does the family go for health and illness care?
- Is the family engaged in a dental program?
- How does the family describe previous experiences with nurses and other health care professionals?

Environment also influences family health and well-being. The home is considered the family's natural environment with the additional environments of neighborhood and community.

Exploration during the assessment of the home environment includes the following areas:

- What type of dwelling is it (condominium, single dwelling, low-income apartment, or temporary shelter)?
- Does the family own or rent their housing?
- Are the interior and exterior of the home in good or poor repair (glass, trash, broken stairs, peeling paint, inadequate insulation, inadequate lighting on stairs, or broken fixtures)?
- Are the number and type of rooms adequate for the size of the family?

- Is there adequate furniture to meet the needs of the family (enough chairs, beds, and a kitchen table)?
- Is the dwelling warm in winter and cool in summer?
- Is the lighting adequate for reading, sewing, and other activities?
- Is there an adequate water supply? Is it fluoridated or polluted?
- Is there a telephone? Are emergency numbers listed?
- Does the kitchen have safe sanitation facilities and adequate refrigeration?
- Does the bathroom have adequate sanitation facilities, water supply, toilet, and towels and soap?
- Are the sleeping arrangements adequate for family members, considering age, gender, relationships, and spatial needs?
- Are there smoke detectors and an escape route and plan inside the home?
- Are first-aid directions posted for poisons, burns, lacerations, and other first aid needs?
- Are signs of vermin present inside or outside the home?
- What are the family's impressions about their home? Do they consider the living space adequate for privacy, their own interests, and status?

Areas to explore for neighborhood assessment are as follows:
- Are dwellings and streets maintained or deteriorated?
- How and when is the garbage collected?
- What is the incidence of violent crime, burglaries, and auto accidents?
- What kinds of industry are nearby and do they produce air pollution or toxic waste?
- What are the social class and ethnic characteristics of the neighborhood?
- What are the occupations and interests of the families in the neighborhood?
- What is the population density?
- Is public transportation available? Is it used?

Exploration during assessment of the community includes the following areas:
- Are resources, such as schools, church, transportation, shopping, and recreational facilities, available for the family's use?
- How accessible are the health facilities, such as physician's office, clinic, hospital, gym, swimming pool, natural food store, and weight-reduction clinic?

By driving or walking around the area, the nurse can obtain neighborhood and community data. Other sources of information include the family, health professionals, teachers, business people, and others who work in the area. Official resources, such as the reports from the U.S. Census Department (*http://www.census.gov/*) or statistics from the city or state health departments and libraries, are also helpful in describing a neighborhood and community.

Nutritional-Metabolic Pattern

The nutritional-metabolic pattern depicts characteristics of the family's typical food and fluid consumption. Included are growth and development patterns, pregnancy-related nutritional patterns, and the family's eating patterns. Dietary habits are learned within the context of the family and involve behavioral patterns central to daily life. A useful way to determine a family's pattern of food and fluid intake is to have them keep a diary of what they eat and drink for a week. Distinctions should be made between family meals and additional consumption by individual members.

Exploration during nutrition pattern assessment includes the following areas:

- Does the family eat together?
- Is food used as a reward or punishment?
- Are there adequate storage and refrigeration?
- Who purchases the food?
- Who prepares the food?
- What kinds of foods are typically consumed?

Elimination Pattern

The elimination pattern describes characteristics of regularity and control of the family's excretory functions. Bowel and bladder function and environmental factors such as waste disposal in the home, neighborhood, and community that influence family life are considered in this pattern.

Questions are phrased according to the age-specific developmental stage of the family. For example, in determining whether there is a problem in the preschool stage, it would be appropriate to ask whether the child is being toilet trained. In families with adolescents, the nurse may ask how often individuals have bowel movements and whether there have been any changes from usual patterns. The nurse may ask elderly members whether they have any problems with constipation.

Activity-Exercise Pattern

The activity-exercise pattern represents characteristics of the family that require energy expenditure. Daily activities, exercise, and leisure activities are reviewed. Families establish the setting for individual members to be physically active, sedentary, or apathetic toward physical activity.

Exploration during assessment of this pattern includes the following areas:

- Does the family believe regular exercise and physical fitness are necessary for good health?
- What types of daily activities include physical exercise and who does what with whom?
- What does the family do to have fun (Figure 7-1)?

Sleep-Rest Pattern

Rest habits characterize the sleep-rest pattern. Without the restorative function of sleep, individuals exhibit decreased performance, bad temper, and reliance on substances, such as alcohol or other chemicals, to induce sleep. Regular, sufficient sleep patterns are linked to better mental status. Most families have sleeping patterns, although in some families these patterns may not be readily apparent. It is impor-

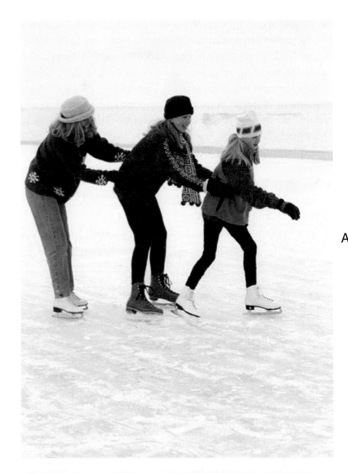

A

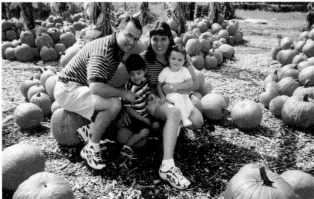

B

Figure 7-1   Family outings can be **A,** adventurous and exciting or **B,** leisurely and restful.

tant to elicit the data about sleep and rest from the family's perspective.

Assessment of the sleep-rest pattern includes the following:

- What are the usual sleeping habits of the family?
- Are they suitable to age and health status?
- Are regular hours established for sleeping?
- Who decides when children go to sleep?
- Do family members take naps or have other regular means of resting or relaxing?

- Does the family rise early and go to bed early or rise late and go to bed late?
- Do all family members have the same general sleep-rest pattern?
- Is there a family member with sleep disruption?

Cognitive-Perceptual Pattern

The cognitive-perceptual pattern identifies characteristics of language, cognitive skills, and perception that influence desired or required family activities. Specifically, this pattern concerns how families make decisions, how concrete or abstract the thought processes are, and whether decisions focus on present or future issues. Decision making in the family is associated with power in family functioning. Highly educated families have greater repertoires for problem solving. Power and ability to solve problems are linked to leadership; the family's leader must be acknowledged if nursing interventions are to be implemented.

Cognitive-perceptual pattern assessment includes the following:
- How does the family usually make decisions about health promotion and disease prevention?
- Do all members contribute to the decision-making process, or is one person responsible for all decisions?
- How knowledgeable is the family about risk factors and developmental milestones?
- How are choices made regarding lifestyle? Are these choices made based on correct information?
- Do family members know whether their health behavior is constructive or destructive?
- Are signs and symptoms of deteriorating health recognized?
- When medical attention is necessary, is there a delay from time of onset to time of treatment? If so, how long is it?
- Are over-the-counter medications taken or home remedies used?

Self-Perception–Self-Concept Pattern

The self-perception–self-concept pattern identifies characteristics that describe the family's self-worth and feeling states. Rapport between the family members and the nurse facilitates disclosure. Families have perceptions and concepts about their image, their status in the community, and their competencies as a family unit. Families manifest these perceptions through shared aspirations, values, expectations, fears, successes, and failures. Relationships in families determine the amount of sharing that occurs. Situations affecting one member influence perceptions of the entire family group. How each member describes the family often gives clues to the family self-concept.

Exploration during assessment includes the following:
- What makes this family different from others?
- What special assets does each member contribute to the family?
- What changes would each member like to see occur in the family?

- What kinds of feelings do family members have for each other?
- Describe the general tone of feelings in the family. Is the tone indifferent, secretive, angry, or open?
- How does the family think it assimilates into the neighborhood?
- Does the family believe it is operating at its maximal potential?
- How does the family handle crisis situations?
- How does the family experience changes in the way it feels about itself?
- How does the family describe the events that led to a change?

Roles-Relationships Pattern

This pattern identifies characteristics of family roles and relationships. Both structural and functional aspects of the family are assessed.

Structural aspects of families include each member's name, age, sex, education, occupation, and role in the family. Traditionally, families have been described as nuclear and extended. The traditional nuclear family consists of husband, wife, and children, with an extended family that would include aunts, uncles, cousins, and grandparents. When families consist of other nontraditional configurations, they are often referred to as the *family of choice*. Exploration of the family's origin and genetic heritage complete family identification data collection. Cultural practices in the home may or may not reflect the family's genetic heritage; therefore, it is important to explore cultural and ethnic practices. Traditional nuclear family structure has been influenced by societal changes, such as the women's movement, employment of mothers, divorce, and remarriage. Since the 1990 census was gathered, the number of nontraditional family households increased by 11%. The number of nontraditional households, on the other hand, rose faster, with a 23% increase (Simmons & O'Neill, 2001; U.S. Census Bureau, 2000). These changes indicate the need to recognize the needs of families with nontraditional structures, such as those listed in Table 7-2. Family structures influence child-rearing and individual development and pose a challenge to the nurse in health promotion and disease prevention.

Allender and Spradley (2001) have classified **divergent family structures** in three types that are of particular relevance to the nurse. The first type is the growing number of adolescent unwed mothers whose developmental needs and lack of parenting skills pose particular challenges for the nurse (Connelly, 1998). The second type refers to couples who, after widowhood or divorce, have remarried and merged two families. Merged families require considerable adjustment to roles, tasks, communication patterns, and relationships. The third type is made up of older couples or older individuals, usually women who live alone. People in this third group often need assistance adjusting to functions and developmental tasks necessary to experience aging in a positive way (Johansson, 2002).

Table **7-2** Variety of Family Structures

Configuration	Positions in Family
Single parent (separated, divorced, or widowed)	Mother or father Son(s), daughter(s)
Unmarried single parent (never married)	Mother or father Son(s), daughter(s)
Unmarried couple	Two adults
Unmarried parents	Mother and father Son(s), daughter(s)
Commune family	Mothers and fathers Shared son(s), daughter(s)
Stepparents	Mother and father Son(s), daughter(s) from previous marriages
Adoptive parents	Mother and father Adopted son(s), daughter(s)

CASE STUDY

Mark and Jennifer

Mark and Jennifer had been married for over 10 years. They both had children from a previous marriage. Jennifer's children, Maureen and Catherine, lived with Mark and Jennifer. The girls were 7 and 9 years old. Mark's children, Jacob and Benjamin, lived with their mother in another city. Mark's children were ages 10 and 12, respectively. The boys lived with Mark and Jennifer for extended periods during the summer and holidays. During one summer visit, Jacob and Benjamin reported to their father that their mother, Deborah, was abusing alcohol and drugs. Deborah often left the two boys alone for the weekend. During these times, their mother was unavailable by telephone and they did not know where she was. When confronted with these reports, Deborah denied everything.

During the boys' extended visit with Mark and Jennifer when they reported Deborah's abnormal behavior, Deborah was hospitalized with a documented cocaine overdose. Mark returned to court to seek custody and lost. Deborah relocated even farther from Mark and Jennifer. Despite persistent efforts, Mark was unable to maintain the same amount of visitation time after this incident.

Reflective Questions
1. How do you think this situation reflects motherhood status?
2. Do you think the concept of the biological family restricted the court's view of the issues facing this family?

Divorce and remarriage involve a complex transition that requires the disintegration of one family structure and organization of another. Developmental levels of the children, their individual temperaments, and the quality of their environmental support all contribute to the family response (Borell, 2003). Addressing the needs of the children may be difficult for the parents, who are at the same time experiencing an adjustment to each other. How parents cope during the situational crisis, as well as after the divorce, is a significant variable in long-term individual and family adjustment. See the Case Study for presentation of a stepfamily situation.

In a study conducted by Rogers, investigators examined factors related to resilience in over 2000 adolescents who belonged to intact, blended, and divorced single-parent families. The authors discussed the merits of using a resilience framework to explore factors associated with family well-being. Findings demonstrated that resilience within the family may be a way to explore family well-being that will allow for different types of family structures (Rogers, 1970). **Family resilience** generally arises from three domains: family belief systems, organizational patterns, and communication–problem solving. This framework may be useful to promote strategies for prevention efforts aimed at strengthening families as they face life challenges (Rogers, 1970; Walsh, 2003).

Using resilience as a framework may help to address the marginalization of families that Jones (2003) describes. Families with structures that are different from the dominant nuclear-based family paradigm are generally left with little support from society. Society tends to support biological families with laws and policies that are less applicable to the more complex nonnuclear family. Jones suggests that values that stem from moral responsibility and bonding are better suited to the current diversity of family types than methods traditionally used to assess biologically structured nuclear families.

Family organization influences performance of health-promotion and disease prevention functions. For example, a single parent without an extended family network may be in need of community resources to help raise the children. A two-parent family living near its extended family may have all the support needed to raise children, but members may need to become aware of growth and developmental stages and immunization schedules.

Individuals may experience a variety of family structures in one lifetime. A person may be part of a nuclear family as an infant, a single-parent family after the parents are divorced, a stepparent family when the mother or father remarries, and an unmarried couple family when the person is one of two adults who share a household. The person brings the values and beliefs about disease prevention and health promotion that were practiced in previous unions to each new family configuration. Divergent values may result in conflicting expectations unless the new union forms a set of integrated values and beliefs. The current trend away from the nuclear family with extended family may influence the general direction of the health care system and the strategies used to promote health with other family configurations.

Certain health-promotion issues are of particular concern to the nurse while assessing family health promotion and disease prevention. Violence is a health problem that threatens the integrity of families. Family violence includes child abuse, spouse abuse, and elder abuse, with women being victimized more often during pregnancy. Health promotion and violence prevention requires a complex set of skills. Nurses use approaches to reduce violence-related injuries and deaths by acquiring the role of advocate and helping to eliminate victim blaming (Gance-Cleveland, 2001; Rugala & Isaacs, 2002) (Research Highlights box).

---

research highlights

Domestic Violence: Resilience in Sheltered Battered Women

Some women respond with less severe outcomes than others to physical and psychological distress related to battering situations. Prevalence of battering is estimated to be 20% to 40% in the general population. The concept of resilience refers to the individual's ability to adapt to and restore equilibrium after an overwhelming event.

This study used a convenience sample of 50 women residing in battered women's shelters. Psychological distress was measured using a symptom checklist, and the frequency of abuse was determined using a scale with established construct validity. Resilience was measured using a 25-item scale.

All participants had been abused by their spouse or partner. Eighty-two percent of the women had children. Only 8% of the participants reported no severe assaults, and 70% reported 10 or more severe assaults. Psychological distress was highly correlated with the frequency and severity of battering the women had experienced. Sheltered battered women in this study reported higher levels of resilience than participants in other studies that measured resilience in caregivers of Alzheimer's patients, female graduate students, first-time mothers during the postpartum period, and public housing residents.

Nurses may use this study to determine how to organize thoughts, actions, and feelings toward clients who have been battered. By focusing on resilience strategies, nurses build upon survival strategies and strengths of the battered women.

Data from Humphreys, J. (2003). Resilience in sheltered battered women. *Issues in Mental Health Nursing, 24*(2), 137-152.

Exploration to assess families for health promotion and violence prevention includes the following:
- What formal positions and roles does each of the family members fulfill?
- Are fulfilled roles acceptable and consistent with the family's expectations?
- What kind of flexibility in roles takes place when needed?
- What informal roles exist? Who plays informal roles and with what consistency? What purpose do the informal roles serve?
- Who were the role models for the couples or single people as parents?
- Who were the role models for marital partners and what were their characteristics?
- How does the family manage daily living? How are the household tasks divided?
- How are problems handled? How are problems with children handled?
- Who is employed outside the home?
- Who takes care of the children when both parents are employed outside the home?
- How does the family care for its ill members? Its elderly members?
- Are behaviors appropriate for family stages of development?
- Is decision making allocated to the appropriate members?
- Does the family respond appropriately to its members' developmental needs?
- Is there fair distribution of tasks among family members?
- Is the family's emotional climate conducive to growth and development?

Genogram

Drawing a **genogram,** or family diagram, views the family from identification data that depicts each member of the family with connections between the generations. This useful technique gathers data on at least three generations, including the current one, their parents, grandparents, aunts, uncles, and their children. The family genogram extends in order to explore clues leading to the family history of health problems. Figure 7-2 depicts the accepted genogram symbols and Figure 7-3 depicts a sample genogram of the Jeddi family. This genogram shows a variety of family structures, including family changes resulting from marriage, divorce, death, and childbearing. This type of information highlights a family's health patterns and enables the nurse to provide related anticipatory health guidance, such as strategies to prevent coronary artery disease.

Ecomap

The **ecomap,** which is similar to the genogram, documents the family's organizational patterns with visual clarity. A genogram is constructed for a family or household. Preceded by the family name, the genogram is placed in a circle in the center of the page. Outside the circle, smaller circles are

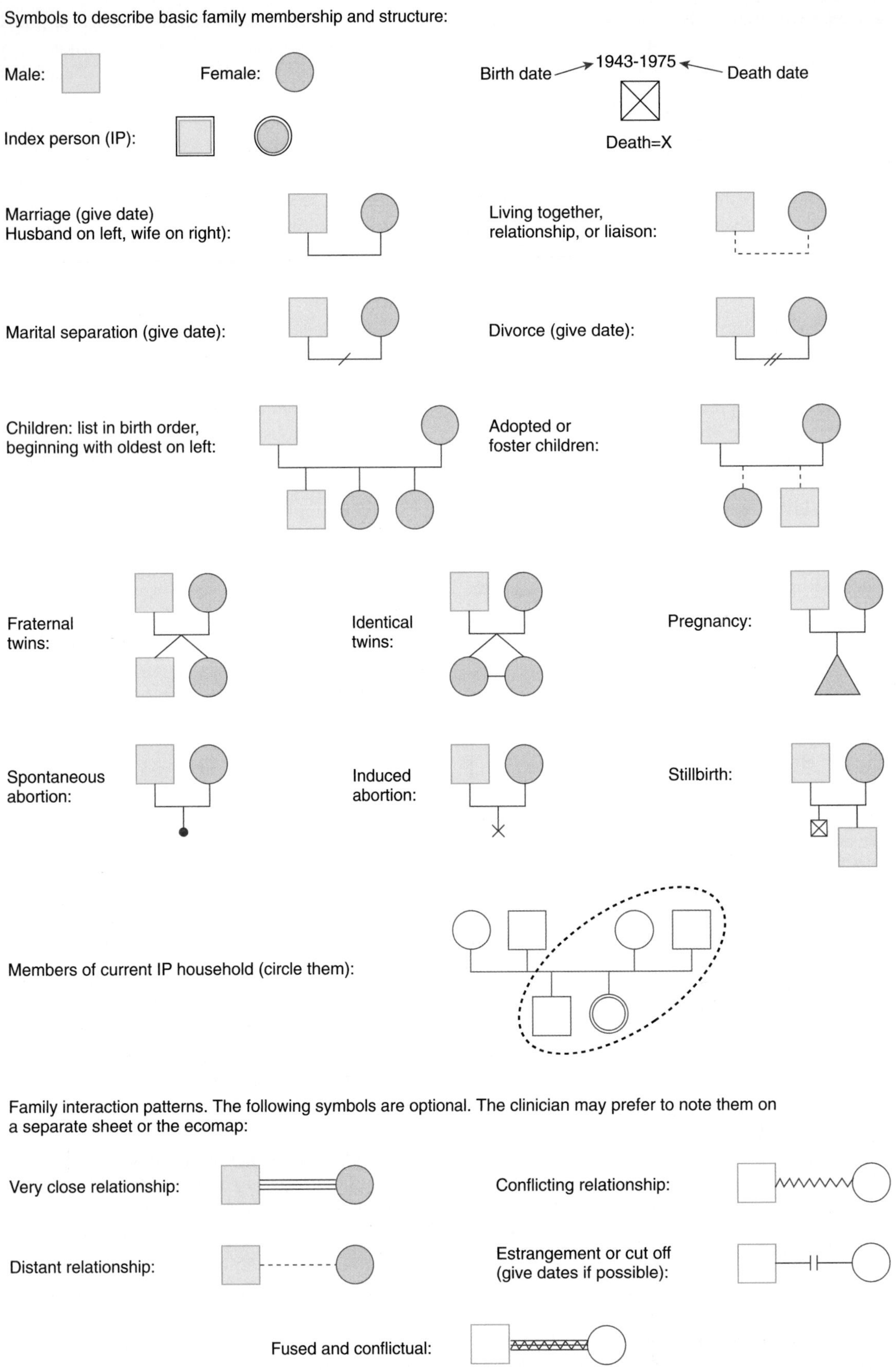

Figure 7-2 Genogram symbols. (Modified from McGoldrick, M., & Gerson, R. [1985]. *Genograms in family assessment.* New York: Norton.)

Date _____ Completed by _____

Family name _____ Jeddi Family _____

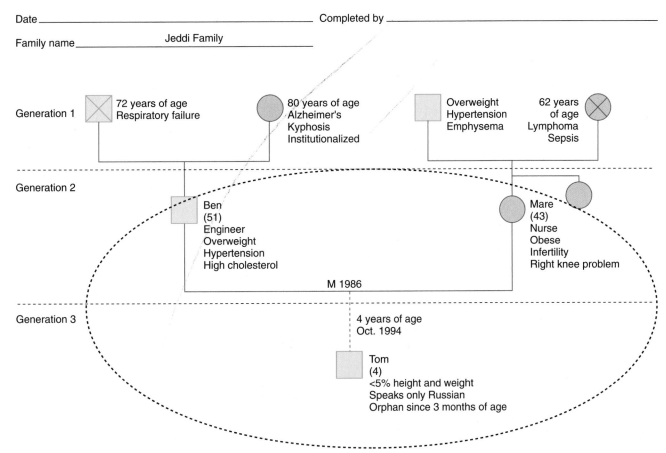

Figure 7-3   Genogram of the Jeddi family. (From Stanhope, M., & Lancaster, J. [2004]. *Community and public health nursing* [6th ed.]. St. Louis: Mosby.)

drawn and labeled with the names of significant people, agencies, and institutions in the family's social environment. Lines are drawn from the family-household to each circle. Straight lines indicate strong connections; a wider line indicates a strong relationship. Dotted lines reflect fragile or tenuous connections. Slashed lines signify stressful relationships. Arrows can be drawn parallel to the lines to indicate the flow of energy or resources. Figure 7-4 shows an ecomap for the Jeddi family.

Sexuality-Reproductive Pattern

Sexuality is the expression of sexual identity. The sexuality-reproductive pattern describes "patterns of satisfaction or dissatisfaction with sexuality" (Gordon, 1994, p. 91), including behavioral patterns of reproduction. This pattern also includes perceptions of satisfaction or disturbances in sexuality, sexual relationships, reproduction, and developmental changes throughout the life span, such as menopause (Hot Topics box). The sexuality-reproductive pattern "includes a couple's level of satisfaction with their sexual relationship, any problems they perceive, how the problems are managed, and the results of actions taken to resolve the problems. Sexual identity develops during childhood; therefore, it is important to know what information

about sexual subjects is taught to the children in the family" (Gordon, 1994, p. 92).

Topics to explore during the assessment include the following areas:

- Is the couple's sexual behavior mutually satisfying?
- Is the couple able to communicate needs to each other?
- Is there a sense of commitment, love, obligation, responsibility, and care for each other?
- Is the couple realistic in their expectations of marriage and parenthood and about their relationship as lovers?
- Are birth control measures used?
- Is the type of contraceptive used satisfactory to both partners?

If a complete pregnancy history is warranted, that information is collected, including sexual practices and partners, number and ages of children, number and outcome of pregnancies, and birth control methods in use. The nurse also observes the level of comfort the adults have when the discussion involves their own sexuality, or if the adult seems uninformed when discussing sexual subjects with their children. Particularly important is the nurse's responsibility to provide appropriate health assessment and information considering the variety of sexual practices within heterosexual,

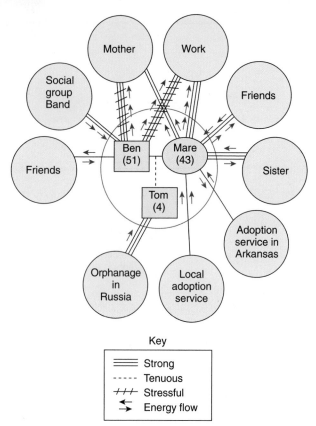

Key

═══	Strong
-----	Tenuous
+++	Stressful
⇆	Energy flow

Figure 7-4   Ecomap of the Jeddi family. (From Stanhope, M., & Lancaster, J. [2004]. *Community and public health nursing* [6th ed.]. St. Louis: Mosby.)

homosexual, and bisexual relationships, with one or more partners (Giami, 2002).

Coping–Stress Tolerance Pattern

The coping–stress tolerance pattern helps to depict the family's adaptation to both internal and external pressures.

Energy for this adjustment develops from within the family. On a day-to-day basis family members generate the energy necessary to face evolving need. Society continually compels families to adapt to new situations. Families face these external demands as they move from stage to stage in their development. Survival and growth are dependent upon this coping mechanism. The family's ability to cope with the demands of everyday living determines its level of success. Family relationships may support coping or lead to stress. Life events such as divorce, moving, or developmental stages of the life cycle and economic hardships, such as loss of a job, are stressful and the strategies a family uses to cope with these stressors help to depict this pattern.

Exploration for assessment of coping and stress tolerance includes the following:

- How does the family cope with stressful life events?
- What strengths does the family have and use to counterbalance the stresses?
- How does the family make appraisals of the situations and are they realistic?
- Is the family able to make decisions based on an objective appraisal of the situation?
- Describe the family's resources? How do family members use knowledge or links to family networks or community resources?
- What kinds of dysfunctional adaptive strategies are used, such as violence?

Values-Beliefs Pattern

The values-beliefs pattern characterizes the family's attitudes and how behavior is affected. Assessment, diagnosis, and intervention are based on these attitudes. Assessment of this pattern enhances the interpretation of family behavior.

Exploration of values and beliefs includes the following:

HOTtopics — TELEVISION, AGGRESSIVE BEHAVIOR, SEXUALITY, AND OBESITY

Television is one of the most pervasive influences in American society. During formative stages of development, children and adolescents view thousands of hours of television. This sedentary activity involves viewing scenes that depict violence and sexual relationships that are rapid, casual, and frequent. These scenes often convey status without depicting responsibility or consequences of actions. Although more research is needed, evidence shows that mass media influences aggressive behavior as well as beliefs about sexual behavior. In addition, as time viewing television programs increases, physical activity levels decrease.

In a study of more than 2000 children, the relationship between body mass index (BMI) and television habits were explored. Children who were identified as overweight or obese generally viewed more television than those with normal BMI (Wake, Hesketh, & Waters, 2003).

The American Academy of Pediatrics (AAP) has described the negative health effects of television viewing on children

and adolescents. Among these effects are aggressive behavior, substance use, sexual activity, obesity, poor body image, and worse school performance. The AAP Committee on Public Education recommends that health professionals remain informed about these issues and use the resources available from AAP, such as the AAP Media Matters campaign and Media History Form. Strategies to ensure appropriate entertainment options should be available in agency waiting rooms and play rooms (AAP, 2001).

In addition to the role that television plays with regard to obesity, sedentary activity has been linked to earlier age of menarche. Body fat mass may play a role in accelerating puberty; however, it is clear that prepubertal activity and nutrition contribute to sexual maturation at some level (Wu, Mendola, & Buck, 2002).

- What are the values and beliefs held by the family? How flexible are rules? Are the rules aggressive, competitive, or rigid?
- Describe the cultural or ethnic group that the family identifies with. What family practices are consistent with the norms of that ethnic group? How are the practices inconsistent with these norms?
- What are the family's traditions and practices?
- How do the significant cultural beliefs affect health or illness?
- Describe the role that religion plays in the family on a regular basis and during times of stress. How does the family rely on religious practices?
- How does the family perceive its competency during crisis?
- What are the family goals and do members perceive that they are attaining these goals?
- Are value conflicts evident within the family?
- How do identified family values affect the health status of the family?

Data collected in the 11 functional patterns reveal ideas about the family's health-promotion and disease prevention practices. Risks to healthy family functioning may be identified in each pattern. Some risk factors may be found in more than one area. For example, passive smoke from one family member's cigarettes may be identified as an environmental risk factor in the home. However, the family's reaction to passive smoking determines their perceived susceptibility, their perceived severity of the problem, and whether they will make a change in the environment to promote family health. The pattern indicates high risk if chronic obstructive lung disease is found in the family history, if many adult members of the family smoke, or if research findings are ignored. In this situation, several other pattern areas support the finding. The nurse determines each risk behavior along with its effects on the others.

ANALYSIS AND NURSING DIAGNOSIS
Analyzing Data

After completing the data collection, the nurse and the family analyze it. Several approaches are used to analyze health data, including systems theory, developmental theory, and risk-estimate theory.

From a systems approach, families are categorized as open or closed, with permeable or rigid boundaries. The systems approach determines both the structural and functional components of the family as a system. The 11 functional patterns organize baseline assessment data **(Web Site Resource 7D).**

Developmental theory approaches families from the perspective of tasks and progression through cycles. The nurse analyzes data to identify the stages of the family life cycle and the tasks the family must accomplish to function successfully. Family developmental needs are determined, considering the wide variety of family structures and functions in society. Analysis of structures other than the nuclear family is indicated based on current population trends, even though most models are based on couples and children (Denham, 2003; Wertlieb, 2003).

Stages of family development guide the analysis of the baseline data. If gaps are noted, missing data or conflicting information is obtained and clarified.

Couple Family

The first stage of family development may or may not begin with marriage. Legal marriage may not be the basis of the relationship; nonetheless, the adults may define themselves as a family unit. Married or not, two individuals move from their family of orientation to an unfamiliar couple relationship. Adaptation to the role expectations of the partner is a developmental task for each individual. One family developmental task is to establish a mutually satisfying adult relationship that converges with the kinship network. Adjustment for the couple includes learning how to mesh two personalities, two life histories, and two aspirations of growth. Decisions in this stage resolve whether both partners work, how they manage money, where they live, how they cope with other family members, and whether to bear children. Other decisions, consciously or unconsciously made, include sharing the household tasks of cooking, washing, cleaning, and shopping.

The developmental task of integrating health practices and habits into the couple's lifestyle requires consideration during analysis. Health behavior constitutes particular actions taken toward promotion of health and prevention of disease. Examples of health-promotion and disease prevention activities that might be considered include participating in well-balanced programs of rest, exercise, and balanced diet, attending smoking-cessation classes, wearing seat belts, and directing activities toward the attainment of self-actualization. Each individual brings values and beliefs to the relationship. Practices from the family of origin and values from personal experiences combine to form the adult beliefs of the individual.

Achieving a mutually satisfying relationship depends on how the couple manages conflicts and differences. When strategies are congruent with each individual's values, the couple adjusts. If the strategies used are quite different, problem solving tends to be less effective.

The decision to adopt or give birth to a child commits the couple to more long-term responsibilities. Those responsibilities focus the family's development and primary health needs. To analyze learning needs of the pregnant couple, the nurse considers aspects of the couple's decision and motivations involved with the pregnancy. With single-parent families becoming increasingly common through divorce, death, adoption, or the choice to have a child out of wedlock, the data analysis should consider the needs of these family structures (Denham, 2003; Simmons & O'Neill, 2001; U.S. Census Bureau, 2000; Wertlieb, 2003).

Attitudes and practices in society regarding sexuality have influenced the incidence of sexually transmitted diseases such as genital herpes, gonorrhea, and syphilis. Acquired immunodeficiency syndrome (AIDS), the most recent sexually transmitted disease, was first described in 1981. AIDS poses a threat to the family and society, as well as to the affected individual. Human immunodeficiency virus (HIV) is transmitted through heterosexual, homosexual, or oral sexual intercourse and through direct contact with infected blood, shared needles during intravenous drug use, and perinatal transfer from infected mothers to their infants. Prevention of HIV transmission requires abstinence and modification of relevant behaviors.

Risk factors associated with sexuality include lack of knowledge about safe sexual practices, the reproductive system, and personal hygiene; lack of prenatal care; pregnancy before age 16; pregnancy after age 35; a history of hypertension or infection during pregnancy; and unplanned or unwanted pregnancy.

Risk factors for premature pregnancies and unsatisfying marriage consist of ignorance about, or values regarding, family planning; adolescence; and knowledge deficit concerning sexuality and role adjustment. In unplanned adolescent pregnancies, parents put their developing child at risk. Lack of knowledge about prenatal care, birthing, and child-rearing practices compounds risks for both the mother and the child. Parents who are unable to perform the parenting role risk an unsatisfying relationship and inappropriate developmental growth for this beginning stage of the family life cycle.

If the couple decides to remain childless, learning needs include information about contraception.

Childbearing Family

Birth or adoption of a child begins a new family unit. Family members adjust to new roles as the unit expands in function and responsibility. The parents' history as a dyad and their experiences in other groups, particularly their families of origin, influence the development of the triad (Multicultural Awareness box).

Accommodating the new member into the group disrupts family equilibrium. As a group, the three individuals explore ways to meet each others' needs, to minimize differences, and to work together. First-time parents often feel a lack of emotional support during the first several months of parenthood. Without a family network or friends, the first days after the birth or adoption proceed with particular difficulty. Needs analysis facilitates new parenting skills. Parents may care for the child proficiently, but they may need assistance to grow in the parenting role. If the mother was employed outside the home, she may encounter difficulty with the routines of baby care and being in the house all day. Anxiety about the adequacy of one income may cause the father to increase his workload. Exhaustion for both parents from working full time and providing child care is common. Single parents, usually mothers, carry these same burdens alone. Emotional support for each other may be limited, particularly if one of the individuals has not found satisfaction in parenthood. The family of origin or other support system, such as self-help groups, neighbors, or friends, assists the family members as they struggle to adapt

MULTICULTURAL AWARENESS

Preconception Care

Preconception care is a significant health-promotion opportunity for the whole family. The importance of this care has been recognized by *Healthy People 2010*, the Institute of Medicine, and the Public Health Services Expert Panel on the Content of Prenatal Care.

One important area of preconception care is evaluating a couple's genetic history as documented on the standard family genogram. Further evaluation should be considered for couples who are related outside marriage or who have ethnic backgrounds such as Mediterranean, black, or Ashkenazi Jew, and for women older than 35 years of age or younger than 16 years of age who have preexisting medical conditions. Couples who have family histories of any of the following health problems should be referred for further genetic testing and counseling: cystic fibrosis, hemophilia, phenylketonuria, Tay-Sachs disease, thalassemia, sickle cell disease or trait, birth defects, or mental retardation.

to a new member (Becker et al., 2002; Cronin, 2003; Friedman et al., 2003). The nurse facilitates this process to promote health in the newly forming family unit.

Some parents thrive during the period when an infant needs almost total constant care and nurturing. These parents find support in a network of family and friends. Couples who find satisfaction in parenthood seem to realize that parental influence begins at birth and is the single most important factor in the child's physical, emotional, and cognitive development. The parents' ability to assume responsibility depends on a complex array of factors: their own maturity; how they were nurtured as children; their conceptions about self, culture, social class, and religion; their relationship with each other; their values and philosophy of life; their perceptions of and experiences with children and other adults; and the life stresses they have experienced.

In analyzing needs of the child-rearing family, the nurse considers many factors, including providing for the physical health, economic support, and nurturing actions that are vital to the child's learning and social development. In analyzing the couple's needs during this stage, the nurse recognizes the importance of interactions among the triad. Observing decision making will help the nurse determine how the family functions, what roles each member has, and how effectively the family meets the needs of all its members.

Risks associated with role relationships include working parents with insufficient resources for child care, abuse or neglect of children, multiple closely spaced children, low family self-esteem, children used as scapegoats for parental frustration, immature parents who are dependent and unable to handle responsibility, and strong beliefs about physical punishment or obedience.

Family With Preschool Children

Families may have more than one child, each growing and developing at an individual pace. Preschool children place great demands on families. Families adjust to each new member with space and equipment for expansion.

The needs and interests of preschool children influence home environments. Whether the child has stimulation-promoting opportunities to experience and explore influences the quality of the home environment. Safety balanced with outlets for exploration by the child result in a home that promotes the health of the child. Rather than removing children from the kitchen or garden, finding ways to include them in a cooking or planting activity provides learning experiences. Other environmental influences affecting the child's rate and style of development include religious practices, ethnic background, education, and discipline techniques.

Increasing evidence demonstrates the link between environment and health. The home environment that contains contaminated air, water, or food increases health risks. For example, lead poisoning, a preventable disease that continues to affect thousands of children, often results from lead paint and other factors in the home. Although restrictions exist in the United States to limit lead-based paint to the exterior, many homes have lead within the interior. Both the home and the automobile should be considered possible sources of exposure to the poisonous agent carbon monoxide. The nurse also reviews data for safety in the home, including storage of dangerous materials, such as detergents, insecticides, and medications.

Developmental tasks for the family include adjusting to fatigue resulting from the demands of parenthood. The nurse explores alternatives for relief from parenting for the couple. Parents need time for themselves, but they need to know their children are safe with a responsible person. Economic restraints may limit relaxation time away from the children.

Awareness of the health-promotion habits for the preschooler, such as proper foods, exercise, sleep, and dental hygiene, are numerous. Parents teach the preschooler through modeling their own routines and use of positive reinforcement.

Family With School-Aged Children

The family with children in school may have reached its maximal size in numbers and interrelationships. The parents' major problem during this stage is the dichotomy between self-interest and finding fulfillment in producing the next generation. The family's developmental tasks revolve around the goals of reorganization to prepare for the expanding world of school-aged children. School achievement is one of the critical tasks in their socialization. Viewing social and educational goals in terms of family culture and the parents' defined goals is particularly important during this stage of development. For example, many opportunities for health education exist in schools, opportunities to influence children to develop desirable health habits and to acquire positive health beliefs. However, health education in the school usually is oriented toward problems such as tobacco and substance abuse. Messages usually address problems and crises instead of positive aspects of healthy behaviors. Families influence health at home and in school by teaching children how to assess situations for risks and how to manage them, and what benefits to expect when practicing healthy behaviors.

As children's activities broaden away from the home, another important developmental task for both parent and child is to let go. Parents are likely to be involved in community groups such as the parent-teacher association, scout groups, sports teams, and other volunteer organizations. The mother may enter the workforce or renew educational opportunities. Encouraging children to join in family discussions to establish policies and make decisions fosters their positive self-concepts. The group's position on health practices is included in family policies and decisions.

During this stage, families are vulnerable to risks related to safety and stimulation, such as repeated infections, family violence, neglect, poverty, and low family self-esteem. Children exposed to an unsafe home environment risk behavior disturbances, school problems, and learning disabilities. Parents who cannot manage their children in growth-promoting ways soon experience energy depletion and may turn to dysfunctional ways of finding relief from parenting.

Family With Adolescents

Parents with adolescent children may experience a late pregnancy, which means the parents are caring for an infant while other children in the family are in school. A new member at this stage may be a source of joy or frustration for the family. The overall goal with adolescent members is to loosen family ties to allow greater responsibility and freedom in preparation for releasing young adults. Although each member of the family strives to achieve individual developmental tasks in the midst of social pressures, the family as a whole has tasks to accomplish. Strengthening the marital relationship to build a foundation for future family stages is a critical task during this time.

Open communication is often difficult during this stage, partly because of the differing developmental tasks of adolescents and adults. Adolescents are seeking their own identities, and adults are attempting to assist in their decision-making processes. Choices about values and lifestyles may differ. Adolescents may challenge family values and standards. Although the parents maintain some power, adolescents have their own desires and needs to consider. Adolescents want to do what their friends do, have their own cars, and make their own money to spend in ways that they see fit. Parents who give adolescent members opportunities to experience social, emotional, and ethical situations with others are providing learning opportunities to enhance their sense of autonomy and responsibility (Figure 7-5).

As adolescents mature and emancipate themselves, families face the task of balancing freedom with responsibility.

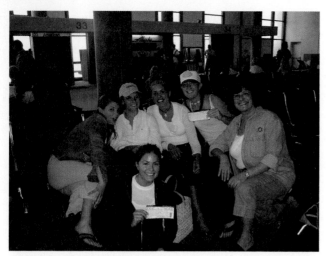

Figure 7-5 Although the parent needs to maintain some responsibility, an adolescent who is given opportunities to experience things with friends will gain an enhanced sense of autonomy and responsibility.

Health problems in this age group include violent deaths, injuries, and alcohol and drug abuse. Contributing risk factors include lack of problem-solving skills, family values of aggressiveness and competition, socioeconomic factors, peer relationships, rigid and inflexible family values, daredevil risk-taking attitudes, and conflicts between parents and children. Environmental risk–related violent deaths and injuries are influenced by the highway system, automobile manufacturers, and the legislation of standards of safety. Families rely on the efforts of nurses as advocates, public health officials, and others to help reduce these environmental risks.

Families support adolescents in this stage of development by including them in the decision-making process and by allowing them to experience positive and negative consequences of their choices. Family values of winning at all costs, aggressiveness, and competition may need to be explored during this period. The adolescent may discard these values if they are no longer applicable. Considerable change in values in the adolescent produces conflict and poses a threat to family cohesiveness. The family may place pressure on the adolescent to conform to family values. In matters of life and death, parents must be firm and take a stand, for example, in regard to driving rules.

When the family stage involves adolescents, there is an identity crisis in the adolescents, the adults, and the family as a whole. Adolescents are moving from childhood to adulthood while the adults are progressing beyond parenthood. Adolescents struggle to find an independent identity that remains connected to the family. Adults are in midlife and must resolve their own adolescent fantasies to move toward their identities for their remaining lives.

Family With Young Adults

The family with young adults acts as a launching center when children begin to leave home. As children leave home, parents relinquish their parenting roles of many years to return to the marital dyad. The couple builds a new life together while maintaining relationships with aging parents, children, grandchildren, and in-laws.

Couples focus on redefining relationships during this stage. For a woman, the role as mother changes, because children no longer need their mother in the same way that they did during their childhood. If the mother devoted 20 years to raising children, she must realize a changed role and purpose within the family. She may reenter the workforce or enter for the first time. Transition from a life with children as the priority to a career may require assistance and support. Men at this stage reach stability in their careers, and further progress is often limited. In addition to individual changes occurring within the couple, the family with young adults may experience other pressures. Aging parents and adult children may require financial or emotional support. Financial and emotional responsibilities to other family members hinder a couple's ability to focus on the marital relationship during this developmental phase.

Health-promoting activities to focus on during this stage include coping with pressures of social roles, occupational responsibilities, maintaining health habits, aging, and reassessing life goals.

Family With Middle-Aged Adults

Families consisting of only two members are able to enhance self-concept and support the marital relationship during middle age. Usually the children have left home and the parents experience a sense of freedom and well-being. Some marriages, by this stage, have reached a level of security and stability; husband and wife meet each other's needs. Parenting pressures diminish, allowing them to enjoy the accomplishments of their children and grandchildren. Couples have acquired a network of friends. Long-time acquaintances seek participation from the couple in neighborhood rituals and events. Economic security and personal self-esteem may be at a peak.

In contrast, some marriages falter at this time. The departed children create a quiet house with less activity, known as the *empty nest*. When unprepared for this stage, individuals might seek opportunities to enhance self-concept from outside of the marriage. The husband, thinking that his father role is now complete, may develop another relationship and begin a new family. The wife, with feelings of inadequacy, may resort to alcohol, drugs, or other self-support.

Health tasks in this developmental stage require a new awareness of susceptibility or vulnerability to health problems. Couples adjust their lifestyle and habits to cope with health risks. Losses promote health problems, and at this stage couples begin to cope with deaths among family and friends, along with declining income.

If the husband or wife has developed a physical or mental illness, then the other may have to adjust to resultant physical and mental impairments. A redefining of self-concept may be necessary.

Middle-aged families are susceptible to a host of risk factors leading to the three most prevalent causes of death: (1) heart disease, (2) cancer, and (3) cerebrovascular accident (stroke). The family lifestyle may help to decrease risks by placing a high value on physical activity, not smoking, maintaining adequate and sound nutritional habits, and consuming moderate amounts of alcohol. Lifestyle habits that are transmitted through role modeling have a greater influence on the younger members of the family than any verbal edict. When possible, middle-aged members can be instrumental in choosing an environment that is free or low in water pollution and air pollution and free from crippling stress factors such as excessive noise, traffic, and overcrowding. Family members can also apply pressure on key members of the community to decrease risks in the environment.

Family With Older Adults

Adjustment to retirement is one of the crucial tasks of the family with older adults. Retirement affects many aspects of a person, including relationships with others (Figure 7-6). Besides a loss of work, retirement also means a sharp reduction in income for most people. Adjusting living standards to retirement income and being able to supplement this income with wage-earning activity is a task of the family with aging members. Other tasks during this stage include making the home environment safe and comfortable and adjusting to the loss of a spouse, which may require the surviving member to look to the family for support and satisfaction (Kahana, Kahana, & Kercher, 2003; Zeiss & Kasl-Godley, 2001). Illness may create further dependence on family members (Kahana et al., 2003).

Health promotion is directed toward maintaining functional ability, limiting the effects of disabling conditions, and maintaining the quality of life. Older adults may fear being helpless and useless and unable to care for themselves. In analyzing risk factors in the aging family, the nurse looks

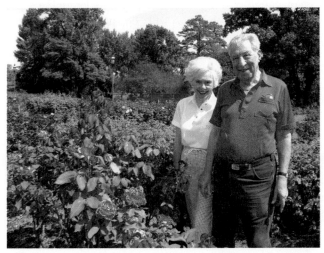

Figure 7-6 Retirement gives the older adult an opportunity to share a new interest with his or her spouse.

at the couple's ability to function well enough to carry out normal roles and responsibilities. As with all people, older adults hope for a state of well-being that will allow them to function at their highest capacity physically, psychologically, socially, and spiritually. Many older adults remain in their own homes, and most of these individuals are vigorous and completely independent. Only 5% of older adults reside in institutions, and many of these people are temporary residents who are recovering from illness and who expect to return to the community.

Ego integrity (the union of all previous phases of the life cycle) is the challenge in this stage and demands successful aging through continued activity. Having gone through the various stages of family development, the couple accepts what they have done as their own. At this time, they may need family or professional support to pursue other interests or maintain former activities to feel needed and useful.

As another approach to data analysis, the nurse and family compare the information to documented norms of health promotion and disease prevention in older adults. Norms or expected values can be derived from the family's baseline information of 11 functional pattern areas, knowledge of growth and development for all age groups and the family as a whole, risk-factor estimates, and population norms.

Population norms specify a range of normal limits for these groups. For example, age is associated with various risk factors; some disorders are so common that they are referred to as *diseases of the older person*. In certain diseases, such as lung cancer, there is a long period of exposure. Risk increases with cumulative exposure; therefore, the incidence and prevalence of diseases increase with age. Gender is a risk factor for various diseases, such as breast cancer in women.

Analysis of data about values, beliefs, self-perception, or role relationships with general population norms may not be easy; the nurse must also consider cultural, ethnic, and religious factors. Analysis may have to be based on whether the family perceives the situation to be a problem or a potential problem. What the nurse identifies as a problem may not be perceived as one by the family (Denham, 2003). The family's baseline information is important because it provides comparative criteria in the analysis. Reviewing records of the family might also be useful in obtaining this data. When no record exists, the information taken on first contact provides criteria for subsequent measurement of progress.

In developing increased awareness or consciousness of a family's health (by the family and the nurse), the nurse may want to reflect on Newman's definitions of family health, which are based on a synthesis of disease and nondisease (Newman, 1995). These are presented in **Web Site Resource 7E.**

Formulating Family Nursing Diagnoses

The purpose of writing a **family nursing diagnosis** is to help the family promote health through the life cycle and prevent disease through low risk–taking behaviors. The nurse derives the diagnosis from assessed validated data. As a concise summary statement of a problem or potential problem, the diagnosis provides direction for outcomes and interventions by identifying the negative health state and the factors that must be changed to alleviate or prevent it (see Chapter 6). Examples of family nursing diagnoses using developmental and risk-factor approaches are presented in **Web Site Resource 7F.**

Describing the health of the family and validating the potential or actual health problems with them are important; cooperation occurs only when the nurse and family agree on the situation. If the family does not agree, then further assessment or negotiation may be needed. The two parties must also agree on the sequence of problem resolution.

The **cultural competence** of the nurse is an essential component of the nursing process. Respect for familial beliefs forms a foundation for nurses. With the changing trends in families and the shifts in heritage within society, cultural competence becomes a priority within nursing practice (Burchum, 2002; Dennis & Small, 2003; Leininger & McFarland, 2002; Parish, 2003). This knowledge increases the efficacy of health promotion for all families, especially those from extraordinarily vulnerable populations.

PLANNING WITH THE FAMILY

A plan of intervention is designed after completion of the assessment, analysis, and nursing diagnosis. The purpose of the plan is to bring about some behavioral change in the family that will promote health or prevent dysfunction. As in the assessment phase, the family is an active participant in the planning process; the degree of responsibility that the family assumes for personal health status is important to the success of behavioral change outcomes. The planning process involves several steps with the nurse and family identifying the following:

1. Order of priority for problems or potential problems
2. Items that can be handled by the nurse and the family and items that must be referred to others
3. Actions and expected outcomes

The planning phase is completed with the nursing plan, which provides direction for implementation of the plan and the framework for evaluation (Care Plan).

As mentioned, a family's health status can be diagnosed as functional, potentially dysfunctional, or dysfunctional. When the family's health status is considered functional, the nurse verifies the situation and a plan for periodic reevaluation is formulated jointly. Plans to continue healthy living behaviors are reinforced and specific information that the family requests or requires is given, such as immunization schedules, growth and development milestones, and recommended dietary allowances. The family is instructed to seek further assistance when necessary. In working with healthy families, the nurse controls the assessment and analysis phases of the nursing process. If the health status is judged functional, then the planning of health education

materials, the scheduling of periodic examinations, and the accessibility of the nurse are all professional responsibilities. Implementation and evaluation of the health-promotion activities are the family's responsibilities.

In setting priorities in health promotion and disease prevention, a life-threatening situation is rarely encountered. However, when the family's data reveal this type of situation, the identified problem receives the highest priority for intervention. For other identified potential or actual problems, the nurse relies on the family to decide which problem or potential problem to approach. After the ordering of priorities is established, the family and nurse determine who will work on the problem.

Problems or potential problems that can be resolved by the nurse are identified separately from those that need referral or the family's intervention. Problems that the family can handle or those with which the family is already involved are considered strengths and should be acknowledged and supported by the nurse. For example, when there is consistency among values and actions, physical fitness, weight management, and ability to cope with stress, the family is already taking informed and responsible action in these areas. The extent to which family members can provide their own health promotion and disease prevention will depend on their knowledge, skills, motivation, and orientation toward health.

Problems that need medical, legal, or social attention should be referred to appropriate agencies. The nurse should have a directory of resources in the community when referrals are needed.

Problems that need nursing interventions must be stated as nursing actions that are clear, purposeful, moral, capable of being accomplished, and adapted to the particular life situation, beliefs, and expectations of the family.

Goals

A goal is a statement describing a desired outcome. Included in the family outcome are expected behaviors of the family, the circumstances under which the behaviors will be demonstrated, and the criteria by which to determine when and how the behaviors will be performed. Health-promotion goals reflect a desire to function at a higher level of health and to grow beyond maintaining health or preventing disease.

IMPLEMENTATION WITH THE FAMILY

Implementation is putting the nursing plan into action. The implementation phase is not to be considered unchangeable. As the nurse and family work together, new information is used to adapt and change the plan, as necessary. **Family nursing interventions** are aimed at assisting the family in carrying out functions that the members cannot perform for themselves. In health promotion and disease prevention, the nurse assists the family in improving their capacity to act on their own behalf (Hatrick, 2000).

Families may know that they are taking risks by smoking, drinking, and engaging in a stressful lifestyle. As the nurse

---

CARE PLAN

Family Member With Alzheimer's Disease

Nursing Diagnosis Risk for Ineffective Role Performance Related to Caring for a Family Member With Alzheimer's Disease

DEFINING CHARACTERISTICS

- Feeling exhausted
- Inability to complete caregiving tasks
- Feeling loss of usual or expected relationship with care receiver
- Increased stress or nervousness about the future
- Preoccupation with care routine
- Withdrawal from social contacts or change in leisure activities

RELATED FACTORS

- Illness severity of care receiver
- Increasing needs of care receiver
- Addiction or codependency of caregiver or care receiver
- Conflicting role demands
- Caregiver health impairment
- Unpredictable illness course or instability in the care receiver's health
- Psychological or cognitive problems in the care receiver
- Caregiver not developmentally ready for caregiving role
- Developmental delay or retardation of the care receiver or caregiver
- Marginal family adaptation or dysfunction before caregiving situation began
- Marginal coping patterns of caregiver
- Providing direct, ongoing in-home care
- History of poor relationship between caregiver and care receiver
- Care receiver who exhibits deviant, bizarre behavior
- Incontinence in the care receiver

EXPECTED OUTCOMES

- Caregiver distinguishes obligations that must be fulfilled from those that can be controlled or limited.
- In conjunction with the nurse, the caregiver develops a plan of care for the client.
- Caregiver receives and accepts appropriate levels of support from family members, friends, and others.
- Caregiver describes help available from informal and formal support systems in the community and takes steps to obtain help.

INTERVENTIONS

- Assess the level of the caregiver's stress.
- Assist the caregiver in developing a realistic plan of care, considering the care receiver's abilities and limitations; the plan will require modification as the person decompensates.
- Instruct the caregiver to encourage the person to participate, to the greatest extent possible, in social and self-care activities such as bathing, dressing, dining out with friends, and playing cards.
- Facilitate a family meeting to help the primary caregiver seek assistance from other family members.
- Support the caregiver and family members as they adjust to the degenerative nature of the disease; be aware that over time the stress associated with caring for the person increases.
- Identify community resources that may offer the caregiver relief from constant supervision of the individual (home health aides, respite care, and adult day care).
- Help the caregiver contact informal sources of support, such as church groups, extended family, and community volunteers.
- Encourage the caregiver to attend an Alzheimer's support group.
- Refer the caregiver to the Alzheimer's Association.

Modified from Carpenito-Moyet, L. J. (2004). *Handbook of nursing diagnosis* (10th ed.). Philadelphia: Lippincott Williams & Wilkins.

---

explains the rationale behind the proposed changes, the family may choose to deny that they are jeopardizing their future health and may simply continue with their risk-taking behaviors. This situation tests the nurse's ingenuity; factors that the nurse has not considered may cause the family's resistance. For example, the family may have more pressing basic needs such as food, clothing, and housing. Health promotion and disease prevention may not have been part of the family's life experiences, giving the nurse the educational task of trying to change attitudes and values so that the family will be more open to considering health needs.

In health promotion and disease prevention, four types of nursing interventions are found: (1) increasing knowledge and skills, (2) increasing strengths, (3) decreasing exposure, and (4) decreasing susceptibility.

Increasing knowledge and skills so that families can improve their capacity to act on health-promotion and disease-prevention behaviors may be the primary strategy. Inherent in this strategy is assisting families to make informed choices about healthful lifestyle behaviors and to eliminate harmful environmental influences that affect their health. The first step is creating awareness, which is accomplished in the first three steps of the nursing process as the nurse and family work together to uncover actual or potential problems. The second step is to recognize particular families at risk. The third step offers families at risk the benefits of nursing knowledge about motivating and supporting behavioral change. The Innovative Practice box presents an example of a program that provides education and support to people with cancer and their families.

The Wellness Community

Local chapters of The Wellness Community are found throughout the United States, offering free educational and support programs for people with cancer and their families. Weekly support groups help family members support one another, explore new ways of coping with the stresses of cancer, and learn ways to become the most effective partners possible with their health care teams.

Wellness communities offer a wide variety of workshops and programs (Gentle Strength and Stretch, Meditation and Guided Imagery, Nutrition Matters, Nutrition and the Immune System, Nutrition at Midlife: Preventing Heart Disease and Osteoporosis, Tai Chi, Yoga, Mindfulness, and Feng Shui). Social events are organized (Comfort Food Potluck Dinner, Couples Networking Groups, Singles Networking Group, Family and Friends Networking Group).

Although each chapter of The Wellness Community does not charge for its services, donations are appreciated and necessary to help serve the thousands of people living with cancer and their families. The Wellness Community's mission is to provide hope to these individuals and to help them regain a sense of control over their lives.

Contact Information:
The Wellness Community (national office)
919 18th Street, NW
Washington, DC 20006
toll-free: 888-793-WELL (-9355)
phone: 202-659-9709
Fax: 202-659-9301
Web site: http://www.wellness-community.org

Family strengths or forces that contribute to family unity and solidarity foster the development of inherent family potential (Ratliffe, Harrigan, Haley, Tse, & Olson, 2002). These factors include the following:

- Physical, emotional, and spiritual factors
- Healthy child-rearing practices and discipline
- Meaningful and clear communication
- Support, security, and encouragement
- Growth-producing relationships and experiences
- Responsible community relationships
- Growth with and through children
- Self-help and acceptance of help
- Flexibility in family functions and roles
- Mutual respect for individuality
- Crisis as a means for growth
- Family unity and loyalty and intrafamily cooperation
- Adaptability of family strengths

In recent years, a shift of family health care from an illness or problem and deficiency focus to a strength-based focus has occurred. Both the McGill model of nursing (Feeley & Gottlieb, 2000) and the Calgary family assessment and intervention model (Wright & Leahey, 2000) are examples of frameworks used by nurses to assess, develop, and use the strengths and resources of families. For example,

Denham (1999) describes how family members use communication, cooperation, and caregiving to develop and maintain health-promotion behaviors. Hatrick (2000) identifies corresponding nursing interventions to support and further develop the family dynamics of socialization, support, and nurturance. Additionally, Plager (1999) describes the importance of understanding the significance of family legacy to a family's health and related health practices.

Families with significant strengths may need to learn new, unfamiliar skills for mastering a specific technique, such as meditation, and to apply new tools for decision making. These families rarely require ongoing supervision or support of sustained interventions aimed at changing their coping patterns, communication, or role behavior. They may be highly capable of seeking and using information.

Assisting functional families may simply involve providing information in terms that can be understood and offering them opportunities to ask questions and clarify information.

Decreasing exposure to risk factors may include making parental behaviors more in tune with the child's behaviors. Poorly educated parents may not respond as constructively to a child's attempt to communicate and in their behavior toward the child than parents in a functional family or those with more education. This tendency may lead to significant differences in the child's intellectual ability. For example, using adequate restraints in automobiles and protecting the toddler from wandering into dangerous streets or places conducive to falls are means of reducing exposure to fatal accidents.

Although no substitute can be found for continuous supervision of a child, homes can be made less hazardous by moving common hazards out of children's reach. This effort includes putting all cleaning solutions and medications beyond their reach; erecting barriers in front of exposed heaters, high windows, and stairways; keeping pots and pans turned inward on the stove; fencing in a yard or a swimming pool; and teaching children to avoid dangerous areas. Becoming aware of peeling paint and toxic chemicals that parents might carry home from the job on their clothing can also protect the child.

Decreasing susceptibility means educating the family about the principles of prevention. The family must realize how diseases are spread, from person to person; through air, water, and food; and by insects and the rodents on which insects live. The role of personal hygiene and cleanliness in avoiding infections must be recognized. The family should know which signs and symptoms need medical attention and learn how to take care of minor illnesses.

Pender cites several research studies that demonstrate that perceived susceptibility is a predictor of preventive behavior (Pender et al., 2001). Perceived susceptibility is the family's estimated subjective probability that a specific health problem will be encountered. Family perceptions of health risks and their susceptibility to them will determine

Table **7-3** Possible Nurse's Roles in Health Promotion and Disease Prevention Through Stages of Family Development

Stage	Possbile Nursing Role
Couple	Counselor on sexual and role adjustment
	Teacher of and counselor on family planning
	Teacher of parenting skills
	Coordinator for genetic counseling
	Facilitator in interpersonal relationships
Childbearing family	Monitor of prenatal care and referrer for problems of pregnancy
	Counselor on prenatal nutrition
	Counselor on prenatal maternal habits
	Supporter of amniocentesis
	Counselor on breast feeding
	Coordinator with pediatric services
	Supervisor of immunizations
	Referrer to social services
	Assistant in adjustment to parental role
Family with preschool or school-age children	Monitor of early childhood development; referrer when indicated
	Teacher of first-aid and emergency measures
	Coordinator with pediatric services
	Counselor on nutrition and exercise
	Teacher of dental hygiene
	Counselor on environmental safety in home
	Facilitator in interpersonal relationships
Family with adolescents	Teacher of risk factors to health
	Teacher of problem-solving issues regarding alcohol, smoking, diet, and exercise
	Facilitator of interpersonal skills with adolescents and parents
	Direct supporter of, counselor on, or referrer to mental health resources
	Counselor on family planning
	Referrer for sexually transmittable disease
Family with young or middle-age adults	Participant in community organizations involved in disease control
	Teacher of problem-solving issues regarding lifestyle and habits
	Participant in community organizations involved in environmental control
	Case finder in the home and community
	Screener for hypertension, Pap smear, breast examination, cancer signs, mental health, and dental care
	Counselor on menopausal transition
Family with older adults	Facilitator of interpersonal relationships among family members
	Referrer for work and social activity, nutritional programs, homemakers' services, and nursing home
	Monitor of exercise, nutrition, preventive services, and medications
	Supervisor of immunization
	Counselor on safety in the home
	Counselor on bereavement

how they change their behavior. If the overweight family believes obesity is a threat to their health and if the nurse works with them in changing their eating habits to reduce weight and maintain weight norms, then the family is likely to react positively to the change. Nurses who introduce threat as a motivator to action are morally obligated to reduce the threat by meaningful and purposeful interventions. Table 7-3 lists various nursing roles used in the implementation stage.

EVALUATION WITH THE FAMILY

The purpose of evaluation is to determine how the family has responded to the planned interventions and whether these interventions were successful. Goals and objectives that are stated in specific behavioral terms will make evaluation much easier than when they are given in general terms. Criteria used to evaluate interventions, such as weight change, increased lung capacity from an exercise program, and lower pulse rate as a result of relaxation exercises, are simple to measure. Other results of health promotion and disease prevention are not as easy to measure but must be considered in the evaluation step of the nursing process. As stated, when considering these factors as values, beliefs, self-perceptions, or role relationships, the nurse may base the evaluation on whether the family indicates that the interventions were successful. Additionally, the family's baseline data are used as comparative criteria in evaluation. The nurse reassesses the situation and compares the new information with that on the original assessment to determine whether change has occurred.

Leavitt (1982) identified the following five measures of family functioning that can be used to determine the effectiveness of interventions:

1. Changes in interaction patterns
2. Effective communication
3. Ability to express emotions
4. Responsiveness to needs of members as individuals
5. Problem-solving ability

Using these measures, the nurse returns to the original assessment of the family's functioning and compares current observations with previous data. These characteristics of family functioning continue to provide a useful framework even today, when trends in family structure are diverse and moving away from the nuclear family (Denham, 2003; Wertlieb, 2003).

When during the planning phase of the nursing process the nurse has identified the criteria (norms and standards) for the desired outcomes, these outcomes are the basis of evaluation. Data from the family that describe their behavior relative to the desired outcomes determine whether the nursing care was successful. With the criteria stated, the goals and objectives outline how the family can demonstrate a successful outcome and the behavior change expected to result from nursing intervention. The more objective and measurable the desired outcome is, the more reliable the results of evaluation will be.

After the goals and objectives are reached, the problem no longer exists. If evaluation shows the nursing actions did not achieve the goals or objectives, then the nurse must review the nursing process to determine whether there were gaps in the assessment data, errors in analysis or nursing diagnosis, or alternative interventions that might have been considered. The nurse also needs to review the process with the family to determine whether they have contributed to outcome failure. Finally, the agency employing the nurse may be another factor; if intervention is costly or a shortage of staff exists, then health promotion and disease prevention may have low priority.

SUMMARY

Learning about health promotion and disease prevention begins at birth, with the family providing the stimulus for incorporating health in the value system of its members. From a systems perspective, the family has both structure and function; relevant functions include values and practices placed on health. The effective execution of health-related functions involves the family's progression through its developmental tasks and its ability to generate low risk–producing behaviors associated with disease prevention.

Developmental and risk-estimate theories can be applied effectively to the nursing process with the family. The nurse uses functional patterns (an inherent part of both theories) to collect data for assessment. After organizing information on family life cycle stages for analysis with the family, the nurse writes the nursing diagnosis and plans, implements, and evaluates the interventions used to promote health and prevent disease in the family.

ADDITIONAL STUDY MATERIAL

Study Questions in the back of the book, see page 663.

evolve WEB SITE MATERIALS

These materials are located on the book's Web site at http://evolve.elsevier.com/Edelman/.

- WebLinks
- Content Updates
- Web Site Resources

7A Nurse's Roles in Health Promotion and Disease Prevention Through Stages of Family Development
7B Developmental Tasks of the Family at Critical Stages
7C Six Progressive Stages in the Natural History of Chronic Diseases
7D Eleven Functional Health Pattern Guidelines for Family Assessment
7E Newman's Definitions of Family Health
7F Examples of Family Nursing Diagnoses

REFERENCES

Allender, J. A., & Spradley, B. W. (2001). *Community health nursing: Concepts and practice* (5th ed.). Philadelphia: Lippincott Williams & Wilkins.

American Academy of Pediatrics. (2001). Children, adolescents, and television. *Pediatrics, 107*(2), 423.

American Academy of Pediatrics. (2003). Family pediatrics report of the Task Force on the Family. *Pediatrics, 111*(6), 1541.

Becker, D., Hogue, A., & Liddle, H. A. (2002). Methods of engagement in family-based preventive intervention. *Child & Adolescent Social Work Journal, 19*(2), 163.

Borell, K. (2003). Family and household. Family research and multi-household families. *International Review of Sociology, 13*(3), 467.

Brannigan, A., Gemmell, W., Pevalin, D. J., & Wade, T. J. (2002). Self-control and social control in childhood misconduct and aggression: The role of family structure, hyperactivity, and hostile parenting. *Canadian Journal of Criminology, 44*(2), 119.

Burchum, J. L. R. (2002). Cultural competence: An evolutionary perspective. *Nursing Forum, 37*(4), 5.

Clark, M. E., Gironda, R. J., & Young, R. W. (2003). Development and validation of the Pain Outcomes Questionnaire-VA. *Journal of Rehabilitation Research & Development, 40*(5), 381.

Connelly, C. D. (1998). Hopefulness, self-esteem, and perceived social support among pregnant and non-pregnant adolescents. *Western Journal of Nursing Research, 20*(2), 195-209.

Cronin, C. (2003). First-time mothers—Identifying their needs, perceptions and experiences. *Journal of Clinical Nursing, 12*(2), 260.

Denham, S. A. (1999). Family health in an economically disadvantaged population. *Journal of Family Nursing, 5*(2), 184-213.

Denham, S. A. (2003). Familial research reveals new practice method. *Holistic Nursing Practice, 17*(3), 143.

Dennis, B. P., & Small, E. B. (2003). Incorporating cultural diversity in nursing care: An action plan. *ABNF Journal, 14*(1), 17.

Duvall, E. M., & Miller, B. (1985). *Marriage and family development* (7th ed.). New York: Harper Collins.

Endo, E., Nitta, N., Inayoshi, M., Saito, R., Takemura, K., Minegishi, H., et al. (2000). Pattern recognition as a caring partnership in families with cancer. *Journal of Advanced Nursing, 32*(3), 603.

Erikson, E. H. (1994). *Identity: Youth in crisis* (Austen Rigg Monograph, Reissue ed.). New York: W. W. Norton.

Feeley, N., & Gottlieb, L. N. (2000). Nursing approaches for working with family strengths and resources. *Journal of Family Nursing, 6*(1), 9-24.

Friedman, M. M., Bowden, V. R., & Jones, E. G. (2003). *Family nursing: Research, theory, and practice* (5th ed.). Upper Saddle River, NJ: Prentice Hall.

Gance-Cleveland, B. (2001). Pediatric nurses: Advocates against youth violence. *Journal of the Society of Pediatric Nurses, 6*(3), 133.

Giami, A. (2002). Sexual health: The emergence, development, and diversity of a concept. *Annual Review of Sex Research, 13,* 1.

Gordon, M. (1994). In Gordon M. (Ed.), *Nursing diagnosis: process and application* (3rd ed.). St. Louis: Mosby.

Gordon, M. (2002). *Manual of nursing diagnosis* (10th ed.). St. Louis: Mosby.

Hatrick, G. (2000). Developing health-promoting practices with families. *Journal of Advanced Nursing, 31*(1), 27-34.

Johansson, C. (2002). Integrity versus despair: An Eriksonian framework for geriatric rehabilitation. *Topics in Geriatric Rehabilitation, 17*(3), 1.

Jones, A. C. (2003). Reconstructing the stepfamily: Old myths, new stories. *Social Work, 48*(2), 228.

Kahana, E., Kahana, B., & Kercher, K. (2003). Emerging lifestyles and proactive options for successful ageing. *Ageing International, 28*(2), 155.

Leavitt, M. B. (1982). *Families at risk: Primary prevention in nursing practice.* New York: Little, Brown & Co.

Leininger, M., & McFarland, M. R. (2002). *Transcultural nursing: Concepts, theories, research and practice* (3rd ed.). New York: McGraw-Hill.

Leppink, H. (1982). Health risk estimation. In M. M. Faber & A. M. Reinhardt (Eds.), *Promoting health through risk reduction.* New York: Macmillan.

Newman, M. (1995). *A developing discipline: Selected works of Margaret Newman.* New York: National League for Nursing.

Newman, M. A. (2002). The pattern that connects. *ANS Advances in Nursing Science, 24*(3), 1.

North American Nursing Diagnosis Association. (2003). *NANDA nursing diagnosis 2003-2004: Definitions and classifications.* Chicago: North American Nursing Diagnosis Association.

Parish, T. G. (2003). Cultural competence: Do we agree on its meaning and should it be considered a core competency in training programs? *Internet Journal of Academic Physician Assistants, 3*(2), 10.

Pender, N. J., Murdaugh, C., & Parsons, M. A. (2001). *Health promotion in nursing practice* (4th ed.). Saddle River, NJ: Prentice Hall.

Plager, K. A. (1999). Understanding family legacy in family health concerns. *Journal of Family Nursing, 5*(1), 51-71.

Pratt, L. (1976). *Family sturucture and effective health behavior: The energized family.* Boston: Houghton Mifflin.

Ratliffe, C. E., Harrigan, R. C., Haley, J., Tse, A., & Olson, T. (2002). Stress in families with medically fragile children. *Issues in Comprehensive Pediatric Nursing, 25*(3), 167.

Rogers, M. (1970). *An introduction to the theoretical basis of nursing.* Philadelphia: F. A. Davis.

Rossi, L. R. (2003). Family health: A pattern that connects. *Holistic Nursing Practice, 17*(1), 5.

Rugala, E. A., & Isaacs, A. R. (2002). *Workplace violence: Issues in response* (Government Report). Washington D. C.: U.S. Department of Justice, Federal Bureau of Investigation.

Simmons, T., & O'Neill, G. (2001). *Households and families 2000: Census 2000 brief* (Publication No. C2KBR/01-8). Washington, DC: U.S. Census Bureau.

U.S. Census Bureau. (2000). *Census 2000: Household and family structure.* Retrieved May 5, 2004, from: *http://www.censuss cope.org/us/print_chart_house.html.*

Wake, M., Hesketh, K., & Waters, E. (2003). Television, computer use and body mass index in Australian primary school children. *Journal of Paediatrics & Child Health, 39*(2), 130.

Walsh, F. (2003). Family resilience: A framework for clinical practice. *Family Process, 42*(1), 1.

Wertlieb, D. (2003). Converging trends in family research and pediatrics: Recent findings for the American Academy of Pediatrics Task Force on the Family. *Pediatrics, 111*(6), 1572.

Wright, L. M., & Leahey, M. (2000). *Nurses and families: A guide to family assessment and intervention* (3rd ed.). Philadelphia: F. A. Davis.

Wu, T., Mendola, P., & Buck, G. M. (2002). Ethnic differences in the presence of secondary sex characteristics and menarche among US girls: The Third National Health and Nutrition Examination Survey, 1988-1994. *Pediatrics, 110*(4), 752.

Zeiss, A. M., & Kasl-Godley, J. (2001). Sexuality in older adults' relationships. *Generations, 25*(2), 18.

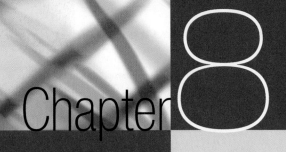

Chapter 8

ANNE RATH RENTFRO

Health Promotion and the Community

objectives

After completing this chapter, the reader will be able to:

- Describe the 11 functional health patterns and explain how they are used as a basis of data collection in assessment of the community.

- Identify characteristics of the community to consider for risk factors and developmental aggregates of potential or actual dysfunctional health patterns.

- Identify methods of community data collection and sources of information.

- Describe a method of planned change for the community.

- Discuss planning, implementing, and evaluating nursing interventions in health promotion with communities.

- Develop a health-promotion plan based on community assessment, nursing diagnosis, and contributing factors.

key terms

Community	Community pattern	Measurement
Community diagnosis	Community risk factors	Observation data
Community evaluation	Demography	Risk factor theory
Community health promotion	Developmental theory	Structure of a community
Community nursing intervention	Function of a community	Systems theory
Community outcome	Interview	Windshield survey
	Interview data	

THINK About It

Teenagers: Drinking and Driving

In a small rural community, seven teenagers have died in alcohol-related car accidents within the past 3 months. Alcohol and drug education is taught during the first year at the local high school, but driver's education classes are not offered because the school cannot afford the program. Parents within this community are extremely concerned.

1. What other information must be acquired before making a diagnosis?
2. What health-promotion ideas could be recommended, based on the information provided?

Over the last 2 decades, several social trends in the United States have increased public interest in health promotion and disease prevention. The landmark documents the U.S. Department of Health and Human Services (2000) published (see Chapter 1) have been helpful in changing the focus of health care from a reactive stance to a proactive stance that emphasizes prevention of disease and promotion of health. By stating national health objectives in relation to age-specific risks to good health, these documents set a course to reduce the percentage of risk factors, thereby reducing the incidence of disease.

Another social trend creating interest in these issues is the changing population of the United States. The U.S. Census Bureau estimates that by the year 2025, there will be 60 million people in the United States over the age of 65 (20% of the population) (U.S. Department of Health and Human Services [USDHHS], 2000). Older people tend to have more chronic diseases and consume a larger portion of health care services than do people in other age groups. It is also anticipated that the aging population will require more home health care and nursing home services than previous generations, because they will experience increasing longevity and illnesses of a chronic nature. A growing number of articles in the literature propose that the major improvements in the population's health will be derived from self-care and strategies of health promotion and disease prevention, not from medical technology and services.

The term **community** is used in various contexts with various meanings, depending on the frame of reference. In this text, the definition of community is the same definition used by *Healthy People 2010* and the *Health Promotion Glossary* of the World Health Organization (WHO), "A specific group of people, often living in a defined geographical area, who share a common culture, values, and norms and who are arranged in a social structure according to relationships that community has developed over a period of time" (USDHHS, 2000, p. 5; World Health Organization, 1998). The community includes workplaces (Workplace Health Strategies Bureau, 2002) and schools (USDHHS, 1993).

School nurses serve the youth in our nation's schools and provide a link to community resources. "The school nurse has a central management role . . . for all children and youth in the school," and collaboration occurs "with primary care physicians, specialists, and local public health and social service agencies to ensure a full spectrum of effective and quality services that sustain children, youth, and their families" (Taras et al., 2001, p. 1231). Results from the School Health Policies Programs Study indicate support for the *Healthy People 2010* Objective 7-4: "Increase the proportion of the Nation's elementary, middle, junior high, and senior high schools that have a nurse-to-student ratio of at least 1:750" (Brener et al., 2001, p. 294; U.S. Department of Health and Human Services, 2000).

People are integral to any concept of community; human beings give it shape, character, and form. An individual's health is reflected in the community through the person's contribution to its statistical rates and cultural and psycho-logical makeup. Conversely, the community is reflected in the individual through similar modes of expression.

This chapter focuses on the application of the nursing process to the community. The nurse's role is inherent in independent, interdependent, and dependent activities. Methods of data collection and sources of information about a community are provided because they may differ from individual sources. Systems theory, developmental theory, and risk factor theory are used to guide the nursing process. Developmental theory refers to a variety of explanations of phases of human development—physical, psychosocial, cognitive, and spiritual dimensions—based on descriptive research studies. Similarly, risk factor theory is an identification of human characteristics and behaviors that increase the likelihood of the manifestation of health problems. Gordon's (1994) typology of 11 functional health patterns is used to provide a database for assessment. An example of a data collection guide is presented to facilitate the comprehension, synthesis, and application of observation, interview, and measurement data. An example of data analysis, nursing diagnosis, planning, implementation, and evaluation follow along with a description.

THE NURSING PROCESS AND THE COMMUNITY

As stated previously, Gordon's 11 functional health patterns (1994) are used to collect a database for assessment. The health-related patterns can provide a useful framework for collecting observation, interview, and measurement data. The health-related patterns that the nurse chooses for an assessment depend on the community setting, the focus of the assessment, and the nurse's preference. Assessing all pattern areas provides a basic set of data that can be analyzed and used for comparison purposes in evaluation (see Chapter 6).

Risk and developmental factors also influence health patterns. For example, a health concern might be identified in one pattern area, such as an increase in an age-related factor of teenage pregnancy (sexuality-reproductive pattern). Data from other areas might reveal the containment of sex education in the home (coping–stress tolerance pattern) and the unacceptability of sex education in the school from parental opposition (values-beliefs pattern). Limiting sex education to the home and ignoring it in the school may be factors that young people of childbearing age in the community share, placing them at risk for unwanted pregnancies. Factors from several pattern areas may form a cluster that can put certain groups at risk (see Chapter 6).

THE NURSE'S ROLE

Community health nursing is seen as a synthesis of nursing practice and public health concepts applied to promote the health of populations. It is not limited to any particular individual or group of individuals (Smith & Bazini-Barakat, 2003). The nursing concerns are the community's responses to existing and potential health-related problems, including such health-supporting responses as monitoring and teaching population groups. The nurse may supply a community at risk with the educational information necessary to develop health-oriented skills, attitudes, and related behavioral changes.

The nurse's role is also concerned with the relationships that are essential to accomplish the community's health-related mission. The complexity and dynamic nature of communities and the increasing public involvement in health and health policy highlight the importance of the human interactions that are inherent in the nurse's responses to potential health problems, needs, and expectations. Therefore nursing practice with communities requires a broad knowledge base derived from the natural, behavioral, and humanistic sciences and the application of intellectual, interpersonal, and technical skills through the nursing process.

The nurse's role can be seen as independent, interdependent, and dependent functions, and these frequently overlap. Independent functions include assessing, analyzing, diagnosing, planning, implementing, and evaluating nursing activities such as health promotion and health education. Interdependent functions include collaboration with community members and interdisciplinary teamwork functions that are crucial to effective community health. Dependent functions include implementing the therapeutic plans of team members.

Community health promotion includes all of the following:

- Community participation, with representatives from at least three community sectors including government, education, business, faith organizations, health care, media, voluntary agencies, and the public
- Assessment guided by a community assessment and planning model to determine health problems, resources, perceptions, and priorities for action
- Targeted and measurable objectives to address health outcomes, risk factors, public awareness, services, and protection
- Comprehensive, multifaceted, culturally relevant interventions that have multiple targets for change
- Monitoring and evaluation of the processes to determine whether the objectives are reached (USDHHS, 2000)

METHODS OF DATA COLLECTION

The nurse obtains community assessment data through observation, interviews, and measurement. These three methods are used most frequently in various combinations to ensure the validity of the information.

Obtaining data through observation—often referred to as the **windshield survey** approach to assessment—includes the use of the senses (sight, touch, hearing, smell, and taste) to determine community appearances. These appearances include the type and state of residential dwellings, the people, and the physical and biological characteristics, such as animal and plant life, temperature, transportation, sounds, and odors. Some communities have a characteristic

"flavor." The community's physical characteristics can influence health. What type of space is available? Children need space in which to run and play; young and middle-aged adults require space for recreation and exercise. What spatial barriers exist? The community nurse can obtain a great deal of subjective data just by walking or riding around a community and using the senses. The data obtained by observation can provide important clues about the community, its actual or potential health problems, and its strengths. When **observation data** are analyzed, hypotheses can be generated that are further assessed by using interview and measurement data.

The second method, the **interview,** is probably the most common approach for collecting information from people. **Interview data** include verbal statements from community residents, key community officials, health care personnel, and various community agency staff. This method is a useful way to obtain information about how members perceive their community. Key community leaders can provide important information about community health concerns, necessary health resources, and community strengths. Particular health beliefs and community health goals can also be ascertained.

Community residents can provide useful information about their perceptions of health, health concerns and needs, and the availability, accessibility, and acceptability of health services. Health agency personnel can provide data on health resources, who they serve, when they are available, and their perceptions of concerns and needs. Developing a basic set of questions in advance will enhance the relevance of interview data.

Measurement, the third method, uses instruments to quantify data in information collection. Measurement data include population statistics, pollution indices, morbidity and mortality rates, census statistics, and epidemiological data. These data can be found in community libraries, health departments, environmental protection agencies, schools, police and fire departments, local health system agencies, and town, city, or state planning offices. Publicly supported agencies are required by law to share their information with interested people, and community nurses should not hesitate to request such data.

SOURCES OF COMMUNITY INFORMATION

Census information found in libraries and public agencies is the most complete source for population information. Because the U.S. Census is completed once every 10 years at the beginning of a decade, the data for most communities become less accurate as the decade progresses. Community agencies, such as the chamber of commerce and local planning commissions, work with census data to develop projection statistics and developmental trends, which the nurse can use to gain an understanding of population patterns and dynamics. Health data are usually available from town, city, or state public health departments and community health–related organizations.

Environmental measurement data can be obtained from the local branch of the U.S. Environmental Protection Agency. Generally the sanitation department of the local health department is in charge of monitoring the community's water, food, and sanitation systems. School health information is available from the health department, school nurse, or school administration.

Information on land use, boundaries, housing conditions, utilities, and community services is generally available from the town, city, or county administration. Community newspapers can be an excellent source of information on community dynamics, health-related concerns, cultural activities, and community decision makers. Recording community observation, interview, and measurement data are approached in the same manner as data on an individual or family. A triple-column format that separates the data of each method can facilitate recording.

COMMUNITY FROM A SYSTEMS PERSPECTIVE

Systems theory provides an overall framework in which otherwise unconnected parts can be integrated. A system is an entity composed of interrelated, interacting parts or components within a boundary that filters both the type and the rate of input and output (Von Bertalanffy, 1976). Just as families are considered systems (see Chapter 7), a community that is viewed as a system has both structure and function. These aspects of a population within a specific geographical area are explored when assessing a community.

Structure

The **structure of a community** system or subsystem can be seen as the formal or informal arrangement of its parts at any given time, including both animate and inanimate properties. The population, schools, fire department, and health resources are examples of structural parts. Nursing, which operates within the context of the health system, can be considered a component of a community system.

The parts of a community are viewed as subsystems, each of which is in itself a system. The suprasystem, often a county or state, is the larger system of which the community is a part. Figure 8-1 shows a hierarchical arrangement of a community system.

The arrangement and organization of a community system's parts, such as the age distribution of the population and the types of health-promotion and health-protection programs and their availability and accessibility, can change over time. The parts may remain relatively stable for long periods, based on the state of the environment and the processes that occur within the parts and between the parts and the larger environment.

The existence, arrangement, and assimilation of a community's parts play a major role in providing direction to both health-promotion and health-protection activities. Therefore, when conducting an assessment, the nurse must consider the various community parts or systems as they relate to health. Viewing the community structure as a population (collection of people) and considering the arrangement of the community's health care parts (existing health services) are especially important.

The study of a population is referred to as demography. **Demography** provides information on population characteristics (size, age distribution, gender ratio, racial composition, marital status ratio, nationality, language, religious grouping, and educational and occupational distributions).

Obtaining demographic data of a population living in a specific area provides an important basis for analysis and a means for identifying developmental concerns of various population groups that might be at risk. Such information can also provide clues for the direction of health strategies. For example, an examination of age distribution over the past several years reveals important population shifts and a need for additional health-promotion activities; the large increase in the population over age 65 may require changes in community health priorities to reflect this group's needs. Demographic information is so vital that generally it is considered first in any community assessment.

Comparison statistics about population characteristics, which also need to be considered in community structure, enable the nurse to make inferences about the community. Comparisons are made among three systems: (1) the town, which is a part of the county, (2) the county, which is a part of the larger system, and (3) the state. Comparisons typically are made between communities of similar population size.

Function

The **function of a community** refers to the process of dynamic change or adaptation in the system's parts and the way the community system and its subsystems interact. How community members make decisions and allocate health-promotion and health-protection resources are important considerations. Nurses have traditionally used the role of health educator to interact with the community to promote

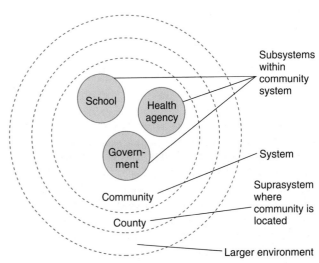

Figure 8-1 Hierarchical nature of a community system.

health. Whitehead (2001) argues that the nurse as health promoter in the community involves a more complex array of responsibilities. To fulfill this role, the nurse acts as an advocate and community liaison, uses proactive planning, collaborates with other disciplines and agencies, establishes priorities for programming, matches resources with needs determined by a community needs assessment, empowers community members, and facilitates social, environmental, and political change.

These multifaceted functions require expertise in communication and interpersonal relations, requiring a slow but deliberate approach. Using such a process, while maintaining the community's vision, can produce effective change within the community.

Interaction

Interaction is an important concept in systems theory. Through dynamic interaction with the environment, a system exchanges matter, energy, and information (in such communication forms as verbal and behavioral) and uses information to make decisions. Interaction is also important if the community system is to survive, protect, and promote the health of its members. Through environmental interactions, a community system uses mechanisms of adaptation. The nurse must determine how the community applies these mechanisms toward health services.

Various health-related patterns emerge from these interactions. For example, certain human activity patterns can negatively alter the natural environmental patterns, which influence human health patterns. Gordon's (1994) assessment framework focuses on 11 health-related functional patterns; community and environment interaction is assumed in each. The framework used, such as the systems theory described, dictates the approach used in assessing these patterns.

COMMUNITY FROM A DEVELOPMENTAL PERSPECTIVE

A framework based on developmental theory can be used to identify existing or potential health problems for a particular age group in a community. A population group is defined as an aggregate of people who share similar personal or environmental characteristics. Community nurses are interested in the total community population; therefore, they use a developmental, age-correlated approach to identify health-promotion and health-protection activities for all age groups.

At each stage of life, age-related risks can be identified and steps taken to maximize wellness and promote health as a lifelong concern (USDHHS, 2000). For example, adolescent single mothers of infants are at high risk both emotionally and physically, and they require help with parenting skills. Accidents are the greatest threat to children's health; therefore, accident-prevention activities are a priority for this age group. Many age-related risk factors (see Chapters 6 and 7) associated with individuals and families can be extended to include community groups.

COMMUNITY FROM A RISK FACTOR PERSPECTIVE

Risk factors are associated with a community's disease, illness, and death rates (USDHHS, 2000). A risk factor does not necessarily play a causal role in these rates but helps to predict the likelihood of a particular adverse health condition.

Risk factors may include a combination of demographic, psychological, physiological, or environmental characteristics (or they may include a single characteristic). For example, age, gender, race, geographical location, consumption pattern, or lack of health services may be considered risk factors, because one or more may contribute to disease or death and place the population sharing them at risk (Research Highlights box). The degree of influence of various risk factors differs from person to person and group to group because of genetic makeup, geographical location, lifestyle patterns, resources, socioeconomic status, level of education, or environmental variation. Some groups may be at high risk from a single risk factor such as insufficient immunizations or exposure to asbestos. However, synergism does operate. A combined potential for adverse health effects exists when many risk factors are present, because they interact in many ways and can potentiate each other (USDHHS, 2000). As a result, communities can experience substantial variability in both the incidence of and susceptibility to adverse health conditions. The **risk factor theory**

---

research highlights

Bicycle Injuries and Safety Helmets in Children

The purpose of this research was to summarize "the current state of research on bicycle injuries and helmet uses" (p. 9) along with an analysis of "legislation and injury prevention strategies" (p. 9). Bicycle injuries cause the most serious, but preventable, head injuries in children. However, children must wear helmets to prevent these injuries.

In this study, literature about bicycle injury prevention published between 1995 and 2001 was summarized, using helmet wearing rates and injuries as outcome measures. Eighteen studies were reviewed. The outcomes reported in the studies indicate that helmets help to decrease the number and severity of injuries in the children. Helmet promotion campaigns and legislation are effective methods to increase helmet use. The role of the nurse as community advocate and community facilitator is instrumental in promoting positive community change. "Nurses have access to the total picture of injury including injury severity and the potential for prevention" (p. 9). Effective injury prevention programs need to be analyzed to better describe the patterns of injury, the needs of children in their community, and the interventions that would be most effective to promote more positive outcomes. The author concludes that, "Nurses can participate both at the institutional level and in community advocacy groups to promote bicycle safety for children" (p. 9).

From Coffman, S. (2003). Bicycle injuries and safety helmets in children. *Orthopaedic Nursing, 22*(1), 9-15.

is based on disease and, conversely, health because it is multifactorial in genesis; the essential cause frequently cannot be attributed to any single risk factor. For example, risk factors such as air pollution, smoking, and forms of radiation in various combinations may be related to high rates of lung cancer, emphysema, and bronchitis in a community. The potential to control many or just a few risk factors and to have relevant health-related resources available is the basis of health-promotion and health-protection activities.

A general description of the 11 functional health patterns and the guidelines for posing questions in observations and interviews are provided in **Web Site Resource 8A**. A variety of functional health pattern assessments are used with communities. The nurse may use Gordon's (1994) functional health reference assessment as exemplified in this chapter or other assessments described in the literature (Anderson & McFarlane, 2004; Clark, 2003).

FUNCTIONAL HEALTH PATTERNS: ASSESSMENT OF THE COMMUNITY
Health Perception–Health Management Pattern

This pattern identifies data about the community's health status, its health-promotion and disease prevention practices, and its members' perceptions of health (Gordon, 1994). Some residents might perceive a substance abuse problem in adolescents or a high rate of unwanted pregnancies, breast cancer, or sexually transmitted disease as a concern. Valuable information can be elicited from interviewing key community members about their health concerns and issues. Mortality and morbidity statistics and other public health information sources can provide measurement data (see Chapter 2).

Nutritional-Metabolic Pattern

This pattern identifies data relevant to a community's consumption habits as reflected in the accessibility and availability of food stores and subsidized food programs for infants, children, and older adults. Community well-being rests on adequate dietary habits, food intake, and supply of nutrients, all of which can be influenced by culture and the presence or absence of kitchen facilities and adequate plumbing.

Obtaining data by a drive or a walk through the community and using the five senses can provide information about grocery stores, fast-food establishments, ethnic shopping facilities, and street corner vendors. Government programs, private soup kitchens, and food donations by houses of worship also provide information about the nutritional pattern of a community.

Elimination Pattern

This pattern identifies data about the environmental factors of a community and includes exposure to pollutants in the community through such media as contaminated soil, water, air, and the food chain. It further classifies environmental factors into two broad areas: (1) physical and (2) biologi-

cal. Alterations in environmental processes can threaten the health and integrity of a community, necessitating health-promotion and health-protection activities.

Physical agents include geological, geographical, climatic, and meteorological aspects of the community. Certain population groups are particularly susceptible to acute respiratory disease and aggravated asthmatic episodes when the air quality is poor. The geographical location of a community and major waterways, highways, or mountains located within it can act as barriers to health facilities. Inaccessibility of health care services can also be a barrier to groups who are at risk for potential health problems. Knowledge of the community's climatic conditions, although obvious to many, can provide clues to a population's susceptibility to illness resulting from temperature or humidity.

Biological agents include living things, such as plants, animals and their waste products, disease agents, microbial pathogens, and toxic substances that can be hazardous to health. For example, Lyme disease, viral hepatitis, pneumonia, influenza, and the large number of diseases associated with childhood continue to be threats to a community's health.

Information concerning elimination patterns can be elicited through observation and interviews with key community people. The Environmental Protection Agency and the Centers for Disease Control and Prevention are excellent resources.

Activity-Exercise Pattern

This pattern identifies a community's physical activities and recreational options. In some communities, science and technology have had an increasing influence on productivity while simultaneously reducing and, in some cases, eliminating the amount of physical work required by the labor force. As a result, physical activity can no longer be attained on the job, and leisure hours represent the only viable time for it. During leisure time, people can choose from literally dozens of activities that are sufficiently different from one another, so that almost anyone can find a physical activity that is enjoyable and challenging. Physical activity reduces the risk of many diseases, including heart disease, hypertension, cancer, osteoporosis, and diabetes mellitus.

Physiological evidence shows that physical activity improves many biological measures associated with health and psychological functioning. Regular physical activity and musculoskeletal fitness are important to healthy, independent living as people grow older.

Observation and interviews provide clues to a community's ability to provide cultural and recreational activities (Figure 8-2).

Sleep-Rest Pattern

This pattern identifies a community's rhythm of sleeping, resting, and relaxing. Some towns never shut down; that is, stores, traffic flow, and recreational facilities are open day and night. These situations can produce disturbances, such

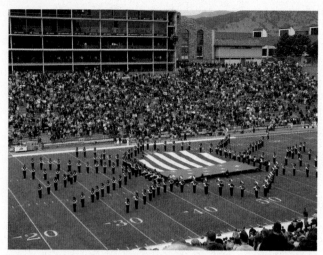

Figure 8-2 The activity-exercise pattern identifies a community's physical activities and recreational options.

as unwanted noise, that are disagreeable or harmful to a community's well being. Excessive noise from highways or airplanes can produce a physiological or psychological problem and can elicit a response ranging from mild irritation to pain or permanent hearing loss. Although noise cannot be eliminated from a community, much can be done to minimize or control it. Observation and interviews will provide clues to this pattern.

Cognitive-Perceptual Pattern

This pattern identifies information about a community's ability to solve problems and make decisions. A community's decision-making and resource allocation processes are necessary for a system's survival and relevant to health promotion and protection. A community must have a functional decision-making body to ensure that its rules are followed and its goals are achieved. Individual patterns connect with environmental patterns in ways that have important implications for community health. The community can be assessed for how it interacts with the environment and whether the strategies used are effective in meeting health concerns and needs (Newman, 2002).

One strategy, bargaining, obtains compliance by offering the community an exchange. For example, one community may have a radiograph machine for mammography but no primary care facility; it might negotiate with another community to provide mammography in return for receiving primary care services.

Strategies using outside authority (legal bureaucratic methods) ensure compliance through rules and structures. For example, the state may mandate that the community maintain certain health standards. Therefore all school children must be immunized against specific diseases before entering public school.

Cooperative strategies persuade members to share common goals. For example, community residents may oppose a chemical dumpsite within the area because they believe it will be detrimental to their health.

Convincing people to comply because they hold some loyalty in the situation or relationship is another method used to mobilize communities. For example, community residents might expend a great deal of effort and money fighting for the retention of a health clinic because they feel loyal to it.

Identifying the various decision-making patterns used by a community can provide clues about its priorities and value system related to health activities, about matches and mismatches between what exists and what are the health goals, and about whether planning is performed. Data can best be obtained by observation and interviews.

Self-Perception–Self-Concept Pattern

This pattern identifies the self-worth and personal identity of a community. Image, status, and perceived competency to deal with problems are characteristics that can be noted about a community. Community image may be reflected in housing conditions, buildings, and cleanliness. Community perception of self-worth may relate to school systems, crime rates, accidents, and whether residents and outsiders consider it a good place to live. Competency in dealing with social and political issues and community spirit will create a positive self-evaluation. Knowing the level of community pride may assist in creating innovative health programs. The emotional tone (fear, depression, or positive emotional outlook) can usually be related to findings in other pattern areas. For example, tensions in the cognitive-perceptual pattern (conflict between groups concerning health issues) may explain a general feeling of fear in the residents. Data are obtained through observation and interviews.

Roles-Relationships Pattern

This pattern identifies communication styles and formal and informal relationships. Of particular concern are roles and relationships that affect the community's ability to realize its health potential. Patterns of crime, racial incidents, and social networks are indices of human relationships in a community. Patterns of official communication are important to know so that health-promotion activities can be publicized; prominent communicators can make or break a health-related program. Key community leaders may not always be identified easily, but community members can help in this area.

Use of the media and other mass information programs can improve communication, the flow of health information, and the number of community members reached. Interviews, television, and newspapers are examples of ways in which information can be obtained.

Sexuality-Reproductive Pattern

This pattern identifies the reproductive data of a community, as reflected in live birth statistics and mothers' ages and marital status. This information provides clues to the health-promotion needs of a particular community group.

The reproductive pattern of a community is also reflected in premature infant rates, abortion rates, and neonatal, infant, and maternal death rates. Such information identifies groups that are at risk based on particular characteristics associated with these rates. Health concerns are also identified when a mismatch is found between existing health services, health education programs, and community health statistics. Other areas to be identified are the availability of sex education in the schools, spouse and child abuse, and sex-related crimes. Minutes of meetings, health records, statistical data, and public documents are examples of places where these data can be found.

Coping-Stress Tolerance Pattern

This pattern identifies the community's ability to cope or adapt. Communities respond in different ways, some of which might threaten their integrity. The way in which a community responds is its coping pattern. The ability of individuals and groups to give and take goods, services, goals, values, and ideals to survive and to promote and protect the community's health is inherent in the community.

Community efforts to obtain goods from the environment, contain goods within the environment, retain goods within the community, and dispose of goods can play a significant role in influencing health. Examples of goods that a community might obtain from the environment to promote health include local, state, or federal funding, health services, a health-related workforce, and new knowledge and technological advances. Some communities have obtained an abundance of health care institutions and services. However, when examined closely, primary services are frequently inadequate or nonexistent. The lack of available health services, or the lack of ability to obtain them, constitutes community health needs.

Examples of goods a community might attempt to contain because a threat to community integrity, values, and health exists include sex-related crimes, diseases, substance abuse, industry, hazardous waste in the water supply, and noxious chemicals in the air.

The community's coping efforts might be geared toward retaining within its boundaries certain health-protection services, such as immunization services for children and adequate health facilities. Coping efforts may also include strict zoning laws and housing codes or certain values such as sex education within the home.

An example of goods that a community might dispose of into the environment include industrial and human wastes. Data can be obtained through minutes of meetings, public documents, health surveys, statistical data, and health records.

Values-Beliefs Pattern

This pattern identifies the values and beliefs of a community. Such information can provide clues to the health-promotion and health-protection efforts that the community values and is willing to support.

Values underlie decisions about whether the community should have health education in the schools, hypertension

---

CASE STUDY

Community Efforts to Decrease Adolescent Pregnancy Rates

The community health nurse is facilitating a grassroots community group that is determined to decrease the adolescent pregnancy rate in the city. The community population hovers around 100,000. It is a community that lies on the Mexican border of the United States. The population is predominantly Mexican American, and there is a high poverty rate.

The schools offer health courses twice between seventh and twelfth grades. The only formal sex education provided occurs within the context of these two health courses. There is community opposition to increasing the amount of sex education in the curriculum. A community group that has researched the problem has decided to use a social marketing approach because of this community resistance.

Most of the materials reviewed do not address the cultural needs of the region. Many of the Spanish language materials use Spanish from countries other than Mexico. The situations posed in the audiovisual materials show people who the adolescents will perceive as different from themselves.

Reflective Questions

1. How could the community group approach their goal to decrease the adolescent pregnancy rate in a manner that will be culturally competent?
2. How might the community group approach this issue without the support of the school district?

---

screening for the general public, prevention programs, or well-child clinics and how much of the community's tax money will be allocated for health-related activities. Traditions, norms, and cultural and ethnic groups all share in identifying the values and beliefs of a community. Data can be obtained through interviews with key community members and health-related personnel.

ANALYSIS AND DIAGNOSIS WITH THE COMMUNITY

Analysis refers to the categorization of data and the determination of patterns. Once information about a community is obtained, the data must be organized and synthesized in a meaningful way to ascertain patterns of health activities and trends. An example of a clinical scenario about a particular community is presented in the Case Study. Decision making and judgment inherent in the nursing process are particularly significant during the analysis and diagnostic phases. Community data can be grouped and organized in several ways. Table 8-1 presents an example of one way to organize community data using Prochaska's stages of change.

Organization of Data

Data can be synthesized using various techniques, such as charts, figures, and tables. Graphic presentations of population distributions, morbidity and mortality data, or vital

Table **8-1** Stages of Change	
Stages	**Interventions**
Precontemplation	Provide information (identify risk factors)
	Raise doubts about current behaviors and future outcomes
Contemplation	Discuss risks of not changing
	Discuss benefits of changing
Action	Help plan phases of change
	Help implement phases of change
Maintenance	Help develop strategies to prevent relapse, emphasizing self-efficacy
	Offer encouragement
Relapse	Highlight past successes and future benefits

Modified from Norcross, J. C., & Prochaska, J. O. (2002). Using the stages of change. *Harvard Mental Health Letter, 18*(11), 11-13.

statistics can be most effective in pinpointing significant community concerns and actual or potential health problems. The data are then compared with the community health-related responses to these concerns.

Mapping is another valuable technique that facilitates data analysis. For example, data that change with time can be followed with a series of maps; several variables that may be spatially identical and contiguous can be analyzed simultaneously, such as the location of environmental hazards, densely populated areas, health-promotion services, and major highways. Poor environmental conditions; the distribution of illness, disease, and death rates; and the accessibility of health-protection and health-promotion activities for the population can be determined at a glance with dotted scatter maps. When maps are used, the population base of the community must be identified. For example, a less populated geographical area might have fewer health facilities for its residents than another area; one community might have fewer neonatal deaths than another because it has fewer women of childbearing age.

The use of theoretical frameworks and the 11 pattern areas will facilitate the organization and analysis of community data. Several guidelines are presented to help the community nurse analyze population data. Analysis often supports the need for further data collection.

Guidelines for Data Analysis
Check for Missing Data

The community nurse cannot obtain all possible facts about the health-related pattern areas because of the complexity, size, and number of community characteristics that must be considered. However, missing or insufficient data that indicate areas in need of further assessment should be identified. Additional assessment may be necessary to determine specific approaches or a particular community diagnosis. Missing data in a community assessment might include pollution indices, links between health resources and population groups, accessibility to resources, and morbidity

statistics, all of which may be necessary to determine actual or potential health concerns. Census data may not be current, which should be noted. Missing data are generally indicated in a nursing diagnosis.

The nurse examines community data for incongruities; it is common to obtain conflicting information. For example, a key community official might deny the existence of pollutants in the water supply, whereas newspaper reports of the health department's water analysis findings indicate otherwise. The nurse validates such inconsistencies before identifying existing or potential health concerns.

Identify Patterns

The subjective and objective data of the assessment are examined for clues to determine whether a **community pattern** emerges or a clustering of information occurs. During this stage, the community nurse makes decisions and begins to formulate diagnostic hypotheses (ideas and tentative judgments about possible health concerns), identify community groups that might be at risk, and establish probable causes and relationships. This activity directs the search for additional clues in the data to confirm, reject, or revise the hypotheses generated. Judgments or hypotheses are generated constantly in the selection of clues that could form patterns in the data or relationships. For example, in obtaining interview data, the community nurse may have generated hypotheses that directed the search for additional information or may have determined the need for education programs within the community.

Community nurses can become overwhelmed by the data collected. They must narrow the huge list of possible community health-promotion and health-protection concerns. One approach is to formulate broad problem statements based on the health-related pattern areas (Gordon, 1994). For example, does the community have an elimination problem (noxious chemicals), a coping and stress-tolerance problem (inability to obtain a particular health education program), or a health perception–health management problem (high teenage mortality rate from motor vehicle accidents)? Asking such broad questions will help direct the nurse to clues in the database.

Apply Theories, Models, Norms, and Standards

Analyzing community data requires a broad knowledge of developmental and age-related risks and theories and concepts of nursing, public health, and epidemiology. This base enables the nurse to search for additional clues in the health-related patterns to develop community nursing diagnoses amenable to nursing interventions.

The developmental approach can be used as a basis for identifying groups with potential health concerns. Different age groups vary in susceptibility; therefore, the nurse must examine the community's resources to determine if they are directing services to highly susceptible groups. For example, community data may indicate an increase in live births among older women, which may indicate a need for additional health-promotion services for this group. If community data show an increasing number of aging citizens, the nurse should explore the availability and accessibility of existing health services.

Data are also analyzed for population groups according to common personal or environmental characteristics. For example, the nurse may identify select groups at risk based on a shared health concern, such as substance abuse, lack of immunizations, unsafe housing conditions, high exposure to asbestos or noxious chemicals, or inadequate health services. A shared characteristic, such as race, may provide clues to susceptible groups in need of particular screening activities. A black population may need screening for hypertension if such services are lacking, and children may be susceptible to dental caries and require screening if fluoridated water systems are lacking.

Other groups may suffer from illiteracy. The literacy of a community is critical to health-promotion activities, because it determines the methods used by nurses in establishing educational programs. These factors may limit the nurse's ability to use all available resources to promote health. Environmental information is readily available on the Internet. Databases and search engines may provide useful information about environmental hazards or other environmental problems in communities. Prevention of disease worldwide depends on the dissemination of global environmental health information (USDHHS, 2000).

Standards are used to analyze data (USDHHS, 2000; Workplace Health Strategies Bureau, 2002). For example, community data regarding air can be compared with state or national ambient air quality standards to determine health. The term *ambient* in this context refers to outside air in a town, city, or other defined region. Air-monitoring stations are generally located in urban and rural areas within each state. One source for air quality information is the Center for Health Policy Studies at the University of Texas Health Science Center at the Houston School of Public Health. The goal of this center is to serve as a resource for information for health policy analysis and research. The Web address is *http://www.sph.uth.tmc.edu/library/charting_ onestop.htm.* The data and links to other sites are continually monitored and updated.

After exploring data concerning health perception–health management, the nurse determines the community resources that are directed toward preventing risk factors and health problems. In this way, gaps in health-promotion and health-protection services can be identified more readily.

Identify Strengths and Health Concerns

Community data are analyzed and interpreted in light of community strengths and concerns and within obtainable limits of certainty. This requires making judgments and inferences about the community's health, responses to health situations and conditions, and population needs. One approach is to assume that health concerns exist unless the assessment data indicate otherwise (Gordon, 1994).

Table 8-2 Examples of Community Strengths and Concerns

Strengths	Concerns
Well-child clinic available	Unavailable
Elderly feeding program accessible	Inaccessible
Sex education in schools acceptable	Unacceptable
Family planning services accessible	Inaccessible
Fluoridated water system	Nonfluoridated water system
Open communication	Dysfunctional communication
Interagency cooperation	Dysfunctional transactions
Adequate kitchen and plumbing facilities	Inadequate
High interest of key leaders in health promotion	Lack of interest

To make a diagnosis, the community nurse summarizes the data and then uses the nursing process first posed by Yura and Walsh (1983) to make one or more of the following judgments:

1. No problem exists, but providing health-promotion or health-protection services may affect a potential health concern. For example, providing health education in the high school could offset a potential for increased sexually transmitted disease in the high school population.
2. A problem exists but is recognized by community members or health-related professionals and is being handled effectively.
3. A problem exists that has been recognized by the community, but resources are inadequate or the community has not responded. Assistance is needed.
4. A problem exists that the community recognizes but cannot cope with at this time, such as a lack of fluoridated water systems. Dentists, nurses, and nutritionists could be assigned to assist the community in resolving actual problems of dental caries.
5. A problem or potential health concern exists that needs further study.

A community may have much strength. Identifying strengths is important, because they can be integrated into plans for health-promotion and health-protection activities. For example, a community may have many nutritional feeding programs for its older adults, women, and children. On the other hand, they may be underutilized. Community members may not know about them because communication is inadequate. Examples of community strengths and concerns are shown in Table 8-2.

Identify Causes and Risk Factors

In this step, the data are examined for those factors or characteristics that contribute to the list of identified potential and existing health-related concerns. The nurse makes inferences about various population groups, identifying factors that place them at risk. For example, children entering elementary school may be at risk for rubella and mumps

Comparing Poverty Rates by Racial and Ethnic Categories

Comparisons must take into account that racial and ethnic census categories were redefined in 2002. Blacks constitute 12.9 % of the population (reported as black or African American). This number and those that follow include the 0.6% of the population who reported as black as well as one or more other races. Although blacks are represented in every socioeconomic group, 24.1% live in poverty. This is a rate 3 times higher than the non-Hispanic white American rate (8.0%). Among people who reported themselves as being Asian American, 10.3% lived in poverty. Poverty rates have remained the same for non-Hispanic whites and Asians when compared to the closest available data groupings from 2001. However, the poverty figures among people who reported being black in 2002 show that there was an increase (U.S. Census Bureau, 2003).

Based on these figures, it seems that poverty is rising in the black population. Most of the black population (54%) lived in the South according to Census 2000. The remaining 46% was spread out over the rest of the United States. In areas other than the South, concentrations of the black population were located in urban areas (McKinnon, 2000).

From McKinnon, J. (2000). *The black population 2000: Census briefs* (No. C2KBR/01-5). Washington, DC: U.S. Census Bureau; and U.S. Census Bureau. (2003). Current population survey: Poverty: 2002 highlights. Retrieved May 14, 2004, from: *http://www.census.gov/hhes/poverty/poverty02/pov02hi.html.*

related to inadequate health-protection services in the community (a health-management deficit in the community). Identification of the risk factors gives direction to community nursing actions. Some risk factors may signify an immediate health concern for a population group, such as polluted water supplies; others may indicate a potential health problem if they are not altered, such as a lack of knowledge about childhood disease prevention.

In identifying **community risk factors,** the nurse must consider what risk factors have the potential to be altered, eliminated, or controlled through nursing actions. Some factors, such as the age, race, and gender of a population, cannot be altered; others, such as a lack of health education programs, can be altered to lower a particular group's risk to potentially harmful health situations or conditions (Multicultural Awareness box).

Community Diagnosis

A community assessment, as previously described, culminates in a nursing diagnosis or diagnoses. The process of determining a **community diagnosis** includes (1) a community situation or state within a population or population group, (2) data collection using some combination of observation, interview, and measurement, (3) a framework, (4) existing or potential health concerns, (5) risk factors related to the health concerns, and (6) a requirement for nursing actions. A diagnosis becomes the basis for planning and

implementing interventions and nursing actions and for making evaluative judgments about health concerns (North American Nursing Diagnosis Association [NANDA], 2003; Sparks, 2004). The Hot Topics box and the Health Teaching box discuss a diagnosis of violence and some recommendations to reduce the problem.

A community diagnosis is stated in a clear and concise manner to facilitate communication among community health professionals, team members, and laypeople. Lists of community diagnostic categories specific to certain populations are being developed (Anderson & McFarlane, 2004; NANDA, 2003; Sparks, 2004). Community health nurses need to continue developing diagnostic statements that are community and population centered, specific, accurate, and amenable to nursing interventions. A diagnosis may be written or stated according to the structural and functional aspects of a community.

Structural aspects include those related to the population, such as the demographic characteristics of groups that have similar characteristics (preschool children, adolescents, or a high school population). Functional aspects include those related to the psychosocial, physiological, or spiritual health patterns, such as decision making (cognitive-perceptual pattern) or communication links among health care resources (roles-relationships pattern). Information about health concerns and risk factors is obtained from the 11 functional health patterns. The structural and functional aspects of the community provide a framework from which diagnostic statements can be made (see Chapter 6).

PLANNING WITH THE COMMUNITY

The community health planning phase begins with the nursing diagnosis. The desired goals are expected to resolve existing or potential health concerns. For example, if a high rate of childhood diseases in the community is the problem, decreasing the rate is the goal. Identification of the specific or potential health concern and planned actions to achieve the desired **community outcome** become the framework and data for **community evaluation.** Therefore, health planning can be viewed as a problem-solving approach that has several purposes.

Purposes

The four major purposes of the planning phase are the following:
1. To prioritize the problems diagnosed from the assessment phase
2. To differentiate problems that nursing actions can resolve from those that others can handle best
3. To identify immediate, intermediate, and long-term goals, behavior objectives oriented to community behavior and derived from the goals, and the specific actions to achieve the objectives
4. To write the problems, actions, and expected behavioral outcomes in a community nursing care plan (Care Plan)

WORKPLACE VIOLENCE

HOTtopics

The terrorist attacks on September 11, 2001, or 9/11, were a tragic reminder that targets often chosen by the terrorists are not military in nature. Targets may be places where people work to support their families. Workplace violence was put in a new context that day. Before then, workplace violence was considered as isolated unplanned incidents that fell under the jurisdiction of the federal Occupational Safety and Health Administration (OSHA). Since 9/11 workplace violence prevention and preparation has included external threats of terrorism. With these new issues in mind a document called *Workplace Violence: Issues in Response* was prepared to assist in prevention and management of potential workplace violence. The recommendations from this report included the following general categories:

1. Public awareness campaigns
2. Workplace policies and plans
3. Preventive law enforcement
4. Government agencies making workplace violence a priority
5. Training
6. Protection of the abused person when domestic violence or stalking occurs in the workplace
7. Development and distribution of clear and comprehensive legal and legislative guidelines
8. Evaluation of programs and strategies
   Suggestions for approaches included the following strategies:
   • Educational efforts should reflect cooperative efforts by government agencies, major corporations, unions, and advocacy groups, with OSHA acting as a facilitator and coordinator.

• Put multidisciplinary no-threats–no-violence policies and prevention plans in place.
• Violence prevention training should occur regularly and include practicing the plan.
• Work space and policies should provide a physically secure work environment.
• Preventive measures should be in place including documenting incidents, antiviolence planning, and conducting threat assessments.
• Systems should be developed for monitoring incidents of workplace violence.
• Resource lists should be maintained and include social service, mental health, legal, and other agencies that provide assistance.
• Training programs should extend community policing concepts to workplace violence.
• Government or private organizations should develop training materials for small employers.
• Employers should keep the abuser out of the workplace (e.g., screening telephone calls, making the victim's work space physically more secure, instructing security guards or receptionists).
• Employers should provide resources for emotional, financial, and legal counseling.
• Clear, comprehensive, and uniform legal guidelines should be distributed widely.
• Incentives for employers should be identified and instituted.

From Rugala, E. A., Isaacs, A. R., Hinojosa, I. (2002). *Workplace violence: Issues in response.* Washington, DC: U.S. Department of Justice, Federal Bureau of Investigation. Retrieved May 14, 2004, from: *http://www.fbi.gov/publications/violence.pdf.*

HEALTH TEACHING   Intervention Techniques to Prevent and Diffuse Workplace Violence

Recognize warning signs, which include changes in mood, personal hardships, mental health issues (e.g., depression, anxiety), negative behavior (e.g., untrustworthy, lying, bad attitude), verbal threats, and history of violence. Do not limit at-risk behavior to a standard profile. Environments should be designed to detect signs of impending violence and to prevent violence with security cameras, key card access, administrative controls, and behavioral strategies. Reporting systems should be confidential and seamless.

• Stay calm; create a relaxed environment and speak calmly.
• Separate the individual from the group, if possible.
• Use nonthreatening body language; build trust and strengthen the relationship.

• Keep your verbal communication simple, clear, and direct; be open and honest.
• Reflect on the person's message to allow time for clarification, allow the person to verbalize, listen attentively, and stop what you are doing and give full attention.
• Ask for examples to help illustrate the points that are being made. Carefully define the problem, exploring with open-ended questions.
• Silence allows the individual time to clarify thoughts.
• Monitor the tone, volume, rate, and rhythm of your speech.
• Seek opportunities for agreement.
• Be creative and open to new ideas.

Compiled from Kohn, C., Henderson, C.W. (2003). Critical warning signs of workplace violence are not what employees expect. *Managed Care Weekly Digest;* DelBel, J. (2003). De-escalating workplace aggression. *Nursing Management, 34(9);* Occupational Safety and Health Administration. (2004). *Preventing workplace violence for health care and social service workers.* Washington, DC: U.S. Department of Labor. Retrieved February 20, 2005, from: *http://www.osha.gov/Publications/osha3148.pdf;* and Crisis Prevention Institute. (2003). Retrieved February 20, 2005, from: *http://www.crisisprevention.com/index.html.*

CARE PLAN

Community Efforts to Decrease Adolescent Pregnancy Rates

(Related to Case Study About Community Efforts to Decrease Adolescent Pregnancy Rates)

Nursing Diagnosis Ineffective Community Coping Related to Increased Levels of Teen Pregnancy

DEFINING CHARACTERISTICS

- Absence of education or support for sexually active teenagers
- Absence of programs for pregnancy testing, counseling, or teaching young women to care for infants
- Absence of sex education in the home, school, and community
- Community conflicts over what to teach adolescent and preadolescent children about sex
- Failure of teenagers to perceive long-term effects of having babies
- High incidence of infants who are born prematurely or with health problems
- High rate of teen pregnancy
- Lack of access to birth control pills or devices for teenagers
- Lack of community support for preventive sex education

RELATED FACTORS

- Community members' lack of knowledge about causes and contributing factors in teen pregnancy
- Inadequate community resources for preventing teen pregnancy
- Lack of adequate communication patterns and community cohesiveness regarding strategies to prevent teen pregnancy

EXPECTED OUTCOMES

- Community members express awareness of the seriousness of the high adolescent pregnancy rate in their community.
- Community members express the need for a plan to reduce the prevalence of teen pregnancies.
- Community members develop and implement plans to prevent teen pregnancy.
- Community members evaluate the success of the plan in meeting goals and objectives.
- Community members continue to revise the plan to prevent teen pregnancy as necessary.

INTERVENTIONS

- Assess teenagers' knowledge about sex and sexuality to determine their educational needs.
- Work with schools to develop pregnancy prevention programs that provide adolescents with information about the risks, problems, and complications of early pregnancy.
- Work closely with individual adolescents who are pregnant to assess their needs and provide care.
- Implement an outreach and health-promotion program to raise community members' awareness of the need to approach teen pregnancy as a community problem. Consider taking the following five steps:

1. Work with teachers, school psychologists, counselors, school nurses, students, and the parent-teacher association to determine the extent of the teen pregnancy problem.
2. Encourage local youth groups, churches, and social service organizations to feature presentations on pregnancy prevention at their meetings.
3. Contact representatives of local corporations to ask for funding for educational programs.
4. Help community members (school nurses, counselors, and teachers) recognize adolescent girls who need counseling regarding such issues as peer pressure to be sexually active and the long-term consequences of pregnancy. Remind community members of the importance of listening attentively and remaining nonjudgmental.
5. Provide education on birth control measures (including abstinence from sex) and make this information available at school.

- Establish clubs for adolescent girls in the community. The goal of these clubs is to foster self-esteem. During club meetings, members should have the opportunity to openly discuss difficult questions, such as why girls consider a baby a status symbol and how to respond to peer pressure to be sexually active. Improved self-esteem has been found the most effective way to reduce teen pregnancy rates.
- Encourage adolescents to participate in peer support networks where they can openly discuss social and dating pressure and other issues related to teen pregnancy, to allow them an opportunity to express their feelings openly and obtain support from peers.
- Encourage community members to establish school-based clinics in which teens can have access to reproductive system models, pregnancy tests, and nonprescription birth control measures to support the teenagers who make the decision to protect themselves from unwanted pregnancies.
- Develop a list of referrals for teenagers, such as hospitals with human sexuality courses, charities that provide prenatal care and childbirth services, women's clinics, and Planned Parenthood, to compensate for restricted access to information in the adolescent's home or school.
- Encourage community members to implement an information campaign to educate adolescents, parents, and community members about the problems associated with teen pregnancy.
- Work with community members to evaluate the effectiveness of the teen pregnancy prevention program and assist in modifying it as needed to ensure its effectiveness and promote the program as a model for preventive health.
- Collect statistical data from the schools to analyze the teen pregnancy rates, to help evaluate the effectiveness of the prevention program.

Modified from Carpenito-Moyet, L. J. (2004). *Handbook of nursing diagnosis* (10th ed.). Philadelphia: Lippincott Williams & Wilkins.

The planning phase culminates in a nursing plan that provides the framework for evaluation. Once developed, the plan is implemented.

The cost of delivering health services, the kinds of personnel involved, and the financial resources available will influence the priority given to health concerns, as will community values and the nurse's philosophy about people, health, the community, and nursing. Examples of problems to be given high priority in some communities are infectious agents, sexually transmitted disease, alcohol and drug use, smoking, inadequate nutrition, inadequate infant and child care, high death rate from motor vehicle accidents, and unwanted teenage pregnancies.

Community participation in health planning is essential to help assign priorities. As recipients of health-related services, members can help ensure that the services being planned are of reasonable cost and high quality. Community residents can help ascertain the benefits sought by groups in need and determine whether the planned health services will be appropriate to the needs and concerns of the population for whom they are intended. If community members and the nurse differ in setting priorities, communication and a statement of the reasons for designating a particular priority can help resolve the difference.

When planning, the nurse must differentiate those problems that **community nursing intervention,** a behavior implemented by the nurse to fulfill a health goal of the community, can resolve from those health concerns that could best be handled by community members, referred to health-related professionals, or handled with community support. Rodents, poor sanitation conditions, or the absence of community recreational facilities should be referred to appropriate community leaders or agencies.

Developing goals, measurable behavioral outcomes, or objectives and designating those actions that will achieve the expected outcomes are important nursing activities. Outcomes are projected before the actual implementation of planned actions and are stated in terms of the individual behaviors that are expected to result from nursing actions. The effectiveness of nursing actions must be evaluated.

Health planning emphasizes promoting and protecting the health of population groups within the community; therefore, problems, solutions, and actions are defined on this level. Community nurses who plan and implement health plans for one community population group, such as school-aged children, help the community to begin developing health-promotion services for all residents. Nurses frequently act as agents of change by taking responsibility for influencing and changing existing and potential health patterns and behavior. Decisions and plans for health interventions are based on the community nurse's awareness and understanding of human behavior and principles of planned change. **Web Site Resource 8B** offers guidelines for interventions with one population group: ethnic elders.

Planned Change

Planned change is the result of efforts by individuals or groups and involves fundamental shifts in their behavior (Prochaska, Norcross, & DiClemente, 1994). Individuals can be the agents of their own health conditions; health is often determined more by what the person does than by what some outside infectious agent can do. Some important community health objectives depend partly on individuals deciding to change their lifestyles (reducing alcohol consumption or giving up smoking).

Efforts to influence and reinforce changes in community health behavior are the central focus if risk reduction programs are to be effective. Any change effort by community nurses and groups can be viewed as a process.

Many studies have tried to explain why some groups of people effectively participate in certain health programs or make lifestyle changes, whereas others do not. The early health belief model proposed by Rosenstock (1974) and more recent models developed by Pender (Pender, Murdaugh, & Parsons, 2001) and Norcross and Prochaska (2002), among others, identify concepts that are critical to understanding how individuals undergo a change in health behavior. In Rosenstock's model, the following four steps are identified:

1. Perceiving the behavior as a threat to health in terms of susceptibility and seriousness
2. Believing the behavior is a threat to health
3. Taking action to adopt preventive health behaviors
4. Reinforcing the new behavior

In this model, the consumer at first takes a passive role; the transition from passive to active occurs between steps two and three (belief to action). If the ultimate goal is to improve the health of a community through risk reduction programs, community members need to be influenced so that they will assume more responsibility for their health and become more active in adopting healthy lifestyles and behaviors. In planning health-promotion activities, the nurse must consider effective strategies to motivate and support the community's transition from a passive to an active state.

Once the plan is developed, it becomes a guide to nursing actions. The nurse must make additions and changes based on the community's problems, resources, and resolution of these problems to keep the plan viable. Table 8-3 gives an example of a community-oriented, health-promotion plan based on the goals recommended by the surgeon general's report on health promotion and disease prevention. As shown, several specific objectives have been derived from a broad goal. The objectives' direction is based on the nursing diagnosis, which includes risk factors that can be altered.

Examples of various rationales in Table 8-3 show how the nurse can incorporate important concepts of planned change into a community-based health-promotion plan.

Communicating the plans to other health professionals, community members, and key officials should not be over-

Table **8-3** Implementation of Community Health Plan With Objectives and Rationale

Nursing Diagnosis: Potential for increasing the incidence of fatal motor vehicle accidents in high school population related to alcohol use and driving. *Goal:* North High School population will have reduced incidence (at least 20%) of fatal motor vehicle accidents related to alcohol use and abuse by December.

Objective	Plans	Rationale
1. Community will have access to information about the incidence of fatal motor vehicle accidents and drunken driving arrests of its high school population for the past 5 years by March.	Interview local police about the incidence of fatal auto accidents and substance abuse in the community. Interview parents of deceased high school students, students, teachers, physicians, clergy, and emergency room personnel about the incidence of the problem and suggested measures for decreasing the incidence; suggest that interviews be broadcast over the high school radio station. Have several people write to the community newspaper commenting on the broadcast and the problem.	*Unfreezing:* For change to occur, the community has to become dissatisfied with status quo and sense a need for change. *Empiric-rational strategy:* People are rational; discussion of facts can bring about support for change. Important elements for preventing the problem include educating the public and having key community leaders discuss their views; concern lends credibility and is necessary for action. People tend to listen to those with informal power. Keeping the issue before the community can raise consciousness.
2. Community will take action to inform the population at risk about responsible drinking and driving by June.	Suggest to school principal and school board the creation of a task force of community residents to plan a health program on individual responsibility and alcohol use in high school. Task force should include teachers, students, parents, clergy, police, nurse, and physician. Task force will examine ways to determine and teach content, integrate it into the curriculum, and recommend that community members, such as a nurse, be involved in teaching content.	*Changing:* Moving to a new level; community involvement will influence acceptability of changes. Community residents like to be involved in decision making. It is important to establish trust and collaboration between community groups; this opens communication channels between adolescents and the health community. Community involvement facilitates acceptance of change.
3. Community will implement an educational program for its high school population related to the use of alcohol and individual responsibility.	Implement educational plan.	*Refreezing:* Moving to the level of change brought about by community forces. Educational strategies built around the concept of individual responsibility are essential elements in promoting the health of young adults.

looked; this is an essential aspect of planning. An article describing the educational plan can be published in local newspapers and bulletins, and school officials can send letters to students' parents.

Other community-based actions in which the nurse may become involved to change alcohol abuse in the community are listed in Box 8-1. The various plans have been categorized according to the health patterns to show that a community problem can be approached from many directions. Plans that are feasible and well formulated help prepare for implementation (USDHHS, 1993).

Box **8-1** Plan Options for Community-Based Action: Alcohol Abuse

COPING–STRESS TOLERANCE PATTERN

Identify community alcohol treatment resources.

Develop local alcohol control laws oriented toward prevention of abuse; develop consistent state regulation and control laws.

ROLES-RELATIONSHIPS PATTERN

Increase communication among community control agencies, the school, residents, and health-related agencies.

Restrict community advertisements for alcohol in local newsletters and newspapers.

Table 8-4 Potential Sources of Resistance to Health-Promotion Programs, With Agent Responses	
Source of Resistance	**Response**
Lack of communication about the implementation of the program	Communicate through community newsletter, newspapers, high school radio station, and posters
Misinformation regarding time and place of health activity	Disseminate valid information
Fear of the unknown	Inform and encourage
Need for security	Clarify intentions and methods
No desired need to change behaviors	Demonstrate opportunity for change
Cultural or religious beliefs or vested interests threatened	Enlist key community leaders in planning change
Inaccessibility	Focus activities near the largest target population and in an area accessible by public transportation

IMPLEMENTATION WITH THE COMMUNITY

Once the plan for health-promotion and health-protection activities has been developed, implementation of the nursing process begins. The plan may be implemented by the community nurse alone or with team members and community residents and tested for viability. Its success or failure will depend on the nurse's intellectual, interpersonal, and technical skills and the plan's acceptability to community members.

Resistance to change usually must be overcome for the planned intervention to be successful. However, resistance to new health-promotion and health-protection activities is feedback that can be used constructively. People generally resist change when they are defending something important that appears to be threatened by the change. Table 8-4 lists several factors identified as deterrents to community participation in health programs. An informed nurse takes steps to deal with such factors to ensure the successful implementation of the plan. The nurse recognizes that community members may resist the type of planned activities or the individuals promoting them. Others resist changing their own attitudes or lifestyle behaviors.

Community nurses implement health-promotion and health-protection plans in a variety of community settings (including schools, industry, public and private health agencies, and ambulatory care settings) where various population groups are relatively healthy. Nursing centers provide nursing faculty, staff, and students some unique opportunities to assess health and plan, implement, and evaluate care (including holistic health promotion and primary health care) to individuals, families, and communities with unmet health care needs (Chiverton, Votava, & Tortoretti, 2003; Johnson, 2001; Schoneman, 2002; Van Zandt, D'Lugoff, & Kelley, 2002). The simplicity or complexity of implementing health actions will vary from one community or population group to another. As the nursing plan is implemented, nurses also learn more about the community and their own responses, strengths, limitations, and abilities to cope and adapt.

Although the implementation phase has an action focus, it also includes assessment, planning, and evaluation activities to monitor the actions taken to resolve, reduce, eliminate, or control the health concern.

EVALUATION WITH THE COMMUNITY

Evaluation is the phase of the nursing process in which the community nurse learns whether the actions designated in the nursing plan actually achieved the desired outcomes. The community and the nurse determine the community's progress or lack of progress toward goal achievement (American Nurses Association, 2003). The nurse is responsible for the evaluation data, although community members or health team members may participate in the process. For example, if a reduction in the incidence of fatal motor vehicle accidents is expected to result from nursing actions, the nurse is responsible for obtaining the community's behavioral outcomes data, which should show that a reduction has occurred and that nursing actions helped bring about these outcomes.

The nursing plan, which includes the nursing diagnosis, expected outcomes, and interventions, provides the framework for evaluation. The community is the focus; its goals and objectives define what is evaluated, and they are considered in terms of how the community responded to the planned actions. For example, if a reduction in childhood disease rates is expected after nursing actions, the nurse compares community responses before and after the actions. This also determines whether nursing actions are completely effective, partly effective, or ineffective in achieving the desired goal.

Evaluation is an ongoing process and is approached in a purposeful, goal-directed manner (Rootman, 2001; USDHHS, 2000). Determining the effect of nursing actions during and after implementation is an important element in evaluating the degree to which goals are achieved. The frequency of evaluation will depend on the situation, the changes expected, and the objectives. For example, an individual who is bleeding may need to be evaluated every 15 minutes for signs of change, whereas evaluation of behavioral changes in community groups is not usually so immediate. In any population group, existing or potential health problems will be resolved or controlled within different intervals. Evaluation is determined by immediate, intermediate, and long-range goals; the process is continued until the goals are realized.

The results of the community nursing plan evaluation are also important because they may indicate the need to reassess, revise, or modify the plan. Community planning and nursing actions are not always effective in achieving the goals related to the health concerns and needs of the community (as noted, resistance to change may play an important role). As a result, the community nurse reassesses the situation and plans a new approach, then implements and evaluates the revised plan. The nursing process is a continual cycle.

Equally important is the community nurse's self-evaluation to determine strengths and weaknesses or how the nursing plan might have been implemented more effectively or efficiently. The quality of health-promotion and health-protection services to a community depends on the professional qualities of those providing the services and their effective use of the nursing process.

Effective programs of community health promotion are needed. However, skyrocketing health care costs limit resources. During this time of dramatic health care reforms, nurses need to increase the support for community health-promotion programs by demonstrating their effectiveness. Schoneman's study (2002) examines surveillance as an intervention provided by nurses and documents its efficacy. Effectiveness is determined through research studies, such as this one, that include analyses and outcome evaluation of home-based and community-centered nursing interventions designed to meet needs of high-risk families, geographical communities, and vulnerable populations. Evidence-based practice and research are needed to gain support from legislators for community health-promotion programs. In addition, *Healthy People 2010 Toolkit: A Field Guide to Health Planning* (Baker, Conrad, Bechamps, & Barry, 2002) includes examples of national and state partnerships setting health objectives and sustaining the initiatives.

SUMMARY

Illness, disability, and disease are not inevitable events that are experienced equally among a community's members.

Understanding the dynamic and complex nature of communities is an important function of the community nurse if planning, delivery, and coordination of health-promotion and health-protection activities for high-risk populations are to be effective.

The nurse uses various theoretical frameworks to assess the community's health-related patterns, health concerns, and health action potential and to implement the nursing process. Community data are collected and analyzed so that subpopulations at risk can be identified and so that health-promotion and health-protection services can be directed most profitably. These activities are enhanced through the nursing process.

Many communities have obvious deficiencies in health services that warrant health planning action. Community nurses play a significant role in health planning that is directed toward reducing risks associated with disease, premature death, and injury and promoting the health of community members. Principles of planned change are used to increase the community's awareness of health, healthy behavior, and participation in preventive health services.

The simplicity or complexity of applying the nursing process will vary from one community or geographical area to another. Community nurses must research the relation of particular health-promotion actions to specific community phenomena to provide the necessary scientific evidence to support the benefits of nursing actions.

ADDITIONAL STUDY MATERIAL

Study Questions *in the back of the book, see page 663.*

evolve **WEB SITE MATERIALS**

These materials are located on the book's Web site at http://evolve.elsevier.com/Edelman/.

- WebLinks
- Content Updates
- Web Site Resources

8A Functional Health Patterns: Data Collection Guide to Community Assessment
8B Guidelines for Nursing Interventions for Ethnic Elders

REFERENCES

American Nurses Association. (2003). *Nursing's social policy statement* (2nd ed.). Washington, DC: American Nurses Association.

Anderson, E. T., & McFarlane, J. (2004). *Community as partner* (4th ed.). Philadelphia: Lippincott Williams & Wilkins.

Baker, S., Conrad, D., Bechamps, M., & Barry, M. (2002). *Healthy people 2010 toolkit* (Government Rep.). Washington, DC: Public Health Foundation.

Brener, N. D., Burstein, G. R., DuShaw, M. L., Vernon, M. E., Wheeler, L. & Robinson, J. (2001). Health services:

results from the school health policies and programs study 2000. *Journal of School Health, 71*(7), 294.

Chiverton, P. A., Votava, K. M., & Tortoretti, D. M. (2003). The future role of nursing in health promotion. *American Journal of Health Promotion, 18*(2), 192.

Clark, M. J. (2003). *Community health nursing: Caring for populations* (4th ed.). Upper Saddle River, NJ: Prentice Hall.

Gordon, M. (1994). *Nursing diagnosis: Process and application* (3rd ed.). St. Louis: Mosby.

Johnson, M. O. (2001). Meeting health care needs of a vulnerable population: perceived barriers. *Journal of Community Health Nursing, 18*(1), 35.

Kohn, C., & Henderson, C. W. (2003, December 23). Critical warning signs of workplace violence are not what employees expect. *Managed Care Weekly Digest,* 100.

McKinnon, J. (2000). *The black population 2000: Census briefs* (No. C2KBR/01-5). Washington, DC: U.S. Census Bureau.

Newman, M. A. (2002). The pattern that connects. *ANS Advances in Nursing Science, 24*(3), 1.

Norcross, J. C., & Prochaska, J. O. (2002). Using the stages of change. *Harvard Mental Health Letter, 18*(11), 5.

North American Nursing Diagnosis Association. (2003). *NANDA Nursing diagnosis 2003-2004: Definitions and classifications.* Chicago: North American Nursing Diagnosis Association.

Pender, N. J., Murdaugh, C., & Parsons, M. A. (2001). *Health promotion in nursing practice* (4th ed.). Saddle River, NJ: Prentice Hall.

Prochaska, J. O., Norcoss J. C., & Diclemente, C. C. (1994). *Changing for good.* New York: Avon.

Rootman, I. (2001). I. Rootman, M. Goodstadt, B. Hyndman, D. V. McQueen, L. Potvin, J. Springett, et al. (Eds.), *Evaluation in health promotion: principles and perspectives.* Copenhagen: World Health Organization.

Rosenstock, I. (1974). The health belief model and preventive health behavior. *Health Education Monographs, 2,* 354.

Schoneman, D. (2002). Surveillance as a nursing intervention: Use in community nursing centers. *Journal of Community Health Nursing, 19*(1), 33.

Smith, K., & Bazini-Barakat, N. (2003). A public health nursing practice model: Melding public health principles with the nursing process. *Public Health Nursing, 20*(1), 42.

Sparks, S. M. (2004). *Nursing diagnosis reference manual* (6th ed.). Springhouse, PA: Springhouse Publishing.

Taras, H. L., Frankowski, B. L., McGrath, J. W., Mears, C., Murray, R. D., & Young, T. (2001). The role of the school nurse in providing school health services, *Pediatrics, 108*(5), 1231.

U.S. Census Bureau. (2003). *Current population survey: Poverty—2002 highlights.* Retrieved May 14, 2004, from: *http://www.census.gov/hhes/poverty/poverty02/pov02hi.html.*

U.S. Department of Health and Human Services. (1993). *Planned approach to community health: Guide for the local coordinator* (Government Rep.). Atlanta, GA: U.S. Department of Health and Human Services, Centers for Disease Control and Prevention.

U.S. Department of Health and Human Services. (2000). *Healthy people 2010: Understanding and improving health* (Publication No. 017-001-001-00-550-9). Washington, DC: U.S. Government Printing Office, Superintendent of Documents.

Van Zandt, S. E., D'Lugoff, M. I., & Kelley, L. (2002). A community-based free nursing clinic's approach to management of health problems for the uninsured: the hepatitis C example. *Family & Community Health, 25*(3), 61.

Von Bertalanffy, L. (1976). *General systems theory: Foundations, development, applications* (Rev. ed.). New York: George Braziller.

Whitehead, D. (2001). Health education, behavioural change and social psychology: nursing's contribution to health promotion? *Journal of Advanced Nursing, 34*(6), 822.

Workplace Health Strategies Bureau. (2002). *Literature review on evaluations of workplace health promotion programs* (Publication No. K1A 0K9). Ottawa, ON: Workplace Health Strategies Bureau. Retrieved May 9, 2004, from: *http://www.hc-sc.gc.ca/hecs-sesc/workplace/pdf/Literature_Review.PDF.*

World Health Organization. (1998). *Health promotion glossary* (Conference Resource Document No. WHO/HPR/HEP/98.1). Geneva: World Health Organization.

Yura, H., & Walsh, M. B. (1983). *Human needs and the nursing process* (3rd ed.). New York: Appleton-Century-Crofts.

Three

Unit

Interventions for Health Promotion

9 Screening

10 Health Education

11 Nutrition Counseling for Health Promotion

12 Exercise

13 Stress Management

14 Holistic Health Strategies

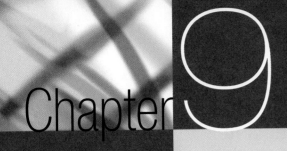

Chapter 9

MARIE TRUGLIO-LONDRIGAN
MARGARET K. MACALI

Screening

objectives

After completing this chapter, the reader will be able to:

- Discuss screening and its relationship to preventive health care intervention.

- Identify the advantages and disadvantages of the screening process.

- Analyze the criteria that determine a screenable disease.

- Discuss the health care and economic issues related to the screening process that result in ethical implications.

- Explain sensitivity and specificity as they relate to the efficacy of screening.

- Identify the broad range of community resources included in and affected by the screening process.

- Describe the nursing role in the screening process.

- Explore critical questions pertaining to culture in relation to screening.

- Discuss how a collaborative partnership may assist a community in the development and implementation of a screening program.

key terms

Cost-benefit ratio analysis
Cost-effectiveness analysis
Cost-efficiency analysis
Ethical issue
False-negative test results
False-positive test results

Group or mass screening
Individual screening
Interobserver reliability
Intraobserver reliability
Multiple test screening
Natural history

One-test disease-specific screening
Reliability
Sensitivity
Specificity
Validity

THINK About It

Screening to Identify Risk Factors

Ms. Lukas is a 55-year-old account executive for a leading advertising firm. This high-power, high-pressure position requires her attention 14 hours a day. There is little time for rest, relaxation, or exercise. Ms. Lukas frequents take-out restaurants because she is unable to find time to cook or shop for healthy food. A recent increase in job pressures has provoked her to resume smoking two to three packs of cigarettes a day.

Ms. Lukas and a colleague visited a health fair one afternoon. Ms. Lukas' blood pressure was 200/110 mm Hg. Her nonfasting serum cholesterol measurement revealed a level of 265 mg/dl. Her colleague, who is 20 years younger and leads a similar lifestyle with similar habits, had a blood pressure reading of 130/82 and a cholesterol level of 215 mg/dl. The counselor evaluated the risk factors for both individuals. This analysis revealed similar risks for both women.

Although Ms. Lukas did benefit from the early identification of hypertension and hypercholesterolemia, she does not reap the benefits of early risk factor analysis like

Continued

THINK About It

Screening to Identify Risk Factors cont'd

her younger colleague. If counseling and education prove successful, Ms. Lukas' colleague will demonstrate increased wellness through appropriate behavioral changes that could prevent the realization of disease.

1 Research supports the need for screening in an attempt to identify disease at early stages. However, if this is the case, does it not support the notion of screening to identify risk factors that have been associated with disease processes?

2 Will this identification of risk factors dramatically affect the onset of disease?

3 How can nurses use their expertise to help individuals achieve the desired behavioral changes necessary for risk factor reduction?

Screening has received growing recognition as a valuable tool for health care professionals, particularly as health care delivery moves toward preventive interventions. Although health education about screening comes under the rubric of primary prevention (see Chapter 1), the actual process of screening is a form of secondary prevention. The primary objective of screening is the detection of a disease in its early stages, to treat it and deter its progression. The basic assumption guiding this process is that detection during the early asymptomatic period allows treatment at a time when the course of the disease can be altered significantly. The screening concept is based on the principle that disease is preceded by a period of asymptomatic pathogenesis (disease development) when risk factors predisposing a person to the pathological condition are building momentum toward manifestation of the disease. Screening takes advantage of the early pathogenic state. The administration of tests (often simple in form) during this stage identifies specific variables that distinguish individuals who most likely have the condition from those who do not. Screening is not considered a diagnostic measure; it is seen as a preliminary step to direct a health care provider in assessment of the ostensibly healthy individual's chances of becoming unhealthy. The ultimate goal could be curative, but more often it is to prevent further development of the disease or to ameliorate the possible outcomes. A second, but equally important, objective of screening is to reduce the costs of managing the disease by avoiding the more vigorous interventions required during its later stages. The added attraction of a cost-conscious approach to health care mandates that health care professionals at all levels acquire a basic understanding of the screening process and its application.

This chapter describes the screening process and the strengths and weaknesses of its implementation. The presentation allows the nurse to (1) analyze the screenability of a particular disease and (2) determine the means of implementing a screening program specific to the population, the disease, and the system of health care delivery.

ADVANTAGES AND DISADVANTAGES OF SCREENING

Preclinical illness and previously unrecognized disease in individuals may be detected via screening efforts (Anderson & McFarlane, 2000). Screening tests offer several advantages. They are often simple, inexpensive, and frequently a trained technician can administer them. The simplicity of the screening procedure decreases the time and cost of involved health care personnel and enables less skilled technicians to administer the test. This also reduces cost and permits the more appropriate use of highly skilled, costly professionals at the definitive, diagnostic stage.

A second advantage is the ability to apply the screening process to both individuals and large groups. In an **individual screening** program, one person is tested by a health professional who has designated the individual as high risk. The practitioner can make this selection independently, the health care agency can define a specific policy, or a legislative body can require the screening by law as in the case of phenylketonuria (PKU) or lead-screening programs. **Group or mass screening** occurs when a target population is selected on the basis of an increased incidence of a condition or a recognized element of high risk within the group. An example of this would be lower-income populations or cultural groups that exhibit a significant prevalence of a particular condition, such as hypertension. The target population may be invited to a central location on a designated day to be tested for the selected disorder.

A third advantage is the ability to provide one-test specific screening or multiple test screenings. A **one-test disease-specific screening** is the administration of a single test that searches for a characteristic that indicates a high risk of developing a disorder. An example of this would be blood pressure screening to evaluate the risk of hypertension. **Multiple test screening** is the administration of two or more tests to detect more than one disease. In some cases, one sample can be used to evaluate the possibility of several conditions, saving time and money and making the process efficient and economical. For example, a blood sample can be evaluated for both elevated glucose and cholesterol levels. Ultimately, the combination of the relatively low cost of a screening test and flexibility makes screenings adaptable to all levels of the health care delivery system.

The disadvantages of screening stem largely from the imperfection of modern science, which results in a margin of error for most instruments and tests. When program effectiveness depends on the test's ability to distinguish those who probably do have the disease from those who do not, the margin of error can precipitate serious consequences. Some individuals who do not have the condition will be referred for further tests and some who do have the disease will not. Those incorrectly referred suffer needless anxiety while awaiting more definitive diagnostic procedures. They must also bear the burden of the cost, follow-up visits, lost time, and inconvenience.

The effects on those whose disorders have been missed are even more important. These individuals leave with a false sense of a healthful state that will be shattered eventually, and they lose the opportunity to receive early treatment that could prevent irreversible damage. The difficulty of balancing the benefits to some against the losses to others is an **ethical issue** of most screening programs. The significance of this disadvantage can vary; therefore, it should be assessed for each project, disease, and population.

SELECTION OF A SCREENABLE DISEASE

The selection of a screenable disease goes beyond examination of the disease alone. The selection process must also encompass less tangible factors, such as the emotional and financial impact of the disease's detection on the screened population. Even after gathering data and reviewing the critical issues, the final decision to screen or not to screen must often be reached with incomplete evidence or with answers that raise ethical issues. The potential uncertainties confounding the decision emphasize the need to conduct an exhaustive analysis of available material to obtain a decision that is as objective and scientific as possible. The answers to the following three questions provide a basis for designating a disease as screenable or not screenable:

1. Does the significance of the disorder warrant its consideration as a community problem?
2. Can the disease be detected by screening?
3. Should screening for the disease be done?

As simplistic as these questions may appear, the answers or lack of answers may expose numerous complex issues that determine whether or not a well-informed decision can be made on screenability.

Significance

The significance of a disease refers to the level of priority assigned to the disease as a public health concern. Although the opinions of political and public interest groups may enter into the evaluation, significance generally is determined by the quantity and quality of life affected by the disorder. The greater the physical and psychological harm experienced by the population, the greater is the need to designate the disease as a priority health problem. The first step in assessing screenability is evaluation of this significance to decide if the disorder warrants the time, effort, and funds that must be allocated.

Estimating the quality of life affected by a disease presents a problem. The perception of quality is subjective and individual evaluations may differ. For example, not all people equally perceive the disability resulting from a disease; some make adjustments and cope, whereas others do not. Those who do not would be more likely to say that the quality of their lives is significantly lower than that of the people around them.

By contrast, measures of the quantity of life affected by the disease are more readily obtainable. Disease-specific mortality rates present one picture of this effect, whereas prevalence and incidence rates provide another. Prevalence is the proportion of existing cases during a specific time; incidence is the frequency of new cases during a specified period (Lundy & Janes, 2001). Usually chronic conditions are measured by their prevalence, whereas acute conditions are assessed by their incidence.

In this era of cost-conscious health care, a new dimension has been added to the evaluation of significance: the cost required to treat the disease. In some cases the prevalence of the disorder may not be great, but the problem requires disproportionate amounts spent on maintenance or management after the condition is fully expressed. For example, with PKU the incidence is not significant, but the cost of a case undetected at birth is a lifetime of case management. Given the costly outcome if undetected and the reasonable price of the test itself, the cost of screening all newborns is nominal.

Can the Disease Be Detected by Screening?

With the relative significance of the disease established, the next step is to determine if health professionals can screen for the disease. Do well-documented diagnostic criteria for the disorder exist? Is there a screening instrument? Are sufficient community resources and treatment modalities available to support a screening program?

Diagnostic Criteria

Detection of a disease requires knowledge of characteristics that indicate its presence or, as in screening, its early pathogenic, asymptomatic state. Selected diagnostic criteria should be well documented; they should not be merely accepted or commonly used indicators. The impact of uncertainty in detecting disease is amplified when considering the application of the screening design. Some diseases, such as sickle cell anemia, are defined by the presence or absence of a single, isolated factor. Other conditions, such as hypertension, are indicated by the measurement of statistically derived numerical values for which a normal range has been set. Disagreement over the parameters of the normal range, combined with contentions that what is abnormal for one individual may not be abnormal for another, make these conditions more controversial to designate as screenable diseases.

Screening Instruments

The next step is to determine if methods exist to detect the disease during early pathogenesis. If instruments are available, a careful analysis should determine if any of them fulfill the requirements for the screening process: safe, cost-effective, and accurate. Ultimately the question is how well the instrument can distinguish those individuals who probably do not have and will not develop the condition from those who are likely to develop it. The variables that aid in instrument evaluation include reliability and validity.

Reliability. Reliability is an assessment of the reproducibility of the test's results when different individuals with the same level of skill perform the test during different periods and under different conditions. If the same result emerges when two individuals perform the test, **interobserver reliability** is shown. If the same individual is able to reproduce the results several times, **intraobserver reliability** is shown. Therefore testing for instrument reliability can yield data on the accuracy and quality of the test (Polit, Beck, & Hungler, 2001).

From these data, the health professional can determine the amount of training that is required for health care technicians or personnel who administer the test. For example, if interobserver reliability is low, additional training might be required to work toward a more consistent method of delivering the test. This is frequently necessary in hypertension screening. If intraobserver reliability is low, the health professional might surmise that the instrument, and not the individual, is at fault.

Validity. Validity reflects the test's ability to distinguish correctly between diseased and nondiseased individuals, or the accuracy of the test (Sackett, Straus, Richardson, Rosenberg, & Haynes, 2000). In a controlled setting, validity is evaluated by testing the instrument on a group of individuals who have positive or negative results. The ideal result is to have the instrument pick out 100% of the diseased people (positive reactions) and 100% of the nondiseased people (negative reactions). Such accuracy rarely occurs in practice; therefore, the measure of validity has been divided into two components that quantify the margin of error in the screening instrument. **Sensitivity** measures the first component. This refers to the proportion of people with a condition who correctly test positive when screened. A test with poor sensitivity will miss individuals with the condition and there will be a large number of **false-negative test results;** individuals actually have the condition but were told they are disease free. Specificity is the second component. **Specificity** measures the test's ability to recognize negative reactions or nondiseased individuals. A test with poor specificity will result in **false-positive test results.** Individuals with false-positive test results are told that they have a condition when in actuality they do not.

Application of sensitivity and specificity data to the actual outcome of the program raises some interesting points. Consider the issues that a public health nurse must face when given a newly developed screening test with low specificity and moderate sensitivity. Low specificity means few true-negative and more false-positive test results. The nurse and other health professionals must then consider the cost, inconvenience, and psychological stress experienced by the people with false-positive reactions during the period after their incorrect screening test, the unnecessary additional referrals, and the ability of the existing follow-up services to meet these needs. With only moderate sensitivity, a number of false-negative results could occur, which

may send away individuals who could benefit from treatment. The issue raised here is ethical; that is, should a screening program be implemented when it is known that the tests deliver false-positive and false-negative results?

Another broader issue concerns large health fair screening programs where a targeted population is sought for a mass screening. The efficiency and efficacy of such programs must be analyzed. Questions that address efficiency and efficacy include: (1) Is the targeted population prepared in an appropriate way before engaging in the screening tests? (2) Are the health care practitioners who are administering the test all educated according to the standard protocols of test administration? and (3) Are follow-up measures instituted in the program? Answers to these questions will challenge the health care providers in the development, implementation, and follow-up processes identified so that efficiency and efficacy will be enhanced.

The issues emerging from investigation of the screening instrument demonstrate the significant influence it has on the entire process. Data on the reliability and validity of the test and screening programs in general provide valuable information to evaluate, anticipate, and ideally control these influences, enabling the program to work effectively toward its goal.

Community Resources

Implementing a screening program depends on availability of appropriate community resources, such as funds, health care workers, follow-through, treatment sources, and administrative personnel. Judicious organization of the overall program is key to its success. Knowledge of the disease's characteristics and the screening instrument are useless without financial and organized human support to apply it. The overall approach is complex, requiring intense efforts in the area of partnership development.

A lead agency is identified to oversee the development process of the community health program. Origins of the lead agency vary from a community service organization to the local public health department responding to a mandate from the state. Regardless of its origin, the agency must perform a self-evaluation to compare its level of expertise with that required to oversee the process inclusive of the screening effort. Early identification of the lead agency, along with potential partnerships, allows for the effective use of talents and the division of labor.

For the lead agency to develop and oversee the development process of the community health program and the delivery of a screening program, partnerships are essential. The agency must contact and organize necessary stakeholders. Examples of stakeholders include key community individuals, hospitals, health and social service agencies such as primary health care centers, and community organizations including houses of worship, community centers, schools, transportation agencies, and volunteer organizations. Key community individuals are those people who are considered leaders within the community. The primary rule is: never assume that what is appropriate and effective for one community will be appropriate and effective for another.

The members of the partnership carry out the community assessment together. A community assessment is a systematic method of data collection that provides a detailed account regarding the type, quantity, and quality of resources. It includes recreation, physical environment, education, safety and transportation, politics, government, health, social services, communications, and economics, the core components of demographic, vital statistics, and morbidity and mortality data (Anderson & McFarlane, 2000).

After completing the assessment, the data analysis will reveal the target community or high-risk population, available health care resources, and the high-risk population health need. The identified partners collaborate, review, and analyze the data leading to the development of health improvement strategies (in this case a screening program), with methods of implementation to move the target population smoothly through the screening process. Finally, monitoring and evaluating outcomes is essential to determine the effectiveness of the program and the achievement of stated goals. Evaluation is inclusive of monitoring the entire process, including the successful workings of the partnership. Figure 9-1 presents a model of collaborative partnership: community health program development.

Constraints affecting the operation of a screening program include financial concerns, political issues, cultural constraints, follow-up and referral services, and accessible treatment facilities. All partners are aware that responses from the target community are affected partly by their experience with other screening programs, such as the means used to inform them, the accessibility of the location, the availability of transportation, the convenience of the program's hours, and the cultural sensitivity of the delivery and design of the program. A public health nursing approach identifies the necessary community resources and defines how these resources interact and may be mobilized to achieve maximal benefits and positive outcomes. One example of this is presented in the Community Care Plan Collaborative Partnership Between a County Department of Health and Hospital Clinic: Breast and Cervical Cancer Screening Program (Care Plan).

Financial support of the screening program is a constraint that can influence all points in the system. Although some programs are delivered entirely on a voluntary basis, organizers of others must submit grant proposals to local, state, or federal departments when consideration of medical and economic ethics is involved. Planners must look beyond the screening day and investigate financial resources for follow-up care and treatment.

In addition to financial accessibility, follow-up services should be accessible in terms of convenient locations and open hours. For example, an evening clinic may reach those who are reluctant or financially unable to miss work. An efficient referral system links the follow-up resources to the screening program, providing continuity of care. A method must be devised to encourage the participant to take positive action on the referral. Public health nurses will facilitate this process with a variety of communication techniques, such as telephone or in-person counseling, mailings, and home visits.

Should Screening for the Disease Be Done?

After determining that the disease is significant and can be screened for, establishing whether health professionals should do so is the final step. Screening for a particular disorder and ultimately treating those with the early-identified disorder should improve the chances of a favorable outcome in comparison with those whose disorder is not found until signs and symptoms become evident. Therefore, several questions must be considered. If a test is accurate in the identification of a condition in the early stages, is there any benefit to the individual? Are there effective treatment modalities for the condition?

Interventions and Treatment Modalities

Screening is based on the disease's asymptomatic period; therefore, adequate information must exist concerning (1) the optimal time for screening, (2) specific intervention during this time, and (3) knowledge as to the effect of early detection and treatment on the prognosis. Without this knowledge, health care professionals are unable to explain how the consequences of the detected disease differ from those of the undetected. They can neither evaluate nor explain the health benefits derived from the screening program.

Not intervening can be almost as detrimental as the adverse effects of a disorder. In this situation, not only has

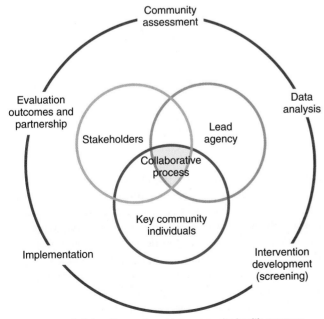

Figure 9-1   Collaborative partnership: community health program development.

CARE PLAN

Community Care Plan Collaborative Partnership Between a County Department of Health and Hospital Clinic: Breast and Cervical Cancer Screening Program

Planning and development of any screening program warrants partnering agencies to address and analyze one primary area of importance: their working relationship and the problems and potential complications that may have an effect on the successful implementation and outcome of the program.

With this information in hand, partnering agencies will know what issues may have to be addressed during the planning process of the screening program. By targeting potential issues, the partnering agencies will be better able to deliver an efficient, reliable, and valid screening program, thereby assisting the participants, and ultimately enhancing health outcomes. (The participant may be an individual, a family, or a targeted group.)

Nursing Diagnosis Regarding Partnering Agencies: Ineffective Management of Interagency Agreements Regarding Screening, Follow-Up, and Treatment Related to Complexity of Partnership and Communication Difficulties.

DEFINING CHARACTERISTICS

- Communication between hospital clinic nurses and public health nurses is not taking place in a timely and efficient manner.
- Public health nurses are experiencing difficulty contacting clinic nurses to ensure that the process of the screening program from planning to follow-up is taking place in an efficient manner and that the screening is reliable and valid.
- Public health nurses have difficulty gaining access to client clinic charts throughout the screening process.
- Nurses in both agencies "double check" outcomes thereby increasing cost, creating a barrier to time efficiency, and increasing length of time to contacting clients with outcomes.
- Outcome reports are not timely; screening results are posted 48 to 72 hours later than initially planned.
- Clients express confusion over self-management of positive screening test results.

- Clients receive bills at home after being counseled there would be no charge.

RELATED FACTORS

- Multiple organizational structures, cultures, and philosophies
- Lack of experiential history of working together in a partnership
- HIPAA and confidentiality concerns
- Reimbursement and insurance realities regarding uninsured clients
- Medical provider reluctance to treat

EXPECTED OUTCOMES

- Clinic and public health nurses freely communicate with each other.
- Client charts are mutually available.
- Public health nurses manage the intake and follow-up; clinic nurses manage the actual screening process.
- Nurses for both agencies view each other as professional peers.
- Clinical outcomes are reported in a timely fashion.
- Billing is handled properly according to grant reimbursement; clients do not receive bills.
- Seamless screening process is in place, with individuals moving effortlessly throughout the program, including follow-up.

INTERVENTIONS

- Develop organizational maps outlining lead agency, stakeholders, and key community individuals in the collaborative partnership.
- Clearly define and document roles and responsibilities.
- Develop mutually agreed upon policies and protocols.
- Establish clear lines of communication within all systems.
- Develop technology systems to assist with communication, documentation, reimbursement, and surveillance.
- Clearly abide by HIPAA, confidentiality, and reimbursement realities.

HIPAA, Health Insurance Portability and Accountability Act.

the program misled the screened population that a health benefit will result from their efforts, but the development and implementation of the screening program has used both personal and community resources that can not possibly alter the course of a particular disease.

Follow-up is critical to determine if intervention strategies prescribed are in fact taking place. The prescribed regimen may be very broad and include a wide variety of intervention strategies such as diet, exercise, and drug therapy. Follow-up may include an evaluation and review of the literature that discusses evidence-based practice per-

taining to a particular drug, as well as the identification of intervention characteristics that impair follow-up, such as cost, inconvenience, or side effects. Consideration must also be given to those factors that enhance follow-up. For example, nurses can provide ongoing counseling and education about a medication and assist individuals in a lifestyle transformation that includes health-promoting behaviors.

Safety of the intervention is a concern when considering the widespread application of a remedy after a screening program. Risks or harmful side effects can be costly in terms of human health and the increased medical care required to correct the iatrogenic effects resulting from the intervention. Health care professionals must decide if these risks significantly diminish the success of the treatment and outweigh the benefits derived from the treatment.

ETHICAL CONSIDERATIONS

A step taken toward improving health usually is deemed a just and moral act within the health care system's values. However, when approaching health care practices with a more critical eye and realizing that not all the results of a well-intended practice are beneficial, the need to balance the benefit against the detriment becomes an issue. The resulting decision process becomes a value judgment and an ethical issue.

Health Care Ethics

A screening program is in a catogory separate from interventions offered for established disease processes. Rather than receiving those who have performed a self-assessment and elected to enter the system, a screening program invites apparently well individuals to be tested to determine disease risk and the need for follow-up. The request for participation implies that a health benefit will be derived, although at this stage nothing is said about what it will be or what the consumer must do to obtain it. Program planning that attempts to clarify this implication and inform participants of the issues develops the basis for an ethically sound project and enhances the screenability of the disease.

Most screening programs are called *hypertension screening* or *diabetic screening*; therefore, it is not surprising that participants enter them assuming the results received are diagnostic and will classify them as disease free or disease laden. This is untrue, because the screening goal is only identification and referral of individuals at risk or who may need further follow-up or evaluation. The initial presentation of and contact with the program implies a benefit not being delivered. To alleviate this problem, the planning committee should develop a method of informing participants of the meaning and limitations of the results. Participants need to know whether the ultimate benefit is preventive, ameliorative, or curative and, most importantly, what responsibility they must assume to secure this outcome.

Misinterpretation caused by the screening instrument is of even greater ethical concern than human misperception. As the information on sensitivity and specificity indicates, false-positive and false-negative results occur with any screening instrument. One of the more difficult ethical issues in screening is to evaluate whether the benefits received by those who receive correct results are worth the problems experienced by those who receive incorrect results. What obligation does the project have to the latter? What is an acceptable number of people with false-negative test results, all of whom will both miss the benefit of early treatment and be misled about the need for tests in the near future? What will be the response of an individual who has a false-positive reaction? Answers to these questions are value judgments that vary according to the disease.

Additional issues that confound the medical ethics of screening are cutoff points for the screening instrument and borderline cases. How precisely do the instrument's numerical values define the high-risk disease state? The goal of a screening program, identifying an individual as high risk or not, depends on this numerical value. When the parameter for this distinction is not clear, a cutoff point is set. Above this point, the person is considered disease positive; below this point, the individual is disease negative. Consequently, readjusting the cutoff point becomes a highly controversial issue, because it controls the percentage of positive and negative results. If the disease were potentially life threatening, an increase in false-positive results (lower cutoff point) would be preferred to missing individuals who may have the disease. In addition, if a disease is relatively benign in terms of potential stigmatization, anxiety, and problems with treatment, lowering the cutoff point could again be safe and ethical.

A problem closely related to the cutoff point is defining a policy for borderline cases. Hypertension is a common disease in which a variance of 5 to 10 mm Hg can make the difference in labeling a person as high risk or not. A more sophisticated approach may be taken to discriminate between a borderline case that should be referred and one that should not. The health professional can specify other risk factors associated with hypertension, such as family history, diet, and smoking, as criteria contributing to the decision to refer an individual. With the increasing interest in and knowledge of risk factors, the effectiveness of this method has improved.

The medical ethics of screening will continue to demand review of the same questions and issues; however, the answers may change as more is discovered about the various conditions and their treatments. An updated literature review is imperative before reviewing these issues in relation to a particular screenable disease.

Economic Ethics

Associating a monetary value with health care outcomes is generally against the nature and ideals of health care professionals. In the past the tendency was to place no limits on the cost of promoting a healthy, disease-free or disease-controlled status, resulting in a philosophy that all care should be given to all people at all costs. This philosophy has evolved to one of conscious recognition of the costs of screening programs. Allocating community funds to a screening program could result in a lack of funds for other projects. Those benefiting from a screening test will be countered by those suffering from a lack of service for other medical or social needs. These trade-offs result in ethical decisions demanding careful analysis by the screening administration (Hot Topics box).

Screening can be a costly project for both organizers and consumers. Initial operational costs must be considered, including buying or renting the screening instruments,

ECONOMIC ETHICS OF SCREENING

Economic ethics have been discussed within this text to include the consideration of cost-benefit ratio, cost-effectiveness, and cost-efficiency analyses when developing selective screening programs. Those working in the health care system are currently struggling to devise program guidelines that are ethically and economically sound. Questions give way to still more questions as nurses grapple with issues of cost, quality, technological benefits in screening, and service rationing. Managed care models continue to be a key force in important decision making in health care.

1. How does this affect a health care provider's decision to deliver care?
2. Do health care providers have the autonomy to make decisions that they deem necessary regarding screening and treatment?
3. How does this affect screening protocols?
4. Will the quality of care deteriorate if screening programs are not implemented?

renting floor space, engaging professionals or technicians to administer the tests, and interpreting the results.

These costs are encountered again when people are referred for further evaluation. Consumer costs include follow-up visits, treatment, time, and income that is lost while complying with each. Given the combined operational and consumer costs, several questions are raised. Do the costs result in the desired health outcome to the individual, group, or community? Are the benefits reaped worth the expenditures required? The answer is determined partly by what values (other than monetary ones) are attributed to the benefit, such as saving a life. A strictly economic approach, however, generally eliminates the intangible variables, demanding the use of more objective data for decision making.

When program designs are being considered with screening, three main approaches may be used to evaluate the economic resources affected: (1) cost-benefit ratio, (2) cost-effectiveness, and (3) cost-efficiency analyses. Once far from the thoughts of health care workers, the current relevance and use of such concepts require a basic understanding of their role in the selection of a screenable condition. Although presented here in successive fashion, they are entirely separate methods and most frequently are used independently of one another.

Cost-Benefit Ratio

Cost-benefit ratio analysis is performed first, because it allows the comparison of various outcomes in monetary values (Sackett et al., 2000). This comparison is necessary in health planning when the initial consideration is which health outcome, such as reduction of cardiovascular disease, decreased infant mortality, or reduction of a visual problem,

will be most beneficial to the community at the most reasonable cost.

Cost-Effectiveness

If the reduction of cardiovascular disease is chosen as the desired outcome, the next step is a **cost-effectiveness analysis,** which determines the optimal use of resources to reach a predetermined, constant end point or the desired health outcome (Sackett et al., 2000). The outcome remains the same; the best method of deriving it is the issue. For example, considering the selected health outcome, such as the reduction of cardiovascular disease, various methods might be used. These methods include screening for hypertension, performing electrocardiograms on all individuals aged 25 or older who are admitted to the hospital, beginning an antismoking campaign, or obtaining nutrition counseling. Implementation of all these options would be ideal, but with limited resources a choice must be made.

Cost-Efficiency

The last approach to help bring the economic resources into perspective is **cost-efficiency analysis.** The purpose is to be efficient and budget a limited amount of money toward achieving as much of the desired outcome as possible. The funds are the central issue, not the health benefit.

SELECTION OF A SCREENABLE POPULATION

The selection of a screenable population is as important as the selection of a screenable disease. The objective is to identify a high-risk group that, when tested, will yield a significant number of diseased individuals. With such results, the efforts and cost of screening the population are minimized and the health benefit received is maximized. The main criterion used to define an appropriate population is the definitive presence of risk factors related to the disorder. To ensure a thorough examination of possible risk factors, both person-dependent and environment-dependent factors should be reviewed.

Person-Dependent Factors

One characteristic related to the person, age, is increasingly important because its distribution changes throughout the population (Tables 9-1 and 9-2). Practice has always placed a high priority on screening the vulnerable, at-risk infant population, partly because of the health outcomes that affect the child's growth and development. As the average life span increases, however, the effects of longer-range risk factors are becoming apparent, making certain prevalent and costly chronic conditions equally important to control. Therefore ideal populations for screening can be found in senior citizen housing projects or elderly day-care settings. Middle-aged adults are also being recognized as a screenable group for certain conditions, such as breast cancer, glaucoma, and heart disease, which commonly appear during this period.

Table 9-1 Recommended Guide to Health Tests and Screenings for Females

Test	Purpose	Age	Frequency
Guthrie	Early detection of PKU	Newborns	Once, unless done before 24 hours of age, when it should be repeated by 2 weeks of age
Blood lead and free erythrocyte (or zinc) protoporphyrin levels	Early detection of lead levels	12 months	At least once for children at risk
Breast self-examination	To detect changes in breast tissue or appearance	Undetermined	Insufficient evidence to recommend for or against
Clinical breast examination	To detect changes in the breast that go unnoticed by self-examination	40 and over	There may be some benefit with screening mammography, but its benefit as a screening tool alone is undetermined
Mammogram	To detect changes in breast tissue that are too small to be felt	40 and over	Every 1 to 2 years
The actual absolute benefit increases with age
Papanicolaou smear	To detect cervical abnormalities, including cancer	Within 3 years of onset of sexual activity or 21 years of age; 65 and over routine screening not recommended for women not at high risk	At least every 3 years; with individual recommendations by primary health care practitioner based on individual risk factors
Digital rectal examination	To detect early signs of colorectal cancer	50 and over	Periodically; at the time of fecal occult blood test, sigmoidoscopy, and colonoscopy
Fecal occult blood test	To detect traces of blood in stool, an early sign of colorectal cancer	50 and over	Annually
Sigmoidoscopy	To detect early signs of colorectal cancer	50 and over	Every 5 years with fecal occult blood test
Colonoscopy	To detect early signs of colorectal cancer within the proximal colon	50 and over	Every 10 years
Serum cholesterol	To determine risk of heart disease	45 to 65; 65 and over review case by case	Once every 5 years if levels are within normal range
Blood Pressure	To detect hypertension, a major risk factor for cardiovascular disease	18 and over	As directed by health care provider
1. Tonometry
2. Ophthalmoscopic evaluation
3. Perimetry	To detect early signs of glaucoma	High-risk individuals	As directed by specialists
Fasting serum glucose test and oral glucose tolerance test	Early detection of type 2 diabetes	Adults with hypertension or hyperlipidemia	Screening of high-risk individuals every 3 years as determined by health care provider

Modified from U.S. Preventive Services Task Force. (1996). *Guide to clinical preventive services* (2nd ed.). Baltimore: Williams & Wilkins; U.S. Preventive Services Task Force. (2002). *Guide to clinical preventive services: Colorectal screening.* Retrieved March 1, 2004, from: *http://www.ahrq.gov/clinic/uspstfix.htm;* U.S. Preventive Services Task Force. (2002). *Guide to clinical preventive services: Breast screening.* Retrieved March 1, 2004, from: *http://www.ahrq.gov/clinic/uspstfix.htm;* U.S. Preventive Services Task Force. (2003). *Guide to clinical preventive services: Hypertension screening.* Retrieved March 1, 2004, from: *http://www.ahrq.gov/clinic/uspstfix.htm;* U.S. Preventive Services Task Force. (2003). *Guide to clinical preventive services: Diabetes screening.* Retrieved March 1, 2004, from: *http://www.ahrq.gov/clinic/uspstfix.htm;* and U.S. Preventive Services Task Force. (2003). *Guide to clinical preventive services: Cervical screening.* Retrieved March 1, 2004, from: *http://www.ahrq.gov/clinic/uspstfix.htm.*
PKU, phenylketonuria.
Note: Due to the time-sensitive nature of this material, readers are advised to search the referenced Web sites for the most recent updates to the information cited here.

Table **9-2** Recommended Guide to Health Tests and Screenings for Males

Test	Purpose	Age	Frequency
Guthrie	Early detection of PKU	Newborns	Once, unless done before 24 hours of age, when it should be repeated by 2 weeks of age
Blood lead and free erythrocyte (or zinc) protoporphyrin levels	Early detection of lead levels	12 months	At least once for children at risk
Prostate digital rectal examination	Early detection of prostate cancer	The recommended age for prostate digital examination not yet determined	The recommended frequency for prostate digital examination is not yet determined: clinical trials in progress
PSA	Early detection of prostate cancer	The recommended age for the PSA is not yet determined	The recommended age for the PSA is not yet determined: clinical trials in progress
Digital rectal examination	To detect early signs of colorectal cancer	50 and over	Periodically; at the time of each screening fecal occult blood test, sigmoidoscopy, and colonoscopy
Fecal occult blood test	To detect traces of blood in stool, an early sign of colorectal cancer	50 and over	Annually
Sigmoidoscopy	To detect early signs of colorectal cancer	50 and over	Every 5 years with fecal occult blood test
Colonoscopy	To detect early signs of colorectal cancer within the proximal colon	50 and over	Every 10 years
Serum cholesterol	To determine risk of heart disease	35 to 65; 65 and over case-by-case review	Once every 5 years if levels are within normal range
Blood Pressure	To detect hypertension, a major risk factor for cardiovascular disease	18 and over	As directed by health care provider
1. Tonometry 2. Ophthalmoscopic evaluation 3. Perimetry	To detect early signs of glaucoma	High-risk individuals	As directed by specialists
Fasting plasma glucose test and oral glucose tolerance test	Early detection of type 2 diabetes	Adults with hypertension or hyperlipidemia	Screening of high risk individuals every 3 years as directed by the health care provider
EIA	Early detection of HIV	Individuals at risk	Individually determined

Modified from U.S. Preventive Services Task Force. (1996). *Guide to clinical preventive services* (2nd ed.). Baltimore: Williams & Wilkins; U.S. Preventive Services Task Force. (2002). *Guide to clinical preventive services: Colorectal screening*. Retrieved March 1, 2004, from: *http://www.ahrq.gov/clinic/uspstfix.htm*; U.S. Preventive Services Task Force. (2002). *Guide to clinical preventive services: Prostate screening*. Retrieved March 1, 2004, from: *http://www.ahrq.gov/clinic/uspstfix.htm*; U.S. Preventive Services Task Force. (2003). *Guide to clinical preventive services: Hypertension screening*. Retrieved March 1, 2004, from: *http://www.ahrq.gov/clinic/uspstfix.htm*; U.S. Preventive Services Task Force. (2003). *Guide to clinical preventive services: Diabetes screening*. Retrieved March 1, 2004, from: *http://www.ahrq.gov/clinic/uspstfix.htm*.
EIA, enzyme immunoassay; *HIV*, human immunodeficiency virus; *PKU*, phenylketonuria; *PSA*, prostate-specific antigen.
Note: Due to the time-sensitive nature of this material, readers are advised to search the referenced Web sites for the most recent updates to the information cited here.

Gender has obvious implications for screening programs. For example, women are tested commonly for two conditions, breast cancer and cervical cancer. Men are tested for prostate cancer and testicular cancer.

A population representing a particular ethnic or racial group is also appropriate to consider when planning screening programs (Multicultural Awareness box).

Race refers to a biologically related group of people whose features are inherited (Allender & Spradley, 2001). It is known that some disorders occur more frequently in certain racial or ethnic groups (Case Study). For example, African Americans have a higher prevalence of and mortality rate from hypertension and cancer of the prostate than whites, and Native Americans have higher rates of diabetes than do other cultural groups (U.S. Department of Health and Human Services [USDHHS], 2000).

Although these health disparities are of great concern, their cause is not easy to ascertain. It is believed that these differences are actually the result of complex interactions among genetic variations, environmental factors, and

MULTICULTURAL AWARENESS

Eliminating Health Disparities among Ethnic Groups

The United States has been referred to frequently as a *melting pot*. Diversity has been acknowledged as a strength, but it is apparent that disparities exist among the various racial and ethnic groups in the attainment and maintenance of health. The minority populations of the United States have been categorized as African Americans, Hispanics, Asian-Pacific Islanders, American Indians, and Alaskan Natives. These categories oversimplify the reality of the multicultural nature of assessing health status, screening, and making plans to improve health. These particular racial groupings are not absolute, because there are subgroups within each (U.S. Department of Health and Human Services, 2000).

Over the past decade racial and ethnic health disparities have become increasingly apparent. The second goal of *Healthy People 2010* is to eliminate as many as possible.

These disparities and factors such as access to care need to be taken into consideration when planning screening programs. In order to plan, implement, and evaluate a screening program that targets a specific population, the provider must have an awareness of that population that includes components such as lifestyle, socioeconomic characteristics, education, heredity, environmental factors, values, religious and cultural beliefs, communication style, and language. Partnering with key individuals and organizations in the community through the entire process is important for any screening program to be successful, as the following scenario illustrates.

Hospital administrators in a town located outside a city in the Northeast are concerned about the health status of a new immigrant population. Recent census data indicate that the number of immigrants from Guatemala has grown. The census data also reveal that this population is primarily young adults, male and female. The officials of the town and the hospital are aware that most of the men are day laborers, many of whom gather each morning in the town square to be transported to their jobs. The young women are mothers who work in small, privately owned businesses or are hired by local house-cleaning services.

Based on these data, the hospital officials decide to plan a health and screening day for this population. The hospital sends out flyers into the community in the primary native language of the target population. The day of the screening arrives and the number of participants is very low. The hospital officials are very concerned. They had good intentions. They do not know what to do next.

1. What critical actions did the hospital officials perform that might be considered positive in the planning of the health and screening day?
2. What critical actions did the hospital officials not perform that might have contributed to the poor turnout at the health and screening function?
3. What might the hospital officials consider in their planning for the next health and screening day?
4. How might they engage the community and the target population in planning the health and screening day?
5. What local community agencies and groups might be invited to participate as partners when planning and implementing the health and screening day?
6. Can you identify any creative ways to bring the health and screening day to the targeted population, making the program more accessible?

health behaviors (USDHHS, 2000). The need to identify the causes of these health disparities has been of central importance. This is evident by the proliferation of research being conducted to identify and describe the possible reasons for these differences. When health care professionals have a better understanding as to why these disparities exist, it will be possible to develop effective and efficient plans to counteract them (Research Highlights box).

Income level has been associated repeatedly with the presence or absence of a healthy state, and it underlies many health disparities. Often lower-income groups have the least education. Such differences in both income and education are associated with disparities in the occurrence of disorders, including heart disease, diabetes, obesity, elevated blood lead levels, and low birth weight (USDHHS, 2000). Poverty accompanies poor environmental conditions, inadequate housing, occupational hazards, violence, unemployment, and limited access to health care (Lundy & Janes, 2001).

Personal behavioral characteristics related to lifestyle may suggest the need to screen an individual or group. When health care practitioners consider lifestyle, they are looking at daily habits that affect health and wellness, such as diet, exercise, smoking, alcohol and drug use, stress

CASE STUDY

Prostate Screening

A hospital offered a comprehensive, free prostate screening for men aged 50 and over in a community with a diverse population. The overall goal was to bring in individuals from lower socioeconomic and diverse cultural groups who ordinarily would not be able to access screening. Publicity, including press releases and advertisements, was run in all the local papers, and screening was conducted at various hours and several days of the week to accommodate the target group. Despite this, the results indicated that the targeted group did not use the service as hoped, and the predominant user group was white, middle class, insured men.

Reflective Questions

1. What was wrong with the presentation of this screening?
2. What were possible reasons for this problem?
3. If you are the public health nurse assigned to plan and implement the screening the following year, what would you do differently?
4. What other community organizations and key individuals or groups would you include in the process?
5. How might a school of nursing and its students assist with the screening process?

management, and use of seat belts. Engaging in some of these behaviors while avoiding others is essential for living a healthy life. Therefore screening for those personal behavioral characteristics that are considered risky suggests the

---

Differences in Factors Related to Breast Cancer Screening Behavior in Mexican-Born and United States–Born Women of Mexican Descent

A survey was completed by 179 female U.S. residents of Mexican heritage who were born in Mexico ($n = 76$) or the United States ($n = 103$). The emphasis of the survey pertained to factors related to breast cancer screening. The women born in the United States had significantly higher levels of income, education, and acculturation. In addition, these women were significantly more likely to be covered by health insurance and to receive health professional interventions and education such as breast self-examination instruction. These factors influenced the women born in the United States to engage in breast self-examination more frequently than did the other group.

In comparison, the Mexican-born women identified significantly more beliefs that breast cancer is a serious illness and that they were relatively more susceptible to the disease than were Americans. The locus of control for these Mexican-born women was geared toward powerful others and chance factors. These factors suggest that Mexican-born women face more breast cancer screening barriers than the U.S.-born women of Mexican descent.

Data from Borrayo, E., & Guarnaccia, C. (2000). Differences in Mexican-born and U.S.-born women of Mexican descent regarding factors related to breast cancer screening behaviors. *Health Care for Women International, 21*(7), 599-613.

---

likelihood of a longer, disease-free life. Once screening suggests those behaviors that are considered risky, the development of healthy behaviors via programming and a conscious transformation in lifestyle is key.

Health care providers bear a responsibility to educate individuals about the next step in the evaluation of their potential condition once a screening is completed. Those being screened bear a responsibility to seek treatment, follow-up, and ultimately engage in behavioral change toward a healthy lifestyle if the screening is to serve a purpose (Health Teaching box).

Environment-Dependent Factors

The area of environmental health and protection has expanded over the years and is becoming more complex. Environmental health and protection has been defined as that science which is concerned with elements of the environment that influence people's health and well-being. These factors include conditions of the workplace, home, and communities including chemical, physical, and psychological forces (Allender & Spradley, 2001). Environment-related risk factors relevant to screening designs are derived from an individual's surroundings. Areas that may be considered include overpopulation; indoor and outdoor air pollution; water pollution; safe drinking water; noise pollution; radiation exposure; biological pollutants; hazardous waste management and disposal of garbage; vector and pesticide control; deforestation, wetlands destruction, and desertification; energy depletion; inadequate housing; contaminated food and foods with toxic additives; safety in the home, worksite, and community; and psychological hazards (Allender & Spradley, 2001).

HEALTH TEACHING Pender's Health Promotion Model

A health care provider's responsibility is to assess, plan, implement, and evaluate a screening program. Part of this responsibility includes teaching individuals, families, and populations about the importance of participating in these programs and ultimately engaging in behavior that enhances health. The health promotion model is a useful guide for practice (Pender, 2002). The model presents the interrelationship among behavior-specific cognitions and affective factors and individual characteristics and experiences that motivate individuals to engage in behaviors that promote health. The health care provider may find that the application of this model in practice influences the relationship between the provider and the individual in a positive way. The model is a framework that assists the provider in assessing factors believed to influence health behavioral changes. Once the provider has an accurate assessment, obtained via questions, decisions may be made concerning factors that inhibit health-promoting behaviors and, ultimately, potential interventions to assist individuals in achieving positive health outcomes. This information will assist the provider to develop appropriate teaching methods.

Health Promotion Assessment Questions
1. How do you define health?
2. What does health mean to you?
3. How would you describe your health now?
4. Do the choices you make and actions you take affect your health?
5. Can you give examples when choices and actions created a positive change in health for you?
6. Can you give examples when choices and actions created a negative change in health for you?
7. What factors facilitated choices and actions that created a positive change in health?
8. What factors created barriers to choices and actions that led to a negative change in health?
9. Are there any supportive personal influences in your life that would assist you in choices and actions that would create a positive change in your health (i.e., family, friends, and health care providers)?
10. Are there any supportive situational influences, such as more than one plan of action, pertaining to the health change available to you?

Modified from Pender, N., Murdaugh, C., & Parsons, M. A. (2002). *Health promotion in nursing practice* (4th ed.). Upper Saddle River, New Jersey: Prentice Hall.

In occupational health, a legitimate population for screening is in the high-risk work area, where harmful chemicals, airborne particles, or high-decibel machinery put the worker at risk of cancer, respiratory conditions, or auditory problems. At the other extreme is the sedentary executive work life, in which stress and lack of exercise are prevalent. The use of an occupational health nurse to provide individual and mass screening for such problems is recognized as an integral role by both the health professions and the business world.

Environment-dependent factors have long been associated with the presence or absence of certain conditions. Primary prevention would be the preferred mode of protection; however, considering the shortsightedness of present society, secondary prevention appears to be the preferred choice. Screening must be focused on the short-term results of certain environmental conditions and on monitoring the long-term trends.

COMMONLY SCREENED CONDITIONS

The following section reviews several commonly screened diseases to demonstrate the complexity of issues that may surround the screening process. Ultimately a systematic approach, in which decision making is collaborative, will move the targeted population toward health improvement and the attainment of the two central goals of *Healthy People 2010* (USDHHS, 2000):

1. Increased quality and years of healthy life
2. Elimination of health disparities

For more specific objectives related to screening see the *Healthy People 2010* box.

Phenylketonuria

PKU is a condition characterized by the genetically determined lack of phenylalanine hydroxylase, an enzyme necessary to metabolize an important amino acid, phenylalanine. In its absence, blood levels of phenylalanine increase, causing irreversible damage to the brain and central nervous system, resulting in severe mental retardation. The significance of PKU screening, therefore, is in its identification of the condition so as to prevent the long-term effects.

Knowledge of PKU's **natural history,** or the progression of the disease from prepathogenesis to pathogenesis, defines the optimal time to administer the test, which is for all newborns before discharge from the nursery (U.S. Preventive Services Task Force, 1996).

The U.S. Preventive Services Task Force (1996) also recommends a repeat screening test by 2 weeks of age if the infant was tested before 24 hours of age. This effective screening method is an individually administered, disease-specific blood test for phenylalanine level, known as the *Guthrie test*. This sample often is used to test for other conditions, reducing the cost of detecting PKU. Dietary control of phenylalanine intake is a safe, effective way to manage PKU. With this diet, individualized according to the infant's rate and point of growth and development, mental

Healthy People 2010
Objectives Related To Screening

1. Ensure appropriate newborn bloodspot screening, follow-up testing, and referral to services.
2. Increase the proportion of sexually active females aged 25 years and under who are screened annually for genital *Chlamydia* infections.
3. Increase the proportion of pregnant females screened for sexually transmitted diseases (including HIV infection and bacterial vaginosis) during prenatal health care visits, according to recognized standards.
4. Increase the proportion of women who receive a Pap test.
5. Increase the proportion of newborns who are screened for hearing deficit by age 1 month, have audiologic evaluation by age 3 months, and are enrolled in appropriate intervention services by age 6 months.
6. Increase the proportion of preschool children aged 5 years and under who receive vision screening.
7. Increase the proportion of people who have a dilated eye examination at appropriate intervals.
8. Increase the proportion of adults who receive a colorectal cancer screening examination.
9. Increase the proportion of women aged 40 years and older who have undergone a mammogram within the preceding 2 years.
10. Increase the proportion of people living in pre-1950s housing who have been tested for the presence of lead-based paint.
11. Increase the proportion of adults who have had their blood pressure measured within the preceding 2 years and can state whether their blood pressure was normal or high.
12. Increase the proportion of adults who have had their blood cholesterol levels checked within the preceding 5 years.
13. Increase the proportion of adults with tuberculosis who have been tested for HIV.
14. Increase the proportion of adults in publicly funded HIV counseling and testing sites who are screened for common bacterial STDs (chlamydia, gonorrhea, and syphilis) and are immunized against hepatitis B virus.

From U.S. Department of Health and Human Services. (2000). *Healthy People 2010* (Conference ed.). Washington, DC: The Department.
HIV, human immunodeficiency virus; *Pap,* Papanicolaou; *STDs,* sexually transmitted diseases.

retardation can be avoided. PKU therefore fulfills the basic law of screening: early intervention can affect a disease's progress. Medically and economically, PKU screening is almost a model screenable disease.

Breast Cancer

In the United States the most common cancer among women is breast cancer (USDHHS, 2000). A malignant lesion in the breast indicates the disease; severity is based on the size of the lesion and the length of time that it has been present. Screening for asymptomatic cases and finding unnoticed and presumably smaller masses permit more successful and conservative treatments, because the stage is less severe.

In American women, the incidence of breast cancer increases with age. Nulliparous women, who have never given birth, run a high risk of breast carcinoma; women who had their first child before the age of 20 constitute the lowest risk group. Women who start menstruating at an earlier age than average and reach menopause at a later age than average also have a somewhat higher risk, as do those who bore their first child in their late 30s. Additional risks may include women with fibrocystic disease of the breast, family history of breast cancer, extended use of estrogen supplements, obesity, and a diet high in fat.

Screening tests that have been considered appropriate for early detection include (1) screening mammography, (2) clinical breast examination (CBE), and (3) breast self-examination.

The U.S. Preventive Services Task Force (2002a) recommends screening mammography every 1 to 2 years, with or without the CBE. The task force report indicated that evidence suggests the benefit is fairly strong, in that screening mammography has a significant impact on reducing breast cancer mortality, and concluded that harms from screening mammography (false-positive results, unnecessary biopsies, cost, and anxiety) tend to decrease in woman aged 40 and over; that is, the benefit-to-harm ratio becomes more favorable to older women. The nurse is often the health care provider who teaches a woman about breast health.

Although breast self-examination has been encouraged and considered an important aspect of breast health education, data regarding its efficacy is weak (U.S. Preventative Task Force, 2002a). Moreover, there has been an associated increase in false-positive findings that result in unnecessary biopsies (U.S. Preventive Services Task Force, 2002a).

The U.S. Preventive Services Task Force (2002a) has not been able to determine whether there are any screening benefits to the CBE alone, and although there may be "incremental benefit" of combining CBE with screening mammography, the data are insufficient for specific recommendation. Screening for breast cancer every 1 to 2 years, with mammography alone or mammography and CBE, is recommended for women aged 40 and older (U.S. Preventive Services Task Force, 2002a).

Cervical Cancer

The tenth most common cancer among women in the United States is cervical cancer (USDHHS, 2000). The principal screening test for cervical cancer is the Papanicolaou (Pap) smear. Although all sexually active women are at risk for cervical cancer, the disease is more common among women of low socioeconomic status, women with a history of multiple sex partners, women with early first sexual intercourse, smokers, and women with certain types of human papilloma virus and human immunodeficiency virus (HIV).

The incidence of invasive cervical cancer has decreased dramatically since the implementation of early detection programs involving the Pap smear. The official guidelines for Pap smear testing include the following:

1. Screening should be performed on all women, aged 21 years and older, or within 3 years of the onset of sexual activity and at least every 3 years thereafter.
2. Routine screening is not recommended for women who are not at high risk, aged 65 and older, whose recent Pap smears have been normal.
3. Screening is not recommended for women with a history of total hysterectomy as a result of benign disease.
4. There is insufficient evidence to recommend for or against the use of the new techniques for routine screening (U.S. Preventive Services Task Force, 2003a).

Colorectal Cancer

Colorectal cancer is the second leading cause of cancer deaths in the United States (USDHHS, 2000). A campaign for early detection of colorectal carcinoma continues to be widely publicized by the American Cancer Society. The U.S. Preventive Services Task Force (2002b) strongly recommends periodic colorectal screening for men and women beginning at age 50. They have concluded that the benefit-to-harm ratio is highly favorable, with the magnitude of each having a different variation with each screening method.

The American Cancer Society (2000) developed guidelines for both men and women who, at the age of 50, should undergo one of the following procedures: (1) an annual fecal occult blood test plus a flexible sigmoidoscopy every 5 years, (2) a colonoscopy every 10 years or double-contrast barium enema every 5 to 10 years, and (3) a digital rectal examination (DRE), which should be performed at the time of each screening. Most organizations recommend the more intensive screening, which includes barium enema and colonoscopy, for those in at-risk groups. Principal risk factors include a history of inflammatory bowel disease, family history of first-degree relative with colorectal cancer, previously diagnosed colorectal cancer, adenomatous polyps, and history of endometrial, ovarian, or breast cancer.

Prostate Cancer

Prostate cancer is the most commonly diagnosed cancer in males and the second leading cause of death among males in the United States (USDHHS, 2000). However, according to the U.S. Preventive Services Task Force (2002c), of the approximately 1 in 6 men who are diagnosed with the disease, only about 1 in 29 will die of it. The risk increases with age, beginning at 50 years, and is considerably higher among black men.

Screening tests commonly used for prostate cancer include DRE and PSA, the analysis for the serum tumor marker prostate-specific antigen (U.S. Preventive Services Task Force, 2002c). However, prostate cancer screening continues to be controversial. Although DRE is easily taught and cost-effective, its effectiveness in reducing prostate cancer death rates has not been determined (National Cancer Institute, 2004), and data are inconclusive to prove that early detection actually improves outcome. In addition, there are considerable harms associated with both the screenings and the treatments for some cancers that might never have altered a person's health (U.S. Preventive Service Task Force, 2002c). False-positive results leading to unnecessary biopsies and anxiety are not uncommon, nor are treatment complications of sexual dysfunction or incontinence. A possible exception to the benefit-to-harm ratio may exist among black men, because both incidence and mortality rates are higher in this group. The best age and intervals for PSA and DRE screenings are not known (National Cancer Institute, 2004b). Clinical trials in progress may provide a more definitive answer (U.S. Preventive Services Task Force, 2002c).

Cholesterol

One of the major modifiable risk factors for coronary heart disease is elevated blood cholesterol levels (USDHHS, 2000). Extensive research, educational programs, and media attention have increased the knowledge and understanding of the implications of high cholesterol levels and of the role of cholesterol in a healthy lifestyle. Cholesterol screening can identify high-risk individuals who are most likely to benefit from individualized risk factor counseling, dietary instruction, and drug therapies. Indeed, the strongest support for cholesterol screening is the ability of cholesterol-lowering interventions to reduce the risk of coronary heart disease in those with high cholesterol levels (U.S. Preventive Services Task Force, 1996).

Screening for total cholesterol and high-density lipoprotein cholesterol (HDL-C) levels can be obtained in fasting or nonfasting individuals from finger stick or venipuncture samples (U.S. Preventive Services Task Force, 1996).

The U.S. Preventive Services Task Force (1996) advises that because a single cholesterol value does not accurately assess an individual's true cholesterol level, intervention decisions must be based on a minimum of two measurements along with assessment of the individuals cardiovascular risk factors.

Recommendations are for periodic screening for high blood cholesterol levels for all men aged 35 to 65 and women aged 45 to 65. Intervals for this periodic screening are not known, but the recommendation remains at every 5 years, with longer intervals for those considered at low risk and more frequently for those considered at high risk. Screening of children, adolescents, and young adults is not recommended, because there is insufficient evidence as to the effectiveness of such actions. Any such considerations must be made on a case-by-case review, depending on risk factors. Screening of people over age 65 must also be done on a case-by-case review (U.S. Preventive Services Task Force, 1996).

Hypertension

According to the Seventh Report of the Joint National Committee on Prevention, Detection, Evaluation, and Treatment of High Blood Pressure (USDHHS, 2003), hypertension is a leading risk factor for congestive heart failure, stroke, heart attack, and renal disease. Detecting high blood pressure is a primary prevention strategy for coronary heart disease, cerebrovascular disease, and peripheral vascular disease; it is a secondary prevention strategy for hypertension. Criteria for referral may vary according to the level of elevation and risk factors. At the very least, the individual will be advised to have a recheck in 2 years; at most the person would be referred for follow-up care immediately.

Periodic screening is recommended for everyone 18 years of age and older, but the optimal interval of screening has yet to be determined and is presently left to the clinician's judgment (U.S. Preventive Services Task Force, 2003c). Currently there are insufficient data to recommend screening intervals for children or adolescents (U.S. Preventive Services Task Force, 2003c).

People with systolic blood pressure readings from 120 to 139 mm Hg and diastolic readings from 80 to 89 mm Hg are classified as prehypertensive (U.S. Department of Health and Human Services, National Institutes of Health, 2003). For people over 50 years of age, the Joint National Committee, VII (USDHHS, 2003) guidelines indicate that systolic pressure has greater impact on health outcome than the diastolic pressure. Therefore, treatment is recommended when systolic pressure is equal to or greater than 140 mm Hg, regardless of the diastolic readings. Assessment of other cardiovascular risk factors, such as diabetes, may modify these guidelines and clinical discretion is always key.

When hypertension is treated effectively, there are important long-term implications for decreased mortality and morbidity from end-organ damage. Therefore it should be a part of any comprehensive screening program.

Glaucoma

Glaucoma is the second leading cause of irreversible blindness in the United States. An estimated 2 million people suffer from this disease and more that 50% are unaware of their condition (Lewis, Heitkemper, & Dirksen, 2004). The prevalence of glaucoma is fourfold to sixfold higher in the black population than the white population, and it increases steadily with age. The prevalence of glaucoma is higher in individuals with diabetes mellitus, myopia, and a family history of glaucoma. The natural history of the disease is explained by increased intraocular pressure, which is caused by an obstruction of the outflow of aqueous humor from the eye's interior and damages the optic nerve, causing loss of vision. Visual deficits that are caused by glaucoma are not generally reversible, but early treatment is widely believed to prevent or delay the progression to more serious problems.

Three diagnostic criteria exist for the screening of glaucoma: (1) an increase in intraocular pressure as measured by a tonometer, (2) damage to the optic nerve, which is assessed through ophthalmoscopic evaluation, and (3) visual field loss, as measured by perimetry. Although the presence of all three criteria is indicative of glaucoma, experts disagree whether one variable alone is indicative of the disease. In addition, the accuracy of testing depends on the choice of test, experience of the examiner, and the variables of the individual. Sufficient evidence does not exist to recommend for or against routine screening. However, at-risk individuals should be referred to experienced specialists who have access to the equipment that is necessary to evaluate the optic disc and measure the visual fields.

Human Immunodeficiency Virus

As of November 1999, human immunodeficiency virus (HIV) and acquired immunodeficiency syndrome (AIDS) have been reported in every racial and ethnic population, in every age and socioeconomic group, in every state, and in most large cities throughout the United States (USDHHS, 2000). HIV is now the leading cause of death for those in the black population aged 25 to 44, and it dropped to eighth place for all others in this age group by 1997 (USDHHS, 2000). *Healthy People 2010* (USDHHS, 2000) reports that infection rates appear to have stabilized to a slower growth rate of approximately 40,000 new infections per year. In addition, recent therapies have reduced the severity of illness and prolonged survival. However, the need for HIV screening to increase the numbers of individuals who know their HIV status continues to be important. The goal is to detect infection at the earliest possible time and decrease transmission when the potential is greatest, and to increase access to early care, prevention, and treatment, including highly active antiretroviral therapy (USDHHS, 2000).

Health care providers need to assess the risk factors for HIV infection in all individuals by obtaining a careful sexual history and inquiring about past or present drug use. Periodic screening for HIV should be offered to all individuals who are at increased risk for the infection. Included are those seeking treatment for sexually transmitted diseases, men who have had sex with men, past or present intravenous drug users, individuals with multiple sexual partners, people who engage in sex for money or drugs, people with a history of transfusion between 1978 and 1985, and men or women whose past or present sex partners were infected with HIV (U.S. Preventive Services Task Force, 1996).

The basic screening test for HIV is the enzyme immunoassay (EIA). Screening is recommended for all people at increased risk of infection, including at-risk pregnant women. There is limited information to recommend for or against routine HIV screening in individuals without risk factors. (U.S. Preventive Services Task Force, 1996).

Lead

Community initiatives have proved successful in the prevention of lead poisoning. The National Health and Nutrition Examination Surveys, conducted by Centers for Disease Control and Prevention's (CDC) National Center for Health Statistics, has been tracking blood lead levels at the national level. Trends indicate a steady decline. Although trends point to positive outcomes, state and local surveillance presents evidence demonstrating that some children tested have high lead levels, depending on the counties and states they live in. Although a known normal blood lead level does not exist, the CDC has reported children's blood lead levels less than 10 μg/dL as normal (CDC, 2004a). Elevated blood lead levels and the threat of lead toxicity continue to be a prevalent, yet preventable, health threat in both children and adults. Childhood lead intoxication can result in serious illness with lifelong consequences, such as developmental delay, behavior problems, seizures, coma, and even death (CDC, 2004a). Childhood lead poisoning often comes from the home itself, such as from lead-based paint and dust, or from items in the home, such as lead-based glass and make-up.

Ninety to ninety-five percent of adults who have elevated lead levels are exposed occupationally. They may demonstrate anemia, nervous system dysfunction, kidney problems, hypertension, decreased fertility, and more miscarriages. In addition, there is always the danger that individuals who experience occupational exposure may bring the lead into their homes (CDC, 2004b).

Two screening tests are used for detecting lead exposure: (1) blood lead and (2) free erythrocyte or zinc protoporphyrin levels. Blood lead level is the more sensitive test, but it can easily be affected by environmental lead contamination during blood collection. Erythrocyte protoporphyrin is an indirect measure of lead exposure and is not affected by environmental contamination. It is not, however, as sensitive to modest lead elevations as the blood lead test. Screening for elevated blood lead levels is recommended at least once at 12 months for all children at risk for exposure. In communities where there is a low prevalence of levels requiring intervention, a lead risk factor questionnaire would identify at-risk children for targeted blood testing.

Diabetes Mellitus

Diabetes mellitus is a group of disorders that have glucose intolerance as the common factor, characterized by hyperglycemia and other disturbances of carbohydrate, protein, and fat metabolism (Huether & McCance, 2000). Onset of symptoms in type 1 diabetes is acute, and symptoms are detected soon. This type occurs because of the body's failure to produce insulin. A person with type 2 diabetes is often asymptomatic in the early stages, and the disease may remain undiagnosed for many years. This type results from insulin resistance. Undiagnosed type 2 diabetes is associated with long-term damage to multiple organ systems. The risk of developing type 2 diabetes increases with age, obesity, and lack of exercise. Individuals with a family history, hypertension, dyslipidemia, delivery of babies weighing more than 9 pounds, or who are members of particular racial or ethnic groups also have increased risk of developing this disease. Other types of diabetes include gestational diabetes and prediabetes (American Diabetes Association, 2004).

The U.S. Preventive Services Task Force (2003b) recommends screening for type 2 diabetes in adults with hypertension or hyperlipidemia. Early detection via screening, in this population, will result in prompt treatment, ultimately reducing the burden of this disease. However, mass screening of all individuals (even all individuals considered at high risk) is not recommended, because there is no evidence to suggest that beginning diabetic management as a result of a mass screening provides an incremental benefit compared with initiating treatment after clinical diagnosis (U.S. Preventive Services Task Force, 2003b). The decision to screen or not to screen should be made based upon expert clinical judgment of the health care practitioner. Screening of high-risk individuals should be considered at 3-year intervals. The fasting plasma glucose test and the oral glucose tolerance test are preferred and recommended tests.

THE NURSE'S ROLE

The need for nursing involvement exists at all levels of the collaborative partnership process. Being some of the many important stakeholders, nurses play a role in every aspect of the screening program development process, including assessment, data analysis, planning, implementation, evaluation of the health outcomes, and the evaluation of the process (including the workings of the partnership). One aspect of this health process is the development and implementation of screening programs for targeted groups. As nurses become more involved in decision making they will be faced with the question, "Should this condition be screened for or not?" In the role of decision maker and planner, the nurse is responsible for reviewing all the issues concerning a screenable disease, including (1) the criteria specific to the disease, (2) the medical and economic ethics, and (3) the community resources that are affected. If the choice is to screen, the participation of nurses and other partnering groups is essential in the development of a care plan (see Care Plan). The last step is the planning and development of an efficient referral system to enhance continuity of care and to ensure follow-up.

Nurses have long been responsible for screening individuals. As in any nursing intervention, adequate knowledge of the method of administration and the potential side effects is needed. Teaching individuals the meaning and limitation of the test results is an important element of this role, as is informing them of their part in obtaining the implied benefit.

The combined health educator and screener component means that the nurse continues to educate individuals about risk factors and teach them ways to alter and reduce risks generally through lifestyle changes, such as proper diet, exercise, and stress management, and by limiting the use of alcohol, drugs, and tobacco. The role as educator is essential in the screening process, because nurses provide individuals with the information necessary for choices that are made regarding healthy behavioral change. The nurse is actually practicing primary prevention interventions, but it is in coordination with a secondary preventive role.

SUMMARY

As a method of preclinical secondary prevention, screening is the rapid administration of a simple test to distinguish individuals who may have a condition from those who probably do not have a condition. It can be an effective, efficient tool in preventive health care if used for conditions applicable to the screening model and directed toward an at-risk population. A unique characteristic and significant advantage of screening is that it can be applied to individuals or groups.

Three questions provide a means of analyzing the screenability of a disease:
1. Is the condition significant?
2. Can screening for the condition be done?
3. Should screening for the condition be done?

Screening programs are not appropriate for all conditions or all communities. Alternative methods of reaching the desired health outcome should always be considered. Screening in health care presents numerous roles for nurses and provides them with a valuable preventive tool in the care of healthy individuals.

ADDITIONAL STUDY MATERIAL

Study Questions in the back of the book, see page 663.

evolve WEB SITE MATERIALS

These materials are located on the book's Web site at http://evolve.elsevier.com/Edelman/.

- WebLinks
- Content Updates

REFERENCES

Allender, J., & Spradley, B. (2001). *Community health nursing: Concepts and practice* (5th ed.). New York: Lippincott.

American Cancer Society. (2000). *Colorectal cancer: Early detection* (On-line). Retrieved March 1, 2004, from: *http://www.cancer.org/docroot/home/index.asp.*

American Diabetes Association (2004). *All about diabetes.* Retrieved March 1, 2004, from *http://www.diabetes.org/about_diabetes.JSP*

Anderson, E. T., & McFarlane, J. M. (2000). *Community as partner: Theory and practice in nursing* (3rd ed.). New York: Lippincott Williams & Wilkins.

Centers for Disease Control and Prevention. (2004a). Lead fact sheet. Retrieved June 4, 2005, from: *http://www.cdc.gov/exposurereport/2nd/lead_factsheet.htm*.

Centers for Disease Control and Prevention. (2004b). *The adult blood lead level epidemiology and surveillance program.* Retrieved June 4, 2005, from: *http://www.cdc.gov/niosh/ablesh.html*.

Huether, S. E., & McCance, K. L. (2003). *Understanding pathophysiology* (3rd ed.). St. Louis: Mosby.

Lewis, S. M., Heitkemper, M. M., & Dirksen, S. R. (2004). *Medical-surgical nursing: Assessment and management of clinical problems* (6th ed.). St. Louis: Mosby.

Lundy, K., & Janes, S. (2001). *Community health nursing: Caring for the public's health.* Boston: Jones and Bartlett.

National Cancer Institute. (2004b). *Prostate cancer: Screening and testing.* Retrieved June 4, 2005, from: *http://www.nci.nih.gov/cancerinfo/screening/prostate*.

Pender, N., Murdaugh, C., & Parsons, M. A. (2002). *Health promotion in nursing practice* (4th ed.). Upper Saddle River, New Jersey: Prentice Hall.

Polit, D., Beck, C., & Hungler, B. (2001). *Essentials of nursing research: Methods, appraisal, and utilization* (5th ed.). New York: Lippincott.

Sackett, D., Straus, S., Richardson, W., Rosenberg, W., & Haynes, R. (2000). *Evidence-based medicine: How to practice and teach EBM* (2nd ed.). New York: Churchill Livingston.

U.S. Department of Health and Human Services. (2000). *Healthy people 2010* (Conference ed.). Washington, DC: The Department.

U.S. Department of Health and Human Services. National Institutes of Health, National Heart, Lung and Blood Pressure. (2003). *Seventh report of the Joint National Committee: On prevention, detection, evaluation, and treatment of high blood pressure.* Retrieved March 1, 2004, from: *http://nhlbi.nih.gov/guidelines/hypertension*.

U.S. Preventive Services Task Force. (1996). *Guide to clinical preventive services* (2nd ed.). Baltimore: Williams & Wilkins.

U.S. Preventive Services Task Force. (2002a). *Guide to clinical preventive services: Breast screening.* Retrieved March 1, 2004, from: *http://www.ahrq.gov/clinic/uspstfix.htm*.

U.S. Preventive Services Task Force. (2002b). *Guide to clinical preventive services: Colorectal screening.* Retrieved March 1, 2004, from: *http://www.ahrq.gov/clinic/uspstfix.htm*.

U.S. Preventive Services Task Force. (2002c). *Guide to clinical preventive services: Prostate screening.* Retrieved March 1, 2004, from: *http://www.ahrq.gov/clinic/uspstfix.htm*.

U.S. Preventive Services Task Force. (2003a). *Guide to clinical preventive services: Cervical screening.* Retrieved March 1, 2004, from: *http://www.ahrq.gov/clinic/uspstfix.htm*.

U.S. Preventive Services Task Force. (2003b). *Guide to clinical preventive services: Diabetes screening.* Retrieved March 1, 2004, from: *http://www.ahrq.gov/clinic/uspstfix.htm*.

U.S. Preventive Services Task Force. (2003c). *Guide to clinical preventive services: Hypertension screening.* Retrieved March 1, 2004, from: *http://www.ahrq.gov/clinic/uspstfix.htm*.

Chapter 10

SUSAN A. HEADY

Health Education

objectives

After completing this chapter, the reader will be able to:

- Define health education.
- Describe the aims of health education.
- Discuss learning principles that affect health education.
- Apply teaching and learning concepts to teaching the family.
- Describe the health belief model and behavior change process.
- Describe the use of social marketing in planning health education programs.
- Identify the steps in preparing a health-teaching plan.
- Select content and learning strategies appropriate to the health learning needs of a target audience.
- List ways to evaluate a person's progress.
- Discuss personal plans for developing teaching skills.

key terms

Behavior change
Disease prevention
Health behaviors
Health belief model

Health counseling
Health education
Health promotion
Social cognitive theory

Social learning theory
Social marketing

THINK About It

The Challenges of Health Education

An analysis of a nursing assessment often leads to a nursing diagnosis related to the individual's lack of knowledge in the areas of health promotion or health-promotion strategies. The nurse may recognize certain risk factors in a person, such as a lack of knowledge, possession of incorrect knowledge, misinterpretation of information, or reliance on harmful myths and folk medicine. Additionally, the individual may demonstrate little or no interest in learning, a lack of motivation to learn, or a cognitive or perceptual inability to learn.

The success of any health activity or goal will depend on the individual's perception of the situation and responsiveness to teaching. The success of health teaching depends on a person's ability to learn and process information and the motivation to change behaviors to improve the present condition or move toward better health. The nurse must assist each person in a process of self-understanding and self-direction, so the individual will experience the desire and motivation to change. Frequently, major life decisions must be made in the process of learning. If through education and counseling the nurse can elicit logical and clear thinking, then the individual's decision-making abilities and progress in meeting life's needs will be developed further. To encourage critical thinking by an individual, the nurse may pose some of the following questions:

Continued

THINK About It

The Challenges of Health Education cont'd

1   What do you know about the health problem or concern?

2   What were you told?

3   What do you think will help you deal with the problem or concern?

4   How do you explain this problem or concern to yourself?

5   How do you see yourself in 6 months?

6   What types of efforts have worked for you in the past with this problem or concern?

7   How does the problem or concern affect your daily life?

8   What one aspect would indicate an improvement in your condition?

9   How much control do you think you have over this situation?

10 What is one goal that you would like to set for yourself?

Scenario

Ronald is a successful executive in a local business. In his annual physical examination, an irregular heartbeat was noted on the electrocardiogram. Ronald's father died of a heart attack at age 50; therefore, the physician scheduled Ronald for a thallium stress test. The stress test indicated a need for further evaluation with a cardiac catheterization. A 60% blockage in one artery was detected during this process. Ronald's condition will be handled conservatively at this point. He recognizes that some lifestyle changes are necessary. He is overweight and eats in restaurants frequently. He has not been active in regular exercise. He and his wife live in a condominium. They have grown children and grandchildren. One of their sons has a serious drug problem, so they have not seen him for several years and hear from him only rarely.

1   How might the nurse begin working with Ronald?

2   How likely is he to be motivated to learn and change?

3   What are some barriers to change in his behaviors?

Healthy People 2010 provides objectives to improve the health of individuals, groups, and communities in the United States (U.S. Department of Health and Human Services, 2000). Implementation of *Healthy People 2010* seeks to improve life expectancy and quality of life by "helping individuals gain the knowledge, motivation, and opportunities they need to make informed decisions about their health" (Lee & Estes, 2003, p. 58). Achievement of these objectives provides challenges and opportunities for health promotion. Although health is influenced significantly by social, economic, physical, and political factors, many health goals are affected by individual lifestyle prac-

tices. *Healthy People 2010* objectives related to educational programs appear in the *Healthy People 2010* box.

Behavior patterns account for 40% to 50% of early deaths among Americans and represent the single most controllable area of influence over the health forecast (McGinnis, 2003). Nursing, with its unique contributions to health care, represents a professional resource that can help facilitate these changes through health education strategies. Nurses, in partnership with other health care professionals, can be the link between the philosophy of *Healthy People 2010* and the people who need to hear its messages and act on those messages.

NURSING AND HEALTH EDUCATION

Nurses as educators play a key role in improving the health of the nation. Educating people is an integral part of the nurse's role in every practice setting—schools, communities, work sites, health care delivery sites, and homes. Health education involves not only providing relevant information, but also facilitating health-related **behavior change.** The nurse, using health education principles, can assist people in achieving their health goals in a way that is consistent with their personal lifestyles, values, and beliefs.

The *Standards of Clinical Nursing Practice* describes education as a primary nursing responsibility. This includes educating people to make informed decisions about their health care and treatment, health promotion, **disease prevention,** and achieving peaceful death (American Nurses Association, [ANA], 1998). Health teaching and **health counseling** are included in the ANA's social policy statement (ANA, 2003). This responsibility to teach individuals is balanced by their right to know about diagnosis, treatment, risks, benefits, costs, and alternatives. The nurse's role is to support the right of individuals to know their health status and to assess and assist a person's physical, psychosocial, and spiritual response to that knowledge. The nurse also provides health teaching and health counseling based on individual interest and decisions (Bandman & Bandman, 2002).

Nurses usually function as health care coordinators for individuals in their care. Depending on the interest and needs of a person, nurses establish a partnership to guide the individual in the selection and use of relevant health services. Principles of health education provide the nurse with strategies and tools for assessing an individual's readiness for health teaching, with technical information and with help in practicing health care techniques at home. These strategies also help the nurse facilitate behavior change, while satisfying the person's right to relevant health information and the freedom for people to make decisions about their own health. Health education encourages self-care, self-empowerment and, ultimately, less dependence on the health care system.

Nurses have long been involved in public health education, taking on the full-time role of coordinating the educational services provided by a health agency or institution. As a health educator, the nurse may use marketing strate-

Healthy People 2010

Selected Health-Promotion and Disease Prevention Objectives Related to Educational and Community-Based Programs

Goal: To Increase the Quality, Availability, and Effectiveness of Educational and Community-Based Programs Designed to Prevent Disease and Improve Health and Quality of Life

School Setting

- 7-1. Increase the rate of completion of high school.
- 7-2. Increase the proportion of middle, junior high, and senior high schools that provide comprehensive health education to prevent problems in the these areas: (1) unintentional injury, violence, and suicide, (2) tobacco use, (3) alcohol and other drug use, (4) unintended pregnancy and sexually transmitted infections, (5) unhealthy dietary patterns, and (6) inadequate physical activity.
- 7-3. Increase the proportion of college and university students who receive information for the institution of each of the six priority health-risk behavior areas listed above.
- 7-4. Increase the proportion of elementary, middle, junior high, and senior high schools that have a nurse-to-student ratio of at least 1:750.

Work Setting

- 7-5. Increase the proportion of work sites that offer a comprehensive employee health-promotion program to their employees.
- 7-6. Increase the proportion of employees who participate in employer-sponsored health-promotion activities.

Health Care Setting

- 7-7. Increase the proportion of health care organizations that provide patient and family education.
- 7-8. Increase the proportion of people who report that they are satisfied with the patient education that they receive from their health organization.
- 7-9. Increase the proportion of hospitals and managed care organizations that sponsor community disease prevention and health-promotion activities that address the priority health needs identified by their community.

Community Setting and Select Populations

- 7-10. Increase the proportion of tribal and local health service areas that establish community health-promotion programs.
- 7-11. Increase the proportion of local health departments that establish culturally appropriate and linguistically competent community health-promotion and disease prevention programs.
- 7-12. Increase the proportion of older adults who have participated during the preceding year in at least one organized health-promotion activity.

Modified from U.S. Department of Health and Human Services. (2000). *Healthy people 2010.* Washington, DC: U.S. Government Printing Office.

---

gies to enhance the effectiveness of health education programs that are focused on certain target populations. The health education specialist helps other nurses and health professionals improve their skills in developing and delivering teaching plans.

Definition

Health education is "any combination of planned learning experiences based on sound theories that provide individuals, groups, and communities the opportunity to acquire the information and the skills needed to make quality health decisions" (Wurzbach, 2004, p. 6). This process involves several key components. First, health education involves the use of teaching-learning strategies. Second, learners maintain voluntary control over the decision to make changes in their actions. Third, health education focuses on behavior changes that have been found to improve health status.

Health education facilitates the development of health knowledge, skills, and attitudes through the application of theories or models. Two commonly used theories, behavioral theory and social learning theory, will be discussed later in this chapter. Generally, health education strategies help ensure that individuals, as consumers of health services, are

satisfied and have received the health care that is most relevant to their problems. From a public health perspective, health education programs are intended not only to enhance individuals' abilities to make positive lifestyle changes, but also to support social and political actions that promote health and quality of life in communities.

The following scenario is an example of a therapeutic situation in which a health education approach may be used to meet an individual's health needs.

Sada Thompson, a 21-year-old university senior, visits university health services because she wants to change her method of birth control. She has experienced side effects from the birth control pill that she has been taking for the past year and knows little about other options. She has recently started dating John after breaking up with Steven 3 months ago. Having decided to be sexually active with John, Sada is feeling uncertain about what she needs to do to take care of herself and how to discuss this uncertainty with John. She is aware of all the talk about acquired immunodeficiency syndrome (AIDS) on campus and she knows that John is popular and has dated several other women in school, which concerns her.

Sada needs to learn new information, she may need to acquire new skills, and she must clarify any feelings or attitudes that affect her decision to use a new birth control method and ensure her continued safety. After recording her health assessment history and arranging for a gynecological examination and laboratory tests, the nurse develops a teaching plan. Selecting one or more strategies for helping Sada review all the birth control options, the nurse establishes an environment in which Sada can choose to try a new method or request a change in her prescription for oral contraceptives. Together they identify actions that Sada can take to use the method properly. They also anticipate and identify ways that Sada can solve problems of adjusting to the new method.

The nurse answers Sada's immediate questions about safe sex, gives her several pamphlets written for college students about this topic, and suggests that she participate in the peer counseling night on sexually transmitted diseases that will be held on campus in 2 weeks. The peer counseling hotline number and drop-in hours are given to her, and the nurse explains that these students are trained to help other students talk about and deal with this important issue. The nurse invites Sada to call or come back to the office for additional help, information, and problem-solving discussion.

This example illustrates that educational interventions, in addition to direct health services, are necessary to meet the individual's goal. Although health care providers and nurses prefer that people choose to take actions that will promote health and not detract from it, the individual controls the at-home application of health recommendations.

Goals

The goal of health education is to help individuals, families, and communities achieve, through their own actions and initiative, optimal states of health. Health education should facilitate voluntary actions to promote health.

Health education encourages positive, informed changes in lifestyle behaviors that prevent acute and chronic disease, decrease disability, and enhance wellness. Another goal of health education that may foster successful changes in health behavior is empowerment. People who believe that they can make a difference in health and who are involved in decision making are more likely to make changes (Anderson, Ward, & Hatton, 2004).

Changes in health behaviors that are related to health education help prevent disease and disability. Two main objectives of health education and counseling are to change health behaviors and to improve health status. Information alone does not change behavior.

Health education and health counseling are mutually supportive activities. Health educators often use one-to-one and group counseling techniques as strategies for active health learning. Counselors may refer people to health education resources or assist them in acquiring information pertinent to solving a health problem. The following example helps illustrate the goals of health education.

Kate Hanson, 22 years old, visits the local family health center for fatigue and symptoms similar to influenza. During the assessment with the nurse, Kate discloses that she has missed her last two periods.

The physical examination, the laboratory tests, and the health assessment pattern confirm Kate's suspicions of pregnancy. Psychosocial evaluation reveals that Kate works part time as a secretary for a temporary agency and lives in an apartment with her recently unemployed husband, Jim. Further interviewing reveals that Kate has minimal knowledge of prenatal care; she has a diet of take-out food that is high in fat, sodium, and sugar, with infrequent consumption of fresh fruits or vegetables; and she has three or four beers on the weekends. Kate has never taken vitamins, she leads a sedentary lifestyle, and she obviously is overwhelmed by the news that she is pregnant.

The nurse first takes steps to create a safe and trusting atmosphere in which Kate can feel free to share her concerns and apprehensions. Finding that Kate needs counseling for telling her husband about the pregnancy, the nurse discusses this with her. Kate is then taught the importance of taking a multiple vitamin with an iron supplement daily, discontinuing the use of alcohol, checking with her doctor before taking medications, and making time for more rest during the day. Sensing that this is all that can be accomplished at this time, the nurse gives Kate two pamphlets on prenatal care and makes an appointment for her to return in a week with her husband. Kate acknowledges that she understands the instructions, and the nurse documents the teaching and recommendations in Kate's chart.

During the next visit, the nurse meets with Kate and Jim, explores the meaning of the pregnancy in their lives, and helps them identify actions they will need to take. The recommendations that were made during Kate's first visit are reviewed and reinforced. The nurse then details specifics of dietary changes, the need for proper rest and exercise, and helps them solve problems as they adjust to these new responsibilities. Most importantly, the nurse gives them information on the clinic's weekly prenatal classes and explains that because the classes are partially covered by local community funding, the charge is minimal. The classes include information about physical changes, psychosocial changes, and nutritional needs during the pregnancy, the labor and delivery, and the newborn and postpartum periods. A nurse practitioner conducts the classes at the clinic, which are given in a group format to facilitate social support and problem solving among expectant parents.

The nurse gives them several other pamphlets to read at home, makes an appointment for Kate to see the physician in a couple of weeks, and encourages her to call if she has questions or concerns in the interim. A schedule of the prenatal classes is reviewed and a date for the next session is made. The couple is encouraged to meet with the social worker to explore their financial needs and options because Jim was recently laid off. Kate and Jim acknowledge that they understand what they need to do, and the nurse documents what was taught and discussed in Kate's health care record.

This example illustrates the goal of health education: to help individuals achieve optimal health and well-being through their actions and initiative. Through health education, individuals can learn to make informed decisions about personal and family health practices and to use health services in the community. The individual in this example receives educational assistance from the nurse that will promote better health and well-being for herself and her baby.

Learning Assumptions

Individual chapters in this text address the factors to consider when teaching different age groups and the learners' respective characteristics to consider when developing a teaching plan. The general principles of learning that are found in Box 10-1 are fundamental to the planning of successful health education programs (Wurzbach, 2004).

The nurse considers the developmental stage, cognitive level, and interests of the individual. The level of information to be conveyed and the skills and abilities of the individual will guide the methods and resources used. Children deserve special planning for health teaching (Health Teaching box).

Family Health Teaching

The family is the unit for the caregiving of its members; therefore, the family must often learn specific tasks of illness care and is responsible for teaching health promotion. Family members learn healthy behaviors in the home (Friedman, Bowden, & Jones, 2003). Skills in family interviewing and assessment are valuable tools for nurses. Family health assessment and health teaching are closely related.

The assessment model in the chapter on family health promotion provides a comprehensive approach to identifying problems, strengths, and health-education needs. The goal is to help the members achieve optimal states of health while guiding them through problem solving and decision making. This process empowers them. Members believe they can make a difference in their own health.

Box 10-1 How to Facilitate Learning

- Use methods that stimulate a variety of senses.
- Involve the person actively in the learning process.
- Establish a comfortable, appropriate learning environment.
- Assess the readiness of the learner, which may be affected by physical and emotional factors.
- Make the information relevant by connecting with the existing needs and interests of the learner.
- Use repetition. Review and reinforce concepts several times in a variety of ways.
- Make the learning encounter positive. Structure it to achieve progress recognizable by the individual and provide frequent, positive feedback.
- Start with what is known and proceed to what is unknown, moving from simple to complex.
- Apply the concepts to several settings to facilitate generalization.
- Pace the learning appropriately for the individual.

HEALTH TEACHING Teaching Health Promotion to Preschoolers and School-Aged Children

Teaching the principles of health promotion to young children can influence their behaviors now and in the future and may affect family health. "Childhood is an ideal time to help children begin to establish behaviors that will promote a healthy lifestyle" (Morotz, Cross, & Rush, 2001, p. 3).

Useful Principles for Teaching Children

- Children learn best by using all their senses.
- Learning activities should be interesting and meaningful.
- Teachers should show love and respect for all children.
- Good teaching is based on theory, philosophy, goals, and objectives.
- Children's learning is enhanced through the use of concrete materials.
- Teaching should be centered on the child.
- Teaching should move from the concrete to the abstract.
- Teaching should be based on the children's interests (Morrison, 2004).

Other Factors

In all planning, the children should be considered. When possible, the particular group should be observed and the learning experience should be as individualized as possible. The approach should be planned for the specific group of children with the following factors considered:

- The children's developmental level
- Any special considerations of the children
- The children's attention span
- The children's past experiences, interests, and abilities
- Activities that create enthusiasm and interest
- Activities that stimulate many senses
- Activities that leave the child with something to take home (Bastable & Rinswalske, 2003)

Suggested Teaching Activities

- Games
- Dialogue and interaction with children
- Hands-on practice
- Role playing and dramatic play
- Showing items, objects, and examples
- Puppets, dolls, stories, and books
- Drawing and painting (Bastable & Rinswalske, 2003)

The nurse may wear a costume or a special item of clothing that is related to the topic. The children will enjoy receiving a certificate of completion of a health lesson. Having something to take home to discuss with their parents is also meaningful.

The health teaching should emphasize skills that children can use or develop immediately. Experiences should be selected with their cognitive abilities in mind. For example, preschool children cannot understand cause and effect; they cannot anticipate the effects of dangerous situations, poor nutrition, and unsound health practices.

In clarifying the health teaching needs of a family, the nurse might ask herself, "Who is in this family? What tasks should they be performing? How are they functioning and how are they meeting each others' needs? How well are they communicating? What does this family need to know? What do they need to know now? What do they think they need to know? How can they learn what they need to know?"

The nurse sets a broad health-promotion goal for the family but directs the health teaching toward a more specific area. Most importantly, the family should be in agreement with the goal and teaching needs. As the family participates in the assessment interview, perhaps members can identify their own health teaching needs. Some broad goals for family teaching include:

- Better family functioning
- Achieving developmental tasks
- Better family communication
- Improved self-concept
- Increased self-esteem
- Reduced health risks
- Healthier lifestyle behaviors (improved diet and health habits)
- Improved energy level within the family
- A sense of control
- Adaptation to change in family structure
- Adaptation to change in family situation or life state

Health teaching includes all family members, with learning activities appropriate for each individual. The general teaching goal will be the same for all members, but the approaches and specific goals for each member or subsystem will be different. Children, adolescents, and elderly members pose special challenges to the nurse, who may be geared toward teaching young or middle-aged adults.

Health Behavior Change

The process of health education directs people toward voluntary changes of their health behaviors. This section examines (1) the use of the health belief model to analyze the probability that a person will make changes to improve health or prevent disease and (2) the application of social learning theory to clarify environmental and social factors that affect learning of new health behaviors.

Beliefs, attitudes, values, and information contribute to motivation and behavior and are underlying factors in making any decision to change behavior (Richards, 2003). **Health behaviors** are any activities that an individual undertakes to enhance health, prevent disease, and detect and control the symptoms of a disease. Identifying and teaching people about lifestyle behaviors that need to be changed is only the first step in the process of assisting individuals in moving from knowledge to action. The nurse uses the health belief model and social learning theory as subsequent steps in formulating an action plan that meets the needs and capabilities of each person in making healthy behavior changes.

Health Belief Model

The **health belief model** is a paradigm used to predict and explain health behavior. The health belief model was developed to describe why people failed to participate in programs to detect or prevent disease. The model has been expanded to explain responses to symptoms, disease, prescribed treatments, and potential health problems (Glanz, Rimer, & Lewis, 2002). The health belief model and social learning theory assist the nurse in formulating an action plan that meets the needs and capabilities of the individual making health behavior changes.

The following components of the health belief model provide guidelines for nurses to analyze factors that contribute to a person's perceived state of health or risk of disease and to the individual's probability of making an appropriate plan of action:

- Individual perceptions or readiness for change
- The value of health to the individual compared with other aspects of living
- Perceived susceptibility to a health problem, disease, or complications
- Perceived seriousness of the disease level threatening the achievement of certain goals or aims
- Risk factors to a disease attributed to heredity, race or culture, medical history, or other causes
- Perceived benefits of health action
- Perceived barriers to promotion action (Becker, 1974; Janz & Becker, 1984; Rosenstock, Strecher, & Becker, 1988)

The health belief model does not specify the interventions that will influence an individual's likelihood of taking action; rather, it explains the role of values and beliefs in predicting treatment outcomes and adherence, while generating data that guide nurses in choosing effective educational strategies. The most appropriate interventions for a particular person must be negotiated between the individual and the health care professional.

Social Learning Theory

Social learning theory, recently renamed **social cognitive theory,** is another model that adds to the understanding of the determinants of health behavior. Bandura (1997) emphasizes the influence of self-efficacy, or efficacy beliefs, on health behavior. Self-efficacy refers to an individual's belief in being personally capable of performing the behavior required to influence one's own health (Case Study). Social cognitive theory also describes the roles of reinforcement and observational learning in explaining health behavior change. Modeling, or providing opportunities for imitating the behavior of others, can be used to demonstrate the desired behavior.

Opportunities to observe others performing the behavior in question, such as in a local Young Men's Christian Association (YMCA) risk factor–reduction program in which individuals exercise together and report on health behavior changes of smoking cessation and eating a low-fat diet, can enhance expectations of mastery. To affect a person's self-efficacy, the model should provide examples of how to change, increase confidence in ability to change behavior, and convince the person of positive benefits of change (Galavotti, Pappas-DeLuca, & Lansky, 2001).

Regardless of nurses' best assessment methods and educational strategies, research in the area of health education indicates that people do not always make the choices recommended to them by health professionals (Rankin & Stallings, 2001). Nurses often label these people *noncompliant*, a term that suggests that the individual has not followed their instructions. Naturally health professionals want people to choose the recommended course of action, but each individual has the right to choose not to follow advice. Enlisting the individual's partnership or cooperation rather than compliance achieves better results.

Attempts to influence a person's behavior through education are not always successful. Attempting to persuade people to change their behavior to something that might make them, their friends, and their family healthier can be discouraging and sometimes futile. An individual's values, beliefs, and life stresses may present obstacles to these changes. Effective health education requires an understanding of the influential factors affecting the individual's decision making (values, beliefs, attitudes, life stresses, religion, previous experiences with the health care system, and life goals).

Many health professionals tend to view a person's cooperation with the medical regimen as a single choice, when this cooperation often involves many choices every day. For example, following a low-fat, low-cholesterol diet involves constant, and often inconvenient, choices throughout the day. The expectation is that people will do this every day for the rest of their lives, even when the nurse cannot guarantee freedom from angina, myocardial infarctions, or other complications.

Ultimately, the nurse must respect a person's right to choose. However, nurses can increase an individual's motivation and capabilities to change by involving the individual in planning and goal setting, providing information that is understandable and acceptable, and assisting the person in developing new skills.

After clarifying behaviors that may need to be changed, the nurse can use the following framework based on a cognitive behavioral approach for developing interventions for behavior change:

- Assess the behavior
- Educate about the need for and benefits of change
- Motivate using personalized messages
- Assess and increase self-efficacy
- Decrease barriers to change
- Modify behavior
- Maintain behavior change (Saarmann, Dougherty, & Riegel, 2002)

Theories of health behavior change are at the heart of health education. The theories presented in this section help the nurses to assess an individual's stage in the behavior change process and to develop appropriate teaching plans. The goals of the teaching plans and the strategies selected will differ depending on the factors affecting the individual's readiness to learn and to change.

Ethics

The nurse upholds democratic principles such as respect for human dignity and the right to self-determination. However, when planning health education to promote health, nurses experience several ethical dilemmas.

Although the focus of health education may be on the behavior change process, the nurse must be certain that tactics of coercion, persuasion, and manipulation have not been used (Bandman & Bandman, 2002). The role of the nurse is to facilitate a communicative environment in which people can exercise their right to make informed free choices. Individuals must participate in the decision-making process when their lives may be influenced by a change.

Although each person's state of health affects family members and the community, individuals are responsible for their own health maintenance. Health professionals must accept and welcome individual differences in meeting this responsibility. By selecting interventions that create an environment of open communication and risk taking, individuals can better develop the problem-solving skills to direct their own growth and development.

Cultural Considerations in Health Teaching

Another challenge for health professionals is to apply health education strategies with people from other cultural backgrounds, people who do not speak English as their native language, and people who cannot read at elementary levels. The health professional must take the time to assess cultural beliefs that influence social and health practices and must make an effort to analyze educational interventions that are

MULTICULTURAL AWARENESS

Cultural Aspects of Health Teaching

WHEN THERE IS A LANGUAGE BARRIER

- Use courtesy and a formal approach.
- Address the person by his or her last name.
- Introduce yourself, pointing to yourself as you give your name.
- Project a friendly attitude with a smile and a handshake.
- Speak with a moderate tone and volume.
- Attempt to use words in the person's language, which indicates respect for the individual's culture.
- Use simple, everyday words rather than complex words, medical jargon, or colloquialisms.
- Use hand gestures to help the person understand.
- Instruct the person in small increments.
- Have the person demonstrate understanding of the message.
- Write down the instructions for the person to take home.
- Involve others who can serve as interpreters.
- When available, use flash cards and phrase books in other languages.

AREAS TO CONSIDER IN CULTURAL ASSESSMENT

- Individual's identification with a particular cultural group
- Habits, customs, values, and beliefs
- Language and communication patterns
- Cultural sanctions and restrictions
- Healing beliefs and practices
- Cultural health practices
- Kinship and social networks
- Nutritional beliefs, food preferences, and restrictions
- Religious beliefs and practices related to health
- Attitudes, values, and beliefs about health (Andrews & Boyle, 2004)

acceptable and satisfying to the individual. Social marketing processes discussed in the next section help identify characteristics, interests, and concerns of target populations.

When teaching people of different cultural, racial, and ethnic groups, the nurse should endeavor to provide culturally sensitive client education. Nurses should recognize that the person's or group's background, beliefs, and knowledge may differ significantly from their own and seek to understand and show respect for these differences (Degazon, 2004) (Multicultural Awareness box).

SOCIAL MARKETING AND HEALTH EDUCATION

When nurses begin to teach groups of people, they automatically enter a program planning and administrative process. When an organization wants to offer an ongoing health education program for a target population, social marketing provides a strategy for reaching members of the group and implementing a service that will satisfy these

members as consumers. Principles of social marketing and health education strategies are combined to promote population-based changes in behavior to improve health.

Social marketing is defined as "the application of commercial marketing technologies to the analysis, planning, execution, and evaluation of programs designed to influence the voluntary behavior of target audiences in order to improve their personal welfare and that of their society" (Andreasen, 1995, p. 7). The primary objective of social marketing is to change behavior. Key attributes of a social marketing approach are the offering of benefits and the reduction of barriers to influence market members' behavior. Social marketers attempt to modify the attractiveness of specific behavioral options to favor one choice over competing alternatives. It is a consumer-oriented process which tends to be culturally sensitive (Maibach, Rothschild, & Novelli, 2004). For example, social marketing strategies could be used in designing smoking-cessation programs for ethnic minorities. Health-related social marketing offerings may include physical goods such as nutritious lunches, services such as stress management workshops, or ideas and concepts such as encouraging safer sex or preventing heart disease (Bensley & Brookins-Fisher, 2003). Any information about the target population that is generated by social marketing strategies will improve the nurse's ability to develop effective educational interventions.

TEACHING PLAN

Preparation for teaching a group program, such as a seminar or course, begins after the marketing and administrative plans are well underway. These activities ensure that there are enough participants for the program, and they provide the structure for developing the teaching plan—the program objectives, available time, human and material resources, and so on. When the marketing and administrative functions have been provided by others and when educational strategies are developed for one person at a time, the nurse can concentrate efforts on developing the teaching plan.

A health-teaching plan may emphasize a phase of the behavior change process that is related to the individual's health-promotion needs or problems. The written teaching plan represents a package of educational services provided to a consumer or student. The plan should be written from the learner's point of view.

The process of generating a teaching plan helps the nurse recognize and use methods of learning that involve the individual as an active participant. The plan should include a list of specific actions or abilities that the person may perform at intervals during and at the end of the educational intervention. Teaching plans help nurses clarify these outcomes. Preparing a teaching plan involves the steps of the teaching-learning process outlined in Box 10-2.

Assessment

Assessment, the first step in the process, involves determining the characteristics of the learner and identifying learning needs. The following characteristics of the learner are important for the nurse to identify and consider in planning:

- Age, developmental stage in the life cycle, and level of education
- Health beliefs
- Motivation and readiness to learn
- Health risks and problems
- Current knowledge and skills
- Barriers and facilitators to learning

The reader is encouraged to refer to the chapters about individual development (see Unit 4).

Assessment of the learner can be accomplished by answering the following five questions:

1. What are the characteristics and learning capabilities of the individual?
2. What are the learner's needs for health promotion, risk reduction, or health problems?
3. What does the person already know and what skills can the person already perform that are relevant to the health needs?
4. Is the learner motivated to change any unhealthy behaviors?
5. What are the barriers to and facilitators of health behavior change?

When preparing a teaching plan for one person in a primary care setting, the nurse may learn background infor-mation about the individual from that person's record and agency reports that include descriptions of the person's population group. Nurses often agree to teach health classes that others have organized. In this case, the nurse should ask for project reports that provide marketing and needs-assessment information about the students who are expected to attend the classes (Care Plan).

Determining Expected Learning Outcomes

To determine the expected learning outcomes of a health education intervention, the nurse answers the following questions:

Box 10-2 Steps in the Teaching-Learning Process

I. Assessment
   A. Learner characteristics
   B. Learning needs
II. Development of expected learning outcomes
III. Development of a teaching plan
   A. Content
   B. Teaching strategies, learning activities
IV. Implementation of the teaching plan
V. Evaluation of expected outcomes
   A. Achievement of learning outcomes
   B. Evaluation of the teaching process

CARE PLAN

Preparing a Teaching Plan

Nursing Diagnosis Knowledge Deficit (Specify Area)

DEFINING CHARACTERISTICS

- Verbalization of inadequate information or an inadequate recall of information
- Verbalization of misunderstanding or misconception
- Request for information
- Instructions followed inaccurately
- Inadequate performance on a test
- Inadequate demonstration of a skill

RELATED FACTORS

- Pathophysiological states
- Sensory deficits
- Memory loss
- Intellectual limitations
- Interfering coping strategies (denial or anxiety)
- Lack of exposure to accurate information
- Lack of motivation to learn
- Inattention
- Cultural or language barriers

EXPECTED OUTCOMES

- The individual will express an interest in learning.
- The individual will correctly state the information on the specific topic.
- The individual will correctly demonstrate skills needed to practice health-related behavior.
- The individual and family will explain how to incorporate new information into their lifestyle.
- The individual will modify health behavior based on the acquisition of new knowledge.
- The individual will list resources for more information or support.

INTERVENTIONS

- Provide accurate and culturally relevant information related to the specific topic.
- Select teaching techniques appropriate to the individual's learning needs.
- Explore the individual's interpretation of the information and its meaning in the context of the person's life.
- Demonstrate and then have the individual practice new skills.
- Assist the person in identifying and implementing alternative strategies when initial choices are not successful.
- Include the family or significant others as appropriate.
- Provide names and telephone numbers of resource people or organizations.

1. What broad public health and social goals guide the proposed educational program?
2. What are the participant's learning goals?
3. What must the learner know, do, and believe to progress through the behavior change process?

Program Goals

The program goals of a health education project should reflect the desire to facilitate improvement in some health problem or social living condition. Program goals are broad statements on long-range expected accomplishments that provide direction; they do not have to be stated in measurable terms (Porche, 2004).

Learning Goals

Learning goals are best established when the student and the nurse work together. These goals reflect the health behavior or health status change that the person will have achieved by the end of an educational intervention. Learning goals should relate to the program goals.

Learning Objectives

Learning objectives indicate the steps to be taken by the individual toward meeting the learning goal and may involve the development of knowledge, skill, or change in attitude. Objectives are most useful when stated in behavioral terms and when they contain these components: (1) the learner and a precise action verb that indicates what the learner should be able to do, (2) the conditions under which the task is performed, and (3) the level of performance expected (Bastable, 2003). Learning objectives guide the selection of content and methods and help narrow the focus of a teaching plan to more achievable steps; they also aid in setting standards of performance and suggesting evaluation strategies.

Selecting Content

To select appropriate content for a health education program, the nurse considers what information, skills, and attitudes need to be taught and the level of learning to be achieved.

Three Domains of Learning

Content is commonly divided into three domains: (1) cognitive, (2) psychomotor, and (3) affective. Cognitive learning refers to the development of new facts or concepts, and building on or applying knowledge to new situations. Psychomotor learning involves developing physical skills from simple to complex actions. Affective learning alludes to the recognition of values, religious and spiritual beliefs, family interaction patterns and relationships, and personal attitudes that affect decisions and problem-solving progress.

To learn or change a health behavior, a person may need to acquire new information, practice some physical techniques, and clarify the ways in which the new behavior may affect relationships with others. The nurse's role is to select a combination of content from the three domains that is appropriate to meet the behavioral objective. To find samples of content for a teaching plan, the nurse researches resource materials, such as books, teaching guides, journal articles, pamphlets, and flyers created by nonprofit agencies and professional organizations. The nurse should be careful about giving students materials with technical vocabulary that is too complex for the audience.

Levels of Learning

The level of learning to be achieved depends on how the nurse anticipates that the content will be used. Taxonomies developed by Bloom and others (Bloom, Englehart, Furst, Hill, & Krathwohl, 1956; Krathwohl, Bloom, & Masia, 1964) are widely accepted as the standard tools for arranging levels of learning objectives according to type and complexity. For example, in the cognitive domain, levels of learning include the following:

- Knowledge: person recalls facts and the concept
- Comprehension: person understands the meaning of the concept
- Application: person uses the concept
- Analysis: person can examine or explain the concept
- Synthesis: person integrates the concept with other learning
- Evaluation: person judges or compares the concept (Bastable, 2003)

When preparing a teaching plan, the nurse differentiates between information the individual must know and information considered helpful to know to develop appropriate learning objectives. This process provides cues to the nurse for planning effective strategies for the necessary level of learning. As the level of learning to be achieved becomes complex, the educational strategies and methods selected should involve the individuals in more active application and analysis of the content.

Designing Learning Strategies

Designing the learning strategies for an educational intervention means selecting the methods and tools and structuring the sequence of activities. The teaching plan to this point provides the foundation on which to base the activity selection and sequence. The following questions should guide the design of learning strategies:

1. What are some basic considerations for selecting teaching methods for health education programs?
2. How does the nurse, as instructor, establish and maintain a learning climate?
3. What actions can the nurse perform to increase the effectiveness of the learning methods?
4. What are the appropriate methods for each learning domain?
5. What methods tend to promote behavior change?

Considerations for Selecting Methods

The nurse's first consideration is to promote an environment and use methods that foster self-directed learning. An active participant usually learns more.

There will be many learning styles in a group audience; therefore, the nurse varies the teaching methods used in a given session. Taking into consideration the characteristics of the population (developmental stage, age, and knowledge of the topic), the nurse selects teaching methods that best support the goals and theme of the educational program. The order of content should proceed from simple ideas and skills to the more complex concepts, from known material toward lesser-known data. The nurse must be sensitive to the energy level and anxiety of the audience when presenting content that requires strong concentration or causes anxiety.

Learning Climate

For group presentations, the nurse addresses several activities when seeking to establish an environment that is conducive to health behavior change. The first activity is creating a sense of preparedness and organization by providing physical facilities with adequate furnishings and suitable audiovisual materials and handouts. Even the instructor's appearance will lend credibility or distraction to the presentation.

The second activity involves anticipating the needs of the group and communicating information about the schedule and the facilities. This action alleviates the group's apprehension and makes them more comfortable.

The third activity focuses on the nurse's assessment of the individual and group learning needs, possibly through questions and dialogue. Members of the group must believe that the program will be beneficial and relevant to their situations. The instructor should watch for and reinforce signs of motivation to participate in the experience.

Fourth, having established a positive learning climate, the nurse seeks to maintain a high level of motivation, a sense of individualized attention, and a progression. As a reality check, the nurse might ask for periodic feedback from the group about the effectiveness of the program and its relevance to group needs.

Finally, the nurse works with the group to maintain the learning climate. This process involves observing group interactions, helping individuals to participate, intervening to help the group deal with controlling its members, and remaining cognizant of dynamics in the group process that will facilitate or inhibit learning.

Teaching for Each Learning Domain

As mentioned, teaching is directed toward one or more of three learning domains: (1) cognitive, (2) psychomotor, and (3) affective. Methods appropriate for cognitive instruction are lecture, programmed instruction, simulations and games, computer-assisted programs, and modules (Figure 10-1). For psychomotor learning, methods include demonstration, drill and practice, games, role-playing exercises, and peer teaching. Strategies for affective learning are discussion, simulations, role playing, and field experiences (Redman, 2001).

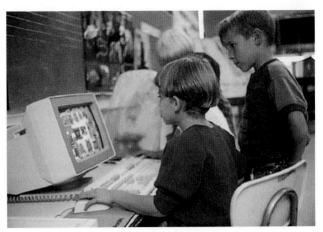

Figure 10-1 School-aged children engaged in computer learning activities. (From Hockenberry, M., Wilson, D., and Winkelstein, M. [2005]. *Wong's essentials of pediatric nursing* [7th ed.]. St. Louis: Mosby.)

Evaluating the Teaching-Learning Process

The teacher can evaluate the learning, or measure achievement of learning objectives, in all domains through the use of written or oral testing, demonstrations, observation, self-reports, and self-monitoring. Teaching methods for one domain may overlap those for another domain.

The nurse can incorporate written, verbal, and nonverbal techniques into the teaching plan for obtaining feedback about teaching performance. Postprogram questionnaires are the usual method for obtaining written feedback. The nurse may ask for verbal feedback at various times from the group, from individual students, and from observers of the class. Nonverbal communication cues from participants may indicate their satisfaction, fatigue, or frustration with the educational intervention.

The overall process of the teaching-learning experience needs to be evaluated. The procedures used to organize and promote an educational program can affect its ultimate success. The nurse (or a program administration committee) records activities such as advertising, registration, fee collection, and availability and repair of equipment and materials. This evaluative information can then be used to improve subsequent programs. Surveys by telephone or by postprogram questionnaires help obtain the consumer's opinion about these implementation procedures (Research Highlights). Word-of-mouth referrals to future programs and support from other community agencies and professionals may also indicate approval of the program format.

Occasionally the nurse is asked to justify a health-education program in terms of its effect on the community's public health goals or social problems. **Health promotion** involves a combination of health-protection activities, preventive health services, and health-education programs; therefore, drawing a direct correlation between an educational intervention and the statistical improvement of the health problem can be difficult.

Health Promotion Via the Telephone

Telephone interventions have been used by nurses, especially ambulatory care nurses, for many years. Research documents the effective use of telephone nursing interventions in several areas. These areas include primary, secondary, and tertiary prevention strategies promoting physical and mental health. The specific interventions include:

- Promoting safety of abused women (McFarlane, 2004)
- Increasing adherence to mammography screening (Champion, 2003)
- Enhancing smoking cessation rates in low-income smokers (Wadland, Soffelmayr, & Ives, 2001)
- Increasing exercise and physical activity among older women (Conn, Burks, Minor, & Mehr, 2003)
- Improving HbA_{1C} levels and adherence to diet and blood glucose testing in people with diabetes (Kim & Oh, 2003)
- Improving health-related outcomes for newly injured clients with spinal cord lesions (Phillips, 2001)
- Improving health-related outcomes for clients newly diagnosed with cancer (Rawl et al., 2002)
- Supporting people with chronic mental illness (Hunter, 2000)
- Reducing depressive symptoms in clients with a major depressive disorder or dysthymia (Hunkeler et al., 2001)
- Preventing hospital readmission and reducing length of stay if readmission occurred in clients with schizophrenia (Beebe, 2001)
- Decreasing the costs of care in clients with congestive heart failure by preventing hospital readmissions and emergency visits (Jerant, Azari, & Nesbitt, 2001)
- Decreasing the costs of care by providing family grief support following the death of a member (Kaunonen, Aalto, Tarkka, & Paunonen, 2000)

Safety-promoting behaviors of abused women who were part of a telephone intervention were compared with the those of women receiving standard care. The intervention group received six 9-minute phone calls over a period of 8 weeks, in which safety-promoting behaviors were discussed. Both groups of women received follow-up calls to assess safety-promoting behavior at 3, 6, 12, and 18 months after intake. Analysis showed that the telephone intervention group practiced significantly more safety-promoting behaviors at each assessment and continued to do so for 18 months (McFarlane, 2004).

A clinical trial was conducted to investigate the impact of nurse telephone calls on HbA_{1C} levels and adherence to diet and blood glucose testing in people with diabetes. The intervention group received continuing education and reinforcement of diabetes control recommendations for 12 weeks. Their adherence to a diet and blood glucose testing regimen was better than that of the control group and HbA_{1C} levels decreased, indicating improved blood glucose control (Kim & Oh, 2003).

Advantages of telenursing are believed to include decreased cost of therapeutic interactions, increased access to rural and other distant people (including international clients), and cost savings resulting from direction of individuals to more appropriate use of health care services, such as avoiding unnecessary after-hours visits to the emergency room. With the growth of managed care financing for health care, telephone nursing is expected to increase. Additional research is needed to describe telephone nursing interventions and to evaluate their effectiveness. Standards of practice for telenursing have been developed by the American Academy of Ambulatory Care Nursing (1997). These standards are likely to facilitate studying the outcomes of telephone interventions by nurses.

HbA_{1C}, glycosylated hemoglobin.

Nurses often can describe the theoretical influence of an educational intervention on health behaviors, health problems, and social problems. Statistics such as the number of people served each year, the percentage of the target population reached, the number of service providers used, and the number and cost of programs are important and must be preserved. As these statistics change over time, the data will provide cues to program successes and problems.

Referring Individuals to Other Resources

The end of a teaching plan should include resources for people to use for continuing education, counseling, peer support, and health services. Nurses should encourage people to view health education as a lifelong learning process. Each person has different developmental needs and health concerns through the life cycle. Moreover, any one educational intervention may help a person move only from one phase of the behavior change process to the next. Additionally, many variables aside from learning may influence a person's health practices (Hot Topics box).

TEACHING AND ORGANIZING SKILLS

To develop teaching and organizing skills in health education, the nurse often must learn new behaviors. A systematic guide can be used for learning these professional skills. To perform these steps, the nurse does the following:

- Seeks self-assessment opportunities
- Identifies, lists, and prioritizes learning needs
- Begins to identify the resources that are available for reading, instructor training, and practice teaching
- Drafts an initial set of learning goals
- Selects the target population and the general topic
- Works through steps of the teaching-learning process, including the development of a teaching plan
- Identifies other people or a project team to help

After implementing the educational intervention, the nurse sets time aside to discuss what took place. Did the program go as planned? What changes were made in the teaching plan? What should be changed for the next program? The nurse reviews the self-developed learning goals and determines new ones.

THE INTERNET AS A HEALTH EDUCATION TOOL

HOTtopics

The availability of health information on the Internet has far-reaching implications for health education. The Internet provides access to information from numerous sources on a broad range of topics to an increasing number of individuals and families. Examples of these topics include well-child care, women's health, nutrition, and information regarding disease treatment and provision of home care for the terminally ill.

Consumers have access to a wealth of valuable information, but they may be overwhelmed by the number and types of resources. Some resources may be useful and accurate; others may be biased, inaccurate, misunderstood, and potentially problematic. Nurses need to develop skill in using the Internet as a client education tool and in guiding individuals' selection of health information sources.

Guidelines are available for selecting sources. One that is useful is *How to Evaluate Health Information of the Internet: Questions and Answers* from the National Cancer Institute. This can be found on the institute's Web site at *https://cissecure.nci.nih.gov/ncibpubs/searchResults.asp?Subject2=General*.

Before recommending Internet sources, nurses should determine if the source is reputable and reliable and if the information is current, accurate, understandable, and appropriate for the target audience. The nurse should identify sites that may be useful to the target group and check them before recommending them. Encouraging people to discuss information obtained from Internet resources is essential to establish an opportunity to clarify their understanding and direct them to sources that are more appropriate, when necessary.

Web sites that provide access to general health information include:
http://www.mayoclinic.com
http://www.healthfinder.gov
http://www.intelihealth.com
http://www.medlineplus.gov
http://www.health.gov
http://www.aoa.gov
http://www.nutrition.gov

Although Internet access is expanding rapidly, it is important to recognize that not everyone has it in their homes. This is particularly true for those with lower levels of income or education.

As additional programs on either an individual or group basis are provided, the nurse will be able to clarify specific instructor teaching and organizing skills that come naturally. These skills tend to improve a program's effectiveness and enable the logistics to run smoothly. The teacher is first a learner; this is true in health education and any other form of education.

SUMMARY

Of all health professionals, nurses spend the most time in direct contact with individuals; they have many opportunities to recognize a need for knowledge and a readiness to learn new information and behaviors. Nurses often coordinate group programs. The more accurate the analysis of the educational aspects of a health-promotion program and the assessment of characteristics and learning needs of the target audience is, the more effective an educational intervention will be in influencing health behaviors.

The principles of health education form a generic basis for implementing a variety of health topics, such as accident prevention and first aid, expectant parent education, hypertension education, nutrition and fitness, stress management, substance abuse, sex education, and client educa-tion in areas including diabetes and arthritis. The two scenarios described in this chapter provide insights into the nurse's role in conducting educational interventions about family planning and prenatal care.

Planning to teach one person is different from planning to teach a group. One-to-one interventions tend to follow a counseling or problem-solving approach. Group interventions can range from guided discussions on concerns that evolve from the group to a more structured learning experience involving presentations, skill practice, and attitude-awareness exercises. The range of health education strategies provides nurses and all health care professionals with techniques and methods applicable in health service settings, schools, work sites, and other community facilities.

ADDITIONAL STUDY MATERIAL

Study Questions in the back of the book, see page 663.

evolve WEB SITE MATERIALS

These materials are located on the book's Web site at http://evolve.elsevier.com/Edelman/.

- WebLinks
- Content Updates

REFERENCES

American Nurses Association. (1998). *Standards of clinical nursing practice* (2nd ed.). Washington, DC: The Association.

American Nurses Association. (2003). *Nursing's social policy statement.* Washington, DC: The Association.

Anderson, D. G., Ward, H., & Hatton, D. C. (2004). In M. Stanhope & J. Lancaster (Eds.), *Community & public health nursing* (6th ed.). St. Louis: Mosby.

Andreasen, A. R. (1995). *Marketing social change: Changing behavior to promote health, social development, and the environment.* San Francisco: Jossey-Bass.

Andrews, M. M., & Boyle, J. S. (2004). *Transcultural concepts in nursing care* (4th ed.). Philadelphia: Lippincott.

Bandman, E. L., & Bandman, B. (2002). *Nursing ethics through the life span* (4th ed.). Upper Saddle River, NJ: Prentice Hall.

Bandura, A. (1997). *Self-efficacy: The exercise of control.* New York: W. H. Freeman.

Bastable, S. B. (2003). Behavioral objectives. In S. B. Bastable (Ed.), *Nurse as educator: Principles of teaching and learning for nursing practice.* Sudbury, MA: Jones and Bartlett.

Bastable, S. B., & Rinswalske, M. A. (2003). Developmental stages of the learner. In S. B. Bastable (Ed.), *Nurse as educator: Principles of teaching and learning for nursing practice.* Sudbury, MA: Jones and Bartlett.

Becker, M. H. (1974). *The health belief model and personal health behavior.* Thorofare, NJ: Charles B. Slack.

Beebe, L. H. (2001). Community nursing support for clients with schizophrenia. *Archives of Psychiatric Nursing, 15*(5), 214-222.

Bensley, R. J., & Brookins-Fisher, J. (2003). *Community health education methods: A practical guide.* Sudbury, MA: Jones and Bartlett.

Bloom, B. S., Englehart, M. S., Furst, E. J., Hill, W. H., & Krathwohl, D. J. (1956). *Taxonomy of educational objectives: The classification of educational goals—Handbook 1: Cognitive domain.* White Plains, NY: Longman.

Champion, V. (2003). Comparison of tailored interventions to increase mammography screening in nonadherent older women. *Preventive Medicine, 36*(2), 150-158.

Conn, V. S., Burks, J. J., Minor, M. A., & Mehr, D. R. (2003). Randomised trial of 2 interventions to increase older women's exercise. *American Journal of Health Behavior, 27*(4), 380-388.

Degazon, C. E. (2004). Cultural diversity and community-oriented nursing practice. In M. Stanhope & J. Lancaster (Eds.), *Community & public health nursing* (6th ed.). St. Louis: Mosby.

Friedman, M. M., Bowden, V. R., & Jones, E. G. (2003). *Family nursing: Research, theory, & practice* (5th ed.). Upper Saddle River, NJ: Prentice Hall.

Galavotti, C., Pappas-DeLuca, K. A., & Lansky, A. (2001). Modeling and reinforcement to combat HIV: The MARCH approach to behavior change. *American Journal of Public Health, 91*(10), 1602-1607.

Glanz, K., Rimer, B. K., & Lewis, F. M. (2002). *Health behavior and health education: Theory, research, and practice* (3rd ed.). San Francisco: Jossey-Bass.

Hunkeler, E. M., Meresman, J. F., Hargreaves, W. A., Fireman, B., Verman, W. N., Kirsch, A. J., et al. (2001). Efficacy of nurse telehealth care and support in augmenting treatment of depression in primary care. *Archives of Family Medicine, 9*(8), 700-708.

Hunter, E. F. (2000). Telephone support for persons with chronic mental illness. *Home Healthcare Nurse, 18*(3), 172-179.

Janz, N. K., & Becker, M. H. (1984). The health belief model: A decade later. *Health Education Quarterly, 11*(1), 1-47.

Jerant, A. F., Azari, R., & Nesbitt, T. S. (2001). Reducing the cost of frequent hospital admissions for congestive heart failure: A randomized trial of a home telecare intervention. *Medical Care, 39*(11), 1234-1245.

Kaunonen, M., Aalto, P., Tarkka, M., & Paunonen, M. (2000). Oncology ward nurses' perspectives of family grief and a supportive telephone call after the death of a significant other. *Cancer Nursing, 23*(4), 314-324.

Kim, H. J., & Oh, J. A. (2003). Adherence to diabetes control recommendations: Impact of nurse telephone calls. *ANS Advances in Nursing Science, 44*(3), 256-261.

Krathwohl, D. R., Bloom, B. S., & Masia, B. B. (1964). *Taxonomy of educational objectives: The classification of educational goals—Handbook 2: Affective domain.* New York: David McKay.

Lee, P. R., & Estes, C. L. (2003). *The nation's health* (7th ed.). Sudbury, MA: Jones and Bartlett.

Maibach, E. W., Rothschild, M. L., & Novelli, W. D. (2004). Social marketing. In K. Glanz, B. K. Rimer, & F. M. Lewis (Eds.), *Health behavior and health education: Theory, research, and practice* (3rd ed.). San Francisco: Jossey-Bass.

McFarlane, J. (2004). Increasing the safety-promoting behaviors of abused women.

American Journal of Nursing, 103(3), 40-51.

McGinnis, J. M. (2003). A vision for health in our new century. *American Journal of Health Promotion, 18*(2), 146-150.

Morotz, L. R., Cross, M. Z., & Rush, J. M. (2001). *Health, safety and nutrition for the young child* (5th ed.). New York: Delmar.

Morrison, G. W. (2004). *Early childhood education today* (9th ed.).Upper Saddle River, NJ: Pearson Prentice Hall.

Phillips, V. L. (2001). Telehealth: Reaching out to newly injured spinal cord patients. *Public Health Report, 116,* 94-102.

Porche, D. J. (2004). *Public and community health nursing practice: A population-based approach.* Thousand Oaks, CA: Sage.

Rankin, S. H., & Stallings, K. D. (2001). *Patient education: Issues, principles, policies* (4th ed.). Philadelphia: Lippincott Williams & Wilkins.

Rawl, S. M., Given, B. A., Given, C. W., Champion, V. L., Kozachik, S. L., Kozachik, S. L., et al. (2002). Intervention to improve psychological functioning for newly diagnosed patient with cancer. *Oncology Nursing Forum, 29*(6), 967-975.

Redman, B. K. (2001). *The practice of patient education* (9th ed.). St. Louis: Mosby.

Richards, E. (2003). Motivation, compliance, and health behaviors of the learner. In S. B. Bastable (Ed.), *Nurse as educator: Principles of teaching and learning for nursing practice.* Sudbury, MA: Jones and Bartlett.

Rosenstock, I. M., Strecher, K. J., & Becker, M. H. (1988). The social learning theory and health belief model. *Health Education Quarterly, 15,* 175-183.

Saarmann, L., Dougherty, J., & Riegel, B. (2002). Teaching staff a brief cognitive-behavioral intervention. *MEDSURG Nursing, 11*(3), 114-151.

U.S. Department of Health and Human Services. (2000). *Healthy people 2010* (Vols. 1-2, Conference ed.). Washington, DC: U.S. Department of Health and Human Services.

Wadland, W. C., Soffelmayr, B., & Ives, K. (2001). Enhancing smoking cessation of low-income smokers in managed care. *Journal of Family Practice, 50*(2), 138-144.

Wurzbach, M. E. (2004). *Community health education and promotion: A guide to program design and evaluation* (2nd ed.). Boston: Jones and Bartlett.

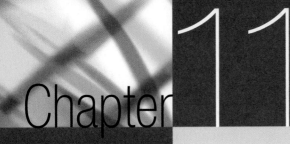

Chapter 11

LINDA SNETSELAAR

Nutrition Counseling for Health Promotion

objectives

After completing this chapter, the reader will be able to:

- Identify *Healthy People 2010* nutrition objectives.

- Analyze the leading nutrition-related causes of death in the United States and identify the dietary factors associated with each cause.

- Summarize the nutrition recommendations contained in the Dietary Guidelines for Americans.

- Compare the number of servings and serving sizes recommended in the Food Guide Pyramid with serving features currently in the marketplace.

- Compare the current Food Guide Pyramid with other suggested versions.

- Analyze U.S. food aid programs for the poor and older adults.

- Plan a 1-day menu that is consistent with recent dietary guidance for a person at any stage of the life cycle.

key terms

Cancer	Food Guide Pyramid	Osteoporosis
Cardiovascular disease	Human immunodeficiency virus	Overweight
Cholesterol		Serving sizes
Coronary heart disease	Hypertension	Stroke
Dietary Guidelines	MyPyramid	Sugar
Fat	Nutrition screening	Type 2 diabetes
Fiber	Obesity	Underweight

THINK About It

Nutritional Self-Assessment

Begin thinking about your food and health and the food and health of people around you. Check each statement that describes the way you usually eat. Add the number of statements that you have checked and compare that number with the scores listed after the questions.
The way I usually eat:

- *I eat whole grain or enriched breads, cereals, rice, or pasta daily.*
- *I eat 2 to 3 pieces or more of fruit daily.*

- *I eat 2 to 3 cups or more of raw or cooked vegetables daily.*
- *I drink skim milk and eat low-fat or fat-free dairy products daily.*
- *I trim fat from meat and take the skin off chicken and turkey or I do not eat meat.*
- *I eat small servings (no larger than the size of a deck of cards) of meat, poultry, and fish or I do not eat meat.*
- *Most food and snacks that I eat are not fried or are made with no added fat.*

Continued

The author wishes to acknowledge the assistance of Amy Greene and Debra Kirch in the preparation of the chapter. She also acknowledges the work of Arlene Spark and Qalvy Grainzvolt in the previous edition as the foundation of this chapter.

Nutritional Self-Assessment *cont'd*

- I add very little fat (butter, margarine, oil, or salad dressing) to my food.
- Most desserts and snacks that I eat contain no added sugar.
- Most of what I drink is made without sugar or contains no added sugar.
- I rarely cook with salt or add salt at the table.
- I do not drink alcohol or I drink no more than 1 to 2 beers, 1 to 2 glasses of wine, or 1 to 2 mixed drinks daily.

  Number of statements checked

  Score: 9 to 12. Evaluation: Great job! **Recommendation:** While reading this chapter, you will be reminded of all the things you are doing that contribute to your healthy lifestyle. You are an excellent role model for others. The best nutrition educators practice what they teach.

  Score: 5 to 8. Evaluation: Okay. **Recommendation:** You do make some good choices, but a number of changes in your food habits would be of great value to you personally and professionally. Hopefully, you will be motivated by some of the ideas presented in this chapter.

  Score: 0 to 4. Evaluation: Improvement needed. **Recommendation:** The first steps toward good eating are the hardest to take, but making healthy choices is worth the investment. You are investing in your education and planning a career in the health professions. Now, begin investing in your own health, also. Improved health is a natural dividend of your training. This chapter will help you focus on improving your own diet and health and the well-being of others.

NUTRITION IN THE UNITED STATES: LOOKING FORWARD FROM THE PAST
Classic Vitamin-Deficiency Diseases

Food and nutrition have always been vitally important to health. Until as recently as the 1940s, many nutrient-deficiency diseases, such as rickets, pellagra, scurvy, beriberi, xerophthalmia, and goiter, were still prevalent in the United States (Carpenter, 2000). Although these conditions still persist in developing countries, they have virtually disappeared from developed areas of the world. Why? An abundant food supply, fortification of some foods with critical nutrients, and better methods of determining and improving the nutrient contents of foods have contributed to the decline of the nutrient-deficiency diseases that are summarized in Table 11-1.

The introduction of iodized salt in the 1920s, for example, contributed greatly to eliminating iodine-deficiency goiter as a public health problem. Similarly, pellagra disappeared after the discovery that inadequate niacin levels contribute to the condition. Today, nutrient deficiencies rarely are reported in the United States. The few cases of protein-energy malnutrition that are listed annually as causes of death generally occur as secondary results of severe illness or injury, premature birth, child neglect, problems of the homeless aged, alcoholism, or some combination of these factors. Although undernutrition still occurs in some groups of people in the United States, including isolated or economically deprived people, these once-prevalent diseases of nutritional deficiency have been replaced by diseases of dietary excess and imbalance (Table 11-2).

Dietary Excess and Imbalance

Problems resulting from overconsumption now rank among the leading causes of illness and death in the United States. The four leading causes of death directly associated with diet are **coronary heart disease** (CHD), some types of cancer, stroke, and diabetes mellitus. In fact, heart disease, cancers, and stroke account for almost two thirds of all deaths every year in America. Four more major causes of death—accidents, cirrhosis of the liver, suicide, and homicide—are associated with excessive alcohol intake.

The number of American children who are overweight is currently 15.5% among 12 to 19 year olds, 15.3% among 6 to 11 year olds, and 10.4% among 2 to 5 year olds (total = 41.2%) (Ogden, 2002) compared with 10.5%, 11.3%, and 7.2%, respectively from 1988 to 1994 (National Center for Health Statistics, 1999). Childhood obesity is the critical health issue of our time. Reducing the incidence of obesity is an important public health goal (National Institutes of Health, 2001; U.S. Department of Health and Human Services [USDHHS], 2001). The cause of excess weight and obesity is an imbalance between energy intake and expenditure (Hill & Peters, 1998), resulting in positive energy balance and fat deposition. Researchers express concern that overweight or obesity in childhood will lead to health-related problems in adulthood.

Encouraging healthy choices in diet, exercise, and weight control is one of the major themes of *Healthy People 2010* (U.S. Department of Agriculture [USDA] and USDHHS, 2000) (Figure 11-1). As dietary factors contribute substantially to the burden of preventable illness and premature death, *Healthy People 2010* is aimed at bringing American dietary patterns into line with current dietary recommendations, especially the Dietary Guidelines for Americans (USDA and USDHHS, 2000).

HEALTHY PEOPLE 2010: NUTRITION OBJECTIVES

As discussed throughout this text, the 28 focus areas in *Healthy People 2010* contain 467 specific national health-promotion and disease prevention objectives. Many *Healthy People 2010* nutrition-related objectives target interventions designed to reduce or eliminate illness, disability, and premature death among individuals and communities. Each objective has a target for specific improvements to be achieved by 2010. The topics covered by these objectives reflect the array of critical influences that determine the health of individuals and communities. For example, individual behaviors and environmental factors are responsible

Table 11-1 Nutrient-Deficiency Diseases

Key Nutrient Involved	Deficiency Disease	Typical Disease Symptoms	Major Dietary Sources for the Nutrient
Protein	Kwashiorkor, protein-calorie malnutrition	Growth failure in children (60% to 80% weight for age), edema, fatty liver, changes in hair texture, apathy, and anorexia	Egg white, beef, fish, poultry, milk, cheese, legumes, and nuts
Thiamine	Beriberi	Nerve degeneration, poor muscle coordination, enlarged heart, and abnormal heart rhythms	Pork, sunflower seeds, dried beans, and wheat germ
Niacin	Pellagra	The 3 Ds (diarrhea, dermatitis, and dementia) and anorexia	Wheat bran, beef, mushrooms, salmon, and tuna
Vitamin C	Scurvy	Impaired wound healing, bleeding gums and skin, and frequent infections	Citrus fruits, broccoli, strawberries, and cabbage
Vitamin A	Xerophthalmia	Blindness, poor growth, infections, and cracks in teeth	Liver, fortified milk, sweet potatoes, pumpkin, and mustard greens
Iron	Iron deficiency anemia	Poor growth, reduced resistance to infection, and impaired learning ability in children	Red meats, oysters, clams, tofu (soybean curd), and spinach
Iodine	Goiter and cretinism	Enlarged thyroid gland, weight gain, and mental and physical retardation in infants	Seafood, crops grown in iodine-rich soil (coastal areas), and iodized salt

Table 11-2 Health Problems Related to Poor Nutrition

A number of health problems are caused or exacerbated by poor nutrition. Health care professionals strive to prevent or delay these health problems.

Health Problem	Questionable Practices
Anemia	Inadequate iron and folate intake
Cancer (breast, cervical, and colon)	Excessive fat intake; low fiber intake
Cirrhosis	Excessive alcohol intake
Constipation	Inadequate fiber or fluid intake; high fat intake; sedentary lifestyle
Dental caries	Excessive, frequent consumption of concentrated sweets; lack of fluoride; poor hygiene
Type 2 diabetes	Excessive energy intake
Hypercholesterolemia	Inadequate fiber intake
Hypertension	Obesity; excessive energy intake; excessive sodium intake in sodium-sensitive individuals
Infection	Malnutrition
Obesity	Excessive energy intake; excessive fat intake; sedentary lifestyle
Osteoporosis	Inadequate calcium intake; inadequate vitamin D intake or inadequate exposure to the sun; sedentary lifestyle
Underweight and growth failure	Inadequate energy intake

for approximately 70% of all premature deaths in the United States. Understanding these influences and how they relate to one another are crucial for achieving *Healthy People 2010* goals.

The report also contains 10 leading health indicators: (1) physical activity, (2) overweight and obesity, (3) tobacco use, (4) substance abuse, (5) mental health, (6) injury and violence, (7) environmental quality, (8) immunization, (9) responsible sexual behavior, and (10) access to health care. By monitoring these measures, states and communities can assess their current health status and follow it over time. Overweight and obesity are supported by two specific measurable objectives:

- 19-3c. Reduce the proportion of children and adolescents who are overweight or obese.
- 19-2. Reduce the proportion of adults who are obese.

The *Healthy People 2010* box presents nutrition-related objectives related to the diseases discussed later in the chapter.

Nutrition-Related Health Status

Overweight and high serum **cholesterol** levels, hypertension (high blood pressure), and osteoporosis (decreased bone mass) increase the risk of CHD, stroke, and bone fracture, respectively. The following statements describe the health status of Americans:

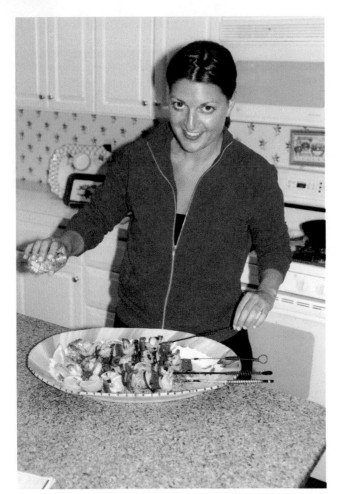

Figure 11-1 Choosing a healthier diet may mean learning new recipes and new ways of cooking.

- More Americans are overweight now than in the late 1970s. Many adults also report sedentary lifestyles. Being overweight is associated with many chronic diseases and health outcomes; therefore, its increased prevalence is a cause for public health concern.
- Although the number of adults with desirable serum total cholesterol levels is increasing steadily, many people still have high levels. A high serum cholesterol is a major risk factor for CHD.
- Hypertension remains a major public health problem in middle-aged and older adults. Blacks have a higher age-related prevalence of hypertension than whites and Hispanic Americans. Hypertension is the most important risk factor for stroke and a major risk factor for CHD.

Nutrition Objectives for the United States

Although Americans are slowly changing their eating patterns toward more healthful diets, a considerable gap exists between public health recommendations and consumers' practices. The overarching goal for nutrition in the begin-

ning of the millennium is that food intake change in the direction of the targeted goals recommended in *Healthy People 2010*, the Food Guide Pyramid, and the Dietary Guidelines for Americans.

FOOD AND NUTRITION RECOMMENDATIONS

Food and nutrition guidelines are introduced in this chapter. A goal of this discussion is to heighten people's interest in the health-promotion power of good nutrition to inspire their gradual adoption of the dietary recommendations presented here.

The kinds and amounts of food that are required to obtain the necessary energy and nutrients are defined in these reports:

- Dietary Reference Intakes (National Research Council [NRC], 1997, 2000a, 2000b), including the Recommended Dietary Allowances (NRC, 1989)
- *Dietary Guidelines for Americans*, sixth edition (USDA/USDHHS, 2005)
- MyPyramid, a new food guidance system introduced by the USDA in 2005 (USDA/CNPP, 2005).

Dietary Reference Intakes

The Dietary Reference Intakes (DRI) is a set of values for the dietary nutrient intakes of healthy people in the United States and Canada. These values are used for planning and assessing diets, including the recommended daily allowance (RDA), adequate intake, estimated average requirement, and Tolerable Upper Intake Level (Box 11-1).

The DRI recommends intake levels for U.S. and Canadian individuals and population groups and it sets maximal level guidelines to reduce the risk of adverse health effects from overconsumption of a nutrient. The understanding of the relationship between nutrition and chronic disease has progressed to the extent that intakes can now be recommended that are thought to help people achieve measurable physical indicators of good health. The DRI represents a major leap forward in nutrition science—from a primary concern for the prevention of deficiency to an emphasis on beneficial effects of healthy eating. The new recommendations focus on decreasing the risk of chronic disease through nutrition.

The old RDA, which existed before 1997, established the minimal amounts of nutrients needed to protect against nutrient deficiency. In contrast, the DRI is designed to reflect the latest understanding about nutrient requirements based on optimizing health in individuals and groups. Collectively called the DRI, the new recommendations include four categories of reference intakes that were established by examining the results of hundreds of nutritional studies on both the beneficial aspects of nutrients and the hazards of consuming too much of a nutrient. When the scientific evidence allows, recommendations are made to help individuals at different stages of life to obtain enough of a nutrient to promote health and to maintain normal nutritional status.

Healthy People 2010
Objectives for Selected Diseases

Heart Disease

Goal: Reduce CHD deaths

- 12-12. Reduce the mean total blood cholesterol levels among adults from 206 mg/dl to 199 mg/dl.
- 12-13. Reduce the proportion of adults with high total blood cholesterol levels.
- 19-8. Increase the proportion of people aged 2 years and older who receive less than 10% of calories from saturated fat.
- 19-9. Increase the proportion of people aged 2 years and older who receive no more than 30% of calories from fat.

Hypertension

- 12-7. Reduce the number of stroke deaths.
- 12-9. Reduce the proportion of adults with high blood pressure.
- 12-11. Increase the proportion of adults with high blood pressure who are taking action (losing weight and reducing sodium intake).
- 19-10. Increase the proportion of people aged 2 years and older who consume 2400 mg or less of sodium daily.

Osteoporosis

Goal: Prevent illness and disability related to arthritis and other rheumatic conditions, osteoporosis, and chronic back conditions

- 2-9. Reduce the overall number of cases of osteoporosis as measured by low total femur BMD.
- 19-11. Increase the proportion of individuals aged 2 years and older who meet dietary recommendations for calcium.

Obesity

Leading health indicators: reduce the proportion of adults who are obese from 23% to 15% and reduce the proportion of children and adolescents who are overweight or obese from 11% and 12% to 5% (objective numbers 19-2 and 19-3).

- 19-1. Increase the proportion of adults who are at a healthy weight from 42% to 60%.

Diabetes

Goal: Through prevention programs, reduce the disease and economic burden of diabetes and improve the quality of life for all people who have or are at risk for diabetes

- 5-1. Increase the proportion of people with diabetes who receive formal diabetes education from 40% in 1998 to 60% in 2010.
- 5-2. Prevent diabetes, from 3.1 new cases per 1000 people in 1994 to 1996 to 2.5 new cases per 1000 in 2010.

Human Immunodeficiency Virus

Goal 13: Prevent HIV infection and its related illness and death

- 13-15. Expand the interval between an initial diagnosis of HIV infection and AIDS diagnosis to increase years of life of an individual with HIV.
- 13-17. Reduce the number of new cases of perinatal-acquired HIV infection.

AIDS, acquired immunodeficiency virus; *BMD,* bone mineral density; *HIV,* human immunodeficiency virus.

Box 11-1   Dietary Reference Intakes

Recommended Dietary Allowance. RDA is the intake that meets the nutrient needs of nearly all healthy individuals in a specific age and gender group. It should be used to guide individuals in achieving adequate nutrient intake aimed at decreasing the risk of chronic disease. The RDA is based on estimating an average requirement in addition to an increase or decrease to account for variations within a particular group.

Adequate Intake. When sufficient scientific evidence is unavailable to estimate an average requirement, AIs are set. Individuals should use AIs as a goal when no RDAs exist. AI is derived through experimental or observational data that show a mean intake that appears to sustain a desired level of health, such as calcium retention in bone for most members of a population group. For example, AIs have been set for infants through 1 year of age using the average observed nutrient intake of populations of breast-fed infants as the standard.

Estimated Average Requirement. EAR is the intake that meets the estimated nutrient need of one half of the individuals in a specific group. It is used as a basis for developing the RDA and by nutrition policy makers in evaluating adequacy of nutrient intakes of the group and for planning how much the group should consume.

Tolerable Upper Intake Level. This is the maximal intake by an individual that is unlikely to pose risks of adverse health effects in almost all healthy individuals in a specified group. UL is not intended to be a recommended level of intake, and no established benefit exists for individuals to consume nutrients at levels above the RDA or AI. For most nutrients, this figure refers to total intakes from food, fortified food, and nutrient supplements.

AI, adequate intake; *EAR,* estimated average requirement; *RDA,* recommended dietary allowance; *UL,* tolerable upper intake level.

Dietary Guidelines for Americans

The influence of the **Dietary Guidelines** for Americans is wide ranging. First issued in 1980 in response to the public's desire for authoritative, consistent guidance on diet and health, the dietary guidelines form the foundation of federal nutrition policy in the United States. Each federally sponsored nutrition program in the United States uses these guidelines as a part of its nutrition standard; therefore, every day they directly influence the lives of millions of Americans in food stamp, school lunch, and school breakfast programs and those receiving benefits under the Special Supplemental Nutrition Program for Women, Infants, and Children (WIC). These guidelines also form the basis for nutrition education messages for the general public of adults and children beginning at 2 years of age. The National Nutrition Monitoring and Related Research Act of 1990 mandates that the guidelines be reviewed every 5 years by the U.S. Department of Agriculture (USDA) and the U.S. Department of Health and Human Services (USDHHS).

Consumption patterns based on the Dietary Guidelines for Americans will lead to major improvements in public health and nutrition for the United States (Johnson & Kennedy, 2000). Nursing professionals play a key role in promoting the guidelines as one component of healthful lifestyles (Multicultural Awareness box). For convenience, the entire dietary guidelines report is available on the Internet. Although the document is lengthy, the report is an excellent source of background information for health care professionals. Individual sections are available to photocopy for use as education materials.

The 2005 *Dietary Guidelines for Americans* have been recently released. The new 2005 guidelines place a stronger emphasis on calorie control and physical activity. A total of 41 key recommendations are grouped under nine interrelated focus areas. The recommendations are based on scientific evidence that points to ways to lower the risk of chronic disease and promote health. The nine focus areas are listed below, and the 41 key recommendations are presented in Box 11-2 (USDA, 2005).

- Adequate nutrients within calorie needs
- Weight management
- Physical activity
- Food groups to encourage
- Fats
- Carbohydrates
- Sodium and potassium
- Alcoholic beverages
- Food safety

These guidelines for a healthy diet are intended for healthy Americans 2 years and older. By following this advice, individuals can benefit from better health and reduce the chance of falling prey to certain diseases such as CHD, high blood pressure, stroke, certain cancers, osteoporosis, and type 2 diabetes. Representing the best and most up-to-date advice from nutrition experts, these guidelines are intended to help people select foods and beverages that will constitute a healthy diet (Box 11-2).

MYPYRAMID: A NEW FOOD GUIDANCE SYSTEM
Food Guide Pyramid

The **Food Guide Pyramid** was introduced in 1992 as a means for the USDA and the USDHHS to translate nutrition recommendations into terms that consumers would understand. As the twentieth century anthropologist Margaret Mead once said, "People eat food, not nutrition." Nutrition recommendations stated in terms of grams of total fat and saturated fat, or milligrams of vitamin C, are useless unless people are advised as to what types and what quantities of foods should be consumed to obtain the recommended nutrients. The Food Guide Pyramid was a graphic representation of dietary balance and variety. Foods were classified into six food groups, each of which contained a variety of nutritionally similar foods.

MyPyramid

In April 2005 the USDA unveiled **MyPyramid**, a new, interactive food guidance system that replaces the 1992 Food Guide Pyramid. Figure 11-2 presents the graphic representation of MyPyramid. The new food guidance system remains based on the pyramid approach, with the base representing five different food groups: grains, vegetables, fruits, milk, and meat and beans. MyPyramid was developed to be a personalized approach to healthy eating and physical activity (USDA/CNPP, 2005). Individuals can obtain a personalized food plan at the Web site *http://www.mypyramid.gov.*

DIETARY SUPPLEMENTS AND HERBAL MEDICINES

The popularity of supplemental vitamins, minerals, proteins, fiber, and herbs has, in recent decades, earned a high profile in the health field. A vast array of these products is available without a prescription. All people are entitled to know exactly what they are ingesting, whether it is necessary, and whether it is safe.

Traditionally dietary supplements were products composed of one or more of the essential nutrients (vitamins, minerals, and proteins) that were ingested to enhance the usual diet. Through the 1994 Dietary Supplement Health and Education Act the definition of dietary supplement has been expanded to include any product intended for ingestion as a supplement to the diet, including vitamins, minerals, herbs, botanicals and other plant-derived substances, amino acids (individual building blocks of protein) and concentrates, metabolites, constituents, and extracts of these substances (U.S. Food and Drug Administration, 2004).

Drugs can also be of plant origin. Drugs are used in Western medicine as agents intended to diagnose, cure, mitigate, treat, or prevent diseases. Before marketing, drugs must undergo clinical trials to determine their effectiveness, safety, possible adverse interactions with other substances,

MULTICULTURAL AWARENESS

Food and Culture

The reasons why people eat the way they do are numerous. Although it is true that without food people cannot survive, food is much more than a tool of survival. Food is also a source of pleasure ("Let's eat out tonight"), a source of comfort ("Right now, I could use some of my mother's chicken soup"), a symbol of hospitality ("Please come to my house for brunch on Sunday"), and an indicator of social status (consider an expensive T-bone steak versus a hamburger). Food has ritual significance, also. Drinking champagne to celebrate an important event, the bride and groom saving the top layer of their wedding cake, or people of the Jewish faith sharing *challah* (braided bread) at their Sabbath (Friday evening) meal are examples.

To a large extent, the environment determines what people typically eat. For example, wheat that is plentiful in the heartland of the United States is the principal grain in North America, whereas rice enjoys a similar status in Asian countries. Typical wheat-based staples in the United States and Canada include a slice of wheat bread, a bowl of wheat cereal, wheat crackers, pastries made from wheat flour, and pasta made from wheat. Rice-based foods form the backbone of the Chinese diet.

Every culture has its particular food ways, or activities related to food. Food ways include the activities that surround procuring, distributing, storing, consuming, and disposing of food, all of which define what is fit to eat, or what is edible. The factors that affect everyone's food choices and factors that affect food selections of new arrivals to a community should be examined.

Food is often believed to promote health, cure disease, or contain other medicinal qualities. Health beliefs, which can have a great influence on food choices, may be beneficial, neutral, and sometimes dangerous. When actions that are based on these beliefs cause no harm, they should be encouraged. For example, in the United States Americans consume vitamin C in the belief that it might help prevent or cure the common cold. Although large doses (500 to 1000 mg per day) have no significant effect on incidence of the common cold, vitamin C provides a moderate benefit in terms of the duration and severity of cold symptoms in some groups of people. The often reported improvement in the severity of colds after ingesting vitamin C may be a result of the antihistaminic action of the vitamin at these large doses (National Research Council, 2000a).

Among traditional Chinese people, health and disease are believed to relate to the balance between the forces of yin and yang in the body. Diseases that are caused by yang forces may be treated with yin forces to restore balance. Yin foods include low-caloric density, low-protein foods, such as fresh fruits and vegetables. Yang foods are high in calories, cooked in oil, irritating to the mouth, or are red, orange, or yellow in color. Examples include most meats, chili peppers, tomatoes, garlic, ginger, and alcoholic beverages. The hot-cold theory in Puerto Rico follows the same basic principles as do yin and yang, but the food groupings differ somewhat.

Religious beliefs affect the food choices of millions of people worldwide. Many religions, including Buddhism, Hinduism, Islam, Judaism, and Seventh Day Adventism, specify the foods that may be eaten and how they should be prepared. The following is a summary of the principal dietary practices of these five major world religions (Barer-Stein, 1979; Kittler & Sucher, 2000).

- Many Buddhists practice vegetarianism. Foods of plant origin are viewed as the most appropriate for consumption, except pungent foods (garlic, leeks, scallions, chives, and onions), which are believed to generate lust when eaten cooked and rage when eaten raw. For most Buddhists, however, dietary rules such as these are observed on a voluntary basis. What characterizes all Buddhists is the belief that all forms of life share a common link and are thus sacred. Therefore rather than the specific type of food eaten, more important is the attitude of the person receiving the food and the person's sincere gratitude for the lives of the plants and animals contained in the meal that have served to sustain and further enhance the life of the individual.
- Many Hindus are vegetarians, but those who come from the cold northern areas of India eat meat (except for beef, which is prohibited).
- Islamic food laws prohibit the consumption of foods believed to be unclean, such as carrion or already-dead animals, swine, animals slaughtered without pronouncing the name of Allah on them, carnivorous animals with fangs (dogs, cats, and lions), birds of prey, and land animals without ears (frogs and snakes). Alcohol is also prohibited.
- Judaism prohibits the consumption of swine, carrion, carrion eaters (scavengers), shellfish, animals with a cloven (split) hoof and those that do not chew their cud (horses), and animals not slaughtered by the appropriate ritual method. According to Jewish dietary laws, meat (beef, lamb, veal, and poultry), fish, and meat products (eggs) cannot be served at the same meal or cooked in the same vessels as dairy products.
- The dietary practices of Seventh Day Adventists focus on health, with vegetarianism as the foundation of their dietary standard. Seventh Day Adventists also abstain from alcohol and many do not drink caffeine-containing beverages.

and appropriate dosage amounts. The U.S. Food and Drug Administration (FDA) reviews the data collected on a studied drug and, depending on the outcome of the review, officially authorizes it as safe for the general public.

Supplements are sold in the pharmaceutical section of retail stores in a variety of forms (tablets, capsules, powders, soft gels, gel caps, and liquids) that make them resemble drugs. Many people use supplements as if they were drugs, because they are marketed in the same manner as over-the-counter medications. Nevertheless, supplements are unregulated by the FDA.

A dietary supplement can be distinguished from an over-the-counter drug by the words *dietary supplement*, which must appear on the product label. A claim that the

Box **11-2** Dietary Guidelines for Americans 2005: Key Recommendations for the General Population

ADEQUATE NUTRIENTS WITHIN CALORIE NEEDS

- Consume a variety of nutrient-dense foods and beverages within and among the basic food groups while choosing foods that limit the intake of saturated and *trans* fats, cholesterol, added sugars, salt, and alcohol.
- Meet recommended intakes within energy needs by adopting a balanced eating pattern, such as the U.S. Department of Agriculture (USDA) Food Guide or the Dietary Approaches to Stop Hypertension (DASH) Eating Plan.

WEIGHT MANAGEMENT

- To maintain body weight in a healthy range, balance calories from foods and beverages with calories expended.
- To prevent gradual weight gain over time, make small decreases in food and beverage calories and increase physical activity.

PHYSICAL ACTIVITY

- Engage in regular physical activity and reduce sedentary activities to promote health, psychological well-being, and a healthy body weight.
  - To reduce the risk of chronic disease in adulthood: engage in at least 30 minutes of moderate-intensity physical activity, above usual activity, at work or home on most days of the week.
  - For most people, greater health benefits can be obtained by engaging in physical activity of more vigorous intensity or longer duration.
  - To help manage body weight and prevent gradual, unhealthy body weight gain in adulthood: engage in approximately 60 minutes of moderate- to vigorous-intensity activity on most days of the week while not exceeding caloric intake requirements.
  - To sustain weight loss in adulthood: participate in at least 60 to 90 minutes of daily moderate-intensity physical activity while not exceeding caloric intake requirements. Some people may need to consult with a health care provider before participating in this level of activity.
- Achieve physical fitness by including cardiovascular conditioning, stretching exercises for flexibility, and resistance exercises or calisthenics for muscle strength and endurance.

FOOD GROUPS TO ENCOURAGE

- Consume a sufficient amount of fruits and vegetables while staying within energy needs. Two cups of fruit and 2½ cups of vegetables per day are recommended for a reference 2000-calorie intake, with higher or lower amounts depending on the calorie level.
- Choose a variety of fruits and vegetables each day. In particular, select from all five vegetable subgroups (dark green, orange, legumes, starchy vegetables, and other vegetables) several times a week.
- Consume 3 or more ounce-equivalents of whole-grain products per day, with the rest of the recommended grains coming from enriched or whole-grain products. In general, at least half the grains should come from whole grains.
- Consume 3 cups per day of fat-free or low-fat milk or equivalent milk products.

FATS

- Consume less than 10 percent of calories from saturated fatty acids and less than 300 mg/day of cholesterol, and keep *trans* fatty acid consumption as low as possible.
- Keep total fat intake between 20 to 35% of calories, with most fats coming from sources of polyunsaturated and monounsaturated fatty acids, such as fish, nuts, and vegetable oils.
- When selecting and preparing meat, poultry, dry beans, and milk or milk products, make choices that are lean, low-fat, or fat-free.
- Limit intake of fats and oils high in saturated and/or *trans* fatty acids, and choose products low in such fats and oils.

CARBOHYDRATES

- Choose fiber-rich fruits, vegetables, and whole grains often.
- Choose and prepare foods and beverages with little added sugars or caloric sweeteners, such as amounts suggested by the USDA Food Guide and the DASH Eating Plan.
- Reduce the incidence of dental caries by practicing good oral hygiene and consuming sugar- and starch-containing foods and beverages less frequently.

SODIUM AND POTASSIUM

- Consume less than 2300 mg (approximately 1 teaspoon of salt) of sodium per day.
- Choose and prepare foods with little salt. At the same time, consume potassium-rich foods, such as fruits and vegetables.

ALCOHOLIC BEVERAGES

- Those who choose to drink alcoholic beverages should do so sensibly and in moderation—defined as the consumption of up to one drink per day for women and up to two drinks per day for men.
- Alcoholic beverages should not be consumed by some individuals, including those who cannot restrict their alcohol intake, women of childbearing age who may become pregnant, pregnant and lactating women, children and adolescents, individuals taking medications that can interact with alcohol, and those with specific medical conditions.
- Alcoholic beverages should be avoided by individuals engaging in activities that require attention, skill, or coordination, such as driving or operating machinery.

FOOD SAFETY

- To avoid microbial foodborne illness:
  - Clean hands, food contact surfaces, and fruits and vegetables. Meat and poultry should not be washed or rinsed.

Box **11-2**	**Dietary Guidelines for Americans 2005: Key Recommendations for the General Population** *cont'd*

- Separate raw, cooked, and ready-to-eat foods while shopping, preparing, or storing foods.
- Cook foods to a safe temperature to kill microorganisms.
- Chill (refrigerate) perishable food promptly and defrost foods properly.

- Avoid raw (unpasteurized) milk or any products made from unpasteurized milk, raw or partially cooked eggs or foods containing raw eggs, raw or undercooked meat and poultry, unpasteurized juices, and raw sprouts.

From U.S. Department of Agriculture. (2005). *Dietary guidelines for Americans 2005: Key recommendations for the general population.* Washington, DC: U.S. Department of Agriculture. Retrieved May 31, 2005, from *http://www.health.gov/dietaryguidelines/dga2005/recommendations.htm.*

supplement is formulated to treat or cure a specific disease or condition cannot appear on the label. However, structure-function claims about certain common conditions associated with aging, pregnancy, menopause, and adolescence that do not relate to disease are permitted. These include health maintenance claims ("maintains a healthy circulatory system"), other nondisease claims ("for muscle enhancement" or "helps you relax"), and claims for common, minor symptoms associated with life stages ("for common symptoms of premenstrual syndrome" or "for hot flashes").

Considerable research on the effects of dietary supplements has been conducted in Asia and Europe where these plant products have a long tradition of use. However, the overwhelming majority of supplements have not been studied scientifically. Therefore the National Institutes of Health (NIH) Office of Alternative Medicine and Office of Dietary Supplements are promoting the scientific study of the benefits and risks of dietary supplements, including medicinal herbs, in health maintenance and disease prevention.

Health care professionals are often asked, "Should I take a nutrient supplement?" Many people in the United States take dietary supplements but not necessarily to meet nutrient requirements. Although the adverse effects of large doses of certain nutrients (such as vitamin A) have been recognized for years, there are no documented reports that daily vitamins and mineral supplements that provide up to the recommended intake for a particular nutrient are either beneficial or harmful for the general population. Low-dose supplements that contain the recommended intakes for micronutrients (vitamins and minerals) appear to be generally safe. Although the desirable way for the general public to obtain recommended levels of nutrients is by eating a variety of foods, when people take dietary supplements they should avoid taking them in excess of the recommended intake on any given day.

Circumstances When Nutrient Supplementation Is Indicated

Nutrient supplements and fortified foods are sometimes necessary for specific populations to obtain desirable amounts of particular nutrients (American Dietetic Association, 2001). Some examples follow:

- Folic acid for females who could become pregnant, to help prevent neural tube defects
- Iron during pregnancy
- Calcium for individuals who do not meet the recommended intake
- Vitamin D for elderly people who do not drink generous quantities of fortified milk or who do not manufacture sufficient vitamin D from sunlight
- Vitamin B_{12} for elderly people with atrophic gastritis who do not absorb enough from the food they eat

Vitamin Toxicity

An important point of concern for many health professionals is the excessive use of vitamin and mineral supplements. Toxic levels of certain micronutrients may result and can cause a host of health problems. For example, it is important to advise clients not to overuse vitamins of the fat-soluble class (vitamins A, D, E, and K). Of particular concern is vitamin A, an excess of which may be teratogenic during pregnancy. On the other hand, water-soluble vitamins such as vitamin C and the B-complex vitamins pose less danger, because the body is able to excrete them through the urine.

Nutrient imbalances and toxicities are less likely to occur when nutrients are derived from foods. Most nutrient toxicities occur through supplementation. Estimated toxic doses for daily oral consumption of vitamins and minerals by adults are as low as 5 times the recommended intake for selenium, and as high as 25 to 50 times or more the recommended intakes for folic acid and vitamins C and E. The toxicities of high doses of nutrients such as vitamins A, B_6, and D, niacin, iron, and selenium are well established. Iron supplements intended for other household members are the most common cause of pediatric poisoning deaths in the United States (American Dietetic Association, 2001).

Large doses of vitamin A may be teratogenic. Because of this risk, supplementation with preformed vitamin A should be avoided during the first trimester of pregnancy unless there is evidence of deficiency. Excess preformed vitamin A (more than 10,000 international units) during the first trimester of pregnancy has been linked to cranial neural crest defects (Rothman et al., 1995). Such a risk in early pregnancy raises a need for caution about general vitamin

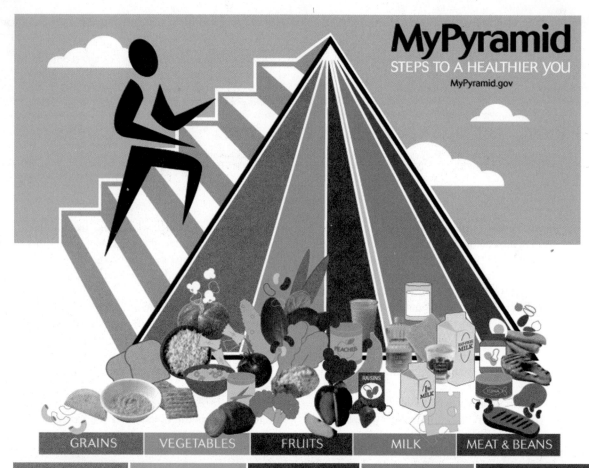

MyPyramid
STEPS TO A HEALTHIER YOU
MyPyramid.gov

GRAINS	VEGETABLES	FRUITS	MILK	MEAT & BEANS
GRAINS Make half your grains whole	**VEGETABLES** Vary your veggies	**FRUITS** Focus on fruits	**MILK** Get your calcium-rich foods	**MEAT & BEANS** Go lean with protein
Eat at least 3 oz. of whole-grain cereals, breads, crackers, rice, or pasta every day 1 oz. is about 1 slice of bread, about 1 cup of breakfast cereal, or 1/2 cup of cooked rice, cereal, or pasta	Eat more dark-green veggies like broccoli, spinach, and other dark leafy greens Eat more orange vegetables like carrots and sweetpotatoes Eat more dry beans and peas like pinto beans, kidney beans, and lentils	Eat a variety of fruit Choose fresh, frozen, canned, or dried fruit Go easy on fruit juices	Go low-fat or fat-free when you choose milk, yogurt, and other milk products If you don't or can't consume milk, choose lactose-free products or other calcium sources such as fortified foods and beverages	Choose low-fat or lean meats and poultry Bake it, broil it, or grill it Vary your protein routine — choose more fish, beans, peas, nuts, and seeds

For a 2,000-calorie diet, you need the amounts below from each food group. To find the amounts that are right for you, go to MyPyramid.gov.

Eat 6 oz. every day	Eat 2 1/2 cups every day	Eat 2 cups every day	Get 3 cups every day; for kids aged 2 to 8, it's 2	Eat 5 1/2 oz. every day

Find your balance between food and physical activity
- Be sure to stay within your daily calorie needs.
- Be physically active for at least 30 minutes most days of the week.
- About 60 minutes a day of physical activity may be needed to prevent weight gain.
- For sustaining weight loss, at least 60 to 90 minutes a day of physical activity may be required.
- Children and teenagers should be physically active for 60 minutes every day, or most days.

Know the limits on fats, sugars, and salt (sodium)
- Make most of your fat sources from fish, nuts, and vegetable oils.
- Limit solid fats like butter, stick margarine, shortening, and lard, as well as foods that contain these.
- Check the Nutrition Facts label to keep saturated fats, *trans* fats, and sodium low.
- Choose food and beverages low in added sugars. Added sugars contribute calories with few, if any, nutrients.

MyPyramid.gov
STEPS TO A HEALTHIER YOU

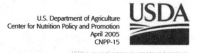

U.S. Department of Agriculture
Center for Nutrition Policy and Promotion
April 2005
CNPP-15

USDA is an equal opportunity provider and employer.

Figure 11-2 MyPyramid, the new food guidance system developed by the USDA. (From U.S. Department of Agriculture, Center for Nutrition Policy and Promotion, April 2005.)

and mineral supplement use by women of childbearing age.

Besides problems with direct toxicity of some individual nutrients, nutrient supplementation can cause problems related to nutrient imbalances or adverse interactions with prescribed medication. Many problems associated with high doses of a single nutrient may reflect interactions that result in a relative deficiency for another nutrient. Some examples follow:

- High doses of vitamin E can interfere with vitamin K action and enhance the effect of coumarin anticoagulant drugs.
- Large amounts of calcium inhibit absorption of iron and possibly other trace elements.
- Folic acid can mask hematological signs of vitamin B_{12} deficiency which, if untreated, can result in irreversible neurological damage. Folic acid can also interact adversely with anticonvulsant medications.
- Zinc supplementation can reduce copper status, impair immune responses, and decrease high-density lipoprotein cholesterol levels.

FOOD SAFETY

Food safety is vitally important in promoting health and remains in the limelight as severe food-borne illnesses sweep across the nation. In this section the importance of safeguarding food, the different types of contamination that endanger the food supply, and steps that can be taken to avoid falling victim to food-borne illness are considered.

Every organization and individual connected to the food chain, from food production to the table, share responsibility for the safety and integrity of the food supply. This chain includes people who produce or grow, process, ship, sell, and prepare food and the consumer who makes up the final link in the chain. The USDA establishes and monitors guidelines and standards to be followed by all groups involved. When the safeguards built into this system fail, however, consumers themselves must serve as the final and sometimes most important guardian against unsafe food. Therefore being informed and educated about the potential dangers of food-borne illness and how to avoid these complications to stay healthy is essential.

Causes of Food-Borne Illness

A food-borne illness is classified according to the source of its contamination (the unintended presence of harmful substances or microorganisms). Food contaminants may be categorized as biological, chemical, or physical. Biological contaminants include bacteria, viruses, parasites, and fungi (yeasts and mold). Chemical contamination refers to the presence of pesticides, kitchen cleaning supplies, and toxic chemicals in food that have been leached out of worn metal cookware and equipment. Physical contamination includes dirt, glass chips, crockery, wood, splinters, stones, hair, jewelry, and metal shavings from dull can openers.

Mad Cow Disease

The highly active surveillance on beef from Europe and particularly the United Kingdom is a prime example of the effect unsafe food can have on entire populations. The problem known as *bovine spongiform encephalopathy* (BSE), or more commonly as *mad cow disease,* is traced back to unsafe practices of certain producers in the meat industry. Cows who eat sheep products and waste meat contaminated with an infectious proteinlike particle known as a *prion* develop a fatal neurological disease. These cows become uncontrollable and wild, much different from their usual docile nature. Humans who eat contaminated beef suffer from a similar fatal neurological degeneration called new variant Creutzfeldt-Jakob disease (nvCJD). The prion cannot be destroyed by heat, radiation, or disinfectants. Cooperation among the entire food safety network, especially the consumer, is therefore important for special cases like this one to be controlled. To reduce the risk of acquiring nvCJD, travelers to Europe should be advised to consider either avoiding beef and beef products altogether, or selecting beef or beef products as solid pieces of muscle meat (versus ground products such as burgers and sausages) that have a reduced opportunity for contamination with tissues that might harbor the BSE agent. Milk and milk products from cows are not believed to pose any risk for transmitting the prion (Centers for Disease Control and Prevention [CDC], National Center for Infectious Diseases, 2001).

Food Safety Practices

Hand washing is one of the most important practices in the prevention of food-borne illness. Hands should be washed thoroughly before food preparation and before eating. The accepted method of hand washing entails running warm water over the hands, applying soap, and generating friction and agitation for approximately 20 to 30 seconds. Young children should be taught to wash their hands for as long as it takes them to sing the alphabet song twice. Nearly one half of all cases of food-borne illness might be avoided completely if people were to wash their hands more often when preparing and handling food.

Raw, cooked, and ready-to-eat foods should be separated while shopping, preparing, or storing foods. Separating foods prevents cross-contamination, which is the transfer of harmful substances or microorganisms from one location to another. Cross-contamination can occur when unwashed hands come in contact with food, when a microorganism-carrying food comes in contact with another food, or when food comes in contact with a contaminated surface. To prevent cross-contamination, follow these additional safety measures:

- Wash fresh fruits and vegetables thoroughly.
- Drink pasteurized juices.
- Do not consume raw (unpasteurized) milk or cheeses made with raw milk.
- Eat food that has been chilled and refrigerated properly.

- When eating out, make sure that food requiring refrigeration is served chilled.
- When shopping, buy perishable foods last and take them straight home.
- Follow the label. Always read and follow safety instructions on the package, such as, "keep refrigerated" and "safe handling instructions."
- Eat food that is served safely. Keep hot foods hot (140° F or above) and cold foods cold (40° F or below). Between these temperatures is the danger zone in which harmful bacteria can grow rapidly, even exponentially.
- Whether raw or cooked, never leave meat, poultry, eggs, fish, or shellfish out at room temperature for more than 2 hours (1 hour in hot weather that is 90° F and above). Be sure to chill leftovers as soon as you finish eating.

These guidelines also apply to carryout meals, restaurant leftovers, and home-packed meals to go. If in doubt, throw it out.

Making a food safe after it has been handled improperly may not always be possible. Therefore the best practice is to discard food when there is a doubt as to the safety of food preparation, service, or storage. For example, certain bacteria found in food that has been left at room temperature too long may produce a heat-resistant toxin that cannot be destroyed by cooking. Therefore the bottom line is to be careful in preparing food, which includes keeping track of the time the food is exposed to certain temperatures and being vigilant when eating out. If there is any doubt about the safety of the food, then caution is urged; it is better not to eat it.

Without exception, everyone should exercise their best judgment and care when eating out, when handling their own food, or when handling the food of others. Prevention through education is the key to promoting healthy lives that are unscathed by the potentially severe and life-threatening effects of food-borne illness. People who do not have healthy immune systems (individuals with various health problems and many older adults) and people with immune systems that are not fully developed (infants) are at the greatest risk of developing food-borne illnesses.

Because food is shipped to the United States from all over the world, and because effective antibiotics are not available to meet the challenge of ever-changing and mutating microbial agents, it is imperative to follow the basic food safety guidelines outlined in this chapter.

On a more positive note, normal healthy adults with healthy immune systems are able to ward off most of the contaminants from the environment and from food without much effort most of the time. Nevertheless, everyone should follow standard safety procedures when eating out and when handling food.

FOOD, NUTRITION, AND POVERTY

Healthy People 2010 Goal: promote health and reduce chronic disease associated with diet.

- 19-18. Increase food security in U.S. households from 88% in 1995 to 94% by 2010.

Poverty and Income Distribution

For most people in the United States, income has risen over time, providing more options for personal consumption expenditures, including expenditures on food. However, growth in income has not increased equally for all households. Poverty still exists in the United States.

According to official 2003 poverty statistics (U.S. Census Bureau, 2004) 12.5% (35.9 million) of people live below the poverty level—a level of income set annually by the government to determine eligibility for various types of government programs as discussed in this section. In 2003, groups with particularly high poverty rates included Hispanics and African Americans, with statistically equivalent poverty rates of 22.5% and 24.4%, respectively. In contrast, the poverty rate was 8.2% for white non-Hispanic people. Children, who make up 35.9% of the poor but only 25.6% of the total population, have a 17.6% poverty rate, which is higher than the rate of any other age group (U.S. Census Bureau, 2004). In 2003 approximately 12.9 million children were poor. People living in families headed by single women have a poverty rate of over 28%.

Food Assistance for the Poor

For people who are poor, obtaining a nutritious diet without assistance can be a challenge. Federal, state, and local governments and private charitable organizations mitigate this problem by providing billions of dollars annually in food assistance. Overall the bulk of food aid in the United States is financed at the federal level by the USDA. In 2003 federally funded outlays for food assistance programs amounted to almost $41.6 billion (*http://www.ers.usda.gov/ briefing/foodnutritionassistance/*), as detailed below:

- Food Stamps: almost $20.5 billion
- Child nutrition (mostly for the School-Based Partnerships and the National School Lunch Program [NSLP]): almost $9.5 billion
- WIC: over $4.5 billion
- Food donations (e.g., to Native American communities, the Nutrition Program for the Elderly [NPE], the Emergency Food Distribution Program): almost $500 million

One in six people in the United States receives federally funded food assistance at some point every year. The Food Stamp Program, NSLP, School-Based Partnerships, WIC, and NPE are the main programs that provide domestic food and nutrition assistance. Table 11-3 contains information on identifying low-income people who need help getting enough food and referring them to the appropriate program.

Food Stamp Program

Food coupons or food stamps are used to supplement the food-buying power of eligible low-income people. The program provides monthly allotments to help low-income families purchase nutritionally adequate foods. Although

Table 11-3 Referral Guide for Federal Food Assistance Programs

Program	Target Population	Indicators of Need	Where to Call
School lunch	Children of school age	Poor nutritional status	Local school district
School breakfast	Children unlikely to eat before school	Harried household, low-income, poor nutritional status	Local school district
Summer food program	Children who live in low-income neighborhoods	Economic stress, poor nutritional status	Local social services office
WIC	Low-income pregnant and lactating women; infants and children up to age 5	Risk of existing health or nutritional problem	Local health department or community action agency
Congregate dining	Elderly adults, especially low-income minority and frail	Few social contacts, poor quality or quantity diet	Local office on aging
Home-delivered meals	Frail, homebound, elderly adults	Unable to shop for or prepare food, no available caretaker	Local hospital or office on aging

From Splett, P. L. (1994). Federal food assistance programs: A step to food security for many. *Nutrition Today, 29*(2), 6-13.
WIC, Special Supplemental Nutrition Program for Women, Infants, and Children.

there is no requirement that food stamps be used to purchase high-quality food, the goal of the food stamp nutrition education program is to increase the likelihood that recipients will make healthy food choices within their limited food budget. Households can use food stamps to buy any food or food product for human consumption and seeds and plants for use in home gardens. Restaurants can be authorized to accept food stamps from qualified homeless, elderly, or disabled people in exchange for low-cost meals. Among the items that recipients cannot buy with food stamps are alcoholic beverages, tobacco, hot ready-to-eat foods, lunch counter items, foods to be eaten in the store, vitamins, medicines, and pet foods. Food stamps cannot be exchanged for cash. The program is administered nationally by the Food and Nutrition Service (FNS) and locally by state welfare agencies. To qualify, households must meet eligibility criteria, including a gross income at or below 130% of the poverty guidelines issued by the USDHHS. Most able-bodied adult applicants must also meet certain work requirements. Households may own certain resources. In addition to income, the food stamp allotment is also based on family size. In 2002 the Food Stamp Program provided benefits to 19 million people: 51% children, 40% adults, and 9% seniors. In 2003 the average monthly benefit per person was approximately $83 and almost $194 per household (U.S. Census Bureau, 2004).

National School Lunch Program

The federally funded NSLP is administered by FNS, an agency within the USDA. On the state level, the NSLP usually is administered by the U.S. Department of Education, which contracts with local schools to provide balanced, low-cost or free lunches. The NSLP reaches about 24 million children each school day.

- Children from families with incomes at or below 130% of the poverty level are eligible for free school meals.

- Children from families with incomes at 130% to 185% of the poverty level are eligible for reduced-price school meals.
- Children from families with incomes over 185% of the poverty level are eligible for full-price school meals.

Schools that choose to take part in the lunch program are provided with cash subsidies and donated commodities from the USDA. Donated foods include meats, canned and frozen fruits and vegetables, fruit juices, vegetable shortening, peanut products, vegetable oil, and flour and other grain products. Free or reduced-price lunches must meet these federal minimum pattern requirements:

- Must provide one third of the recommended nutrient intake
- To the extent possible, must be consistent with the Dietary Guidelines for Americans recommendations for reducing sugar, salt, and fat intake

To help meet the goal of healthier school meals, the USDA launched Team Nutrition, an initiative designed to help make implementation of the new policy in schools easier and more successful.

School Breakfast Program

Skipping breakfast can adversely affect children's performance in math and reading. A study of low-income elementary school students indicated that children who participated in the School Breakfast Program had greater improvements in standardized test scores and reduced rates of absence and tardiness than did children who qualified for the program but did not participate (CDC, 2004). The School Breakfast Program provides assistance to states to initiate, maintain, or expand nonprofit breakfast programs in eligible schools and residential child care institutions. The program is administered by the FNS. Any child attending a participating school may receive a free, reduced-price, or full-price breakfast based on the same income criteria used by the NSLP.

Women, Infants, and Children

Food, nutrition counseling, and access to health services are provided to low-income women, infants, and children under the WIC program, which is administered by the FNS. This grant program provides supplemental foods and health care referrals and nutrition education at no cost to the recipient. Low-income pregnant or postpartum women and children younger than 5 years old who are at risk nutritionally are eligible for WIC. The eligibility level is an income less than 185% of the poverty level. Nutritional risk is determined by federal guidelines. Three major types of nutritional risk are recognized: (1) high-priority, medically based risks, such as anemia, being underweight, low maternal age, history of pregnancy complications, (2) diet-based risks, such as inadequate dietary patterns, and (3) conditions such as alcoholism or drug addiction that predispose people to medically based or diet-based risks.

WIC participants receive coupons redeemable for foods that are rich in protein, calcium, iron, vitamin A, and vitamin C. Also included are iron-fortified infant formula and infant cereal, iron-fortified adult cereal, fruit or vegetable juice rich in vitamin C, eggs, milk, cheese, and peanut butter or dried beans. Special therapeutic formulas are provided when prescribed by a physician for a specific medical condition. Each WIC participant is designated to receive one of six different food packages that is specially designed for: (1) infants from birth through 3 months, (2) infants from 4 months through a year, (3) women and children with special dietary needs, (4) children 1 to 5 years of age, (5) pregnant and breast-feeding women, and (6) non–breast-feeding postpartum women. In 2002 more than 1.9 million infants participated in WIC, which is almost one third of the infants born in the United States (*http://www.fns.usda.gov/wic/FAQS/faq.htm#3*).

Two major types of nutritional risk are recognized for WIC eligibility:

- Medically based risks, such as anemia, underweight, maternal age, history of pregnancy complications, or poor pregnancy outcome
- Diet-based risks, such as inadequate dietary pattern as determined by 24-hour recall, food frequency questionnaire, or diet history

Children have always made up the largest category of WIC participants. An average monthly participation for 2004 was approximately 24 million people (*http://usfoodpolicy.blogspotcom/2005/02/foodstamp-high-performance-bonus.html*).

Financial constraints preclude WIC from serving all eligible people; therefore, a system of priorities has been established for filling program openings. After a local WIC agency has reached its maximal caseload, vacancies generally are filled in the order of the following priority levels:

- Pregnant women, breast-feeding women, and infants determined to be at nutritional risk from serious medical problems

- Infants up to 6 months of age whose mothers participate in WIC or are eligible to participate and have serious medical problems
- Children up to age 5 at nutritional risk from serious medical problems
- Pregnant or breast-feeding women and infants who are at nutritional risk from dietary problems
- Children up to age 5 at nutritional risk from dietary problems
- Non–breast-feeding postpartum women with any nutritional risk
- Individuals at nutritional risk only because they are homeless or migrants and current participants who would likely continue to have medical or dietary problems without WIC assistance

In most WIC state agencies, participants receive checks or vouchers monthly to purchase specific foods to supplement their usual diets. These nutrients frequently are missing in the diets of the program's target population. Food packages are provided for various categories of participants. A few WIC state agencies distribute foods through warehouses; some agencies deliver foods to participants.

The WIC Farmers' Market Nutrition Program, established in 1992, provides additional coupons to WIC participants to use for purchasing fresh fruits and vegetables at participating farmers' markets. The program has two goals: (1) to provide fresh, nutritious, unprepared, locally grown fruits and vegetables from farmers' markets to WIC participants and (2) to expand consumers' awareness and use of farmers' markets. In 1998, this program was offered in 50 states, the District of Columbia, and 33 Indian tribal organizations.

The WIC program is effective in improving the health of its participants. Medicaid costs for women who participate in the program during pregnancy and their infants are lower than those for women who do not participate. WIC participation is also linked to longer gestation periods, higher birth weights, and lower infant mortality rates.

Nutrition Program for the Elderly

Nutrition Program for the Elderly (NPE) helps provide elderly adults with nutritionally sound meals. These are provided by Meals on Wheels programs or in senior citizen centers and similar congregate feeding settings, in which meals provide the focal points for activities that have the dual objective of promoting better health and reducing the isolation that may occur in old age. Age is the only factor used in determining eligibility. People 60 years or older and their spouses, regardless of age, are eligible for NPE benefits. Native American tribal organizations may select an age below 60 for defining an *older* person for their tribes. Additionally, disabled people who live in elder care housing facilities, people who accompany elderly participants to congregate feeding sites, and volunteers who assist in the meal service may also receive meals through NPE.

There is no income requirement for NPE meals. Each recipient may contribute as much as desired toward the cost of the meal, but they are free to people who cannot make any contribution. In 1996, more than 3 million people participated, about one third of whom received home delivery. The NPE is administered by the Administration on Aging, a component unit of the USDHHS. However, the NPE receives commodity foods and financial support from the USDA's FNS. This program is administered at the state level; therefore, the local state distribution agency should be contacted for information about local programs.

NUTRITION SCREENING

Nutrition screening is the process of discovering characteristics or risk factors that are known to be associated with dietary or nutrition problems. Its primary purpose is to identify individuals (such as older adults and the poor) who are potentially at high risk from complex and involved problems that relate to nutrition. To serve this purpose, screening criteria must be simple, relatively straightforward, and easy to administer. Screening is also helpful in establishing priorities for the most efficient use of valuable time and money.

The single largest demographic group at disproportionate risk of malnutrition is elderly Americans. Nutrition screening holds a tremendous preventive health potential for older adults. The nurse should provide nutrition counseling or a referral to a registered dietitian for an older person who has food-related problems. A dietitian or community nutrition program might be appropriate if any of the following are identified in the individual:

- Inappropriate, inadequate, or excessive food intake
- Problems complying with a special diet
- Need for nutrient-specific counseling or counseling related to a disease
- Weight of more than 20% above what is desirable
- Serum cholesterol level of more than 240 mg/dl
- Functional dependency for eating or for food-related activities of daily living

The health care professional should refer the individual to a physician when there has been an involuntary decrease in weight of more than 10 pounds during the previous 6 months. Additional anthropometric measurements suggesting malnutrition include the following:

- Triceps skin-fold thickness less than 10th percentile
- Midarm muscle circumference less than 10th percentile
- Serum albumin level less than 3.5 g/dl
- Evidence of osteoporosis or mineral deficiency (indicated by a history of bone pain or fractures, particularly in housebound older women)
- Evidence of vitamin deficiency (indicated by inadequate fruit and vegetable intake; angular stomatitis, glossitis, or bleeding gums; pressure sores in bedridden individuals)

Otherwise healthy older people can be provided with the 70+ Pyramid, which they can use as a quick screening tool to assess their own food intake.

NUTRITION AND DISEASE

In any assessment of the role that diet plays in the prevention of heart disease, cancers, stroke, and other diseases, an understanding is required that a combination and interaction of environmental, behavioral, social, and genetic factors cause these conditions. The exact number of factors that can be attributed directly to the diet is unknown. Although suggestions are such that dietary factors overall are responsible for at least one third of all cases of cancer and CHD, these estimates are based on interpretations of research studies that cannot completely distinguish dietary factors from genetic, environmental, and behavioral causes. Many dietary components are involved in the relationship between diet and health. Chief among them is the disproportionate consumption of foods high in fats, often at the expense of foods that are rich in nutrients and the complex carbohydrates and dietary fibers that may be more conducive to health.

This section examines the role of nutrition in the etiology and prevention of the leading nutrition-related chronic diseases: heart disease, stroke, some forms of cancer, osteoporosis, obesity, and type 2 diabetes, and in the early treatment of people who are recently diagnosed with the human immunodeficiency virus.

Each disease discussed contains references to Web sites to which clients can be referred if they have access to the Internet, or the information can be downloaded to customize educational materials.

Understanding the Hispanic culture is particularly important in any review of nutrition and disease in the United States, because Hispanics or Latinos account for about 13% of the people in the United States (35.3 million from the total population of 281.4 million). Hispanic Americans are the largest minority group, outnumbering African Americans, who account for about 12.9% of the population (Grieco & Cassidy, 2001). Aside from cultural and language barriers, Hispanic Americans challenge the health care industry because they are twice as likely to have diabetes than members of the white population of similar age. Additionally, since 1989 the rate of acquired immunodeficiency syndrome among Hispanic Americans has been higher than that of the white population.

Cardiovascular Diseases

Cardiovascular disease (CVD), principally CHD and **stroke,** are among the nation's leading killers of both men and women and among all racial and ethnic groups. Approximately one fourth of the nation's population has some form of CVD, including high blood pressure, CHD, and stroke.

Heart Disease
Diet Intervention

In an attempt to reduce CVD, the American Heart Association (AHA) recommends that people over the age of 2 years adopt an overall healthy diet and achieve and maintain an appropriate body weight, cholesterol level, and blood pressure level (Krauss et al., 2000). (The AHA did not set guidelines for those under 2 years of age.)

To achieve an overall healthy eating pattern, include a variety of fruits, vegetables, grains, low-fat or nonfat dairy products, fish, legumes, poultry, and lean meats. Specifically:

- Choose an overall balanced diet with foods from all major food groups, emphasizing fruits, vegetables and grains.
- Consume a variety of fruits, vegetables, and grain products.
- Consume at least 5 daily servings of fruits and vegetables.
- Consume at least 6 daily servings of grain products, including whole grains.
- Include fat-free and low-fat dairy products, fish, legumes, poultry, and lean meats.
- Eat at least 2 servings of fish every week.

To achieve and maintain an appropriate body weight, match the energy intake to energy needs, with appropriate changes to achieve weight loss when indicated. Specifically:

- Avoid excess intake of calories.
- Maintain a level of physical activity that achieves fitness and that balances energy expenditure with caloric intake; for weight reduction, expenditure should exceed intake.
- Limit foods that are high in calories and low in nutritional quality, including foods with a large amount of added **sugar**.

To achieve and maintain a desirable cholesterol level, limit foods high in saturated fat and cholesterol and substitute unsaturated fat from vegetables, fish, legumes, and nuts. Specifically:

- Limit foods with a high content of saturated fat and cholesterol. Substitute these foods with grains and unsaturated fat from vegetables, fish, legumes and nuts.
- Limit cholesterol to 300 mg a day for the general population and 200 mg a day for people with CVD or its risk factors.
- Limit *trans*-fatty acids. *Trans*-fatty acids are found in foods containing partially hydrogenated vegetable oils, such as packaged cookies, crackers, and other baked goods, commercially prepared fried foods, and some margarines.

To achieve and maintain a desirable blood pressure level, limit salt and alcohol, maintain a healthy body weight, and enjoy a diet with emphasis on vegetables, fruits, and low-fat or nonfat dairy products. Specifically:

- Limit salt intake to less than 6 g (2400 mg sodium) per day, slightly more than 1 teaspoon a day.
- If you drink, limit alcohol consumption to no more than 1 drink per day for women and 2 drinks per day for men. A drink is defined as 12 ounces of beer, 5 ounces of wine, or 1.5 ounces of distilled spirits.

Many children, adolescents, and adults who already have undesirable levels of lipids in their blood should receive nutrition counseling when their total **cholesterol** level is elevated. In children ages 2 to 20, an acceptable level of cholesterol is less than 170 mg/dl.

Individuals with low-density lipoprotein (LDL) cholesterol levels that are above 2000 National Cholesterol Education Program (NCEP) targets for primary or secondary prevention should be advised to reduce their intake of dietary saturated fat and cholesterol to levels below the levels recommended for the general population (Expert Panel on Detection, Evaluation, and Treatment of High Blood Cholesterol in Adults, 2001). The upper limit for these individuals is less than 7% of the total energy for saturated fat and less than 200 mg of cholesterol per day. In both cases, however, even lower intake levels can be of further benefit in reducing LDL cholesterol levels. After the program is outlined, follow-up sessions are scheduled to monitor lipid levels and dietary compliance. After 3 to 6 months, if acceptable lipid levels have not been achieved, then the individual should be referred to a registered dietitian.

The NCEP develops new guidelines periodically, as warranted by research advances. Their first and second guidelines were issued in 1988 and 1993. The most recent set of guidelines was released in 2001, Third Report of the NCEP Expert Panel on Detection, Evaluation, and Treatment of High Blood Cholesterol in Adults, also known as Adult Treatment Panel (ATP) III. The ATP guidelines are expected to result in about 6.5 million Americans being treated for high cholesterol through Therapeutic Lifestyle Changes (TLC) (Table 11-4).

The ATP recommends that healthy adults have a lipoprotein analysis once every 5 years. A lipoprotein profile

Table 11-4 ATP-III Classification of Serum Lipid Levels* in Adults Age 20 and Older

Classification	LDL-Cholesterol, mg/dl	Total Cholesterol, mg/dl	Triglycerides, mg/dl	HDL-Cholesterol, mg/dl
Optimal/desirable	<100	<200	<150	≥60
Near optimal/above normal	100-129	—	—	—
Borderline high	130-159	200-239	150-199	—
High	160-189	—	200-499	—
Very high	≥190	≥240	≥500	—
Low	—	—	—	≤40

From Expert Panel on Detection, Evaluation, and Treatment of High Blood Cholesterol in Adults. (2001). Executive summary of the third report of the National Cholesterol Education Program (NCEP) expert panel on detection, evaluation, and treatment of high blood cholesterol in adults (adult treatment panel III). *Journal of the American Medical Association, 285,* 2486-2497.
*Measured in milligrams (mg) of lipid per deciliter (dl) of blood.
ATP, Adult Treatment Panel; *HDL,* high-density lipoprotein; *LDL,* low-density lipoprotein.

measures levels of LDL, total cholesterol, high-density lipoproteins (HDL), and triglycerides (another fatty substance in the blood). The level at which low HDL becomes a major risk factor for heart disease is <40 mg/dl.

In addition to a low HDL, there are other major risk factors for CHD:

- Clinical forms of atherosclerotic disease (peripheral arterial disease, abdominal aortic aneurysm, and symptomatic carotid artery disease)
- Age (55 for men and ≥65 for women)
- Cigarette smoking
- Hypertension (BP ≥140/90 mm Hg or taking antihypertensive medication)
- Diabetes (fasting blood glucose ≥110 mg/dl)
- Family history of premature heart disease (heart disease in a first-degree relative at age ≤55 for men or at age ≤65 for women)

HDL cholesterol ≥60 counts as a negative risk factor.

Therapeutic Lifestyle Changes
Treatment Plan

The TLC treatment plan of nutrition, physical activity, and weight control is recommended for treating people who present with type 2 diabetes, elevated LDL, or metabolic syndrome.

Metabolic syndrome describes the presence of a cluster of risk factors that often occur together, which dramatically increases the risk for coronary events. The syndrome is diagnosed when an individual has three or more of these factors:

- Excessive abdominal fat, as indicated by too large a waist measurement (over 35 inches or 88 centimeters in women and over 40 inches or 102 centimeters in men)
- Elevated blood pressure (≥130 mm Hg systolic or ≥85 mm Hg diastolic)
- Low HDL level (<40 mg/dl)
- Elevated triglyceride level (≥150 mg/dl) which is significantly linked to the degree of heart disease risk. (The guidelines recommend treating even borderline high triglyceride levels with therapy that includes weight control and physical activity.)

The dietary component of the TLC includes daily intake of:

- Less than 7% of calories from saturated fat
- Less than 200 mg of dietary cholesterol
- Up to 35% of calories from total fat, provided most of the fat is from unsaturated fat, which does not raise cholesterol levels (A higher fat intake may be needed by some clients with high triglycerides or a low HDL or both to keep their triglyceride levels or HDL status from worsening.)
- Intake of certain foods to boost the diet's LDL-lowering power: 2 g/day of plant stanols and sterols found in cholesterol-lowering margarines and salad dressings, and 10 to 25 g/day of foods high in soluble fiber, such as cereal grains, beans, peas, legumes, and many fruits and vegetables

A primary treatment goal of the TLC is reducing elevated LDL to:

- <100 mg/dl in the presence of CHD or other forms of atherosclerotic disease
- <130 mg/dl in the presence of two or more risk factors for CHD
- <160 mg/dl in the presence of fewer than two risk factors for CHD

The final goal of the TLC includes weight control (to enhance LDL lowering and raise HDL) and physical activity that lasts at least 30 minutes, expending at least 200 calories per day on most days (to improve HDL and, for some, LDL levels).

Removing Barriers to Compliance

To improve client adherence to ATP-III goals, treatment barriers can be eliminated by developing protocols to encourage long-term client compliance and follow-up, such as establishing clinic policy and developing computerized client databases, establishing management algorithms, reinforcing and rewarding adherence, and enhancing third party reimbursement. The nurse should use behavioral theories to identify a client's level of readiness to change and focus on counseling strategies to match that level of readiness (Snetselaar, 2004).

Hypertension

Blood pressure, the force of blood against the walls of arteries, is recorded as the systolic pressure (as the heart beats) over the diastolic pressure (as the heart relaxes between beats). The measurement is written one above (or before) the other, with the systolic number on top and the diastolic number on the bottom. For example, a blood pressure measurement of 120/80 mm Hg (millimeters of mercury) is expressed verbally as "120 over 80." Normal blood pressure is less than 130 mm Hg systolic and less than 85 mm Hg diastolic. Optimal blood pressure is less than 120 mm Hg systolic and less than 80 mm Hg diastolic.

Epidemiology

Hypertension (high blood pressure) killed 46,765 Americans in 2001 and contributed to the deaths of approximately 251,000 people. As many as 50 million Americans aged 6 and older have high blood pressure, which represents 20% of the total population and 25% of all adults in the United States (based on National Health and Nutrition Examination Survey III data). Of the 50 million people, only two thirds know they have high blood pressure, and of these, only about 59% receive adequate therapy (diet alone or diet and drugs). Untreated hypertension can damage arteries and increase the risk of stroke and congestive heart failure. High blood pressure is also responsible for many cases of kidney failure requiring dialysis and increases the risk of kidney failure in diabetics.

African Americans and Hispanic Americans are more likely to suffer from high blood pressure than are white non-Hispanic Americans. Additionally, people with lower educational and income levels tend to have higher blood pressure levels. In 2002 the death rates per 100,000 population from high blood pressure were 14.4 for white non-Hispanic men, 49.6 for African American men, 13.7 for white non-Hispanic women, and 40.5 for African American women.

Diet Intervention

The modifiable nutrition-related risk factors for stroke include obesity, habitual high alcohol intake, and high intake of sodium. No certain method exists for identifying susceptible people or ascertaining how many of them become hypertensive as a result of excessive salt intake; therefore, the conservative preventive health approach recommends a salt intake limited to 6 g or less per day for adults. Sodium chloride is approximately 40% sodium by weight; therefore, a diet with 6 g salt contains about 2.4 g of sodium. This amount is regarded as mild sodium restriction. Table 11-5 lists the approximate sodium content of representative foods.

The three major sources of sodium in the U.S. diet are:

Table 11-5 Sodium Content of Foods

Food Group	High	mg Na⁺	Low	mg Na⁺
Grain products	English muffin	300	White rice, 1 cup	6
	Waffle, 1 frozen	275	Popcorn, 3 cups	3
	Potato chips, 10	200	Puffed rice, 2 cups	2
	White bread, 1 slice	115	Oatmeal, ¾ cup	1
	Saltine crackers, 2	70	Wheat germ, toasted, ¼ cup	1
Meat, poultry, and fish	Herring, 3 oz, smoked	5235	Codfish, 3 oz	65
	Frankfurter, 1 oz	310	Chicken, 3 oz	60
	Ham, 3 oz, baked	280	Beef, 3 oz	55
	Bacon, 2 strips	275	Turkey, 3 oz	50
	Bologna, 1 slice	220		
	Scallops, 3 oz	215		
	Lobster, 3 oz	180		
	Shrimp, 3 oz	115		
Dairy products	Cottage cheese, ½ cup	460	Yogurt, ½ cup, frozen	60
	American cheese, 1 slice	405	Ricotta, 1 oz, whole milk	24
	Buttermilk, 1 cup	240	Cottage cheese, ½ cup, dry curd	10
	Gouda cheese, 1 oz	230		
	Cheddar cheese, 1 oz	175		
	Yogurt, 1 cup, low-fat	175		
	Milk, 1 cup	120		
	Butter, 1 tbsp	100		
Fruits and vegetables	Sauerkraut, 1 cup	1555	All fresh fruits	0 to 20
	Mushrooms, 1 cup, canned	800	Brussels sprouts, 1 cup	15
	Spinach, 1 cup, canned	780	Mushrooms, 1 cup, fresh	10
	Creamed corn, 1 cup, canned	670	Potato, 1 medium	5
	Tomato juice, 1 cup	500	Corn, 1 cup, fresh or frozen	2
	Tomatoes, 1 cup, canned	430		
	Peas, 1 cup, canned	490		
	Corn, 1 cup, canned, whole kernel	385		
	Celery, 1 cup, diced	130		
	Orange drink, 1 cup	80		
	Lemonade, 1 cup	60		
Miscellaneous	Garlic salt, 1 tsp	1850	Peanuts, 1 cup, unsalted	8
	Dill pickle, 1 large	1430	Jam or jelly, 1 tbsp	2
	Soy sauce, 1 tbsp	1030	Vinegar, ½ cup	1
	Baking soda, 1 tsp	1000	Lemon juice, 1 tsp	1
	Olives, 10 small green	685	Yeast, 1 package dry	1
	MSG, 1 tbsp	490	Honey, 1 tbsp	1
	Bouillon, 1 cube	425	Garlic powder, 1 tsp	1
	Baking powder, 1 tsp	370	Vegetable oil, 1 tbsp	0
	Catsup, 2 tbsp	355		
	Margarine, 1 tbsp	135		

MSG, monosodium glutamate.

1. Salt added by consumers to food during cooking or at the table
2. Salt added by food processing companies as an ingredient in almost all processed foods (including many foods that do not taste salty, such as baked goods); most processed foods are high in sodium content.
3. Salt from all animal products, which are a natural source of sodium

The following recommended food tips are designed to reduce salt and sodium intake:

- Sodium occurs naturally in many foods and is also added to most processed foods; therefore, added salt should be used only sparingly in home cooking and at the table.
- Consume fewer foods that have high sodium levels, such as many cheeses, processed meats, most frozen dinners and entrees, packaged mixes, most canned soups and vegetables, salad dressings, and condiments such as soy sauce, pickles, olives, catsup, and mustard.
- Before warming canned vegetables, rinse them first.
- Salty, highly processed salty, salt-preserved, and salt-pickled foods should be eaten sparingly.
- Check labels for the amount of sodium in foods and choose products lower in sodium.

According to the study presented in the Research Highlights box, the DASH eating plan makes consuming less salt and sodium easier because the plan includes abundant fruits and vegetables, which are lower in sodium than other foods. The DASH clinical study found that elevated blood pressure can be reduced with an eating plan low in saturated fat, total fat, and cholesterol and rich in fruits, vegetables, and low-fat dairy foods. The plan is rich in magnesium, potassium, calcium, and protein and fiber. The amounts of the nutrients vary by caloric intake. At approximately 2000 calories a day, the nutrients include 4700 mg of potassium, 500 mg of magnesium, and 1240 mg of calcium. These totals are approximately 2 to 3 times the amounts most Americans receive.

When blood pressure is normal, the DASH eating plan may help prevent blood pressure problems. If blood pressure is only slightly elevated, then the plan may actually eliminate the need for medication. For more severe high blood pressure, the plan may allow a reduction in medication. Other steps to control or prevent hypertension should continue to be encouraged, including exercising, losing excess weight, not smoking, and limiting alcohol. DASH may improve health in other ways, also. Fruits and vegetables

---

research highlights

Dietary Approaches to Stop Hypertension

This research is supported by grants from the NHLBI, the Office of Research on Minority Health, and the National Center for Research Resources of the NIH. From the disproportionate burden of hypertension in minority populations, particularly among blacks, one of the goals of the trial was to recruit a cohort in which two thirds of the subjects were members of a racial or ethnic minority.

METHODOLOGY

This study was a multicenter, randomized controlled, clinical trial of three experimental diets given to 459 adult participants (approximately one half of whom were women and 60% were black). All three diet plans contained about 3000 mg of sodium daily (approximately 20% below the U.S. average for adults). None of the plans was vegetarian or used specialty foods.

For 3 weeks the subjects consumed a control diet that was low in fruits, vegetables, and dairy products, with a fat content typical of the average diet in the United States. The subjects were then randomly assigned for 8 weeks to receive the control diet; a diet rich in fruits and vegetables; or the DASH eating plan, rich in fruits, vegetables, and low-fat dairy products with reduced saturated and total fat. All food for the experimental diets was provided to the participants. Body weights of participants were maintained at constant levels.

RESULTS

At baseline, the mean systolic and diastolic blood pressures were 131.3 ± 10.8 mm Hg and 84.7 ± 4.7 mm Hg, respectively.

DASH reduced S/D blood pressure by 5.5 and 3.0 mm Hg more, respectively, compared with the control diet; the fruits-and-vegetables diet reduced systolic blood pressure by 2.8 mm Hg more and diastolic blood pressure by 1.1 mm Hg more than the control diet. Among the 133 subjects with hypertension (systolic pressure greater than or equal to 140 mm Hg, diastolic pressure greater than or equal to 90 mmHg, or both), the combination diet reduced S/D blood pressure by 11.4 and 5.5 mm Hg more, respectively, compared with the control diet; among the 326 subjects without hypertension, the corresponding reductions were 3.5 mm Hg ($P < 0.001$) and 2.1 mm Hg. All results are statistically significant.

CLINICAL APPLICATION

Both the fruit-and-vegetable and DASH plans reduced blood pressure, but DASH had the greater effect, reducing blood pressure by an average of 6 mm Hg for systolic and 3 mm Hg for diastolic. The DASH plan worked even better for people with high blood pressure (on average, the systolic dropped 11 mm Hg and the diastolic dropped approximately 6 mm Hg). Furthermore, the reductions came quickly, within 2 weeks of starting the eating plan. The dietary patterns are constructed with commonly consumed food items; therefore, the positive results may be implemented conveniently in dietary recommendations to the general public.

Modified from Appel, L. J., Moore, T. J., Obarzanek, E., Vollmer, W. M., Svetkey, L. P., Sacks, F. M., et al. (1997). A clinical trial of the effects of dietary patterns on blood pressure. DASH Collaborative Research Group. *New England Journal of Medicine*, 336, 1117-1124.
DASH, dietary approaches to stop hypertension; *NHLBI*, National Heart, Lung, and Blood Institute; *NIH*, National Institutes of Health; *S/D*, systolic/diastolic.

may reduce the risk for some cancers; the calcium in dairy products can lower risk for osteoporosis; and a diet low in saturated fat and cholesterol can reduce CVD risk.

Cancer
Epidemiology

In 2000 approximately 1,220,100 cases of **cancer** were diagnosed in the United States, and approximately 552,200 Americans died of this disease. Overall, blacks were more likely to develop cancer than were people of any other racial or ethnic group. During the period from 1990 to 1996, incidence rates were 442.9 per 100,000 among blacks, 402.9 per 100,000 among whites, 275.4 per 100,000 among Hispanic Americans, 279.1 per 100,000 among Asian Americans, and 153.4 per 100,000 among Native Americans. During these same years, cancer incidence rates decreased among whites (down 1.2% per year), Hispanic Americans (down 1.7% per year), and Native Americans (down 0.7% per year), and remained relatively stable among blacks and Asian Americans. The incidence of breast cancer in women is highest among white women (113.2 per 100,000) and lowest among Native American women (33.9 per 100,000). Black women have the highest incidence rates of colon and rectal cancer (44.9 per 100,000) and lung and bronchial cancer (46.2 per 100,000) followed by whites, Asian Americans, Hispanic Americans, and Native Americans.

Blacks are approximately 33% more likely to die of cancer than whites and are 2 times more likely to die of cancer than Asian Americans, Native Americans, and Hispanic Americans. During the period from 1990 to 1996, cancer mortality rates were 223.4 per 100,000 among blacks, 167.5 per 100,000 among whites, 104.9 per 100,000 among Hispanic Americans, 103.4 per 100,000 among Asian Americans, and 104.0 per 100,000 among Native Americans. Cancer mortality rates for many racial and ethnic groups have begun to decline recently. During the period from 1990 to 1996, mortality rates decreased among whites (down 0.5% per year), blacks (down 0.9% per year), and Hispanic Americans (down 0.6% per year), remained relatively stable among Asian Americans, and increased slightly among Native Americans (up 0.9% per year). Black women are more likely to die of breast cancer (31.4 per 100,000) and colon and rectal cancer (20.0 per 100,000) than are women of any other racial or ethnic group (American Cancer Society [ACS], 2005b).

Approximately 40% of cancer incidence among men and 60% among women is related to diet. The introduction of a healthy diet and exercise practices at any time from childhood to old age can promote health and likely reduce cancer risk.

Diet Intervention for Risk Reduction

Many dietary factors can affect cancer risk: types of foods, food preparation methods, portion sizes, food variety, and overall caloric balance. An overall dietary pattern that includes a high proportion of plant foods (fruits, vegetables, grains, and beans), limited amounts of meat, dairy, and other high-fat foods, and a balance of caloric intake and physical activity can reduce the risk of cancer.

Based on its review of the scientific evidence, the American Cancer Society (ACS) updated its nutrition guidelines in 1999. The ACS recommendations are consistent in principle with the 1992 Food Guide Pyramid, the Dietary Guidelines for Americans, and dietary recommendations of other agencies for general health promotion and for the prevention of CHD, diabetes, and other diet-related chronic conditions. Although no diet can guarantee full protection against any disease, the ACS believes that the following recommendations offer the best nutrition information currently available to help Americans.

Choose Most of the Foods You Eat From Plant Sources. Eat 5 or more servings of fruits and vegetables every day; eat other foods from plant sources, such as breads, cereals, grain products, rice, pasta, or beans several times every day. Many scientific studies show that eating fruits and vegetables (especially green and dark yellow vegetables, foods in the cabbage family, soy products, and legumes) can protect against cancers at many sites, particularly for cancers of the gastrointestinal and respiratory tracts. Grains are an important source of many vitamins and minerals, such as folate, calcium, and selenium, which have been associated with a lower risk of colon cancer in some studies. Beans (legumes) are especially rich in nutrients that may protect against cancer.

Since 1991 the 5 A Day for Better Health Program has raised public awareness about the importance of fruits and vegetables in disease prevention. The program is jointly sponsored by the National Cancer Institute (a division of the USDHHS) and the Produce for Better Health Foundation (a nonprofit consumer education foundation representing the fruit and vegetable industry). Through its unique national public-private partnership, 5 A Day for Better Health Program seeks to increase consumption of fruits and vegetables to 5 or more servings each day. The program gives Americans a simple, positive message: eat 5 or more servings of fruits and vegetables every day for better health.

In The New American Plate, the American Institute for Cancer Research recommends reducing the portion size of meat, fish, or chicken to 3 ounces and filling the rest of the dinner plate with dishes composed of vegetables, fruits, whole grains, and beans. The program urges people to reverse the traditional American plate and think of meat as a side dish or condiment rather than the primary ingredient. In terms that laypeople can understand, this regimen translates into vegetables, fruits, whole grains, and beans covering two thirds (or more) of the plate, with animal-source foods covering one third (or less) (American Institute for Cancer Research, 2000).

The National Cancer Institute recommends that adult diets contain 20 to 30 g of **fiber** daily (not to exceed 35 g because of possible adverse effects). Typical diets in the United States contain approximately 11 g of fiber. The recommended fiber intake is proportionally lower for children. The recommended fiber intake for children older than 2 years can be determined by using the handy formula: age plus 5 (add 5 g of fiber per day to the child's age in years) (Williams, 1995; Williams, Bollella, & Wynder, 1995). Therefore the dietary fiber recommendation for an 8-year-old child is 13 g of fiber per day (8 + 5 = 13). If the child needs more fiber because of obesity or hypercholesterolemia, then the recommendation may be calculated by adding as much as 10 g to the child's age (age plus 10), which is 18 grams of fiber for an 8-year-old child. By the time a child reaches the age of 18, the fiber recommendation becomes 23 g per day, which is within the range of intake recommended by the National Cancer Institute. Foods that are high in fiber are usually low in fat; the only source of fiber-containing foods is the plant kingdom.

Limit Intake of High-Fat Foods, Particularly From Animal Sources. Choose foods low in fat and limit consumption of meats, especially high-fat meats. High-fat diets have been associated with an increased risk of cancers of the colon and rectum, prostate, and endometrium. The association between high-fat diets and the risk of breast cancer is weaker. Two studies funded by NIH are ongoing to identify the causal relationship of low-fat diets and eventual breast cancer. One study, the Women's Health Initiative, focused on primary prevention of breast cancer through low-fat diet in women who currently have no disease. The second, Women's Intervention Nutrition Study, will look at secondary prevention of breast cancer through low-fat diet in women who currently have breast cancer, with the goal being prevention of recurrence of disease. Whether these associations are caused by the total amount of fat, the particular type of fat (saturated, monounsaturated, or polyunsaturated), the calories contributed by fat, or by some other factor in food fats has not been determined. Consumption of meat, particularly red meat, has been associated with an increased risk of cancer at several sites, most notably the colon and prostate.

Be Physically Active: Achieve and Maintain a Healthy Weight. Physical activity can help protect against some cancers, either by balancing caloric intake with energy expenditure or by other mechanisms. An imbalance of caloric intake and energy output can lead to being overweight or obese and an increased risk for cancers at several sites, such as the colon and rectum, prostate, endometrium, breast (among postmenopausal women), and kidney. Both physical activity and controlled caloric intake are necessary to achieve or maintain a healthy body weight.

Limit Consumption of Alcoholic Beverages. Alcoholic beverages, along with cigarette smoking and the use of snuff and chewing tobacco, cause cancers of the oral cavity, esophagus, and larynx. The combined use of tobacco and alcohol leads to a greatly increased risk of oral and esophageal cancers; the effect of tobacco and alcohol combined is greater than the sum of their individual effects. Studies also have shown an association between alcohol consumption and an increased risk of breast cancer. The mechanism of this effect is not known, but the association may be related to carcinogenic actions of alcohol or its metabolites, to alcohol-induced changes in levels of hormones such as estrogens, or to some other process. Regardless of the mechanism, studies show that the risk of breast cancer increases with an intake beginning at only a few drinks per week. Reducing alcohol consumption is a good way for women who drink regularly to reduce their risk of breast cancer (ACS, 2005a).

Osteoporosis
Epidemiology

In the United States in 2001, 10 million individuals had decreased bone mass, known as osteoporosis, and 34 million more people had low bone mineral density (BMD), placing them at increased risk for osteoporosis. Of the people with hip fractures, 20% die within a year, and one half of the survivors never walk again. Direct financial expenditures for management of osteoporotic fracture alone are estimated at $15 billion to $17 billion annually. These figures underestimate significantly the true costs of osteoporosis, because they fail to include the costs of treatment for individuals without a history of fractures or the indirect costs of lost wages or productivity of either the individual or the caregiver.

The prevalence of osteoporosis and the incidence of fracture vary by gender and race-ethnicity. The probability that a 50-year-old individual will have a hip fracture during a lifetime is 16% to 18% for a white woman and 5% to 6% for a white man. The risk for blacks is much lower, at 6% and 3% for a 50-year-old woman and man, respectively.

- White postmenopausal women have a one in seven chance of having a hip fracture during their lifetimes.
- Black women have higher BMD than white women throughout life, and they experience lower hip fracture rates.
- Some Japanese women have lower peak BMD than white women, but they have a lower hip fracture rate, the reasons for which are not fully understood.
- Hispanic American women have bone densities between those of white women and those of black women.
- Limited information on Native American women suggests they have lower BMD than white women.

Pathophysiology

Osteoporosis is a slowly developing condition that causes loss of bone mass and fractures, especially in the wrist, hip, and spinal areas. **Osteoporosis** is defined as a skeletal disorder characterized by compromised bone strength predisposing to an increased risk of fracture. Bone strength reflects the integration of two main features: (1) bone density and (2) bone quality. Bone density is expressed as grams of mineral per area or volume and, in any given individual, is determined by peak bone mass and amount of bone loss. Bone quality refers to architecture, turnover, damage accumulation (microfractures), and mineralization. Osteoporotic bone fractures more easily than normal bone; therefore, osteoporosis is a significant risk factor for fracture.

Factors Involved in Building and Maintaining Skeletal Health Throughout Life. Growth in bone size and strength occurs during childhood, but bone accumulation is not completed until the third decade of life, after the cessation of linear growth. The bone mass attained early in life is perhaps the most important determinant of lifelong skeletal health. Individuals with the highest peak bone mass after adolescence have the greatest protective advantage when the inevitable declines in bone density associated with increasing age, illness, and diminished sex-steroid production take their toll.

Genetic factors exert a strong and perhaps predominant influence on peak bone mass, but physiological, environmental, and modifiable lifestyle factors can also play a significant role. Among these factors are adequate nutrition and body weight, exposure to sex hormones at puberty, and physical activity. Therefore maximizing BMD early in life presents a critical opportunity to reduce the effect of bone loss related to aging. Childhood is a critical time for development of lifestyle habits conducive to maintaining good bone health throughout life. Additionally, cigarette smoking, which usually starts in adolescence, may have a deleterious effect on bone mass.

Prevention

Once thought to be a natural part of aging among women, osteoporosis is no longer considered age dependent or gender dependent and is largely preventable, thanks to the recent progress in the understanding of its causes, diagnosis, and treatment. Optimization of bone health is a process that must occur throughout the life span in both men and women. Factors that enhance bone health at all ages are essential to prevent osteoporosis and its devastating consequences. Calcium is the nutrient most important for attaining peak bone mass and for preventing and treating osteoporosis.

Good nutrition is essential for normal growth. A balanced diet, adequate calories, and appropriate nutrients are the foundation for developing all tissues, including bone. Adequate and appropriate nutrition is important for all individuals, but not everyone follows a diet that is optimal for bone health.

Dietary calcium intake recommendations for various stages of life include:

- Young children, 3 to 8 years: 800 mg per day
- Children and adolescents, 9 to 17 years: 1300 mg per day (Only 25% of boys and 10% of girls meet these recommendations. Supplementation of calcium and vitamin D may be necessary. Excessive pursuit of thinness, in particular, may affect adequate nutrition and bone health.)
- Adults: 1000 to 1500 mg per day (Only 50% to 60% meet this recommendation.)

Factors contributing to low calcium intake are restriction of dairy products, a generally low level of fruit and vegetable consumption, and a high intake of low-calcium beverages such as soft drinks. Lactose and vitamin D enhance calcium absorption and exercise enhances calcium balance. Calcium is absorbed best from dairy foods. It is the only source of the disaccharide lactose.

Vitamin D is synthesized in the body when the skin is exposed to the ultraviolet rays of the sun. Commonly added to milk, other food sources of vitamin D include fatty fish (salmon and mackerel), margarine, eggs, and some fortified, ready-to-eat cereals. Most infants and young children in the United States have adequate vitamin D intake from the supplementation and fortification of milk. During adolescence, when consumption of dairy products decreases, vitamin D intake is likely to be inadequate, which may affect calcium absorption adversely. Other nutrients have been evaluated relative to bone health. High dietary protein, caffeine, phosphorus, and sodium can adversely affect calcium balance; however, their effects appear to be unimportant in individuals with adequate calcium intakes.

Food should be selected to provide adequate calcium, paying special attention to that eaten by adolescents, who normally have high mineral requirements, and by women who are susceptible to inadequate dietary calcium because of low caloric intake. Women of all ages should be concerned about adequate calcium intake. A means for increasing individual consumption of calcium includes educating consumers to eat more calcium-rich foods, including calcium-fortified foods such as orange juice, and recommending dietary supplements. Individuals who wish to increase their calcium intake can consume more low-fat or nonfat dairy products or fortified food products. Supplementation with calcium tablets may be appropriate for people at high risk of health problems from inadequate calcium intake.

Although maintaining a proper daily calcium intake through food is preferable, calcium supplements are available for people who do not get enough of the mineral through their regular diets. Calcium carbonate (40% elemental calcium), calcium citrate (24%), calcium lactate (14%), and calcium gluconate (9%) are preferred. (Dolomite and bone meal are not recommended, because they may be contaminated with lead.) Calcium supplement absorption is most efficient for individuals with adequate gastric acid production at individual doses no greater than 500 mg when taken between meals.

The mandate is clear for nursing professionals interested in preventive health: encourage increased consumption of calcium-rich foods. Milk and dairy products deliver the most calcium of any food group, but they are also among the richest sources of fat in the American diet. Low-fat and fat-free milk, yogurt, and low-fat cheeses are the dairy products of choice. Other good sources of calcium include sardines, canned salmon (if the bones are eaten), and some dark green leafy vegetables, especially collard greens. Orange juice and milk fortified with calcium are also good sources. The calcium content of some common foods is summarized in Table 11-6.

Table **11-6** Calcium Content of Foods

Calcium Sources	Calcium (mg)
1 cup plain, low-fat yogurt	400
3 oz sardines, with bones	370
1 cup low-fat fruit yogurt	345
¼ of 14-inch cheese pizza	330
1 cup fluid milk (whole, fat-free skim milk, 1% [low-fat], 2% [reduced fat], buttermilk)	330
1 cup calcium-fortified soy milk	300
1 cup calcium-fortified orange juice	300
1 oz Swiss cheese	270
1 oz cheddar cheese	200
½ cup cooked collard greens	180
1 oz American cheese	170
4 oz tofu (soybean curd)	145
1 tbsp blackstrap molasses	140
1 5-inch stalk broccoli	100
½ cup kale, cooked	100
2 oz cornbread, enriched	95

From Pennington, J. A. T. (1997). *Bowes and Church's food values of portions commonly used* (17th ed.). Philadelphia: Lippincott.

Anyone under 25 years of age who ingests less than the recommended intake of calcium should be urged to develop strategies for increasing it. Children, particularly preadolescent girls, should take care to receive the proper amount. By modeling appropriate behaviors, health care professionals can help prevent or delay the onset of osteoporosis in themselves, their families, and the people who are in their care.

Obesity

As almost everyone in health care in the United States knows, a paradox exists in modern America. On the one hand, many people who do not need to lose weight are trying to do so, and on the other hand, many who actually need to lose weight are not trying; those who are trying are unsuccessful in losing the weight and maintaining their weight loss.

Overweight, defined as about 10% to 20% over healthy weight, can seriously affect health and longevity and is associated with the leading nutrition-related causes of death in the United States: type 2 diabetes, CVD, and some cancers. **Obesity,** about 20% or more overweight, is also associated with gout and gallbladder disease and may contribute to the development of osteoarthritis in the weight-bearing joints.

Epidemiology

Overweight and obesity are found worldwide and the prevalence of these conditions in the United States ranks high with that of other developed nations. Approximately 30,000 adult deaths in the United States each year are attributable to obesity. Two thirds of the nation's adults are overweight (including people who are obese) (USDHHS,

CASE STUDY

Janie

Janie is a 25-year-old black woman who works 5 days a week as a kindergarten teacher. She weighs 175 pounds and is 5 feet, 4 inches tall. Her father died of a heart attack at 50 years of age. Janie lives with her 55-year-old mother, who is confined to a wheelchair as a result of a massive stroke she suffered 6 months ago. Born and raised in Atlanta, Janie's mother prides herself as an excellent "soul food" cook. In fact, she is still able to prepare most of the family's meals.

Janie recently joined the health maintenance organization, which covers one complete physical per year. She was referred to a dietician because she is engaged to be married and wants to lose 16 pounds by her wedding day, which is 2 months from now.

NIH, National Institute of Diabetes & Digestive & Kidney Diseases, [NIDDK], 2004). **Web Site Resource 11A** presents a table of healthy weight, overweight, and obesity among people 20 years of age and over.

The prevalence of being overweight has increased steadily over the years among nearly all racial and ethnic groups. From 1960 to 2000 the prevalence of overweight increased from 31.5% to 33.6% in adults in the United States. The prevalence of obesity during this same period increased from 13.3% to 30.9%—a relative increase of more than 50%, with most of this increase occurring during the 1990s. The prevalence of overweight and obesity increases with advancing age until people reach their 60s, when it starts to decline. From 1991 to 1998, obesity increased in every state of the United States, in both genders and across all races and ethnicities, age groups, educational levels, and smoking statuses, with the exception of white non-Hispanic men in their 20s to 40s, in whom the prevalence of obesity decreased from the early 1970s to late 1970s (USDHHS, NIH, NIDDK, 2004).

Obesity is more common in women than in men. Among men there is a modest ethnic variation in the prevalence of being overweight, the greatest difference occurring between white men and Hispanic American men. Among women, the ethnic variation is substantial. Almost 25% of white women are overweight; Hispanic American and Puerto Rican women have a greater prevalence of being overweight than their white counterparts; and more than 45% of black women are overweight. Potential contributing factors to the greater propensity for adult black women to become obese include a more sedentary lifestyle, higher energy intake, earlier menarche, earlier age of first childbirth, and less loss of weight gained during gestation (Burke et al., 1992) (Case Study and Care Plan).

Excess body weight is 7 to 12 times more frequent in women from lower social classes than in women from upper social classes. In men, social class has a significantly less pronounced relationship (Bray, 1996).

CARE PLAN

Obesity/Overweight

(Related to Janie Case Study)

Nursing Diagnosis Alteration in current weight related to diet modification and weekly monitoring.

DEFINING CHARACTERISTICS

- Increase in blood pressure: 25-year-old black woman with a blood pressure reading of 139/80
- Works 5 days a week as a kindergarten teacher
- Weighs 175 pounds and is 5 feet, 4 inches tall
- Father died of a heart attack at 50 years of age
- Lives with 55-year-old mother, who is confined to a wheelchair due to massive stroke 6 months ago
- Most of the family's meals prepared by Janie's mother, an excellent soul food cook
- Recently joined the health maintenance organization, which covers one complete physical per year
- Engaged to be married and wants to lose 16 pounds by her wedding day 2 months hence

EXPECTED OUTCOMES

- Janie will decrease her weight and blood pressure in the next 2 months.
- Weight loss will progress at 2 pounds per week.

INTERVENTIONS

- Over a 2-month period document weight and blood pressure.
- Work with Janie's mother to modify her style of food preparation.
- Use reduced-fat and lower carbohydrate foods; increase water consumption.

Body Mass Index for Adults

Based on an adult's height and weight, body mass index (BMI) (wt/ht^2) is a helpful indicator of obesity and being **underweight** (Garrow & Webster, 1958). A person's BMI can be determined by referring to the table in **Web Site Resource 11B,** by using a calculator on the Internet (the CDC's online BMI calculator) *(http://www.cdc.gov/nccdphp/dnpa/bmi/calc-bmi.htm),* or by using a hand-held calculator and the following formulas:

Body Mass Index Formulas.
English Formula

$$BMI = \text{weight in pounds} \div \text{height in inches}$$
$$\div \text{height in inches} \times 703$$

Example: For a 6-foot-tall person weighing 210 pounds: BMI = 210 pounds divided by 72 inches divided by 72 inches multiplied by 703 = 28.5.
Metric Formulas

$$BMI = \text{weight in kilograms} \div (\text{height in meters})^2$$

and

$$BMI = (\text{weight in kilograms} \div \text{height in cm} \div \text{height in cm})$$
$$\times 10,000.$$

Example: For a person who is 182.9 centimeters tall and weighs 95.3 kilograms: BMI = 95.3 kg divided by 182.9 cm multiplied by 10,000 = 28.5.

BMI is a good indicator of body fat, but it cannot be interpreted as a specific percentage of body fat. Age and gender influence the relationship between fat and BMI. For example, women are more likely to have a higher percentage of body fat than men have for the same BMI. At the same BMI, older people have more body fat than do younger adults (Gallagher et al., 1996). BMI is used to screen and monitor a population to detect the risk of health or nutritional disorders. In an individual, other data must be used to determine whether a high BMI is associated with increased risk of disease and death for that person; BMI alone is not diagnostic (Willett, Dietz, & Colditz, 1999).

BMI ranges are based on the effect body weight has on disease and death. A BMI value from 19 to 25 is a healthy target range for adults. BMI values greater than 25 are associated with increasing risks for developing CVD, gallbladder disease, high blood pressure, and non–insulin-dependent diabetes mellitus. A high BMI value is predictive of death from CVD (Calle, Thun, Petrelli, Rodriguez, & Heath, 1999).

BMI values for adults are expressed with one number, regardless of age or sex, using the following guidelines:
- Underweight: BMI less than 18.5
- Healthy weight: BMI of 18.5 to 24.9
- Overweight: BMI of 25 to 29.9
- Obese: BMI of 30 or more

Body Mass Index Growth Charts for Children

Many parents are familiar with the original growth charts used by pediatric health care providers since 1977. Those charts were used widely by pediatricians, nurses, and nutritionists to track growth and development in children and assist in signaling potential developmental problems. The charts consist of a series of percentile curves that illustrate the distribution in growth of children across the United States.

In 2000 the Centers for Disease Control and Prevention (CDC) released new pediatric growth charts that more accurately reflect the nation's cultural and racial diversity and track children and young people through age 20. The new charts will be used to monitor children's growth and help identify weight problems early in childhood. The charts include an assessment of BMI. The BMI is an early warning signal that is helpful as early as age 2 to help identify children who have the potential to become overweight. Early identification of obesity risk gives parents the opportunity to modify their children's eating habits before a weight problem develops.

The CDC's new charts are based on data gathered through the National Health and Nutrition Examination Survey, the only survey that collects data from actual physical examinations on a cross-section of Americans from all over the country. This survey shows that since the 1980s the number of overweight children and adolescents has doubled. Additionally, it shows that over one half of all American adults are overweight and that the number of obese adults has doubled. It is expected that the new BMI charts will help address this nationwide problem. The growth charts indicate that, in general, children are heavier today than in 1977, but height has remained virtually unchanged. The new charts are available on the CDC Web site at *http://www.cdc.gov/growthcharts*.

Diet Intervention

"Please help me lose weight" is one of the most common requests heard in the health field. As discussed, a balanced diet is important and must include the appropriate serving sizes for the recommended daily intake of each food group. Additionally, exercise is particularly necessary from the outset, because with exercise there is less need to restrict food. Exercise also favors long-term maintenance of body weight (as described in Chapter 12).

Nurses should make referrals to supervised or unsupervised programs as appropriate. People expect this type of advice on maintaining their health. Therefore nurses can play an important role, although not supervising individuals' weight loss efforts directly. (For more information on obesity among adults, see USDHHS, National Heart, Lung, and Blood Institute, 1998).

There are many positive effects of only relatively small amounts of weight loss (5% to 10% of body weight) for people who are obese:
- Decreased blood pressure (decreased risk of a heart attack and stroke)
- Reduced abnormally high levels of blood glucose associated with diabetes
- Reduced elevated levels of cholesterol and triglycerides associated with CVD
- Reduced sleep apnea (irregular breathing during sleep)
- Decreased risk of osteoarthritis in the weight-bearing joints
- Decreased depression
- Increased self-esteem

The acronym LEARN has been suggested as a mnemonic device for health professionals. LEARN refers to the steps nurses can take to help the person who needs to improve health-related behavior (Brownell, 2000). LEARN is particularly useful as a guideline for communicating with the clinically obese client who has indicated dissatisfaction with current weight:

L: Listen with sympathy and understanding to the client's perception of the problem.

E: Explain personal perceptions of the problem.

A: Acknowledge and discuss differences and similarities.

R: Recommend treatment.

N: Negotiate an agreement.

In 1992 an NIH-sponsored technical support conference identified the following characteristics of voluntary weight loss and weight control in the United States (USDHHS, 1992):
1. Obesity is a chronic disease.
2. Obesity has many causes.
3. Cure is rare; palliation is realistic.
4. Weight loss is slow.
5. Recidivism is common.
6. Weight regain may be slow, but it is often rapid.
7. Management is often more frustrating than the underlying disease.

The conference noted significant adverse effects for obese dieters who regain lost weight:
- Repeated weight gain and loss may have adverse psychological and physical effects; for example, evidence suggests that mildly to moderately overweight women who are dieting may be at risk for binge eating without vomiting and purging.
- Although data on the health effects of repeated weight gain and loss (weight cycling) are also inconclusive, weight cycling appears to affect energy metabolism and may cause faster regaining of weight.
- Depression and decreased self-esteem occur.

According to some radical nurses, nutritionists, social workers, physicians, and lay advocates, a new model for health care is needed for people who cannot maintain a BMI under 30. The new paradigm, health at any size, is described in the Hot Topics box. Fad diets do not provide the best way to lose weight and should be avoided (see Health Teaching box).

Diabetes
Prevalence and Incidence

Diabetes is becoming more prevalent. The numbers of existing cases (prevalence) and new cases (incidence) are increasing, and most of this increase is not a result of aging of the U.S. population. Trends show that minority and elderly populations are disproportionately affected by diabetes. An estimated 13.8 million Americans had the disease in 2003 (CDC, 2005).

Previously called non–insulin-dependent diabetes mellitus or adult-onset diabetes, **type 2 diabetes** accounts for 90% to 95% of all diagnosed cases of diabetes. Risk factors include older age, obesity, family history of diabetes, history of gestational diabetes, impaired glucose tolerance, physical inactivity, and race and ethnicity. Blacks, Hispanic Americans, Native Americans, and some Asian Americans are at particularly high risk.

Type 2 diabetes is one of the leading causes of death among Americans and the leading cause of new cases of blindness, kidney failure, and lower extremity amputations, plus it greatly increases a person's risk for a heart attack or stroke. In 2002 diabetes accounted for more than $132 billion in direct and indirect medical costs and lost pro-

HEALTH AT ANY SIZE: THE SIZE ACCEPTANCE NONDIET MOVEMENT

HOTtopics

The new paradigm has replaced the question, "How can fat people lose weight?" with the question, "How can fat people be healthy?" (Spark, 2001). The following tenets are the foundation of the movement:

- Good health is a state of physical, mental, and social well-being. People of all sizes and shapes can reduce their risk of poor health by adopting a healthy lifestyle, which includes (1) eating a variety of healthy foods, (2) being physically active because it is fun and feels good, and (3) appreciating the body as it is.
- Human beings come in a variety of sizes and shapes; size diversity is a positive characteristic of the human race. Respect the bodies of others, although they might be quite different.
- There is no ideal body size, shape, BMI, or body composition that every individual should strive to achieve.
- Self-esteem and body image are strongly linked. Helping people feel good about their bodies and about who they are can help motivate and maintain healthy behaviors.
- People are responsible for care of their own bodies.
- Appearance stereotyping is wrong. Their weight notwithstanding, all people deserve to be treated equally in the job market and on the job, to be treated equally in the media, and to receive competent and respectful treatment by health care professionals.

How to Become a Size-Sensitive Health Professional

- On the intake form, include a question asking whether the person is satisfied with the body size. If the answer is "yes," then try to avoid the issue in the future.

- When the person asks not to be weighed, the request is acknowledged without complaint and automatically taken into account on follow-up office visits. (There are a few cases in which weighing is necessary, such as when administering certain medications, chemotherapy, or anesthesia.)
- A size-sensitive health care professional does not necessarily avoid mentioning weight but should avoid making an issue of weight, avoid lectures and humiliation, and respect the individual's wishes with regard to weight discussions.
- When weight contributes to a problem, the professional mentions this situation but also considers other diagnoses and recommends tests to determine the actual diagnosis when appropriate. If weight loss is a recommended treatment for a problem, then the compassionate professional may mention this, but at minimum, and recommend and prescribe other treatments. Accept the individual's wish not to use weight loss as a treatment.
- Some health care professionals believe that overweight and obesity are not necessarily unhealthy. However, other professionals who believe that fat is unhealthy may acknowledge that weight loss is usually ineffective or that the clients have the right to direct their own treatment.
- Ideally the waiting area, examining suite, and consultation room are equipped with armless chairs, large blood pressure cuffs, large examination gowns, and other equipment suitable for large people. If this is not the case, then the office staff acknowledges the importance of these items when told.

BMI, body mass index.

---

ductivity (CDC, 2004). Much of the burden of diabetes can be prevented with early detection, improved delivery of care, and better education on disease self-management.

Type 2 Diabetes in Children

Although diabetes mellitus in children and adolescents was believed to be exclusively type 1, type 2 diabetes in children and adolescents is now considered a sizeable and growing problem among Native Americans and an emerging public health problem among other North American ethnic groups. The epidemic of obesity among children and adolescents, the decreasing level of physical activity during adolescence, and the increased exposure to diabetes in utero are likely contributors to the increase in type 2 diabetes during childhood and adolescence.

Although some children and adolescents are symptomatic, others do not enter the clinical arena until they are in severe ketoacidosis and may have a transient insulin requirement. Diabetic complications (dyslipidemia and hypertension) have been observed among Pima Indians as early as the teenage years. No evidence-based guidelines for treatment of type 2 diabetes in children and adolescents are available, and oral agents have not been tested or approved for this age group. Generally, children and adolescents with type 2 diabetes have poor glycemic control. Population mobility, lack of symptoms, denial, absence of family support, and inadequate health care insurance coverage have all been identified as major barriers to adherence to treatment and follow-up and to successful clinical management. Because of a longer duration of disease (from earlier onset) and because glucose control and compliance are challenging during the teenage years, the lifetime complications (microvascular and macrovascular diseases and decreased quality of life) in this population will probably be considerable (Fagot-Champagna et al., 2000).

Diet Intervention

Medical nutrition therapy (MNT) is the most critical and pivotal component of diabetes care. At the minimum, MNT involves the team efforts of a physician, a registered nurse or registered dietitian, and in some practice settings a mental health professional. The purpose of MNT for people with type 2 diabetes is to delay or prevent the development of diabetic complications (blindness, CHD, nephropathy, and neuropathy). No single diabetic diet or American Dia-

HEALTH TEACHING   Types of Fad Diets

Food-Specific Diets

Certain diets focus on one food (such as grapefruit), class of foods (such as fresh fruit), or combination (such as kelp and vinegar) that has purported special properties that facilitate weight loss. Following a plan by which only one type of food is eaten while others are excluded results in weight loss, the reason being that eating the same food becomes monotonous and results in reduced eating, causing a loss of weight. These food-specific diets fail to teach healthy eating habits and are usually nutritionally unbalanced.

Liquid Diets

Liquid diets include over-the-counter liquid meal replacements. Each 8-ounce single serving provides approximately 300 calories and approximately one quarter of the recommended intake for most nutrients. When limited to 4 cans per day, a liquid diet will provide 1200 calories and will therefore result in weight loss. Many people have reported that removing the temptations of usual food and beverages and the social trappings of traditional mealtime makes adhering to a reduced-calorie regimen easier. Liquid diets fail to teach portion control and provide no guidance for healthful eating after the desired amount of weight is lost. Although liquid diets have been used for large weight losses (more than 100 pounds) in clinical settings with medical supervision and psychological support, regaining the lost weight is common.

High-Fiber Diets

Fiber-rich foods are an essential part of a healthy diet and can be especially beneficial to people trying to lose weight. Fiber-rich foods are filling and because fiber cannot be digested, it contains no calories. Conversely, eating too much fiber is not necessarily better. Consuming more than 50 or 60 grams of high-fiber foods every day can lead to bloating, cramping, diarrhea, and loss of minerals from the body. However, enjoy-ing 30 to 35 grams per day of fiber-rich foods is likely to result in weight loss, because the fiber-containing choices displace other high-calorie foods from the diet.

High-Protein Diets

High-protein, low-carbohydrate diets lead to weight loss, although the weight loss may be temporary. If an individual needs to lose weight quickly and decides to accomplish this task with a high-protein, low-carbohydrate diet, this is how it will work.

- A portion of potential calories from the protein-rich food is absorbed by the process of metabolizing the large amount of nitrogen in the protein; therefore, the energy is not available to the body for any other use.
- The diet can be monotonous from eating the same high-protein foods over and over again, ultimately leading to a decreased food intake.
- High-protein intake causes an increased water loss to carry the nitrogen from the body, therefore the dieter should drink enough water to compensate.

Fasting

Fasting has been recommended for decades to cleanse the body of impurities or to embark on a weight-loss plan. Most people who undergo fasts use their common sense: they drink liquids that can supply some energy and nutrients, set safe time limits as to how long they will abstain from solid foods, and educate themselves on the basics of safe fasting. However, fasting deprives the body of nutrients. A person undergoing an especially prolonged fast experiences not only weight loss, but also low energy, weakness, poor nutritional status, and lightheadedness. Additionally, when carbohydrates are not available for energy, ketones can accumulate (as the body's carbohydrate substitute), causing stress for the kidneys, which can be harmful to overall health.

Modified from Kirby, R. (1998). *Dieting for dummies.* New York: IDG Publishing.

---

betes Association diet exists. The recommended diet can be defined only as a nutrition prescription based on assessment and treatment goals and outcomes. Nutrition advice for people with type 2 diabetes is essentially the same as for the general population; they should be following the Dietary Guidelines for Americans. MNT for people with diabetes should be individualized, with consideration given to usual eating habits and other lifestyle factors. Nutrition recommendations are then developed and implemented to meet treatment goals and desired outcomes. Monitoring metabolic parameters, including blood glucose levels, glycosylated hemoglobin levels, lipid values, blood pressure, body weight, renal function (when appropriate), and quality of life is crucial to ensure successful outcomes. The American Diabetes Association further recommends ongoing nutrition self-management education for these individuals.

For people with hyperglycemia, hyperlipidemia, obesity, or suboptimal nutrition, start with this nonpharmacological management:

1. Recommend an appropriate tailored meal plan. Determine daily energy needs based on healthy body weight and then use the client's daily energy needs to determine the appropriate number of choices from the food groups in MyPyramid, the new food guidance system.
2. Encourage regular aerobic exercise.
3. Evaluate the individual using outcome measures in Table 11-7. People who have been counseled regarding diet and exercise but who have not responded satisfactorily after 4 to 6 weeks should be referred to a registered dietitian or nurse who is a registered diabetes educator. Refer to a physician a client with acute complications of diabetes, such as hypoglycemia, exercise-related problems, renal disease, autonomic neuropathy, hypertension, or CVD.

A nurse should know as much as possible about the individual and the condition of the individual before writing a nutrition prescription. (This requirement is comparable to the physician's need to complete a physical and medical assessment before writing a medication prescription.) The nutrition prescription may be general, but it should reflect the person's therapy goals. The following are some sample orders the nurse might write for the dietitian:

- Diabetic meal plan to achieve clinical goals of diabetes MNT

Table **11-7** Desired Outcomes After 4 to 6 Weeks of MNT for Individuals With Type 2 Diabetes

Index	Goal	Desired Outcome After 4 to 6 Weeks of Initial MNT
FBS	80-120 mg/dl	Downward trend (down 10%) or at target goal
HbA$_{1c}$	60-75%	Downward trend (down 10%) or at target goal
Weight change	Maintain reasonable weight	Loss of 1.5-3 kg (3-6 lb)
Food and meal planning	Meals and snacks eaten on a regular basis; appropriate food choices and amounts	Positive changes in food selection and amount, frequency, and timing of meals
Exercise	If no medication limitations, physical activity for at least 10 minutes, 3 times a week	Physical activity level gradually increased or continued at target goal

FBS, fasting blood sugar; *HbA$_{1c}$*, glycosylated hemoglobin; *MNT*, medical nutrition therapy.

- MNT to achieve as near-normal blood glucose as possible
- Meal plan to improve diabetes control and blood lipid levels
- Diet for improved glycemia
- Diet for diabetes and hypertension

The prescription may be defined further by the registered dietitian with a summary of the planned nutrition intervention. For example, the dietitian might write:

- Weight-reduction meal plan based on general eating guidelines, 1200 to 1500 calories, 3 meals, and 1 snack
- 2400 mg sodium meal plan with weight maintenance
- Cholesterol-counting meal plan, adjusting cholesterol and meal timing to achieve target glucose goals

Human Immunodeficiency Virus and Acquired Immunodeficiency Syndrome
Epidemiology

In 2003 the estimated number of persons diagnosed with acquired immunodeficiency syndrome (AIDS) was 43,171. The cumulative estimated number of persons in the United States diagnosed through 2003 with AIDS was 929,985 (CDC, 2003)

Diet Intervention

Attention to nutrition in early HIV intervention is essential for several reasons. AIDS produces nutritional consequences; therefore, good dietary habits early in the disease may have benefits for end-stage developments such as severe weight loss. The person diagnosed as HIV positive usually becomes depressed. Depression leads to loss of appetite; therefore, attention to nutrition is critical as soon as a diagnosis is made.

An initial nutritional assessment is necessary, suggesting the extent to which nutrition education is needed and providing valuable baseline information for evaluating the disease's progression. Nurses should involve the person's significant others in early discussions of optimal nutrition. A nutrient-dense, protein-rich, well-balanced diet that includes a vitamin and mineral supplement should be stressed. Information on food sanitation should also be provided because people with HIV have altered immune function and will get sicker with food-borne organisms. The

aims of nutrition therapy and counseling specifically for HIV and AIDS follow:

- Determine how the person appeared physically before becoming HIV positive. Was the client obese or heavily muscled? A couch potato or an athlete? Eating a good diet?
- Help meet or exceed the amount of muscle the person had before becoming HIV positive. Introduce the person to proper eating and exercise.
- Help get the person back to the original weight or maintain the current weight.
- Teach about food and water safety.
- Advise on the ability of food to ease some of the gastrointestinal side effects of medications.
- Teach the importance of maintaining eating and medication schedules to ensure maximal absorption of medications.
- When the individual is diabetic or hyperlipidemic, teach about the dietary management of these conditions. Viewing HIV as a terminal illness is no longer appropriate. HIV is now considered a chronic disease, because infected people are living many years (Krales, 2000).

Breastfeeding should be avoided to prevent vertical transmission of HIV from mother to child. This objective is fairly easy to implement in the United States, which has had a long history of safe breast milk substitutes in the form of milk-based and soy-based infant formulas. In many developing countries, however, the risks attached to feeding an infant with something other than breast milk are greater than the 20% risk of vertical transmission of the virus that causes AIDS.

SUMMARY

This chapter introduces a wide range of subjects, including the Healthy People 2010 nutrition objectives, the most current diet recommendations to reduce the risks of developing nutrition-related diseases, FDA regulations for food labeling, government food aid programs for the poor and elderly Americans, and primary and secondary prevention strategies related to the most common nutrition-related chronic diseases. Together these topics form the basis of what is known as preventive nutrition, a requisite for the promotion of the nation's public health. All of the topics examined in this chapter can be studied further using the Internet. High quality, up-to-date materials and continuing nutrition education literature for professionals are free and on-line. **Web Site Resource 11C** discusses the varied sources of nutrition information. See the Web links on the book's Web site to access live links to numerous Internet resources.

ADDITIONAL STUDY MATERIAL

Study Questions in the back of the book, see page 663.

evolve **WEB SITE MATERIALS**

These materials are located on the book's Web site at http://evolve.elsevier.com/Edelman/.

- WebLinks
- Content Updates
- Web Site Resources

11A   Healthy Weight, Overweight, and Obesity Among People 20 Years of Age and Over

11B   Body Weight in Pounds According to Height and Body Mass Index

11C   Sources of Nutrition Information

REFERENCES

American Cancer Society. (2005a). *Facts sheet: Nutrition and cancer.* Retrieved March 29, 2005, from: *http://www.cancer. org/docroot/PRO/content/PRO_1_1_220_Fa ct_Sheets.asp?*

American Cancer Society. (2005b). *Cancer Statistics Presentation 2004: Cancer death rates by race and ethinicity.* Retrieved March 29, 2005, from: *http://www.cancer. org/docroot/PRO/content/PRO_1_1_Cancer _Statistics_2004_presentation.asp?*

American Dietetic Association (2001). Position of the American Dietetic Association: Food fortification and dietary supplements. *Journal of the American Dietetic Association, 101,* 115-125.

American Institute for Cancer Research. (2000). The new American plate, 2000 (On-line). Retrieved February 26, 2005, from: *http://www.aicr.org/nap2.htm.*

Barer-Stein, T. (1979). Multiculturalism and nutrition counseling. *Journal of the Canadian Dietetic Association, 40,* 112-116.

Bray, G. A. (1996). Obesity. In E. E. Zeigler & L. J. Filer, Jr. (Eds.), *Present knowledge in nutrition* (7th ed.). Washington, DC: International Life Sciences Institute Press.

Brownell, K. (2000). *The LEARN program for weight management 2000.* Dallas: American Health Publishing.

Burke, G. L., Savage, P. J., Manolio, T. A., Sprafka, J. M., Wagenknecht, L. E., Sidney, S., et al. (1992). Correlates of obesity in young black and white women: The CARDIA study. *American Journal of Public Health, 82,* 1621-1625.

Calle, E. E., Thun, M. J., Petrelli, J. M., Rodriguez, C., & Heath, C. W., Jr. (1999). BMI and mortality in a prospective cohort of U.S. adults. *New England Journal of Medicine, 341,* 1097-1105.

Carpenter, K. J. (2000). *Beriberi, white rice, and vitamin B: A disease, a cause, and a cure.* Berkeley, CA: Berkeley University Press.

Centers for Disease Control and Prevention. (2003). *Divisions of HIV/AIDS Prevention.* Retrieved on March 29, 2005 from *http:// www.cdc.gov/hiv/stats/htm.*

Centers for Disease Control and Prevention. (2004, June). School Breakfast Program, Child Nutrition and WIC Reauthorization Act of 2004. Retrieved February 26, 2005, from: *http://www.frac.org/html/federal_food_ programs/programs/sbp.html.*

Centers for Disease Control and Prevention, National Center for Infectious Diseases (2001). Bovine spongiform encephalopathy and new variant Creutzfeldt-Jakob disease (On-line). Retrieved February 26, 2005, from: *http://www.cdc.gov/ncidod/ diseases/cjd/bse_cjd.htm.*

Centers for Disease Control and Prevention. (2005). *National Diabetes Surveillance System: Prevalence of diabetes.* Retrieved July 2, 2005, from *http:www.cdc.gov/ diabetes/statistics/prev/national/index.htm.*

Expert Panel on Detection, Evaluation, and Treatment of High Blood Cholesterol in Adults. (2001). Executive summary of the third report of the National Cholesterol Education Program (NCEP) expert panel on detection, evaluation, and treatment of high blood cholesterol in adults (adult treatment panel III). *Journal of the American Medical Association, 285,* 2486-2497.

Fagot-Champagna, A., Pettitt, D. J., Engelgau, M. M., Burrows, N. R., Geiss, L. S., Valdez, R., et al. (2000). Type 2 diabetes among North American children and adolescents: An epidemiologic review and a public health perspective. *Journal of Pediatrics, 136,* 664-672.

Gallagher, D., Visser, M., Sepulveda, D., Pierson, R. N., Harris, T., & Heymsfield, S. B. (1996). How useful is BMI for comparison of body fatness across age, sex and ethnic groups? *American Journal of Epidemiology, 143,* 228-239.

Garrow, J. S., & Webster, J. (1958). Quetelet's index (W/H²) as a measure of fatness. *International Journal of Obesity, 9,* 147-153.

Grieco, E. M., & Cassidy, R. C. (2001). *Census 2000 brief: Overview of race and Hispanic origin* (p. 11). Washington, DC: U.S. Department of Commerce, Economics and Statistics Administration, U.S. Census Bureau.

Hill, J. O., & Peters, J. C. (1998). Environmental contributions to the obesity epidemic. *Science 208,* 1371-1390.

Johnson, R. K., & Kennedy, E. (2000). The 2000 dietary guidelines for Americans: What are the changes and why were they made? *Journal of the American Dietetic Association, 100,* 769-774.

Kittler, P. G., & Sucher, K. P. (2000). *Cultural foods: Traditions and trends.* Belmont, CA: Wadsworth.

Krales, E. (2000, April 13). Setting standards: The expert panel for developing national HIV/AIDS nutrition guidelines. Body positive (13, On-line). Retrieved February 26, 2005, from: *http://www.thebody.com/bp/ apr00/standards.html.*

Krauss, R. K., Eckel, R. H., Howard, B., Appel, L. J., Daniels, S. R., Deckelbaum, R. J., et al. (2000). AHA dietary guidelines. Revision 2000: A statement for healthcare professionals from the Nutrition Committee of the American Heart Association. *Circulation, 102,* 2284-2299. Retrieved February 26, 2005, from: *http://circ.ahajournals.org/ cgi/content/full/4304635102.*

National Center for Health Statistics. *Prevalence of overweight among children and adolescents: United States, 1999-2001.* Retrieved August 25, 2005, from *http:// www.cdc.gov/products/pubs/pubd/hestats/over wght99.htm.*

National Institutes of Health. (2001). *NHLBI task force report on research in prevention of cardiovascular disease.* Washington, DC: U.S. Department of Health and Human Services. Retrieved August 25, 2005, from *http://www.nh/bi.nih.gov/resources/docs/cvdr pt.htm.*

National Research Council, Food and Nutrition Board. (1989). *Recommended dietary allowances* (10th ed.). Washington, DC: National Academy Press.

National Research Council, Institute of Medicine, Food and Nutrition Board. (2000a). *Dietary reference intakes for thiamin, riboflavin, niacin, vitamin B₆, vitamin B₁₂, pantothenic acid, biotin, and choline.* Washington, DC: National Academy Press.

National Research Council, Institute of Medicine, Food and Nutrition Board. (2000b).

Dietary reference intakes for vitamin C, vitamin E, selenium, and carotenoids. Washington, DC: National Academy Press.

National Research Council, Institute of Medicine, Food and Nutrition Board, Standing Committee on the Scientific Evaluation of Dietary Reference Intakes. (1997). *Dietary reference intakes for calcium, phosphorous, magnesium, vitamin D, and fluoride.* Report of the Subcommittee on Calcium and Related Nutrients. Washington, DC: National Academy Press.

Ogden, C. L., Flegal, K. M., Carroll, M. D., & Johnson, C. L. (2002). Prevelance and trends in overweight among US children and adolescents, 1999-2000. *JAMA 288* (14):1728-1732.

Rothman, K. J., Morre, L. L., Singer, M. R., Nguyen, U. D. T., Mannino, S., & Milunsky, A. (1995). Teratogenicity of high vitamin A intake. *New England Journal of Medicine, 333,* 1369-1373.

Snetselaar, L. (2004). Counseling for change. In L. K. Mahan & S. Escott-Stump (Eds.), *Krause's food, nutrition, and diet therapy* (11th ed., pp. 519-530). St. Louis: Elsevier.

Spark, A. (2001). Health at any size: The size acceptance nondiet movement. *Journal of the American Medical Women's Association, 56,* 69-71.

U.S. Census Bureau. (2004). *Income, poverty, and health insurance, coverage in the United States: 2003* (Current Population Rep., pp. 60-226). Washington, DC: U.S. Government Printing Office.

U.S. Department of Agriculture and U.S. Department of Health and Human Services. (2005). *Dietary guidelines for Americans* (6th ed.). Washington, DC: U.S. Government Printing Office. Retrieved May 31, 2005, from *http://www.health.gov/dietaryguidelines/dga2005/documents/.*

U.S. Department of Agriculture, Center for Nutrition Policy and Promotion. (2005). *MyPyramid.* Retrieved May 31, 2005, from *http://www.mypyramid.gov.*

U.S. Department of Health and Human Services. (1992). *10. Methods for voluntay weight loss and control.* Retrieved June 2, 2005, from *http://consensus.nih.gov/ta/010/010_statement.htm.*

U.S. Department of Health and Human Services, National Institutes of Health, National Heart, Lung, and Blood Institute. (1998). *Clinical guidelines on the identification, evaluation, and treatment of overweight and obesity in adults.* Bethesda, MD: U.S. Department of Health and Human Services. Retrieved August 25, 2005, from *http://www.nhlbi.nih.gov/guidelines/obesity/ob_home.htm.*

U.S. Department of Health and Human Services. (2001). *The Surgeon General's call to action to prevent and decrease overweight and obesity, 2001.* Rockville, MD: U.S. Department of Health and Human Services, Public Health Service, Office of the Surgeon General.

U.S. Department of Health and Human Services, National Institutes of Health, National Institute of Diabetes & Digestive & Kidney Diseases. (2004). *NIDDK: Recent advances and emerging opportunities.* Retrieved on April 14, 2005 from *http://www.niddk.nih.gov/federal/advances/2004/entire_book.pdf.*

U.S. Food and Drug Administration, Center for Food Safety and Applied Nutrition. (2004). *Dietary Supplement Health and Education Act of 1994.* Washington, DC: U.S. Food and Drug Administration. Retrieved September 26, 2004, from: *http://www.fda.gov/opacom/laws/dshea.html.*

Willett, W. C., Dietz, W. H., & Colditz, G. A. (1999). Primary care: Guidelines for healthy weight. *New England Journal of Medicine, 341,* 427-434.

Williams, C. L. (1995). Importance of dietary fiber in childhood. *Journal of the American Dietetic Association, 95,* 1140.

Williams, C. L., Bollella, M., & Wynder, E. L. (1995). A new recommendation for dietary fiber in childhood. *Pediatrics, 96,* 985-988.

Exercise

objectives

After completing this chapter, the reader will be able to:

- Explain the physical activity and fitness goals of *Healthy People 2010* and the progress made toward these goals.

- Describe how physical activity positively influences physical and psychological health.

- Identify the benefits of physical activity throughout the aging process.

- Describe the prescriptions for and benefits of daily physical activity, aerobic exercise, and resistance training.

- Discuss how exercise can be combined with mindfulness to facilitate body awareness and self-inquiry.

- Explain the interventions to promote exercise adherence and compliance.

key terms

Aerobic exercise
Anaerobic exercise
Cardiorespiratory fitness
Cool-down period
Exercise

Flexibility
Muscular fitness
Physical activity
Physical fitness
Relaxation response

Resistance training
Warm-up period
Yoga

THINK About It

Knowing Versus Doing

Having the knowledge about the benefits of exercise does not correlate well with long-term exercise compliance. Confidence in the ability to exercise and a sense of the meaning and purpose (core desire) of exercise in life ensures better success.

1 What motivates putting the effort into developing and maintaining an active lifestyle?

2 Why is being active and physically fit important?

Regular physical activity and exercise enhance both physical and psychological health. Generally people who exercise regularly, or those who naturally include physical activity in their daily routine, feel better mentally and physically, improve their health profiles, and safeguard their

The author wishes to acknowledge the contributions of James S. Huddleston as author of the previous edition's exercise chapter.

functional independence as they go through the aging process. A holistic approach to physical activity involves exercise for cardiorespiratory health (endurance), exercise for musculoskeletal health (strength, flexibility, and bone density), and body awareness. Body awareness and mindfulness during exercise facilitate self-inquiry and self-acceptance, helping to relieve psychological stress and preventing physical injury (Box 12-1). Not only is an active

Box **12-1** Health Impact of Physical Activity

- Improves mood and promotes a sense of well-being
- Improves flexibility
- Builds muscle strength
- Increases endurance
- Increases the efficiency of the heart
- Increases bone density
- Decreases risk of stroke
- Helps with weight reduction

lifestyle an important component of primary prevention, but regular physical activity is also an essential modality in the treatment of chronic disease, which sets up the potential for benefit in all aspects of the biopsychosocial and spiritual model of health.

DEFINING PHYSICAL ACTIVITY IN HEALTH

To fully understand the *Healthy People 2010* objectives regarding exercise, the following definitions will be used:

- **Physical activity:** bodily movement that is produced by the contraction of skeletal muscles and that substantially increases energy expenditure; includes transportation and vocational and leisure-time activity. Leisure-time activity can be further categorized into sports, recreational activities, and exercise training.
- **Exercise** (exercise training): planned, structured, and repetitive bodily movement performed to improve or maintain one or more components of physical fitness.
- **Aerobic exercise:** activity that uses large muscle groups in a repetitive, rhythmic fashion over an extended period to improve the efficiency of the oxidative energy-producing system and improve cardiorespiratory endurance; uses stored adipose tissue as major fuel source.
- **Anaerobic exercise:** high-intensity, short-duration activity that improves the efficiency of the phosphocreatine and glycolytic energy-producing systems and increases muscle strength, power, and speed of reactivity; uses phosphagens and glucose-glycogen as major fuel sources.
- **Physical fitness:** a set of attributes (cardiorespiratory fitness, muscular fitness, and flexibility) that people have or achieve that relates to the ability to perform physical activity without undue fatigue or risk of injury.
- **Cardiorespiratory fitness** (aerobic capacity, functional capacity, and oxygen uptake [V_{O_2}]): the ability to deliver and use oxygen throughout the body to allow physical activity over an extended period without excessive fatigue.
- **Muscular fitness:** the strength and endurance of muscles that allows for participation in daily activities with low risk of musculoskeletal injury.
- **Flexibility:** adequate muscle length and joint mobility to allow free and painless movement through a wide range

of motion (ROM) (American College of Sports Medicine [ACSM], 1998; U.S. Department of Health and Human Services [USDHHS], 2000).

HEALTHY PEOPLE 2010 OBJECTIVES

Unfortunately only 23% of the adult population performs enough regular, sustained exercise to gain any significant health benefit, and slightly over 10% of the population exercises at an intensity necessary to promote cardiorespiratory fitness. A full 70% to 75% of adult Americans are sedentary, reporting no leisure-time activity or are not regularly active (USDHHS, 2000).

The importance of physical activity in the nation's health is reflected in the *Healthy People 2010* physical activity objectives (USDHHS, 2000). These objectives take into account the demonstrated relationship between physical activity and an improvement in the biological markers associated with health, and they identify the reasons for the trend toward a more sedentary lifestyle. The *Healthy People 2010* box provides a summary of the physical activity objectives set for 2010.

Physical Activity Objectives: Making Progress

The *Healthy People 2010* objectives (USDHHS, 2000) provide evidence of the progress that has been made toward achieving the original objectives. Figure 12-1 shows that progress has been made in decreasing the number of people who die from coronary heart disease (CHD). The number of people who engage in regular moderate and vigorous physical activity and strength training activities has also increased. However, despite solid gains (indicating that the message regarding the benefits of physical activity is reaching some segments of the population), the improvements fall short of the objectives set for the year 2010. The new goals set for *Healthy People 2010* reflect the work that remains (USDHHS, 2000).

The one area in which considerable improvement has been demonstrated, and actually exceeds the objective, is providing work site fitness programs. The significant increase in work site programs may be contributing to the increase in the number of people who are performing regular physical activity.

On a less positive note, Figure 12-1 indicates that little progress has been made in mobilizing the population out of a sedentary lifestyle. Although only 10.4% of adolescents report no leisure-time physical activity, the percentage increases throughout the life span from approximately 31% for men and women 18 to 24 years of age to 65% for individuals 75 years and older (USDHHS, 2000). The tendency to be sedentary continues to increase with age, increasing the risk of premature morbidity, mortality, and disability and limiting functional independence.

The prevalence of obesity has increased in all age groups in the United States. One in five teens and one in three adults are overweight. The number of adults who combine good dietary practice with regular physical activity in an

Healthy People 2010
Objectives for Physical Activity

- Increase the proportion of people appropriately counseled about health behaviors.
- Increase the proportion of physicians and dentists who counsel their at-risk clients about tobacco use cessation, physical activity, and cancer screening.
- Increase the proportion of middle, junior high, and senior high schools that provide school health education to prevent problems in these areas: unintentional injury, violence, suicide, tobacco use and addiction, alcohol and other drug use, unintended pregnancy, HIV/AIDS and other sexually transmitted disease infection, unhealthy dietary patterns, inadequate physical activity, and environmental health.
- Increase the proportion of college and university students who receive information from their institution on each of the six priority health-risk behavior areas.
- Increase the proportion of local health departments that have established culturally appropriate and linguistically competent community health-promotion and disease prevention programs.
- Increase the proportion of adults with high blood pressure who are taking action (e.g., losing weight, increasing physical activity, and reducing sodium intake) to help control their blood pressure.
- Increase the proportion of public and private schools that require use of appropriate head, face, eye, and mouth protection for students participation in school-sponsored physical activities.
- Reduce the proportion of adults who engage in no leisure-time physical activity.
- Increase the proportion of adults who engage regularly, preferably daily, in moderate physical activity for at least 30 minutes per day.
- Increase the proportion of adults who perform physical activities that enhance and maintain muscle strength and endurance.
- Increase the proportion of adults who perform physical activities that enhance and maintain flexibility.
- Increase the proportion of adolescents who engage in moderate physical activity for at least 30 minutes on 5 or more of the previous 7 days.
- Increase the proportion of adolescents who engage in vigorous physical activity that promotes cardiorespiratory fitness 3 or more days per week for 20 or more minutes per occasion.
- Increase the proportion of the nation's public and private schools that require daily physical education for all students.
- Increase the proportion of adolescents who participate in daily school physical education.
- Increase the proportion of adolescents who spend at least 50% of school physical education class time being physically active.
- Increase the proportion of adolescents who view television for 2 or fewer hours on a school day.
- Increase the proportion of the nation's public and private schools that provide access to their physical activity spaces and facilities for all people outside of normal school hours (that is, before and after the school day, on weekends, and during summer and other vacations) (developmental).
- Increase the proportion of work sites offering employer-sponsored physical activity and fitness programs.
- Increase the proportion of trips made by walking.
- Increase the proportion of trips made by bicycling.

From U.S. Department of Health and Human Services. (2000). *Healthy People 2010*. Washington, DC: Centers for Disease Control and Prevention, President's Council on Physical Fitness and Sports.

attempt to attain an appropriate body weight has decreased. This decidedly negative trend may be related to the decline in physical activity in the schools. The number of students involved in daily school physical education decreased from 42% in 1991 to 27% in 1997, and only 32% of students are physically active for 20 minutes or more in daily physical education classes (USDHHS, 2000). Physical activity habits tend to track (be consistent) during early childhood, and less active children tend to remain less active over time, increasing their risk of becoming sedentary adults (Pate, Baranowski, Dowda, & Trost, 1996). If a standard is to be set for the importance of physical activity throughout the life span, then it needs to start with children, who have the potential to develop lifelong healthy habits.

As the health care system moves toward a preventive model, primary care providers must facilitate a wellness atti-

tude in their clients, which involves not only encouraging individuals to be physically active, but also leading by example. Recommending regular exercise and espousing the benefits from personal experience can have a significant influence on individual involvement. Nurses are in a position to inquire about and provide counseling for exercise habits of their clients. Although some progress has been made in providing this service, especially with nurse practitioners, data through 1997 indicate a shortfall in reaching the goal set for 2010 of 50% of people (USDHHS, 2000). Although there has been some improvement in some areas, overall the proportion of the population reporting physical activity has remained essentially unchanged and progress is limited. Obviously the progress that has been made toward physical activity objectives for the year 2010 does not reflect a significant shift in the attitude of the general population

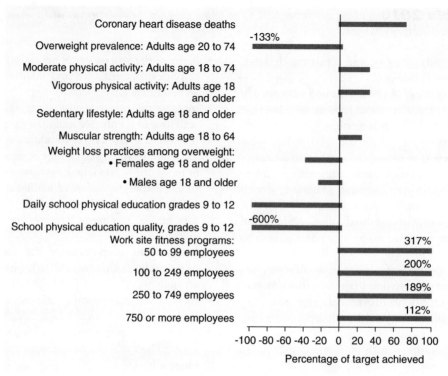

Coronary heart disease deaths
Overweight prevalence: Adults age 20 to 74
Moderate physical activity: Adults age 18 to 74
Vigorous physical activity: Adults age 18 and older
Sedentary lifestyle: Adults age 18 and older
Muscular strength: Adults age 18 to 64
Weight loss practices among overweight:
• Females age 18 and older
• Males age 18 and older
Daily school physical education grades 9 to 12
School physical education quality, grades 9 to 12
Work site fitness programs:
50 to 99 employees
100 to 249 employees
250 to 749 employees
750 or more employees

-133%
-600%
317%
200%
189%
112%

-100 -80 -60 -40 -20 0 20 40 60 80 100
Percentage of target achieved

Figure 12-1 The status of physical activity and fitness objectives. Tracking data for the objective concerning community involvement are unavailable.

Box 12-2 Populations With Low Rates of Physical Activity

- Women generally are less active than men at all ages.
- People with lower incomes and less education are typically not as physically active as those with higher incomes and education.
- African Americans and Hispanics are generally less physically active than whites.
- Adults in northeastern and southern states tend to be less active than adults in north central and western states.
- People with disabilities are less physically active than people without disabilities.
- By age 75, one in three men and one in two women engage in no regular physical activity.

From U.S. Department of Health and Human Services. (2000). *Healthy people 2010.* Washington, DC: Centers for Disease Control and Prevention, President's Council on Physical Fitness and Sports.

or the health care profession. There are still populations at risk (Box 12-2).

AGING

The biological changes attributed to aging closely resemble the effects of physical inactivity. The list for both aging and inactivity includes an increase in body fat and a decrease in aerobic capacity, muscle mass, metabolic rate, strength and flexibility, bone mass, sexual function, mental performance, immune function, and sleep quality.

Among older adults, exercise can improve health, prevent disability and hospitalizations, improve blood lipid profiles, and reduce body fat.

Exercise is especially important for older women, who make up the majority of the older population, because it may help prevent osteoporosis (Schneider, Mercer, Herning, Smith, & Prypah, 2004).

In 1991 an estimated 31.8 million older adults resided in the United States, consisting of 19 million elderly women and 12.8 million elderly men. In addition it is estimated that by the year 2030, more than 22% of all Americans will be 65 or older (Ourania, Yvoni, Christos, & Ionannis, 2003).

By maintaining an active lifestyle or by increasing the level of activity in previously sedentary individuals, older people can maintain relatively high levels of cardiovascular and metabolic functions, including skeletal muscle function and aerobic capacity (Kohrt et al., 1991). Several researchers have reported significant improvements in strength and in flexibility. Consequently, they can improve functional mobility and the ability to live independently. Elderly people with more muscle mass can eat more calories and take in more nutrients because their metabolic rate is higher. As a result the potential for malnutrition, a common problem for older adults, is decreased (Fiatarone, O'Neill, Ryan, Clements, Solares, & Nelson, 1994).

The health of the musculoskeletal system depends on movement and activity. Bone is a dynamic tissue, constantly changing and adapting to the stresses to which it is subjected. Bone strength is dependent on stresses applied by muscular and weight-bearing activity (mechanical stress during active movement). Exercise enhances bone mineralization and helps prevent bone loss over time (Aisenbrey, 1987). To stay healthy, joints must do what they are designed to do—move and bear weight. The health of the cartilage covering the joint surfaces is vital for maintaining proper joint function. The only way the cartilage can receive nourishment is through the manufacture and distribution of synovial fluid, which delivers nutrients, removes waste products, and lubricates joint surfaces (Schatz, 1985). Movement is vital for creating this environment of blood and lymph in and out of joint structures and the adjacent soft tissues. Without the stress of weight-bearing activity, normal bone and cartilage metabolism and repair become dysfunctional, resulting in injury and disease.

Effects of Exercise on the Aging Process

Everyone needs physical activity to be healthy. Human physiology has evolved in preparation for physical exertion. Until recently, survival through the vigor of daily living depended on a moderate degree of physical fitness. However, with mechanization and the style of living in today's society, daily life has become too sedentary. A lifestyle of inactivity places the population at risk for mortality and morbidity, and the literature supports exercise as an essential element of health.

Regular physical activity can help maintain functional independence and improve the quality of life throughout the aging process (USDHHS, 2000). Physical and psychological benefits of increased physical activity have been documented widely in healthy and in chronically ill older adults (Geffken et al., 2001; USDHHS, 2000). Only 12% of adults aged 75 and older engage in 30 minutes of moderate physical activity 5 or more days per week, and 65% report no leisure physical activity (USDHHS, 2000). Considerable research has tested interventions to increase activity by younger adults and by populations of all ages. Interventions-research with older adults is being reported more frequently. The most common interventions are self-monitoring, general health education, goal setting, supervised center-based exercise, problem solving, feedback reinforcement, and relapse prevention education. A few studies inadvertently have adapted motivational interventions, used mediated intervention delivery, and integrated multiple theoretical frameworks into the intervention. Lifestyle activity in an older adult recommends the accumulation of minutes of physical activity spread over the entire day. Some evidence suggests potential beneficial effects of lifestyles activity and the probability that some aging adults may be more receptive to lifestyles activity changes that include episodic exercise (Brawley, Rejeski, & Lutes, 2000).

CORONARY HEART DISEASE

Of particular importance is the role of physical activity in preventing CHD, the leading cause of death in the United States. Physical inactivity affects more people in the devel-

Table **12-1** Major Coronary Risk Factors	
Positive Risk Factors	**Defining Criteria**
Age	Men over age 45; women over age 55 or at early menopause without estrogen replacement therapy
Family history	MI or sudden death under age 55 in father or under age 65 in mother (or other first-degree relative)
Current cigarette smoking	—
Hypertension	BP >140/90 mm Hg (measured on two separate occasions) or on antihypertension medications
Hypercholesterolemia	Total serum cholesterol >200 mg/dl (5.2 mmol/l) (if lipoprotein profile is unavailable) or HDL <40 mg/dl (0.9 mmol/l)
Diabetes mellitus	People 1 to 30 years old with IDDM or who have had it for >15 years, and people with NIDDM >35 years
Sedentary lifestyle	Sedentary job and no regular exercise or leisure-time activity

Modified from American College of Sports Medicine. (1995). *Guidelines for exercise testing and prescription* (5th ed.). Media, PA: Williams & Wilkins.
BP, blood pressure; *HDL*, high-density lipoproteins; *IDDM*, insulin-dependent diabetes mellitus; *MI*, myocardial infarction; *NIDDM*, non–insulin-dependent diabetes mellitus.

opment of CHD than any other risk factor, making it a significant public health problem. Until recently, physical inactivity was not considered one of the most powerful risk factors; hypertension (HTN), smoking, obesity, and hyperlipidemia were considered to have greater influence. However, at any level or combination of risk factors, sedentary individuals are at an even greater risk (Table 12-1).

All of these studies reveal the value of exercise in the primary prevention of CHD. Exercise also plays a role in secondary prevention (recurrence). Increased physical activity appears to benefit individuals with cardiovascular disease (CVD), including myocardial infarction (MI), angina pectoris, and congestive heart failure, and their status after coronary artery bypass surgery or percutaneous transluminal coronary angioplasty or stent placement. Benefits include reduction in cardiovascular mortality rates, reduction of symptoms, improvement in exercise tolerance and functional capacity, and improvement in psychological well-being and quality of life (National Institutes of Health [NIH], 1996). In an analysis of 10 large studies involving more than 4000 people who had had an MI, individuals who participated in cardiac rehabilitation exercise programs had 25% fewer deaths from CHD. People who include regular exercise in their lives after an MI have improved rates of survival.

The 1990 statement on exercise by the Committee on Exercise and Cardiac Rehabilitation (McHenry et al., 1990) concurs with these findings. The consensus is that regular dynamic physical activity plays a role in both the primary and secondary prevention of CHD. Regular moderate or vigorous leisure-time or occupational physical activity may protect against CHD. Additionally, exercise may improve the likelihood of surviving an MI and reduce the chances of recurrence in some individuals. Although heavy physical exertion can trigger an MI, habitual physical activity lowers the relative risk of suffering an MI during heavy physical exertion (Mittleman et al., 1993).

The literature strongly demonstrates that the risk of CHD decreases as physical activity increases and that a plausible relationship between the decreased risk and a number of potential physiological and metabolic mechanisms exists:

- Increasing high-density lipoprotein (HDL) cholesterol
- Decreasing serum triglyceride (TRG) levels
- Decreasing high blood pressure
- Improving glucose tolerance and insulin sensitivity
- Decreasing obesity; altering distribution of body fat
- Reducing the sensitivity of the myocardium to the effects of catecholamines, thereby decreasing the risk of ventricular arrhythmias
- Enhancing fibrinolysis and altering platelet function (Pate et al., 1995)

High-Density Lipoprotein and Serum Triglyceride Levels

Exercise has a major influence on lipoprotein metabolism, primarily affecting plasma levels of HDL and TRG. There is a powerful negative correlation between CHD and plasma HDL levels. Increases in HDL lower the total cholesterol-to-HDL ratio, thereby reducing CHD risk. Exercise also has a potent lowering effect on levels of plasma TRG that is evident within hours after a bout of exercise (Haskell et al., 1992). Exercise training increases activity of lipoprotein lipase, an enzyme that removes cholesterol and fatty acids from the blood (Stefanick & Wood, 1994). TRG levels are lower and HDL levels are higher in physically active people than in the sedentary population. A dose response relationship between amounts of physical activity and HDL levels appears to exist, with endurance-trained athletes having 20% to 30% higher HDL levels and lower TRG levels than do healthy, age-matched, sedentary people (Leon, 1991). In a study of women runners, Williams (1996) identified a significant incremental dose response relationship between increased weekly running distance and increased HDL concentrations.

The effect of exercise on lipid metabolism may be related more to the volume (duration and frequency) than to the intensity of the exercise. Although single episodes of physical activity result in an improved blood lipid profile that can last for several days (Durstine & Haskell, 1994), regular repeated bouts of activity are needed for long-term benefits. Short periods of exercise training result in modest increases in HDL, but longer periods of training produce larger increases in HDL (Haskell et al., 1992). Exercise's lowering effect on TRG is cumulative; therefore, frequent bouts of exercise result in a progressive decrease in TRG. Changes in lipid profiles are most significant with moderate exercise over a prolonged period (1 year). On the average, exercise training has the potential to increase HDL approximately 2 mg/dl. Although this benefit may not appear significant, a 1 mg/dl increase in HDL is associated with a 2% decrease in CHD risk. More exercise may provide even more benefit. In the study by Williams (1996), the 9.6 mg/dl difference in HDL between the groups running the shortest distances and the longest represents a 29% reduction in CHD risk. However, exercise is not a quick fix. At best, exercise appears to involve a commitment to regular, moderately intense physical activity over an extended period—a lifetime commitment to an active lifestyle.

Hypertension

Studies by Paffenbarger, Wing, Hyde, and Jung (1983) and Blair and others (1989) suggest that habitual activity and physical fitness may reduce the risk of developing HTN. In these studies, people who did not engage in vigorous sports play or who were at low levels of fitness were at 35% to 52% greater risk for developing HTN. Although these studies reflect the long-term effect of exercise on control of HTN, studies by Roman, Camuzzi, Villalon, and Klenner (1981) and Kiyonaga, Arakawa, Tanaka, and Shindo (1985) demonstrate that regular bouts of aerobic exercise (3 times a week for 30 to 60 minutes at a moderate intensity for 3 months) result in a significant reduction of both systolic blood pressure (SBP) and diastolic blood pressure (DBP) at rest. The benefits of aerobic exercise on lowering blood pressure are supported by two analyses (Arroll & Beaglehole, 1992; Kelly & McClellan, 1994); both SBP and DBP decreased approximately 6 to 7 mm Hg with aerobic exercise (of parameters similar to those listed previously). Fagard and Tipton (1994) report that endurance training decreases resting blood pressure (RBP) an average of 7 to 10 mm Hg for both SBP and DBP in individuals with HTN. Keleman, Effron, Valenti, and Stewart (1990) suggest that exercise may be as strong a treatment modality for HTN as some medications. The need for making exercise part of a habitual lifestyle change is reflected in the study by Roman and colleagues (1981); RBP increased again when training was discontinued.

Low– to moderate–intensity endurance exercise appears to be most effective in lowering blood pressure. Circuit weight training also has a positive effect on HTN, whereas resistance training (designed primarily to increase strength) and high-intensity aerobic training appear to have minimal benefit. Mechanisms underlying the exercise-training effect on lowering blood pressure are not completely clear but may involve attenuation of sympathetic nervous system activity. This attenuation results in the dilation of peripheral blood vessels, which decreases systemic vascular resistance. Decreasing sympathetic nervous system activity may have a beneficial effect on the insulin resistance that is often observed in hypertensive people. Reductions in circulating insulin levels decrease the potential for insulin-mediated sodium reabsorption by the kidneys and increased blood pressure (Tipton, 1984).

Hyperinsulinemia and Glucose Intolerance

Hyperinsulinemia and glucose intolerance account for the various types of diabetes. Diabetes mellitus (DM) encompasses a group of metabolic disorders that have in common an increase in blood glucose levels and associated metabolic dysfunction. Insulin-dependent diabetes mellitus (IDDM) involves elevated blood glucose levels that are a result of a deficiency of circulating insulin caused by destruction of the pancreatic β cells, and non–insulin-dependent diabetes mellitus (NIDDM) involves elevated blood glucose levels from insulin resistance (decreased insulin sensitivity)—largely in skeletal muscles—or impaired insulin secretion. Approximately 90% of those with diabetes have NIDDM.

Exercise training is associated directly with improved insulin sensitivity (Holloszy et al., 1986). Prospective cohort studies demonstrate that physical activity is related to a reduced incidence of NIDDM (Helmrich, Ragland, Leung, & Paffenbarger, 1991; Manson et al., 1999). These findings are supported by population studies of various ethnic groups (Multicultural Awareness box). Physical activity is inversely related to the incidence of NIDDM, a relationship that is most evident in men at high risk for developing diabetes (those with a high body mass index [BMI], a history of HTN, or a family history of DM). A dose response relationship was noted: each 500 calories of additional leisure-time physical activity per week was associated with a 6% reduction in the risk of developing NIDDM (Helmrich et al., 1991).

During physical activity, contracting skeletal muscles work with insulin to enhance glucose uptake into the cells. Insulin resistance impedes glucose mobilization into cells, increasing plasma glucose levels and setting the potential for developing NIDDM. Although insulin resistance in skeletal muscles may be the primary defect, the development of disease appears to be related to elevated insulin levels, a result of the body's response to the need to mobilize glucose into the cells. Additionally, this syndrome often also involves elevated TRG levels and HTN, which contribute to the potential for disease. Exercise increases insulin sensitivity, improves the inherent effect of endoge-

MULTICULTURAL AWARENESS

Walk Away From Ethnic Glucose Intolerance

The Pima Indians of the Gila River Indian Community in Arizona have the highest documented incidence rates of NIDDM in the world. On the island of Mauritius in the southwest Indian Ocean, all four ethnic groups (Hindu and Muslim Asian Indians, African Creoles, and Chinese) have unusually high rates of NIDDM. In the United States, NIDDM is 30% more prevalent in blacks than in whites. The presence of NIDDM in each of these ethnic groups provides strong support for the existence of one or more modifiable risk factors in the cause of the disease.

Excessive weight gain is a strong independent predictor of NIDDM. The development of NIDDM (characterized by insulin resistance, hyperinsulinemia, and glucose intolerance) is related to weight gain in adults, particularly in fat accumulation around the waist, abdomen, and upper body (android or apple shape). This type of fat distribution is also associated with a higher risk of developing CHD. Adipose tissue is a major site for insulin insensitivity, and most obese individuals have increased insulin resistance or some degree of glucose intolerance, or both.

Physical activity has an important role in the prevention and treatment of NIDDM. By helping to maintain a proper lean-to-fat body mass, either by losing weight or preventing weight gain, physical activity may indirectly protect against the development of NIDDM. The modulating effect of physical activity on fat stores helps to improve insulin sensitivity and glucose tolerance. Additionally, physical activity may directly affect glucose metabolism. The acute effect of exercise can lower plasma glucose levels by enhancing the effect of insulin; long-term exercise improves insulin action and glucose tolerance.

Epidemiological studies of ethnic groups indicate that physical inactivity is also a risk factor for NIDDM. In the United States, blacks and Native Americans have a disproportionate number of poor, unemployed, and disadvantaged individuals who lack access to the health care system. The least active individuals within these populations should be given the most attention, because they have the most to gain. The methods and programs that are used to get information on the importance of physical activity out to the public need to be varied, depending on the socioeconomic and cultural factors specific to the ethnic populations. Promotion of physical activity by schools, communities, and government and health agencies, with these factors in mind, will significantly help achieve the goal of improving lifestyles and decreasing the incidence of NIDDM.

Data from Harris, M. I., Flegal, K. M., Cowie, C. C., Eberhardt, M. S., Goldstein, D. E., Little, R. R., et al. (1988). Prevalence of diabetes, impaired fasting glucose, and impaired glucose tolerance in U.S. adults. The Third National Health and Nutrition Examination Survey, 1988-1994. *Diabetes Care, 21*, 518-524; Helmrich, S. P., Ragland, D. R., & Paffenbarger, R. S. (1994). Prevention of non-insulin-dependent diabetes mellitus with physical activity. *Medicine and Science in Sports and Exercise, 26*, 824-830; Kriska, A. M., LaPorte, R. E., Pettitt, D. J., Charles, M. A., Nelson, R. E., Kuller, L. H., et al. (1993). The association of physical activity with obesity, fat distribution and glucose intolerance in Pima Indians. *Diabetologia, 36*, 863-869; Pereira, M. A., Kriska, A. M., Joswiak, M. L., Zimmet, P. Z., Gareeboo, H., Chitson, P., et al. (1995). Physical inactivity and glucose intolerance in the multi-ethnic island of *Mauritius. Medicine and Science in Sports and Exercise, 27*, 1626-1634.

nous insulin, decreases obesity, and plays a role in lowering TRG levels and blood pressure; therefore, it is recommended in the management of NIDDM. With diet, weight control, and exercise, preventing or decreasing the need for oral antiglycolytic agents and insulin is possible while maintaining normal blood glucose levels. Physical activity may be most beneficial in preventing the progression of NIDDM during the earlier stages of the disease process, before insulin therapy is required (Holloszy, 1986). Overall, physical activity has a significant positive effect on a chronic disease that is associated with a high risk of developing CHD. Wei, Gibbons, Kampert, Nichaman, and Blair (2000) reveal that cardiorespiratory fitness and physical activity lower mortality rates in men with NIDDM. Low-fitness men are 7.4 times more likely to die from their diabetes and twice as likely to die from CHD.

OBESITY

Obesity is not often considered an independent risk factor for CHD, because its effects are exerted through other risk factors such as HTN, hyperlipidemia, and DM. Nevertheless obesity should be considered an independent target for intervention in health promotion. Being overweight and obese are major contributors to many preventable causes of death. On average, higher body weights are associated with higher death rates (USDHHS, 2000). The prevalence of obesity in women exceeds that of men in seven out of nine ethnic groups. Obesity increases in prevalence with aging and is associated with an increased risk of HTN, type 2 diabetes, cardiovascular disease, certain types of cancer, and other illness (Dennis, 2004).

In the United States, the incidence of adult obesity has increased from 25% in the 1970s to 64.5% in 2004 (Kuczmarski, Flegol, Campbell, & Johnson, 1994). Obesity is generally defined as an excess of adipose tissue, corresponding to a weight that is equal to or greater than 120% to 125% of the ideal body weight (Kuczmarski et al., 1994). Fat mass (body fat percentage) is most important in determining the ideal body weight. The recommended body fat levels for men and women are approximately 15% to 16% for men and 23% to 24% for women (ACSM, 1997). The average American man and woman tend to exceed the recommended body fat level. An increase in fat mass and the development of obesity occur when energy intake exceeds total daily energy expenditure for a prolonged period (Leibel, Rosenbaum, & Hirsch, 1995). Decreased physical activity may be both a cause and a consequence of weight gain over a lifetime.

Maintaining fitness and health is closely related to controlling weight. Literature supports the positive influence that physical activity has on body weight and obesity (USDHHS, 1996). Physical activity does the following:

- Promotes a negative energy balance (burns calories)
- Increases metabolic rate for an extended period after the activity

- Increases metabolic efficiency for burning calories by increasing lean body mass
- Helps counteract the decrease in metabolic rate associated with low-calorie diets by preserving lean body mass
- Is a good alternative to eating when eating is a response to stress rather than to hunger (Williford, Scharff-Olson, & Blessing, 1993)

Unfortunately most overweight people ignore exercise as a means of weight loss or they exercise at rates below federal health guidelines (Centers for Disease Control and Prevention, 2000).

Management of obesity involves a comprehensive program of nutrition management, behavior modification, and physical activity or exercise. The key to normalizing body fatness is long-term adherence and permanent lifestyle changes, not dieting or short-term exercise trials.

Increasingly sophisticated obesity treatments that demonstrate the best outcomes emphasize five components: behavioral techniques, cognitive strategies, social support, nutrition, and exercise. The effectiveness of physical activity is related to the frequency and duration of each activity session and the longevity of the activity program. Recommended thresholds for exercise include the following:

- A program of low-impact aerobic exercise, increase in daily activities, and resistance training
- A frequency of 5 to 7 times a week
- A length of 40 to 60 minutes a day or 20 to 30 minutes twice daily (ACSM, 1997)

As long as calorie expenditure is similar, moderate lifestyle activity may be as effective as structured exercise (Andersen et al., 1999). Moderate intensity appears to be most effective for total and fat calorie consumption during the activity (Health Teaching box).

Women tend to have a 5% to 10% lower resting metabolic rate than men and a higher percentage of body fat than men of similar weight. Consequently, women have a lower percentage of lean body mass and may not be as metabolically active as are men during exercise. Women may expend up to 40% fewer calories than do men during the same exercise protocol at the same relative intensity (Tremblay, Despres, & Bouchard, 1985).

Fat in men is stored primarily in the upper body or upper abdominal region. Fat in women is primarily stored in the lower half of the abdomen, the hips, and the thighs. Adipose tissue metabolism tends to be different in various regions. The fat-metabolism response to exercise appears to be less in the femoral-gluteal region than in the upper body–abdominal region. Femoral-gluteal adipose tissue serves as an important source of energy during lactation. Women may not lose fat as easily as do men in response to exercise, because genetic differences are related to where and how fat is stored and metabolized (Williford et al., 1993). Consequently women who need to lose weight may need to be more diligent about increasing the duration of their exercise training sessions and to make resistance training a priority to facilitate maximal energy expenditure.

In the April 2004 issue of *Obesity in Children and Teens,* the American Academy of Child and Adolescent Psychiatry reported on a survey of 83 parents, 23% of whom had overweight children. Only 10.5% of parents with overweight children perceived their children's weight accurately compared with 59.4% of other parents. "Focus on healthy lifestyles and on the person's strength. Talk about the advantages of exercise: improved strength, athletic abilities," suggests Daniel Bronfin, MD, Vice Chairman of Pediatrics at New Orleans Ochsner Clinic.

OSTEOPOROSIS

Osteoporosis is the most common bone disease, affecting 28 million Americans. It is characterized by decreased bone mass and structural weakness of bone tissue, leading to bone fragility and increased risk of fractures. Eighty percent of those affected are women (Berarducci, 2000). Some loss of bone occurs naturally after age 30. Twenty to thirty percent of bone mass development is regulated by environmental factors, such as nutrition and physical activity. In addition to the importance of optimizing physiological intake of calcium, vitamin D therapy, and maintaining normal menstrual cycles for maximizing peak bone mass, physical activity plays a significant role in developing bone mass during childhood and adolescence and in maintaining skeletal mass into adulthood and old age (Williams & Eickhoff, 2002). Using environmental changes and lifestyle modification during the third and fourth decades of life, women can increase their bone mass and effectively retard osteoporosis (Berarducci, Burns, Lengacher, & Sellers, 2000).

Physical activity increases the potential for increased peak bone mass and provides for a stronger skeletal foundation throughout aging (USDHHS, 2000).

Several empirical referents support the belief that adequate intake of calcium from dietary sources during the developmental years of skeletal growth is imperative for achieving peak bone mass (Packard & Hearney, 1997). Although dietary sources are the preferred means of achieving adequate calcium intake, foods fortified with calcium are becoming more prevalent and are manufactured to provide approximately 300 mg of calcium in each serving (see Chapter 11).

Bone mass increases during childhood and adolescence and peaks during the third decade of life. When a person reaches approximately age 30, age-related bone loss occurs throughout the skeletal system, in all races, and in both sexes. However, there are significant differences in bone loss patterns between the sexes. Women have less bone mass than men at all ages and by their mid-30s can expect age-related bone loss at approximately 1% annually. The rate of bone loss accelerates rapidly during the first 5 postmenopausal years, with annual losses of 3% to 5% common. By the fifth decade, or during their 40s, women can anticipate a 10% loss of vertebral bone mass. Cumulative bone loss can approach 40% of peak bone mass over a woman's lifetime (DeCherney, 1996). Therefore it is important to detect women at risk early in the natural course of the disease and to target interventions toward lifestyle-oriented health promotion.

Maintenance of bone mass may be related to the intensity of the physical activity and the degree to which the activity stresses the bone. Weight-bearing actions that stress

research highlights

Resistance and Agility Training Reduce Fall Risk in Women Aged 75 to 85

Objectives: To compare the effectiveness of group resistance- and agility-training programs in reducing fall risk in community-dwelling older women with low bone mass.

Design: A randomized, controlled, single-blind 25-week prospective study with assessments at baseline, midpoint, and trial completion.

Setting: Community center.

Participants: Community-dwelling women aged 75 to 85 with low bone mass.

Intervention: Participants were randomly signed to one of three groups: resistance training ($n = 32$), agility training ($n = 34$), and stretching (sham) exercises ($n = 32$). The exercise classes for each study arm were held twice weekly.

Measurements: The primary outcome measure was fall risk (derived from weighted scores from tests of postural sway, reaction time, strength, proprioception, and vision), as measured using a Physiological Profile Assessment. Secondary outcome measures were ankle dorsiflexion strength, foot reaction time, and Community Balance and Mobility Scale Score.

Results: Attendance at the exercise sessions for all three groups was excellent: resistance training (85.4%), agility training (87.3%), and stretching program (78.8%). At the end of the trial, Physiological Profile Assessment fall-risk scores were reduced by 57.3% and 47.5% in the resistance and agility training groups, respectively, but by only 20.2% in the stretching group. In the resistance and agility groups, the reduction in fall risk was mediated primarily by improved postural stability, where sway was reduced by 30.6% and 29.2%, respectively. There were no significant differences between the groups for the secondary outcomes measures. Within the resistance-training group, reductions in sway were significantly associated with improved strength, as assessed using increased squat load used in the exercise sessions.

Conclusion: These findings support the implementation of community-based resistance- and agility-training programs to reduce fall risk in older women with low bone mass. Such programs may have particular public health benefits because it has been shown that this group is at increased risk of falling and sustaining fall-related fractures.

Liu-Ambrose, T., Khan, K. M., Eng, J. J., Janssen, P. A., Lord, S. R., McKay, H. A. (2004). Resistance and agility training reduce fall risk in women aged 75 to 85 with low bone mass: A 6-month randomized, controlled trial. *Journal of the American Geriatric Society, 52,* 657-665.

the skeleton (walking, stair climbing, and aerobic dance) have a positive effect on bone density. Weight-bearing exercise is an important component of reducing osteoporosis risk and occurs from exercise that increases mechanical stresses on the skeleton. These exercises should be performed for 30 minutes or more, at least 3 to 4 times per week (Slemeada, 1997). In younger women the goal of exercise is to increase bone density; in elderly women who are already 30 to 40 years past menopause a more realistic goal would be to decrease the risk of fractures through fall prevention (Research Highlights box).

ARTHRITIS

Arthritis upsets the balance of joint health. Although rheumatoid arthritis and osteoarthritis have different causes and attack different parts of the joint, impaired joint function is the result. Cartilage is worn away and irregularities occur in the bone ends. As normal movement is altered, proper joint alignment fails, normal ROM is decreased, and disfigurement and dysfunction occur with the imbalance of altered muscle activity. Although there is an ongoing progression in arthritis that cannot be healed by exercise, physical activity nevertheless helps to restore health to synovium and cartilage, improve strength and flexibility, decrease joint vulnerability, and delay the onset of dysfunction.

One of the chief goals of exercise and physical activity for the individual with arthritis is to counter the effects of inactivity (ACSM, 1998). Although researchers have concluded that regular exercise cannot improve or cure arthritis, exercise has quality-of-life benefits for people with arthritis:

- Improvement in joint function and ROM
- Increase in muscle strength and aerobic fitness that enhance daily activities of living
- Improvement in psychological state
- Decrease in loss of bone mass
- Decrease in the risk of chronic disease (Nieman, 2000)

Consequently, exercise programs based on individual needs and interests should emphasize exercises to develop joint ROM and flexibility (daily) and should also include muscle strengthening (2 to 3 times per week), aerobic exercise (30 to 45 minutes most days of the week), and recreational activities that are enjoyable (ACSM, 1998).

LOW BACK PAIN

Low back pain is a common medical and social problem frequently associated with disability and absence from work (La Forge, 2004). Most causes of low back pain can be traced to lifelong histories of poor posture, weak muscles, poor body mechanics, and a sedentary lifestyle. However, exercise can have a positive influence on back pain. Staal and colleagues (2004) concluded that graded activity was more effective than usual care in reducing the number of days of absence from work because of low back pain.

The spinal column is made up of a series of vertebrae stacked one on another, forming natural curves that allow the bony column to function with the resiliency of a spring. The intervertebral disks help with mobility and shock absorption. The health of the bony vertebrae and the cartilaginous disks depends on movement. The cartilage gets its nutrients from the compression of bearing weight, and this same weight-bearing activity stimulates vertebral bone integrity.

Muscles are intimately involved in the support and function of the spinal column. Maintaining the proper curves (anterior and posterior convexities) of lordosis in the cervical and lumbar vertebrae and kyphosis in the thoracic vertebrae is vital for sustaining the spring and shock-absorption qualities of the spine. The lumbar curve is especially influenced by three sets of muscles that are attached to the pelvis and the lumbar vertebrae. By altering the tilt of the pelvis, these muscles can increase (iliopsoas muscle) or decrease (abdominal and hamstring muscles) the lumbar curve (Schatz, 1985). In addition, the deep muscles of the back (paraspinal muscles) work in controlled synergistic and antagonistic fashions to control spinal planes of motion; they are also influential in supporting the spinal curves in posture. Weakness, overstretching, or tightening of any of these muscles can negatively affect posture and increase wear and tear on the back. The result can be back pain from muscle strain, altered joint function (facet joints), and abnormal force on the intervertebral disks.

The goal of exercise programs for individuals with low back pain is to prevent debilitation as a result of inactivity and to improve endurance, strength, and flexibility, allowing for a return to usual functional activities. Exercise recommendations and progression of activity are highly individualized based on origin, duration, and severity of pain. Strengthening exercises for trunk and extremity musculature are useful in people with chronic—but not acute—low back pain. Aerobic conditioning, such as walking, swimming, and stationary bicycling, is recommended to maintain endurance and prevent debilitation from inactivity (ACSM, 1997).

Advanced age, osteoporosis, arthritis, and low back pain are not reasons to exclude exercise from anyone's lifestyle. In fact, the opposite is true. These conditions are reasons to remain as physically active as possible to facilitate the ability to function throughout the aging process.

IMMUNE FUNCTION

The relationship between exercise and immune function has a fairly long history of study, but renewed interest has grown out of the human immunodeficiency virus (HIV) epidemic. Several studies demonstrate that people with impaired immune function can exercise safely without risk to their health status and can enhance their physiological and psychological well-being with regular exercise (LaPerriere, Fletcher, Antoni, Klimas, & Schneiderman, 1991; Rigsby, Dishman, Jackson, MacLean, & Raven, 1992; Spence, Galentino, Mossberg, & Zimmerman, 1990). Changes in immune markers, such as CD4 and CD8 cell counts and the number and activity of natural killer (NK) cells, indicate that moderate exercise may help bolster an impaired immune system (LaPerriere et al., 1991).

Evidence also suggests that regular exercisers do not get sick as often as do less active people. Epidemiological studies indicate that a J-curve relationship exists between the intensity of exercise and the risk of upper respiratory tract infection (URTI) (Figure 12-2).

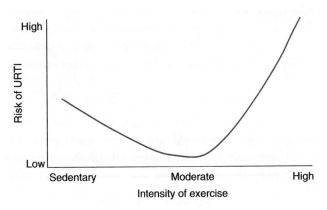

Figure 12-2 Relationship between exercise and the risk of upper respiratory tract infection (URTI). This relationship is often referred to as a *J curve.* (Modified from Nieman, D. [1994]. Exercise, upper respiratory tract infection, and the immune system. *Medicine and Science in Sports and Exercise, 26,* 128-139.)

Moderate exercise may decrease the risk of URTI below that of a sedentary individual, but high-intensity exercise may raise the risk above average. Ultramarathoners and high-intensity marathoners have a significantly higher incidence of URTI symptoms than control subjects. Female and elderly subjects who perform moderate exercise have less than one half the incidence of URTI than do sedentary control subjects (Neiman, 1994; Nieman et al., 1990).

Immune system changes that are apparently related to the intensity of exercise have been identified. Moderate-endurance exercise stimulates the neuroendocrine system, which causes changes in the function and numbers of various immune system cells, such as the NK, CD4, and CD8 cells as mentioned. Evidence also indicates that moderate exercise is associated with a prolonged improvement in the killing capacity of neutrophils (one of the most efficient phagocytes). Several immune marker changes suggest increased risk for illness in those who engage in high-intensity exercise, including low level of salivary immunoglobulin (antibodies), low serum complement levels, low lymphocyte count, depressed NK cell activity, low helper and suppressor T-cell ratio, and decreased neutrophil phagocytic capacity (Mackinnon, 1992; Nieman, 1994; Pedersen & Ullum, 1994).

Changes in immune cell counts and activity may be related to hormonal immunoregulation. Moderate exercise increases the release of immunostimulatory hormones, such as growth hormone and endogenous opiates (β-endorphin and methionine-enkephalin). The increase in β-endorphins with exercise seems to have a positive effect on NK cell activity. Conversely, intense exercise is associated with increases in catecholamine and corticosteroid (cortisol) levels, which have immunosuppressive characteristics (Mackinnon, 1992). High-intensity exercise is also associated with muscle cell damage and inflammation. The immune system is involved in tissue repair. It is theorized that while immune cells are busy with the repair process, host protection may suffer. A window of opportunity for infection during recovery from high-intensity exercise appears to exist. Accordingly, rest is recommended after vigorous exercise to allow the body to recover, and moderate exercise may be the better choice for enhancing health and well-being.

Research on occupational and leisure-time activity strongly suggests that physical activity has a protective effect against colon cancer (Lee, 1994). Data from the Nurses' Health Study indicate that women who are more physically active in adulthood have a lower risk of breast cancer than those who are less physically active (Rockhill et al., 1999). Physical activity during adolescence and young adulthood may protect women from the later development of breast cancer (Bernstein, Henderson, Hanisch, Sullivan-Halley, & Ross, 1994). Researchers argue that lifetime physical activity is the critical variable affecting breast cancer risk. A large prospective study of over 12,000 men suggests that cardiorespiratory fitness and higher levels of physical activity may protect against prostate cancer (Oliveria, Kohl, Trichopoulos, & Blair, 1996).

NK cells and microphages are involved in the first-line defense against the development and spread of malignancies. Exercise can help increase NK cell cytotoxicity, change the influx of macrophages into tissue, and promote the release of cytokines with antitumor properties (Woods & Davis, 1994). In helping to prevent colon cancer, exercise increases intestinal motility by altering local prostaglandin synthesis and decreases gastrointestinal transit time, thereby decreasing length of contact between colon mucosa and carcinogens (Lee, 1994).

MENTAL HEALTH

People who exercise regularly generally state that they feel better, have increased self-esteem, and have a more positive outlook on life. Not only do they feel better physically, they also feel better mentally. Epidemiological research with both men and women suggests that physical activity may be associated with reduced symptoms of depression and anxiety and improvements in positive affect and general sense of well-being (USDHHS, 2000). A Canadian survey (Stephens & Craig, 1990) suggests that higher levels of daily energy expenditure are associated with a more positive mood compared with lower levels of expenditure, and an inverse relationship exists between physical activity and symptoms of depression in people aged 25 years and older. Paffenbarger, Lee, and Leung (1994) revealed the same inverse relationship in a Harvard alumni cohort study.

Intervention studies have supported the positive influence of physical activity on mental health. Folkins (1976) found that after 12 weeks of exercise, the exercise group showed significant improvement in all levels of cardiovascular fitness and decreases in measures of anxiety and depression. In aerobic exercise studies (Berger & Owen, 1988; Blumenthal, Williams, Williams, & Wallace, 1980) the exercise groups experienced reductions in anxiety, tension, depression, and fatigue and an increase in vigor and clear-mindedness. A recent study by Blumenthal and colleagues (1999) demonstrates that exercise is as effective as antidepressant medication in reducing levels of depression in older clients with major depressive disorder. These findings suggest that improvements in physical health are associated with improvements in psychological health.

Jin (1989) found that mood states become more positive during and for a short time after Tai Chi. The psychological changes include a decrease in depression, tension, anger, fatigue, confusion, and anxiety and an increase in vigor. Brown and colleagues (1995) determined that exercise combined with a cognitive activity (low-intensity walking with the relaxation response, or modified Tai Chi) appears to be more effective in improving mood states than exercise alone.

Physical activity helps to improve the mental health of both clinical and nonclinical populations. Although suggestions are that the greatest benefits from conditioning are experienced by the least fit and the most anxious and depressed (Goff & Dimsdale, 1985), Blumenthal, Williams, Williams, and Wallace (1980) conclude that basically healthy, well-adjusted people who exercise can increase their sense of well-being more than healthy people who do not exercise. Even when no change is observed in objective mental health measures with older people in relatively good physical and mental health, they report feelings of improved physical, psychological, and social well-being after regular physical activity (Blumenthal et al., 1989).

Kobasa (1985) has performed extensive work on the stress-illness relationship. Exercise is considered one of the moderating variables (resistance resources)—in addition to hardiness and social support—that affects the relationship. Exercise likely protects through decreasing the physical strain of stressful events. In support of these findings, Dyer and Crouch (1988) conclude that exercise not only improves regular participants' feelings about coping with stress, it also enhances their overall feeling of well-being. Physical activity and exercise should be encouraged in an attempt to maximize their associated benefits of enhanced sense of personal achievement, self-esteem, and social participation (Goff & Dimsdale, 1985).

HOW MUCH EXERCISE IS ENOUGH?

Literature certainly reflects both the physiological and psychological benefits that can be experienced with commitment to an active lifestyle. In short, regular physical activity or exercise can help people feel better, look better, and perform better. Unfortunately, as discussed, Americans have failed to embrace the concept and health value of an active lifestyle. Many have been overwhelmed by the misperception that to gain health benefits they must perform vigorous, continual exercise. The result has been discouragement in getting started and poor compliance in staying with it.

LESS PAIN, MORE GAIN

In an attempt to encourage increased participation in physical activity, a panel of scientists from the Centers for Disease Control and Prevention and the American College of Sports Medicine came together to review the evidence related to physical activity and to issue a public health message concerning the recommended types and amounts of physical activity (Pate et al., 1995). The evidence clearly indicates that the protective effects of exercise can be achieved at more moderate levels of intensity than had been recommended previously. The health and fitness benefits of exercise appear to be related more to the total amount of exercise accomplished (calories expended) rather than to the specific exercise intensity, frequency, and duration. The recommendations are as follows:

- Adults should accumulate 30 minutes or more of moderate-intensity (brisk) physical activity on most (or all) days of the week, for a weekly total of 3 to 4 hours.
- The activity need not be continuous; benefits can be realized with short bouts of activity (a minimum of 10 minutes) over the course of the day.
- This amount of activity will expend about 150 to 200 calories per day (the equivalent of walking 2 miles briskly) or 1000 to 1400 calories per week.
- All types of activity can be applied to the daily total (raking leaves, dancing, or gardening).
- Lower-intensity activities should be performed more often, or for longer periods, or both. More vigorous activities should be performed for shorter periods or less frequently.

Because most adults do not meet these standards, they have the most to gain by incorporating a few minutes of increased activity into their day, gradually building up to 30 minutes a day. People who are active on an irregular basis should strive to be more consistent. People who prefer more formal exercise can choose to participate in more vigorous, organized exercise regimens, sports, and recreational activities. A dose-response curve best represents the relationship between physical activity (dose) and health benefit (response).

Sedentary individuals gain the most by increasing their activity to the recommended level. However, any person who already meets the standards can derive some additional benefit by becoming more active.

People who do a little bit of exercise are better off than those . . . who do none. Those who do a little more are better off still. (Franklin, 1993, p. 476)

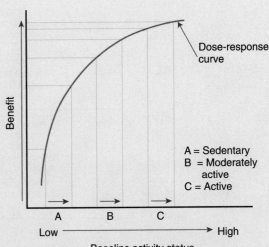

The dose-response curve represents the best estimate of the relationship between physical activity (dose) and health benefit (response). The lower the baseline physical activity status, the greater the health benefit associated with a given increase in physical activity (arrows **A, B,** and **C**). (From Pate, R. R., Pratt, M., Blair, S. N., Haskell, W. L., Macera, C. A., Bouchard, C., et al. [1995]. Physical activity and public health: A recommendation from the CDC and the ACSM. *Journal of the American Medical Association, 273,* 402-407.)

"No pain, no gain" has been an unfortunate, common refrain (Hot Topics box).

People should be reminded that many of their daily physical activities are actually forms of exercise (Figure 12-3). This approach to physical activity serves as a good foundation to a healthy lifestyle. However, when possible, individuals should also be encouraged to include more formal exercise training in their overall activities to promote optimal cardiorespiratory fitness and significantly improve muscle strength and endurance. How much exercise is required to achieve these goals is determined by the parameters of an exercise prescription:

F (Frequency)   3 to 5 times a week of aerobic exercise
2 to 3 times a week of resistance training
I (Intensity)   Moderate to vigorous, by heart rate and perceived exertion

Able to complete each resistance exercise, 8 to 12 repetitions, without strain
T (Time)   20 to 60 minutes, plus warm-up and cool-down periods
15 to 30 minutes to complete a series of 8 to 10 resistance exercises
T (Type)   Aerobic (walking, jogging, biking, swimming, rowing, cross-country skiing, NordicTrack, StairMaster, aerobics, dancing, skating, or rollerblading)
Resistance training (weight machines, free weights, and calisthenics such as push-ups, sit-ups, or pull-ups) (ACSM, 1998; Westcott, 1993)

Aerobic Exercise

The benefits of aerobic exercise are cumulative; therefore, a frequency of 3 to 5 times a week is recommended. Every

PHYSICAL ACTIVITY PYRAMID

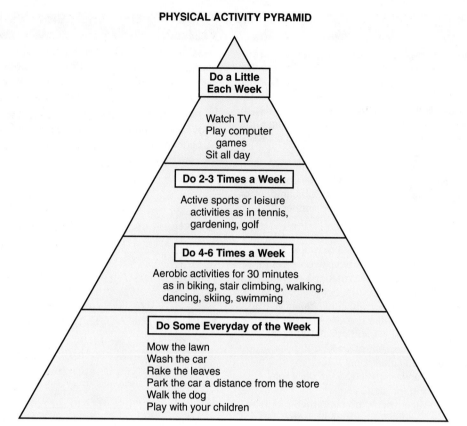

Figure 12-3   Physical activity pyramid.

other day is a good frame of reference. The benefits of exercising more than 5 times a week are outweighed by the risk of injury, especially with higher-impact activities. When more frequent exercising is a goal, cross-training is recommended. Cross-training means performing different types of exercise on different days of the week or performing different types of exercise within one session. The benefits of cross-training include a decreased risk of musculoskeletal injury, an increased potential for total body conditioning, and improved long-term compliance because variety decreases boredom and eliminates the exercise barrier of limited choices.

The intensity of exercise that results in health and fitness benefits ranges from moderate to vigorous and is comfortable, but challenging (brisk). Intensity is defined by the objective measure of heart rate (HR) and the subjective measure of perceived exertion.

The increase in HR during exercise has a strong linear relationship with exercise intensity and aerobic capacity. Resting heart rate (RHR) is the HR measured at rest. Maximum heart rate (MHR) is the rate measured at the highest workload tolerated during exercise. MHR also decreases with age; therefore, a generic formula for determining MHR is 220 minus age. Formulas for determining appropriate exercise HRs have been developed that take RHR and MHR into consideration.

The Borg Scale for rating perceived exertion (RPE) is a psychophysical category scale for the subjective rating of sensations associated with the intensity of physical work (Borg, 1973, 1982) (Figure 12-4). The scale uses ratings based on the individual's overall feeling of exertion and physical fatigue. These ratings correspond well with metabolic responses to exercise, such as HR and oxygen consumption. The strong linear relationship between HR and RPE was originally suggested by Borg and has been verified by subsequent studies. Correlation coefficients from 80% to 90% have been reported consistently using a variety of work tasks and exercise conditions (Borg, 1973, 1982; Skinner, Hustler, Bergsteinova, & Buskirk, 1973). However, perceptions of exertion and the relationship to HR are influenced by both physiological and psychological factors (aches, cramps, pain, fatigue, shortness of breath, anxiety, depression, and introversion or extroversion) (Morgan, 1973; O'Sullivan, 1984). Smutok, Skrinar, and Pandolf (1980) noted that some subjects are more accurate in regulating exercise intensity by RPE than are others and that this variability may be more the result of psychological rather than physiological factors. Other factors that may alter the strong relationship between HR and RPE are drug-related situations (β-blockers), age, and disease states (O'Sullivan, 1984).

Despite this potential for variability in perception, RPE correlates well with HR clinically, and together they form

6	
7	Very, very light
8	
9	Very light
10	
11	Fairly light
12	Somewhat hard
13	
14	Hard
15	
16	Very hard
17	
18	
19	Very, very hard
20	

Figure 12-4 Borg scale for rating perceived exertion (RPE). (From Borg, G. A. [1982]. Psychophysical basis of perceived exertion. *Medicine and Science in Sports and Exercise, 14*, 377-381.)

a complementary means of helping individuals determine a comfortable, beneficial level of exercise intensity. An RPE of 11 to 14 corresponds well with 50% to 85% MHR. Subjective parameters include being slightly short of breath, but not out of breath; able to talk without difficulty, but unable to sing a song easily; being pleasantly fatigued, but not exhausted; and having mild musculoskeletal discomfort, but no pain.

Attention to RPE helps a person develop a sense of body awareness and an appreciation for the body's response to the stress of activity. Awareness of RPE helps people listen to their bodies and to become aware of how it feels to move, where they carry tension, and where they have discomfort. With this increased awareness, individuals can choose how they want to respond, adjusting their exercise practice on a day-to-day basis, making the activity more enjoyable, decreasing the risk of injury, and improving long-term exercise compliance.

The recommendation for the duration of aerobic conditioning exercise is generally 20 to 60 minutes. Less than 20 minutes usually provides minimal benefit. However, for people who are unaccustomed to exercising or for those who are greatly deconditioned, short durations are permissible, gradually increasing to a beneficial, comfortable level as tolerance and confidence improve. Everyone has to start somewhere and doing a little is much better than doing nothing at all.

The benefit of sessions longer than 45 to 60 minutes is again outweighed by the potential for injury. Exercising more than 60 minutes on occasion (such as an extended bike ride with friends or a leisurely walk on a beautiful day) is certainly not wrong, but a person who increases duration should consider decreasing intensity. Improvements in cardiorespiratory fitness can also be accrued from intermittent bouts of moderate to vigorous exercise (10-minute segments) on a workout day (DeBusk, Stenestrand, Sheehan, & Haskell, 1990; Jakicic, Wing, Butler, & Robertson, 1995). As discussed, longer bouts of exercise are more beneficial for weight loss. The range of acceptable duration allows for greater flexibility, giving reassurance of benefit to the individual who varies exercise choices daily based on capability, interests, and life demands.

As mentioned, many different choices for aerobic exercise are available. The question is often asked, "What is the best aerobic exercise?" The answer is, "the one that the individual is willing to do on a regular basis." Different aerobic exercises have different benefits; they all have their advantages and disadvantages. From a cardiovascular point of view, with relative intensity, frequency, and duration being equal, the benefit is about the same for all modes. Probably the best scenario is cross-training, which results in the best all-around benefits. However, the most important recommendation is that people get out and start moving. The type of exercise they prefer and will continue doing is the best one for them to do.

Walking is probably the most accessible and popular form of aerobic exercise. Done briskly, walking provides a good cardiorespiratory challenge in 60% to 80% of the adult population (Blair et al., 1989). Walking is also an activity that nearly everyone can do, requires little equipment or cost, can be done almost anywhere (even on vacation), and can be a social or a solitary activity, depending on individual needs. For people who are unaccustomed to exercising, walking is a great place to start.

Walking is often the recommended exercise of choice for people who are greatly deconditioned or for those who have physical limitations. Considered a low-impact activity, walking can be easily regulated to accommodate a wide range of fitness levels and motor abilities. Cycling, rowing, and swimming (or water walking or other water aerobics) are also non–weight-bearing to low weight-bearing activities that may be good choices for individuals with physical limitations. Water activities are a good exercise alternative for individuals with musculoskeletal limitations who need some weight relief with exercise. Although the buoyancy of the water provides this weight relief, the water also provides resistance to the limbs as they move, encouraging an increase in intensity and conditioning. Individuals should be encouraged to do the types of aerobic exercise that best fit their needs, interests, and lifestyles while providing reasonable benefits.

Warm-Up and Cool-Down Periods

In addition to the endurance phase of exercise, warm-up and cool-down periods should be a regular part of the exercise session. The **warm-up period** usually lasts 5 to 10 minutes and may include light stretching, calisthenics, or performance of the chosen aerobic activity at a low intensity. This approach prepares both the musculoskeletal and cardiorespiratory systems for the transition from rest to exercise by increasing blood flow, respiration, body temperature, and muscle flexibility. The warm-up period decreases the risks of injury and heart irregularities.

The **cool-down period** follows the endurance phase and usually lasts 5 to 10 minutes. This phase allows the body to readjust gradually from the demands of exercise back to baseline. Stretching and slow, rhythmical movement help to increase muscle elasticity, prevent blood pooling and hypotension, and facilitate dissipation of body heat and removal of lactic acid. The result is the prevention of injury, light-headedness, fatigue, and muscle soreness.

Yoga is an excellent form of exercise to use during warm-up and cool-down periods. The word **yoga** means union or "established in being," which implies a mind-body connection. Simply defined, yoga is mindful stretching. The mind is quiet and awareness is focused on feeling the body as it moves. Movement into and out of yoga postures (called *asanas*) provides the necessary stimulation of weight-bearing activity to help keep bones strong, provides the movement to increase joint ROM, and stretches and tones muscles. The sun salute (surya namaskar), a series of 12 flexion-extension yoga postures linked together as one fluid movement by the breath rhythm, is a wonderful practice to include in the warm-up and cool-down phases of exercise, providing both physiological and mind-body benefits.

Yoga also helps develop an appreciation for the experience of the basic resting state, a mindfulness of how it feels to be relaxed physically and mentally during the activity. In this form, exercise becomes an inner experience; that is, quiet and settled on the inside, dynamic and lively on the outside. The yoga philosophy encourages an appreciation of bodily sensations, slow stretching, and maintenance of proper posture, all of which help to prevent injury and promote health.

Flexibility

Flexibility is a basic component of physical fitness. Warm-up and cool-down periods provide the opportunity to work on stretching muscles and increasing joint ROM. A safe stretch is one that is gentle and relaxing; a little discomfort may be felt as the muscle stretches, but the discomfort should never reach the point of pain. Stretching mindfully, as in yoga, will ensure a safe stretch. Holding the position for 10 to 20 seconds and repeating the stretch 3 to 5 times will encourage optimal flexibility (ACSM, 1998).

Resistance Training

Studies suggest that people who maintain or improve their flexibility and strength are better able to perform daily activities and avoid injury and disability (Pate et al., 1995). **Resistance training** increases muscle strength and endurance, increases muscle mass, improves metabolic effi-

ciency, maintains or increases bone density, prevents limitations in performance of everyday tasks, decreases the effort required to perform these tasks, and decreases the potential for injury during physical activity.

On the average, after their early 20s people lose about one half a pound of muscle every year through lack of use. This reduction in muscle mass is largely responsible for a decrease in resting metabolic rate, which may translate into weight gain. Resistance training is recommended for the general population because it has a positive effect on many of the degenerative problems associated with the aging process (Westcott, 1993).

Every individual should try to perform activities throughout the day that stimulate muscle strength and endurance. Activities that involve lifting, carrying, or performing repetitive movement against a resistance (vacuuming, raking, shoveling, or baking bread) help preserve lean body mass. If these types of activities are not performed on a regular basis, then the guidelines for resistance training provided in Box 12-3 are suggested. These guidelines are not meant to represent workouts performed by bodybuilders and competitive weight lifters; they are not meant to result in "bulking up." The purpose of weight training from a health perspective is (1) to develop toned, healthy muscles that provide the strength to do daily activities without risk of injury and (2) to stimulate bone health.

The figures in Box 12-3 demonstrate several suggested resistance exercises for upper body strengthening. Resistance training for all major muscle groups is appropriate, but individuals often choose to concentrate on the upper body, because these muscles tend to be neglected in daily activity and other exercise regimens. Although many people believe that they need to do three sets of each exercise, excellent results can be attained by doing one set (Hass, Garzarella, De Hoyos, & Polloch, 2000; Westcott, 1993). The weight that is lifted should result in near muscle fatigue at the end of each set (8 to 12 repetitions) and should be performed without strain and while maintaining proper form. Once 12 repetitions can be completed easily, the resistance can be increased (by 5% or less), or the same weight can be used to do another set of 8 to 12 repetitions (ACSM, 1998). The movements should be made slowly, preferably coordinated with the breath. Slow, controlled movements result in greater benefits, lower risk of injury, and an appreciation of how the body feels as its muscles are challenged.

EXERCISE THE SPIRIT: RELAXATION RESPONSE

Exercise should not be considered merely a physical regimen with objective outcomes (calories burned and repetitions completed). Exercise is also a process of challenging the body and the mind to gain a sense of well-being and a feeling of accomplishment, an opportunity to learn about who we really are.

The body mirrors the mind and soul and is much more accessible than either. If you can become proficient at

Box **12-3** **Resistive Training Exercises**

CHEST PRESS (FIGURES 1 AND 2)

a. Lie on bench with feet flat on bench, or lie on the floor with knees bent, feet flat, whichever is more comfortable.

b. Hold weights near shoulders with elbows out and palms facing away from body.

c. Exhale while extending arms straight up, following an "A" pattern with weights touching at peak.

d. Slowly lower weights back to original position while inhaling

e. Repeat 8 to 12 times.

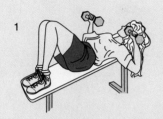

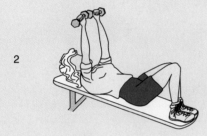

CHEST FLY (FIGURES 3 AND 4)

a. Lie on bench with feet flat on bench, or lie on the floor with knees bent, feet flat, whichever is more comfortable.

b. With palms facing each other, extend arms above chest, keeping elbows slightly bent at all times.

c. Inhale and lower arms perpendicularly away from body until arms are out of peripheral vision.

d. Exhale while returning to starting position by visualizing arms hugging a barrel that is lying on the chest.

e. Repeat 8 to 12 times.

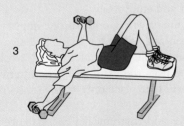

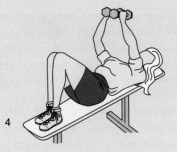

BENT OVER ROW (FIGURES 5 AND 6)

a. Bend at waist while supporting body with one hand (on table, bench, etc.) and holding weight with other in an overhand grip.

b. Keep knees bent while weight is hanging perpendicular to torso.

c. Slowly pull weight up to chest as if starting a lawn mower, exhaling and keeping elbow away from body.

d. Slowly lower weight back to starting position while inhaling.

e. Repeat 8 to 12 times on each side.

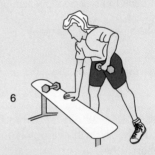

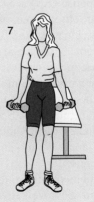

DUMBBELL CURL (FIGURES 7 AND 8)

a. Stand or sit with weights held at sides in an underhand grip, keeping elbows close to body and upper arms stationary.

b. Curl weight to chin or upper chest while exhaling.

c. Inhale while slowly lowering weights.

d. Keep back straight through duration of motion.

e. Repeat 8 to 12 times.

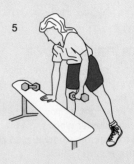

Box **12-3** Resistive Training Exercises *cont'd*

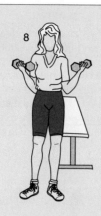

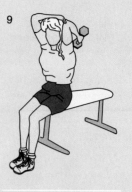

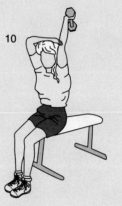

TRICEPS EXTENSION (FIGURES 9 AND 10)
a. While seated or standing in neutral back position, lift hand holding weight straight above head and in alignment with ear.
b. Keeping upper arm tight, slowly bend elbow to lower weight between shoulder blades.
c. Use free hand to support elbow and to prevent movement in upper arm.
d. Raise weight back to its original position by straightening arm and exhaling.
e. Repeat 8 to 12 times on each side.

listening to your body, you will eventually hear from your whole self (Sheehan, 1994).

Most people understand the physical benefits of exercise and some people enjoy the challenge of being physically active, but few realize the learning potential inherent in physical activity. Success in embracing a physically active lifestyle may involve a change in focus from the mechanics of exercise to an appreciation for how it feels and what it means to move. Physical activity can be time spent in meditation that fuels both the body and the spirit.

The **relaxation response** (RR) is an inborn set of physiological changes that offset those of the fight-or-flight (stress) response. When elicited, the RR results in a "letting go" of physical, emotional, and mental tension. The RR is a physiological response inborn in everyone and, although it can sometimes occur without the individual being aware of it, people generally need to develop techniques that help them let go on a more regular basis. Some techniques that are used commonly to elicit the RR include diaphragmatic breathing, meditation, imagery, mindfulness, yoga stretching, and repetitive exercise.

The RR can be combined with exercise to facilitate the release of tension and improve self-awareness and the feeling of well-being. However, a shift in attitude about exercise is also involved, with the focus becoming the process and awareness of movement. Successful elicitation

of the RR involves two basic components: (1) a repetitive focus (the breath, a mantra, and the cadence or rhythm of physical activity) and (2) a nonjudgmental attitude (about everyday thoughts and the quality of performance) (Benson & Stuart, 1992). Berger and Owen (1988) have developed exercise characteristics that facilitate stress reduction and support an exercise environment that allows the successful elicitation of the RR. Activities must:

- Be pleasant and enjoyable
- Be noncompetitive (Competition implies judgment about the self and others.)
- Be predictable (Elicitation of the RR involves a shift in awareness from the external to the internal environment that will take place only with a sense of safety and reliability.)
- Be repetitive and rhythmical (The cadence of activity provides a focus for awareness.)
- Facilitate abdominal breathing (Watching the breath serves to anchor thoughts in the moment; in combination with cadence, it provides a focused awareness.)
- Continue for 20 to 30 minutes at a comfortable intensity on most days of the week (This continuity restores a sense of serenity.)

All forms of exercise can be used to gain this experience. As discussed, yoga involves mindful stretching with a breathing focus, providing an environment for successful elicitation of the RR. Tai Chi is another exercise practice with roots in Eastern philosophy. Known as *moving meditation*, Tai Chi combines movement with focused awareness, involving a physical and cognitive focus for moving in choreographed forms that become a meditation.

The quality of body awareness can also be brought into a more traditional exercise practice. Aerobic exercise lends itself well to the elicitation of the RR, because it has rhythmical and repetitive form and because it facilitates abdominal breathing. The practitioner can focus on the breath rhythm, the step cadence of walking or jogging, the pedaling cadence of bicycling, or the stroke cadence of swimming. Mantras can be used to create a positive mind-set and to focus the mind in the present moment as the experience unfolds. Resistance training takes on new meaning when coordinated with the breath. Focusing on the muscles and how it feels to move through the ROM enhances the knowledge of what feels good and what does not, providing feedback on accepting physical challenge.

Exercise focus can and should vary on a day-to-day basis depending on need, mood, and intent. Some days it feels right to focus on the more physical aspects of the activity, appreciating the challenge of working harder or longer. Other exercise sessions may be more contemplative, letting creativity run, working through the tension of a lingering stressor, quieting the mind for relaxation, listening to music, or appreciating nature. Focusing on the process rather than the outcomes brings meaning and purpose to the activity and helps achieve something more valuable than mere physical outcomes.

When exercise integrates mind and body, it stops being something that has to be done and instead becomes something desired. Being mindful during physical activity and exercising in the moment increases awareness. With awareness comes choices in the possibilities of self-care. Exercise for fitness of the spirit, walk for the soul, and just let the body do the work.

MONITORING THE INNER AND OUTER ENVIRONMENT

The primary purpose of exercise is to enhance health. However, because exercise involves stress to the body, the potential to cause or exacerbate health problems is inherent. When a person is not feeling well, the exercise effort should be decreased or stopped until the individual is feeling better. With an infection, a cold, or influenza, the body is under stress and overexertion will only increase that stress and possibly lengthen the healing time. The level of activity should be adjusted to accommodate how the individual feels, slowly progressing to normal workout levels until strength and energy return. This philosophy also holds true for chronic diseases such as arthritis and HIV. During an acute exacerbation, activity should be limited to necessary activities of daily living (ADLs), but on a regular basis staying active is important, adjusting activity levels as tolerated. Exercise can be a useful tool in coping with chronic illness.

Missing an occasional workout will not affect the fitness level; choosing to stop or cut back on exercise when not feeling well is the right choice. However, after missing workouts for 2 weeks, a decline in fitness is inevitable. When starting up again, resuming the activity should be slow, gradually working back to the usual level of activity. Inactivity for 3 to 5 months results in the loss of all conditioning benefits gained, and resumption of exercise involves starting over (ACSM, 1998). Being aware of the external exercise environment is also important. Extremes of heat and cold affect performance as the body adjusts to different temperatures and wind conditions. Changing the time of day for exercise (early morning or later evening are better choices for humid days), adjusting fluid intake, and varying the length of warm-up and cool-down periods will improve tolerance for environmental conditions and enhance exercise safety.

Fluid News

Proper hydration is an important component of a good fitness program. Extra fluid is needed to support physiological homeostasis during exercise, especially during hot weather. Drinking a cup of water 15 to 30 minutes before exercise is recommended. If the weather is hot or the indoor exercise area is very warm, then 5 to 12 ounces of fluid should be taken in every 15 or 20 minutes during exercise (Applegate, 1996, 2000). "Fitness water" is new on the market and is a good fluid replacement during exercise periods lasting less than 1 hour. Propel (Gatorade) and Ultima are low in calories and contain small amounts of electrolytes to help retain fluid, with flavors to encourage drinking more (Applegate, 2000). For exercise routines lasting longer than 1 hour, a sports drink with carbohydrates and electrolytes enhances performance and is recommended. This type of liquid provides muscles with energy and helps delay fatigue while meeting fluid needs. Sports drinks containing a 4% to 6% carbohydrate concentration are designed to replace carbohydrates at the proper rate during exercise. They also contain sodium, which promotes fluid retention, enhances flavor, and protects against hyponatremia, which can occur with lengthy exercise sessions. Most sports drinks provide 14 to 20 grams of carbohydrate per 8-ounce serving. The recommended intake is 5 to 12 ounces every 15 to 20 minutes. Which sports drink is the best? Several brands should be tried to determine personal preference in taste, but one should be chosen that contains approximately 50 to 80 calories per 8-ounce serving; any more and the carbohydrate concentration will inhibit fluid absorption (Applegate, 2000). Table 12-2 provides choices for sports drinks that both hydrate and energize.

SPECIAL CONSIDERATIONS

Most adults do not need to consult a physician before starting a moderate-intensity physical activity program. However, men older than 40 years of age and women older than 50 years of age who plan a vigorous program (intensity more than 60% of MHR or Vo₂ maximum) or who have either chronic disease or risk factors for chronic disease should consult an appropriate health care provider before starting exercise (Table 12-3 and Box 12-4).

People with CHD or diabetes have special exercise needs. Earlier in this chapter the ways in which exercise and physical activity positively affect primary and secondary prevention in both disease processes were discussed. Limitations in the ability to exercise are related to the severity of the disease and the signs and symptoms of intolerance. For people with CHD and DM, safety with starting a new exercise program requires supervision and guidance from knowledgeable health care providers. Before starting, these individuals should have a medical evaluation, including an exercise tolerance test (ETT) to determine functional capacity and severity of disease.

Coronary Heart Disease

Exercise plays a strong role in rehabilitation after a cardiac event such as MI, coronary artery bypass surgery, percutaneous transluminal coronary angioplasty or stent placement, and angina. Increased physical activity appears to benefit individuals from all of these groups. Benefits include the following:

- Reduction in cardiovascular mortality
- Reduction of symptoms
- Improvement in exercise tolerance and functional capacity
- Increase in the confidence and ability to carry out usual ADLs
- Improvement in psychological well-being and quality of life (Schneider, Eveker, Bronder, Meiner, & Binder, 2003; USDHHS, 2000)

Generally, people with CHD demonstrate a reduction in Vo₂ maximum and the ability to do submaximal levels of work. With exercise training, the increase in Vo₂ maximum in clients with CHD averages approximately 20% after 3

Table 12-2 Sports Drinks That Hydrate and Energize

Brand	Calories	Carbohydrates (grams)
All Sport	70	19
Cytomax	80	19
Endura	62	16
Gatorade	50	14
Hydra Fuel	70	17
Isostar	70	16
Met-Rx ORS	75	19
Perform	60	16
Powerade	70	19
PowerSurge	80	20
Race Day	63	15
XLRB	62	15

From Applegate, L. (2000). Liquid assets. *Runner's World, 35,* 30-32.

Box 12-4 Symptoms and Signs Suggestive of Cardiopulmonary Disease

1. Pain, discomfort (or other anginal equivalent) in the chest, neck, jaw, arm, or other areas that may be ischemic in nature
2. Shortness of breath at rest or with mild exertion
3. Dizziness or syncope
4. Orthopnea or paroxysmal nocturnal dyspnea
5. Ankle edema
6. Palpitations or tachycardia
7. Intermittent claudication
8. Known heart murmur
9. Unusual fatigue or shortness of breath with usual activities

These symptoms must be interpreted in the clinical context in which they appear, because they are not all specific for cardiopulmonary or metabolic disease.

From American College of Sports Medicine.(2001). *Guidelines for exercise testing and prescription* (6th ed.). Media, PA: Williams & Wilkins.

Table 12-3 ACSM Recommendation for Medical Examination and Exercise Testing Before Beginning an Exercise Program

Medical Examination and Clinical Exercise Test Recommended Before	Apparently Healthy		Increased Risk*		
	Younger[‡]	Older	No Symptoms	Symptoms	Known Disease[†]
Moderate exercise[§]	No	No	No	Yes	Yes
Vigorous exercise[¶]	No	Yes	Yes	Yes	Yes

From American College of Sports Medicine. (1995). *Guidelines for exercise testing and prescription* (5th ed.). Media, PA: Williams & Wilkins.
ACSM, American College of Sports Medicine.
*Persons with two or more risk factors or one or more signs or symptoms (see Box 12-4).
[†]Persons with known cardiac, pulmonary, or metabolic disease.
[‡]Younger implies ≤40 years of age for men, ≤50 years of age for women.
[§]Moderate exercise defined by an intensity of 40% to 60% of Vo₂ maximum, or if intensity uncertain, an effort well within the individual's current capacity and that can be comfortably sustained for a prolonged period (60 minutes), slow progression, and generally noncompetitive.
[¶]Vigorous exercise is defined by an intensity >60% of Vo₂ maximum, or if intensity is uncertain, exercise intense enough to represent a substantial cardiorespiratory challenge or result in fatigue within 20 minutes.

months. This improvement in conditioning is the result of both central (cardiac) and peripheral (muscular) changes (Thompson, 1988). Some of the most significant improvements in exercise tolerance have been noted in clients with angina. With a decrease in submaximal HR or a decrease in SBP resulting from conditioning, myocardial oxygen demand is decreased and clients are able to do a greater amount of work before reaching the anginal threshold. This boost is reflected in an observed increase in rate pressure product (RPP; HR × SBP) at the anginal threshold (Thompson, 1988). An increase in functional capacity allows for progression of exercise tolerance and progression with daily activities and leisure or vocational activities.

Appropriately prescribed and conducted exercise training programs improve exercise tolerance and physical fitness in clients with CHD. Moderate and vigorous regimens are of value, but care must be taken to determine safe exercise parameters for each individual. The parameters of the exercise prescriptions are the same as those for the general population, including frequency, intensity, duration, and mode of exercise.

Aerobic exercise improves cardiorespiratory fitness and functional capacity. Any of the aforementioned aerobic exercises are acceptable for this population, depending on the level of fitness and musculoskeletal limitations. Traditionally, resistance training was not commonly recommended for clients with CHD. The belief was that lifting weights resulted in a disproportionate rise in blood pressure, increased the myocardial oxygen demand, and increased risk of angina and MI. However, data from several studies indicate that moderate, supervised weight training is feasible, tolerable, and beneficial for clients with HTN and CHD. Strength training can keep the heart healthy by helping to control body weight, reduce cholesterol levels, and control blood sugar levels. Guidelines for determination of appropriate individual training include an aerobic capacity of at least 4 to 5 metabolic equivalents, or METS, an ejection fraction of greater than 30%, and no severe, symptomatic aortic stenosis (Merrill, 1997). However, clinical experience demonstrates that people with more severe disease can use small hand weights to increase muscle tone without risk of cardiovascular compromise.

The exercise intensity for clients who have had a cardiac event but who have not had a symptom-limited ETT should be kept at a low level based on an elevated heart rate (EHR) of 20 to 30 beats per minute above the RHR and an RPE rating of less than 12. After an ETT has been performed, intensity should then be prescribed based on 50% to 85% MHR, an RPE of 11 to 14 or below the ischemic, anginal, or arrhythmic threshold. Duration and frequency recommendations are similar to those for the general population. People who are the most deconditioned may need to exercise at lower intensities, for short durations, and more frequently throughout the day. Generally, a reasonable goal is 3 to 5 times per week for 20 to 40 minutes, plus 5 to 10 minutes each for warm-up and cool-down.

Diabetes

Exercise has long been regarded as part of the triad in the management of diabetes in conjunction with diet and medication (insulin or oral medication). In the early 1900s it was determined that exercise lowers the blood glucose concentration of people with diabetes. After the introduction of insulin, studies revealed that exercise can potentiate the hypoglycemic effect of injected insulin. More recently, findings suggest that in individuals who are in poor control (excessive blood glucose levels), exercise may induce a further increase in blood glucose levels, resulting in ketosis. On the average, people with diabetes have a lower MHR, achieve a lower cardiac output at maximal exercise, and have a higher blood pressure during exercise, resulting in lower maximal oxygen consumption (McMillan, 1975). However, these individuals can improve their exercise capacity with training and can experience the benefits related to overall fitness and cardiorespiratory training similar to the benefits gained by people without diabetes.

Apparently, both benefits and risks from exercise exist for people with diabetes. The overall goals regarding physical activity should be to teach individuals to incorporate activity into their daily life, pursue an exercise program if they wish, and develop strategies to avoid the complications of exercise (Horton, 1988).

As discussed, in addition to diet and weight loss, regular physical activity is an important modality in the prevention and treatment of NIDDM. People with NIDDM should monitor their blood glucose levels and determine their responses to exercise. However, individuals with NIDDM usually can follow the same exercise prescription parameters as those of the general population. Although the same exercise benefits can be appreciated by people with IDDM, the inherent behavior and function of endogenous insulin makes exercising a more difficult proposition for them. The major functions of insulin are to promote glucose uptake into the cells and control metabolic homeostasis during exercise, working in synergy with the counter-regulatory hormones. With exercise, insulin secretion decreases slightly and the concentration of counter-regulatory hormones increases. This increase stimulates hepatic glucose production, which balances the increased use of glucose by the working muscles, maintaining normoglycemia. However, with injected insulin the plasma insulin concentration does not decrease with exercise, hepatic glucose production does not keep up with glucose use, and a decrease in blood glucose results. In contrast, people who have poorly controlled diabetes with decreased plasma insulin concentrations already have elevated blood glucose levels, because there is insufficient insulin to assist glucose transport into cells. During exercise the liver is stimulated to produce more glucose, which causes a further elevation in blood glucose levels, worsening the hyperglycemic condition. Ketosis may also result from increased mobilization and incomplete combustion of free fatty acids in muscle cells and accelerated ketone body formation in the liver (Franz, 1987; Zinman & Vranic, 1985).

Although each person with diabetes should be evaluated and given individual exercise recommendations, the goals of an exercise program are universal:

1. Maintain or improve cardiovascular fitness to prevent or minimize long-term cardiovascular complications
2. Improve flexibility that is impaired as muscle collagen becomes glycosylated
3. Improve muscle strength, which may deteriorate as a result of neuropathy
4. Allow people with IDDM to safely participate in and enjoy physical activities or sports
5. Assist with weight control for people with NIDDM
6. Allow people with diabetes to experience and gain the same benefits and enjoyment from regular exercise as do people without diabetes (Franz, 1989)

Box 12-5 presents a list of recommendations and precautions for people with diabetes who are interested in regular physical activity and exercise.

BUILDING A RHYTHM OF PHYSICAL ACTIVITY

Participation in regular physical activity increased gradually from the 1960s to the 1980s but seems to have plateaued in recent years. The progress made toward *Healthy People 2010* physical activity goals indicates that most of the population has not embraced a physically active lifestyle (USDHHS, 2000). Although the benefits of physical activity are common to all people, patterns of physical activity vary among population subgroups defined by gender, age, racial background, income, and body fat. The following generalities are true:

- Men are more active than are women.
- Physical activity declines with age.
- Ethnic minorities are less active than are white Americans.
- Higher education and income are associated with more leisure-time activity.
- People who are obese are usually less active than their leaner counterparts (Pate et al., 1995).

| Box **12-5** | **Recommendations and Precautions for People With Diabetes Who Are Interested in Regular Physical Activity and Exercise** |

1. Notify primary care physician, ophthalmologist, and podiatrist of intent to exercise.
2. Monitor blood glucose level before and 20 to 30 minutes after exercise to determine the response to exercise.
3. Be sure blood glucose level is less than 300 mg/dl in those with IDDM or less than 400 mg/dl in those with NIDDM, and urine test results are negative for ketones (if blood glucose level is greater than 240 mg/dl). If blood glucose level is consistently equal to or greater than 250 mg/dl, improved control must be established before continuing exercise.
4. If possible, exercise approximately 1 hour after meals when blood glucose level is highest. This plan helps with weight loss, because extra food will not have to be eaten to ward off hypoglycemia. When exercising before meals, a snack may be necessary. (See Table 12-4 for suggestions on food adjustments to maintain blood glucose balance with exercise.)
5. Know the action and peak times of insulin dosage and avoid exercising at peak.
6. Consider adjusting oral medication or insulin dosage to prevent low blood glucose level during exercise. Table 12-5 shows several ways to adjust insulin for exercise. The adjustment will depend on the intensity of the exercise, how long the exercise session lasts, and the type of insulin that is acting during exercise.
7. Watch out for the hypoglycemic lag effect that may occur 12 to 24 hours after vigorous exercise; an extra snack after exercise will help.

8. Avoid injecting insulin into a muscle area that will be active during exercise; the pumping action of the muscle may speed up absorption of the insulin and cause a rapid decrease of blood glucose.
9. Use proper footwear and make frequent foot inspections.
10. Avoid high-impact activity when prone to neuropathy in the legs or feet or when there is a history of neuropathy.
11. Keep SBP below 180 to 200 mm Hg in the presence of eye or kidney disease.
12. Exercising every day is best, but at least 3 to 4 times per week. Start with 10 to 20 minutes and gradually increase to 30 to 40 minutes at 50% to 75% MHR. Continuous aerobic activity helps maintain good blood glucose control better than stop-and-go activities. Do not forget the 5-minute to 10-minute warm-up and cool-down periods.
13. Avoid high-intensity anaerobic exercise, but low- to moderate-intensity resistance training is acceptable.
14. Carry a concentrated form of carbohydrate (sugar packets, glucose tablets, or hard candy) when exercising.
15. Wear some form of diabetes identification.
16. People with NIDDM need to test blood glucose levels with exercise and potentially adjust oral medications. Consider decreasing medication if blood glucose level is less than 80 mg/dl after exercise. For weight loss, plan the best time to exercise so that snacks can be avoided (Beaser & Hill, 1995).

IDDM, insulin-dependent diabetes mellitus; *MHR,* maximum heart rate; *NIDDM,* non–insulin-dependent diabetes mellitus; *SBP,* systolic blood pressure.

Table **12-4** Food Adjustments

Duration and Intensity	Blood Glucose (mg/dl)	Suggested Food Adjustment
<30 Minutes of moderate activity **Examples: walking a mile or bicycling <30 minutes**	<100 100 to 180 >180	1 Fruit + 1 bread + 1 meat 1 Bread or 1 fruit May not need snack
30 to 60 Minutes of moderate activity **Examples: tennis, swimming, jogging, bicycling, yard work or housework**	<100 100 to 180 >180 to 240 >240	1 Fruit + 1 bread + 1 meat 1 Bread or 1 meat 1 Bread or 1 fruit May not need snack
60 Minutes of moderate- to high-intensity activity **Examples: sports, strenuous bicycling, long-distance running, heavy shoveling**	If doing strenuous activity or playing sports, consult a physician or exercise physiologist for advice on blood glucose management. Insulin adjustment may be required in addition to food adjustments (see Table 12-5). Blood glucose should be tested hourly: 1 bread or 1 fruit per hour unless blood glucose is ≥180 (snack may not be needed for that hour).	

Modified from Beaser, R. S., & Hill, J. (1995). *The Joslin guide to diabetes*. New York: Simon & Schuster.

Table **12-5** Insulin Adjustment Guidelines for Exercise

Duration of Exercise	Intensity of Exercise	% to Decrease Peaking Insulin
<30 Minutes	Low, moderate, or high	0%
30 to 60 Minutes	Moderate	10%
>60 Minutes	Moderate	20%
>60 Minutes	High	30% or more

Modified from Beaser, R. S., & Hill, J. (1995). *The Joslin guide to diabetes*. New York: Simon & Schuster.
Intensity of exercise:
Low = casual, easy (below exercise heart rate range)
Moderate = comfortable but challenging, brisk (low end of exercise heart rate range)
High = challenging, hard (high end of exercise heart rate range)
Regular insulin peak action = 2 to 4 hours
NPH/lente insulin peak action = 6 to 12 hours
Ultralente insulin peak action = 18 to 24 hours (do not adjust Ultralente insulin)

Adherence and Compliance

Physiological, behavioral, and psychological variables all influence the decision to be physically active. Each person is unique, and success with exercise over the long term comes from recognition of personal motivation or core desire and support from the social environment. Core desire defines the purpose behind putting the effort into developing and maintaining an active lifestyle; it is what motivates the individual to exercise. People should be encouraged to spend some quiet time meditating on why being physically fit is important to them.

Finding meaning and purpose in an active lifestyle can enhance behavior. Biopsychosocial and spiritual variables need to be considered in promoting physical activity. An individual's biopsychosocial factors and spiritual beliefs affect the behavioral and attitudinal factors that influence the motivation and ability to adhere to an active lifestyle. Generally, however, physical activity is more likely to be initiated and maintained if the individual:

- Perceives a net benefit
- Chooses an enjoyable activity
- Feels competent doing the activity
- Feels confident in overcoming barriers that may interfere with the activity
- Feels safe doing the activity
- Can access the activity easily on a regular basis
- Perceives no significant negative financial or social cost
- Experiences minimal musculoskeletal discomfort
- Is able to address competing time demands
- Is readily able to fit the activity into the daily schedule
- Balances the use of labor-saving devices with activities that involve physical exertion (NIH, 1998)

Educating the public about physical activity helps to provide guidelines for safe and effective exercise, to reinforce potential benefits, and to alleviate misperceptions that may interfere with the decision to change behavior. However, knowledge about exercise and the intent to exercise do not correlate well with long-term compliance. Confidence in the ability to be physically active—and the confidence that overcoming barriers produces positive benefits that are related to personal goals (self-efficacy) (Bandura, 1989)—is strongly related to participation and compliance (Figure 12-5). Exercise self-efficacy is increased when people perform exercise successfully, receive positive feedback about success, view exercise role models, and learn more about the relationships among exercise, health, and body awareness (Schlicht, Godin, & Camaione, 1999) (Case Study and Care Plan).

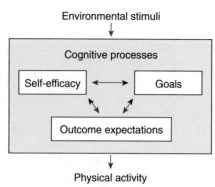

Figure 12-5 Three interacting cognitive processes of Bandura's social cognitive theory. (Modified from Dzewaltowski, D. A. [1995]. Physical actively determinants: a social-cognitive approach. *Medicine and Science in Sports and Exercise, 26,* 1395-1399.)

Creating a Climate That Supports Exercise

Clearly exercise and fitness need to be social norms. A climate that supports and encourages physical activity should be fostered. Other people and organizations in the individual's social environment can influence the adoption and maintenance of physical activity (NIH, 1996, 1998; USDHHS, 1996).

Health Care Professionals

People are more likely to increase physical activity if counseled to do so by clinicians. Clinicians should inquire about exercise habits, communicate the benefits of increased activity, assist the person in initiating activity, and provide adequate follow-up. Challenging perceived individual barriers to exercise and offering alternative viewpoints can help create new exercise paradigms. Clinicians should also serve as role models by demonstrating enthusiasm for being physically active.

Recognizing the stages of behavioral change helps in meeting people at their stage of readiness to change behavior (Prochaska, Norcross, & DiClemente, 1994). Marcus et al. (1992) demonstrated that providing information on physical activity that is designed for specific stages of readiness enables people to move from stages of contemplation and preparation into action. An individual in precontemplation is not ready to actively change behavior.

CASE STUDY

Ms. G.

Ms. G. is a 53-year-old account executive who is 2 years post-menopause, complains of insomnia, and has chronic LBP and knee pain.

History: Motor vehicle accident (2000), resulting in bone graft to left leg (her left leg is shorter than her right leg). As part of rehabilitation, Ms. G. started jogging, which was more comfortable than walking with chronic right-sided sacroiliac joint pain. She started running marathons in 2002 and continued until 2003. In 2003, she began to add more variety into exercise and decreased her running, but she still identified herself as being an athlete.

In 2004, she suffered a fall that resulted in chronic LBP and was unable to continue aerobic exercise. She began to experience depression and insomnia; exercise had been a significant coping mechanism in the past and now her whole sense of well-being is being affected. As Ms. G. attempted to rebuild her exercise practice, she would alternate between doing too much, exacerbating symptoms, and then having to stop and recuperate, reinforcing her negative self-image.

MRI showed mild arthritis in her knees.

Questions
1. What are some of her barriers to exercise?
2. How will a regular practice of mindfulness and the RR benefit her exercise practice?
3. How would she benefit from cross-training?
4. What exercise is she doing that is beneficial for helping to prevent osteoporosis?

Answers to Questions
1. Barriers to exercise:
   - Past image of self as high-level exerciser
   - Current negative self-image
   - Musculoskeletal limitations
   - Exacerbation of symptoms with excessive exercise
   - Outcome oriented versus process oriented
2. With practice of RR, mindful stretching (yoga), and being more mindful with regular exercise, Ms. G. is able gradually to accept herself in the present and let go of expectations related to past experiences. She is able to accept decreased level of exercise intensity and to adapt the idea of "less is more," listening to her body and not to mental messages. She is now enjoying the experience of being physically active rather than focusing on specific accomplishments.
3. Cross-training provides overall body conditioning and decreases risk of injury (or exacerbating existing conditions) by decreasing repetitive stress to body parts. Cross-training also provides a greater variety of choices, eliminating barriers and improving enjoyment and compliance.
4. Weight-bearing activities, such as walking, low-impact aerobics, and weight training, stress the skeleton and help stimulate bone density preservation.

After a 3-month period, Ms. G. demonstrates the following improvements:
- Frequency of low back and knee pain has decreased from constant to 2 to 4 times per week; although she still has some discomfort, the intensity is less and it interferes less with her life.
- Insomnia is decreased from 2 to 3 times per week to once per month; she has stopped taking sleep medications.
- She experiences decreased depression and anxiety.
- She is less unhappy about weight gain and more accepting of who she is.

LBP, low back pain; *MRI,* magnetic resonance imaging.

CARE PLAN

Exercise Self-Efficacy

(Related to Ms. G. Case Study)

Nursing Diagnosis Altered Sleep Pattern related to low back pain, depression, and recent weight gain.

MEDICATIONS

- Serax (oxazepam) 30 mg, 4 to 6 times a week; Ginkgo biloba

DEFINING CHARACTERISTICS

- Insomnia
- Chronic low back and knee pain
- Depression
- Upset about recent weight gain of 10 lbs ($61\frac{1}{2}$ inches, 118 lbs); sees ideal body weight as 108 lbs

EXPECTED OUTCOMES

- Walking, treadmill, bicycling, and low-impact aerobics (30 minutes, 3 to 4 times per week)
- Weights 3 to 4 times per week
- Stretching 3 to 4 times per week
- Daily RR
- Build mindfulness into exercise practice

EXERCISE PRACTICE

- Treadmill and walking daily for 30 minutes
- Weights 2 to 3 times per week
- Yoga and stretching daily

RR, relaxation response.

This person may respond better to support and information about the benefits of changing behavior rather than being placed in an action environment. The decision to change may come gradually. After a person has made the commitment to change, the action phase lasts about 6 months. Continued follow-up throughout the action phase into maintenance is valuable in helping the individual stay committed until the termination phase is reached and the behavior is secure.

Family and Friends

Social support can be a valuable resource for behavioral change. Significant others or friends can serve as buddies, providing a source of companionship and motivation. These people can offer to share daily responsibilities (household chores) to free up time for exercise. Parents can support their children's activity by having family outings and providing transportation, praise, and encouragement. Joining a fitness club or an exercise group at work provides various forms of stimulation and socialization, which increases the potential for new friendships grounded in an appreciation of the rewards of exercise.

Work Sites

In reviewing progress toward *Healthy People 2010* goals, fitness opportunities at the work site are one of the few bright spots. Employers can provide space for fitness facilities or offer payroll deductions for affiliated health facilities. Companies can make time and programs available to encourage people to be active during work hours. Motivational signs can be placed strategically around the facility that encourage stair climbing and walking or bicycling to work. Secured areas for bikes and shower facilities encourage people to take advantage of building exercise into their work-related schedules.

Schools

Schools are one of the most important resources for increasing physical activity. Strategies must be developed to facilitate increased activity in children, because it is clear that children are becoming less active and more obese. Schools are providing less opportunity and poorer quality time for physical activity during school hours. All schools should provide opportunities for physical activity that:
- Are appropriate and enjoyable for children of all skill levels and are not limited to competitive sports or physical education classes
- Appeal to girls and boys and to children from diverse backgrounds
- Are offered on a daily basis
- Can serve as a foundation for activities throughout life (NIH, 1996a)

Schools can also serve as a resource for the community. Expanding operating hours at either end of the school day creates a safe, indoor environment for hall walking.

Communities

Participation in regular physical activity at the community level depends in large part on the availability and proximity of facilities and safe environments. Community government agencies, local health agencies, schools, and places of worship have the potential to provide activity resources to the population at large. Churches seem to have been particularly successful in reaching ethnic minorities and elderly adults. Making neighborhoods safe for outdoor activities can have a major effect on improving activity habits, especially among low socioeconomic and disadvantaged populations, who report lower levels of daily physical activity.

Recognizing that many of the previous recommendations require a financial commitment, government agencies must respond to reports by health agencies and establish public policies that support the importance of physical activity for the general population. Individuals should make a personal commitment to be physically active, but that commitment needs to be supported by a social and political environment that values this type of lifestyle choice.

SUMMARY

It is important that people incorporate increased activity into their lifestyles on a long-term basis; exercise in the short term is of little overall benefit. Helping them gain the knowledge (benefits of exercise and recommended parameters for exercise), skills (self-monitoring), and attitude (core desire) improves compliance. People need to be motivated enough to start, enjoy the activity enough to want to continue, and appreciate the value enough to start again if they lapse. Lapses should be anticipated to avoid the unrealistic sense of total success or total failure. Behavioral change is cyclical rather than linear; success often comes with repeated movement through stages of change (Prochaska et al., 1994), and it helps to explore the reasons for the lapse and to view the lapse as a learning experience rather than a failure. The goal is to prevent a relapse that results in a more permanent noncompliance.

The benefits and enjoyment derived from a physically active lifestyle have a significant effect on the quality of life. However, this lifestyle is successful only when it is supported by a degree of self-awareness and self-care. People must realize that they are worth the effort of doing something good for themselves, that they have the perceived right to be happy and healthy, and that exercise can help them achieve that end. By adding a mind-body component to physical activity and not regarding it solely as a physical regimen, people can experience true health rather than mere fitness. A great deal of bodily exercise is not required; 30 minutes a day can make a significant difference. Success comes with building a rhythm of physical activity into everyday life. Suggestions for a lifestyle approach to exercise include:

- Something is better than nothing.
- Attempt small changes over time (gradualism).
- Emphasize moderate intensity.
- Make activity an integral part of life.
- Focus on the process rather than the outcome.
- Clinicians can provide a knowledgeable, supportive, and enthusiastic environment to encourage the change to a healthier, more active way of life.

ADDITIONAL STUDY MATERIAL

Study Questions in the back of the book, see page 663.

evolve WEB SITE MATERIALS

These materials are located on the book's Web site at http://evolve.elsevier.com/Edelman/.

- WebLinks
- Content Updates

REFERENCES

Aisenbrey, J. (1987). Exercise in the prevention and management of osteoperosis. *Physical Therapy 67*, 1100-1104.

American Academy of Child and Adolescent Psychiatry. (2004). Obesity in Children and Teens, No. 79. Retrieved April 18, 2005, from http://www.aacap.org/publications/factsfam/79.htm.

American College of Sports Medicine. (1997). *Exercise management for persons with chronic diseases and disabilities*. Champaign, IL: Human Kinetics.

American College of Sports Medicine. (1998). The recommended quantity and quality of exercise for developing and maintaining cardiorespiratory and muscular fitness, and flexibility in healthy adults. *Medicine and Science in Sports and Exercise, 30*, 975-986.

Andersen, R. E., Wadden, T. A., Bartlett, S. J., Zemel, B., Verde, T. J., & Franckowiak, S. C. (1999). Effects of lifestyle activity vs. structured anaerobic exercise in obese women. *Journal of the American Medical Association, 281*, 335-340.

Applegate, L. (1996). Fluid news you can use. *Runner's World 31*, 26-28.

Applegate, L. (2000). Liquid assets. *Runner's World, 35*, 30-32.

Arroll, B., & Beaglehole, R. (1992). Does physical activity lower blood pressure? A critical review of the clinical trials. *Journal of Clinical Epidemiology, 45*, 439-447.

Bandura, A. (1989). Human agency in social cognitive theory. *The American Psychologist, 9*, 1175-1184.

Bean, A. (1996). The truth about burning fat. *Runner's World, 31*, 47-50.

Beaser, R. S., & Hill, J. (1995). *The Joslin guide to diabetes*. New York: Simon & Schuster.

Benson, H., & Stuart, E. (1992). *The wellness book*. New York: Simon & Schuster.

Berarducci, A., Burns, P. A., Lengacher, C. A., Sellers, E. (2000). Health-promoting educational practices related to osteoporosis. *Applied Nursing Research, 13*(4), 173-180.

Berger, B., & Owen, D. (1988). Stress reduction and mood enhancement in four exercise modes: Swimming, body conditioning, hatha yoga and fencing. *Research Quarterly for Exercise and Sport, 59*, 148-159.

Bernstein, L., Henderson, B. E., Hanisch, R., Sullivan-Halley, J., & Ross, R. K. (1994). Physical exercise and reduced risk of breast cancer in young women. *Journal of the National Cancer Institute, 86*, 1403-1408.

Blair, S. N., Kampert, J. B., Kohl, H. W., Barlow, C. E., Macera, C. A., Paffenbarger, R. S., & Gibbons, L. W. (1996). Influences of cardiorespiratory fitness and other precursors on cardiovascular disease and all-cause mortality in men and women. *Journal of the American Medical Association, 42*, 289-296.

Blair, S. N., Kohl, H. W. III, Paffenburger, R. S., Clark, D. G., Cooper, K. H., and Gibbons, L. W. (1989). Physical fitness and all-cause mortality: A prospective study of healthy men and women. *Journal of the American Medical Association, 262*, 2395-2401.

Blumenthal, J., Babyak, M. A., Moore, K. A., Craighead, W. E., Herman, S., Khatri, P., et al. (1999). Effects of exercise training on older patients with major depression. *Archives of Internal Medicine, 159*, 2349-2356.

Blumenthal, J., Emory, C. F., Madden, D. J., George, L. K., Coleman, R. E., Riddle, M. W., et al. (1989). Cardiovascular and behavioral effects of aerobic exercise training in healthy older men and women. *Journal of Gerontology, 44*, 147-157.

Blumenthal, J., Williams, R. S., Williams, R. B., & Wallace, A. G. (1980). Effects of exercise on the type A (coronary prone) behavior pattern. *Psychosomatic Medicine, 42*, 289-296.

Borg, G. A. (1973). Perceived exertion: A note on history and methods. *Medicine and Science in Sports and Exercise, 5*, 90-93.

Borg, G. A. (1982). Psychophysical basis of perceived exertion. *Medicine and Science in Sports and Exercise, 14*, 377-381.

Brawley, L., Rejeski, W., & Lutes, L. (2000). A group-mediated cognitive-behavior intervention for increasing adherence to physical activity in older adults. *Journal of Applied Biobehavioral Research, 5*, 47-65.

Brown, D. R., Wang, Y., Ward, A., Ebbeling, C. B., Fortlage, L., Puleo, E., et al. (1995).

Chronic psychological effects of exercise and exercise plus cognitive strategies. *Medicine and Science in Sports and Exercise, 27,* 765-775.

Centers for Disease Control and Prevention. (2000). Overweight need to step up exercise regimens. *Morbidity and Mortality Weekly Report, 49,* 326-330.

DeBusk, R. F., Stenestrand, V., Sheehan, M., & Haskell, W. L. (1990). Training effects of long versus short bouts of exercise in healthy subjects. *American Journal of Cardiology, 65,* 1010-1013.

DeCherney, A. (1996). Bone-sparing properties of oral contraceptives. *American Journal of Obstetrics and Gynecology, 174,* 15-20.

Dennis, K. E. (2004). Weight management in women. *Nursing Clinics of North America, 39,* 231-241.

Durstine, J. L., & Haskell, W. L. (1994). Effects of exercise training on plasma lipids and lipoproteins. *Exercise and Sport Sciences Review, 22,* 477-521.

Dyer, J., & Crouch, J. (1988). Effects of running and other activities on moods. *Perceptual and Motor Skills, 67,* 43-50.

Fagard, R. H., & Tipton, C. M. (1994). Physical activity, fitness, and hypertension. In C. Bouchard, R. J. Shephard, & T. Stephens (Eds.), *Physical activity, fitness and health: International proceedings and consensus statement.* Champaign, IL: Human Kinetics.

Fiatarone, M. A., O'Neill, E. F., Ryan, N. D., Clements, K. M., Solares, G. R., & Nelson, M. E. (1994). Exercise training and nutritional supplementation for physical frailty in very elderly people. *New England Journal of Medicine, 330,* 1769-1775.

Folkins, C. H. (1976). Effects of physical training on mood. *Journal of Clinical Psychology, 32,* 385-388.

Franklin, B. (1993). How much exercise is enough? (p. 471-476). *Encyclopedia Britannica.* Encyclopedia Britannica, Inc.

Franz, M. (1987). Exercise and the management of diabetes mellitus. *Journal of the American Dietetic Association, 87,* 872-880.

Franz, M. (1989). Conclusions. *Diabetes Spectrum, 1,* 247-250.

Geffken, D., Cushman, M., Burke, G., Polak, J., Sakkinen, P., & Tracy, R. (2001). Association between physical activity and markers of inflammation in a healthy elderly population. *American Journal Epidemiology, 153,* 242-250.

Goff, D., & Dimsdale, J. (1985). The psychological effect of exercise. *Journal of Cardiopulmonary Rehabilitation, 5,* 234-240.

Haskell, W. L., Leon, A. S., Caspersen, C. J., Froelicher, V. F., Hagberg, J. M., Harlan, W. (1992). Cardiovascular benefits and assessment of physical activity and physical fitness in adults. *Medicine and Science in Sports and Exercise, 24*(6 Suppl.), S201-S220.

Hass, C. J., Garzarella, L., De Hoyos, D., & Polloch, M. (2000). Single versus multiple sets in long-term recreational weightlifters. *Medicine and Science in Sports and Exercise, 32,* 235-242.

Helmrich, S. P., Ragland, D., Leung, R., & Paffenbarger, R. (1991). Physical activity and reduced occurrence of non-insulin-dependent diabetes mellitus. *New England Journal of Medicine, 325,* 147-152.

Holloszy, J. O., Schultz, J., Kusnierkiewicz, J., Hagberg, J. M., & Ehsani, A. A. (1986). Effects of exercise on glucose intolerance and insulin resistance. *Acta Medica Scandinavica Supplementum, 711,* 55.

Horton, E. (1988). Role and management of exercise in diabetes mellitus. *Diabetes Care, 11,* 201-211.

Jakicic, J. M., Wing, R. R., Butler, B. A., & Robertson, R. J. (1995). Prescribing exercise in multiple short bouts versus one continuous bout: Effect on adherence, cardiorespiratory fitness and weight loss in overweight women. *International Journal of Obesity, 19,* 893-901.

Jin, P. (1989). Changes in heart rate, noradrenaline, cortisol and mood during Tai Chi. *Journal of Psychosomatic Research, 33,* 197-206.

Keleman, M. H., Effron, M., Valenti, S., & Stewart, K. (1990). Exercise testing combined with anti-hypertensive drug therapy. Effects on lipids, blood pressure, and left ventricular mass. *Journal of the American Medical Association, 263,* 2766-2771.

Kelly, G., & McClellan, P. (1994). Antihypertensive effects of aerobic exercise: A brief meta-analytic review of randomized controlled trials. *American Journal of Hypertension: Journal of the American Society of Hypertension, 7,* 115-119.

Kiyonaga, A., Arakawa, K., Tanaka, H., & Shindo, M. (1985). Blood pressure and hormonal responses to aerobic exercise. *Hypertension, 7,* 125-131.

Kobasa, S. (1985). Effectiveness of hardiness, exercise and social support as resources against illness. *Journal of Psychosomatic Research, 29,* 525-533.

Kohrt, W. M., Malley, M., Coggan, A., Spina, R., Ogawa, T., Ehsani, A. (1991). Effects of gender, age, and fitness level on response of Vo_2 max to training in 60-71 year olds. *Journal of Applied Physiology, 71,* 2004-2011.

Kuczmarski, R. J., Flegol, K. M., Campbell, S. M., & Johnson, C. L. (1994). Increasing prevalence of overweight among U.S. adults: The National Health and Nutrition Examination Surveys, 1960 to 1991. *Journal of the American Medical Association, 272,* 205-211.

La Forge, R. (2004). Can exercise heal low-back pain? *Idea Health & Fitness Source, 16.*

LaPerriere, A., Fletcher, M. A., Antoni, M. H., Klimas, N. G., & Schneiderman, N. (1991). Aerobic exercise training in an AIDS risk group. *International Journal of Sports Medicine, 12*(Suppl 1), S53-57.

Lee, I. M. (1994). Physical activity, fitness, and cancer. In C. Bouchard, R. J. Shephard, & T. Stephens (Eds.), *Physical activity, fitness and health: International proceedings and consensus statement.* Champaign, IL: Human Kinetics.

Leibel, R. L., Rosenbaum, M., & Hirsch, J. (1995). Changes in energy expenditure resulting from altered body weight. *New England Journal of Medicine, 332,* 621-628.

Leon, A. S. (1991). Effects of exercise conditioning on physiologic precursors of coronary heart disease. *Journal of Cardiopulmonary Rehabilitation, 11,* 46-57.

Mackinnon, L. T. (1992). *Exercise and immunology.* Champaign, IL: Human Kinetics.

Manson, J. E., Hu, F. B., Rich-Edwards, J. W., Colditz, G. A., Stampfer, M. J., Willet, W. C. (1999). A prospective study of walking as compared with vigorous exercise in the prevention of coronary disease in women. *New England Journal of Medicine, 341,* 650-658.

Marcus, B. H., Banspach, S. W., Hefebvre, R. C., Rossi, J. S., Carleton, R. A., & Abrams, D. B. (1992). Using the stages of change model to increase the adoption of physical activity among community participants. *American Journal of Health Promotion, 6,* 424-429.

McHenry, P. L., Ellestad, M. H., Fletcher, G. F., Froelicher, V., Hartley, H., Mitchell, J. H., & Froelicher, E. S. S. (1990). A special report: Statement on exercise. *Circulation, 81,* 396-398.

McMillan, D. (1975). Deterioration of the microcirculation in diabetes. *Diabetes, 24,* 944-957.

Merrill, J. (1997). Resistance training in cardiac rehabilitation. *Fitness Management Magazine, 13,* 35-37.

Mittleman, M. A., Maclure, M., Tofler, G. H., Sherwood, J. B., Goldberg, R. J., & Miller, J. E. (1993). Triggering of acute MI by heavy physical exertion: Protection against triggering by regular exertion. *New England Journal of Medicine, 329,* 1677-1683.

Morgan, W. (1973). Psychological factors influencing perceived exertion. *Medicine and Science in Sports and Exercise, 5,* 97-103.

Morganti, C. M., Nelson, M. E., Fiatarone, M. A., Dallal, G. E., Economos, C. D., Crawford, B. M., et al. (1995). Strength improvements with 1 year of progressive resistance training in older women. *Medicine and Science in Sports and Exercise, 27,* 906-912.

National Institutes of Health. (1998). *Clinical guidelines on the identification, evaluation, and treatment of overweight and obesity in adults,* Vol. 8, Pub. No. 98-4083. Bethesda, MD: Dept of Health and Human Services, National Institutes of Health, National Heart, Lung, and Blood Institute.

National Institute of Health, Concensus Development Panel. (1996). Physical activity and cardiovascular health. *Journal of the American Medical Association, 276,* 1909-1914.

Nieman, D. (1994). Exercise, upper respiratory tract infection, and the immune system. *Medicine and Science in Sports and Exercise, 26,* 128-139.

Nieman, D. (2000). Exercise soothes arthritis. *ACSM's Health and Fitness Journal, 4,* 20-27.

Nieman, D., Nehlsen-Cannarella, S. L., Markoff, P. A., Balk-Lamberton, A. J., Yang, H., Chritton, D. B. (1990). The effects of moderate exercise training on natural killer cells and acute upper respiratory tract infections. *International Journal of Sports Medicine, 11,* 467-473.

Oliveria, S. A., Kohl, H., Trichopoulos, D., & Blair, S. (1996). The association between cardiorespiratory fitness and prostate cancer. *Medicine and Science in Sports and Exercise, 28,* 97-104.

O'Sullivan, S. B. (1984). Perceived exertion: A review. *Physical Therapy, 64,* 343-346.

Ourania, M., Yvoni, H., Christos, K., & Ionannis, T. (2003). Effects of a physical activity program. The study of selected physical abilities among elderly women. *Journal of Gerontological Nursing, 29*(7), 50-55.

Packard, P. T., & Hearney, R. P. (1997). Medical nutrition therapy for patients with osteoporosis. *Journal of the American Dietetic Association, 97*(4), 414-417.

Paffenbarger, R. S., Lee, I. M., & Leung, R. (1994). Physical activity and personal characteristics associated with depression and suicide in American college men. *Acta Acta Psychiatrica Scandinavica Supplementum, 89*(377 Supp.) 16-22.

Paffenbarger, R. S., Wing, A. L., Hyde, R. T., & Jung, D. C. (1983). Physical activity and incidence of hypertension in college alumni. *American Journal of Epidemiology, 117,* 245-257.

Pate, R. R., Baranowski, T., Dowda, M., & Trost, S. (1996). Tracking of physical activity in young children. *Medicine and Science in Sports and Exercise, 28,* 92-96.

Pate, R. R., Pratt, M., Blair, S. N., Haskell, W. L., Macera, C. A., Bouchard, C., et al. (1995). Physical activity and public health: A recommendation from the Centers for Disease Control and Prevention and the American College of Sports Medicine. *Journal of the American Medical Association, 273,* 402-407.

Pedersen, B., & Ullum, H. (1994). NK cell response to physical activity: Possible mechanisms of action. *Medicine and Science in Sports and Exercise, 26,* 140-146.

Pereira, M. A., Kriska, A. M., Joswiak, M. L., Zimmet, P. Z., Gareeboo, H., Chitson, P., et al. (1995). Physical inactivity and glucose intolerance in the multi-ethnic island of Mauritius. *Medicine and Science in Sports and Exercise, 27,* 1626-1634.

Prochaska, J. O., Norcross, J. C., & DiClemente, C. C. (1994). *Changing for good.* New York: William Morrow.

Rigsby, L., Dishman, R., Jackson, A., Maclean, G., & Raven, P. (1992). Effects of exercise training on men seropositive for the human immunodeficiency virus. *Medicine and Science in Sports and Exercise, 24,* 6-12.

Rockhill, B., Willett, W. C., Hunter, D. J., Manson, J. E., Hankinson, S. E., & Colditz, G. A. (1999). A prospective study of recreational physical activity and breast cancer risk. *Archives of Internal Medicine, 159,* 2290-2296.

Roman, O., Camuzzi, A., Villalon, E., & Klenner, C. (1981). Physical training program in arterial hypertension: A long-term prospective follow-up. *Cardiology, 67,* 230-243.

Schatz, M. P. (1984). Living with your lower back. *Yoga Journal,* 36-45.

Schatz, M. P. (1985). Yoga relief for arthritis. *Yoga Journal,* 29-34.

Schlicht, J., Godin, J., & Camaione, D. N. (1999). Build self-efficacy to promote exercise adherence. *ACSM's Health & Fitness Journal, 3*(6), 27-31.

Schneider, J. K., Eveker, A., Bronder, D. R., Meiner, S.E., & Binder, E. F. (2003). Exercise training program for older adults. *Journal of Gerontological Nursing, 29,* 21-31.

Schneider, J. K., Mercer, G., Herning, M., Smith, C., & Prypah, M. D. (2004). Promoting exercise behavior in older adults. *Journal of Gerontological Nursing, 30*(4), 45-53.

Sheehan, G. (1994). The best of Sheehan: Changing course. *Runner's World, 29,* 16.

Skinner, J. S., Hustler, R., Bergsteinova, V., & Buskirk, R. (1973). The validity and reliability of a rating scale of perceived exertion. *Medicine and Science in Sports and Exercise, 5,* 94-96.

Slemeada, C. W. (1997). Prevention of hip fracture: Risk factor modification. *American Journal of Medicine, 103*(2A), 658-735.

Smutok, M., Skrinar, G., & Pandolf, K. (1980). Exercise intensity: Subjective regulation by perceived exertion. *Archives of Physical Medicine and Rehabilitation, 61,* 569-574.

Spence, D., Galentino, M. L., Mossberg, K., & Zimmerman, S. (1990). Progressive resistance exercise: Effect on muscle function and anthropometry of a select AIDS population. *Archives of Physical Medicine and Rehabilitation, 71,* 644-648.

Staal, J. B., Hlobil, H., Twist, J. W., Smid, T., Koke, A. J., & van Mechelen, W. (2004). Graded activity for low back pain in occupational health care. *Annals of Internal Medicine, 140*(2), 77-84.

Stefanick, M. L., & Wood, P. D. (1994). Physical activity, lipid and lipoprotein metabolism, and lipid transport. In C. Bouchard, R. J. Shephard, & T. Stephens (Eds.), *Physical activity, fitness and health: International proceedings and consensus statement.* Champaign, IL: Human Kinetics.

Stephens, T., & Craig, C. L. (1990). *The well-being of Canadians: Highlights of the 1988 Campbell's survey.* Ottawa: Canadian Fitness and Lifestyle Research Institute.

Thompson, P. D. (1988). The benefits and risks of exercise training in patients with chronic coronary artery disease. *Journal of the American Medical Association, 259,* 1537-1540.

Tipton, C. M. (1984). Exercise and resting blood pressure. In H. M. Eckert & H. J. Montoye (Eds.), *Exercise and health.* Champaign, IL: Human Kinetics.

Tremblay, A., Despres, J. P., & Bouchard, C. (1985). The effects of exercise training on energy balance and adipose tissue morphology and metabolism. *Sports Medicine, 2,* 223-233.

U.S. Department of Health and Human Services. (1996). *Physical activity and health: A report of the surgeon general.* Atlanta: U.S. Department of Health and Human Services, Centers for Disease Control and Prevention, National Center for Chronic Disease Prevention and Health Promotion.

U.S. Department of Health and Human Services. (2000, Jan.). *Healthy people 2010* (Vol. 1 and 2, Conference ed.). Washington, DC: Centers for Disease Control and Prevention, President's Council on Physical Fitness and Sports.

Wei, M., Gibbons, L. W., Kampert, J. B., Nichaman, M. Z., & Blair, S. N. (2000). Low cardiorespiratory fitness and physical activity as predictors of mortality in men with type 2 diabetes. *Annals of Internal Medicine, 132,* 605-611.

Westcott, W. L. (1993). Strength for everyone. *Fitness Management,* 32-36.

Williams, P. T. (1996). High density lipoprotein cholesterol and other risk factors for coronary heart disease in female runners. *New England Journal of Medicine, 334,* 1298-1303.

Williams, M. A., & Eickhoff, J. (2002). Exercise prescription for older women. *Women's health in primary care, 15*(10), 640.

Williford, H. N., Scharff-Olson, M., & Blessing, D. (1993). Exercise prescription for women. *Sports Medicine, 15,* 299-311.

Women's health in primary care. (2002). Vol. 5, No. 10.

Woods, J. A., & Davis, J. M. (1994). Exercise, monocyte/macrophage function, and cancer. *Medicine and Science in Sports and Exercise, 26,* 147-156.

Zinman, B., & Vranic, M. (1985). Diabetes and exercise. *Medical Clinics of North America, 69,* 145-157.

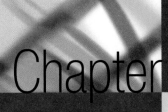

Chapter 13

JUNE ANDREWS HOROWITZ
CAROL LYNN MANDLE

Stress Management

objectives

After completing this chapter, the reader will be able to:

- Define stress and stressor.
- Differentiate eustress and distress.
- Evaluate potential physical, psychological, social, and behavioral stressors.
- Identify pathophysiology of the stress response and effects on health and illness.
- Analyze primary and secondary appraisals of stress.
- Propose stress management interventions that can be used in clinical practice.
- Discuss the nurse's role in stress management.
- Develop a nursing care plan for stress management.

key terms

Affirmation	Healthy diet	Social support
Assertive communication	Healthy pleasures	Spiritual practice
Cognitive restructuring	Humor	Stress
Coping	Journal writing	Stress management
Distress	Mini-relaxations	Stress warning signs
Empathy	Primary appraisal	Stressor
Eustress	Relaxation response	Values clarification
Exercise	Secondary appraisal	
Goal setting	Sleep hygiene	

THINK About It

Do We Live to Work or Work to Live?

When asked about yourself, what is your first response? Do you say what you do for work or do you describe your characteristics? For most of us, our work roles, including being students, define us to a great extent. For most adults in the United States and many other societies, employment is a primary source of income and social connection; working also contributes to a personal sense of accomplishment. However, how much work is too much? Americans take fewer yearly vacation days than their counterparts in other industrial countries, and workplace pressures can increase risk for a variety of disorders. Work-related stress can be a real problem.

1. What aspects of work typically create stress?
2. How do people manage work-related stress? Which strategies are effective and which strategies increase health risks?
3. What health-promotion strategies could you implement to reduce your own work-related stress?
4. What could you do to promote workers' health in your own practice?

Stress is an excellent paradigm for understanding the relationships among the determinants of health, the leading health indicators, and health outcomes. Stress has been shown to cause or exacerbate many of the leading health problems in the United States today, such as those related to obesity, alcohol and drug abuse, and sexually transmitted diseases (U.S. Department of Health and Human Services [USDHHS], 2000). Consequently, helping individuals, families, and communities to find more effective ways to respond to stress is an important health-promotion goal.

Stress management has been an effective intervention for health promotion, disease prevention, and symptom management. Stress management strategies such as relaxation and imagery, self-monitoring, goal setting, cognitive restructuring, and problem solving have long been the staple of community programs, including Alcoholics Anonymous, Smoke Enders, and Weight Watchers. These strategies help people to modify health risk behaviors and thereby improve quality of life. However, current national health data indicate the need for continued and expanded use of these modalities across the life span. Unfortunately, although the United States' health care system provides excellent, expensive, heroic care, it provides poor quality low-cost preventive care, including stress management. Moreover, to ameliorate many harmful effects of stress, community-level health promotion is essential. Even though shifting focus from providing acute care for individuals to enhancing health of communities requires a revolution in our health care delivery systems and outlook, successful community health-promotion initiatives hold promise for the future (Easterling, Gallagher, & Lodwick, 2003).

The goal of **stress management** is to improve quality of life by increasing healthy, effective coping, thereby reducing unhealthy consequences of distress. This process produces a dynamic interaction of mind, body, and spirit, which affects not only physical health and well-being, but also cognitive and emotional states and behavior; therefore, stress management is an essential tool for expert nursing practice. Nursing's perspective on the human being that recognizes mind, body, and spirit and use of critical reasoning to examine multiple factors contributing to symptom development provides a valuable contribution to meeting the goals of *Healthy People 2010*. Stress management has strong potential for influencing all of the following leading health indicators in *Healthy People 2010*: physical activity, obesity, tobacco use, substance abuse, responsible sexual behavior, mental health, injury and violence, environmental quality, immunization, and access to health care (USDHHS, 2000). (See Chapter 1 for additional discussion of *Healthy People 2010*.) This chapter outlines the psychophysiological aspects of stress, examines strategies shown to mediate its harmful effects, reviews clinical situations in which stress management has been effective, and explores the unique perspective nurses bring that help clients identify healthy stress management strategies.

SOURCES OF STRESS

A **stressor** is any psychological, environmental, or physiological stimulus that disrupts homeostasis (Bartol & Courts, 2000; Black & Garbutt, 2002), thereby requiring change or adaptation. This definition underscores two important ideas: even welcome events are stressors because they precipitate change, and stress is not intrinsically bad or unhealthy. Stress is an essential component of being alive.

Individuals encounter a variety of physical, psychological, social, spiritual, and environmental stressors. Stressors range from health and illness experiences such as childbirth, physical illness, trauma, or blood loss; to activities of daily living such as caring for children, meeting work deadlines, and cleaning or repairing the house; to less common events such as taking a critical examination, experiencing the death of a relative, losing possessions in a fire, losing a job, getting a divorce, or getting married. Stressors can be organized into three categories, (1) stressors over which people have no control (extrinsic factors), such as the weather, a traffic jam, or the death of a spouse, (2) stressors that individuals can modify by changing their environment, social interactions, or behaviors, and (3) stressors created or exacerbated (intrinsic factors) by poor time management, procrastination, poor communication, catastrophic negative thinking (expecting the worst), or struggling with self-defeating behaviors. Stress is a person-environment process in which the person appraises a situation as taxing or as exceeding an individual's resources and endangering well-being (Stuart & Wells-Federman, 2000). Appraisal is an important concept that helps to explain why two people react in different ways to the same situation.

The example of Ms. Smith and Ms. Jones is a case in point. Both individuals are about to become residents of the nursing home in their hometown. Ms. Smith perceives this move as an opportunity to increase the ease of her socializations and activities of daily living and is looking forward to making new friends and participating in new recreational activities. In contrast, Ms. Jones views this move as an abandonment by her family and fears the care will be inadequate. Although the event is the same for both Ms. Smith and Ms. Jones, the physiological and psychosocial consequences will not be the same because there are differences in the way in which each perceives the situation.

Stress is the physical, psychological, social, or spiritual effect of life's pressures and events. Stress is an interactive process that involves "recognition, perception, and adaptation to the loss or the threat of loss of homeostasis or well-being" (Cahill, 2001, p. 230). Canadian physiologist Dr. Hans Selye (1982) demonstrated that, to a certain extent, stress can be challenging and useful, which he identifies as **eustress.** Selye also observed that when stress becomes chronic or excessive, the body is unable to adapt and maintain homeostasis and thus coined the term **distress.** Stress can be both useful and harmful. As stress increases, efficiency and performance also increase, but not endlessly. As illustrated in Figure 13-1, at a certain point performance

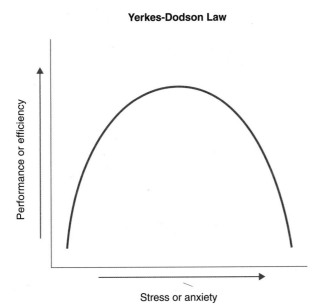

Figure 13-1 Yerkes-Dodson law. (Modified from Benson, H. [1987]. *Your maximum mind.* New York: Times Books.)

HOT Topics

RELATIONSHIP BETWEEN STRESS AND DEVELOPMENT OF BREAST CANCER AND SURVIVORSHIP

Nurses appreciate the multiple factors in the development of breast cancer and other diseases. Studies exploring the relationship between stress and breast cancer demonstrate a relationship among stress (personality traits, stressful life events, and responses to stress), the immune system, genetics, and environmental factors. The physiological influences of stress in breast cancer may be mediated by the immune system. Although women may be unable to prevent stress in their lives, they can learn stress management strategies. Dealing positively with stress may improve the quality of life for individuals and their families with or at risk for breast cancer.

Surviving breast cancer poses ongoing challenges. Uncertainty about recurrence can persist long after diagnosis and conclusion of treatment. Triggers of uncertainty include social and environmental factors, such as hearing about someone else's cancer and learning about contradictory research findings, and personal factors such as a new ache or pain. This kind of uncertainty has been found across ethnic and racial groups. Sensitivity to chronic uncertainty stress after diagnosis and conclusion of treatment can assist nurses to help clients to identify, monitor, and manage problematic signs of emergent stress.

From Bryla, C. M. (1996). Relationship between stress and the development of breast cancer: A literature review. *Oncology Nursing Forum, 23*(3), 441-448; Gil, K. M., Mishel. M. H., Belyea. M., Germino, B., Porter, L. S., LaNey, I. C., et al. (2004). Triggers of uncertainty about recurrence and long-term treatment side effects in older African American and Caucasian breast cancer survivors. *Oncology Nursing Forum, 31*(3), 633-639.

and efficiency start to decrease significantly if stress continues unabated. It is important to understand the many causes of stress and the negative physical, psychosocial, and spiritual consequences of distress. Understanding many-sided sources of stress provides the rationale for a multifaceted approach to its management. (See Hot Topics Box.)

PHYSICAL, PSYCHOLOGICAL, SOCIOBEHAVIORAL, AND SPIRITUAL CONSEQUENCES OF STRESS
Physiological Effects of Stress

An individual's response to stress provides a model to examine changes across the biopsychosocial-spiritual domains. In response to a perceived threat (i.e., stressor), the body prepares to meet the challenge. Perception of threat stimulates a physiological pattern of neuroendocrine activation and behavioral changes mediated by the central nervous system (Figure 13-2) (Bartol & Courts, 2000; Black & Garbutt, 2002; Cahill, 2001; Wells-Federman et al., 1995). In most cases this reaction is an adaptive, short-term, acute response to a stressor. First termed the fight-or-flight response (Cannon, 1914) and later called the stress response (Selye, 1982), the individual's reaction to a real or imagined threat prepares the body for emergency reaction and fosters survival in circumstances of immediate, time-limited threat. The hypothalamus signals the sympathetic nervous system to release epinephrine and norepinephrine, along with other related hormones. A state of arousal results that is characterized by increased metabolism, pulse, blood pressure, respiration, and muscle tension (The Mind Body Medical Institute, n.d.b). This physiological arousal proceeds along three main pathways: (1) the musculoskeletal

system, (2) the autonomic nervous system, and (3) the psychoneuroendocrine system.

The musculoskeletal system responds by increasing tension and tone. At the same time, the autonomic nervous system, via the sympathetic branch, orchestrates a generalized arousal that includes increases in heart rate, blood pressure, and respiratory rate. Additionally, a heightened awareness of the environment is triggered, and blood shifts from the visceral organs to the large muscle groups. Concurrently the psychoneuroendocrine system stimulates the hypothalamic–pituitary–adrenal axis and the secretion of corticosteroids (primarily cortisol) and other neuroendocrine substances into the systemic circulation, increasing blood glucose levels, influencing sodium retention and, in the acute phase, increasing the antiinflammatory response. Proinflammation associated with stress is emerging as a common pathway in a variety of diseases (Black & Garbutt, 2002; Esch & Stefano, 2002). Nitric oxide pathways involved in proinflammation may have cytotoxic and detrimental effects (Esch, Stefano, Fricchione, & Benson, 2002). Additionally, other hormones regulated by the psychoneu-

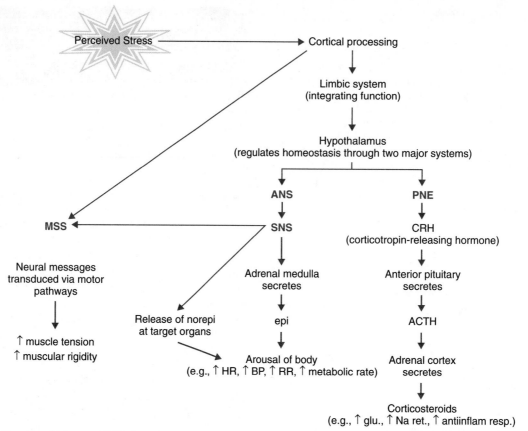

Figure 13-2 The stress response. *ACTH,* adrenocorticotropic hormone; *ANS,* autonomic nervous system; *antiinflam resp.,* antiinflammatory response; *BP,* blood pressure; *CRH,* corticotropin-releasing hormone; *epi,* epinephrine; *glu.,* blood glucose level; *HR,* heart rate; *MSS,* musculoskeletal system; *Na ret.,* sodium retention; *norepi,* norepinephrine; *PNE,* pituitary-neuroendocrine system; *RR,* respiratory rate; *SNS,* sympathetic nervous system. (From Wells-Federman, C., Stuart-Shor, E., Deckro, J., Mandle, C. L., Baim, M., & Medich, C. [1995]. The mind/body connection: The psychophysiology of many traditional nursing interventions. *Clinical Nurse Specialist, 9,* 60.)

roendocrine system system, such as reproductive and growth hormones, endorphins, and enkephalins, can be affected by chronic stress (Chapman & Gavrin, 1999; Shelby & McCance, 1998).

As mentioned, in most cases the stress response is a beneficial adaptive pattern that increases efficiency and quality of performance (The Mind Body Medical Institute, n.d.a), but it can prove maladaptive when a stressor continues indefinitely. Maladaptive stress is an enduring and sometimes self-sustaining cascade of responses that degenerate physical, psychosocial, and spiritual well-being. Studies show that maladaptive stress can cause or exacerbate disease or symptoms of diseases, such as angina, cardiac arrhythmias, pain, tension headaches, insomnia, and gastrointestinal complaints. This influence is well documented in comprehensive experimental and clinical literature (Bartol & Courts, 2000; Chapman & Gavrin, 1999; Esch & Stefano, 2002; Shelby & McCance, 1998). Not surprisingly, stress has been found to have a harmful influence on susceptibility, progress, and outcomes of cardiovascular disease (Black & Garbutt, 2002; Esch et al., 2002). The Research Highlights box presents a study of nurses' experiences as cancer survivors.

Psychological Effects of Stress

The psychological effects of stress are best illustrated by its contributory role in negative mood states, including anxiety, depression, hostility, and anger. Depressed individuals have elevated cortisol levels (Cahill, 2001). Cortisol concentration is frequently above normal in urine, plasma, and cerebrospinal fluid of clients with depression. Further investigations indicate that when a depressed individual returns to good health, cortisol secretion returns to normal (Chapman & Gavrin, 1999). These observations suggest that continual stress may cause an excessive neuroendocrine response.

At the same time, a growing body of literature documents the relationship between sustained negative mood states and increased morbidity and mortality in certain diseases. A chronic state or repeated episodes of psychological stress may trigger an inflammatory process leading to atherosclerosis. This stress-related inflammatory process may be responsible for as much as 40% of atherosclerosis among people without other known risk factors (Black & Garbutt, 2002). Clinical studies provide mounting evidence of links between psychological state and disease. For example,

research highlights

Nurses' Experiences as Cancer Survivors

The purpose of this study was to uncover dimensions of nurses' experiences of cancer survivorship. The researchers interviewed 25 registered nurses diagnosed with cancer who lived in a metropolitan area in the northeastern United States. The method was interpretive and phenomenological. The mean age was 50 years, and 20 participants had been diagnosed less than 5 years before. Five themes of cancer survivorship emerged: role ambiguity, increased compassion for clients and others, use of self-disclosure as an intervention, advocacy for change, and volunteerism. Nurses' experiences as cancer survivors shaped their clinical practice. Being a client themselves changed their practice by increasing their compassion and use of self-disclosure. Implications for practice include the value of inviting nurse cancer survivors to share their two-world perspective on compassionate care, disclosure, advocacy, volunteering, and dialogue.

Picard, C., Agretelis, J., & DeMarco, R. F. (2004). Nurse experiences as cancer survivors: Part II. *Oncology Nursing Forum, 31*(3), 537-542.

Frasure-Smith et al. (2000) reported an association between depression and increased risk for morbidity and mortality from cardiovascular disease, and Williams et al. (2000) found a relationship between increased anger and increased risk of coronary artery disease.

Research results concerning health effects of stress on frail elderly and on terminally ill individuals and family members further underscore the influence of stress on quality of life. For example, transition from rehabilitation care to a nursing home was associated with significantly more depression symptoms than transition back to living alone or with others (Loeher, Bank, MacNeill, & Lichtenberg, 2004). Qualitative research with clients who had terminal cancer defined suffering as experiences of violence, deprivation and being overwhelmed, and apprehension (Daneault et al., 2004). Family members of decedents reported the following sources of stress in relation to changes in their loved ones prior to death: loss of bodily functions, being dependent, and being a burden. Findings indicate that worries about loss of quality of life, independent of level of symptom severity of loved ones, contributed to suffering (Hickman, Tilden, & Tolle, 2004). Thus stressful aspects of illness experiences can produce negative psychological health effects for clients and family members.

Sociobehavioral Effects of Stress

In response to stress, individuals often revert to or increase their reliance on less healthy behaviors, such as overeating, excessive use of alcohol or drugs, and smoking. Recognizing that such behaviors are inconsistent with the healthy behaviors needed to cope with stress is easy; however, stopping these behaviors and using health-promoting strategies is not. Risky behaviors and traits such as a sedentary lifestyle, obesity, overeating high-fat foods, smoking, drug use, and social isolation have been linked to morbidity and

mortality (USDHHS, 2000). Conversely, exercise, healthy diet, smoking cessation, healthy weight maintenance, and social interaction have been identified as leading indicators of health in this country (USDHHS, 2000). Furthermore, encouraging these health behaviors supports goals of *Healthy People 2010*. Strategies that help break the cycle of stress-disinhibition in response to stress are important to mediate unhealthy patterns (Davis, Eshelman, & McKay, 2000).

Spiritual Effects of Stress

Interest in the connection between spirituality and health is significant. In response to stress, people often feel disconnected from life's meaning and purpose; harmful effects on their health and well-being can result. Finding meaning and connection through religion or spirituality can protect against negative outcomes of stress, at least to some extent. After large-scale community disasters such as September 11th and the Oklahoma City bombing, turning to religion, as well as engaging in open discussion and community activities, helped people to cope with their reactions to these events (Marshall, 2002). Research demonstrates a variety of associations between religious activity or spirituality and stress reduction. For example, religiosity among a sample of women with fibromyalgia had protective effects against stress (Dedert et al., 2004), Difficulty forgiving oneself and negative religious coping were related to depression, anxiety, and posttraumatic stress disorder symptom severity among a sample of veterans (Witvliet, Phipps, Feldman, & Beckham, 2004). Among a group of African American heterosexuals with human immunodeficiency virus infection, religious and existential well-being explained 32% of variance in depression (Coleman, 2004). Thus research now affirms what nurses have known since the writings of Florence Nightingale (1859, 1992) over a century ago; that is, helping people use interventions that influence or restore connection with life meaning and purpose has important health-promoting benefits.

The previous section provided information that stress can adversely affect biological activity, cognition, emotions, behavior, and spiritual well-being. This understanding of the psychophysiology of the mind-body-spirit connection is fundamental to the application of stress management in nursing and provides an obvious rationale for a multifaceted approach. Further support is provided from research endorsing the health-promoting effects of managing stress.

HEALTH BENEFITS OF MANAGING STRESS

A growing body of evidence underscores the importance of controlling stress to promote health and quality of life for people with a variety of health problems. Immune system diseases have responded to interventions that reduce the stress response (Cruess et al., 2000). For example, continuous labor support reduces the stress response, promotes a woman's positive memory of the experience, and affects various desired health outcomes (Pascali-Bonaro & Kroeger,

2004). Psychotherapeutic approaches, such as interpersonal and cognitive-behavioral psychotherapies that focus on perception and management of life stressors, are effective treatments for depression and related mental health disorders (Markowitz, 2004; Power, 2004).

Promoting a positive attitude and development of skills to cope with stress is foundational to many stress management interventions. Kobasa, Maddi, and Kahn (1982) made a groundbreaking contribution to understating the stress-illness relationship when they identified characteristics of hardiness. They described individuals with stress-hardy characteristics who, when exercising and accessing social support, were less vulnerable to stress-related symptoms and diseases. The characteristics of stress hardiness are control, challenge, and commitment. For stress-hardy individuals, stress is viewed as a challenge rather than a threat; they feel in control of situations in their lives, and they are committed to rather than alienated from work, home, and family.

Research outcomes support the role of stress-hardy characteristics in promoting better health. Pengilly and Dowd (2000) found that hardiness moderates the relationship between stress and depression. When individuals do not possess hardiness attributes, stress is more likely to result in symptoms. For example, Kenney and Bhattacharjee (2000) found that women with medium or high stressors and low assertiveness, low hardiness, or the inability to express their feelings were more likely to report physical symptoms than were women who were stronger in these personality traits. However, other researchers found that hardiness buffered effects of stress on illness for males, but not for females (Klag & Bradley, 2004). This finding indicates that possible gender influences merit consideration.

Investigators also have found links between health and explanatory style. For example, a pessimistic explanatory style has been associated with early mortality (Manuta, Colligan, Malinchoc, & Offord, 2000). In a study of people undergoing cardiac rehabilitation, optimism contributed to positive health outcomes directly, as well as indirectly, through mediation of less engagement in harmful coping and fewer depression symptoms (Shen, McCreary, & Myers, 2004). Recognizing the influence of explanatory style on health and well-being furthers the understanding of how thoughts, feelings, behaviors, and physiological activity interact. Furthermore, nurses can identify people with high stressors and unhealthy personality traits that increase their risk for stress-related illnesses and assist them to modify these factors to enhance their health.

The previous section described the bidirectional relationship among thoughts, feelings, behaviors, beliefs, and biological activity and offered a systematic way to understand these interactions. Evidence was presented that perceptions, or the way individuals view situations, can lead to stress and, in turn, adversely affect biological activity, emotions, behavior, and the connection with life meaning and purpose. This, in turn, increases stress and fosters a negative stress cycle. The remainder of this chapter examines the

---

CASE STUDY

John R.

John R., a 29-year-old man separated from his wife, walked into the health maintenance organization (HMO) stating he had a severe sore throat, could not eat, had not worked for a day, and was feeling "awful." He wanted to see the doctor and get a prescription for an antibiotic. The medical record revealed two episodes within the last 9 months of complaints of a sore throat, culture of organism, and antibiotic treatment. The separation from his wife occurred 1 year ago. He had not had a physical in 2 years. During the assessment interview, the nurse gathered the following information: John R. appeared tired, he presented his problem in short, terse statements, he was irritable about the clinic's slow service, and he expressed a need to get back to work. Within the last 3 weeks, he had been required to work overtime because he faced deadline penalties, and his boss said that John R.'s promotion, due in 2 months, depended on his performance now. John R. said that, in general, things were fine. His wife was apparently happy without him and he was too busy to care or to think about that relationship. He made one remark about his boss, "What do you do with a nervous boss?" He described his diet as fast food "taken on the run." He said he obtains about 6 hours of sleep per night and awakens 1 to 2 times near morning. He has infrequent contact with family members, who live in the area.

Reflective Questions
1. Describe how John R.'s nurse will comprehensively assess his health.
2. Discuss several different diagnoses and possible individual, family, and community causes.

---

assessment of stress relating to the physical, psychosocial, and spiritual health and well-being of individuals and introduces the application of a variety of strategies shown to help break the negative stress cycle and mediate its harmful effects across the biological, psychosocial, and spiritual domains.

ASSESSMENT OF STRESS

Assessment of the stress-coping abilities of an individual, family, or community is part of comprehensive health assessment that includes past and present subjective and objective data. Collecting these data enables the client and nurse to determine the status of the person's stress-coping pattern, and actual and potential strengths and weaknesses.

The nurse thoroughly collects data during the history, physical examination, and health patterns assessment (see Chapters 7, 8, and 9). Identifying the stress-coping pattern is especially important. Each individual is the primary data source; no other person can explain accurately the individual's perceptions of the stressors, stress responses, and resources to prevent or alleviate the stress.

Stress is experienced across biological, psychosocial, and spiritual domains; therefore, all perceptions are important to the assessment. Throughout the assessment process, individuals may become aware of information of which they were previously unaware, or they may identify information related to their perceived problems. For example, a man may be aware of the stress of his job but may be unaware that he has high blood pressure caused by this stress.

Lazarus and Folkman (1984) proposed a theory comprising primary and secondary appraisals of stressful events, situations, or demands and the effectiveness of an individual's coping skills (see Chapter 5). **Primary appraisal** of coping includes descriptions of perceived actual and potential positive and negative outcomes. Negative outcomes refer to harm, whereas positive outcomes refer to the challenges resulting from stressors that an individual perceives can be overcome. Examples of negative outcomes are physical injury, disease, loss of a cherished relationship, position or possession, and death. Positive outcomes include graduation, promotion, and development of important relationships (Case Study).

Secondary appraisal follows primary appraisal. Secondary appraisal consists of the individual's identification of choices to cope with the actual or potential harm, threat, or challenge. The choices may be internal or external resources and responses. For example, a social resource in coping with the needs of a toddler might be learning strategies in a parent-effectiveness training course. A coping response to the challenges of parenting a toddler might be restructuring the toddler's and parent's schedules to allow for more frequent cycles of activities and rest.

The individual's primary and secondary appraisals of stress provide opportunities to consider the stress experiences in different ways. Resources that had been forgotten may be remembered, or a threat may be newly viewed as a challenge and an opportunity for enhanced development and status. Stress responses are mediated by the appraisal process.

By using measurement instruments with established reliability and validity, nurses can improve assessment of an individual's stress and coping. Tools can help nurses distinguish between diagnoses that have many signs and symptoms in common. For example, disturbances in thinking and feeling processes can be difficult to distinguish and may have confounding clinical pictures. These disturbances can occur separately or simultaneously in the same person. An example of this complexity is the similarity in symptomatology of depression and dementia. The nurse must determine whether or not one health problem is actually the cause of the other in order to develop an effective plan of care (Care Plan). The Schedule of Recent Experiences (Holmes, 1981) is an example of an instrument used widely

---

CARE PLAN

Plan for Effective Coping

(Related to John R. Case Study)

Nursing Diagnosis Ineffective Individual Coping related to increased stress at work and limited coping strategies.

DEFINING CHARACTERISTICS

- Physiological disturbances
- Abuse of alcohol or drugs
- Participation in potentially dangerous activities
- Engaging in lifestyle with risk to health
- Impairment of social role functioning:
  - Nonproductive lifestyle
  - Failure to function in usual social roles
  - Nonperformance of activities of daily living
  - Inappropriate behaviors in social situations
  - Self-absorption
  - Lack of concern for or detachment from usual social supports

POOR MORALE

- Unhappiness
- Lack future orientation
- Hopelessness
- Unacceptable quality of life
- Pessimism

DEFENSIVE PATTERNS

- Inflexibility
- Hypervigilance

- Avoidance
- Inertia
- Refusal or rejection of help

EXPECTED OUTCOMES

John R. will:

- Report increased information on and consequences to himself of stressors experienced
- Practice the relaxation response for 20 to 30 minutes every day through prayer or contemplation; use multiple mini-relaxations throughout each day
- Report increasing weekly exercise or activity and healthy changes in nutrition and sleep or rest patterns
- Develop effective coping and problem-solving abilities to manage stress, beginning with the stress at work

INTERVENTIONS

- Promote an attitude of openness to new information.
- Enroll client in a cognitive behavioral group program to learn stress management strategies and health promotion.
- Monitor client's daily practice of relaxation response.
- Monitor client's changes in exercise or activity, nutrition, and sleep or rest patterns, and mood.
- Guide client to develop two coping strategies through cognitive-behavioral restructuring.

in clinical assessment to measure the amount of life change and associated stress. This tool was a groundbreaking contribution to knowledge about links among life events, stress, and illness. Davis and colleagues (2000) have found that this inventory can assist people to assess the degree of recent changes in their lives.

A wide variety of tests and questionnaires are available to help nurses assess orientation, attention, cognitive skills and patterns, traits and states of emotions, symptoms of psychiatric disorders, and overall quality of life. For example, instruments are available to assess mental status, anxiety, depression, coping, lifestyle, and quality of life. Prior to use, clinicians and researchers need to check training requirements and copyright restrictions (e.g., purchase requirements) that can affect access to instruments.

Use of standardized instruments promotes accuracy in developing diagnoses and plans of care, and assists in evaluating the effectiveness of care. For example, a nurse may compare an individual's self-evaluation scores before intervention with postintervention scores and revise the plan of care accordingly. Additionally, nurses may analyze population baseline scores for relevant characteristics and develop programs of research and quality improvements aimed at improving outcomes.

STRESS MANAGEMENT INTERVENTIONS

Stress management strategies are beneficial to people across a broad spectrum of chronological, gender, cultural, and ethnic characteristics. Men and women, young and old, from divergent socioeconomic, cultural, and ethnic backgrounds can benefit from stress management interventions. Sensitivity to needs and values of individuals and communities, particularly for high-risk groups, guides modification of assessment and intervention techniques. The language, belief system, and cultural distinctions of individuals guide the choice and alteration of stress management strategies.

Developing Self-Awareness

Self-awareness is one of the most effective stress management tools. Self-awareness helps people learn about interactions among mind, body, and spirit, increases a sense of control, and counters self-defeating perceptions. Interventions that promote self-awareness help people make sense of life events and circumstances that may be bewildering or discomforting. Many experiences in life lead to feelings of emptiness and disharmony, because people are unable to connect the experience with thoughts, feelings, actions, and physiological responses. Self-awareness helps individuals recognize stress that they create through negative, exaggerated, unrealistic thinking. This recognition affords an opportunity to change these negative thought patterns, thereby decreasing stress and increasing control. Strategies that increase self-awareness can empower individuals to make new connections and to reframe and reinterpret their experiences in light of their own inner strengths and wisdom.

Techniques for Developing Self-Awareness

Monitoring Stress Warning Signs. The negative stress cycle can be difficult to interrupt. Recognizing warning signs of stress is a necessary first step. Often individuals have long ignored physical, emotional, or behavioral cues or reactions to a stressor that are **stress warning signs.** The man suffering from chronic intermittent backaches, who ignores the daily muscle tension caused by poor posture that precedes the backaches, provides an example. If he had attended to his early stress warning signs of poor posture and muscle tension, then he might have avoided the backache that kept him from exercising and socializing. Becoming aware of these stress warning signs is the first step. Attending to these cues is the next step. After this connection is made, developing skills to reduce negative mood states, unhealthy behaviors, and physical symptoms becomes much easier. To continue with the previous example, preventing a backache from becoming disabling is easier when the man notices muscle tension and then stops, takes a few deep breaths, corrects his posture, and gently stretches the area, rather than waiting for the backache to become incapacitating before acting.

Nurses teach people to identify their warning signals of stress and to stop, take a few breaths, and break the cycle. Figure 13-3 is a sample form for identifying and recording this information. These signals or cues differ from individual to individual and can be physical, emotional, behavioral, cognitive, relational, or spiritual. When asked to monitor their responses to a particular event, individuals become more consciously aware of these cues. Although this heightened awareness initially may increase an individual's consciousness of physical pain or emotional discomfort, awareness is a necessary first step in recognizing the negative effects of stress and the relationship of thoughts, feelings, behavior, and biological processes.

Try this: ask an individual to identify a stressful experience and the physical or emotional reactions (stress warning signals) to that particular experience. For example, after being instructed to stop, take a breath, and notice the physical and emotional response to a stressful situation, one woman related the following:

> On my way to work yesterday, I sat in a huge traffic jam. I noticed that my heart was racing, my breathing had changed, and my hands were gripping the steering wheel. I felt angry and frustrated because I was going to be late for work.

Although these responses seem quite obvious, most people are unaware of the effects of stress on their minds and bodies. After individuals become aware of these effects, they may be able to release tension more easily, countering the negative effects of stress and increasing a sense of control. Techniques that help to reduce negative effects of stress include using distraction by purposefully shifting focus to pleasant thoughts or engaging in a diversional activity, and using a relaxation technique, as described below.

STRESS WARNING SIGNALS

Physical Symptoms

____ Headaches   ____ Back pain
____ Indigestion   ____ Tight neck and shoulders
____ Stomachaches   ____ Racing heart
____ Sweaty palms   ____ Restlessness
____ Sleep difficulties   ____ Tiredness
____ Dizziness   ____ Ringing in ears

Behavioral Symptoms

____ Excess smoking   ____ Grinding of teeth at night
____ Bossiness   ____ Overuse of alcohol
____ Compulsive gum chewing   ____ Compulsive eating
____ Attitude critical of others   ____ Inability to get things done

Emotional Symptoms

____ Crying   ____ Overwhelming sense of pressure
____ Nervousness and anxiety   ____ Anger
____ Boredom (no meaning to things)   ____ Loneliness
____ Edginess (ready to explode)   ____ Unhappiness for no reason
____ Feeling powerless to change things   ____ Easily upset

Cognitive Symptoms

____ Trouble thinking clearly   ____ Inability to make decisions
____ Lack of creativity   ____ Thoughts of running away
____ Memory loss   ____ Constant worry
____ Forgetfulness   ____ Loss of sense of humor

Spiritual Symptoms   ### Relational Symptoms

____ Emptiness   ____ Isolation
____ Loss of meaning   ____ Intolerance
____ Doubt   ____ Resentment
____ Unforgiving   ____ Loneliness
____ Martyrdom   ____ Lashing out
____ Looking for magic   ____ Hiding
____ Loss of direction   ____ Clamming up
____ Cynicism   ____ Lowered sex drive
____ Apathy   ____ Nagging
____ Needing to "prove" self   ____ Distrust
                                                   ____ Lack of intimacy
                                                   ____ Using people

Figure 13-3   Stress warning signals. (From *Medical symptom reduction clinic patient notebook.* Boston: Division of Behavioral Medicine, Beth Israel Deaconess Medical Center, The Mind Body Medical Institute, Harvard Medical School.)

Learning and Practicing a Relaxation Technique. Eliciting the **relaxation response** is another technique to help people develop awareness and counter the negative effects of stress. Relaxation techniques counter the stress response by reducing sympathetic arousal (Benson, 1975). The immediate physiological effects of relaxation are decreases in heart rate, blood pressure, respiratory rate, and muscle tension. The long-term physiological effect is a decrease in central nervous system arousal with a concomitant decrease in musculoskeletal system, autonomic nervous system, and psychoneuroendocrine system arousal. To the extent that stress causes or exacerbates a symptom, eliciting the relaxation response can break this stress–symptom cycle. In addition to these physiological changes, psychological changes such as improved mood and behavioral changes, including a reduction in risky behaviors, can occur. The relaxation response can counteract stress-related disease processes, particularly processes associated with immunological, cardiovascular, and neurodegenerative disorders (Esch, Fricchione, & Stefano, 2003).

The relaxation response is an innate physiological response (Benson, 1975); therefore, a number of techniques that involve mental focusing can be used. Details on these techniques and guidelines for clinical applications can be found in Chapter 14. All of these techniques have two basic components:

1. The repetition of a word, sound, phrase, prayer, image, or physical activity
2. The passive disregard of everyday thoughts when they occur

Audiotapes are recommended to help guide this process of focusing, especially during the initial learning phase.

Nurses often can introduce individuals to the immediate calming effects of the relaxation response in less than 5 minutes. One effective way is to have the person make a fist and notice what happens to the breathing pattern. Most people have a tendency to hold their breath while tensing a body part. Now ask the person to take a few deep diaphragmatic breaths while making a fist. Most people will notice that the tension is much harder to maintain while taking a deep breath. This awareness helps to recognize the relationship between breath and tension. This connection between breathing and relaxation is the principle behind Lamaze techniques for helping mothers control pain during delivery.

Most people hold their breath when they perceive a threat (stress), feel anxious, or become angry. By stopping and taking a few deep breaths when they become aware of physical changes (holding the breath or clenching the jaw) or emotional changes (feeling anxious or angry), individuals can elicit the relaxation response, reduce sympathetic arousal, calm negative mood states, and gain a sense of control.

Using Mini-Relaxations. Mini-relaxations can be taught quickly and used throughout the day to help develop awareness and to counter the negative effects of stress on the mind, body, and spirit. Individuals can be taught to monitor minor stress warning signs (jaw and shoulder tension) and to use a mini-relaxation to keep these initial symptoms of stress from developing into an incapacitating tension headache. A mini-relaxation exercise can be anything from a few conscious, deep diaphragmatic breaths to several minutes of sitting quietly (Health Teaching box).

Alternative and Complementary Therapies. A variety of alternative and complementary therapies can prevent and reduce harmful effects of stress. These include acupuncture, hypnosis, aromatherapy, reflexology, and chiropractic and herbal therapies. These approaches have developed outside the mainstream of traditional Western medicine; however, developing evidence of efficacy has promoted growing acceptance of some of these approaches (Brennan, 2000). People increasingly are using alternative and complementary practices as self-help measures, and research to study their effects has exploded in recent years (Snyder, 2002). Nurses can assist clients to base their use on evidence of safety and efficacy. In particular, herbal remedies require cautious use because they can have harmful, as well as beneficial, effects, and they sometimes interfere with other treatments. Among the alternative therapies available, there is strong evidence of effectiveness of acupuncture and hypnosis, and they are becoming widely accepted within mainstream health care.

Acupuncture is an ancient Chinese technique used to reduce pain and to prevent and manage various disorders by placement of fine needles at specific meridian points on the body. Acupuncture is not a self-help approach, so seeking treatment from an experienced acupuncturist is required. The Western scientific community cannot explain why acupuncture works but acknowledges its effectiveness. Even the World Health Organization has listed illnesses that can

---

HEALTH TEACHING Mini-Relaxation

Nurses can teach individuals to perform a mini-relaxation exercise through a variety of suggestions, including:

- Count slowly up to 4 as you inhale and slowly back down again as you exhale.
- Change your breathing to diaphragmatic breathing. Try inhaling through your nose and exhaling through your mouth. You should feel your stomach rising about 1 inch as you inhale and falling about 1 inch as you exhale.
- Take a few deep diaphragmatic breaths, and as you do so, begin to recall something that would bring a smile to your

face, which might be the image of your child's face, your favorite pet, or another loved one; or it could be the memory of a favorite place, food, or event in your life.

Nurses can remind people to notice how quickly "minis" help to relieve tension and worry. People can be advised to practice often throughout the day to counter the harmful effects of arousal from the stress response.

Modified from Hoblitzelle, O. A., & Benson, H. (1993). Eliciting the relaxation response. In H. Benson & E. Stuart (Eds.), *The wellness book: The comprehensive guide to maintaining health and treating stress-related illness.* New York: Fireside; The Mind Body Medical Institute. (n.d.). The stress response. Retrieved September 26, 2004, from: *http://www.mbmi.org/pages/mbb_s1.asp*; The Mind Body Medical Institute. (n.d.). Stress and performance. Retrieved September 26, 2004, from: *http://www.mbmi.org/pages/mbb_s2.asp.*

be managed with acupuncture (Brennan, 2000), and some health insurance plans cover it.

Hypnosis comes from a Greek word meaning sleep (Brennan, 2000; Davis et al., 2000). Hypnosis narrows consciousness and elicits relaxation, inertia, and passivity, like sleep, yet awareness is never lost completely and the hypnotized person can respond (Davis et al., 2000). The exact mechanisms through which hypnosis works are not known, although perhaps its ability to induce deep relaxation and its possible action in shifting brain activity from the analytical left side to the nonanalytical right side might be explanatory (Brennan, 2000). Nevertheless, its effectiveness in managing a variety of conditions, notably smoking and anxiety-related problems, and managing pain is well recognized. Trained therapists provide hypnotherapy to manage stress and various mental health problems, including phobias, addictions, and posttraumatic stress disorder. Self-hypnosis, a form of deep relaxation similar to relaxation techniques described in this chapter, can be a useful stress-reduction tool. Self-help guides such as *The Relaxation & Stress Reduction Workbook* (Davis et al., 2000) provide safe and easy-to-follow guidelines. One note of caution is warranted: hypnosis is not recommended for people with organic brain disorders, psychotic disorders, or other severe mental disorders.

Journal Writing. Journal writing—more specifically, self-confessional writing—is useful in processing emotions and in measurably improving physical and mental health (Pennebaker, 2000). Journaling can assist people to reflect upon stressful events and their reactions to these events. Such reflection is an opportunity to reform perceptions and to consider alternative ways to manage stress. Individuals may find resolutions to conflicts that work uniquely for them. These resolutions then may increase a sense of control and mediate negative consequences of stress. This self-reflective process shares elements of cognitive-behavioral therapy (CBT)—an intervention effective in reducing harmful effects of stress.

Nurses can advise people to get a special notebook for a journal and write about a stressful event for 15 minutes a day, in a setting in which they will not be interrupted. From a health perspective, people will be more effective when making themselves the only audience. The nurse should warn that the individual may feel sad or depressed immediately after the writing session, but these feelings usually dissipate within an hour. Exploring deep thoughts and feelings on paper is not a panacea. When an individual is coping with death, divorce, or some other major stressor, feeling better instantly after writing cannot be expected. A person can, however, develop a clearer understanding of feelings and of the situation through journal writing. In other words, journal writing helps people objectify experiences, identify the influence of stress on symptoms, and develop insights into more effective problem solving. Some individuals may recognize the need for psychotherapeutic support through journal writing, and an appropriate referral can then be made.

Healthy Diet

Countering negative effects of stress requires caring for physical health and well-being. The mind and body are connected; therefore, paying attention to one while ignoring the other does not promote overall health. The body requires rest, a **healthy diet** of balanced food choices from the five food groups, and exercise. Over the last few decades, nutrition has moved to the forefront as a major component of health promotion, disease prevention, and symptom management. Food is now viewed as a positive influence on health, physical performance, and state of mind, rather than simply a fuel needed to prevent disease and sustain life (Luck, 2000). Nutrition is becoming an important component of early intervention strategies to improve physical, cognitive, emotional, and social functioning.

However, the American lifestyle has made practicing healthy eating habits increasingly difficult. Americans frequently replace nutritionally balanced meals with readily available high-fat, high-calorie foods. Many times this course of action is an attempt to find immediate gratification to counter feelings of anxiety and depression caused by stress (stress-disinhibition). One of the frustrations that nurses experience is trying to help children and adults develop healthy eating habits. This effort takes planning and correctly choosing a variety of foods, and choosing a diet low in fat, saturated fat, and cholesterol, with plenty of vegetables, fruits, and grain products. The current U.S. dietary guidelines presented in the Food Guide Pyramid (U.S. Department of Agriculture [USDA], n.d.) emphasize that daily food choices should be made from the five food groups. Research confirms this dietary pattern to be associated with a decreased risk of mortality (Kant, Schatzkin, Graubard, & Schairer, 2000). The pyramid is under review, and updated government guidelines may be issued. Yet regardless of adjustments to specific recommendations that may be forthcoming, the pyramid will continue to serve as an outline of what to eat each day, not a rigid prescription, and represents a general guide that helps individuals choose a healthful diet. A detailed discussion of the health benefits of balanced nutrition and guidelines throughout the life span can be found in Chapter 11.

Encouraging healthier dietary choices helps people to recognize that control over their health and well-being is possible. This knowledge, in turn, helps counter the negative effects of stress and lower the stress-disinhibition effect that can influence poor dietary choices. Nurses can encourage people to monitor their daily dietary patterns to gain awareness of how they use food in times of stress. Tools like food diaries help people to monitor the amount and quality of what they eat and drink and to set realistic goals (Davis et al., 2000).

Physical Activity

Combining a healthy diet with a regular exercise routine has many health benefits and can positively affect quality of life. For example, one of the most effective ways to lose

Helping Individuals Increase Physical Activity

Nurses can suggest ways for individuals to increase physical activity throughout the day, including:
- Have fun and play active games with children.
- Engage in a sport.
- Find a friend with whom to walk or jog.
- Take a class in yoga or Tai Chi.
- Get and walk a dog.
- Garden on the weekends.
- Walk or bicycle to school or work.
- Take the stairs, never the elevator.
- Park the car at the farthest point in the parking lot at work, school, or when shopping.

By simply changing a few daily routines, a person can gain enormous physical, psychosocial, and spiritual rewards that promote health and break the negative stress cycle.

weight and improve self-esteem is to combine exercise with nutritious eating. **Exercise** (physical activity that improves strength, flexibility, and conditioning) and balanced nutrition serve as protective factors against several major chronic diseases. Regular physical activity decreases the risk of death from heart disease, lowers the risk of developing diabetes, and is associated with a decreased risk of colon cancer (USDHHS, 2000). Exercise helps prevent high blood pressure and helps lower blood pressure in people with elevated levels. Regular physical activity, even at moderate levels, is associated with lower death rates for adults of any age. Psychological well-being is enhanced and the risk of developing depression can be reduced; regular physical activity appears to reduce symptoms of depression and anxiety and to improve mood.

Additionally, children and adolescents need weight-bearing exercise for normal skeletal development, and young adults need this type of exercise to achieve and maintain peak bone mass (USDHHS, 2000). Regular physical activity also increases the ability of older people, and those with certain chronic, disabling conditions, to perform activities of daily living. Nevertheless, high stress could increase injury risk for athletes, and injured athletes may experience greater stress than noninjured peers when they are sidelined from competition. Chapter 12 provides a comprehensive discussion of the benefits of exercise and clinical application throughout the life span.

Regular physical activity helps people adopt a more active lifestyle as they begin to feel better physically and emotionally, helping to break the negative stress cycle. These positive effects can be obtained with exercise of only moderate intensity. For example, a brisk walk of 30 to 60 minutes, 3 to 5 times a week, promotes fitness and decreases risk of disease. Being physically active on a daily basis is extremely important; therefore, nurses can help individuals increase physical activity by suggesting a variety of activities in which they might engage each day (Box 13-1). An exercise diary can generate a baseline for usual activity to set realistic goals, and monitor progress (Davis et al., 2000). By simply changing a few daily routines, individuals can gain enormous physical, psychosocial, and spiritual rewards that promote health and break the negative stress cycle.

Sleep Hygiene

Good health and the ability to meet life's many demands and manage stress effectively require proper rest. Many people suffer from sleep deprivation that can cause or exacerbate conditions such as depression and fatigue and contribute to poor concentration and ineffective problem solving. Insomnia can be induced by stress or other cognitive-behavioral factors, such as unrealistic expectations, inappropriate scheduling of sleep, trying too hard to sleep, consuming caffeine, getting inadequate exercise, and a number of other factors including illness, alcohol use, or drug use. By determining the extent to which sleep disturbance is the result of behavior or stress-related issues and by counseling people to follow several **sleep hygiene** or behavior guidelines (keeping a sleep diary, having a regular sleep-wake cycle, and making prudent dietary changes), nurses can help individuals improve their sleep patterns (Abascal, Brucato, & Brucato, 2001; Jacobs, 1998). Box 13-2 presents several sleep hygiene strategies.

Overcoming sleep disturbances cannot be done quickly. Changing these behaviors requires patience and persistence. Individuals often will abandon a behavior technique when it does not produce an immediate improvement. Nurses can remind individuals that although these changes may be slower than those produced by sleep aids, these techniques are more enduring and effective (Morin, Colecchi, Stone, Sood, & Brink, 1999). Assisting people to make healthy behavior changes in their sleep habits provides another opportunity for them to increase self-regulation, confidence, and control, thereby reducing stress and improving quality of life.

Cognitive Restructuring

Many stressful situations can be created or exacerbated by negative, exaggerated, catastrophic thinking. Cognitive therapy is a conceptual model for a short-term intervention to modify this thinking and reduce stress. In the context of cognitive therapy, **cognitive restructuring** is a technique or series of strategies that help people evaluate their thoughts, challenge them, and replace them with more rational responses. Appraisal, or the way in which a situation is viewed, can be a major cause of stress. When situations are viewed in a negative, distorted, or illogical manner, this perception can adversely affect emotions, behaviors, beliefs, and physiological parameters. Cognitive restructuring teaches people to recognize that negative thinking often causes emotional distress. This recognition, in turn, reduces the negative consequences of stress and enhances health (Stuart & Wells-Federman, 2000).

Cognitive restructuring does not gloss over or deny misfortune, suffering, or negative feelings. Many circumstances

Box **13-2** Sleep Hygiene Strategies

Nurses find the following suggestions to be helpful for individuals with sleep disturbance resulting from behavioral or stress-related issues:
- Keep a sleep diary, which helps determine sleep patterns more accurately, assess progress, and reinforce behavior change.
- Challenge irrational beliefs.
- Reduce consumption of alcohol and caffeine. (Chapter 11 gives some tips.)
- Avoid use of sleeping pills.
- Have a regular sleep-wake schedule, even on the weekends.
- If unable to fall asleep within 20 to 30 minutes or if waking up and unable to fall back to sleep within that time, get out of bed and do something until groggy and sleepy again.
- Focus on relaxation, not sleep. Use a relaxation tape, practice diaphragmatic breathing. Limit naps during the day to less than 45 minutes. Longer naps reset the biological clock and disturb nighttime sleep.
- Exercise within 3 to 6 hours of bedtime. Exercise improves sleep by producing a significant rise in body temperature, followed by a compensatory drop a few hours later, making it easier to fall asleep and stay asleep. Furthermore, because exercise is a physical stressor, the brain compensates by increasing the amount of deep sleep.
- Take a hot bath 2 hours before bedtime. The temperature drop after the bath helps to induce sleep.
- Sleep in a cool room. Individuals grow sleepier and become less active when body temperature falls.

Modified from Abascal, J. R., Brucato, D., & Brucato, L. (2001). *Stress mastery: The art of coping gracefully.* Upper Saddle River, NJ: Prentice Hall; Jacobs, G. D. (1998). *Say goodnight to insomnia.* New York: Henry Holt and Co.

Box **13-3** The Four-Step Approach to Cognitive Restructuring

To help individuals develop the skill of cognitive restructuring, nurses can teach them to examine a stressful situation using a four-step approach.
1. Stop (break the cycle of escalating, negative thoughts).
2. Take a breath (elicit the relaxation response and release tension).
3. Reflect (ask, "What is going on here? What am I thinking? Is the thought true? Is the thought helpful? Am I jumping to conclusions or magnifying the situation?").
4. Choose a more realistic, rational response.

From Stuart, E., & Wells-Federman, C. L. (2000). Cognitive therapy. In B. Dossey, C. Guzetta, & L. Keegan (Eds.), *Holistic nursing: A handbook for practice* (3rd ed.). Gaithersburg, MD: Aspen.

a variety of other stress-related symptoms, which may exacerbate the headache. To help individuals develop the skill of cognitive restructuring, nurses can teach them to examine a stressful situation using a four-step approach highlighted in Box 13-3 (Stuart & Wells-Federman, 2000).

In the previous example, the woman may reflect that "I am having a migraine headache and I hate that it is on a day that I had made plans, but I will take my medication, listen to my relaxation tapes, and rest. I'll call my friend and see if we can change our plans. Perhaps she can come over to visit me for tea this afternoon if I feel better." Although it is understandable that anyone would be disappointed and upset over this situation, applying the four-step cognitive restructuring technique can help identify healthy choices and gain a sense of control.

Cognitive therapy is an efficacious treatment approach for many stress-related and mental health disorders, particularly depression. For example, researchers have shown that cognitive therapy and CBT are as effective as antidepressant medications in treating postpartum depression (Highet & Drummond, 2004). Peden, Hall, Rayens, and Beebe (2000) tested the effects of a 6-week cognitive-behavioral group intervention on depressive symptoms, negative thinking, and poor self-esteem with 92 college women who were at risk for depression. They randomly assigned participants to either the control or experimental group. Compared with the women in the control group, the women in the experimental group had a significantly greater decrease in both depressive symptoms and negative thinking and increased self-esteem at both 1 month and 6 months after intervention. Thus evidence supports use of cognitive therapy as a stress management approach.

Affirmations

Affirmations can be an effective stress management and cognitive restructuring skill, because they are a method of countering self-defeating negative thoughts and attitudes

exist in peoples' lives for which it is appropriate to feel sad, anxious, angry, or depressed. More accurately, cognitive restructuring is a technique that helps people become unstuck from these moods so that they can experience a broader range of feelings (Wells-Federman, Stuart-Shor, & Webster, 2001). In this structured method, individuals are asked to consider their cognitive appraisal of a situation and how this assessment affects feelings, behaviors, and physiological processes. Reframing, or cognitive reappraisal, educates individuals in monitoring thoughts and replacing those that are negative and irrational with those that are more realistic and helpful.

For example, a woman may have had plans to meet a friend for lunch on a day she woke up with a migraine headache. She might begin to think such thoughts as "This always happens to me when I have plans," "This headache will never go away," "I shouldn't have to deal with this," or "My day is ruined." The result of this negative irrational self-talk is disappointment, frustration, and anger. This emotional arousal will, in turn, increase muscle tension and

(Stuart & Wells-Federman, 2000), in addition to being helpful in addressing spiritual needs. An **affirmation** is a positive thought, in the form of a short phrase or saying, which has meaning for the individual. By reinforcing new ways of thinking or behaving in the present moment, affirmations are statements that people can use to reaffirm new intentions and to clarify goals.

Nurses can coach individuals to create an affirmation as a way of developing a more helpful, realistic belief system. For example, thoughts such as "I can't handle this" and "My day is ruined" can be countered with "I can handle this" and "I know ways to increase my comfort." Repeating an affirmation often throughout the day, perhaps after eliciting the relaxation response or as part of a breathing exercise, can become second nature and can help to enhance self-esteem and reduce stress.

Social Support

Having supportive family, friends, and co-workers is for many individuals an important contributor to effective coping and stress hardiness (Kobasa et al., 1982; Pengilly & Dowd, 2000). Many people believe that confiding in others and talking out problems can be a helpful way to get good advice or uncritical support (Pennebaker, 2000). **Social support** comprises a network of close family, friends, co-workers, and professionals. Social support literature notes that both the number of supports and the quality of the relationships are important (Frasure-Smith et al., 2000).

Research outcomes demonstrate the protective health effects of social support. For example, social support can protect against dementia (Berkman, 2000; Fratiglioni, Wang, Ericsson, Maytan, & Winblad, 2000). Among people participating in a cardiac rehabilitation program, social support contributed to desired health outcomes (Shen et al., 2004). Emotional support during labor and delivery appears to effect positive health outcomes. Delivery by cesarean (C-section), the most common surgical procedure performed in the United States, increases the risk of complications to mother and child and extends hospital stay (USDHHS, 2000). Researchers found that the presence of a supportive woman (*doula*) during labor and delivery reduced the need for many medical procedures, including C-sections, and enhanced breastfeeding success, mother-infant bonding, and mothers' memories of the experience (Pascali-Bonaro & Kroeger, 2004). The Multicultural Awareness box presents information related to the effects of social support on the health of Hispanic Americans.

Nurses can do much to facilitate social support to promote effective coping and reduce stress. Using information available in their local communities or through national organizations, nurses can suggest support groups (see Chapter 8), Web site chat rooms, educational classes, and exercise facilities, to name a few. Individuals and their families are often referred to organizations such as the American Lung Association, American Heart Association, American Cancer Society, and the Arthritis Foundation for resources related to specific health-promotion needs.

MULTICULTURAL AWARENESS

Hispanic American Paradox

For nearly 20 years studies have demonstrated that Mexicans and Mexican Americans typically had lower socioeconomic status, yet their health compared similarly with non-Hispanic white individuals with a higher socioeconomic status—thus the Hispanic American paradox.

Experts suggest the most compelling reasons for this paradox might be diet, social support, and location. Hispanic Americans eat more fruits and vegetables than do most Americans. Additionally, strong social supports exist in Hispanic American families that are more intact, and there is a transplanting of the Mexican environment. These factors are easier to maintain when there is geographical closeness to the country of origin, as there is in Los Angeles County.

As Mexican Americans become more acculturated, rates of smoking, alcohol, and illicit drug consumption tend to increase.

Modified from Ericksen, A. B. (2000). Separate identities. *Minority Nurse*, 20-23; Hajat, A. (2000). *Health outcomes among Hispanic subgroups: Data from the National Health Interview Survey 1992-1995*. Boston: Vital Health and Statistics of the Centers of Disease Control and Prevention; *Medical symptom reduction clinic patient notebook*. Boston: Division of Behavioral Medicine, Beth Israel Deaconess Medical Center, The Mind Body Medical Institute, Harvard Medical School.

Assertive Communication

Effective communication is an important stress-management skill. An important coping and problem-solving skill, communication can be adversely affected by exaggerated negative thoughts and deeply held negative beliefs and assumptions (Stuart & Wells-Federman, 2000). (See Chapter 4 for additional discussion of communication.) People who have difficulty with communication usually have one or all of the following problems:

- Disparity between what they say (statement) and what they want (intent)
- Confusion about or resistance to stating clearly how they feel, what they want, or what they need (assertiveness), with either a tendency to deny their own feelings (passiveness) or indifference toward the feelings of others (aggressiveness)
- Inability to listen (Caudill, 1995)

The importance of matching the statement with intention is illustrated by the following example:

As David is leaving for his basketball game on a Saturday afternoon, his mother tells him, "Remember to be home early tonight." When David arrives home at 9:00 PM, his mother, who is waiting at the front door, yells, "Where were you? Is this your idea of early? You know your father and I had plans tonight. We were counting on you. You think only of yourself. This always happens. You'll never change. You'll always be irresponsible and selfish."

The first principle of effective communication is that people are clear about what they want and what they need (intent) in statements to others. Although it would be wonderful if a son, spouse, friend, or other were a great mind reader, assuming that does little to help with communication. Nurses can help individuals match statements with intentions. This process requires that individuals recognize distorted, exaggerated thoughts and emotions and take responsibility for their part of the conversation. Communicating effectively is an art and a skill.

Reviewing the previous example, if the mother's intention was to have her son home before 8:00 PM, then her statement needed to reflect this. She should have said, "I hope you enjoy the game, but remember your father and I are going out tonight. We need to have you home before 8:00 PM to take care of your sister." It is important that the person understand that the other person in the conversation is not obligated to respond as one would wish. However, a request can be much clearer when the statement reflects the intent.

The next principle of effective communication is to be assertive (Caudill, 1995). **Assertive communication,** in most cases, is the most effective way to communicate. An assertive statement is nonjudgmental, expresses feelings and opinions, and reaffirms perceived rights. The general format of an assertive statement is: I feel [emotion], when you [the behavior], because [explanation].

The formula requires that all three elements be included. Cognitive restructuring facilitates assertive communication, because it requires individuals to identify their thoughts and feelings. In the previous example, David's mother should:
1. Stop (breaking the cycle of escalating, negative thoughts)
2. Take a breath (releasing physical tension; promoting relaxation)
3. Reflect:
   How do I feel emotionally? (frustrated)
   What are my automatic thoughts? ("If he cared about us, then he would have been home on time. He's always selfish and irresponsible. He's never going to change.")
4. Choose:
   A more realistic, helpful way of thinking ("He's not always selfish and irresponsible. Even though it feels like he doesn't care about us when he does this, I know he cares.")

Becoming aware of her automatic thoughts and feelings would help David's mother plan an assertive statement when David comes home. She could then say, "I feel frustrated [emotion] when you are late [behavior], because I expected you would be home in time to care for your sister while your father and I went out, or that you would have called if you were going to be late [explanation]." This statement makes both her feelings clear and explains why she feels this way which, in turn, provides a better opportunity to work on problem solving. When people cannot verbalize both their feelings and their needs, others are forced to figure out what they are. When others fail to do so correctly, individuals may feel victimized and blame the others for not

understanding. Nurses help people recognize that they have a right and a responsibility to speak up and to do so in an assertive manner. The nurse can help individuals in matching their emotion with the explanation (frustration equals unmet expectation). It is important to remind them that this way of communicating may feel awkward and uncomfortable at first. Practicing this technique many times will be required before communication improves. Other people need time to become accustomed to the changes. Effective communication takes both practice and patience with everyone involved (Caudill, 1995; Stuart & Wells-Federman, 2000).

Empathy

Empathy is an effective stress management intervention, because it helps communication (Stuart & Wells-Federman, 2000). **Empathy** is the ability to take another person's perspectives into consideration and to communicate this understanding back to that person. Empathy helps individuals become better listeners.

Empathy can be facilitated through the technique of active listening. Active listening requires conscious, empathic, nonjudgmental awareness. Listening also helps clarify the issues involved and can deescalate many emotional exchanges. For example, during a situation in which a spouse announces, "I'm fed up with you always being late," the response may be important to resolving the issues without promoting further miscommunications and increasing problems. Rather than being caught by a defensive emotional reaction, individuals can learn to communicate empathetically using the four-step approach:
1. Stop (breaking the cycle of escalating, negative thoughts)
2. Take a breath (releasing physical tension; promoting relaxation)
3. Reflect:
   How do I feel emotionally? (hurt, angry)
   What are my automatic thoughts? ("How could [person] say that? It's not my fault. I have things to do. [Person] always accuses me. This is never going to change.")
   What are the thoughts and emotions being expressed by the other person?

The practice of asking this question will provide a different view. The individual can then begin to plan a response:
4. Choose:
   "My feelings are hurt, but I don't have to react defensively."
   "I'm going to try to understand [person's] perspective using this phrase: 'You sound _____ about _____' and listen to [person's] response."

By using this phrase, an individual can gain awareness from another person's perspective (Rogers, 1951). Continuing with the scenario, the response might be, "You sound upset about my being late." Possible responses to this empathetic statement might include, "It's not just about that. Everything went wrong today and this was just one more thing," or, "You're right. I hate having to wait. It feels like you don't respect or value my time."

When one uses active listening, the other person often feels heard. An opportunity to clarify any misunderstanding becomes available. This exercise may help reduce emotional arousal, defensive behavior, and conflict. Active listening allows the individual to buy time and to get a better perspective on what the other person is thinking and feeling. Individuals can then make a choice as to how they want to respond. They may choose to use assertive communication or to step away from the interaction. Active listening promotes empathic, objective, and nonjudgmental communication. Nurses can suggest that individuals use stress management skills that include active listening techniques to facilitate effective communication which, in turn, reduces conflict and stress (Stuart & Wells-Federman, 2000).

Healthy Pleasures

Engaging in **healthy pleasures** (activities that bring feelings of peace, joy, and happiness) is, for most individuals, an important part of life. However, for individuals who are feeling overwhelmed with daily hassles, illness, or loss, this practice may have been lost. Individuals may feel that they do not deserve to have pleasure or that they are waiting for happiness until they feel better, until the stressors are resolved or until they go away. This belief makes breaking the stress cycle even more challenging; however, rewards motivate behavior (Abascal et al., 2001). By asking people to pursue a healthy and pleasurable activity every week, motivating them to become more involved in their lives and break this cycle is often easier. The activity can be simple and it need not cost money. For example, people often find pleasure in watching a sunset, observing birds at a feeder, calling a friend with whom they have not spoken in years, reading a favorite poem or book, or watching a funny movie (Wells-Federman, 2000). Hobbies are purposeful leisure activities that can balance hectic, stressful lives. A hobby should be chosen from interest and/or talent. Many hobbies have added benefits of increasing activity (e.g., gardening) or promoting social engagement (e.g., a book club or chorus). Nurses can suggest that individuals make leisure activities a regular part of the week as a purposeful and conscious plan to break the stress cycle.

Spiritual Practice

In response to stress, people can feel disconnected from life's meaning and purpose which, in turn, affects spiritual health and well-being. Meeting spiritual needs may be facilitated by **spiritual practice** or activities that help people find meaning, purpose, and connection. For example, individuals may choose to elicit the relaxation response through prayer. This focused, relaxed state of mind might help them develop a spiritual perspective that can engender a shift in values and beliefs to help cope with a stressor they cannot change, such as chronic illness or loss of a loved one.

Nurses might suggest a referral to a chaplain or clergy member, provide spiritual music or art work, recommend spiritual reading material, and provide personal presence (Box 13-4).

Nurses can suggest activities that provide a sense of meaning and purpose. Keeping a gratitude journal can be an important strategy to help individuals focus on aspects of life that are more positive and that become clouded from view when feeling overwhelmed by stress. Finding ways of

---

| Box **13-4** | A Stress Management Strategy for Nurses |

Develop the skill of personal presence. Presence is the gift of self through availability and attention to needs. Presence means "being there" for another person. To be available to others in this way, first practice the skill of being present with yourself. One effective way of developing this skill is through mindfulness, which is the ability to focus attention on what you are experiencing from moment to moment. Mindfulness encompasses the abilities of slowing down and bringing your full attention (thoughts, feelings, and bodily sensations) to the action in which you are engaged at the moment. The practice can be particularly useful in allowing yourself to extend the benefits of eliciting the relaxation response in more areas of your daily life.

Some ideas for practicing personal presence (mindfulness) are:

- When you awaken each morning, bring your full attention to your breathing. Allow your awareness to expand gradually into the room and then slowly begin to listen to the sounds of the outdoors.
- On your way to work, focus on how you walk, drive, or ride the transit. Take some deep diaphragmatic breaths and relax your body as you travel.
- Take a moment to attend to your breath, relax your body, and focus your mind before entering a client's room.
- As you eat a meal, carefully examine it through all of your senses, the sight, smell, touch, taste and the sound of each bite. Mindfully enjoy this new experience.
- Recurring events of the day can become cues for a mini-relaxation (the ringing telephone, auscultating a heart beat, answering a call light, before, during, and after rounds or report).
- Make the transition home from work mindful. Leave thoughts and worries of work at work and be conscious of your home environment each day.
- Once again, focus on your breathing and become completely aware of your surroundings as you go to sleep. Practice mindfully letting go of today and tomorrow as you allow your mind and body to get some much needed rest.

Modified from Hoblitzelle, O. A., & Benson, H. (1993). Eliciting the relaxation response. In H. Benson & E. Stuart (Eds.), *The wellness book: The comprehensive guide to maintaining health and treating stress-related illness.* New York: Fireside; The Mind Body Medical Institute. (n.d.). Stress and performance. Retrieved September 26, 2004, from: *http://www.mbmi.org/pages/mbb_s1.asp;* The Mind Body Medical Institute. (n.d.). The stress response. Retrieved September 26, 2004, from: *http://www.mbmi.org/pages/mbb_s2.asp.*

helping others (tutoring children, reading to the blind, or visiting an elderly adult) can have a positive influence on spiritual health and well-being. Altruism, generosity, kindness, and service to others are more than moral virtues. These attributes not only help to make the world a better place, they also help people find meaning and purpose in life. Religious and existential well-being have provided some defense against depression for people living with chronic and life-threatening conditions (Coleman, 2004). Elderly, chronically ill, and homebound people can be encouraged to produce written or oral histories that can be a legacy or, when able, to contact others needing care or to make telephone calls to raise funds for a favorite charity.

Clarifying Values and Beliefs

To manage stress and develop a balanced lifestyle, people must recognize the things that are important to them, reflect on where they are in life, evaluate what needs to be changed, and generate an action plan for that change (Gaydos, 2000) (see Chapter 4). This process is known as **values clarification.** The first step is to identify what is important, meaningful, and valuable so as to assess whether actions are consistent with beliefs. What people believe and value guide their actions by endorsing certain behaviors and changing others. When people assess their values and beliefs, they employ the ability to make their own choices rather than relying on beliefs and values dictated to them by others.

One method nurses can use to help people identify what they value and, ultimately, to help them clarify the relationship between their beliefs and actions is to ask them to identify what is important or meaningful to them. The form in Figure 13-4 is an example of questions used in the Medical Symptom Reduction Clinic at the Division of Behavioral Medicine at the Beth Israel Deaconess Medical Center in Boston. Individuals are asked to identify what is important and meaningful to them in eight domains. Nurses may change the domains to reflect more accurately the values and beliefs of the individuals they are counseling. After reviewing the results, individuals may find that they have not been doing certain things that are important to them (becoming more physically active, eating a healthier diet, volunteering, or spending time with their children). When people detect inconsistencies between their values and their actual living habits, they can begin to develop a working plan for correcting these inconsistencies. This process enables them to make conscious choices and to have more control.

Setting Realistic Goals

Developing an action plan for change to work toward a more balanced health-promoting lifestyle that is consistent with a person's values and beliefs is an important stress management strategy. Setting realistic, attainable goals facilitates this exercise. **Goal setting** is a dynamic process that involves both the individual and the nurse (Stuart & Wells-Federman, 2000). Goals should be specific, concrete, measurable, and achievable. Nurses can facilitate this process by respecting the individual's input, using a values clarification exercise (such as the one mentioned) to facilitate a more complete database to guide individuals to identify and prioritize problems to be addressed, and set mutually agreed upon long-term and short-term goals. Nurses should encourage individuals to challenge themselves when their behaviors are not consistent with what they identified as important and meaningful to them. For example, when an overweight man with hypertension and high cholesterol levels continues to smoke and eat high-fat foods, encourage him to look at these behaviors relative to what is meaningful to him, such as his family. The cost benefit is usually clear and the responsibility for the change is with the individual, not the nurse. Nurses can use the following questions to help individuals clarify long-term goals (Stuart & Wells-Federman, 2000, p. 399):

- What is most important and meaningful in your life?
- What aspects of your life would you like to change most right now?
- How can you begin the first step in that change?
- On what date would you like to achieve that goal?
- How can you reward yourself for success?
- How will your life be different when you succeed?
- How can I help?

When helping people set goals, nurses often advise using the 2×50 rule. The individual is asked to state the goal and then multiply the amount of time needed to accomplish the goal by 2, or reduce its difficulty by 50%. For example, losing 10 pounds in the next month is likely an unrealistic goal; losing 10 pounds in 2 months or losing 5 pounds in the next month is a more attainable goal. Setting realistic, attainable goals helps to create a sense of confidence and achievement and to build enthusiasm to set future goals. This, in turn, increases a sense of control and mediates the negative effects of stress (Stuart & Wells-Federman, 2000).

Humor

Humor is not only enjoyable and one of the best antidotes to stress, it has also been found to have significant health-promoting properties (Wooten, 2000). Laughter creates predictable physiological changes in the body. Similar to how it behaves with other forms of exercise, the body responds in two stages: (1) an arousal phase with an increase in physiological parameters and (2) a resolution phase, during which these parameters return to resting values or lower values. Laughter is a powerful stress reducer (Wooten, 2000).

Humor can be empowering; it gives people a different perspective on their problems and it facilitates objectivity, which increases a sense of self-protection and control in their environment. Finding humor in a stressful situation can help people to reframe perceptions of the event. More and more hospitals are recognizing the value of humor to health promotion. Some hospitals have laughter libraries, humor rooms, comedy carts that can be wheeled into an individual's hospital room, or clowns to bring laughter and

"What Is Important and Meaningful to You in Life?"

In each of the following areas, what do you want for yourself, today, next week, a year from now?

Under each of the following categories, please ask yourself these important questions.

Professional, educational, and intellectual
Today _____
Next week _____
A year from now _____

Relationships
Today _____
Next week _____
A year from now _____

Creative things
Today _____
Next week _____
A year from now _____

Spiritual
Today _____
Next week _____
A year from now _____

Volunteer and altruistic
Today _____
Next week _____
A year from now _____

Health
Today _____
Next week _____
A year from now _____

Fun and play
Today _____
Next week _____
A year from now _____

Material objects
Today _____
Next week _____
A year from now _____

Figure 13-4 What is important and meaningful in life? (From *Medical symptom reduction clinic patient notebook.* Boston: Division of Behavioral Medicine, Beth Israel Deaconess Medical Center, The Mind Body Medical Institute, Harvard Medical School.)

joy to the bedside. Humor is a powerful, inexpensive stress reduction and health-promotion strategy that can offer a valuable perspective for people on their world and on themselves (Box 13-5).

EFFECTIVE COPING

When people believe that they can cope effectively, the harmful effects of stress can be minimized. The stressful situation is perceived as a challenge rather than a threat.

This often elusive difference has vital mind, body, and spirit effects. When people believe that their lives are more balanced and under control, they are productive, but not driven; aroused, but not anxious; and may even be physically or mentally tired, but not exhausted.

Effective coping is what helps people face great adversity (such as illness) and recognize the opportunity that the situation often presents (Stuart & Wells-Federman, 2000). Primarily, individuals must recognize that **coping** is the art

Box **13-5**	Humor Strategies for Stress Reduction

Nurses help individuals use humor for health promotion and stress reduction in a variety of ways, including:
- Keeping a humor journal: looking for the unintentional amusing remark, watching for funny things young children say or do, and looking in the newspaper for humorous grammatical errors or an inappropriate choice of words and writing them down in a journal
- Looking on the Internet for humorous resources
- Creating a scrapbook of humorous cartoons, pictures, stickers, poems, and songs
- Reading a cartoon or joke in the newspaper every day and sharing it with a friend
- Watching funny movies or reruns of old television programs
- Finding and spending time with funny, light-hearted people

of finding a balance, the ability to find a balance between acceptance and action, between letting go and taking control. Many stress management strategies help individuals distinguish these differences by providing a format for observing or objectifying their experiences. Other strategies such as exercise and balanced nutrition help individuals promote physical health and well-being to counter the harmful effects of stress.

Nurses can help individuals improve effective coping by guiding them in the art of choosing the right strategy at the right time. In doing so, people gain a sense of control that minimizes or buffers harmful effects of stress.

When individuals cannot control or influence the situation (extrinsic stressors), nurses can advise them to:
- *Take care of physical health and well-being:* exercise, eat healthy balanced meals, and practice sleep hygiene.
- *Accept:* learn to accept that some situations or people cannot be changed or avoided. Letting go of resentment and forgiveness are often a part of acceptance.
- *Use distraction:* distraction involves putting a worry aside, when necessary, until the situation can be dealt with directly. This prioritizing is quite different from procrastinating or denial, because it is a necessary delay rather than avoidance.
- *Reduce emotional arousal:* practice mini-relaxations, listen to a relaxation tape, use the four-step cognitive restructuring technique, exercise, seek social support, pray, use humor and affirmations, write in a journal, and engage in a healthy pleasure.

When individuals can alter or influence the situation, or when they are contributing to or creating the stress (intrinsic stressors), nurses can advise them to:
- *Take care of physical health and well-being:* exercise, eat healthy balanced meals, and practice sleep hygiene.
- *Reduce emotional arousal:* practice mini-relaxations, listen to a relaxation tape, exercise, seek social support, pray,

use humor and affirmations, write in a journal, engage in a healthy pleasure, and use the four-step cognitive restructuring strategy:
1. Stop (breaking the cycle of escalating, negative thoughts)
2. Take a breath (eliciting the relaxation response and release tension)
3. Reflect (asking, "What is going on here? What am I thinking? Is the thought true? Is the thought helpful? Am I jumping to conclusions or magnifying the situation?")
4. Choose a more realistic, rational response
- Problem solve:
1. Clarify values and beliefs.
2. Gather information.
3. Seek advice, support, assistance, or information.
4. Use assertive communication and empathy.
5. Set realistic goals, design action strategies, and determine the best steps to handle the problem.
6. Take action.

See the Care Plan for John R. for an example of a plan for effective coping.

SUMMARY

Good health and the ability to meet effectively the many demands of life require managing stress. Combining careful assessment and choice of strategies, thoughtful and honest feedback, and continued support, nurses can help people cope more effectively with the innumerable stressors they encounter. Research to discern the interplay of physiological, psychological, social, and spiritual responses to stress has yielded important knowledge for practice. However, uncovering the intricate workings of the brain within the context of human stress and coping experiences is a daunting and critical challenge for today's health researchers (Cahill, 2001).

Stress management strategies provide an opportunity for individuals to acquire the necessary skills to cope more effectively and become confident in self-managing. From this awareness, the individual is able to challenge and change perception, decrease stress reactivity, improve self-management skills, and minimize the harmful consequences of stress. This process positively influences health promotion, disease prevention, and symptom management. Understanding influences of stress on health and illness is essential to all nursing practice.

ADDITIONAL STUDY MATERIAL

Study Questions in the back of the book, see page 663.

evolve WEB SITE MATERIALS

These materials are located on the book's Web site at http://evolve.elsevier.com/Edelman/.

- WebLinks
- Content Updates

REFERENCES

Abascal, J. R., Brucato, D., & Brucato, L. (2001). *Stress mastery: The art of coping gracefully.* Upper Saddle River, NJ: Prentice Hall.

Bartol, G. M., & Courts, N. F. (2000). The psychophysiology of bodymind healing. In B. Dossey, C. Guzetta, & L. Keegan (Eds.), *Holistic nursing: A handbook for practice* (3rd ed.). Gaithersburg, MD: Aspen.

Benson, H. (1975). *The relaxation response.* New York: William Morrow & Co.

Berkman, L. F. (2000). What influences cognitive function: Living alone or being alone? *Lancet, 355,* 1291-1292.

Black, P. H., & Garbutt, L. D. (2002). Stress, inflammation and cardiovascular disease. *Journal of Psychosomatic Research, 52,* 1-23.

Brennan, R. (2000). *Stress: The alternative solution.* London: Foulsham.

Cahill, C. A. (2001). Women and stress. In J. J. Fitzpatrick & D. Taylor (Eds.), *Annual review of nursing research: Vol. 19. Women's health research* (pp. 229-248). New York: Springer.

Cannon, W. (1914). The emergency function of the adrenal medulla in pain and the major emotions. *American Journal of Physiology, 33,* 356-372.

Caudill, M. A. (1995). *Managing pain before it manages you.* New York: Guilford Press.

Chapman, C. R., & Gavrin, J. (1999). Suffering: The contributions of persistent pain. *Lancet, 353,* 2233-2236.

Coleman, C. L. (2004). The contribution of religious and existential well-being to depression among African American heterosexuals with HIV infection. *Issues in Mental Health Nursing, 25*(1), 103-110.

Cruess, D., Antoni, M., Schneiderman, N., Ironson, G., McCabe, P., Fernandez, J. B., et al. (2000). Cognitive-behavioral stress management increases free testosterone and decreases psychological distress in HIV-seropositive men. *Health Psychology, 19,* 12-20.

Daneault, S., Lussier, V., Mongeau, S., Paillé, P., Hudon, É., Dion, D., et al. (2004). The nature of suffering and its relief in the terminally ill: A qualitative study. *Journal of Palliative Care, 20,* 7-11.

Davis, M., Eshelman, E. R., McKay, M. (2000). *The relaxation & stress reduction workbook* (5th ed.). Oakland, CA: New Harbinger.

Dedert, E. A., Studts, J. L., Weissbecker, I., Salmon, P. G., Banis, P. L., Sephton, S. E. (2004). Religiosity may help preserve the cortisol rhythm in women with stress-related illness. *International Journal of Psychiatry in Medicine, 34,* 61-77.

Easterling, D. V., Gallagher, K. M., & Lodwick, D. G. (2003). *Promoting health at the community level.* Thousand Oaks, CA: Sage.

Esch, T., & Stefano, G. (2002). Proinflammation: A common denominator or initiator of different pathophysiological disease processes. *General Medical Science Monitor, 8*(5), HY1-9.

Esch, T., Fricchione, G., & Stefano, G. (2003). The therapeutic use of relaxation-response in stress-related diseases. *Medical Science Monitor, 9*(2), RA23-34.

Esch, T., Stefano, G., Fricchione, G., & Benson, H. (2002). Stress in cardiovascular diseases. *General Medical Science Monitor, 8*(5), RA93-101.

Frasure-Smith, N., Lesperance, F., Gravel, G., Masson, A., Martin, J., Talajic, M., et al. (2000). Social support, depression, and mortality during the first year after myocardial infarction. *Circulation, 101,* 1919-1924.

Fratiglioni, L., Wang, H. X., Ericsson, K., Maytan, M., & Winblad, B. (2000). Influence of social network on occurrence of dementia: A community-based longitudinal study. *Lancet, 355,* 1315-1319.

Gaydos, H. L. B. (2000). The art of holistic nursing and the human health experience. In B. Dossey, C. Guzetta, & L. Keegan (Eds.), *Holistic nursing: A handbook for practice* (3rd ed.). Gaithersburg, MD: Aspen.

Hickman, S. E., Tilden, V. P., & Tolle, S. W. (2004). Family perceptions of worry, symptoms, and suffering in the dying. *Journal of Palliative Care, 20,* 20-27.

Highet, N., & Drummond, P. (2004). A comparative evaluation of community treatments for post-partum depression: Implications for treatment and management practices. *Australian and New Zealand Journal of Psychiatry, 38,* 212-218.

Holmes, T. H. (1981). *The schedule of recent experience.* Seattle, WA: University of Washington Press.

Jacobs, G. D. (1998). *Say goodnight to insomnia.* New York: Henry Holt and Co.

Kant, A. K., Schatzkin, A., Graubard, B. I., & Schairer, C. (2000). A prospective study of diet quality and mortality in women. *Journal of the American Medical Association, 283,* 2109-2115.

Kenney, J. W., & Bhattacharjee, A. (2000). Interactive model of women's stressors, personality traits and health problems. *Journal of Advanced Nursing, 32,* 249-258.

Klag, S., & Bradley, G. (2004). The role of hardiness in stress and illness: An exploration of the effect of affectivity and gender. *British Journal of Health Psychology, 9*(Pt. 2), 137-161.

Kobasa, S. C., Maddi, S. R., & Kahn, S. (1982). Hardiness and health: A prospective study. *Journal of Personality and Social Psychology, 42,* 391-404.

Lazarus, R., & Folkman, S. (1984). *Stress, appraisal, and coping.* New York: Springer.

Loeher, K. E., Bank, A. L., MacNeill, S. E., & Lichtenberg, P. A. (2004). Nursing home transition and depressive symptoms in older medical rehabilitation patients. *Clinical Gerontologist, 27,* 59-70.

Luck, S. (2000). Nutrition. In B. Dossey, C. Guzetta, & L. Keegan (Eds.), *Holistic nursing: A handbook for practice* (3rd ed.). Gaithersburg, MD: Aspen.

Manuta, T., Colligan, R. C., Malinchoc, M., Offord, K. P. (2000). Optimists vs. pessimists: Survival rate among medical patients over a 30-year period. *Mayo Clinic Proceedings, 75,* 140-143.

Markowitz, J. C. (2004). Interpersonal psychotherapy of depression. In M. Power (Ed.), *Mood disorders: A handbook of science and practice* (pp. 183-200). West Sussex, England: John Wiley & Sons.

Marshall, R. D. (2002). If we had known then what we know now: A review of local and national surveys following September 11, 2001. *CNS Spectrums, 7*(9), 645-649.

Morin, C. M., Colecchi, C., Stone, J., Sood, R., & Brink, D. (1999). Behavioral and pharmacological therapies for late-life insomnia: A randomized controlled trial. *Journal of the American Medical Association, 281,* 1991-1999.

Nightingale, F. (1859, 1992). *Notes on nursing: What it is and what it is not* (Commemorative ed.). Philadelphia: J. B. Lippincott.

Pascali-Bonaro, D., & Kroeger, M. (2004). Continuous female companionship during childbirth: A crucial resource in times of stress or calm. *Journal of Midwifery and Women's Health, 49*(4 Supplement), 19-27.

Peden, A. R., Hall, L. A., Rayens, M. K., & Beebe, L. L. (2000). Reducing negative thinking and depressive symptoms in college women. *Image: The Journal of Nursing Scholarship, 32,* 145-151.

Pengilly, J. W., & Dowd, E. T. (2000). Hardiness and social support as moderators of stress. *Journal Clinical Psychology, 56,* 813-820.

Pennebaker, J. (2000). Telling stories: The health benefits of narrative. *Literary Medicine, 19,* 3-18.

Power, M. (2004). Cognitive behavioral therapy for depression. In M. Power (Ed.), *Mood disorders: A handbook of science and practice* (pp. 167-181). West Sussex, England: John Wiley & Sons.

Rogers, C. (1951). *Client-centered therapy.* Boston: Houghton Mifflin.

Selye, H. (1982). History and present status of stress concept. In L. Goldberger & S. Breznitz (Eds.), *Handbook of stress: Theoretical and clinical aspects.* New York: The Free Press.

Shelby, J., & McCance, K. L. (1998). Stress and disease. In K. L. McCance & S. E. Heuther (Eds.), *Pathophysiology: The biologic basis for disease in adults and children.* St. Louis: Mosby.

Shen, J., McCreary, C. P., & Myers, H. F. (2004). Independent and mediated contributions of personality, coping, social support, and depressive symptoms to physical functioning outcome among patients in cardiac rehabilitation. *Journal of Behavioral Medicine, 27,* 39-62.

Snyder, M. (2002). An overview of complementary/alternative therapies. In M. Snyder & R. Lindquist (Eds.), *Complementary/alternative therapies in nursing* (4th ed., pp. 3-15). New York: Springer.

Stuart, E., & Wells-Federman, C. L. (2000). Cognitive therapy. In B. Dossey, C. Guzetta, & L. Keegan (Eds.), *Holistic nursing: A handbook for practice* (3rd ed.). Gaithersburg, MD: Aspen.

The Mind Body Medical Institute. (n.d.a.). The stress response. Retrieved September 26, 2004, from: *http://www.mbmi.org/pages/mbb_s1.asp.*

The Mind Body Medical Institute. (n.d.b.). Stress and performance. Retrieved September 26, 2004, from: *http://www.mbmi.org/pages/mbb_s2.asp.*

U.S. Department of Agriculture. (n.d.) The Food Guide Pyramid. Retrieved September 28, 2004, from: *http://www.pueblo.gsa.gov/cic_text/food/food-pyramid/main.htm.*

U.S. Department of Health and Human Services. (2000). *Healthy people 2010* (On-line). Retrieved March 9, 2005, from: *http://www.health.gov/healthypeople/document/html.*

Wells-Federman, C. (2000). Caring for the patient in chronic pain. Part II. *Clinical Excellence for Nurse Practitioners, 4,* 4-12.

Wells-Federman, C., Stuart-Shor, E., Deckro, J., Mandle, C. L., Baim, M., & Medich, C. (1995). The mind/body connection: The psychophysiology of many traditional nursing interventions. *Clinical Nurse Specialist, 9,* 59-66.

Wells-Federman, C., Stuart-Shor, E., & Webster, A. (2001). Cognitive therapy: Applications for health promotion, disease prevention and disease management. *Nursing Clinics of North America, 36,* 93-133.

Williams, J. E., Paton, C., Siegler, I. C., Eigenbrodt, M. L., Nieto, F. J., & Tyrole, H. A. (2000). Anger proneness predicts coronary heart disease risk: Prospective analysis from the Atherosclerosis Risk in Communities (ARIC) study. *Circulation, 101,* 2034-2039.

Witvliet, C. V., Phipps, K. A., Feldman, M. E., & Beckham, J. C. (2004). Posttraumatic mental and physical health correlates of forgiveness and religious coping in military veterans. *Journal of Traumatic Stress, 17*(3), 269-273.

Wooten, P. (2000). Humor, laughter, and play: Maintaining balance in a serious world. In B. Dossey, C. Guzetta, & L. Keegan (Eds.), *Holistic nursing: A handbook for practice* (3rd ed.). Gaithersburg, MD: Aspen.

Chapter 14

REGINA LOWRY

Holistic Health Strategies

objectives

After completing this chapter, the reader will be able to:

- Define holistic health.
- Contrast holistic health care and conventional health care.
- Describe the philosophical base of energy medicine.
- Describe the origin and practice of selected holistic health strategies.
- Contrast the importance of self-exploration for individuals and health care professionals.

key terms

Acupuncture	Imagery	Reflexology
Aromatherapy	Meditation	Reiki
Centering	Prana	Subtle energy
Chi (Qi)	Prayer	Tai Chi
Energy	Presence	Therapeutic touch
Holism	Qi Gong	Yoga

THINK About It

Please Answer the Following Questions

- When you wake up, does the idea of the day to come excite you?
- Does a lack of energy keep you from doing what you want to do?
- What makes you laugh? Can you laugh at yourself? Do you laugh often?
- Are you confident about the decisions you make?
- Do the choices you make have the outcomes you expect?

- Are you valued and appreciated at home, on the job?
- Are there people you appreciate? Do you tell them so?
- Do you have friends who offer you love, companionship, and support?

   If you answered "no" to any of these questions, you may have identified areas in your life that you want to change. Knowing yourself—the good and not so good—is the first step toward holistic health.

Modified from the American Holistic Health Association. (2003). *Wellness from within: The first step.* Anaheim, CA: Author. Retrieved April, 20, 2005, from: *http://ahha.org/ahhastep.htm.*

HOLISM

Too often in health care practice, an individual seeking care has been viewed as the sick part (the gallbladder) or characterized by the sick function (the insomniac). Consumers are often dissatisfied with conventional health care and perceive that, within the conventional model, they are viewed as machines with parts and pieces. Consumers are seeking an alternative style of health care that will focus on wellness and reduce the number of medications taken (Pelletier, Astin, & Haskell, 1999). Behind the idea of **holism** is the understanding that people are not just physical bodies; people have emotions, spirits, and relationships that combine with the physical body to make a whole person. People have relationships with the earth and their environment, with other people, and with themselves as they attempt to find the meaning and purpose in life (Bright, 2002). The holistic movement in the healing arts reflects the theory of holism and recognizes that all these aspects of the person must be considered when planning and delivering care.

Holistic practitioners believe that health is more than the absence of disease; health is optimal wellness. The individual seeking health defines health. Working toward health and wellness is an ongoing process that includes self-knowledge and self-care. When disease occurs, holistic practitioners seek to support the person's natural healing systems, to consider the whole person, and to consider the environment (both physical and mental) surrounding the person. The holistic practitioner promotes wellness, treats illness, and attempts to look beyond the symptoms to discover the cause of illness (Walter, 2000).

Many of the interventions used in holistic health care practice are backed by centuries of tradition (Thompson, 2000) but are often considered alternative practices and are not currently incorporated into most conventional health care practices. This view is changing; alternative and complementary practices are moving into the mainstream. Several medical and nursing schools are adding courses on alternative therapies to their curricula. Dr. Dean Ornish's Program for Reversing Heart Disease, which incorporates diet, yoga, and meditation, is now available in 19 sites in 4 states (for a list of sites visit the Lifestyle Advantage Web site at *http://www.lifestyleadvantage.org/sites.html*). Under the Medicare demonstration project testing this intervention, 1800 people will qualify for Medicare payment for the program (Lifestyle Advantage, 2002). Alternative therapies can also be used as an adjunct to conventional medical care. Rapidly increasing numbers of managed care groups, insurers, and hospitals are including holistic health practices, because consumers are demanding them (Pelletier et al., 1999). **Web Site Resource 14A** presents a table depicting how many adults in the United States use holistic therapies. Regions Hospital in St. Paul, Minnesota, opened a holistic nursing unit. People on the unit can receive massage, aromatherapy, music therapy, meditation, and relaxation therapy as standard nursing care (Horrigan, 2000). The Van

innovative practice

Connections: A Campus Caring Model

Nursing faculty at Western Michigan University (WMU), Kalamazoo, Michigan, have founded an on-campus healing center called Connections. The original purposes of the healing center were to (1) provide opportunities for healing and stress reduction to students of the WMU community, (2) provide a site to demonstrate holistic nursing interventions to students, and (3) provide an avenue for faculty practice in holistic care.

The Student Housing Manager donated space and furniture for the project; the center is housed in WMU married and international housing. Nursing faculty, an informal practice group of healers who joined to share healing modalities, and campus individuals who were trained in Reiki and massage originally staffed the center. Currently, nursing faculty provide healing touch and auricular acupuncture treatments. The center is open by appointment. There is no charge for services; however, there is a possibility of reaching out to the broader community on a fee-for-service basis.

As with any new project, problems have been encountered in making this center an ongoing reality. Faculty time constraints and changing teaching and practice assignments have been among the biggest hurdles to overcome; maintaining a volunteer staff is another hurdle, as volunteers come into and leave the practice due to other commitments. This idea of the clinic has great possibilities for improving the well-being of a campus community, and this clinic proves that the idea is feasible, if not easily accomplished.

From E. VanArsdale, B. Starke, personal communication, April 17, 2004.

Elslander Cancer Center at St. John Hospital in Detroit, Michigan, has a similar clinic that also offers Qi Gong, Tai Chi, and yoga classes, hypnotherapy, and guided imagery (Lento, 2003). The Innovative Practice box presents a holistic program on a college campus that is staffed partly by nursing faculty. Movements are underway to integrate holistic practices with conventional medical practices; this effort may broaden the opportunity for holistic practitioners even further as some people who might not normally visit an alternative practitioner willingly accept a referral within the same group (Thompson, 2000).

Holistic interventions are used to promote wellness. Holistic interventions are used to manage illness and reduce pain and can help meet the goals of *Healthy People 2010*, including increasing quality and years of healthy life, increasing physical activity and flexibility in all age groups, decreasing pain, and reducing substance abuse. See the *Healthy People 2010* box for selected objectives that relate to holistic interventions. Holistic practices are moving into the mainstream; therefore, nurses should understand the interventions that constitute holistic practice. Nurses must be able to discuss these practices with individuals who are using them. Nurses may wish to make referrals to alternative practitioners. Nurses may also find that holistic inter-

Healthy People 2010
Selected National Health-Promotion and Disease
Prevention Goals and Objectives

- Increase quality and years of healthy life (p. 8)
- Quality of life reflects a general sense of happiness and satisfaction with our lives and environment (p. 10)
- Reduce the proportion of adults who engage in no leisure-time physical activity (p. 22-8)
- Increase the proportion of adults who engage regularly, preferably daily, in moderate physical activity for at least 30 minutes per day (p. 22-9); adolescents for at least 30 minutes on 5 or more of the previous 7 days (p. 22-17)
- Increase the proportion of adults [and adolescents, p. 22-19] who engage in vigorous physical activity that promotes development and maintenance of cardiorespiratory fitness 3 or more days per week for 20 or more minutes per occasion (p. 22-11)
- Increase the proportion of adults who perform physical activities that enhance and maintain muscular strength and endurance (p. 22-11)
- Increase the proportion of adults who perform physical activities that enhance and maintain flexibility (p. 22-15)
- Reduce substance abuse to protect the health, safety, and quality of life for all (p. 26-3)
- Increase the mean number of days without severe pain among adults who have chronic joint symptoms (p. 2-11)
- Reduce the proportion of adults with chronic joint symptoms who experience a limitation in activity due to arthritis (p. 2-11)

From U.S. Department of Health and Human Services. (2000). *Healthy people 2010: Understanding and improving health and objectives for improving health* (2nd ed.). Washington, DC: U.S. Government Printing Office.

ventions such as energy work, bodywork, aromatherapy, prayer, meditation, massage, imagery, music therapy, and the movement arts of yoga, Tai Chi, and Qi Gong provide a useful adjunct to current nursing practice. Nurses interested in certification as holistic practitioners or training in various holistic interventions will find the American Holistic Nurses Association (*http://www.ahna.org/*) a useful resource.

INTERVENTIONS
Energy Work

People are animate beings with **energy,** a life force present in all living and nonliving elements of the universe. This energy is the animating force that flows through the body and extends beyond the body (Krieger, 1998) to interact with the energy in the environment (Rogers, 1970). The human energy field may be detected, assessed, and manipulated by an energy practitioner. Martha Rogers (1970) brought the idea of energy to nursing when she stated, "The fundamental unit of the living system is an energy field"

Box 14-1   Feel Your Own Energy

This exercise will help you feel your own energy, or chi.
- Sit quietly, back straight, feet touching the floor.
- Place your hands in your lap.
- Take a few deep breaths. Become quiet and still.
- Breathe slowly in and out for a few minutes.
- Slowly raise your hands in front of you, palms facing, hands about 15 inches apart. Cup your fingers as though you are holding a basketball between your hands.
- Concentrate on the space between your hands. What is there? Can you feel anything?
- Slowly bring your palms closer together, focusing on the space between your hands.
- Can you feel warmth? Does it feel spongy? Can you move your hands around a shape?
- What you are feeling is the energy coming from the energy centers in your hands. Focus on the energy. Try to increase the sensation of fullness in the space between your hands.
- If you do not feel anything right away, bring your hands back out to 15 inches apart and slowly move your hands together again. Try no more than 3 times each time you attempt the exercise.

(p. 92). Certain types of body energy are well known. Electrical energy in the body is reflected by electrocardiographic and electroencephalographic tracings.

People can be affected by the energy of their environments, including the energy of other people. For example, anxiety is contagious and moves readily and quickly from person to person (Bowman, 2004). There are medical uses for energy that comes from the environment. The energy of radiation is used to shrink tumors; sound energy, in the form of ultrasound waves, is used to break up kidney stones (Gray, 2004). Music, a form of sound energy, can be relaxing or stimulating and has been used to decrease the anxiety of ventilated patients (Thomas, 2003) and to decrease preoperative anxiety and stress (Norred, 2000). Light energy is useful in treating seasonal affective disorder (Levitt, Lam, & Levitan, 2002) and the depression of pregnancy (Oren et al., 2002). Color, another form of light energy, may have an effect on emotions and behaviors (Knez, 2001; Stone, 2003). Lasers, focused light energy, are used in many types of surgery and to treat other disorders (Demarco & Clarke 2001).

Other energies can affect healing. Many cultures believe that an energy flows through the body; this energy nourishes organs and promotes optimal functioning. Chinese call this energy **chi** (or *qi*), Japanese call it *ki,* and East Indians call it **prana.** In the West, this energy is often called **subtle energy,** *life energy,* or *universal energy.* Most of the detailed information on this energy system comes from ancient metaphysical texts and from people who have an ability to see the energy as it moves in and surrounds people. Personal experience may reveal the subtle energy in the body, as demonstrated by the exercise in Box 14-1.

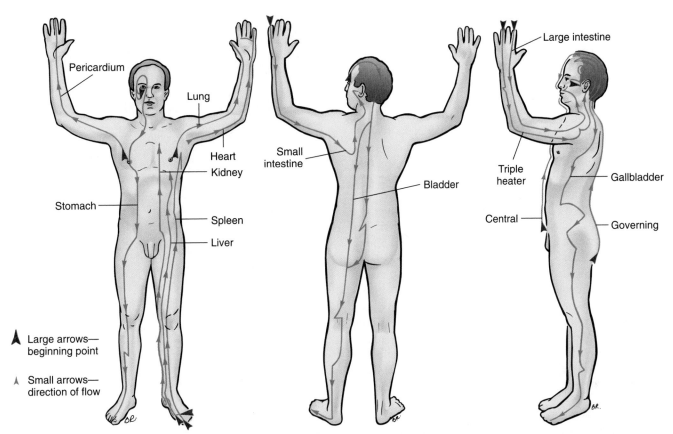

Figure 14-1 Typical locations of meridians. (From Fritz, S. [2004]. *Mosby's fundamentals of therapuetic massage* [3rd ed.]. St. Louis: Mosby.

Illness, stress, emotional upset, or spiritual distress can affect the flow of life energy; the flow can become blocked, unbalanced, or chaotic. These disruptions in the flow of life energy can cause or exacerbate illness in the physical body and can increase emotional and spiritual distress. The basic premise behind energy work is releasing blockages to energy flow, stimulating deficient life energy, and rebalancing life energy. Various modalities are used.

Acupuncture, Acupressure, and Reflexology

Acupuncture. Acupuncture manipulates life energy (chi or qi) by stimulating precisely mapped points on the skin surface. The points overlie the channels, called *meridians*, through which chi travels (Figure 14-1). The channels are named for the organs they affect, such as the lung meridian, heart meridian, and kidney meridian. Stimulation of the points may be accomplished by inserting fine needles into the points, by electrostimulation, by laser, and by light stimulation. The acupuncture points act as valves in the meridian system. When stimulated, the valve may open to release blocked or excess chi. The valve may close to allow chi to collect if it is deficient. Burning herbs can be used on or over the points to increase point stimulation; this technique is known as *moxibustion*. Acupuncture is used to diagnose disharmony; the points become tender to palpation in the presence of disturbance. By stimulating points to manipulate chi, acupuncture becomes a treatment modality.

Acupuncture is a useful treatment for substance abuse; the treatments may stand alone or combined with other forms of therapy. The National Acupuncture Detoxification Association (NADA) protocol for addiction involves general stimulation of five points in each ear. Treatment goals include symptom palliation during withdrawal (Killeen et al., 2002). Many nurses are trained in the NADA program (Jay Renaud, NADA, personal communication, July 13, 2000). Information on training can be found at the NADA Web site *(http://www.acudetox.com/NADA/training/trng-info.htm)*.

Acupuncture is also an effective adjunctive treatment for musculoskeletal pain (Kerr, Walsh, & Baxter, 2001). The National Institutes of Health Consensus Development Panel found acupuncture to be effective on postoperative and chemotherapy-induced nausea and vomiting and postoperative dental pain and found that acupuncture may also be useful for other pain syndromes, addiction, stroke rehabilitation, and asthma (Mayer, 2000). Acupuncture education is available through many schools of traditional Chinese medicine and other sources; a Web search of acupuncture schools provides several sources for education.

Acupressure. The meridian points may also be stimulated by hand pressure. Acupressure involves stimulation of the acupuncture points by pressing, knuckling, rubbing, squeezing, and stretching. No oil is used for acupressure and the treatments may be performed with the person fully clothed. Both shiatsu and Amma therapy use acupressure along with massage to move and balance the body's energies. Education in these methods may be acquired through massage schools. Dibble, Chapman, Mack, and Shih (2000) found that acupressure applied to a point on the inner aspect of the forearm and to a point slightly below the knee decreased the intensity and experience of nausea for the treatment group of patients receiving chemotherapy for breast cancer. Maa and others (2003) found acupuncture and acupressure were both effective in improving quality of life for patients with stable chronic obstructive asthma.

Reflexology. **Reflexology** is another method of moving energy by using hand pressure. Rather than acupuncture points, the reflexologist applies pressure to mapped points on the feet or hands or both. Pressure is applied with the thumbs, pressing deeply into the point to release tension and stimulate circulation of blood, lymph, and energy. Reflexology is more than massage; practitioners believe that the points correspond to the organs of the body and that stimulating the points will stimulate the organs. There are many Web sites related to reflexology. The Association of Reflexologists home page *(http://www.aor.org.uk)* provides information on reflexology history, training, and research.

Touch Therapies

In the touch therapies (therapeutic touch, healing touch, Reiki, pranic healing, Qi Gong healing, and polarity therapy, among others), practitioners use their hands to direct life energies drawn from the environment to the individual in an effort to restore balance and harmony within the human energy system. The mechanism of action for the touch therapies is, at this time, unknown. An actual exchange of physical energy may take place between practitioner and individual (Bruyere, 1994); others believe that the intent and consciousness of the practitioner is the mechanism that causes the effect of the intervention. Still others believe that intention creates an actual exchange of subtle energy (Benor, 1999-2000). During these therapies, the hands can be placed directly on the person's body (contact) or at a distance from the body (no contact).

Therapeutic Touch. **Therapeutic touch** (TT) may be the best known of the touch therapies. Delores Krieger, a registered nurse and professor of nursing, and her friend Dora Kunz, a lay healer, developed TT during the early 1970s. After observing Kunz and others healing by laying on of hands and analyzing their techniques, Krieger trained herself in the technique and began healing patients. Krieger (1979) believes that the ability to transmit universal energy is a natural ability of all humans. She taught a small group of nursing students to perform laying-on-of-hands therapy. This small group became the basis for TT and, since this modest beginning, about 130,000 health care professionals all over the world have been trained in the techniques (D. May, personal communication, March 30, 2004).

TT practice comprises three essential elements. The first element is **centering** by the practitioner. Centering is a

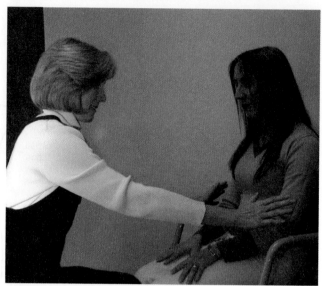

Figure 14-2 The assessment phase of therapeutic touch. The practitioner is attempting to sense disturbances or imbalances in the person's energy field.

process of becoming calm, present in the moment, and connected with the individual being treated, allowing the practitioner to give the person undivided attention. The centered practitioner is able to let go of personal feelings and emotions and is more open to inner perceptions (Krieger, 1998). The practitioner remains centered throughout the treatment. During assessment, the second element, the practitioner's hands move over the individual's body at a height of about 3 inches above the skin in an attempt to sense disturbances or imbalances in the person's energy field (Figure 14-2).

Assessment is performed before treatment begins and continues throughout treatment. Krieger (1993) describes the treatment techniques, the third element of TT practice. These techniques consist of methods to change the patterns in the human energy field (unruffling), to direct energy to the person to replenish depleted energy (modulation), and to balance or redistribute the individual's energies (modulation). The Case Study presents the treatment of one person using TT for neck pain. The Care Plan offers additional information on the techniques of TT; please note that the way this nursing diagnosis is written, there is an inherent requirement in the defining characteristics that the nurse be trained to assess and recognize the energy field disturbance.

Healing Touch. A technique known as healing touch (HT) is a modality similar to TT, developed by Janet Mentgen. HT adds full-body techniques for moving energy and disorder-specific energetic interventions to the modulation phase of TT (Hover-Kramer, 1996). Wardell and Weymouth (2004) reviewed studies of HT and found that the studies indicated "results in reducing stress, anxiety, and pain; accelerated healing . . . and a greater sense of well-

CASE STUDY

Mr. P.

Mr. P., an 82-year-old white man, came to the clinic reporting neck pain and stiffness of approximately 4 months duration. He was previously treated with ibuprofen (Motrin), acetaminophen and oxycodone (Percocet), and physical therapy. At the time of the initial clinic visit, Mr. P. was still taking Motrin but had stopped taking Percocet because the pain "isn't bad enough to take drugs [narcotics]." He rated his neck pain as 5 on a scale of 1 to 10. Neck range of motion (ROM) had improved, but it still caused problems for Mr. P. when driving. Mr. P. lives next to a very busy street and did not feel that he could turn his neck well enough to see the traffic coming. He was afraid to pull out into the street. His daughter had driven him to the clinic. She said, "Pop is still in pain. He has little interest in doing anything. He walks like an old man and he can't work in his garden because of the pain." The goal of treatment for Mr. P. is pain relief and increased ROM.

Reflective Questions

1. What holistic health strategies might be used to relieve Mr. P.'s pain and to help him increase his ROM?
2. After the treatment goals are reached, what holistic health strategies would you recommend to assist Mr. P. in maintaining and improving his health?

Therapeutic Touch (TT) was offered to Mr. P. Although he was skeptical that this treatment would be effective, he agreed to treatment to please his daughter. Increased heat was noted in the neck and shoulder areas. A 30-minute TT treatment was performed, with special attention given to the neck and shoulder area. Immediately following the TT treatment, Mr. P. rated his pain as 0 on a scale of 1 to 10 and reported that he "couldn't remember when he'd been so relaxed"; the excess heat had dissipated. Mr. P. was also given some simple yoga exercises for the neck and advised to perform the exercises twice a day, five gentle repetitions each time. Mr. P. was seen in the clinic a total of 8 times for TT and was given increasingly difficult yoga stretches for the neck and shoulders. His pain rating at the end of treatment remained at 0 on the 10 scale. He had stopped taking Motrin, saying, "I don't need it anymore." His neck ROM had improved, and he was driving and working in his garden again. He continues his yoga stretches and has started performing daily Qi Gong exercises.

CARE PLAN

Techniques of Therapeutic Touch

Nursing Diagnosis Energy Field Disturbance Related to Slowing or Blocking of Energy Flow Secondary to Repetitive Motion Injury

DEFINING CHARACTERISTICS

Perceptions of changes in patterns of the energy flow, such as:

- Temperature change: warmth, coolness
- Visual changes: image, color
- Disruption of the field: vacant, hole, spike, bulge
- Movement: wave, spike, tingling, dense, flowing
- Sounds: tone, words

Related Factors

- Pathophysiological: illness, injury
- Treatment-related: immobility, perioperative experience, labor and delivery
- Situational: pain, fear, anxiety, grieving
- Maturational: related to age-related developmental difficulties or crises

Expected Outcomes

- The person will report increased sense of relaxation.
- The person will report decreased anxiety and tension.
- The person will demonstrate evidence of physical relaxation (e.g., decreased blood pressure, pulse, respiratory rate, muscle tension).
- The person will report an increased sense of well-being.

Interventions

- Provide privacy if possible.
- Explain energy therapy (therapeutic touch, Reiki, healing touch) and obtain permission to treat.
- Position the person comfortably.
- Become quiet and still (centered) and bring the focus to the patient.
- Assess (scan) the energy field for openness and flow.
- Clear the exterior energy field by combing through the field from head to toe (unruffling).

  Move the palms of the hands toward the person, 2 to 4 inches over the person's body, from head to feet in a smooth, light movement.

  Sense the cues to energy imbalance (i.e., warmth, coolness, tightness, heaviness, tingling, emptiness).

- Focus on perceived areas of imbalance to repattern the energy flow.
- Reassess and smooth the exterior energy field, ensuring that the energy flow is open in the feet.
- Gently stop the treatment and provide the person time to rest.
- Encourage the person to discuss the experience.

Modified from Carpenito-Moyet, L. J. (2004). *Nursing diagnosis: Application to clinical practice* (10th ed.). Philadelphia: Lippincott; and Ackley, B. J., & Ladewig, B. G. (1999). *Nursing diagnosis handbook: A guide to planning care* (4th ed.). St. Louis: Mosby.

---

being" (p. 154). Training in TT and HT is readily available. Nurse Healers–Professional Associates International (*http://www.therapeutic-touch.org*) and Healing Touch International (*http://www.healingtouch.net*) provide information on training programs.

Other Touch Therapies. Qi Gong healing, pranic healing, and Reiki are similar modalities from the Chinese, East Indian, and Japanese traditions, respectively. Yoga practitioners may offer training in pranic healing during 1-day workshops. Qi Gong healing is provided primarily by Qi Gong masters and some traditional doctors of Chinese medicine, but others who practice Qi Gong regularly may also use the Qi Gong energy to heal (Cohen, as reported in Horrigan, 2003). Lee, Jang, Jang, and Moon (2003) found decreases in anxiety (significant at $P = 0.014$), depression, fatigue, pain, and blood pressure in a group receiving Qi therapy.

Reiki healing, from the Japanese tradition, requires training by a Reiki master. In addition to teaching the hand placements and symbolic gestures used in Reiki, the master attunes the student. Attunement opens the energy channel, enabling the student to bring universal energy through the body and to the recipient (Shiflett, Nayak, Bid, Miles, & Agostinelli, 2002). Further information on Reiki is available at the Web site for The International Center for Reiki Training (*http://www.reiki.org*) and at numerous other Web sites.

Polarity therapy was created by Randolph Stone, D.C., D.O., as a combination of energy work, caring intention, movement exercises, and dietary regimens. Polarity therapy is aimed at clearing energy blockages and building health (American Polarity Therapy Association, 2003). Information regarding training and treatment may be found at the American Polarity Therapy Association Web site (*http://www.polaritytherapy.org*) as well as other Web sites.

Other skilled people have developed healing schools and training programs. Rosalyn Bruyere and Barbara Brennan are skilled at reading auras (the extension of the energy field beyond the physical body) and the energy flow through the body (Brennan, 1987; Bruyere, 1994). The Brennan school appears to be formally structured; classes, tuition, and other information can be found on the school's Web site (*http://www.barbarabrennan.com*). Rosalyn L. Bruyere, an ordained minister, teaches healing through a series of workshops. Rev. Bruyere also has a Web site (*www.rosalynlbruyere.org*).

Much of the research on touch therapies has examined TT, and not everyone agrees that current research is scientifically valid (Hot Topics box). O'Mathuna (2000) discusses problems noted with the science in literature reviews of TT. Many of the studies had small sample sizes, reducing their power. In many of the studies, the results were not statistically significant; this, too, could be the result of small sample sizes. Hagemaster (2000) reported that TT improved depression scores and scores in various social stressor categories in a group of alcohol and drug abusers involved in a pilot study; no such changes were noted in the two control groups. Newshan and Schuller-Civitella (2003) report that a "majority of inpatients who receive TT have a positive outcome" (p. 191). Olson, Hanson, and Michaud (2003) used Reiki as an adjunct to opiate therapy and found it helpful in reducing the pain of patients with advanced cancer.

Energy healing takes place in many cultures. There are other types of healing and healers. Shamanism has existed in many parts of the world for centuries. As the population of Mexican Americans increases in the United States, the curandero (healer) of Mexican and South American culture is becoming more familiar. Faith healers are associated with

HOTtopics

HOW SHOULD ALTERNATIVE THERAPIES BE EVALUATED?

Those who use Therapeutic Touch (TT) believe strongly that it is an effective intervention, because they have seen it work. Despite an impressive body of research, TT continues to be attacked in the media by people who do not believe that scientific evidence of the effectiveness of the practice exists (Fish, 2005). Much of the research on TT has attempted to test efficacy using a version of the randomized controlled clinical trial (RCT) study design to conform to current scientific paradigms concerning the acceptability of research evidence. Many of the study findings were statistically nonsignificant results. Although this lack of statistical significance could have been due solely to small sample size, it added fuel to the fire of those who question the validity of the practice.

Many alternative therapies, including TT, are tailored specifically to the individual and produce treatment plans that are therefore nonstandardized, which does not fit the requirements of the RCT design. A TT treatment is dictated by the needs of the individual and is finished when the practitioner believes that it is finished, not within a rigid time limit imposed by a study protocol. A TT practioner cannot participate in a blind trial, because intentionality is a large part of the practice. Additionally, healers may be unable to perform identically from day to day, and psychological and physical changes within the healer may affect the ability to heal. Walach, Jonas, and Lewith (2002) suggest using quasi-experimental comparisons, outcomes studies, and prospective documentation designs to study alternative therapies.

1. What standards of proof should the nurse require before adopting an alternative therapy in clinical practice?
2. Have all (or even most) of the alternative therapies commonly used by nurses today been subjected to these standards?

From Fish, S. (2005). *Therapeutic touch: Healing science or psychic midwife?* Retrieved April 21, 2005, from *http://www.equip.org/free/DN105.htm*; and Walach, H., Jonas, W. B., & Lewith, G. T. (2002). The role of outcomes research in evaluating complementary and alternative medicine. *Alternative Therapies in Health and Medicine, 8*(3), 88-95.

many different religions. The trance surgeons of Brazil are discussed in the Multicultural Awareness box.

Movement Arts

The movement arts of Qi Gong, Tai Chi, and yoga have also been found to be helpful for body, mind, and spirit. Similar to energy work practices, the movement arts manipulate life energies.

Qi Gong

Qi Gong (pronounced chee gung), a part of traditional Chinese medicine, combines relaxed movements with a meditative aspect and controlled breathing to move qi

MULTICULTURAL AWARENESS

Trance Surgery

Two field workers visited Brazil to observe and document the work of healer-mediums who perform surgery while in a state of possession trance (Don & Moura, 2000). The healer-mediums believe that during the surgical procedures, the spirit of an intelligent entity possesses their bodies for its own medical purpose. The first trance surgeon began his practice in 1950, possessed by Dr. Fritz, a German physician killed during World War I. He performed surgery and wrote prescriptions under trance until his death in 1971. Since his death several other mediums have begun to practice trance surgery. Although some mediums are controversial, others have been accepted as being truly possessed by Dr. Fritz, other surgeon spirits, or the spirits of saints.

Don and Moura observed the practice of nine healer-mediums as they treated several thousand patients. Most of the trance surgeons actually cut or pierced the body of the patient and many of the incisions were deep; three incisions entered the peritoneal cavity. Only one of the trance surgeons had formal medical training. Antonio, a former laborer whose education ended after the first grade, practices as Dr. Ricardo. Don and Moura, accompanied by a Brazilian orthopedic surgeon, watched Dr. Ricardo work on 35 patients in a 3-hour period. They report:

> There was no major anesthesia or sterile procedure, and the same tray of instruments was used on all patients. Patients showed no evidence of pain, bleeding was minimal, and no patients went into shock. . . . Major blood vessels were not sutured, although we observed spurting of arterial blood during some procedures. . . . Within 1 hour, all patients were ambulatory; some patients who had been cut deeply were strolling on the town streets. . . . The patients often claim to have been healed. (Don & Moura, 2000, pp. 41, 44)

In addition to surgical procedures, Don and Moura report that one healer-medium injected a mixture of alcohol, iodine, and turpentine into both muscles and veins. They witnessed "hundreds of such injections" (p. 41) with no apparent ill effects.

Don and Moura witnessed events that, according to the beliefs of Western medicine, should be impossible. They describe trance surgery as "culturally bounded" (p. 47). Large numbers of Brazilians believe in spirit possession.

From Don, N. S., & Moura, G. (2000). Trance surgery in Brazil. *Alternative Therapies in Health and Medicine, 6*(4), 39-48.

Creamer, Singh, Hochberg, and Berman (2000) noted sustained improvements in pain for 28 patients with fibromyalgia.

Tai Chi

Tai Chi (pronounced tie chee) began as a Chinese martial art. Tai Chi combines physical movement, breath control, and meditation in a dancelike sequence of poses based on the movements of animals. One pose flows into the next in a slow, relaxed, gentle, unbroken rhythm. The slowness of movement and focus on breathing brings an awareness of the moment-to-moment state of the body and produces a meditative state. The sequence of poses is called a *form;* there are both short forms (13 to 18 poses) and long forms, but the focus of all is on relaxation, balance, posture, easy movements, and balancing of energy flow (Lewis, 2000). Tsai and colleagues (2003) found that Tai Chi had beneficial effects on blood pressure, lipid profiles values, and anxiety status when subjects participated in a 12-week program. Wang, Collet, and Lau (2004) present a systematic review of the research literature on the effects of Tai Chi in patients with chronic conditions and conclude that "Tai Chi appears to have physiological and psychosocial benefits . . . [and promotes] balance control, flexibility and cardiovascular fitness" (p. 493). Mills, Allen, and Morgan (2000) noted improvements in depression and balance in patients with multiple sclerosis who participated in Tai Chi sessions.

Yoga

Yoga, from the Hindu tradition, originated as a form of spiritual practice. The word *yoga* means union, and the system of yoga teaches the methods by which the individual can be joined with the Supreme Being and achieve liberation (Iyengar, 1979). There are several types of yoga—several paths to liberation. Karma yoga is the yoga of right action and good works; bhakti yoga, the yoga of devotional practices. Raja yoga is the yoga of meditative practices; jnana yoga, the yoga of the study of spiritual texts. Mantra yoga is the yoga of repetition of a sacred phrase, while laya yoga is the yoga of blending self with the Supreme (Sivananda, 1994).

Hatha yoga, the yoga of physical practice of various postures called *asanas* and of breath control, is most familiar to the Western culture, but ideally an individual's personal practice of yoga includes all methods. Well-known yoga teacher B. K. S. Iyengar (1979, p. 57) states that without the spiritual aspects of practice, yoga practice of the postures is "mere acrobatics." Iyengar (1979) defines health as "a state of complete equilibrium of body, mind, and spirit" (pp. 40-41) and states:

> Asanas [the postures or poses of hatha yoga] have been evolved over the centuries so as to exercise every muscle, nerve, and gland in the body. They secure a fine physique, which is strong and elastic without being muscle-bound, and they keep the body free from disease. They reduce

energy through the energy channels. The goal of this technique is to balance, smooth, and strengthen the individual's own qi energy (Lewis, 2000). Many books and videos explain Qi Gong practice. Qi Gong exercises can be performed by people of all age groups and all body types, regardless of their state of health, because the exercises may be done in either a static or moving manner (Lewis, 2000). Lee, Lee, Choi, and Chung (2003) found decreases in blood pressure and improved ventilatory function in hypertensive middle-aged patients who practiced Qi Gong for 10 weeks.

fatigue and soothe the nerves. But their real importance lies in the way they train and discipline the mind. The yogi [one who practices yoga] conquers the body by the practice of asanas and makes it a fit vehicle for the spirit. (p. 40)

Yoga asanas often have evocative, descriptive names, such as proud warrior, waterfall, runner's pose, downward-facing dog, mountain pose, and eagle pose. Other asana names are simple descriptions of what the body is doing during the posture, such as standing forward bend and spinal twist. Some of the poses are restful and restorative; some require strength and flexibility, which come with regular practice. Asana practice is a process of effortless effort that often involves a letting go and relaxing into the pose rather than forcing the body into the pose. Asana practice should be noncompetitive. The practice should not be about how the person looks in the pose, but rather, about how the person feels in the pose from the inside out. During asana practice, the breath should flow easily in and out through the nostrils. The body should be active, but the mind should be restful and watching, a witness to your actions. The energies of the body should extend equally through all the limbs and in all directions. Relaxation pose should follow the active asanas to allow incorporation of the work that has been done (Teri Landers [yoga teacher], personal communication, May 2000).

Hatha yoga also includes breathing exercises known as *pranayama*. Prana means "breath, respiration, life, vitality, wind, energy, or strength. It also connotes the soul as opposed to the body. . . . Ayama means length, expansion, stretching, and restraint" (Iyengar, 1979, p. 43). Control of the breath helps the yogi to control the mind and keep it focused on the present moment or the Supreme Being or both. Breath control also helps move the subtle energy (prana) through channels in the body (nadis) to nourish the body organs and the spirit (Iyengar, 1979). Yoga is an integral part of Dr. Dean Ornish's Program for Reversing Heart Disease (Ornish, 1990).

Although little research has been done on yoga in the United States, Ornish (1990) states that many well-researched techniques are derived from yoga, including various relaxation techniques, meditation and imagery practice, Lamaze breathing techniques, physical therapy stretches, and athletic stretches. Yoga has been used to help people stop smoking (McIver, O'Halloran, & McGarland, 2004). It improved balance and flexibility while decreasing disability and depression in a small sample of patients with low back pain (Galantino et al., 2004) and decreased self-reported symptoms of depression and anxiety in mildly depressed young adults (Woolery, Myers, Sternlieb, & Zeltzer, 2004).

Self-instructional videos in the movement arts are available from many sources; however, a well-trained teacher can help refine practice. Qi Gong, Tai Chi, and yoga classes are available at many fitness centers and community settings. There are different styles of practice within each discipline; therefore, experience with different teachers might be nec-essary to find one whose practice corresponds to the needs of the student.

Meditation

Blacker (2002) defines **meditation** as descriptive of "many different methods of quiet contemplation or observation . . . a certain kind of paying attention" (p. 105). During meditation, one becomes "still, so that you can discover who you are" (Tigunait, 2003, p. 30). A part of the religious life of many cultures, meditation has become prevalent in the West as a tool to improve physical and mental well-being. Generally, meditation involves the focusing of concentration on a single point. When the mind wanders, the individual consciously brings the mind back to the point of concentration. The focus of concentration can be a burning candle, a word, a phrase, the breath, or simply a quiet awareness of what is happening in the present moment. Centering prayer can be considered a form of meditation as practitioners focus on a sacred word from the Christian tradition. Meditation can be practiced while sitting, walking, or moving.

There are many techniques for meditating. One of the best known is Transcendental Meditation (TM). There are an estimated 5 million TM practitioners worldwide (Maharishi Vedic Education Development Corporation, 2004). The Indian spiritual leader Maharishi Mahesh Yogi brought TM to the United States during the 1960s. The TM technique is repetition of a mantra (a word, sound, or phrase). Practitioners repeat the mantra silently over and over again (for 20 minutes, morning and evening). When other thoughts arise during mantra repetition, the practitioner should notice the thought, let the thought go, and return to the mantra.

Mindfulness meditation is a way of paying attention; the point of focus varies. The individual can choose to focus on thoughts, on actions, or on the activity in the environment. Jon Kabat-Zinn (1990) believes that "knowing what you are doing while you are doing it is the essence of mindfulness practice" (p. 28). As an introduction to mindfulness meditation in his stress-reduction clinic, Kabat-Zinn asks people to eat three raisins, one at a time. He describes the process of eating a raisin:

First we bring our attention to seeing the raisin, observing it carefully as if we had never seen one before. We feel its texture between our fingers and notice its colors and surfaces. We are also aware of any thoughts we might be having about raisins or food in general. We note any thoughts and feelings of liking or disliking raisins if they come up while we are looking at it. We then smell it for a while and finally, with awareness, we bring it to our lips, being aware of the arm moving the hand to position it correctly and of salivating as the mind and body anticipate eating. The process continues as we take it into our mouth and chew it slowly, experiencing the actual taste of one raisin. And when we feel ready to swallow, we watch the impulse to swallow as it comes up, so that even that is experienced consciously. We even imagine, or "sense," that now our bodies are one raisin heavier. (Kabat-Zinn, 1990, pp. 27-28)

HEALTH TEACHING   Teaching the Technique of Breath Meditation

- You may stand, sit, or lie quietly as you begin to focus on your breath.
- Inhale and feel the air come into your nostrils, move down your throat, and into your lungs. Do not try to control the breath. Just observe it.
- Exhale and feel the air move up from your lungs and into your throat. Feel the warmth of the exhaled air in your nostrils.
- Breathe. Feeling the air move in and out. Concentrate on the breath. Do not try to control the breath. Just observe it.

- Continue watching the breath for 5 to 10 minutes. As other thoughts come into focus, notice them and let them go. Focus again on the breath.

As you become comfortable with breath meditation, you may easily add simple imagery to this technique.

- As you inhale, imagine breathing in peace or love or wellness.
- As you exhale, imagine breathing out pain or sorrow or grief.
- As you inhale, breathe in whatever it is that you need.
- As you exhale, breathe out whatever you wish to be free of in your life.

Walking meditation is another form of mindfulness practice; with each step, the person is aware of the movements of the body that make the step possible and of both the external environment and the internal environment. Hanh believes that the true sense of walking meditation is gained when walking "as if one were planting peace with each step" (Anselmo & Kolkmeier, 2000, p. 507).

One of the simplest methods of meditation is concentration on breathing. With breath meditation, there is no need for a special room, a special mat, or a cushion. The breath is an ever-present tool. Breath meditation can evoke the relaxation response (Anselmo & Kolkmeier, 2000). This technique can be taught easily (Health Teaching box) and is useful for anyone who is having a bad day or who wants to be more present with another.

Meditation is an important part of Dr. Dean Ornish's Program for Reversing Heart Disease (Ornish, 1990). The Web site for TM (*http://www.tm.org*) states that over 500 studies have been completed on the technique; findings include fewer chest pain episodes in women diagnosed with cardiac syndrome X (Cunningham, Brown, & Kaski, 2000) and a significant decrease in carotid intima-media thickness (a surrogate measure for coronary atherosclerosis) among African Americans (Castillo-Richmond et al., 2000). Bonadonna (2003) presents a literature review summarizing various studies involving both TM and other types of meditation. Schneider, Alexander, Salerno, Robinson, Fields, and Nidich (2002) offer a review of studies involving Maharishi Vedic Medicine, of which TM is a part.

Prayer and Distant Healing
Prayer

Prayer is one of the oldest forms of therapy (Byrd, 1997). People pray for themselves and they pray for others. Prayer has different meanings to different people; a prayer may be a request for divine intervention, a type of meditation (centering prayer), or a form of intentionality that is useful in healing. Prayer is the basis for Christian Science healing practices (The Church of Christ Scientist, 2001); prayer facilitates healing by causing changes in consciousness that help individuals recognize their innate wholeness.

In one of the first research studies involving prayer, Byrd (1997) studied the therapeutic effects of intercessory prayer on 393 patients in a coronary care unit. The patients were randomly assigned to a prayer group and a control group; none of the participants, patients, staff, or doctors, knew who was assigned to either group. Prayers for rapid recovery and prevention of complications were offered on behalf of the people in the prayer group by 3 to 7 people daily. There was a significant difference between the two groups in several areas. Fewer patients in the prayer group required intubation or ventilation, antibiotics, and diuretics. Fewer patients in the prayer group developed congestive heart failure, went into cardiorespiratory arrest, or developed pneumonia. Severity scores showed that the prayer group had significantly better outcomes.

Bernardi and colleagues (2001) found that recitation of "both [a] prayer and [a yoga] mantra caused striking, powerful, and synchronous increases in existing cardiovascular rhythms . . . and baroflex sensitivity . . . resulting in favorable psychological and possibly physiological effects" (p. 1446). Meisenhelder and Chandler (2000) examined prayer and health outcomes among 1025 church members. People who prayed most frequently had poorer physical health and were older, yet they experienced better mental health than those who prayed less frequently.

Distant Healing

Praying for others may be a form of distant healing; many who practice energy work believe that their efforts are effective over long distances. A review of 23 studies involving distant healing and using randomized trials (Astin, Harkness, & Ernst, 2000) concluded that 13 studies (57%) had statistically significant treatment effects, 9 studies showed no effect over control interventions, and 1 study showed a negative effect. Studies involving TT, prayer, mental healing, and spiritual healing were included.

One method of participating in distance healing is the healing circle. The members of the healing circle join hands. Each member sends healing energy to his or her neighbor on the right until the energy is flowing around the circle. When the energy is flowing readily, each member of the group focuses the energy on one group member, who acts to send the energy to someone they know in need of healing. Each member of the circle may, in turn, receive energy from the group and send it to an individual in need of healing.

Guided Imagery

The physical body may react to sensory images in the mind the same way it responds to the real thing (Naparstek, 1994). To illustrate this point, Naparstek uses the example of a woman whose first dose of chemotherapy caused extreme nausea. Traveling to the clinic for the second dose, the individual remembered the experience and formed an image in her mind of the experience. She became nauseated and began to vomit. Serious illness often brings fears of death or disability with it; people imagine the worst and anxiety increases. These examples demonstrate the negative effects of imagination.

Imagination can have a positive influence on health. **Imagery** can be used to promote a sense of well-being and to help cope with stress, diseases, or pain (Schaub & Dossey, 2000). During imagery practice, the person relaxes and focuses attention on the images chosen or presented. Guided imagery scripts are available from several sources; individuals may also work with the practitioners to develop their own script that is specific to their need (Schaub & Dossey, 2000). Generally the images are presented verbally but are designed to evoke all the senses. For example, imagery for distraction during a painful procedure might involve asking the individual to identify a special place as a retreat. If the person's special place is a beach, then the practitioner might ask the individual to hear the water softly lapping at the shore, to see the white sand (senses of hearing and sight), and to feel the warm sun falling softly on skin (sense of touch) as the smell of orange blossoms drifts through the air (sense of smell).

When people learn and understand some basic principles of anatomy and physiology, imagery can be used to affect physiological functioning: bone healing, wound healing, and immune system enhancement (Schaub & Dossey, 2000). Research on imagery has shown improvements in chronic pain (Lewandowski, 2004), sleep (Richardson, 2003), limb performance in hemiparesis (Stevens & Stoykov, 2003), asthma symptoms (Epstein et al., 2004), and recurrent abdominal pain in children (Ball, Shapiro, Monheim, & Weydert, 2003), as well as decreases in length of stay and medication costs for patients undergoing cardiac surgery (Halpin, Speir, CapoBianco, & Barnett, 2002).

Music Therapy

Music therapy is the use of specific kinds of music (or sounds) to produce desired changes in behaviors, emotions, and physiological processes. Music works as therapy by influencing the limbic system, the area of the brain involved with emotions and feelings (Guzetta, 2000). Various types of music may be used therapeutically. Guzetta (2000) reports that the classical music of Mozart, Haydn, and Bach improves concentration and memory, and classical music of the Baroque period (Vivaldi and Handel) gives a sense of safety and stability. Debussy and Ravel, impressionist composers, evoke dreamlike images and open creativity. Gregorian chants ground the individual in the present moment, eliciting feelings of deep peace; they are also useful for releasing pain. Other types of music have different actions. Some music is composed specifically for therapeutic effect; this music is called *designer music,* which may include sound frequencies that alter brainwave frequencies to achieve a particular brain state or emotion. Because of the emotions that can surface during music therapy, it should be tailored to the individual and the purpose of the therapy (Petterson, 2001). Music can serve as a reminder of past events and be useful in opening communication. Some of the events remembered can be unpleasant. While listening to Gregorian chants during an energy therapy session, one patient reported "I feel like I'm at a mass." This was not something she found soothing, and the feelings that arose while listening to the music interfered with her relaxation.

McRee, Noble, and Pasvogel (2003) write of several studies in which music therapy decreased anxiety and increased pain thresholds in postoperative patients; Brunges and Avigne (2003) found decreased anxiety and shorter lengths of postoperative stays when patients listened to music before and during surgery; and Good, Anderson, Stanton-Hicks, Grass, and Makii (2002) found that relaxation, music, or a combination of relaxation and music were equally effective in reducing pain following gynecological surgery. Labor pain (Phumdoung & Good, 2003) and osteoarthritis pain (McCaffrey & Freeman, 2003) (Research Highlights box) also have responded positively to music therapy. Although music therapy can be used by anyone, the American Music Therapy Association (*http://www. musictherapy.org*) offers training in music therapy and certifies music therapists who have completed formal education programs.

Bodywork
Massage

Massage is the manipulation of soft tissues of the body. Formal massage techniques are variations of rubbing a sore spot after bumping your head or rubbing a friend's back as consolation after a loss. Nurses are taught to give massage (back rubs) to promote sleep and relaxation (Harkreader & Hogan, 2004), and that massage is a useful adjunct therapy for pain control (Ersek & Poe, 2004) and stress reduction (Witek-Janusek, 2004). Massage may involve stroking, kneading, pulling, or pinching the skin. Skin lubrication with oil, lotion, or powder reduces friction, pinching, and hair pulling during the massage.

The benefits of massage are supported by research. Massage has been found to reduce systolic blood pressure in patients going for cardiac catheterization (McNamara, Burnham, Smith, & Carroll, 2003), to reduce the stereotypic behaviors of children with autism (Escalona, Field,

research highlights

Music Therapy and Chronic Osteoarthritis Pain

Osteoarthritis is a common complaint among older people. A Rogerian study tested the effect of listening to music on a convenience sample of community-dwelling elders aged 65 or older with a self-reported diagnosis of osteoarthritis. The sample was randomized to control and experimental groups; there were 22 women and 11 men in each group. Participants in the intervention group were given a cassette player and a cassette of classical music selections prepared by the primary investigator. They were asked to sit quietly and listen to the entire tape each day for 14 days. The control group simply sat in a quiet comfortable place for 20 minutes each day for 14 days.

Both groups were given the short-form McGill Pain Questionnaire to determine the perceived level of pain and a Visual Analogue Scale to measure pain intensity. Mean scores were calculated and t-tests were conducted using a statistical software package. There were significant differences in the means of both measures on day 1, day 7, and day 14 ($P = 0.001$ for all six measures). The authors report that the "study demonstrates that in the group who listened to music, pain continued to decrease across the 14-day study period as compared with the group who did not listen to music and whose pain remained constant" (p. 522).

Data from McCaffery, R., & Freeman, E. (2003). Effect of music on chronic osteoarthritis pain in older people. *Journal of Advanced Nursing*, 44(5), 517-524.

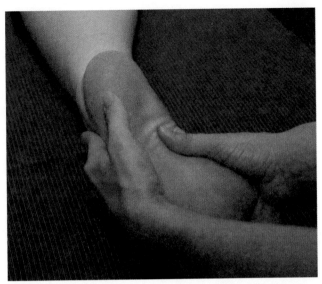

Figure 14-3   Massage can be effective for many areas of the body.

Singer-Strunck, Cullen, & Hartshorn, 2001), and to lessen anxiety and depression and increase muscle strength in a group of patients with spinal cord lesions (Diego et al., 2002). A 10-minute foot massage given on three consecutive evenings provided significant decreases in pain and nausea and increased feelings of relaxation for patients hospitalized with cancer (Grealish, Lomasney, & Whiteman, 2000); this treatment was not a reflexology treatment (Figure 14-3). Many massage therapists, who may be certified by the American Massage Therapy Association after their training, practice a variety of bodywork modalities and may also include forms of energy work in their practices. A brief overview of several additional modalities follows.

Trager Therapy

Trager Psychophysical Integration involves tissue manipulation, relaxation, and movement reeducation. Practitioners work from a meditative state while they rock, jiggle, vibrate, and stretch the body in an effort to set off waves of motion that will lead to deep relaxation and greater mobility. This relaxation and mobility can release long-standing physical and mental patterns. Following treatment, the person is taught a series of exercises and stretches that will reinforce the treatment. Training in Trager therapy is available through schools of massage. A Web search for the topic Trager therapy yields a multitude of sites.

Craniosacral Therapy

Craniosacral therapy originated in osteopathy, a medical practice that adds manipulation of the bones of the body to conventional medical education. Craniosacral therapists believe that the bones of the cranium, spine, and sacrum are moveable and connected and that the cerebrospinal fluid has a pulse that can be felt. The therapist uses gentle pressure to restore free movement of cerebrospinal fluid, allowing for normal functioning. The therapist also believes that emotions are stored in musculoskeletal tissue and can be released through manipulation of the craniosacral system. Craniosacral therapy training is provided through the Upledger Institute (*http://www.upledger.com*).

Bowenwork

Bowenwork is based on the work of Tom Bowen, an Australian natural healer. The therapy involves gentle, rolling moves across physical structures of the body (muscles, tendons, and neurovascular bundles) to "reset the body and allow it to heal itself" (Amato, 2001, p. 2). Treatments may be performed with the patient fully clothed. Bowenwork is helpful for a variety of conditions: pain or numbness from accidents, whiplash, sports injuries, muscular and skeletal problems, scoliosis, neck and shoulder problems, tennis elbow, restricted joints, arthritis, temporomandibular joint (TMJ) problems, stress, tension, emotional depression, respiratory problems, asthma, allergies, fibromyalgia, and chronic fatigue (N. Pierson [Bowenworker and instructor], personal communication, March 10, 2004). Information on training may be found at *http://www.bowtech.com*.

Aromatherapy

Aromatherapy uses aromatic plant materials and the essential oils of plants. There is a long history of the use of plant materials in both ayurvedic medicine and traditional Chinese medicine. The use of aromatherapy without professional clinical training is strongly discouraged; people must have this training to know the specific warnings and contraindications for each oil, to know how to handle the oils, and to be aware of possible allergic reactions to oils (Buckle, 2003). The essential oils have a pharmacological, a physiological, and a psychological effect on the human body. Essential oils may be added to the bath or used in a douche, mixed with carrier oils and used during massage, placed on a cloth and applied as a compress, applied directly to minor injuries to speed healing, or inhaled (Buckle, 2003). Buckle (2003) presents several case studies that demonstrate the use of essential oils to help with the healing of herpetic lesions (eucalyptus oil), reduce the itching of psoriasis (lavender oil), reduce vaginal yeast infection (tea tree oil), and reduce pain in a patient with cancer and bone metastases (rose oil). Aromatherapy research has demonstrated decreased agitation behaviors in patients with dementia (Thorgrimsen, Spector, Wiles, & Orrell, 2004). Soden, Vincent, Craske, Lucas, and Ashley (2004) found improvement in sleep and reductions in depression when aromatherapy (lavender oil) was combined with massage in a hospice setting.

Presence

The way people interact with one another can cause pain or promote healing. **Presence** is defined as "being available in a situation with the wholeness of one's individual being . . . of 'being with' rather than 'doing to'" (McKivergin, 2000, p. 208). A classic study by Halldorsdottir (1991) examined individuals' perceptions of their interactions with nurses. Subjects maintained that nurse interactions followed a continuum from life-destroying to life-sustaining to life-giving. Individuals perceived life-giving nurses as a healing force; they were perceived as being present with—rather than simply being there for—the individuals.

As described by Fredriksson (1999), being there (Table 14-1) would normally be considered acceptable nursing behavior. However, the individuals in the Halldorsdottir (1991) study demonstrate that nurses can be much more than acceptable; the nurse's presence can actually contribute to healing. In examining the differences in being there and being with, Fredriksson (1999) found that when nurses are being with subjects, the nurses' attention was focused rather than merely attentive, their touch was caring rather than task oriented, and nurses did not merely hear, they listened.

When using presence as a holistic intervention and establishing a whole person–to–whole person relationship, the nurse becomes vulnerable to the pain of the individual. Nurses may choose to avoid this pain by walking away, maintaining a professional distance, and being too busy with other tasks to be fully present. Nurses may have personal limitations that prevent the use of presence, such as the need to be in control, a lack of patience, a lack of openness, and a lack of desire to be present (McKivergin, 2000). Many of these barriers can be overcome with self-knowledge and self-care.

Table **14-1** Being There Versus Being With	
The Nurse Who Is BEING THERE for Patients	**The Nurse Who Is BEING WITH Patients**
Is attentive	Is available with whole self
Is task oriented	Enters the patient's world
Does the right thing	Becomes vulnerable
Fulfills a role	Is present as a whole person
Assists with coping	Alleviates suffering
Provides security	Enables growth

SELF-KNOWLEDGE

Holistic health involves a personal commitment to wellness and an exploration of what works for the individual and what does not (Walter, 2000). Additionally, holistic health involves knowing the physical self, the emotional self, the mental self, and the spiritual self, seeking a comfortable balance among these aspects of being, and knowing what changes need to be made to achieve this balance (American Holistic Health Association, 2003).

This knowledge is vital to both the nurse attempting holistic practice and the individual interested in pursuing holistic health. The Think About It questions at the beginning of this chapter can assist both nurse and individual in the exploration of self that begins the process of self-care. An example of a more detailed assessment instrument, a personal health workbook, is presented in **Web Site Resource 14B.** Self-exploration enhances the abilities of the nurse who wants to consider using nursing presence as a holistic healing intervention (McKivergin, 2000). The expanded knowledge of self is valuable because the more that is known about oneself, the more there is of oneself to offer to another, and "the only thing you ever have to offer to another human being, ever, is your own state of being" (Dass, 1976, p. 6).

When self-knowledge is gained, one or more of the holistic health strategies mentioned in this chapter can be useful in helping people achieve optimal wellness. In addition to the strategies mentioned, many other holistic interventions can be helpful. These strategies include homeopathy, flower essences, crystals, and additional forms of bodywork and movement therapies. Every person is a whole, unique being; therefore, each person needs to explore the strategies and decide which modalities are the best methods to achieve an improved state of wellness.

People beginning this self-exploration and the practice of holistic health strategies may find that the practice changes their lives. Using presence and giving the gift of self enhance personal growth in the giver (McKivergin, 2000). Whelan and Wishnia (2003), for example, found that Reiki practice benefits the nurse by reducing daily stress and burnout and increasing intuition, insight, and time spent with patients.

SUMMARY

Holistic health strategies are designed to view the individual as a biopsychosocial-spiritual whole being. Many holistic health strategies have been practiced in other cultures for many years; some began as religious practices. As these practices moved to the West, the health-promoting nature of these therapies came to the forefront and the emphasis on religion waned. Many of these strategies can be used to help nurses and their patients reach the Healthy People 2010 goals of increasing physical activity and flexibility, decreasing substance abuse, reducing pain, and improving quality of life.

A body of research already exists supporting the use of these therapies and more research is being performed. Although the studies to date have been unsuccessful in persuading some health care practitioners of the utility of the practices, holistic health practitioners are convinced that these practices help promote and maintain health.

Every person is a unique, individual being; therefore, some exploration of self, the various strategies, and the practitioner will be necessary before determining which strategy is the right fit for the individual. The right-fit strategy will increase both physical and mental well-being. **Web Site Resource 14C** presents a summary list of definitions of many holistic strategies, most of which were discussed in the chapter. Nurses need to understand holistic health strategies, because patients are using them in increasing numbers. Nurses who begin to practice holistic interventions may find them a useful adjunct to their nursing practice. Additionally, nurses may find that using holistic interventions in their nursing practices changes their practices and their very selves.

ADDITIONAL STUDY MATERIAL

Study Questions in the back of the book, see page 663.

ⓔⓥⓞⓛⓥⓔ WEB SITE MATERIALS

These materials are located on the book's Web site at http://evolve.elsevier.com/Edelman/.

- WebLinks
- Content Updates
- Web Site Resources

14A   Proportions of U.S. Adults Using Holistic Therapies in 2001 and 2002

14B   Example of a Personal Health Workbook

14C   Holistic Practitioners' Specialties and Definitions of Their Practice

REFERENCES

Amato, D. (2001, Oct. 22). Accelerated healing response: The Bowen Technique can complement traditional PT. *Advance for Physical Therapists & PT Assistants,* 1-2.

American Holistic Health Association. (2003). *Wellness from within: The first step* (booklet). Anaheim, CA: Author. Retrieved April 20, 2005, from: *http://ahha.org/ahhastep.htm.*

American Polarity Therapy Association. (2003). About polarity therapy. Retrieved March 20, 2004, from: *http://www.polaritytherapy.org/polarity/index.html.*

Anselmo, J., & Kolkmeier, L. G. (2000). Relaxation: The first step to restore, renew, and self-heal. In B. M. Dossey, L. Keegan, & C. E. Guzetta (Eds.), *Holistic nursing: A handbook for practice* (3rd ed., pp. 497-535). Gaithersburg, MD: Aspen.

Astin, J. A., Harkness, E., & Ernst, E. (2000). The efficacy of "distant healing": A systematic review of randomized trials. *Annals of Internal Medicine, 132,* 903-910.

Ball, T. M., Shapiro, D. E., Monheim, C. J., & Weydert, J. A. (2003). A pilot study in the use of guided imagery for the treatment of recurrent abdominal pain in children. *Clinical Pediatrics, 42*(6), 527-532.

Benor, D. J. (1999/2000, Winter). Intentionality in wholistic spiritual healing. *Bridges, 10*(4), 15-17.

Bernardi, L., Sleight, P., Bandinelli, G., Cencetti, S., Fattorini, L., Wdowczyc, J., et al. (2001). Effect of rosary prayer and yoga mantras on autonomic cardiovascular rhythms: Comparative study. *British Medical Journal, 323,* 22-29.

Blacker, M. (2002). Meditation. In M.A. Bright (Ed.), *Holistic health and healing* (pp. 105-112). Philadelphia: F. A. Davis.

Bonadonna, R. (2003). Meditation's impact on chronic illness (Electronic Version). *Holistic Nursing Practice, 17*(6), 309-319.

Bowman, G. (2004). Test anxiety. Retrieved March 19, 2004, from: *http://www.hsc.edu/counseling/selfhelp/test_anxiety.html.*

Brennan, B. A. (1987). *Hands of light: A guide to healing through the human energy field.* New York: Bantam.

Bright, M. A. (2002). *Holistic health and healing.* Philadelphia: F. A. Davis.

Brunges, M., & Avigne, G. (2003). Music therapy for reducing surgical anxiety. *AORN Journal, 78*(5), 816-818.

Bruyere, R. L. (1994). *Wheels of light: Chakras, auras, and the healing energy of the body.* New York: Simon & Schuster.

Buckle, J. (2003). *Clinical aromatherapy: Essential oils in practice* (2nd ed.). New York: Churchill Livingstone.

Byrd, R. (1997). Positive therapeutic effects of intercessory prayer in a coronary care unit population. *Alternative Therapies in Health and Medicine, 3*(6), 87-90.

Castillo-Richmond, A., Schneider, R. H., Alexander, C. N., Cook, R., Myers, H., Nidich, S., et al. (2000). Effects of stress reduction on carotid atherosclerosis in hypertensive African Americans (Electronic Version). *Stroke, 31*(3), 568-573.

The Church of Christ Scientist (Christian Science). (2001). Retrieved April 21, 2005, from *http://religiousmovements.lib.virginia.edu/nrms/chrissci.html.*

Creamer, P., Singh, B. B., Hochberg, M. C., & Berman, B. M. (2000). Sustained improvement produced by nonpharmacologic intervention in fibromyalgia: Results of a pilot study. *Arthritis Care and Research, 13*(4), 198-204.

Cunningham, C., Brown, S., & Kaski, J. C. (2000). Effects of Transcendental Meditation on symptoms and electrocardiographic changes in patients with cardiac syndrome X. *American Journal of Cardiology, 85,* 653-655.

Dass, R. (1976). *The only dance there is.* New York: Jason Aronson.

Demarco, A., & Clarke, N. (2001). An interview with Alison Demarco and Nichol Clarke: Light and colour therapy explained. *Complementary Therapies in Nursing & Midwifery, 7,* 95-103.

Dibble, S. L., Chapman, J., Mack, K. A., & Shih, A. S. (2000). Acupressure for nausea: Results of a pilot study. *Oncology Nursing Forum, 27*(1), 41-47.

Diego, M. A., Field, T., Hernandez-Reif, M., Hart, S., Brucker, B., Field, T. (2002). Spinal cord patients benefit from massage therapy. *International Journal of Neuroscience, 112*(2), 133-142.

Epstein, G. N., Halper, J. P., Barrett, E. M., Birdsall, E., McGee, M., Baron, K. P., et al. (2004). A pilot study of mind-body changes in adults with asthma who practice mental imagery. *Alternative Therapies in Health and Medicine, 10*(4), 66-71.

Ersek, M., & Poe, C. M. (2004). Pain. In S. M. Lewis, M. M. Heitkemper, & S. R. Dirksen (Eds.), *Medical-surgical nursing: Assessment and management of clinical problems* (6th ed., pp. 131-151). St. Louis: Mosby.

Escalona, A., Field, T., Singer-Strunck, R., Cullen, C., & Hartshorn, K. (2001). Brief report: Improvements in the behavior of children with autism following massage therapy. *Journal of Autism and Developmental Disorders, 31*(5), 513-516.

Fish, S. (2005). *Theraputic touch: Healing science or psychic midwife?* Retrieved April 21, 2005, from *http://www.equip.org/free/DN105.htm.*

Fredriksson, L. (1999). Modes of relating in a caring conversation: A research synthesis on presence, touch and listening. *Journal of Advanced Nursing, 30*(5), 1167-1176.

Galantino, M. L., Bzdewka, T. M., Eissler-Russo, J. I., Holbrook, M. L., Mogck, E. P., Geigle, P., et al. (2004). The impact of modified hatha yoga on chronic low back pain: A pilot study. *Alternative Therapies in Health and Medicine, 10*(2), 56-59.

Good, M., Anderson, G. C., Stanton-Hicks, M., Grass, J. A., & Makii, M. (2002). Relaxation and music reduce pain after gynecologic surgery. *Pain Management Nursing, 3*(2), 61-70.

Gray, M. (2004). Renal and urologic problems. In S. M. Lewis, M. M. Heitkemper, & S. R. Dirksen (Eds.), *Medical-surgical nursing: Assessment and management of clinical problems* (6th ed., pp. 1172-1209). St. Louis: Mosby.

Grealish, L., Lomasney, A., & Whiteman, B. (2000). Foot massage: A nursing intervention to modify the distressing symptoms of pain and nausea in patients hospitalized with cancer. *Cancer Nursing, 23*(3), 237-243.

Guzetta, C. E. (2000). Music therapy: Hearing the melody of the soul. In B. M. Dossey, L. Keegan, & C. E. Guzetta (Eds.), *Holistic nursing: A handbook for practice* (3rd ed., pp. 585-610). Gaithersburg, MD: Aspen.

Hagemaster, J. (2000). Use of therapeutic touch in treatment of drug addictions (Electronic Version). *Holistic Nursing Practice, 14*(3), 14-20.

Halldorsdottir, S. (1991). Five basic modes of being with another. In D. A. Gaut & M. M. Leininger (Eds.), *Caring: The compassionate healer* (NLN Publication No. 15-2401, pp. 37-49). New York: National League for Nursing Press.

Halpin, L. S., Speir, A. M., CapoBianco, P., & Barnett, S. D. (2002). Guided imagery in cardiac surgery. *Outcomes Management, 6*(3), 132-137.

Harkreader, H., & Hogan, M.A. (2004). *Fundamentals of nursing: Caring and clinical judgment* (2nd ed.). St. Louis: Saunders.

Horrigan, B. (2003). Ken Cohen, MA, MSTH. Healing through ancient traditions: Qigong and Native American medicine (Interview). *Alternative Therapies in Health and Medicine, 9*(3), 83-91.

Horrigan, B. J. (2000). Regions Hospital opens holistic nursing unit. *Alternative Therapies in Health and Medicine, 6*(4), 92-93.

Hover-Kramer, D. (1996). *Healing touch: A resource for health care professionals.* Albany, NY: Delmar.

Iyengar, B. K. S. (1979). *Light on yoga: Yoga dipika* (Rev. ed.). New York: Schocken.

Kabat-Zinn, J. (1990). *Full catastrophe living: Using the wisdom of your body and mind to face stress, pain, and illness.* New York: Delta.

Kerr, D. P., Walsh, D. M., & Baxter, G. D. (2001). A study of the use of acupuncture in physiotherapy. *Complementary Therapies in Medicine, 9,* 21-27.

Killeen, T. K., Haight, B., Brady, K., Herman, J., Michel, Y., Stuart, G., et al. (2002). The effect of auricular acupuncture on psychophysiological measures of cocaine craving. *Issues in Mental Health Nursing, 23,* 445-459.

Knez, I. (2001). Effects of colour of light on nonvisual psychological processes. *Journal of Environmental Psychology, 21,* 201-208.

Krieger, D. (1979). *The therapeutic touch: How to use your hands to help or to heal.* New York: Simon & Schuster.

Krieger, D. (1993). *Accepting your power to heal: The personal practice of therapeutic touch.* Santa Fe, NM: Bear.

Krieger, D. (1998). Healing with therapeutic touch (Interview). *Alternative Therapies in Health and Medicine, 4*(1), 87-92.

Lee, M. S., Jang, J., Jang, H., & Moon, S. (2003). Effects of Qi-therapy on blood pressure, pain and psychological symptoms in the elderly: A randomized controlled pilot trial. *Complementary Therapies in Medicine, 11*(3), 159-164.

Lee, M. S., Lee, M. S., Choi, E., & Chung, H. (2003). Effects of Qigong on blood pressure, blood pressure determinants and ventilatory function in middle-aged patients with essential hypertension. *American Journal of Chinese Medicine, 31*(3), 489-497.

Lento, L. (2003). The Healing Arts Center at St. John: Connecting CAM into the traditional hospital setting. *Alternative Therapies in Health and Medicine, 9*(3), 110-111.

Levitt, A. J., Lam, R. W., & Levitan, R. (2002). A comparison of open treatment of seasonal major and minor depression with light therapy. *Journal of Affective Disorders, 71*(1-3), 243-248.

Lewandowski, W. A. (2004). Patterning of pain and power with guided imagery. *Nursing Science Quarterly, 17*(3), 233-241.

Lewis, D. E. (2000). T'ai chi ch'uan. *Complementary therapies in Nursing & Midwifery, 6,* 204-206.

Lifestyle Advantage. (2002). Medicare demonstration to test lifestyle change program to reverse heart disease. Retrieved April 15, 2004, from: *http://www.lifestyleadvantage.org/medicare.html.*

Maa, S. H., Sun, M. F., Hsu, K. H., Hung, T. J., Chen, H. C., Yu, C. T., et al. (2003). Effect of acupuncture or acupressure on quality of life of patients with chronic obstructive asthma: A pilot study. *Journal of Alternative & Complementary Medicine, 9*(5), 659-671.

Maharishi Vedic Education Development Corporation. (2004). The Transcendental Meditation Program. Retrieved April 8, 2004, from: *http://www.tm.org.*

Mayer, D. J. (2000). Acupuncture: An evidence-based review of the clinical literature. *Annual Review of Medicine, 51,* 49-63.

McCaffrey, R., & Freeman, E. (2003). Effect of music on chronic osteoarthritis pain in older people. *Journal of Advanced Nursing, 44*(5), 517-524.

McIver, S., O'Halloran, P., & McGarland, M. (2004). The impact of hatha yoga on smoking behavior. *Alternative Therapies in Health & Medicine, 10*(2), 22-23.

McKivergin, M. (2000). The nurse as an instrument of healing. In B. M. Dossey, L. Keegan, & C. E. Guzetta (Eds.), *Holistic nursing: A handbook for practice* (3rd ed., pp. 207-227). Gaithersburg, MD: Aspen.

McNamara, M. E., Burnham, D. C., Smith, C., & Carroll, D. L. (2003). The effects of back massage before diagnostic cardiac catheterization. *Alternative Therapies in Health and Medicine, 9*(1), 50-57.

McRee, L. D., Noble, S., & Pasvogel, A. (2003). Using massage and music therapy to improve postoperative outcomes. *AORN Journal, 78*(3), 433-447.

Meisenhelder, J. B., & Chandler, E. N. (2000). Prayer and health outcomes in church members. *Alternative Therapies in Health and Medicine, 6*(4), 56-60.

Mills, N., Allen, J., & Morgan, S. C. (2000). Does Tai Chi/Qi Gong help patients with multiple sclerosis? *Journal of Bodywork and Movement Therapies, 4*(1), 39-48.

Naparstek, B. (1994). *Staying well with guided imagery.* New York: Warner.

Newshan, G., & Schuller-Civitella, D. (2003). Large clinical study shows value of therapeutic touch program. *Holistic Nursing Practice, 17*(4), 189-192.

Norred, C. L. (2000). Minimizing preoperative anxiety with alternative caring-healing therapies (Electronic Version). *AORN Online, 72*(5), 838, 840, 842-843.

Olson, K., Hanson, J., & Michaud, M. (2003). A phase II trial of Reiki for the management of pain in advanced cancer patients. *Journal of Pain and Symptom Management, 26*(5), 990-997.

O'Mathuna, D. P. (2000). Evidence-based practice and reviews of therapeutic touch (Electronic Version). *Image: The Journal of Nursing Scholarship, 32*(3), 279-285.

Oren, D. A., Wisner, K. L., Spinelli, M., Epperson, C. N., Peindl, K. S., Terman, J. S., et al. (2002). An open trial of morning light therapy for treatment of antepartum depression. *American Journal of Psychiatry, 159*(4), 666-669.

Ornish, D. (1990). *Dr. Dean Ornish's program for reversing heart disease.* New York: Ballantine.

Pelletier, K. R., Astin, J. A., & Haskell, W. L. (1999). Current trends in the integration and reimbursement of complementary and alternative medicine by managed care organizations (MCOs) and insurance providers: 1998 update and cohort analysis. *American Journal of Health Promotion, 14*(2), 125-133.

Petterson, M. (2001). Music for healing: The Creative Arts Program at the Ireland Cancer Center. *Alternative Therapies in Health and Medicine, 7*(1), 88-89.

Phumdoung, S., & Good, M. (2003). Music reduces sensation and distress of labor pain. *Pain Management Nursing, 4*(2), 54-61.

Richardson, S. (2003). Effects of relaxation and imagery on the sleep of critically ill adults. *Dimensions of Critical Care Nursing, 22*(4), 182-190.

Rogers, M. E. (1970). *An introduction to the theoretical basis of nursing.* Philadelphia: Davis.

Schaub, B. G., & Dossey, B. M. (2000). Imagery: Awakening the inner healer. In B. M. Dossey, L. Keegan, & C. E. Guzetta (Eds.), *Holistic nursing: A handbook for prac-* *tice* (3rd ed., pp. 539-581). Gaithersburg, MD: Aspen.

Schneider, R. H., Alexander, C. N., Salerno, J. W., Robinson, D. K., Fields, J. Z., & Nidich, S. I. (2002). Disease prevention and health promotion in the aging with a traditional system of natural medicine: Maharishi Vedic Medicine. *Journal of Aging and Health, 14*(1), 57-78.

Shiflett, S. C., Nayak, S., Bid, C., Miles, P., & Agostinelli, S. (2002). Effect of Reiki treatments on functional recovery in post-stroke rehabilitation: A pilot study. *Journal of Alternative and Complementary Medicine, 8*(6), 755-763.

Sivananda, S. S. (1994). *Practice of yoga* (7th ed.). Shivanandanagar, India: The Divine Life Society.

Soden, K., Vincent, K., Craske, S., Lucas, C., & Ashley, S. (2004). A randomized controlled trial of aromatherapy massage in a hospice setting. *Palliative Medicine, 18*(2), 87-92.

Stevens, J. A., & Stoykov, M. E. P. (2003). Using motor imagery in the rehabilitation of hemiparesis. *Archives of Physical Medicine and Rehabilitation, 84*(7), 1090-1092.

Stone, N. J. (2003). Environmental view and color for a simulated telemarketing task. *Journal of Environmental Psychology, 23*, 63-78.

Thomas, L. A. (2003). Clinical management of stressors perceived by patients on mechanical ventilation. *AACN Clinical Issues, 14*(1), 73-81.

Thompson, E. (2000, May). The alternative model. *Modern Healthcare, 30*(20), 26-28, 32-34.

Thorgrimsen, L., Spector, A., Wiles, A., & Orrell, M. (2004). *Aroma therapy for dementia* (Cochrane Review). In The Cochrane Library, Issue 3, 2004. Chichester, UK: John Wiley & Sons.

Tigunait, P. R. (2003, Nov.). Dialogue with Pandit Rajmani Tigunait. *Yoga International, 74*, 30-34.

Tsai, J. C., Wang, W. H., Chan, P., Lin, L. J., Wang, C. H., Tomlinson, B., et al. (2003). The beneficial effects of Tai Chi Chuan on blood pressure and lipid profile and anxiety status in a randomized controlled trial. *Journal of Alternative & Complementary Medicine, 9*(5), 747-755.

Walter, S. (2000, July). Holistic health (Online). Retrieved April 20, 2005, from: *http://www.ahha.org/rosen/htm.*

Wang, C., Collet, J. P., & Lau, J. (2004). The effect of Tai Chi on health outcomes in patients with chronic conditions: A systematic review. *Archives of Internal Medicine, 164*, 493-501.

Wardell, D. W., & Weymouth, K. F. (2004). Review of studies of healing touch. *Image: The Journal of Nursing Scholarship, 36*(2), 147-154.

Whelan, K. M., & Wishnia, G. S. (2003). Reiki therapy: The benefits to a nurse/Reiki practitioner. *Holistic Nursing Practice, 17*(4), 209-217.

Witek-Janusek, L. (2004). Stress. In S. M. Lewis, M. M. Heitkemper, & S. R. Dirksen (Eds.), *Medical-surgical nursing: Assessment and management of clinical problems* (6th ed., pp. 112-130). St. Louis: Mosby.

Woolery, A., Myers, H., Sternlieb, B., & Zeltzer, L. (2004). A yoga intervention for young adults with elevated symptoms of depression. *Alternative Therapies in Health & Medicine, 10*(2), 60-63.

Unit Four

Application of Health Promotion

15 Overview of Growth and Development Framework

16 The Prenatal Period

17 Infant

18 Toddler

19 Preschool Child

20 School-Age Child

21 Adolescent

22 Young Adult

23 Middle-Age Adult

24 Older Adult

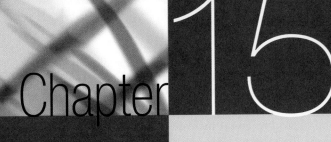

Chapter 15

MARTHA DRIESSNACK

Overview of Growth and Development Framework

objectives

After completing this chapter, the reader will be able to:

- Discuss the importance of growth and development as a framework for assessing and promoting health.

- Contrast the terms *growth* and *development.*

- Discuss factors that influence the rate and pattern of growth of an individual.

- Describe Erikson's theory of psychosocial development.

- Outline the four stages of Piaget's theory of cognitive development.

- Compare and contrast Gilligan's and Kohlberg's theories of moral development.

key terms

Denver Developmental
 Screening Test
Development
Developmental patterns
Erikson's theory of
 psychosocial
 development

Gilligan's theory of moral
 development
Growth
Growth charts
Growth patterns
Kohlberg's theory of moral
 development

Learning
Maturation
Piaget's theory of cognitive
 development

THINK About It

Vaccine Issues and Controversies

A 4½-year-old child begins to scream as the nurse approaches with her "kindergarten shots."

Her mother tries to comfort the child as she turns to the nurse saying "I've heard shots can be dangerous. Is it really necessary to expose her to possible harm? Won't all these shots weaken her natural immune system?"

1 Based on both Piaget's theory of cognitive development and Erikson's theory of psychosocial

development, what approach might the nurse take to gain the child's cooperation?

2 How might the mother's response and questioning influence the child's behavior?

3 What approach and information should the nurse have for the mother?

The author acknowledges the work of Marinda Allender in the previous edition of the chapter.

Unit 4 focuses on growth and development throughout the life span as a framework for health assessment and promotion. An understanding of human growth and development can facilitate accurate assessment of health and health practices in all age groups. Health education is more appropriate when the nurse acknowledges the individual's developmental level and needs.

This chapter sets the stage for the study of health promotion at individual developmental levels by exploring basic concepts of growth and development and by presenting an overview of four representative theories of development. Each of the following nine chapters deals with a specific age group. Health assessment and promotion strategies appropriate to each age group are described. The age groups described are prenatal, infant, toddler, preschool age, school age, adolescent, and young, middle, and older adult (Table 15-1).

OVERVIEW OF GROWTH AND DEVELOPMENT

In today's world the concepts of growth and development have expanded in proportion to advances in all fields of science. The increased ability to observe biophysical and biochemical events during the intrauterine stage of life has led to increased awareness and knowledge of the effects of fetal events on later life. The behavioral sciences have contributed to significant changes in the ways in which children of technological societies are reared, taught, and understood. Discoveries in health care have also yielded the ability to alter the course of human life when deformity or debilitating disease occurs.

Research has revealed that young, middle, and older adults continue to experience normative transitions that are as essential to their continuing development as the normative transitions of childhood. Furthermore, research in gerontology is receiving increased attention and funding as average life expectancy increases and older adults become our fastest growing age group.

Concept of Growth

Growth refers to changes in the structure, reflects an increase in the number and size of cells, and results in an increase in the size and weight of the whole or any of its parts. During childhood, physical changes in head circumference, weight, height, and overall body proportion are readily noticeable and their measurement is a basic component of health care visits. However, growth refers not only to the obvious changes in height and weight, but also to the increases (and in old age, the decreases) in the size of individual organs and systems. The health history and physical assessment of an individual should include all body systems, but should also emphasize systems undergoing the most change. Table 15-2 outlines the growth as it takes place throughout the body systems and life span. The growth of some systems, such as the skeletal and muscular systems, is influenced by gender, whereas the growth of others, such as the nervous and respiratory systems, is independent of gender. Changes that take place in young, middle-aged, and older adults should be noted. The nurse who has studied growth only from the perspective of children can be missing important differences among adults.

Text continued on p. 337

Table **15-1** Developmental Periods

Period	Age	Characteristics
Infancy	0 to 12 months	Infant fully dependent on others for basic needs Ends when child begins walking alone and possesses the beginning speech sounds of language
Toddler period	12 months to 3 years	Motor development progresses significantly Child achieves a degree of physical and emotional autonomy while maintaining a close identity with the primary family unit
Preschool period	3 to 6 years	Child has increased interest and involvement with peers and may have social interactions with many people
School-age period	6 to 10 years	Marked by entrance into elementary school Interests turn away from family and toward peers
Adolescence	11 to 18 years	A period of transition, adjustment, and personal exploration Ends when individual demonstrates readiness to assume full adult responsibilities of financial, emotional, and social independence
Young adulthood	18 to 35 years	Getting started in an occupation or career, finding and learning to live with a partner, and starting and rearing a family
Middle adulthood	35 to 65 years	Being established in a marriage, an occupation or career, and a community May continue to be a time of transition Must adjust to physiological changes of middle age
Older adulthood	Over 65 years	Must adjust to decreased physical strength and health, retirement, reduced income, decreasing independence, and deaths of spouse, friends, and self May be a time of continued involvement in work and active socializing

Table 15-2 Flowchart Showing Directions of Growth Changes Throughout Life Cycle*

Overview of Developmental Changes	Prenatal→	Infancy→	Childhood→	Puberty and Adolescence→	Adulthood→	Middle Age→	Old Age
HEART AND CIRCULATORY SYSTEM							
Action of heart and circulatory system is under control of autonomic nervous system. Throughout life cardiac rate is responsive to organ needs and emotional states (fear, anxiety, tension, depression).	Heart formed and begins to beat about third week	Heart grows somewhat more slowly than rest of body (weight doubled by 1 yr, body weight tripled) Grows steadily during childhood With birth, considerable change in paths and relative volumes of blood flow, reflected in loss of certain fetal structures and changes in heart and major vessels		At puberty, heart takes part in rapid growth, reaching mature size with rest of body	Heart weight remains relatively constant after age 25 (only organ other than prostate that does not decrease in weight with age) Cardiac output decreases 30% to 40% between age 25 and 65 Cardiac strength lessens with age, whereas expenditure of energy is more than in youth Capacity to increase rate and strength of beat during physical work is diminished		
	Heart rate high, approx. 150 beats/min	Heart rate falls steadily throughout childhood 130 beats/min	70 to 80 beats/min	60 beats/min in adolescence, rate differs with gender	After maturity, women have slightly higher pulse rate than men, 65 beats/min (girls' temperature remains stationary, higher than boys'); men maintain same pulse rate in maturity (slightly lower body temperature than women)		
		Heart rate more variable during childhood—regular Not until middle childhood does peripheral blood picture become same as adult					
URINARY SYSTEM							
Parallels growth as a whole. Proportion of bodily water and solids follows pattern related to growth—tendency for human organism to dry out as life progresses. Function of kidneys, with other organ systems, is to help in regulation of internal environment of body.	Young fetus is about 90% water Urinary system begins in first month	Newborn is about 70% water Urinary system does not complete full development until end of first year All renal units immature at birth; thus fluid and electrolyte imbalance occurs readily Kidney function adequate at birth if not subjected to undue stress	Composition of urine in healthy child (after age 2) changes very little as child matures; thus renal function and urinalysis can be used as monitor of well-being		Adult is about 58% water Glomerular filtration rate decreases about 47% from age 20 to 90		

Continued

Table **15-2** Flowchart Showing Directions of Growth Changes Throughout Life Cycle* cont'd

Overview of Developmental Changes	Prenatal→	Infancy→	Childhood→	Puberty and Adolescence→	Adulthood→	Middle Age→	Old Age
DIGESTIVE SYSTEM							
As a whole, grows as total body grows, although evidence suggests that various parts of gastrointestinal system undergo separate periods of growth, maturity, and senescence.	Before birth nutrients are supplied through placental circulation; digestion and absorption do not occur in the GI tract	Stomach size increases rapidly first months, then grows steadily throughout childhood		Spurt of growth at puberty	All actions of the GI tract (food intake, digestion, absorption, elimination) not only respond to physiological needs but from birth to old age are sensitive to tensions and anxiety		
		Digestive apparatus immature at birth (food passes through rapidly, reverse peristalsis common)			Data suggest generalized atrophy of entire GI tract with advancing age		
		Acidity of gastric juices varies over life span; low during infancy, rises during childhood, plateaus about age 10, rises during puberty			Nutritional needs vary according to individual variation—decreasing metabolism → enzyme production ↓ HCl ↓ stomach volume—tone of large intestine may become impaired until decrease with senescence (also diminished taste)		
		Free gastric acid (HCl) more marked in boys					
	Salivary glands small at birth	Increase rapidly during first 3 mo; reach relative adult proportions by age 2					
SPECIAL SENSES							
Most are well developed at birth, although their association with higher centers comes about gradually during early life and diminishes with advancing age.	Begin very early in embryonic development —3 to 6 wk	Sense of touch is developed first, then hearing and vision					
		Vision: infant can perceive simple differences in shape but not complex patterns (greater proportion of total growth before birth); various dimensions of vision develop at various ages, eye muscles function at mature level first year, fusion begins 9 mo until 6 yr; refractive power changes over life cycle—hyperopia increases until eyeball reaches adult size (approx. 8 yr), then reverses trend toward emmetropia—postpubertal years—toward myopia until 30 yr when myopia decreases and hyperopia increases					
ADIPOSE TISSUE							
Although adipose tissue varies greatly from individual to individual, overall lifetime pattern exists. Fat accumulation varies greatly with body build and constitution. Relationship between caloric intake, amount of exercise, and utilization or	Accumulates rapidly before birth; peak at seventh gestational month Premature infant may look wrinkled and scrawny because of lack of adipose tissue	Increases rapidly during first 6 mo	Decreases from first to seventh year in both genders	Then begins to increase slowly to puberty Fat begins to accumulate slowly and continues uninterrupted in girls, producing feminine curves, and accounts for much of weight gain	Some girls slim down after full maturation; many maintain about the same amount of adipose as at puberty	Typically both sexes tend to gain weight in 50s and 60s but do not maintain same body contours of earlier years at same weight (increase deposit on abdomen and hips)	Usually fat stores are lost after seventh decade in both genders Sharpness in contours, increasingly prominent bony landmarks
		(Gender differences are not noted in the body shape of prepubescent children)		Deposition of fat differs in body—	After full maturation, fat		

Table 15-2   Flowchart Showing Directions of Growth Changes Throughout Life Cycle* *cont'd*

Overview of Developmental Changes	Prenatal→	Infancy→	Childhood→	Puberty and Adolescence→	Adulthood→	Middle Age→	Old Age
accumulation of fat is not yet fully understood but is basis of much interrelated research.				amount decreases sharply at time of maximum growth spurt (increased weight caused by increase in muscle mass and bones)	accumulation begins→		

LYMPHOID TISSUE

Lymphoid tissue is scattered widely throughout body and includes lymph nodes, tonsils, adenoids, thymus, spleen, and lymphocytes of the blood; follows unique pattern of growth, rapid in infancy and begins to atrophy at puberty.	Begins during last month of uterine life—cross placenta at levels equal to mother's and remain for several months after delivery	Grows most rapidly during infancy and childhood, reaching maximum size a few years before puberty; parallels development of immunity Thus increased incidence of disease with increasing age of child		Then atrophies and is smaller in volume at full maturity than during childhood			Thymus so small that it is difficult to locate in older people

RESPIRATORY SYSTEM

Growth parallels that of total body growth. Respiratory apparatus is a highly organized system of organs under nervous and hormonal regulation, which functions in coordination with rest of body. Gender difference in gas exchange becomes apparent during puberty.	Before birth, air sacs do not contain air; oxygen supplied through maternal circulation	When umbilical cord is cut, infant must use own breathing apparatus—breathing irregular at first both in rate and depth—fast in infancy—gradually slowing through childhood until maturity is reached			No gender difference in respiratory rate at anytime of life Basal metabolic rate declines (rate higher in men than women)		

Respiratory exchange gradually becomes more efficient as life advances. Actual volume of air inhaled with each breath increases as lung size expands with general body growth. Vital capacity and maximum breathing capacity rise gradually in both genders, increasing more in boys during puberty; adult men have more efficient respiratory exchange, are capable of greater feats of muscular exertion without exhaustion than women.

Continued

Table **15-2** Flowchart Showing Directions of Growth Changes Throughout Life Cycle* *cont'd*

Overview of Developmental Changes	Prenatal→	Infancy→	Childhood→	Puberty and Adolescence→	Adulthood→	Middle Age→	Old Age
SKELETAL SYSTEM							
Bone growth passes through successive stages of development from connective tissue to cartilage to osseous tissue; completion of calcification indicates end of growing period and is thus a useful measure of growth rate and physiological maturity. Most growth ceases during adolescence.	Follows cephalocaudal law of development 70% of head growth before birth; bones of hands and wrist laid down in cartilage	Trunk fastest growing, 60% of total increase	Reserved during growth spurt After first year, legs fastest growing, 66% of total increase in height; longer puberty is delayed, greater the leg length	Length of trunk and depth of chest reach peak growth	Maximum height in early 20s to 30s	Then gradual decline until onset of senescence Thinning of vertebral disks beginning in middle years; most rapid in last decade	
		At birth, shafts of metacarpals are ossified (and visible by radiography); carpal bones begin to ossify	Growth of both genders nearly even until onset of puberty in girls first (approx. 10 yr) Boys begin approx. 2 yr later, but markedly greater Peak in height comes before peak in weight			Spinal column shortens (osteoporosis) with thinning vertebrae—shortening of trunk with long extremities—reversal of growth proportions in infancy	
MUSCLE SYSTEM							
Number of striated muscle fibers is roughly same in all human beings. Tremendous difference in size, not only from fetus to adult, but among adults, is caused by ability of individual muscle fibers to increase in size.	Muscle formation begins early, assuming final shape by end of second month	Increases rapidly during infancy but slowly during childhood Growth in both genders is same in childhood	Increase in muscle size means increasing strength in children; increase in skill is more intimately related to maturation of nervous system	With onset of puberty, muscle strength is greater in boys (when muscle growth is stimulated by testosterone) Greatest increase begins in puberty; muscle size precedes muscle strength in boys	Muscle mass continues to increase gradually—maximum strength in early adulthood—then declines slightly—according to use and genetic constitution Will increase in bulk and strength as used until onset of senescence		Atrophy and loss of muscle tone

Table 15-2   Flowchart Showing Directions of Growth Changes Throughout Life Cycle* *cont'd*

Overview of Developmental Changes	Prenatal→	Infancy→	Childhood→	Puberty and Adolescence→	Adulthood→	Middle Age→	Old Age
NERVOUS SYSTEM							
Growth and maturation of central and peripheral nervous system (brain, cord, peripheral nerves, many sense organs) reflected by changing size of head.	Growth very rapid during intrauterine development; head grows at greater rate than rest of body	Has all the brain cells in first year, which will continue to increase in size; number and complexity of axons, dendrites, and synapses will continue to increase			Function continues with use		Depletion of fully functioning brain cells, whether they are lost, shrink, or lose connections
		All neural tissues grow rapidly during infancy and early childhood		(No neural growth spurt at puberty)			Decrease in myelin sheath, impulses decrease; slow down speed of action and reaction
		Brain grows rapidly after birth, reaching 90% of total size by age 2	By middle childhood almost reaches adult size	Then slow increase to full maturity	Brain weight decreases with age		
		Segmented spinal nerves are mature, fully myelinated, and functioning at term (e.g., knee jerk), but acquisition of myelin in cortex, brainstem, and cord is closely correlated with observed behavior (myelination of this tract follows cephalocaudal, proximodistal law)			Taste less acute, less discriminatory with advancing age		
		Equipment for sense of taste and smell present at birth and perhaps most acute at that time			Structural changes in CNS result in impaired perception		
REPRODUCTIVE SYSTEM							
Organs of reproductive system show little increase during early life but rapid development just before and coincident with puberty. Maturation and fulfillment of reproductive functions of maturity (in female) are followed by involution in later years.	Genital organs form during uterine life; uterus undergoes growth spurt before birth (hormonal stimulation from mother)	Female sex organs well formed but not functioning at birth (but have full quota of sensory nerves)	Quiescent during childhood →	Maturation at puberty (menstruation) →			Involution after menopause
		Uterus undergoes involution to half its birth weight	Regained size by age 10 to 11→	Adult size at puberty→	Maximum increase with pregnancy→		Begin to atrophy with advancing age
		In male— testes, as with ovaries, remain dormant and small, not even growing in proportion to rest of body (with sensory nerves)		Until puberty, interstitial cells of Leydig reappear and secrete testosterone, so testes and penis continue to increase in size; pubic hair appears			

Continued

Table **15-2** Flowchart Showing Directions of Growth Changes Throughout Life Cycle* *cont'd*

Overview of Developmental Changes	Prenatal→	Infancy→	Childhood→	Puberty and Adolescence→	Adulthood→	Middle Age→	Old Age
	Mammary glands develop in both sexes during fetal life	Enlargement of breasts at birth (both sexes)→	Nonsecretory during childhood until puberty→	Development rapid→	Enlarge during pregnancy, developing alveoli→		Atrophy with advanced age
	Sex hormones: until puberty girls and boys produce male hormones (androgens) and female hormones (chiefly estrogens) in small and roughly equal amounts						

INTEGUMENTARY SYSTEM

Includes skin and its appendages and adnexa (nails, hair, sebaceous glands, eccrine and apocrine sweat glands). Although all skin is similar, this organ shows considerable variability in different parts of body (and from individual to individual) and varies greatly during the life span.	Hair, skin, and sebaceous glands fully formed in utero Lanugo begins to decrease before birth and continues regression few weeks postnatally→ Activity of sebaceous glands decreases after birth→	Skin contains all its adult structures at birth but immature in function	Matures slowly until puberty (children prone to rashes) Replaced by body hair, less extensive distribution; marked difference in type and distribution of hair at puberty→	Rapid spurt in maturation of skin and all its structures Increases rapidly at puberty (more prone to acne)			Changes in skin most obvious sign of aging (exposure and environmental conditions) Regenerative and growth power decreases and skin loses elasticity

ENDOCRINE SYSTEM

Consists of number of glandular structures scattered throughout the body. Although small in size, their hormones influence all growth and development of whole organism.	Immaturity of entire endocrine system puts infant at disadvantage if required to adjust to wide fluctuations in concentration of water, electrolytes, glucose, amino acids. All are interrelated, but each organ develops at own rate: Thyroid—increases from midfetal life to maturity; slightly larger in boys than girls; growth spurt at adolescence Adrenals—after birth decrease in size and continue throughout first year, increase again during childhood (but smaller than birth); spurt at puberty, reaching maturity with rest of body; greater increase in male gonads and testes and female ovaries (endocrine glands as well as reproductive organs), follow genital type of growth pattern Hypophysis, or pituitary gland—produces or stimulates hormones that influence growth Parathyroid—produce hormones that maintain homeostasis of calcium and phosphorus Islets of Langerhans—dispersed through pancreas; produce insulin and glucagon					With age, decline occurs in all endocrine gland functions	

Modified from Sutterly, D., & Donneley, G. (1973). *Perspectives in human development: Nursing throughout the life cycle.* Philadelphia: J. B. Lippincott.
CNS, central nervous system; GI, gastrointestinal.
*This chart indicates only general trends and directions of growth and development; it is not all inclusive. No distinct ages, absolute values, or ranges of normal variations are intended in this flowchart.

MULTICULTURAL AWARENESS

Childhood Lead Poisoning in Hispanic Children

Lead poisoning is a major, preventable environmental health problem. Excessive lead exposure affects an estimated 890,000 children annually and can lead to mental retardation, coma, seizures, and death (Mahon, 1997). Chronic low-level exposure results in learning disabilities, impaired growth, poor eye–hand coordination, antisocial behavior, dental decay, and hearing loss (Rothman, Lourie, & Gaughan, 2002). During the last 2 decades, public health and provider efforts have resulted in a 90% decline in the overall number of children affected, although the risk for Hispanic children has remained steady.

In 1997 the Centers for Disease Control and Prevention (CDC, 1997) issued new guidelines for blood lead screening. Children were to be screened if they met any of the following criteria:

1. Receives services from public assistance programs for the poor
2. Lives in an area where more than 27% of the housing was built before 1950
3. Parent or guardian answers yes to any of the following:
   a. Does your child live in or regularly visit a house that was built before 1950?
   b. Does your child live in or regularly visit a house that was built before 1978 with recent or ongoing renovations or remodeling?
   c. Does your child have a sibling or playmate who has or did have lead poisoning?

These screening questions target only children whose exposure is through lead-based paint. However, this is not the primary source of lead exposure for Hispanic children.

Food and culturally defined health practices bring additional risk to this population. Foods packaged or canned outside the United States, in Mexico or South America, foods cooked, stored, eaten or drunk using ceramic containers or pottery made outside the United States, in Mexico or South America, Mexican or South American raisins, and wrapped Mexican candies, specifically tamarind fruit candies and lollipops, all increase lead exposure (MMWR, 2002). *Empacho,* a common Hispanic term for a stomach or intestinal upset or obstruction, is treated with a folk remedy which is 99% lead (Lynch, Boatright & Moss, 2000). It is known by many names, including *Alarcon, Azarcon, Coral, Greta, Liga, Maria Luisa,* and *Rueda.* Another common Hispanic folk remedy containing lead is *Pay looah.* An overlooked risk for Hispanics is the use of warm, hot, or boiled tap water from contaminated pipes. Many Hispanics feel that heating the water rids it of contaminants, although any heat mobilizes the lead and makes it easier to absorb. This is also true of pottery that is heated by cooking in it, placing heated fluids in it, or heating it in the microwave oven (Lynch et al., 2000). A typical instruction sheet for lead poisoning prevention teaches that water should be run for a full minute before it is consumed; however, it fails to say that the water consumed should come only from the cold tap.

When screening for lead poisoning in Hispanic children, the nurse must remember to include questions about the use of folk remedies, pottery, imported foods and candies, as well as the use of boiled or hot tap water. In addition, the nurse should include dietary education that encourages decreasing fat intake, because lead is retained in fat, and increasing vitamin C, calcium, and iron intake, all of which reduce the amount of lead in the body.   •

Influences on an individual's potential for growth include genetic factors, prenatal and postnatal health, nutrition, and the environment. Other less obvious influences are the emotional health of the developing child or adult and the ethnic and cultural practices that influence child-rearing, life style, and health care practices. (See the Multicultural Awareness box for discussion of childhood lead poisoning in Hispanic children.) Although the limits of growth are genetically determined, health and environmental deficits may hamper a person's growth. A developing individual is most subject to the influence of these factors during periods of rapid growth. The timing of exposure to environmental hazards may determine to a great extent the amount and kind of effects of these influences. For example, if a pregnant mother is exposed to the rubella virus, the developing fetus is much more vulnerable than either the mother or an older child, especially during the first trimester when all organ systems are being established. The Care Plan relates to a nursing diagnosis for a family with a chronically ill or disabled newborn.

Growth Patterns

Expected **growth patterns** exist for all people. Growth is not steady throughout life. The periods of extremely rapid growth—prenatal, infancy, and adolescence—are contrasted with slower rates of growth during the toddler, preschool, and school-age periods and the almost imperceptible rate of growth after adolescence. Infants typically double their birth weight by 6 months of age and triple their birth weight by 1 year of age. The well known "growth spurt" in height typically occurs early in adolescence for girls and later in adolescence for boys.

Different parts of the body increase in size at different rates. For example, during early life the head is the fastest growing section, followed by the trunk, and then the arms and legs. Newborns' heads account for one quarter of their overall length, as opposed to adults' heads which account for one ninth of their overall height. The changes in proportion of body parts from infancy to adulthood are demonstrated in Figure 15-1.

Growth Charts

Growth is one of the most important indications of a child's overall health and well-being. Accurate growth assessment depends on precise measurement of growth parameters using proper equipment, correct and consistent techniques, careful plotting of measurements, and thoughtful interpretation of the data (Winch, 2002).

CARE PLAN

Birth of Chronically Ill or Disabled Child

Nursing Diagnosis Altered Family Processes Related to Chronic Sorrow Over the Birth of a Chronically Ill or Disabled Child

DEFINING CHARACTERISTICS

- Parental expression of disparity between reality and desired reality of parenthood
- Parental expression of an ongoing sense of loss or of multiple losses over time
- Parental expression that feelings are periodic and permanent but do not interfere significantly with daily functioning
- Parental expression that resurgence of feelings often is triggered by health care crises or conflict with expected social norms

RELATED FACTORS

- Change in family structure
- Change in parental role expectation
- Parental coping styles
- Goal: Assist family unit to attain, maintain, or regain optimal health

EXPECTED OUTCOMES

- Parents will acknowledge change in family structure and parental role expectations.
- Parents will identify triggers for resurgence of feelings including illness, discovery of new medical problems, and delay in development.
- Parents will identify individual and collective coping mechanisms.

NURSING INTERVENTIONS

- Recognize chronic sorrow as a natural reaction, rather than a pathological response.
- Act as an advocate for the parents and child.
- Identify sources of support and respite.
- Assist parents in mobilizing effective coping strategies.
- Assist parents in maintaining hope and finding meaning in their experience.

Modified from Scornaienchi, J. M. (2003). Chronic sorrow. *Journal of Pediatric Health Care, 17,* 290-294.

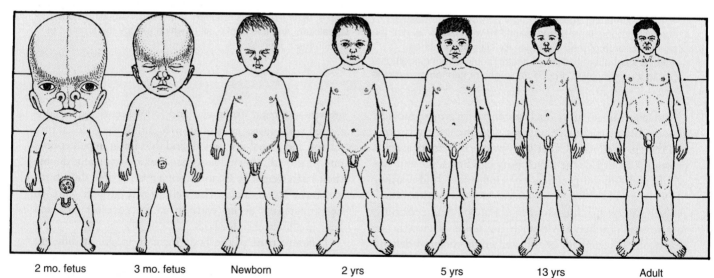

Figure 15-1   Changes in body proportions from birth to adulthood. (Redrawn from Crouch, J. E., & McClintic, J. R. [1976]. *Human anatomy and physiology* [2nd ed.]. New York: John Wiley & Sons.)

2 mo. fetus   3 mo. fetus   Newborn   2 yrs   5 yrs   13 yrs   Adult

The Centers for Disease Control and Prevention (CDC) **growth charts**, released in May 2000, consist of both revised versions of the old growth charts developed by the National Center for Health Statistics (NCHS) in 1977 and the addition of body mass index (BMI)-for-age charts. The BMI is an anthropometric index of weight and height combined with age. These charts are used to identify children and adolescents as underweight, overweight, or at risk of overweight. The CDC recommends that the BMI-for-age charts be used for all children and adolescents 2 to 20 years of age. The revised growth charts are more reflective of ethnic diversity and current feeding practices and also include percentile curves up to 20 years of age, as well as the addition of a 3rd and 97th percentile (Winch, 2002). See the Research Highlights box for more details on the changes.

A single measurement, although helpful, does not allow for the best assessment of a child's growth. Serial measure-

New CDC Growth Charts

In a policy statement issued by the AAP in 2003 outlining the need for widespread, comprehensive prevention efforts to address the increase in prevalence of overweight in children and adolescents, the sequential assessment of BMI was identified as an important strategy. The CDC growth charts (2000) consist of revised growth charts and the newly introduced BMI-for-age charts. Use of BMI-for-age allows significant changes in growth patterns to be recognized and addressed before children become severely overweight. It also facilitates anticipatory guidance for children and adolescents at risk of overweight or for those who are underweight.

An appropriate reference population, accurate measurements, and age calculations are important factors when assessing childhood growth. Comparing body measurements with the appropriate age-specific and gender-specific growth chart enables pediatric health care providers to monitor growth and identify potential problems related to health or nutrition. When the 1977 NCHS growth charts were developed, they were based on a sample consisting primarily of white, middle-class, formula-fed infants and children from southwestern Ohio. The new charts, on the other hand, are based on data that include a nationally referenced population reflective of age, sex, and racial and ethnic composition, as well as breast-fed and formula-fed infants.

The new CDC growth charts furnish health care providers and researchers with an improved tool to assess and track the growth of infants, children, and adolescents up to 20 years of age. They provide one set of growth charts for all racial and ethnic groups and can be used for both breast-fed and formula-fed infants. Condition-specific growth charts are also available for children with special health care needs such as Turner syndrome, achondroplasia, Down syndrome, Marfan syndrome, sickle cell anemia, and myelomeningocele. All growth charts and instructions for their use are available at the CDC Web site (http://www.cdc.gov/growthcharts).

AAP, American Academy of Pediatrics; *BMI,* body mass index; *CDC,* Centers for Disease Control and Prevention; *NCHS,* National Center for Health Statistics.

ments, plotted on a growth chart over time, best reflect a child's pattern of growth. Slowed growth, plateaus, or decreases in height, weight, and head circumference, as well as rapid increases, raise questions for health care providers about the adequacy of a child's nutritional intake, syndromes or disease states, neglect, or emotional problems (Winch, 2002).

Concept of Development

Development refers to gradual change and expansion of ability and advance in skill from lower to more advanced complexity. In contrast to growth, which is a quantitative or precisely measurable change, development is a qualitative change. Qualitative changes are more challenging to describe, because they cannot be measured in precise units. Development has best been conceptualized as a process that can be assessed as it follows certain sequencing or patterns, although the timing of this advancement is individual.

Developmental Patterns

All individuals follow similar **developmental patterns**, with one stage of development building on and leading to the next. Early development proceeds as follows:

Pattern of Development:
1. Cephalocaudal: head to toe
2. Proximodistal: midline to periphery
3. Differentiation: simple to complex; general to specific

Examples:
1. Infants gain neck and head control before controlling the movements of the extremities.
2. Infant central nervous systems develop before the peripheral nervous system.
3. Infants use a whole-hand grasp before learning the finer control of the pincer grasp and coo or babble before they speak.

Although the sequence of development is predictable, the exact timing of the sequencing is individual. Individuals develop at their own rate, on their own schedule. For example, infants creep and crawl before they walk and their primary teeth erupt in a predictable sequence, but each will walk and teethe on an individual schedule. However, there are guidelines or parameters that assist parents and health care providers in assessing whether children are progressing in an acceptable developmental sequence within a reasonable time frame. Areas of assessment usually focus on personal and social, gross and fine motor, and language development. The **Denver Developmental Screening Test,** which was revised in 1992 (now known as Denver II), is a screening tool that assists health care providers in monitoring children's development in each of these areas from birth to 6 years of age. The Denver II is presented in **Web Site Resource 17A**.

Social expectations can influence developmental tasks with expectations that an individual achieve certain landmarks during each period of development. However, the age at which a child is expected to master certain developmental tasks is determined partly by cultural expectations. Some cultures are comfortable with breast-feeding their children well into childhood, while others expect the transition to self-feeding with a cup much earlier. When assessing a child's abilities, one of the areas nurses need to be aware of is that a child who has never been given the opportunity to learn or master a skill may be developmentally capable, but fails when tested. For example, a child who is capable of learning colors or numbers can do so only if taught, just as the child who was breast-fed well into childhood, never having been offered a cup, may well be developmentally capable of drinking from a cup but probably will fail at early tries.

Development is closely interrelated with the concepts of both learning and maturation. **Learning** is the process of

HEALTH TEACHING Anticipatory Guidance

The nurse is often in a position to provide anticipatory guidance to parents, which involves teaching them ways to handle a situation before it becomes an issue or problem. Knowledge of normal growth and development provides a foundation for this teaching. For example, the toddler period is one of intense exploration of the environment, when locomotion is the major gross motor skill acquired. The nurse, knowing the number 1 cause of death in toddlers is accidents, provides the following teaching to the parents of a child who is entering the toddler period as a means of injury prevention:

- Always use a federally approved car restraint and check for proper installation and placement.
- Supervise child closely near any source of water, including buckets, bathtubs, and toilets.

- Turn pot handles toward the back of the stove and use the back burners whenever possible.
- Place all toxic substances in a locked cabinet and have the poison control contact number easily accessible. Avoid the use of syrup of ipecac unless advised by a poison control representative to do so.
- Move toddler from the crib to a bed.
- Provide barriers on open windows.
- Decrease the water heater temperature to avoid scald burns from tap water.
- Avoid foods that pose a choking hazard such as nuts, hard candies, raisins, fresh carrots, whole grapes, chewing gum, hot dogs, and fish with bones.

---

gaining specific knowledge or skills that results from exposure, experience, education, and evaluation. **Maturation** is an increase in competence and adaptability that is reflective of changes in the complexity of a structure that make it possible for that structure to begin to function or to function at a higher level. Maturation of a structure, system, or individual refers to the emergence of the genetic potential of that structure, system, or individual. Learning cannot occur unless the individual is mature enough to be able to understand and control behavior. Children can be toilet trained only when their bodies have matured to the point of developing internal and external sphincter control. Earlier attempts will be frustrating for both child and parent.

Growth and development are complex, interrelated processes that are influenced by and, in turn, influence the health of an individual. The nurse who understands this relationship is aware of the need for age-specific health assessment and promotion strategies (Health Teaching box).

THEORIES OF DEVELOPMENT

Specific aspects of development of the person have been studied for centuries. Many theories of development are used in the study of individuals throughout the life span; the nurse may wish to refer to a text on developmental psychology to become familiar with some of these theories. Four theories are introduced in this unit to gain a holistic view of the progression of individual development throughout the life span. These theories were developed by Erikson, Piaget, Kohlberg, and Gilligan.

Psychosocial Development: Erikson's Theory

Erik Erikson described the development of identity of the self and the ego through successive stages that naturally unfold throughout the life span (Erikson, 1968, 1993; Erikson & Erikson, 1998). Although he studied with Freud and supported the psychosexual theory of development, **Erikson's theory of psychosocial development** is based on

the need of each person to develop a sense of trust in self and others and a sense of personal worth. Erikson described a healthy personality in positive terms, not merely through the absence of disease.

Psychosocial development is based on critical stages, each requiring resolution of a conflict between two opposing forces. Each stage depends on the stage before it and must be accomplished successfully for the person to proceed. Erikson's use of a psychosocial framework acknowledges the influence of other people and the environment but maintains that it is ultimately the individual who must master each of the conflicts. Although each of the conflicts is predominant at a certain stage in life, it is important to recognize that all the conflicts exist in each person, to some extent, at all times and that a conflict, once resolved, may emerge again in appropriate situations. These stages are summarized in Table 15-3 and discussed more fully in the chapters on each developmental age group. See the Case Study about an infant girl and how hospitalization could affect her psychosocial development.

Cognitive Development: Piaget's Theory

Another aspect of development is the progressive acquisition of higher levels of cognitive ability. Jean Piaget, a Swiss psychologist trained in zoology, viewed children as biological organisms interacting with their environment. A child's main goal is to master the environment and establish harmony or equilibrium between it and the self.

Piaget's theory of cognitive development is concerned primarily with structure rather than content, with how the mind works rather than with what it does. Piaget uses the word *scheme* to describe a pattern of action or thought. A scheme is used to take in or assimilate new experiences or may be modified or accommodated by new experiences. Each person is striving to maintain a balance, or equilibrium, between assimilation and accommodation (Phillips, 1969; Piaget, 1950).

Piaget described the stages of cognitive development throughout the developmental years. Through a natural

Table **15-3** Erikson's Eight Stages of Human Development

Age Group	Psychosocial Stage	Lasting Outcomes
1. Infancy	Basic trust versus basic mistrust	Faith and hope
2. Toddler stage	Autonomy versus shame and doubt	Self-control and willpower
3. Preschool stage	Initiative versus guilt	Direction and purpose
4. School age	Industry versus inferiority	Method and competence
5. Adolescence	Identity versus role confusion	Devotion and fidelity
6. Young adulthood	Intimacy versus isolation	Affiliation and love
7. Middle adulthood	Generativity versus stagnation	Production and care
8. Older adulthood	Ego integrity versus despair	Renunciation and wisdom

Modified from Erikson, E. H. (1993). *Childhood and society* (35th anniversary ed.). New York: W. W. Norton; Erikson, E. H., & Erikson, J. M. (1998). *Life cycle completed.* New York: Norton.

CASE STUDY

Samantha

Samantha is a 9-month-old infant who has been admitted to the children's hospital. She must receive intravenous antibiotics for 10 days; however, her mother lives 100 miles away and is a single mother with other children at home. The mother must continue to work to support her family and provide the health insurance. Samantha will therefore be alone in the hospital except on the weekend. As the nurse, you consider promotion of normal growth and development as part of your nursing care.

Reflective Questions

1. What stage of psychosocial development is Samantha experiencing according to Erikson?
2. What are some important nursing interventions to facilitate a successful outcome of this stage?
3. What are some developmentally appropriate toys or transition items that the nurse can provide or request from home?
4. What anticipatory guidance should the nurse provide Samantha's mother?

unfolding of ability, the child acquires sequentially predictable cognitive abilities. Given adequate environmental stimuli and an intact neurological system, the child gradually matures toward full ability to conceptualize. Piaget's theory of cognitive development encompasses the time from birth to approximately 15 years of age. Each of the four distinct stages is summarized in Table 15-4 and discussed more fully in the specific chapters on each developmental age. Piaget suggests that quantitative, but no further qualitative, changes in cognitive function take place after about age 15.

Moral Development: Kohlberg's Theory

One aspect of cognitive development is the development of moral thinking and judgment. Lawrence **Kohlberg's theory of moral development** is based on interviews that focused on hypothetical moral dilemmas such as: Should a man steal an expensive drug that would save his dying wife? From these interviews, Kohlberg developed his theory, which is outlined in Table 15-5 (Kohlberg, 1981; Kohlberg & Kramer, 1969). The three stages of moral development, preconventional, conventional, and postconventional, are based on Piaget's theory of cognitive development and emphasize an ethic of justice. Progression through the successive stages of moral development generally takes place during the school age, adolescent, and young adult years. Beyond the young adult years, stabilization or increased consistency of thought and perhaps an increased correlation between moral judgment and moral action occurs (Kohlberg, 1981).

Moral Development: Gilligan's Theory

Gilligan's theory of moral development (1982, 1990) suggests that there is a different process of moral development in women in society. Carol Gilligan worked with Lawrence Kohlberg as a research assistant. She discovered that Kohlberg's original research was conducted using only men and that women often scored lower in Kohlberg's subsequent investigations. She asserted that women were not inferior in their moral development, just different. After her own research with women, she proposed her own theory of moral development which, like Kohlberg's, has three stages (Table 15-6). However, Gilligan concluded that the transitions between stages are based on changes in one's sense of self rather than on changes in cognitive development, as Kohlberg proposed. She also reported that women think more in terms of caring and relationships than men do, who are more inclined to think in terms of rules and justice. See the Hot Topics box discussion about self-esteem in males versus females.

SUMMARY

Individuals make many choices that affect their health each day, and a multitude of factors influence how these choices are made. Their stage of growth and development can greatly influence how they experience and perceive situations and the choices available to them. The nurse who has studied growth and development has a clearer understanding of what challenges individuals will likely encounter and what skills they will have to address them. Theories of

Table 15-4 Piaget's Stages of Cognitive Development

Stage	Age	Characteristics
Sensorimotor	Birth to 2 years	Begins with a predominance and reliance on reflexes which set the body up to learn Reflexes decrease and voluntary acts develop Imitation predominates Thought is dominated by physical manipulation of objects and events Develops the concept of object permanence and the ability to form mental representations
Preoperational	2 to 7 years	Advancing use of language and movement Development of egocentric, animistic, and magical thinking Uses representational thought to interpret and learn, not in terms of general properties, but in terms of the relationship or use to them No cause-and-effect reasoning Thought is dominated by the senses—what is seen, heard, or experienced
Concrete operations	7 to 11 years	Mental reasoning processes assume logical approaches to solving concrete problems including cause and effect Collecting; mastering facts Can consider other points of view Thought influenced by social contacts Language is perfected
Formal operations	11 to 15 years	True logical thought and manipulation of abstract concepts emerge Morality

Modified from Schuster, C., & Ashburn, S. (1992). *The process of human development: A holistic life span approach.* Boston: Lippincott.

Table 15-5 Kohlberg's Stages of Moral Development

Stage	Age	Goal
Preconventional	Birth to 9 years	Avoiding punishment Gaining reward
Conventional	9-20 years	Gaining approval Avoiding disapproval
Postconventional	20+ years	Agree upon rights Personal moral standards Justice

Compiled from Kohlberg, L. (1981). *The philosophy of moral development, Vol. 1.* San Francisco: Harper & Row.

Table 15-6 Gilligan's Stages of Moral Development (for Women)

Stage	Characteristics	Goal
Preconventional	What is practical and best for self, realizing connection to others	Individual survival
Conventional	Sacrifices wants and needs to fulfill others' wants and needs	Self-sacrifice is goodness
Postconventional	Moral equality of self and others	Principle of nonviolence, do not hurt self or others

Compiled from Gilligan, C. (1982). *In a different voice: Psychological theory and women's development.* Cambridge, MA: Harvard University Press; Gilligan, C., Ward, J. V., & Taylor, J. M. (Eds.) (1990). *Mapping the moral domain: A contribution of women's thinking to psychology and education.* Cambridge, MA: Harvard University Press.

HOTtopics

SELF-ESTEEM IN MALES VERSUS FEMALES

Recent statistics have shown that boys are encountering more difficulties in growing up and succeeding in schools and colleges. Consider the following:

- An increasing number of boys are reared in fatherless homes.
- Boys are less likely to complete high school, attend college, and stay out of jail than are girls.
- Boys commit 75% of suicides in the age group of 10 to 14 years.
- Four times as many boys as girls are prescribed methylphenidate (Ritalin) for attention deficit disorder.
  Concern over many years for the self-esteem of girls has paid off. Gender equity programs in school appear to have

worked to their benefit. A girl can now be a tomboy or feminine; either role is acceptable. Girls have become empowered to become who they want to be. Should boys be socialized to be more like girls? Is the rowdy, aggressive play of boys normal, or is it something to be reined in with discipline and medication? Some researchers believe that violence is a response to pressure placed on boys to conform to a macho stereotype.

- Should boys be allowed to be boys?
- Should boys be encouraged to express their emotions easily?
- What are the consequences of the current education system that seems suited to girls rather than boys?

Modified from Leo, J. (2000, July 17). Boys will be boys. *US News and World Report.*

development provide the nurse with a framework for health assessment, promotion, and care planning.

ADDITIONAL STUDY MATERIAL

Study Questions in the back of the book, see page 663.

evolve WEB SITE MATERIALS

These materials are located on the book's Web site at http://evolve.elsevier.com/Edelman/.

- WebLinks
- Content Updates

REFERENCES

Centers for Disease Control and Prevention. (1997). *Screening young children for lead poisoning.* Atlanta: CDC.

Erikson, E. H. (1968). *Identity, youth and crisis.* New York: Norton.

Erikson, E. H. (1993). *Childhood and society* (35th anniversary edition). New York: Norton.

Erikson, E. H., & Erikson, G. M. (1998). *Life-cycle completed.* New York: Norton.

Gilligan, C. (1982). *In a different voice: Psychological theory and women's development.* Cambridge, MA: Harvard University Press.

Gilligan, C., Ward, J. V., & Taylor, J. M. (Eds.) (1990). *Mapping the moral domain: A contribution of women's thinking to psychology theory and education.* Cambridge, MA: Harvard University Press.

Kohlberg, L. (1981). *The philosophy of moral development: Vol. 1.* San Francisco: Harper & Row.

Kohlberg, L., & Kramer, R. (1969). Continuities and discontinuities in childhood and adult moral development. *Human Development, 12,* 93.

Leo, J. (2000, Jul. 17). Boys will be boys. *US News and World Report.*

Lindeke, L., Rogers, S., & Finley, L. (2002). An update on growth charts, old and new. *Pediatric Nursing, 28*(138), 140-141.

Lynch, R. A., Boatright, D. T., & Moss, S. K. (2000). Lead contaminated imported tamarind candy and children's blood lead levels. *Public Health Reports, 115,* 543.

Mahon, I. (1997). Caregiver's knowledge and perceptions of preventing childhood lead poisoning. *Public Health Nursing, 14*(3), 169-182.

Miller, K. (2001). Evaluating growth in children: Distinguishing between normal and worrisome. *Advances for Nurse Practitioners, 9*(11), 42-46, 49.

MMWR. (2002). Childhood lead poisoning associated with tamarind candy and folk remedies—California, 1999-2000. *MMWR Morbidity and Mortality Weekly Report, 51*(31), 684-686.

Phillips, J. R. (1969). *The origins of intellect: Piaget's theory.* San Francisco: W. H. Freeman.

Piaget, J. (1950). *The psychology of intelligence.* London: Routledge and Kegan Paul.

Rothman, N. L., Lourie, R., & Gaughan, J. (2002). Lead awareness: North Philly style. *American Journal of Public Health, 92*(5), 739-741.

Scornaienchi, J. M. (2003). Chronic sorrow: One mother's experience with two children with lissencephaly. *Journal of Pediatric Health Care, 17,* 290-294.

Winch, A. E. (2002). Obtaining accurate growth measurements in children. *Journal for Specialists in Pediatric Nursing, 7*(4), 166-169.

Chapter 16

CAROLYN SPENCE CAGLE

The Prenatal Period

objectives

After completing this chapter, the reader will be able to:

- Discuss fetal development and the newborn transition to extrauterine life.
- Analyze changes in the maternal system during pregnancy based on their influences on pregnancy adaptation.
- Interpret the role of the nurse in promoting the physical, mental, and spiritual health of the childbearing family.
- Discuss fetal problems caused by maternal drinking, smoking, drug use, and viral exposure during pregnancy.
- Discuss the nursing role during labor and delivery with a focus on the physical, emotional, and educational needs of the delivering woman and her family.
- Analyze the influence of factors such as ethnicity, legislative priorities, and the sociopolitical context of the health care delivery system on childbirth care and the needs of families.

key terms

Acquired immunodeficiency syndrome
Amniocentesis
Apgar scoring system
Bacterial vaginosis
Bradycardia
Candida albicans
Cervix
Chlamydia
Chloasma
Chorionic and amniotic membranes
Chorionic villi
Colostrum
Congenital defect
Cytomegalovirus
Decidua
Dilation
Down syndrome
Effacement
Embryo

Endometrium
Episiotomy
Estrogen
Fertilization
Fetal heart monitor
Fetus
First stage of labor
Fourth stage of labor
Fundus
Gonococcus
Group B Streptococcus
Hepatitis B
Herpes simplex
Human chorionic gonadotropin
Infant mortality rate
Lamaze
Linea nigra
Meconium
Pica
Placenta

Positive signs of pregnancy
Probable signs of pregnancy
Progesterone
Quickening
Rubella
Second stage of labor
Sexually transmitted diseases
Spontaneous abortion
Station
Striae gravidarum
Syphilis
Tachycardia
Teratogen
Thalidomide
Third stage of labor
Toxoplasmosis
Trimester
Ultrasonography
Zygote

First Pregnancy Labor

Laura, currently 41 weeks into her first pregnancy, is admitted at 2:00 AM to St. Jude's Medical Center with uterine contractions occurring every 8 minutes since midnight. Her cervix is dilated to 2 cm and is 80% effaced, and station is –3. Her husband is out of town on a business trip, and Laura's neighbor has accompanied her to the hospital. Although Laura attended Lamaze classes with her husband, she is anxious about the labor. She says to the nurse, "My back is about to break, I have so much bottom pressure, and I wanted to go natural, without medication and all this high-technology stuff, including the monitor."

1 Based on your knowledge of ethical and legal principles of care, how would you as a caregiver appropriately respond to Laura's needs with labor and delivery?

2 What factors in Laura's database would support the use of the fetal heart monitor? What factors would not support use of the monitor?

3 What political, legal, ethical, and other factors might be relevant to the wide use of monitors in American maternity units today?

4 How does the use of fetal heart rate monitoring fit into a health-promotion approach to labor and delivery?

The process of conception, pregnancy, and birth involves a complex interaction of many factors, including the physiological and psychological changes in the woman and family and the development of a fetus into a viable newborn. The focus of this chapter is on the pregnant woman, her family, and the developing fetus; discussing one without the others is impossible. The nurse must consider all three entities when seeking to promote a healthy pregnancy and healthy family system after birth.

PHYSICAL CHANGES IN MATERNAL AND FETAL SYSTEMS

The physical changes during pregnancy include natural processes involving fertilization of the egg by the sperm, implantation of the fertilized egg into the uterus, embryonic or fetal growth and development, placental development and function, and maternal changes related to the pregnancy process.

Duration of Pregnancy

Pregnancy begins with the union of a sperm and egg, a process called **fertilization.** Under normal healthy circumstances, a full-term pregnancy lasts approximately 9 solar months, 10 lunar months, or 40 weeks. An accurate estimated date of delivery is determined by using Nägele's rule. This is done by adding 7 days to the date of the first day of the last normal menstrual period and subtracting 3 months. A usual pregnancy consists of 9 months, divided into three equal periods called **trimesters.** Oftentimes these trimesters form the basis for discussion of expected fetal and maternal changes during pregnancy.

Fertilization

The union of sperm and egg requires several crucial factors, many of which are not fully understood. When a sperm cell penetrates an egg in the fallopian tube, the beginning of a human being called a **zygote** results. Additional division of zygotic cells results in more differentiated structures that eventually produce an **embryo** and subsequently a **fetus.**

An absence of one or more critical factors may cause infertility (failure of the couple to become pregnant despite usual sexual activity over a year's time). For example, both a sperm cell and an egg cell must be mature and in the fallopian tube for approximately 5 hours for union of sperm and egg to occur (the process of conception). The sperm must be of uniform size, be normally formed, possess high motility, and have an ability to secrete enzymes that dissolve the membrane surrounding the egg. The woman attempting pregnancy must have a certain basal body temperature and fallopian tubes free of adhesions or obstructions. A woman will likely conceive within 24 hours after ovulation. However, because sperm live for up to 72 hours in the female reproductive tract, fertilization may take place even if intercourse occurred up to 3 days before ovulation.

Implantation

Transplantation of the fertilized egg in the uterine cavity after its trip through the fallopian tube requires approximately 6 days (Georges, 2000). Once the zygote reaches the uterus, it floats there for an additional 2 to 5 days, receiving nutrition from the **endometrium,** the inner lining of the uterus (Lowdermilk & Perry, 2003a). The cells around the developing zygote secrete enzymes that digest the endometrial lining, which allows the zygote to become attached to the uterine wall and the placenta to develop. Within a week after implantation, the **placenta** provides primary nourishment and protects the baby throughout pregnancy, or gestation. Fertilization triggers the production of large amounts of the hormone **progesterone** (Georges, 2000), which stimulates the formation of endometrial cells known as the **decidua.** The decidua provides nutrition for the *embryo,* a term that defines the growing baby from 2 to 8 gestational weeks.

Fetal Growth and Development

Much is known about the stages of physical development in each structural system of the embryo. However, metabolic functions, particularly those relevant to the endocrine and neurological systems, are less well defined. Appropriate fetal development depends on these events occurring in a specified period and order during each trimester of pregnancy. If this does not occur, an abnormality in structure or function (a **congenital defect**) may result. This defect may be noted at birth, did not occur at conception (called a *genetic defect*), but most likely resulted from some disruption that occurred after conception and during fetal development. **Web Site Resource 16A** presents a summary of fetal growth and development.

Placental Development and Function

After zygotic implantation, the placenta develops through an integration of embryonic and decidual cells. The **chorionic and amniotic membranes,** which surround the fetus throughout gestation, also begin to form. The amniotic fluid, manufactured by the amniotic membrane, supports the developing infant and protects it from injury.

The basic structure of the placenta **(Web Site Resource 16B)** allows maternal–fetal blood exchange to nourish the fetus and allow excretion of fetal waste. Throughout most of gestation, increasing placental development allows maternal blood to flow through the intervillous spaces and fetal circulation to flow through the **chorionic villi** (Cunningham et al., 2001a; Georges, 2000). The unique structure of the placenta permits the exchange of certain molecules but prevents fetal and maternal blood supplies from mixing for most of the pregnancy. Larger and heavier molecules normally do not pass through the placenta to the fetus, but lighter molecules (such as anesthetic gases, oxygen, carbon dioxide, and electrolytes) readily cross the placenta. Other processes, such as diffusion, pinocytosis, facilitated diffusion, and active transport, may operate as transfer mechanisms (Cunningham et al., 2001a; Lowdermilk & Perry, 2003a). Because of the difficulty involved in predicting exactly which substances will cross the placenta, the nurse needs to encourage pregnant women and those contemplating pregnancy to avoid any agent that might cause harm to the fetus early in pregnancy.

Inspection of the placenta after birth reveals important clues to the quality of gestational life. The maternal side of the placenta appears dark red and spongy, and the fetal side is shiny gray with a glassy consistency. The umbilical cord normally arises from near the center of the placenta, and the membranes arise smoothly from the rim. Abnormal insertion of the cord or membranes, necrotic areas in the placenta, or two umbilical vessels rather than three may cause problems during gestation and after birth (Cunningham et al., 2001a).

The fetus, which continues to gain strength and maturity during the later weeks of gestation, generally rests its head in the lower maternal pelvis by the end of pregnancy (Figure 16-1). The membranes protect the fetus from infection and act as a container for the amniotic fluid. As birth begins, the membranes may rupture, causing the loss of amniotic fluid and stronger uterine contractions, or tightenings of the uterus, reflective of the labor process. If the

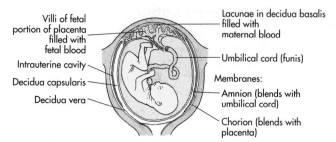

Figure 16-1 Diagrammatic representation of relationship of fetus, placenta, membranes, and uterus during gestation. (From Lowdermilk, D., & Perry, S. [2004]. *Maternity and women's health care* [8th ed.]. St. Louis: Mosby.)

membranes rupture more than 24 hours before delivery, uterine infection and fetal harm may result. If this occurs, a woman may require hospitalization and high-risk assessment for the remainder of her pregnancy because of concerns about maternal and fetal health.

As gestation nears completion, placental function gradually decreases, which may serve as a stimulus for the onset of labor. When pregnancy continues beyond 42 weeks, or 2 weeks beyond the calculated due date, placental function decreases even more, posing concerns about the well-being of the fetus.

This discussion of fetal development provides only half of the story about the prenatal period. Maternal changes and culmination of the prenatal period, labor, and birth are also important to address.

Maternal Changes

A woman experiences various physiological effects based on a combination of hormonal and mechanical changes during pregnancy. Hormonal influences tend to increase as the pregnancy progresses. The mechanical (hemodynamic) changes reach a peak in the seventh or eighth month and then gradually decline as the pregnancy nears completion (Cunningham et al., 2001b).

Signs of Pregnancy

A woman may assume that she is pregnant because she has skipped her menstrual period or experiences nausea and vomiting, changes in breast sensations and size, or increased urinary frequency (presumptive signs of pregnancy). If she suspects she is pregnant, the woman should seek a pregnancy test. The woman should be cautioned against relying on these tests, because concurrent medication or substance use may cause a false result (Pagana & Pagana, 2001). If performed too early, a home pregnancy test may also produce a false-negative result due to a low level of **human chorionic gonadotropin** (HCG). This hormone, produced by the placenta, is found in a pregnant woman's urine and blood. As the pregnancy progresses, the woman may have both **probable** and **positive signs of pregnancy,** objective changes that increasingly verify that a pregnancy exists (Box 16-1). With the advent of first-trimester, sophisticated

Box **16-1** Signs of Pregnancy

PROBABLE

- Enlargement of the uterus
- Softening of the uterine isthmus (Hegar sign)
- Bluish or cyanotic color of cervix and upper vagina (Chadwick sign)
- Softening of the cervix (Goodell sign)
- Asymmetrical, softened enlargement of the uterine corner caused by placental development (Piskacek sign)
- Positive test for HCG in the maternal urine or blood serum
- Changes in skin pigmentation (chloasma and linea nigra)

POSITIVE

- Detection of fetal heart tones by auscultation, ultrasonography, or use of a Doppler instrument
- Palpation of fetal parts using Leopold maneuvers
- Objective detection of fetal movements
- Radiological or ultrasonographic demonstration of fetal parts

HCG, human chorionic gonadotropin.

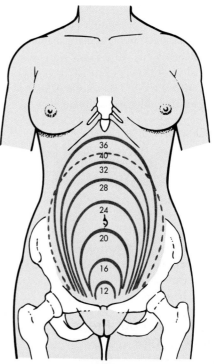

Figure 16-2 Upper level of enlarging uterus by weeks of normal gestation with a single fetus. (From Seidel, H. M., Ball, J. W., Dains, J. E., & Benedict, G. W. [2003]. *Mosby's guide to physical assessment* [5th ed.]. St. Louis: Mosby.)

testing with **ultrasonography** (sonography), health care providers now determine fetal presence and placental adequacy early in pregnancy. This technology, using high-frequency sound waves that bounce off the fetus and are interpreted by a computer, allows visualization of the fetus and gestational structures throughout pregnancy.

Adaptive Changes of Other Systems

In addition to pregnancy-related changes in the reproductive system, adaptive changes in other body systems occur. The urinary system undergoes dramatic changes during gestation; a 50% increase in glomerular filtration rate (Georges, 2000) occurs related to the influences of **estrogen** and progesterone. These hormones also cause smooth muscle relaxation in the gastrointestinal tract, resulting in maternal constipation, heartburn, and increased salivation (Lowdermilk & Perry, 2003b).

Circulatory system changes also begin early in pregnancy, with an increase in cardiac output of 30% to 40% by the end of the first trimester. Total blood volume increases 30% to 45% during pregnancy (Cunningham et al., 2001b; Georges, 2000). Physiological anemia of pregnancy may result because of an increase in the proportion of plasma to red blood cells.

Respiratory system changes include increased tidal volume during pregnancy (Cunningham et al., 2001b), although toward the end of pregnancy the enlarging uterus causes some shortness of breath for many women. This continues until the baby descends into the pelvis during the final weeks of pregnancy.

Increased elasticity and softening of connective tissue of the musculoskeletal system cause relaxation of the joints,

especially the pelvic joints that support the pregnancy but must stretch during labor and delivery. Lumbar and dorsal curves of the spine increase late in pregnancy and contribute to low back pain and the waddle of pregnancy.

Changes in the integumentary system occur. Hormones cause many pregnant women to gain stretch marks on their abdomen and breasts (**striae gravidarum**), a darkened line from the symphysis pubis to the umbilicus (**linea nigra**), and darkening of the skin across the forehead and nose (**chloasma**) (Lowdermilk & Perry, 2003b). The metabolic and endocrine changes that occur with pregnancy to support optimal fetal growth and development are dramatic.

Reproductive System

Effects on the reproductive system include changes in the uterus, breasts, vagina, vulva, and ovaries. The prepregnant uterus is approximately the size of a closed fist. The uterus at term has the capacity to contain a 3.2-kg to 4.5-kg (7-lb to 10-lb) infant and the placenta. As the uterus enlarges, the **fundus** (the upper uterine segment) moves higher in the abdomen (Figure 16-2). The breasts begin enlarging early in the pregnancy, and in late pregnancy they may secrete small amounts of **colostrum,** a precursor of mature breast milk. The vagina and vulva receive a greater blood supply and appear darker (cyanotic) as a result. Some women will notice an increase in vaginal secretions.

Hormones such as HCG and estrogen, secreted by the placenta and the fetus, create an optimal intrauterine environment for the fetus and stimulate many changes in the pregnant woman's body. The developing fetus contributes to the provision of an adequate environment for its own growth and nourishment, despite the possibility of creating discomforts for the pregnant woman.

Normal Discomforts

Changes in the woman's body during pregnancy support a nursing diagnosis of alteration in comfort with relevant interventions for most women (Table 16-1). Women may feel a sense of relief that other pregnant women have these concerns and that interventions exist to increase their comfort at various points during gestation. Particularly for those experiencing a first pregnancy, the nurse serves as a valuable support person to help expectant couples adjust to the challenges and discomforts of pregnancy, a goal for the earlier stated diagnosis.

Teaching Throughout Pregnancy Related to Bodily Changes

In addition to serving as a caregiver, advocate, and support person, the nurse serves as a teacher throughout the pregnancy care process. Active teaching responsive to an individual's concerns about pregnancy may occur in the clinic, physician's office, or other care environments. Nursing intervention should address recommended professional practice guidelines for education during the prenatal period to prevent complications for the family. For example, the nurse may offer textbooks, pamphlets, videotapes, and referrals to Web sites and other media to increase a couple's knowledge of fetal, maternal, and family changes during gestation and then encourage questions based on the material. Going beyond one-to-one teaching, the nurse may also refer couples to early pregnancy and **Lamaze** childbirth preparation classes to enlarge their social support network and increase knowledge about labor and delivery. Throughout the care process, the nurse must be sensitive to the cultural and ethnic beliefs and behaviors of the individual or family. By incorporating knowledge of these beliefs and behaviors, the nurse protects the pregnant woman and her baby by providing individualized care addressing the childbearing rituals held by various cultural groups (Table 16-2).

Total Weight Gain

Total weight gain during pregnancy reflects not only the growth of the baby and placenta, but that of the uterus, breasts, maternal fat storage, and increases in blood and other body fluids. Many practitioners recommend a weight gain of about 25 to 35 lb for a pregnancy involving one fetus (Cunningham et al., 2001c; Institute of Medicine, 1990; U.S. Department of Health and Human Services [USDHHS], 2000). Additionally, a consistent pattern of gain, with most weight gained during the final two trimesters, has been recommended (Georges, 2000; USDHHS, 2000).

Labor and Delivery

Pregnancy culminates with labor and delivery. The process of giving birth elicits a significant emotional response from the delivering family. A description of the events of a usual labor and delivery must occur to establish a background for considering the physiological changes in the mother and the infant.

Several theories offer explanations for the cause of labor. Several factors likely interact, including uterine distention, mechanical irritation, progesterone deprivation, placental aging and hormones, and posterior pituitary activity. Labor usually begins around 40 weeks' gestation, suggesting that hormonal control similar to that regulating the menstrual cycles also contributes to its onset (Cunningham et al., 2001c).

Labor may be divided conveniently into four distinct stages. The **first stage of labor** starts with regular timing of uterine contractions and ends with complete **dilation** (opening) and **effacement** (thinning) of the **cervix.** Signs of beginning labor include those listed in Box 16-2. The cervix, the lower portion of the uterus, must dilate from a closed position (0 cm) to a totally open position (10 cm, or 4 inches, in diameter). During the first stage, the cervix must also completely efface or shorten, from a length of 1 to 2 inches to a barely palpable (paper-thin) thickness. For most women, painless Braxton-Hicks contractions throughout pregnancy cause some cervical dilation and thinning, or at least cervical softening, before the onset of active labor.

During the first stage of labor, the presenting part of the fetus begins to press on the cervix, lower uterine segment, and nerve endings around the cervix and vagina. Women's responses to this process vary; pain thresholds and cultural perceptions of and responses to pain differ among laboring women (see Table 16-2). The fundus, the active contractile part of the uterus, becomes thicker as labor progresses, retracts the lower uterine segment and cervix, and helps push the fetus toward the cervix and eventually through the vagina for birth. Stage one lasts an average of 12 hours for women experiencing a first birth and somewhat less for women having a second or additional child. Based on a laboring woman's needs, various medications, ambulation to decrease the need for medication (Frenea et al., 2004), Lamaze breathing, and other distractive techniques may alleviate the discomfort associated with first-stage labor. Sterile vaginal examinations by the nurse or other health care provider indicate a laboring woman's cervical dilation and effacement and descent of the fetus into the birth canal (a concept called **station**). In a full-term pregnancy, loss of the amniotic membrane usually increases pressure of the fetal head against the cervix, making dilation and effacement more efficient, and represents the irreversibility of the labor process (Piotrowski, 1999).

During the **second stage of labor,** the baby descends through the lower birth canal toward the woman's perineum. The upper uterine segment greatly thickens, and

Table **16-1** Normal Discomforts Experienced During Pregnancy, Probable Cause, and Nursing Suggestions for Relief

Discomfort	Known or Probable Cause	Nursing Suggestions for Relief
Backache	Changes in posture such as increased lumbar curve Excessive bending or lifting	Practice good posture Perform pelvic rocking Wear comfortable, low-heeled shoes Apply ice or heat to lower back Massage Squat to lift Avoid prolonged sitting Sleep on firm mattress Avoid fatigue Do Kegel exercise during the day
Constipation	Pressure of enlarging uterus Slowed peristalsis caused by progesterone Side effect of iron therapy and increased calcium intake with pregnancy	Increase intake of fruits and vegetables Eat high-fiber foods Exercise Drink warm water first thing in morning Only as last resort, take laxative, stool softener, or suppository with doctor's permission
Fatigue	Decreased metabolic rate with pregnancy Extra weight of pregnancy to carry during day	Get full night's sleep Increase exercise over time Share workload when possible Nap or rest during day Eat healthy diet Usually better after first trimester
Hemorrhoids	Constipation Pressure of enlarged uterus Straining with bowel evacuation	Relieve problem with measures discussed previously Take sitz baths Use ice pack or witch hazel for local relief Do perineal tightening exercises Seek out physician advice for problem
Leg cramps	Pressure of uterus on blood vessels Fatigue or chilling Lack of calcium Sudden stretching or overextension of foot Excessive phosphorus in diet	Take calcium supplement or increase calcium-rich foods Practice steady, gentle stretch to relieve cramp Never massage a cramping muscle Avoid toe-pointing when exercising If Homan sign negative, dorsiflex ankles throughout day to prevent cramps
Leukorrhea	Increased vascularity of cervix and vagina	Wear cotton-crotch underpants Wash genital area frequently When infection develops (itching and profuse drainage), call physician Do not douche
Nausea and vomiting	Increase in estrogen and progesterone Changes in blood glucose levels	Eat small, frequent meals Eat dry crackers in the morning before arising Snack at bedtime Drink chamomile or ginger tea Avoid greasy, fried foods
Varicosities	Increased vascularity of pelvic organs Venous return slowed by pressure of uterus Familial tendency Progesterone effect on smooth muscles	Avoid knee socks and tight elastic on underwear Elevate feet for 10 to 15 minutes several times a day Avoid long periods of standing Avoid crossing legs when sitting Wear support stockings Engage in consistent walking during pregnancy
Urinary frequency	Pressure of uterus against bladder during first and third trimesters Nocturia may result from increased extremity venous return when lying down	When interfering with sleep, limit amount of fluids in evening Rest during the day

Table **16-2**	Cultural Values Related to Pregnancy and Birth*
Filipino	Structured prenatal care for those who can afford it
	Pregnancy normal event with family focused on pregnant woman's needs
	Pregnant woman encouraged to eat well, sleep often, and not to work out of home
	Sexual intercourse taboo during last 2 weeks of pregnancy
	Pregnant woman encouraged to eat fresh eggs close to delivery to help baby "slide out" with birth
	Woman very modest about body needs and care during pregnancy
	Father passive with birth process; pregnant woman active participant with birth
	Breast-feeding encouraged until child toddler
American Indian	In many tribes women are expected to seek prenatal care with pregnancy; some tribes accept late care
	Dialogue with women in tribal community important to maximize pregnancy and birth process
	Meditation, self-control practice, and indigenous plants (herbal teas) used for discomforts of pregnancy and birth
	Pregnant woman stoic about birth process; father present but not active participant
	Female kin present to support woman in labor; breast-feeding and bottle feeding encouraged after birth
	Father may avoid hunting immediately after birth or until infant's cord falls off
Arab American	Pregnancy normal event; may not access prenatal care because of that belief
	Much family support given to pregnant woman to allow maximal rest and minimal work
	Present orientation: little preparation for birth, fears labor pains but responds once they come
	Expressive with labor but not active with control of pain; relies on family members for support; father not active, may feel powerless with birth process
	Very modest about care, especially with opposite gender health care provider
	Prefer bottle feeding; colostrum believed to harm baby
Blacks	Most access prenatal care after first trimester or seek care earlier with problems
	Female kin provide most of support with pregnancy and birth; male support less visible
	Open expression of pregnancy and birth discomfort; active participant in birth process
	May self-medicate with cultural remedies for pregnancy complaints
	May avoid being in photographs due to fear of stillbirth
	May crave certain foods: chicken, greens, clay, starch, or dirt (pica)
	If of Muslim faith, may wish to have head covered during labor and birth process
	Breast-feed if given information on the benefits of this method
Mexican American	Often face barriers to prenatal care due to lack of insurance, fear of health care system, lack of transportation to clinic
	May consider prenatal care not needed due to normal life event
	Education and acculturation influence prenatal care access
	Pregnancy considered to follow marriage; familism supports respect and assistance to pregnant woman
	Pregnant woman does not smoke, work, drink alcohol, or use drugs; pregnancy a time to rest, walk, eat well, sleep, drink chamomile tea, and avoid cold air
	Grandmother may move into the home close to delivery time to help and provide folk remedies after birth
	Modest about care and needs; same gender health care provider encouraged
	Generally walks during labor to enhance birth; wants family for support; woman active and father delegates support to female members of family
	Generally breast-feeds for up to 1 year
Vietnamese	Generally early prenatal care unless immigrant status, then depend on family for care
	Encouraged to eat healthy foods, get rest, avoid strenuous activity during last trimester
	Focus on keeping pregnant woman warm, encouraging salt water for oral care, and maintaining good hygiene
	Sexual intercourse taboo with pregnancy
	Father present but not active with pregnancy
	Birth a time of hot and cold imbalance; mother "suffers in silence, may moan or grunt; mother depends on female relatives for support and guidance
	Mother breast-feeds for up to 1 year; avoids cold foods for this period

Data from Spector, R. E. (2004). *Cultural diversity in health & illness* (6th ed., pp. 101-137). Upper Saddle River, NJ: Pearson/Prentice Hall; Ferrales, S. (1996). Vietnamese. In J. G. Lipson, S. L. Dibble, & P. A. Minarik (Eds.), *Culture & nursing care: A pocket guide* (pp. 280-290). San Francisco: UCSF Press; Kramer, J. (1996). American Indians. In J. G. Lipson, S. L. Dibble, & P. A. Minarik (Eds.), *Culture & nursing care: A pocket guide* (pp. 11-22). San Francisco: UCSF Press; Meleis, A. I. (1996). Arab Americans. In J. G. Lipson, S. L. Dibble, & P. A. Minarik (Eds.), *Culture & nursing care: A pocket guide* (pp. 23-36). San Francisco: UCSF Press; Cantos, A., & Rivera, E. (1996). Filipino. In J. G. Lipson, S. L. Dibble, & P. A. Minarik (Eds.), *Culture & nursing care: A pocket guide* (pp. 115-123). San Francisco: UCSF Press; Locks, S., & Boateng, L. A. (1996). African Americans. In J. G. Lipson, S. L. Dibble, & P. A. Minarik (Eds.), *Culture & nursing care: A pocket guide* (pp. 37-43). San Francisco: UCSF Press; de Paula, T., Lagana, K., & Gonzalez-Ramirez, L. (1996). Mexican Americans. In J. G. Lipson, S. L. Dibble, & P. A. Minarik (Eds.), *Culture & nursing care: A pocket guide* (pp. 203-221). San Francisco: UCSF Press.

*General ideas about beliefs and behaviors of each of these cultural groups have been given with no intent to stereotype all persons who represent these groups' beliefs or behaviors. It is hoped that this information will provide direction to the nurse who will continue to assess each client to render care that meets that person's traditional values in a biomedical model of health care in the United States today.

Box **16-2** Signs of Beginning Labor

- Bloody show or loss of the mucous plug that seals cervical canal during pregnancy
- Regular uterine contractions
- Contractions increasing in intensity, duration, and frequency
- Palpable hardening of the uterus during contractions
- Pain in the lower back and front of abdomen

the abdominal muscles assist in the fetus' descent and expulsion. Women who have attended childbirth classes often are better prepared to actively push the baby through the pelvis and perineum during contractions. Cultural practices may support pushing from a squatting or upright position, such as that seen with Hmong women (Gupta & Nikoderm, 2000). For many women, an overwhelming urge to bear down during uterine contractions occurs at this time. The fetal head accommodates to the mother's pelvis and vaginal structure and, finally, the head becomes flush with the vaginal opening on the woman's perineum. At this time, the physician or nurse midwife may perform an **episiotomy,** a surgical incision into the perineum, to allow the baby's head and, ultimately, the entire body to deliver (the time of birth). During stage two, women birthing their first baby may push for up to 2 hours. However, women with a history of childbearing, active coaching during birth, or education about pushing may deliver more rapidly.

The **third stage of labor** begins after the birth and lasts until placental expulsion. Placental separation usually takes place within 5 to 30 minutes after completion of the second stage. After delivery the doctor or midwife examines the placenta to determine that all placental tissue has been delivered and to detect any abnormalities that could affect the infant's condition and adaptation to extrauterine life.

The **fourth stage of labor** generally consists of the first 2 hours after delivery, during which the mother faces the greatest danger of postpartum hemorrhage. An expected blood loss of 250 to 500 ml may cause the mother to experience a moderate decline in blood pressure. She may also demonstrate **tachycardia,** or increased heart rate, to compensate for blood loss during the early postpartum period. The Care Plan on page 352 addresses the nursing role in managing the stages of labor.

Overview of Care

Professional members of the health care team play an important role in labor and delivery, but a woman's family or significant other (i.e., labor attendant, partner) also inherently contributes to her care during labor and delivery, particularly in certain cultures (see Table 16-2). Many practitioners suggest that the expectations and beliefs of a birthing couple have a great effect on how the woman fulfills the mothering role. Therefore the nurse needs to

collaborate with the people who care for the pregnant woman to meet that family's needs during pregnancy, labor, and delivery.

The importance of the nurse's knowledge, caregiving, and support cannot be underestimated during the first stage of labor. Active emotional and physical nursing support decreases the length of many women's labors, analgesia and anesthesia use, and number of operative deliveries and may help women reach their birthing goals (Association of Women's Health, Obstetrical, and Neonatal Nursing [AWHONN], 2000). Independent nursing interventions to increase comfort and as accepted by a woman's culture (e.g., giving backrubs, massages, offering ice or warm fluids by mouth, assisting with ambulation and position changes, and providing a clean and dry environment) may help the laboring woman cope with the challenges of labor. Many women will request medication to diminish the pain of delivery, and the nurse may need to review options for medication with each woman or couple. During the first stage the mother must not bear down, because this may cause cervical swelling; often, active nursing support and distractive techniques, such as breathing and visual refocus, can prevent pushing before the second stage of labor. A woman may depend on the nurse to model breathing techniques to relieve labor discomfort. The nurse may need to explain usual interventions during this stage of labor, including the use of a **fetal heart monitor** (a machine that detects and records fetal heart rate and activity during labor), intravenous fluids, automatic blood pressure machine, and urinary catheterization. Open and clear communication among the health care provider and laboring woman and her significant others, particularly during frequent and difficult uterine contractions, will improve coping before the pushing stage begins.

During the second stage of labor, the woman needs reassurance and support for her pushing work. Constant reinforcement and education by the nurse about labor progress, fetal heart monitor tracings, and other interventions will give the mother and her support system the energy needed to deliver the infant. Throughout labor the nurse considers the cultural and ethnic needs to support nursing assessment and a positive perception of labor by the childbearing family.

Active nursing support during the third and fourth stages of labor includes observing for excessive vaginal bleeding after placental discharge, assisting the woman in breastfeeding her new baby, monitoring vital signs, and implementing uterine massage if the uterus becomes boggy or fails to contract over the placental site. Emotional support during assessments and delivery of information to explain the rationale for assessments are also important nursing roles supported by professional practice standards.

Throughout the entire labor and delivery process, the nurse makes careful observations of the laboring woman and fetus so that she can detect early any difficulties with the progress of labor or with maternal or fetal health. Problems may include unusual fetal or uterine activity, presence of

CARE PLAN

Nursing Management for Stages of Labor

Nursing Diagnosis Ineffective Individual Coping Related to Active Labor Status

DEFINING CHARACTERISTICS

- Initiation of labor at 2:00 AM with SROM
- First-time mother who did not attend childbirth classes
- Supportive spouse
- Current gestational age of 36 weeks
- Contraction pattern defined as moderate intensity, frequency every 2 minutes, 60 seconds in duration
- After 6 hours of labor, 4 cm dilated, 100% effaced, and −2 station
- Moaning, moving around in bed, and stating, "I can't take this much longer; it hurts too much!"

RELATED FACTORS

- Prenatal history of URI and UTIs, currently diagnosed with sore throat as a result of streptococcal infection; client taking amoxicillin 250 mg q 8 hours for 10 days
- Prenatal care since 12 weeks pregnant
- History of depression in college
- Works as engineer with large manufacturing firm
- Gravida 3, para 0 (two losses at 6 to 8 weeks of gestation before current marriage)
- Recent resident of city, moved from East Coast approximately 4 months ago
- 22 years of age, Asian family history, married 1 year

EXPECTED OUTCOMES

- Mother will state level of pain to be less than 4 on a scale of 1 to 10 during labor.

- Mother will successfully use visual imagery techniques, massage, and slow deep breathing for relaxation during labor.
- Mother will state early in labor at least three ways to cope effectively with pain and will implement these strategies as relevant.
- Fetus will demonstrate an expected FHR pattern and will experience no compromise during labor.
- Mother and family will verbalize needs during labor and delivery to health care team.

INTERVENTIONS (BY NURSE)

- Assess level of labor discomfort every 20 to 30 minutes and as needed according to pain scale rating of 1 to 10.
- Implement and document nursing interventions (backrubs, heat and cold, position changes, back pressure and massage, and Jacuzzi therapy, among others) to relieve labor discomforts.
- Assess cultural beliefs with labor and delivery management and implement interventions as needed to meet practice standards.
- Provide teaching about labor and delivery progress and breathing, visual imagery, and massage techniques that may decrease labor discomfort.
- Provide verbal and nonverbal reassurance during labor.
- Teach about fetal response during labor and rationale for nursing interventions to support fetal health, such as left side position to increase placental blood flow.
- Throughout labor, answer any questions from mother and family members about needs and responses to labor process.
- Involve family members as much as possible during labor and as requested by mother to improve her ability to cope.

FHR, fetal heart rate; *SROM,* spontaneous rupture of membranes; *URI,* upper respiratory infection; *UTI,* urinary tract infection.

---

meconium (fetal stool) in the amniotic fluid, fetal tachycardia (heart rate above 160 beats per minute) or fetal **bradycardia** (heart rate below 120 beats per minute) in a full-term infant, and fetal heart rate decreases with uterine activity during labor (AWHONN, 1998; Lowdermilk & Perry, 2003c). These events must be reported immediately to the physician, midwife, or appropriate health care provider, with a complete oral and written description of the event. The nurse must be aware that abnormal fetal and maternal signs and patterns may be related to factors such as maternal diabetes or hypertension; type, timing, or dosage of labor medications; uterine contraction pattern; presence and character of amniotic fluid; bleeding in the pregnant woman or fetus; or gestational age of the infant (Piotrowski, 1999).

CHANGES DURING TRANSITION FROM FETUS TO NEWBORN

Most babies experience a smooth transition from intrauterine to extrauterine life. When difficulty occurs, however, the infant's viability depends on the nurse's understanding of the fine balance of chemical, physiological, and anatomical changes that occur as it makes the transition to extrauterine life (Lowdermilk & Perry, 2003d). **Web Site Resource 16C** presents details about the adaptation of the fetus to extrauterine life.

Nursing Interventions

Nursing activities during this adaptation process include assessment and interventions aimed at specific protection of the infant and prevention of complications. Cold stress should be avoided by keeping the newborn dry, warmly wrapped, and avoiding environments that cause heat loss. Overall, the nurse should minimally disturb, but maximally observe and document, the newborn's behavior during reactive periods. Bathing and bottle feeding, for instance, should be delayed until behavior and physiological mechanisms stabilize, usually between 4 and 8 hours of age.

Mucus

Newborns tend to regurgitate during this period. Mucus is a normal product of intrauterine life and probably originates

Table 16-3   Apgar Scoring

Sign	Score		
	0	1	2
Heart rate	Absent	Slow (under 100)	Over 100
Respiratory effort	Absent	Weak cry, hypoventilation	Good strong cry
Muscle tone	Flaccid, limp	Some flexion of extremities	Active motion, extremities well flexed
Reflex irritability	No response	Grimace	Cry
Color	Blue, pale	Body pink, extremities blue	Completely pink

From Lowdermilk, D. L., & Perry, S. E. (2003). *Maternity nursing* (6th ed., p. 462). St. Louis: Mosby.

in the lung and gastrointestinal tissues. When mucus production reaches a level at which aspiration becomes an obvious hazard, suctioning should be employed. When vomiting occurs, oral suctioning of mucus with a simple bulb syringe may help, but the more effective approach is to remove material from the esophagus, then the stomach.

Apgar Score

Assessment of the newborn after the first few hours of life is essentially the same as assessment of the young infant (see Chapter 17). One technique, specific to timing after birth, is the **Apgar scoring system.** This scoring historically has been used to provide a simple clinical measure to evaluate an infant's general condition at birth. The Apgar score, made at 1 minute and 5 minutes of age, may be repeated until the infant's condition has stabilized. A total score is calculated by adding the values allotted to the categories noted in Table 16-3. The highest possible score is 10. A score of 8 to 10 indicates that the baby is adapting well. Juretschke (2000) notes that the Apgar score does not predict the neurological development of an individual but may relate to the infant's risk of illness or death during the first year of life, important information for parents of an infant with a low Apgar score to know.

Gender

Gender differences occur in fetal growth. Generally boys grow faster than girls in the third trimester, and at birth boys are slightly heavier, longer, and have a larger head circumference than girls (Guyton & Hall, 1997). Although more boys are conceived, they tend to be aborted spontaneously more often than girl embryos; the two X chromosomes possessed by female embryos may protect them from the early hazards of pregnancy. After birth, boys continue to have a lower survival rate than do girls, and by middle age women are more numerous than men.

Race and Culture

Race may affect the fetus' health in several ways. For example, in the United States, nonwhites (mainly blacks) have more fraternal twin pregnancies than whites (Cunningham et al., 2001d). Twin fetuses face an increased risk for premature delivery due to gestational factors in the mother or death because their organs are less mature. Currently the United States is 35th in the world ranking for **infant mortality rate** (IMR), with a rate of 6.75 (GeographyIQ, n.d.). This rate, which reflects the number of infants that die before the end of their first year of life and is the leading indicator of a nation's health, reflects the higher IMRs and low-birth-weight outcomes of blacks and other ethnic minority populations in the United States. This rate illustrates the complex sociopolitical issues that produce birth outcomes in this country and those needing attention to improve the IMR (Smedley, Stith, & Nelson, 2003; USDHHS, 2000).

Race is also a factor in the frequency of certain genetic and congenital malformations. For example, more white babies have cleft palates (an opening in the oral palate) than do black babies (Carlson, 1999). Black babies have higher rates of sickle cell anemia (abnormally shaped red blood cells) than white babies. Interestingly, the total number of malformations tends to be about the same in all races that have been studied (whites, blacks, Hispanics, and Asians) (Creasy & Resnik, 1999).

A woman's ethnic background may also influence her fetus' health based on a link to socioeconomic status. For increasing numbers of homeless pregnant women, income may support family survival needs, but not prenatal care. Minority group pregnant women may have fewer economic resources to obtain a nutritious diet or early and consistent quality prenatal care. These outcomes may relate to access factors or cultural beliefs that do not support recommended foods or prenatal care (*Healthy People 2010* box).

Genetics

Genetic influences affect the survival and later well-being of the child through several known mechanisms. **Down syndrome** (trisomy 21) remains the most recognized and most commonly occurring example of an extra chromosome. Extra chromosomes, deleted chromosomes, or translocations usually cause multiple malformations incompatible with life, causing early loss of the fetus via spontaneous abortion. Single malformations in an otherwise normal fetus (e.g., clubfoot, cleft palate, or neural tube defect) probably result from a combined effect of many genes (Askin, 1999). These defects, found at birth, may be

---

Healthy People 2010

Selected National Health-Promotion and Disease Prevention Objectives for the Prenatal Period

- Reduce the infant mortality rate (28 weeks to 7 or more months after birth) to no more than 4.5 per 1000 live births (baseline: 7.2 per 1000 live births in 1998)

Special Population Targets: Infant Mortality	1997 Baseline	2010 Target
Blacks	13.7	4.5
Native Americans–Alaska Natives	7.9	4.5
Asians	4.6	4.5
Hispanics	6.5	4.5

- Reduce the fetal death rate (20 or more weeks of gestation) to no more than 4.1 per 1000 live births plus fetal deaths (baseline: 6.8 per 1000 live births plus fetal deaths in 1997)

Special Population Target: Fetal Deaths	1997 Baseline	2010 Target
Blacks	12.5	6.8

- Reduce low birth weight to an incidence of no more than 5% of live births and very low birth weight to no more than 0.9% of live births (baseline: 7.6% and 1.4%, respectively, in 1998)

Special Population Target	1998 Baseline	2010 Target
Low Birth Weight		
Blacks	13%	5%
Very Low Birth Weight		
Blacks	3%	0.9%

- Reduce the number of unintended pregnancies to no more than 30% (baseline: 51% of pregnancies for females 15 to 44 years of age in 1995 were unwanted or earlier than intended)

- Reduce the number of pregnancies occurring in girls ages 15 to 17 to no more than 46 per 1000 (baseline: 72 pregnancies per 1000 girls of this age in 1995)
- Increase the number of women who breast-feed during the early postpartum period to at least 75% and increase the proportion who breast-feed for 5 to 6 months after birth to at least 50% (baseline: 64% of women chose to breast-feed during the early postpartum period in 1998; 29% chose to breast-feed for 5 to 6 months in 1998)
- Increase abstinence by pregnant women from tobacco to at least 98%, from alcohol to 94%, and from illicit drugs (cocaine and marijuana) to 100% (baseline: 87% of pregnant women abstained from tobacco, 86% abstained from alcohol, 98% abstained from cocaine, and 98% abstained from marijuana from 1996 to 1997)
- Increase the number of women who receive prenatal care during the first trimester of pregnancy to at least 90% (baseline: 83% of live births in 1997)

Special Population Targets: Prenatal Care	1997 Baseline	2010 Target
Native Americans–Alaska Natives	68%	90%
Asians	85%	90%
Blacks	72%	90%
Whites	85%	90%

- Increase the proportion of mothers who achieve a recommended weight gain during their pregnancies (baseline: 75% of married women delivering at term gained the recommended weight of 25 to 35 lb with pregnancy in 1988)
- Reduce the cesarean delivery rate to no more than 15 per 100 deliveries (baseline: 17.8 per 100 deliveries in 1997; a rate of 15.5 for primary cesareans and 71 for repeat procedures in 1997)

From U.S. Department of Health and Human Services. (2000). *Healthy People 2010: Vol. 1* (Conference edition). Washington, DC: U.S. Government Printing Office.

---

surgically corrected or managed during the child's life. Modern techniques of **amniocentesis,** chorionic villus sampling, and chromosome analysis have expanded genetic counseling options and interventions for women facing possible fetal genetic defects. The nurse needs to work with other members of the health care team to inform these women and couples of genetic and high-risk screening resources when family history or other factors indicate that a fetal genetic defect may be likely.

GORDON'S FUNCTIONAL HEALTH PATTERNS

Box 16-3 provides an example of a pregnancy assessment using Gordon's functional health patterns (1995).

Health Perception–Health Management Pattern

Based on her culture and life experience, a woman may view pregnancy as an illness, as a completely natural and healthy state, or as a combination of the two. This perception will influence her view of her changing body, attitude toward the usual discomforts of pregnancy such as fatigue or backache, choice of health-oriented or illness-oriented care, and her decision to seek prenatal care. The woman who sees herself as healthy and pregnancy as a normal part of her life most likely will seek a health care provider with a similar outlook. Another woman with the same perception may seek help from a socially approved group, as defined by her

Box 16-3 Assessment for Pregnancy According to Gordon's Functional Health Patterns

Health perception–health management pattern: aware of or participates in management of pregnancy, or both; expects an uncomplicated pregnancy based on woman's or significant other's active involvement in her own care; able to state complications of pregnancy that mandate physician notification; engages in health-promotion behaviors specific to pregnancy

Nutritional-metabolic pattern: follows diet changes of pregnancy as recommended by nurse; has appropriate weight for height and has gained adequate weight for gestational age of pregnancy; eats three meals a day and two snacks (afternoon and evening), focusing on increased amounts of vegetables and fruits; drinks healthy fluids involving at least 8 glasses of water per day; has elastic skin turgor

Elimination pattern: experiences occasional constipation from iron therapy of pregnancy—usually corrected by increased fluids, nightly walking, and more diet roughage; voids 7 to 10 times a day, depending on amount of fluids consumed; no known hemorrhoids or difficulty in elimination; voiding without excess frequency, urgency, or burning; understands signs of UTI

Activity-exercise pattern: walks 3 times a week for 20 minutes without complaints of unusual fatigue or soreness; active at home with housework and at work teaching primary school; swam 2 times a week before pregnancy and move to current residence

Sleep-rest pattern: generally sleeps 7 to 8 hours a night; has increased total daily sleep somewhat with fatigue of pregnancy—naps for 1 hour on weekends and 30 minutes after work; sleeps on side and with two pillows for comfort; uses no sleep aids; generally able to relax and initiate sleep without difficulty; occasionally has headache at end of workday and takes acetaminophen (Tylenol) for relief or listens to soft music after work to enhance relaxation

Cognitive-perceptual pattern: realizes the need to decrease work activity and increase rest periods as she nears end of pregnancy; answers questions in appropriate tone and words during pregnancy visits; has intact memory (alert and remote); reads about pregnancy and early parenthood to prepare for the birth

Self-perception–self-concept pattern: states she is excited about pregnancy after a year of trying to conceive; well groomed, wears maternity clothes because "I want to"; believes she looks "nice" due to pregnancy

Roles-relationships pattern: lives with husband of 3 years; visits extended family, 60 miles away, every month; shares family roles with husband, accepts this balance; has many friends who support her pregnancy; perceives extensive employee and employer support with pregnancy and time off after delivery

Sexuality-reproductive pattern: states, "I have a satisfying love life and enjoy my husband"; before pregnancy, engaged in sexual intercourse 4 to 5 times a week with desire to become pregnant; with pregnancy and fatigue, has intercourse generally 2 to 3 times a week, with pattern acceptable to both partners; no known STDs in past or present

Coping-stress tolerance pattern: concerned about fatigue affecting performance as primary school teacher; walks 3 times a week for 20 minutes to "center myself and feel good"; smiles often, good sense of humor; supportive family excited about her pregnancy

Values-beliefs pattern: Protestant religion; prays daily and gains strength from religion

Other Data:
- Medication history:
  Prenatal vitamin (Materna), 1 tablet each morning
  Ferrous sulfate, 1 tablet each morning
  Acetaminophen (Tylenol) 650 mg for occasional headaches
- Physical examination:
  5 feet, 4 inches tall
  Weight 140 lbs (at 14 weeks' pregnancy; weight gain of 5 lbs with pregnancy)
  29 years of age
  PERRLA
  TPR 98.2-76-16
  BP 114/78 right arm (sitting, left arm)
  Peripheral pulses equal, strong bilaterally
  Skin warm, dry, elastic turgor; mucous membranes intact, moist; alert, oriented ×3

Modified from Peterson, R. (2005). *Clinical companion for fundamentals of nursing* (6th ed). St. Louis: Elsevier Mosby.
BP, blood pressure; *PERRLA,* pupils equally round and reactive to light and accommodation; *STDs,* sexually transmitted diseases; *TPR,* temperature, pulse, respirations; *UTI,* urinary tract infection.

culture, and avoid standard Western medicine during pregnancy (e.g., Roma [gypsies]). Generally, both women with a positive view of pregnancy will continue active participation in her respective social circle and career. However, the woman who sees her pregnancy as a time of illness may use this as a reason to withdraw from her work and social obligations.

A woman's acceptance of her pregnancy influences her health management practices and choices. The woman who denies or has strong negative feelings about her pregnancy may fail to eat properly, get enough rest and exercise, breastfeed, or seek prenatal care. A woman may deny a pregnancy because she never intended to become pregnant despite having sexual intercourse without birth control. Approximately 50% of American pregnancies are unintended, par-

ticularly among adolescents, women over age 40, women with low income, and women who lack access, cultural acceptance, education, and financial resources to purchase or use contraception (Kost, Landry, & Darroch, 1998a, 1998b; USDHHS, 2000). These women, faced with an unplanned or closely spaced pregnancy, may expose a fetus to alcohol, tobacco, and **sexually transmitted diseases (STDs),** abuse a child who was never wanted, or fail to get follow-up care for a high-risk child (i.e., experienced complications from delivery) (USDHHS, 2000; U.S. Preventive Services Task Force, 2004c).

The nurse who works with a pregnant population should be sensitive to a wide range of views expressed by these women and work with each to effectively manage their pregnancies. For example, Hispanic women are less likely to get early prenatal care based on a belief that pregnancy is not an illness. The nurse must target interventions that focus on this group's needs and beliefs while adhering to professional practice standards that will improve their outcomes.

Nutritional-Metabolic Pattern

Massive amounts of literature support the importance of optimal nutrition during pregnancy for maternal and fetal well-being. Maternal malnutrition before and during pregnancy may exert a teratogenic effect on the fetus. A **teratogen** is an agent that causes either a functional or structural disability in the organism based on exposure to that agent (Perry, 1999). Teratogens principally affect the central nervous system of the fetus, leading to impaired intelligence and performance later in life. They are discussed more in the Pathological Processes section later in the chapter.

Various factors influence the quality of nutrition needed for positive fetal development and birth outcome. Fetal development suffers in cases of adolescent pregnancy or older women who experience poor nutrition between and during several pregnancies. Maternal nutritional deficiencies during one's own fetal, infant, and childhood periods also contribute to the development of structural and physiological disadvantages to supporting a growing fetus. For example, women who are severely underweight before pregnancy often experience higher rates of low-birth-weight infants and preterm labor than do women of appropriate prepregnant weight (Cunningham et al., 2001e). Inherited maternal stature and pelvic development may influence pregnancy and efficiency of labor and delivery. A lack of income to buy healthy food may also exist, and sometimes cultural values related to food intake influence the quality of nutrition during pregnancy.

To meet increased metabolic, energy, and structural needs for pregnancy, most nutritionists recommend that a pregnant woman increase her intake by approximately 200 to 300 calories each day (USDHHS, 2000). This results in a total weight gain of about 25 to 35 pounds. If at the end of 20 weeks of gestation the woman has not gained at least 10 pounds, she risks delivering an ill infant suffering from intrauterine growth retardation (IUGR). These risks also exist when a woman continues to gain insufficient weight throughout the pregnancy or in one who was underweight or overweight before pregnancy. Although the rate of gain and the total gain during pregnancy vary among women, a correlation exists between an erratic pattern of weight gain or a too-rapid weight gain and a lack of fetal well-being (Lowdermilk & Perry, 2003e). The nurse should advise the pregnant woman to eat a well-balanced diet from the six food groups and according to her appetite to protect herself and the fetus.

A well-balanced diet for a pregnant woman parallels that needed by all human beings, with increases of certain components as recommended by the Food and Nutrition Board of the National Academy of Science (Institute of Medicine,

1990; USDHHS, 2000). The nurse should recommend that the entire family eat a healthy diet. She should also encourage the pregnant woman to drink at least 8 glasses of water per day to develop amniotic fluid and prevent urinary tract infections often seen with pregnancy. The nurse may also need to encourage the woman to modify her diet to include more fiber and roughage to avoid constipation during pregnancy.

Protein requirements during pregnancy increase to about 60 g per day over that required during nonpregnancy. Four glasses of milk a day, which have 32 g of protein, meet one half of this increased requirement. Other protein sources, such as cheese, cream soups, puddings, tofu, and yogurt, may be better tolerated by some women and by those from cultures (Hispanic) that do not drink milk. Animal protein and less expensive legume sources provide protein and, if combined with other healthy food sources, provide high-quality meals (e.g., tuna and rice, peanut butter and whole wheat bread). Protein foods cost more than other foods. Therefore the nurse may need to teach pregnant couples about economical ways to meet protein needs for fetal development.

Mineral intake must also increase during pregnancy. Increased protein intake usually provides the extra needed essential minerals, particularly phosphorus and calcium. The rapid deposit of calcium in fetal bones and teeth during the third trimester of pregnancy requires adequate maternal calcium stores from early pregnancy and continued calcium intake to prevent maternal bone demineralization. One quart (4 cups) of cow's milk each day supplies the needed 1.2 g daily calcium. Other calcium sources include green leafy vegetables and calcium-fortified foods, sources more acceptable to cultures with a history of lactose intolerance (African, Mexican, and some European groups).

A woman who eats a well-balanced diet should gain sufficient vitamins and minerals for maternal and fetal needs during pregnancy. However, most health care providers recommend that the pregnant woman include an additional 30 to 60 mg of iron daily to benefit both mother and fetus, particularly during the last trimester. Iron deficiency anemia is common among pregnant women, and anemia contributes to hemorrhage, postpartum infection, and preterm birth. Anemia occurs more often among pregnant adolescent, black, and older white women (Allen, 2000). Research supports that women planning pregnancy and those in their first trimester take 0.4 mg of folic acid in a daily multivitamin supplement to prevent neural tube defects and anemia. This is particularly important for women with multiple gestations who experience a greater risk of anemia. However, research has shown that only 25% of women of childbearing age consume this amount of folic acid, which is critical for early fetal development (USDHHS, 2000).

Fats and carbohydrates must supply the caloric requirements during pregnancy. Although increased protein intake provides more calories, the body-building requirements of pregnancy and fetal growth demand most of the added protein. Fats and carbohydrates remain the most important sources of energy and essential vitamins and minerals. Supplemental vitamins and minerals, although not known to cause maternal or fetal harm if taken in reasonable dosages, probably cost the pregnant woman more to meet the nutritional needs of pregnancy than does a well-balanced diet.

The practice of **pica** may negatively influence the quality of a pregnant woman's nutrition during pregnancy. This practice, acceptable in some rural Black cultures, involves eating materials such as starch, mud, and other nonfoods instead of more healthy foods. Common in rural pregnant black women, this practice may contribute to iron deficiency anemia, particularly among women of lower economic status. The nurse should complete a nutritional assessment on any pregnant woman to identify instances of pica and suggest a culturally sensitive diet that will better meet the needs of the woman and her developing fetus.

The best time to teach a woman about prenatal nutrition is before she becomes pregnant. Most women do not seek prenatal care until they suspect pregnancy. Therefore the nurse often delivers information about optimal nutrition to the pregnant woman after critical fetal development has already begun. If all school children received nutrition information as part of their kindergarten through twelfth grade curriculum (a primary prevention approach), then women might have better overall personal nutrition established through lifestyle practices that would support quality prenatal nutrition later in their lives. Without such a primary prevention approach, secondary prevention intervention during pregnancy occurs through laboratory monitoring of iron levels, assessment of the woman's feelings of well-being, her actual intake of essential nutrients, and assessment of her pattern and total weight gain during the pregnancy. Many pregnant women work outside the home and may be among the increasing numbers of American families who spend 40% of their food budgets on food eaten outside the home (USDHHS, 2000). The nurse should alert the pregnant woman and her family to the documented high amounts of cholesterol, sodium, and fat and low amounts of iron and calcium that these foods contain so as to improve nutritional intake during pregnancy.

Elimination Pattern
Fetus

The fetus accomplishes all essential elimination functions through the placenta. Carbon dioxide, water, urea, and other waste products pass through the placenta, to be eliminated by the mother's body. By the end of the first trimester, the fetus swallows, makes respiratory movements, and urinates. However, these abilities become truly functional only after birth.

Pregnant Woman

The pregnant woman experiences changes in her elimination pattern because of the enlarging uterus and hormonal influences. These changes (urinary frequency during the first and third trimesters, constipation, and hemorrhoids) cause normal, minor discomforts (see Table 16-1). Anticipatory guidance by the nurse helps the pregnant woman cope with these changes and prevent complications of pregnancy. For example, teaching the pregnant woman commonsense measures (Health Teaching box) may prevent urinary tract infections (UTIs), typically a problem that is more common during pregnancy. With a known correlation between UTIs and premature labor, a focus on preventing and managing these infections must occur during pregnancy.

Activity-Exercise Pattern
Fetus

Early spontaneous movements of the fetus may be reflexive, stimulated by passive uterine movement. Ultrasonographic

---

HEALTH TEACHING   Suggestions for Preventing Urinary Tract Infections and Promoting Genitourinary Health

- Increase fluid intake to approximately 8 to 10 glasses per day; plain water is best to flush the body's systems of potential toxins; drink a glass of water before sexual intercourse to allow urinary output afterward and prevent UTIs.
- Avoid bladder irritants such as caffeine products, alcohol, artificial sweeteners, spicy foods, and carbonated beverages.
- Make urination a regular habit; avoid waiting to urinate until bladder is full.
- Urinate before and after sexual intercourse to cleanse the urethra and empty the bladder.
- Be aware that vigorous or frequent intercourse may contribute to increased risk of UTIs.
- Maintain consistently good perineal hygiene, including wiping from front to back after urination and bowel movements.

- Take all prescription medications given for UTIs, even when the symptoms of the infection have been alleviated.
- Drink cranberry or blueberry juice to acidify the urine or take cranberry pills; these products may relieve some of the symptoms of a UTI.
- Seek health care advice for a vaginal infection, which may contribute to development of a UTI.
- The nurse should assess for increased risk of developing a UTI: congenital or structural abnormalities of the genitourinary system, previous surgery to the genitourinary system; pregnancy; previous UTIs; high intake of carbonated beverages; and poor intake of water.

UTI, urinary tract infection.

observation of fetal movement shows repetitive movements early in pregnancy; at about 16 weeks, the pregnant woman feels these movements, termed **quickening.** By the end of the second trimester, fetal movement occurs less frequently because of lack of space in the uterus. The woman and her partner look forward to the regular daily cycle of movements, indicators of fetal well-being. An absence of or dramatic increase in fetal movements for more than 8 hours may indicate fetal distress. The nurse should routinely teach a pregnant woman to count the number of fetal movements each day and report any changes in fetal activity to the health care provider.

Pregnant Woman

The physical changes during pregnancy and the rigors of labor and delivery require that a pregnant woman be in the best physical condition of her life. Fortunately many pregnant women view pregnancy as a normal, natural state, and they often participate actively in physical activities or sports enjoyed before pregnancy. Generally a woman should avoid high-risk sports, such as sky diving and high-altitude climbing, because these could cause trauma to the fetus from low oxygen pressure or a maternal fall. Nurses should encourage a woman to choose activities based on her interests, comfort, and good judgment. When a sport or activity causes exhaustion or pain, it should be modified or discontinued. Later in pregnancy the woman should be encouraged to choose safe physical activities because of changes in her center of gravity due to the enlarging uterus and in the musculoskeletal system.

The woman with a sedentary lifestyle before pregnancy should slowly increase her activity level during pregnancy. A daily swim or 30-minute walk provides a good introduction to a regular exercise program. Regular exercise contributes to joint flexibility, improved cardiovascular and gastrointestinal fitness, uterine tone for an efficient labor, fewer pregnancy discomforts, weight control and a lower risk for diabetes, and overall feelings of well-being in the pregnant woman (USDHHS, 2000). For the self-directed woman, prenatal class exercises or a consumer-oriented book of exercises will facilitate an adequate exercise program. For most women, group exercise with other pregnant women is more enjoyable than exercising alone. The nurse may encourage women to enter a structured diet and exercise program sponsored by a delivering hospital to help women lose weight after delivery (O'Toole, Sawicki, & Artal, 2003).

In an uncomplicated pregnancy, a couple may continue their usual sexual activity. However, threatened abortion or history of abortion in the first trimester, early rupture of membranes, and other complications may call for restrictions on sexual intercourse or orgasm. In some cases the enlarging uterus will require the couple to modify positions for intercourse, particularly during the latter part of pregnancy. The couple's feelings about the woman's changing body may alter their sexual relationship. (See the section on roles and role changes later in this chapter.) The nurse's first step in primary prevention intervention in this area is to support the couple's needs and relate, in a sensitive fashion, accurate information that facilitates couple intimacy during pregnancy.

Sleep-Rest Pattern
Fetus

Electroencephalographic studies have shown four cyclical states of activity in the fetus: complete wakefulness, drowsy wakefulness, rapid eye movement sleep, and quiet sleep. Evidence suggests that a diurnal (day-night) pattern exists during the fetal period. Generally a healthy baby moves approximately 3 times per hour during waking periods.

Pregnant Woman

Fatigue reflects the significant physical and emotional changes occurring in the pregnant woman. The nurse should counsel a woman that fatigue usually subsides by the fourth month but may return later in pregnancy. Rest breaks during the day and 8 hours of sleep each night help prevent fatigue and increase the pregnant woman's comfort. The nurse must encourage each pregnant woman to rest when her body says so because of the rapidly growing fetus and the woman's needs for physical renewal. This encouragement must be directed particularly toward working women, who may need a doctor's note for their employer that validates the need for rest during the workday.

Many pregnant women do not sleep well because they need to urinate several times a night during the first and third trimesters. In addition, some women experience positional discomfort in late pregnancy that prevents effective sleep and, therefore, increases their fatigue (see Table 16-1). Fatigue may influence a woman's evaluation of her role as a pregnant woman, her body changes, and her cultural beliefs related to her ability to succeed in pregnancy. The nurse should help the woman express her thoughts and feelings and find ways to support better sleep and rest patterns (e.g., sleeping upright in a chair at night for easier breathing).

Cognitive-Perceptual Pattern
Fetus

During the prenatal period, all fetal sensory systems function or nearly function. These systems include vision, hearing, taste, smell, touch, and proprioceptive and vestibular senses (Lowdermilk & Perry, 2003a). Although capable of seeing by 28 to 32 weeks of age, the fetus has little opportunity to use this ability in utero (Cole, 1997; Lowdermilk & Perry, 2003a). After approximately 25 weeks, pregnant women note that their babies respond to a loud, sudden noise. Some pregnant women and their partners offer sensory stimulation to the fetus by singing or rubbing the woman's abdomen. This parental behavior may assist in the bonding process between parent and baby. Thus the nurse may wish to include this kind of information in prenatal teaching sessions.

Pregnant Woman

Physical and psychological processes remain closely intertwined as pregnancy progresses. Psychological stresses and normal emotional growth affect the physical status of the pregnancy, interactions of the family members, and the eventual relationship between mother and infant. When considering the emotional aspects of pregnancy, the nurse must recognize that the woman's personality, environment, physical state, family, and sociocultural and spiritual background affect the ways in which she handles the psychological changes.

Two major categories of psychological influences are (1) normal psychological growth required of parents to emotionally and physically prepare them for parenthood and (2) internal or external stressors on the pregnant woman that decrease her ability to provide the best environment for the developing fetus. The pregnant woman undergoes many cognitive changes that ultimately result in her psychological readiness for motherhood.

Emotional Changes. Hormonal and other physical changes assist the woman in the psychological work of pregnancy. Progesterone level increases affect the woman's general mood, causing her to be more introverted and passive. These mood changes help her to focus her energy on the growing child and her own growth and development. In addition to hormonal changes, the presence, growth, and movements of the fetus become more a part of the woman's experiential self. According to Rubin (1984), the classic researcher on maternal-infant bonding, the pregnant woman receives immediate sensations of touch, motion, and weight from the fetus that she can share only partially with others. These support a maternal feeling of separateness and uniqueness that causes the woman to turn inward. She frequently worries that the shift in energy away from the world toward herself and her child may cause her to lose contact, drift away from valued relationships, and lose feelings of competence in her areas of achievement. She spends time analyzing her experiences and their possible influence on her effectiveness as a future parent. She constantly studies the qualities of human relationships and shows increased sensitivity and perceptiveness to many people. To others, the woman may seem overly sensitive and analytical during pregnancy (Rubin, 1967, 1984).

Although a woman's mood varies based on a variety of factors and at different times during the pregnancy, many women experience wide mood swings, emotional lability, irritability, and changes in sexual desire. Physical discomforts, hormonal changes, feelings about altered body image, cultural considerations, work and relationship adjustments, and demanding cognitive maturational processes may also cause these emotional changes.

Stressors Influencing Development. The mother's age, fears related to a previous fetal loss (O'Leary & Thorwick, 1997), feelings about the pregnancy, life situation, and culture, degree of stress, the presence of other children, and the influence of loved ones may serve as stressors that influence the ways in which she completes the developmental tasks of motherhood. A young pregnant woman facing the additional developmental task of adolescence may have difficulty incorporating the pregnant body or the role of mother into her still undefined self-image. Cognitively, she may still be unable to make plans for the baby or even accept the pregnancy until she feels the baby move. Nursing teaching interventions seem critical when an adolescent faces overlapping developmental challenges of age and pregnancy.

On the other hand, a pregnant woman older than 35 years may feel more isolated by her situation than does the pregnant woman in her 20s. Frequently established in career and family, the older pregnant woman needs to learn to balance her growth and development in these valued areas with her new sense of self. Fears related to being considered at high risk because of age may increase her anxiety and ambivalence about the pregnancy, even if she was previously infertile. As a first-time mother, she may worry about managing the physical demands of labor and delivery, sleeplessness of motherhood, chances of having an abnormal child, and the need to juggle conflicting life responsibilities and relationships.

A woman with other children moves through the developmental tasks differently than does a woman who is pregnant for the first time. Even with a desired pregnancy, the woman may worry about incorporating the new infant into her relationships and managing the time needed for a new baby. She may have fears and anxieties about labor and delivery because of a previous negative experience. She may be much more aware of the problems involved with caring for a new infant and may not be excited about another pregnancy experience that demands a redefinition of motherhood or additional child-rearing expenses.

Developmental Tasks

Rubin (1967, 1977, 1984) describes four major developmental tasks that a woman seeks to accomplish as she learns to become a mother. These include ensuring safe passage through pregnancy and childbirth, ensuring acceptance of the child by significant people in her family, binding into her unknown child, and learning to give of self. According to Rubin, all four tasks must be confronted simultaneously, but each task assumes greater priority at certain times than do other tasks. Each woman works through these tasks based on her unique style, cultural values, and life priorities. At the end of pregnancy, however, all tasks must be integrated to create a presentation, similar to a tapestry (Rubin, 1984).

Ensuring Safe Passage. The woman attempts to ensure safe passage for herself and her infant in many ways. Generally, she engages in a variety of prenatal care options appropriate to her culture and life experience. These options may include seeking health care from a doctor, midwife, or cultural health practitioner, gaining support and information from family and friends, and reading and watching videos. For example, pregnant Cambodian women rely on elderly same-culture women to give prenatal care and advice and rely little on prenatal classes or visits. Some Hispanic American women, based on their view that pregnancy is a healthy, natural experience, may not seek prenatal care but seek a strong matriarchal support system for a positive outcome.

The folklore of pregnancy becomes extremely important to some women, and they attempt to avoid activities believed to harm the baby. Mexican American folklore includes myths that the cord will strangle the infant if the mother raises her arms above her head or that viewing a disabled person will cause the baby to be abnormal. Chinese American women may avoid the zoo during pregnancy for fear that the baby will resemble one of the animals.

As the pregnancy evolves, the woman becomes more protective of herself and the fetus by avoiding crowds, revolving doors, small spaces, and people believed to place the mother at risk. During the third trimester, the pregnant woman may have dreams that echo her fears and desires for delivery and her future child. She tires of being pregnant but fears the effect of delivery on her safety and that of her child (Rubin, 1972, 1984). Although sharing fears and desires with her partner, family, or health care provider helps, only the safe delivery of a normal child can fully free a pregnant woman from her fears to meet this developmental task (Rubin, 1972, 1977).

Ensuring Acceptance of the Child. The woman must believe that her child will be accepted into her family based on her definition of family. According to Rubin (1984), the partner's receptivity to the child is particularly important, and many women fantasize about the gender of their child based on a partner's preference. The woman frequently judges his degree of receptivity to the infant by the amount of love and attention that she, herself, receives from him during her pregnancy. She may desire support from other women, rather than her partner, based on her life experience, values, and cultural background.

Binding Into Her Unknown Child. This task is the most complex cognitive process for the pregnant woman (Rubin, 1984). To accomplish this task, she must integrate the fetus as an integral part of her but also as a separate being. Completion of this task occurs with birth of the baby. Initially, the woman fantasizes about the baby through associative images: when she eats an egg, she thinks of the baby. Fantasies in the second and third trimesters relate more specifically to what the child will be like; the woman may imagine the baby in little girl or little boy clothes. During the eighth month, the woman begins nesting activity by preparing the nursery and thinking increasingly of the baby as an external reality in her home.

Learning to Give of Herself. Although the actual mothering activity occurs after birth, the learning process to become a mother begins during pregnancy. The woman begins the task by examining what she will gain and lose by becoming a mother. She then explores the meaning of giving by examining how others give to her and to others and how she has given to others in the past (Rubin, 1984). Gifts for herself and the baby represent meaningful manifestations of her own and others' acceptance of her motherhood and her ability to give to her child and develop her identify as mother (Rubin, 1967, 1972).

Self-Perception–Self-Concept Pattern

To develop a maternal identity, the woman must first accept the pregnant body image. Initially she may show ambivalence based on her need to "fit" the pregnancy with her perception of self. She may dislike the physical changes of pregnancy or gladly "show off" her pregnant body to others. During the second trimester, however, the woman frequently begins to feel more positive about her changing womanly image as she feels the baby move, and increased estrogen and progesterone increase her sense of vitality, inner peace, and acceptance. Her body begins to look pregnant, and generally others respond positively to this change (Rubin, 1972).

By the third trimester, however, the woman frequently tires of the pregnancy. Her sense of awkward moments supersedes feelings of well-being. She may experience uncomfortable sleepless nights, the constant need to urinate, Braxton-Hicks contractions, and other discomforts. Some women experience infant movement or mild contractions as pleasurable, sensual sensations, whereas others find them extremely uncomfortable. By pregnancy's end, these women yearn to have their former body boundaries back, to hold the baby in their arms, or to have someone else carry the baby.

After birth, the woman gradually sees the infant more and more as a separate individual, dependent on her care. The mother starts to bond with her baby based on her self-perception. If she feels good about herself, she will show love toward the infant; when she feels ugly or unlovable, she may make uncomplimentary remarks about the infant's appearance (Rubin, 1984).

Maternal Role

The pregnant woman's personality, maturity level, and psychological development influence her readiness to assume the role of mother. The way in which society in general and her culture in particular perceive motherhood and the role of women, and the way in which her own views mesh with these perceptions, will affect the ease of the transition. The family situation, the availability of peer role models, and the relationship with her mother are also significant. Internalization of the mother role occurs only after the birth, when the woman interacts with the infant in a reciprocal relationship (Rubin, 1977).

Nursing Interventions

The woman may feel overwhelmed by her feelings and thoughts during pregnancy. Although others acknowledge her physical changes, only she experiences the psychological changes of excitement, ambivalence, or confusion associated with being pregnant. During prenatal assessment, the nurse should address expected cognitive changes and self-image issues with each pregnant woman and respond nonjudgmentally to concerns expressed in this area. In one-to-one sessions or group prenatal classes, women and their partners should be encouraged to discuss their ideas and feelings related to the emotional and relationship changes expected during pregnancy, because these changes influence the future intimate relationship.

Roles-Relationships Pattern

The pregnant family changes throughout the pregnancy and postpartum period as each family member explores and responds to new roles and relationships. A pregnant woman without a partner may feel isolated during pregnancy and depend on family or friends as she adjusts to her situation. Cultural beliefs and traditions may produce stresses during pregnancy, change roles and relationships, or provide emotional and physical support to the pregnant family as it prepares for the baby.

The partner of the pregnant woman faces many new situations that influence that person's parental development. The pregnant woman may seem to be a different person to him because of her emotional response to the pregnancy, introspection, fantasies, need for more rest, and changes in sexual drive. He may feel a rivalry with the fetus and baby, because the woman has a need and desire to divide her time between him and the baby. He may resent the attention that she receives during the pregnancy and the additional demands that she may make on his time. He may experience more financial pressure because of baby expenses and his partner's need to stop working on a short-term or long-term basis. These perceptions may lead him to batter or otherwise abuse his partner, possibly causing a loss of the fetus, preterm labor, or fetal injury (Hot Topics box). The nurse must assess each pregnant woman for abuse and intervene appropriately to protect the safety and health of the family during gestation.

The male partner may be concerned about his ability to fulfill the father role and support his wife or significant other. His fathering role models may be limited because of a lack of contact with his own father or because he spends time with men who are not actively parenting. He may never have held a baby before and may worry that he might drop or harm his own child. If his partner experiences pregnancy complications, he may feel guilty about causing the pregnancy. Table 16-4 gives a more complete list of both the father's and the mother's emotional responses to a first pregnancy. The nurse must work with the pregnant family to help them adapt to a first pregnancy, because this one affects how they will cope with subsequent pregnancies.

HOTtopics

BIRTH OUTCOMES IN ABUSED PREGNANT WOMEN

Nurses and other providers who deliver health care to women must address the issue of abuse of the pregnant woman by an intimate partner. Consider the following research study and the questions that follow to understand the issue further.

The purpose of this study was to explore differences between publicly and privately insured pregnant women with respect to maternal and fetal effects related to recent intimate partner abuse.

Pregnancy may be an optimal time to screen women for abuse by an intimate partner, based on evidence that this is one of the few times in a woman's life when consistent health care may be delivered. An estimated 1 in 6 pregnant women experience abuse from an intimate partner (Curry, Perrin, & Wall, 1998), and research supports that abuse causes infant low birth weight, preterm labor, and increased rates of maternal infection. African American women may face a higher risk of partner abuse than do women of other ethnic backgrounds (Curry, Perrin, & Wall, 1998; Huth-Bocks, Levendosky, & Bogat, 2002). Using this background, the authors of this study used a previously tested tool to assess abuse and analyzed for prenatal and birth outcome data from the medical records of over 2000 women known to have experienced abuse. Women insured through both public and private mechanisms were included in the study.

Findings indicated that more recently abused women were more likely to have public insurance, to be single, to have less than a high school education, and to have medical or obstetrical complications. There was no relationship between ethnicity, number of births, or infant outcome and abuse. Statistical analysis supported that women who received public funding had a greater risk of low infant Apgar scores and more physical complaints than did privately insured abused women.

Overall, study results indicate a need to tailor nursing interventions supportive of pregnant women facing abuse according to the type of insurance these women have. Indicators of abuse may also vary in low income and higher income women, mandating that nurses conduct sensitive abuse screening for all pregnant women.

Questions

1. How do the current health care system and the sociopolitical context of care in this country contribute to the high numbers of pregnant women facing abuse from their intimate partners?
2. What kind of interventions do you believe would be effective for these abused women?
3. How should U.S. health care policy ethically and legislatively address the problem of intimate partner abuse, based on data that indicate that women in European countries experience less abuse during pregnancy?

From Curry, M. A., Perrin, N., & Wall, E. (1998). Effects of abuse on maternal complications and birth weight in adult and adolescent women. *Obstetrics and Gynecology, 92,* 530-534; Huth-Bocks, A. C., Levendosky, A. A., & Bogat, G. A. (2002). The effects of domestic violence during pregnancy on maternal and infant health. *Violence and Victims, 17,* 169-183; Kearney, M. H., Haggerty, L. A., Munro, B. H., & Hawkins, J. W. (2003). Birth outcomes and maternal morbidity in abused pregnant women with public versus private health insurance. *Image: The Journal of Nursing Scholarship, 35,* 345-349.

Table **16-4** Possible Responses to First Pregnancy

Phase of Pregnancy	Father's Response	Mother's Response
First trimester	Fear of losing wife or child Self-doubt as a future father	Loss of interest in coitus Possible less sexual effectiveness Sleepiness and chronic fatigue Nausea Increased dependence
Second trimester	Increased respect Awe as quickening comes Names for fetus coined	Solemnity, hilarity, and playfulness about fetal movements Talks about and with fetus Increased eroticism
Third trimester	Fear of coitus hurting fetus Abstinence difficult Envy or pride or both at wife's creativity Worry about birth Keen awareness of male-female differences	Lessened sexual activity Abstinence (often recommended by physician) Sleepiness Backache Abdominal discomfort Sexual isolation Heightened sense of femininity
Postpartum	Eagerness to resume marital relations Concern over endangering wife's recovery Sense of triumph in becoming a father Tenderness toward wife and baby	Pain and fear of harm from too early coitus Low eroticism Concern about effect on husband of continued abstinence Sense of completion as a mother
Pregnancy as a whole	Increased romanticism Increased nurturance Increased family life participation Anxiety about costs Concern about lack of skills in baby care	Increased romanticism Increased optimism Family roles replacing marital emphases Fear of miscarriage or problems with baby Pride of accomplishment

From Ramer, L., & Frank, B. (2001). *Pregnancy: Psychosocial perspectives* (3rd ed). White Plains, NY: March of Dimes.

Box **16-4** Nursing Strategies to Help Parents Prepare Siblings for the Neonate

- Explain the pregnancy and birth appropriate to the child's age.
- Answer all the child's questions.
- Use relevant literature to educate the child about the coming baby.
- Encourage discussion and questions by talking about the new baby during relaxed family times rather than during busy, rushed times.
- Have the child participate in decisions, such as choosing a name, clothes, and toys for baby.
- When sibling classes are available as part of the childbirth education process, encourage parents and child to attend.
- Suggest that the child go with the mother during clinic or office visits.
- Allow and discuss negative comments about the pregnancy or baby.
- Encourage child to make drawings or give small gifts to the baby when it is born.

Children in the family also experience role changes during and after the pregnancy. The very young child, unaware of the concept of a new baby before the infant arrives, may experience a changed relationship with his pregnant mother. She may have less time to play, be more irritable from fatigue, or limit or stop active play late in pregnancy because of increased awkwardness and concern about her safety. After the baby arrives, the child may be kept away from both baby and mother by well-meaning friends and relatives, have to share parents with others, or may want to breast-feed from the mother as the baby does. When permitted to see the newborn, the child may be admonished to "be careful" or "don't touch the baby." Thus a young child may not accept the baby with open arms.

The older child understands the newborn's significance more clearly but still experiences apprehensions about the effects of the baby on the family. Older children may have been told that they will become a big brother or sister, but does this mean they will lose toys, time with parents, and have to give up a private bedroom? Older children may worry about their mother who seems more tired, less available, and perhaps even sick at times. Her enlarging abdomen may appear frightening. With help from the nurse, parents can make pregnancy an exciting time of learning and growing for the family (Box 16-4). Chapter 18 also discusses the sibling relationship in greater detail.

In extended families, expectant grandparents also experience changes during the pregnancy of their daughter or daughter-in-law. The maternal grandmother, seeing her daughter assume the mother role, may now view her daughter as a rival, because they are both mothers. The grandparents may be reminded of their own aging, resenting when their advice about pregnancy and parenting goes unheeded. A positive outcome of a pregnancy may be a new closeness between woman and mother if the daughter turns to her mother to seek advice and share feelings. The nurse may encourage expectant parents to use pregnancy as a transition time for their own parents, which can enhance extended family cohesion in the future.

During pregnancy and after birth, each family member begins to establish an emotional attachment to the imagined or real new baby. Research shows that when the mother has a strong support system to develop deep feelings of attachment to the fetus, she will most likely attach to the baby after birth. Therefore the nurse should assess the support system of each pregnant woman and implement primary and secondary interventions to increase family bonding with a new baby.

Sexuality-Reproductive Pattern

The pregnant woman's body image and merging of this body image with her definition of femininity greatly influence her feelings about her sexuality. For previously infertile women, achieving pregnancy may be a blessed event, despite the need for technology that affects a woman's concept of self and femininity. The reflections of others, particularly a pregnant woman's partner, helps women to accept their bodies, leading to better adjustment in their sexual relations.

On the other hand, women may experience different sexual feelings during pregnancy. Some women experience an increase in desire, but most worry about intercourse during pregnancy, fearing that it will cause miscarriage, infection, early delivery, or harm to the baby. Sexual dissatisfaction of the couple may result from restrictions in sexual positions, pain on penetration, increased vaginal discharge, breast tenderness, or the other physical discomforts of pregnancy such as fatigue or heartburn. Some women experience a decreased desire for sexual intercourse but an increased desire for holding, touching, and other signs of physical affection from their partners.

Coping-Stress Tolerance Pattern

Physical and psychological adaptations of the woman to pregnancy affect her perception of stressors and her ability to cope. Even normal discomforts of pregnancy may be stressful for a woman, mandating her to modify her usual routine to cope more effectively. Anxiety tends to be high during the first trimester as the woman adapts to pregnancy and anticipated life changes. During the second trimester, the woman feels less anxious, but anxiety returns during the third trimester with impending labor and delivery. Throughout pregnancy women may demonstrate their anxieties through psychosomatic complaints and behaviors, such as nausea and vomiting after the first trimester, excessive eating, food cravings, sleeplessness, and fainting. Realistically, every pregnant woman probably experiences some degree of stress. However, many women have considerable stress or ongoing stress, such as poverty, marital difficulties, or unsatisfactory living or working conditions, which influence their coping abilities.

A pregnant woman's anxieties may be reflected in her dreams and fantasies. Many pregnant women report dreams about their babies being deformed or dead, themselves dying, or a family member being injured. Many women at the end of their pregnancies express fears about body mutilation with delivery. Other women may manifest their anxiety by smoking, drinking, or using drugs (legal or illegal), all of which can harm the fetus. Maternal anxiety may cause increased fetal activity and heart rate, as well as decreased blood flow to the uterus, thus influencing adequate oxygen and food to the fetus (Piotrowski, 1999). The nurse must direct a pregnant woman who is not coping well to relevant resources for assistance. The nurse must also assess each woman's progress in taking on the mothering role as the pregnancy nears term. This information can be shared with the postpartum nursing staff to encourage discussion in this important area.

The nurse may encourage the pregnant woman to use tension-relieving strategies such as listening to soft music, using humor, crying, sleeping, talking to a friend, meditating, exercising, and fantasizing during times of stress. These strategies are safe for the fetus and provide relief from many normal tensions and anxieties during pregnancy and afterward. For women with strong spiritual needs related to their cultural backgrounds, spiritual interventions will help them integrate various dimensions of their lives, develop the ability to parent successfully, and find meaning in the changes and goals of pregnancy. Overall, the nurse plays a key role in nonjudgmental responding and promoting the coping of women during pregnancy.

Values-Beliefs Pattern

Although pregnancy has been described as the fulfillment of the deepest and most powerful wish of a woman, this fulfillment often coincides with a woman's fear of losing part of herself. She gives up some relationships and pleasures to take on other anticipated satisfactions. She may find that she values friendships with other mothers now, whereas before pregnancy her friendships focused on work or school colleagues. She may discover, much to her husband's confusion, that she values different qualities in him than she did before anticipating birth. Her husband may also experience a shift in his values.

Pregnant women and their partners may experience changes in their spiritual values. Seen as a mystical event or miracle, conception may lead to an increased faith in God or a favorite saint. Nonreligious couples may start to attend church after the baby's birth, because they want religion to be part of their child's life. Religious beliefs may influence a woman's decision to undergo certain tests or procedures, such as amniocentesis or abortion. Some women may feel forced to reproduce because their religious or cultural mores forbids contraception or encourages large families. In these groups, each pregnancy may be seen as another unwanted, but unavoidable, burden or may be valued because more children signify a stronger family.

PATHOLOGICAL PROCESSES

A healthy infant is the outcome of most pregnancies. However, genetic abnormalities and environmental hazards may cause fetal harm, **spontaneous abortion** (natural loss of conceptive products), or minor or serious congenital defects. Diagnostic methods that identify an early pregnancy or a fetal loss may assist couples in practicing healthy decisions to prevent loss or congenital abnormalities. Cunningham and colleagues (2001f) note that congenital defects affect 3% to 4% of all live births and contribute to infant mortality rates by causing structural or functional disability incompatible with life. Real-time ultrasonography identifies approximately 85% of fetal anomalies by 36 weeks of gestation (Manning, 1999). This knowledge, gained before delivery, permits expectant couples and the health care delivery team to access resources for improving the baby's life or support family grieving if the baby is not expected to live. With progress made in diagnostic tools and the Human Genome Project, some couples may be able to prevent fetal defects or manage them during pregnancy to improve the quality of their baby's life after birth (Case Study). Unfortunately, even when no genetic or congenital defects exist, the fetus may still be injured during the process of labor and delivery and face a lesser quality of life.

Teratogens are environmental agents that cause spontaneous abortions or congenital defects. Unlike genetic abnormalities, which occur only at conception, environmental agents may affect the developing infant at any point during gestation. Fetal organs have critical periods of development and, if affected at that time by a teratogen, the infant may have a defect in that organ system. **Web Site Resource 16D** depicts the effects of teratogens on the embryo and fetus. Teratogens normally do not cause a congenital defect during the first 14 days after conception. However, the embryo may be lost later but during early gestation (a spontaneous abortion). Therefore, as a primary prevention strategy, any woman contemplating or attempting pregnancy should be counseled to avoid teratogens that might cause fetal loss or damage.

Physical Factors and Diagnostic Tools

Modern diagnostic tools, such as ultrasonography, amniocentesis, chorionic villus sampling, and α-fetoprotein screening, have been used to identify a number of fetal problems. Many of these tools are presented in **Web Site Resource 16E.** Certain risk factors, such as family history, maternal age, maternal illness, or previous fetal abnormalities, may indicate the need for these diagnostic tools during a woman's pregnancy. These tools commonly identify problems related to abnormal size or rate of fetal growth, chromosomal abnormalities, neural tube defects and fetal lung

---

CASE STUDY

Ms. James

Ms. James, a second time 38-year-old black mother, had elevated blood pressure with her first baby 6 years ago. Because of this problem and because the baby weighed 9 pounds, the baby was delivered by cesarean section. Ms. James is interested in having a vaginal delivery this time, but recently her blood pressure has been elevated and the α-fetoprotein level was abnormal at 16 weeks of pregnancy. She is currently 18 weeks pregnant and has been scheduled for ultrasonography to visualize the fetus to rule out an open spinal defect or Down syndrome. Ms. James and her boyfriend disagree about what to do (keep or terminate the pregnancy) if the ultrasonography indicates a spinal problem.

Reflective Questions

1. As the nurse, what priority data would you collect from this couple to help define relevant interventions to meet their needs?
2. How can you help this couple in deciding about termination or continuation of the pregnancy? What are your personal views on both options? How does the database influence your views?
3. With the influence of the recent Human Genome Project and the possibility of predicting open spinal defects earlier in pregnancy, how will maternity care change in the future?

Prediction of Human Disease

Starting in 1990, the federal government and a private agency engaged in genetic research as part of the International Genome Project, a coordinated effort to map the genetic instructions found on human DNA and within the DNA of several model organisms. Initial sequencing of the human genome has been accomplished, so the ability to predict and manage hereditary diseases is on the horizon. Although this knowledge holds much hope for predicting fetal defects and disease in humans, ethicists have expressed concerns about how this information might be used. Will this material be used to discriminate against individuals with predisposition to genetically related diseases? Will couples wanting the perfect baby seek genome technology to decide whether to maintain a pregnancy or to abort a fetus if a child has a disease perceived as causing a lesser quality of life? Will this information be made available to employers and health care insurers, who might then decide to deny insurance to people with existing or future disease that may increase health care costs? Although the Human Genome Project will provide information intended to help individuals have a better quality of life, many ethical questions remain for society to address concerning the use of this information.

From Strauss, R. P. (2003). Beyond easy answers: Prenatal diagnosis and counseling during pregnancy. *Cleft Palate & Craniofacial Journal, 39*(2), 164-168. *DNA,* deoxyribonucleic acid.

immaturity. The nurse, in consultation with the health care team, must participate in providing informed consent to women before these diagnostic tools are utilized.

Biological Agents

Biological processes in the fetal environment, which include infections and other health problems of the mother, may affect fetal growth and development. A pregnant woman who acquires an asymptomatic viral infection may not seek health care because she believes that the fetus will not be harmed. However, viral agents may cause fetal damage early in pregnancy. The woman with a health problem, such as diabetes, may also cause fetal damage if she fails to adhere to her health care provider's directives.

When the nurse discusses with pregnant couples the effects of biological processes on the fetus, she must emphasize that the timing of the maternal infection or illness is critical to predicting fetal defects. Maternal infections during the first trimester of pregnancy may cause severe fetal defects or death, depending on the organism. Infections later in pregnancy may also seriously affect the fetus, but less often. Unfortunately, pregnancy renders many women more susceptible to viral illness, supporting an argument for all women of childbearing age to be fully immunized. Many vaccines (measles, mumps, rubella, and polio) cannot be given during pregnancy due to potential risk to the fetus, but others present no risk (tetanus and diphtheria). Only the infections that tend to cause the most serious problems will be discussed.

Toxoplasmosis

Toxoplasmosis is caused by a protozoan that infects people through undercooked meat, handling of cat feces, and exposure to infected soil in countries outside the United States (Cook et al., 2000). An infected pregnant woman may have flulike symptoms or mild to severe upper respiratory symptoms believed to be unrelated to an infection. About 30% of infants exposed during pregnancy may have skin rashes, enlarged lymph nodes and liver, inflammation of the heart, pneumonia, jaundice, and severe central nervous system damage (Lynfield & Guerina, 1997) after birth or years later. Pregnant women should use good hand washing technique, avoid eating raw meat, and avoid handling cats or cleaning cat litter boxes to avoid exposure to *Toxoplasma*.

Syphilis

An infected mother transfers **syphilis,** an STD that is caused by a protozoan, to her fetus. Although preventable and treatable, the number of congenital and neonatal syphilis cases has increased over the last several years (Askin, 1999). Maternal risk factors for acquiring syphilis include homelessness, human immunodeficiency virus (HIV)-positive status, single marital status, and a history of STDs. Syphilis may cause preterm labor and miscarriage (Cunningham et al., 2001c). Approximately 30% of all affected fetuses die and, if the mother fails to get treatment

during pregnancy, 40% to 50% of live newborns have symptoms of active disease (Carlson & Dattel, 2000). The infant may be born with localized mucocutaneous lesions, nasal congestion, anemia, and generalized septicemia, but may appear healthy at birth only to have symptoms appear later. Routine testing of high-risk women for syphilis at the first prenatal visit and during the third trimester, as well as antibiotic treatment (penicillin) for affected women and their partners, have reduced the number of infants with congenital syphilis (Lowdermilk & Perry, 2003f). Treating the infected mother during the first 18 weeks of pregnancy usually protects the fetus (Askin, 1999).

Rubella

Despite the broad use of the measles, mumps, and **rubella** vaccine, or MMR, and the resulting immunity to rubella, approximately 20% of women reach their childbearing period without immunity to this disease (USDHHS, 2000). The symptoms of rubella may cause the mother to think she has a minor viral infection, but rubella during the first trimester may cause improper fetal development of the ears, eyes, and heart and deafness. No treatment exists for an infected fetus; however, no pregnant woman may receive the vaccine to protect future pregnancies if she has no history of rubella infection. After delivery, new mothers often receive the vaccine with a recommendation to avoid pregnancy for at least 3 months to prevent fetal harm from the vaccine.

Cytomegalovirus

Cytomegalovirus (CMV) is responsible for the most common infection that may cause serious fetal complications. CMV infects an estimated 1% to 2% of all infants born in the United States. Most mothers infected with CMV have mild, often nonspecific symptoms, but their babies may have symptoms similar to those of toxoplasmosis (Brown & Abernathy, 1998; Fanaroff & Martin, 1997). Unfortunately, no means exist to prevent or manage this viral infection. Perhaps an immunization similar to that for rubella will be developed in the future.

Herpes Simplex Virus

Herpes simplex virus infections remain extremely common today, with many people unaware that they have the disease. Herpes simplex may cause spontaneous abortion or fetal neurological damage. Infants infected at birth may show localized or generalized disease with symptoms of vesicular skin lesions, conjunctivitis, seizures, respiratory distress, or gastrointestinal bleeding. These symptoms may cause newborn death. An infant delivered vaginally by a woman with active genital herpes has a 40% to 60% chance of being infected (Fanaroff & Martin, 1997), supporting a decision for a cesarean delivery for any women with active vaginal or perineal herpes lesions. Generally acyclovir is not recommended during pregnancy for treatment of viral lesions. The nurse may educate the affected woman about comfort measures at this time, including ways to keep the lesions dry and to apply oatmeal compresses to alleviate the pain of the lesions (Lowdermilk & Perry, 2003a).

Chlamydia, Gonococcus, Group B *Streptococcus*, Bacterial Vaginosis, and *Candida albicans*

Infections caused by these bacteria and yeast (*Candida albicans*) may occur in the woman's vagina or cervix, infecting the infant during a vaginal delivery. **Chlamydia,** the most common bacterial STD, appears most often among poor women with little access to care. Although few symptoms are seen, infection may cause preterm labor or newborn conjunctivitis or pneumonia. Routine treatment of the newborn's eyes after birth with erythromycin destroys the organisms. Maternal **gonococcus** (GC) infection, which can cause preterm labor, preterm rupture of amniotic membranes, and miscarriage (Cunningham et al., 2001c), may be treated with erythromycin; newborn infants often receive either erythromycin ointment or silver nitrate drops in the eyes to prevent GC infection. Screening at 36 to 37 weeks of pregnancy for **group B *Streptococcus*** infection has been recommended, because this infection causes preterm rupture of the amniotic membranes, premature labor, fetal respiratory distress syndrome, fetal septicemia, and meningitis (Lowdermilk & Perry, 2003f). **Bacterial vaginosis** may also cause premature labor (U.S. Preventive Services Task Force, 2001). *Candida albicans,* cause of a common vaginal fungal infection, may also cause an oral infection called *thrush* in the newborn. Routine assessment of pregnant women, and occasionally their sexual partners (GC), for these bacterial and yeast infections must occur during pregnancy so that treatment can occur and prevent fetal infection at the time of delivery.

Acquired Immunodeficiency Syndrome

With more women, particularly African American and Hispanic (Duff, 2002), testing positive for **acquired immunodeficiency syndrome** (AIDS), the Centers for Disease Control and Prevention (CDC) recommends screening and counseling for this disease both before and as early in pregnancy as possible (Centers for Disease Control and Prevention [CDC], 1998). Any woman in a high-risk group (e.g., an intravenous drug user, one who has bisexual partners, one who has multiple sexual contacts, or black or Hispanic women living in poverty) should be tested for antibodies to HIV. For the HIV-positive woman or one who engages in high-risk sexual practices, counseling must occur before conception. Counseling should include both the effect of the virus on pregnancy and the effect of pregnancy on HIV disease progression. Although unclear, it appears that HIV infection becomes worse during pregnancy because of a woman's altered immune status. Some early pregnancy discomforts, such as fatigue, anorexia, and weight loss, may mask the early symptoms of HIV infection and thus postpone a definitive diagnosis.

Infants born to HIV-positive women have an infection rate of 5% to 60% (Lowdermilk & Perry, 2003g). Affected infants may not be seropositive for HIV for many months after birth and then later develop the disease. Recent use of zidovudine (AZT) protocol treatments throughout pregnancy have improved the prognosis of an HIV-positive woman and have decreased viral transmission to the fetus, although the drug remains expensive and may be inaccessible for women who do not receive prenatal care.

The pregnant woman who has AIDS or who is HIV positive should be carefully monitored by a health care team for opportunistic infections that occur frequently. The nurse can be instrumental in helping this woman coordinate her contacts with care providers, answering her questions, and working as a member of the team to provide optimal care for her and her child. Frequently the pregnant woman with AIDS does not seek care, based on fears of being reported for her disease. Involving the woman in continuous prenatal care decreases her risk of preterm rupture of membranes, problems with fetal growth, postpartum infection, drug and alcohol abuse, and difficulty in addressing sociocultural barriers to a better life (Duff, 2002).

Although important in decreasing the transmission of any disease, astute preventive measures are mandatory for nurses who come in contact with HIV-infected body fluids, such as blood, amniotic fluid, and vaginal secretions (universal precautions). All health care providers must follow hospital and birth center policies regarding the use of gloves, gowns, and the disposal of needles and other potentially contaminated equipment to prevent the transmission of this disease in particular.

Hepatitis B

Hepatitis B virus (HBV) infection remains a significant concern during pregnancy, because it affects the maternal liver and has a high fetal transmission rate (60%) if present during the third trimester. High-risk groups for HBV include women from Asia, Pacific Islands, and sub-Saharan Africa, as well as health care workers, intravenous drug users, and women with multiple sex partners (CDC, 1998). Based on the large number of infected women who fail to show symptoms until liver damage has occurred, all pregnant women early in pregnancy and those at risk should be screened routinely for this virus (U.S. Preventive Services Task Force, 2004a). HBV immunization (three shots over a period of 6 months) may be given before or during pregnancy to a mother who is seronegative (CDC, 1998). According to Fanaroff and Martin (1997), most women harboring the virus transmit it through the placenta to the fetus or through contaminated urine, feces, saliva, or vaginal fluids during birth. Many women carrying the virus deliver prematurely, and some infants may have acute hepatitis or later develop liver cancer.

Other Health Concerns

Pregnant women may also develop any of the infections of nonpregnant women. For example, pregnant women frequently experience upper respiratory and gastrointestinal infections, adding to the discomforts of pregnancy.

However, there is no evidence the viruses causing these infections have a teratogenic effect on the fetus.

Fever frequently occurs with illness. A high, prolonged fever (hyperthermia) in a pregnant woman may harm the fetus, especially during the first trimester. Some literature indicates that high fever is associated with miscarriages, stillbirths, and premature deliveries. Whether the high fever or an underlying illness causing the fever has created the problem must be determined. Some reports have also correlated prolonged use of a sauna or hot tub, causing hyperthermia, with birth defects such as microcephaly, anencephaly, and hypotonia. Until health care providers understand this issue better, the nurse should advise pregnant women to avoid prolonged sauna or hot tub use and people who are ill or carrying disease. When a pregnant woman develops a high fever, she should be advised to contact her health care provider immediately.

Pregnant mothers may have other health problems that influence their physiological processes and thus harm the developing fetus. Black women experience twice the rate of hypertension and diabetes mellitus as do white women. These higher rates may account for the 3 to 4 times higher maternal mortality rate seen among pregnant black women as compared with white women (USDHHS, 2000).

Diabetes. Diabetes may exist before or during pregnancy, affecting both mother and fetus. Pregnancy increases the need for maternal insulin to balance the woman's blood sugar. Currently the American College of Obstetricians and Gynecologists recommends that all pregnant women complete a glucose tolerance test at 28 weeks' gestation to identify abnormal blood glucose utilization and need for additional monitoring. Complications from diabetes during pregnancy include polyhydramnios, acidosis, increased rate of infection, vascular complications, and increased risk of pregnancy-induced hypertension. Because of an increased incidence of intrauterine death after 36 weeks of gestation, early and cesarean delivery of these infants often occurs. Neonatal complications from diabetes include hypoglycemia, respiratory distress syndrome, hyperbilirubinemia, and hypocalcemia. Infants of mothers with diabetes also have a higher incidence of congenital anomalies, such as a heart lesion or meningocele (Creasy & Resnik, 1999). The diabetic pregnant woman needs close health care team supervision and ongoing health teaching, including diet and exercise management, in order to control her disease effectively.

Heart Disease and Hypertension. Heart disease and hypertension are the two serious maternal cardiovascular problems during pregnancy. Rheumatic heart disease, a common problem, contributes to congestive heart failure, threatening both the mother's and fetus' life. The fetus may be premature because of the need for early delivery. Chronic hypertension, seen more frequently in first-time mothers over age 35, increases the chance of stillbirths, premature delivery, and the development of pregnancy-induced hypertension, which increase both maternal and infant mortality

rates. Mothers with these problems must be monitored closely throughout pregnancy to prevent complications (Garrett, 1999).

Rh Blood Group Incompatibility. Rh blood group incompatibility sometimes affects fetal development. This problem usually occurs when the mother has Rh-negative red blood cells and the fetus has Rh-positive red blood cells. Rh incompatibility affects 10% to 15% of white women, 5% of black women, but few Asian women (Lowdermilk & Perry, 2003g). In this disorder maternal antibodies develop, cross the placental membranes, and destroy the Rh-positive red blood cells of the fetus. Based on the severity of the response, the infant may develop varying levels of hyperbilirubinemia after birth or may die in utero from the anemia of erythroblastosis fetalis.

All women should be assessed for blood type, Rh factor, and antibody development to Rh-positive cells at their first prenatal care visit and again at 24 to 28 weeks of pregnancy unless the father of the baby is Rh negative (U.S. Preventive Services Task Force, 2004b). Rh incompatibility between a mother and future fetus may be prevented by administering $Rh_o(D)$ immune globulin (RhoGAM) to an Rh-negative mother at 28 weeks of gestation and within 72 hours after birth. The immunization prevents the mother's sensitization to fetal Rh-negative cells by inactivating fetal red blood cells in the mother before she can develop an antibody response. The ideal injection time is after the mother's first delivery of an Rh-positive infant, miscarriage, or therapeutic abortion. The incompatibility generally does not occur during the first pregnancy, and the immunization prevents problems with later pregnancies.

Chemical Agents

Drugs ingested by the mother may be teratogenic to the fetus. The tragic experience with the tranquilizer drug **thalidomide** during the early 1960s led to a recommendation that medications be avoided almost completely during pregnancy, unless a physician or a midwife approves their use. The fact remains, however, that during the most critical early weeks of fetal development and growth when many women do not know they are pregnant, ingested drugs may seriously affect the fetus. Based on fetal gestational age and drug metabolism, drugs may alter the placenta itself or directly affect development and growth of the fetus. The drugs that most commonly cause congenital defects are prescription medications, over-the-counter (OTC) drugs, street drugs, nicotine (cigarettes), caffeine, and alcohol. The U.S. Food and Drug Administration has labeled some of these drugs with an "X"; this means that scientific studies have shown negative fetal effects when pregnant women take them.

Prescription Medications

Women frequently become pregnant while on medications for illnesses diagnosed before pregnancy, such as hypertension, or they may receive medication to treat an illness acquired during pregnancy, such as a UTI. Some of the more common drugs that have been studied for fetal effects include antibiotics and anticonvulsants.

Most short-term and usual-dose antibiotics do not cause fetal harm. Tetracycline given to a pregnant mother between the fourth month of pregnancy and delivery, however, may cause abnormalities in tooth development, including brown spotting and enamel hypoplasia (Gorrie, McKinney, & Murray, 1994; Spratto & Woods, 2001). Primary teeth seem most affected, but when the antibiotic is given near the time of delivery the permanent teeth may be damaged, also.

The effects of anticonvulsants on the fetus have been documented thoroughly. Women with seizure disorders have carried infants to term while being treated with hydantoin, barbiturates, and other antiseizure medications. Infants born to mothers taking hydantoin (Dilantin) may have fetal hydantoin syndrome, reflected in microcephaly, retardation, cleft lip and palate, and congenital heart disease. Barbiturates, such as phenobarbital, may cause newborn addiction. Women with seizure disorders should discuss their medication requirements with their physicians before becoming pregnant and have close health care team monitoring throughout pregnancy.

Over-the-Counter Drugs

Pregnant women frequently choose to treat minor illnesses with OTC drugs. Research on acetylsalicylic acid (aspirin) and acetaminophen (Tylenol) indicates that both medications are safe in recommended dosages. However, aspirin alters platelet function and may cause maternal and newborn bleeding if taken close to delivery. Acetaminophen can be toxic to the liver. Certain ingredients in common cold remedies have been associated with fetal irritability (Spratto & Woods, 2001). Ibuprofen may prolong labor based on its antiprostaglandin effect. Any drug may harm a fetus, so all drugs should be avoided during pregnancy.

The nurse should include information on the known and probable effects of medications on the fetus in prenatal teaching of couples. Discussion of herbal treatments should also be included, because little research exists on their effects and interactions with more traditional medications. The nurse must recognize that many cultural groups use these nontraditional agents, because they believe that they will effectively manage pregnancy-related concerns. The nurse may need to encourage a client to reconsider the use of herbs when evidence exists that these may harm the fetus or mother.

Drug Abuse

Maternal use of narcotics, tranquilizers, cocaine, amphetamines, marijuana, and other drugs may cause serious health problems to both the mother and unborn child. These drugs represent an enormous cost to society by causing increased risks of low birth weight, preterm birth, and deficits in child development if the mother ingests them during pregnancy (D'Apolito, 1998; Sable & Herman, 1997).

Narcotics. The narcotics heroin and methadone cause infant prematurity, IUGR, respiratory distress at birth, fetal addiction in utero, and neonatal withdrawal after birth. Signs of narcotic withdrawal in the newborn include tremors, irritability, hyperactivity, vomiting, diarrhea, sweating, poor feeding, and possibly convulsions. No evidence suggests withdrawal in infants whose mothers used cocaine or amphetamines, although some animal experiments indicate that these drugs cause impaired fetal growth and increased rates of spontaneous abortion (Bennett, 1999). Frequent maternal marijuana use during pregnancy may cause fetal immunological problems. To avoid these problems, nurses must recognize women who abuse drugs and assist them in seeking appropriate help. This task may be difficult because drug abusers often try to hide their habit, fear being reported to the police, and may be unable to change their lifestyle without extensive intervention.

Alcohol. Many women in today's society drink alcohol regularly. However, alcohol crosses the placenta and may cause fetal death early in pregnancy. Fetal exposure to alcohol throughout pregnancy may cause fetal alcohol syndrome, a collection of symptoms including IUGR, increased risk of anomalies, structural brain abnormalities, attention deficit hyperactivity disorder, and retardation (Stratton, Howe, & Battaglia, 1996). Studies have shown that no safe level of alcohol use exists during pregnancy; therefore, alcohol should be avoided during this time and when attempting conception. Particularly among blacks, Native Americans, and Alaskan Natives, rates of fetal alcohol syndrome have increased over the last decade (D'Apolito, 1998; USDHHS, 2000).

Nicotine. Since the 1940s evidence has existed that cigarette smoking by pregnant mothers causes fetal problems. The U.S. Preventive Services Task Force (2003) recommends screening of all pregnant women for tobacco use and pregnancy-tailored counseling for those who smoke and as proposed by the Association of Women's Health and Obstetric, Neonatal Nurses (AWHONN, 2004) (Innovative Practice box). Evidence indicates that maternal smoking causes increased rates of spontaneous abortion, low birth weight, preterm delivery, placental abnormalities, vaginal bleeding, congenital anomalies, and premature rupture of the membranes (Bennett, 1999; Lee, 1998). These conditions place the fetus at risk for illness or death, as well as learning difficulties during the school years. Even secondhand smoke, gained from exposure to someone else's smoking, may create fetal problems. The best advice for pregnant mothers or women considering pregnancy is not to smoke at all, decrease smoking if one is a heavy smoker, and avoid places where smoking occurs. The nurse needs to understand the context of a smoking woman's life and the complexity of her choice to quit smoking in order to propose solutions to decrease fetal exposure to nicotine (Research Highlights box).

Caffeine. Coffee, cocoa, tea, cola, and chocolate contain caffeine, another addictive drug. Gene mutations have been found in laboratory animals exposed to moder-

Development of Protocol for Smoking Cessation During Pregnancy

Based on a concern about the numbers of pregnant women who smoke and lack of a consistent approach to stopping this habit, AWHONN has proposed testing an evidence-based clinical practice guideline called SUCCESS. This research project will focus on nurses and other health care providers delivering a multifaceted intervention that is expected to increase the success of smoking cessation among childbearing women.

Thirteen clinical sites in the United States and Canada that meet study criteria will participate in the research study involving an expected 6000 women, 1000 of which currently smoke or face the risk of returning to this habit once they give birth. Using research-based practice guidelines, researchers will investigate whether changed smoking practices decrease health-related risks to women and newborns involved in the study.

The study will incorporate previously tested programs from a variety of agencies focused on smoking cessation. Culturally sensitive tools will be used to screen participants. Trained nurses will deliver standard smoking cessation counseling approaches from previously tested programs. Materials such as the U.S. Department of Health and Human Services, Public Health Service's publication, Treating Tobacco Use and Dependence: A Clinical Practice Guideline, *Healthy People 2010*, and patient education materials developed by Smoke Free Families will structure and evaluate the SUCCESS program.

From Association of Women's Health, Obstetrical, and Neonatal Nursing. (2004). SUCCESS: Nursing care for pregnant women who smoke. Retrieved May 19, 2004, from: *http://www.awhonn.org/awhonn/ ?pg=874-2190-6070-6080.*
AWHONN, Association of Women's Health, Obstetrical, and Neonatal Nursing; SUCCESS, Setting Universal Cessation Counseling, Education, and Screening Standards.

Context of Smoking and Smoking Cessation

The purpose of this study was to describe the context of the lives of recently delivered African American women who smoke, related to their smoking and smoking cessation beliefs and behaviors.

The sample included 15 women with an average age of 25.7 years and an educational level of 10.7 years. Most women reported an annual income of less than $10,000 and had previously participated in a smoking cessation program called Smoke Free Families. Sixty percent of the women had pregnancy complications, and most had one or more perinatal risk factors. After receipt of informed consent, individual women responded to interviews that contributed qualitative data for the study. Thematic content analysis occurred to identify themes of the women's responses.

Two predominant themes evolved from the study data, living the stressed life (context theme) and personal accountability for smoking cessation (belief theme). Women related their personal and community stressors, including financial, parenting, lack of social support, violence, and chronic health problems that prevented effective coping. Although most women knew the relationship between smoking and fetal and maternal health problems, they noted that cigarettes were an easily accessible resource that they needed to manage their life stressors. Women noted they could not stop smoking without more personal determination, a behavior that many lacked as a result of their life stressors.

The study displays the context of a sample of African American women's lives and various barriers to their smoking cessation. The authors emphasize that to help these women stop smoking, a focus broader than the individual must be used. They suggest that health care policy must address changing the living environments of these women. Nurses have a responsibility to support organizational and legislative policies that will improve access to care, safer neighborhoods, and additional educational opportunities for these women if the quality of their lives is to improve.

From Pletsche, P. K., Morgan, S., & Pieper, A. I. (2003). Context and beliefs about smoking and smoking cessation. *Maternal Child Nursing, 28,* 320-325.

ate amounts of caffeine; however, these defects have not been found in human beings. At least one study implicates excess caffeine intake (more than 300 mg or more than three cups of coffee per day) during pregnancy with problems such as spontaneous abortions, IUGR, and prematurity (Santos, Victora, Huttly, & Carvalhal, 1998). Until additional research clarifies the relationship between caffeine intake and fetal effects, caregivers should teach pregnant women to avoid excess caffeine intake.

Environmental Chemicals

The influence of these chemicals on human development remains unclear. Some natural substances found to be teratogenic in animals, but not necessarily in human beings, include insect and bacterial toxins, insecticides, herbicides, and fungicides, including dichlorodiphenyltrichloroethane, or DDT. Recent studies involving pregnant women who eat fish with high mercury levels support evidence that mercury negatively affects fetal development, particularly brain development. Some studies report stillbirths, abortions, and

mental retardation in fetuses exposed to lead. This area needs more study, particularly with more women working in traditional male workplaces where there are environmental contaminants. Nurses should assess and provide women in their first trimester with information on environmental agents that are potentially damaging throughout gestation and counsel them on ways to avoid exposure.

Medications Given During Delivery

The final time that the fetus encounters drugs through the mother is during delivery. Many women desire medications for labor discomforts, and usually only medications deemed safe and monitored closely during labor and birth have been used (e.g., epidural anesthesia, meperidine [Demerol] in small doses). Some analgesic drugs administered during labor, such as meperidine, can cause respiratory depression in the fetus and influence the rate and quality of the infant's adaptation to extrauterine life. Studies of visual attentiveness, sucking behavior, and neurological and electroencephalography suggest that fetal depressant effects may last as long as days after birth.

Mechanical Forces

The amniotic fluid reservoir protects the fetus during pregnancy and during mild to moderate trauma to the mother's abdomen. However, major trauma to the mother's abdomen, such as that sustained in a severe car accident, may cause maternal bleeding, preterm labor, and other concerns. The nurse should instruct the pregnant woman in the proper way to wear both a lap belt and shoulder harness to protect her and her fetus while driving. All women in the second and third trimester should be encouraged to seek medical care following an accident believed to influence the health of mother or fetus.

The uterus, another mechanical force, also influences the fetus. Near the end of pregnancy, the fetus outgrows the uterus and becomes molded by it, particularly in cases of multiple pregnancy. Some children have congenitally dislocated hips from uterine pressure and fetal position in utero. Most deformities return to normal either naturally or with repositioning after birth. Fetal malposition cannot be prevented; therefore, the neonate should be assessed for problems and support provided to the parents about the newborn's appearance.

The actual labor and delivery process represents the final mechanical force. Few newborns experience injury during this process, and those who do usually recover with no effect. Some of the more common injuries that occur during this time appear in **Web Site Resource 16F.** Predicting and preventing traumas during birth is difficult, such as when delivery of an infant who is larger than expected requires forceps, which may injure the child. In these cases, based on health care team assessment, the mother may undergo cesarean delivery to protect her and the baby.

Radiation

Scientific evidence indicates that exposure to x-rays, especially early in pregnancy, may cause chromosomal changes that result in fetal loss or malignancy later in life. Literature supports a greater incidence of leukemia in children of women exposed to x-rays during pregnancy compared with children whose mothers were not exposed. Unless the benefits of radiographic information clearly outweigh the risks of exposing the fetus to x-rays, these examinations should not be performed during gestation. If radiography is deemed necessary, a lead apron, as low a radiation dose as possible, and other recommendations made by the National Council on Radiation Protection and Measurements should be used to protect the developing fetus.

SOCIAL PROCESSES
Community and Work

Many more women now work outside the home, either in careers or jobs needed for family economic survival. As each woman considers or experiences pregnancy, she will need to ask herself questions that will optimize her pregnancy outcome. These questions include the following: Is my work strenuous or possibly dangerous to my baby because of exposure to toxic substances? Do I need to work for long periods, influencing my need for rest? Will workplace stressors influence my coping with pregnancy and my family needs?

A safe workplace environment (one that does not involve exposure to hazardous substances or organisms and provides adequate breaks for worker rest and body movement), will allow a pregnant woman to work until her baby is due, unless her health becomes impaired. The nurse can help each woman assess the safety of her workplace and suggest ways to decrease hazards in that setting. These hazards include exposure to viruses, fungi, industrial products (hydrocarbons or pesticides), smoke, radiation emitted by medical diagnostic equipment, air pollutants, asbestos, possibility for workplace violence, mental and physical stress, and even noise pollution. The nurse must also encourage the pregnant worker to consider workplace ergonomics, addressing how the current work space will meet her changing physical needs.

Some employers in this country have been designated creators of "family friendly" work environments, because they have willingly made accommodations to support pregnant workers. These accommodations allow women to prioritize their pregnancy and family needs. Evidence indicates that such approaches reduce pregnancy complications and increase work productivity. Although few in number, family friendly employers offer health-promotion programs focusing on healthy nutrition, stress management, and exercise for employees, who experience better pregnancy outcomes.

As a rule, however, too few employers support flexible work schedules for prenatal care visits, rest periods for pregnant workers, or removal of vending machines to support optimal nutrition for pregnant working class women. Some working women, regardless of status, believe that once they announce their pregnancy, they will face workplace pressure to stop working or change positions in the company based on their gestational needs. Based on experience, some employers fear that their pregnant employees will overuse sick time or seek a reduced workload. The pregnant woman must deal with these situations by being factual and assertive about her ability to continue working. National law dictates that it is illegal to discriminate against a woman because she is pregnant. If a woman believes that she has been treated unfairly because of her pregnancy, then she may pursue the issue legally or become active in local women's rights organizations to gain support. However, when a woman leaves a job that did not support her pregnancy, she often gives up accrued leave time or takes a lower salary at another job. These outcomes influence her choices during pregnancy and early parenting.

Workplaces vary greatly in allowing leave time during and after pregnancy. Federal legislation, the Family and Medical Leave Act, obligates employers of at least 50 people to provide up to 12 weeks' paid leave for new parents or women who have medical problems during pregnancy. Ideally a woman who desires children should explore the issue of leave during a job interview, but many women fail to do this until they are already pregnant. A woman often requires written verification from her physician if she needs a leave of absence from her job due to pregnancy complications. Although she may wish to return to work shortly after delivery, the woman should be counseled to allow sufficient time to regain her strength and adapt to parenting. The nurse may help the woman make reasonable decisions related to locating resources for child care, exploring "shared-time" with other new mothers in the woman's workplace, or for balancing work and family needs.

Culture and Ethnicity

Cultural groups have unique ideas and beliefs related to pregnancy, childbirth, and childbearing that must be understood by the nurse in order to render individualized care to each pregnant woman. **Web Site Resource 16G** presents a list of questions to ask the client to gain this understanding. As part of the assessment, the nurse must also determine the cultural attachment of a woman by asking the following question: Does she think that some or most of the childbearing ideas of her culture are old fashioned, but does she feel obligated to follow these ideas, at least superficially, because of family pressure? In this situation, the nurse may need to be a confidant for the woman who needs to vent her frustrations about cultural restrictions. Nursing support may assist the individual in adjusting both her needs and those of the culture she represents to experience a satisfactory pregnancy.

The nurse has an obligation to read about and seek information on cultures encountered in practice and to become active in community organizations that represent cultures whose members get prenatal care from the nurse. Above all, the nurse must be open to a variety of viewpoints, judging them not against personal beliefs, but rather in relation to the general concept of health promotion and today's goal to provide culturally competent care to a variety of cultural groups (Multicultural Awareness box).

Legislation

Both legislative actions and social movements influence childbearing. In some countries, such as China, the government decrees the number of children a couple may have and imposes economic or social sanctions to enforce these restrictions. Although Americans may have as many children as they desire, various coalitions lobby strongly for families. The recent Family and Medical Leave Act validates the federal government's commitment to prioritizing family issues by giving new parents time off from work during the

---

MULTICULTURAL AWARENESS

Nursing Roles in Providing Culturally Competent Care

Delivery of culturally competent care implies that a nurse acknowledges and acts on the unique history that a pregnant woman and family bring to a health care interaction. The nurse supports culturally competent care by:

- Recognizing that cultural diversity exists and affects the process and outcome of health care
- Respecting people as unique individuals who, by their differences from the majority, bring a broadened definition of appropriate health care
- Using data gained from a cultural assessment for completion of a care plan
- Encouraging cultural behavior that protects the biopsychosocial, spiritual, and safety needs of the individual
- Gaining insight into the nurse's own beliefs and values about people who may be different or have different needs than the majority or those of the nurse's own culture; understanding how these beliefs and values influence the outcomes of health care delivery with childbearing families
- Recognizing the values of the health care system reflected in the customs and practices of birthing facilities and responding to these facilities based on one's value system
- Providing interpreters to improve communication between the individual and health care providers
- Becoming literate in languages, customs, and cultural practices of people commonly seen in the health care environment

---

early months of parenthood, while supporting these individuals' professional work goals and needs.

The U.S. government remains concerned about the health of pregnant women and ways to decrease fetal and infant morbidity and mortality. Historically states have used federal monies from Medicaid and Title V maternal and child health block programs to provide services for pregnant women and children. Many countries provide universal access to prenatal care, but in the United States low-income women rely on Medicaid, a joint federal-state program, to cover most of the cost of prenatal care. With constraints on state and federal budgets, many of which fund community prenatal clinics, concerns have been expressed about whether sufficient money will exist for funding women and children's care programs. Local health departments may offer free or low-cost prenatal care for women who are pregnant, but again, the extent of services depends on state government or local allocation of funds. Despite this free or low-cost care, over 44 million Americans overall lack health insurance and, therefore, face barriers that affect their easy access to prenatal care (covertheuninsured week.org, 2005; (DeNavas, Proctor, & Mills, 2004); USDHHS, 2000). Many ethnically diverse populations and, in particular, Hispanic groups, lack insurance and a level of education that increases their understanding of health-related information for family health promotion. Educating women during the childbearing cycle seems particularly important to increase the chances of families obtaining and understanding health-promotion information for healthier behaviors (USDHHS, 2000).

With the nurse's help, consumers should be encouraged to express their views on pregnancy and parenting topics to their elected governmental representatives (Cobb, 1998). This expression indeed works; many states recently legislated hospital stays of at least 48 hours for women with vaginal deliveries and even longer stays for women with cesarean deliveries. These laws evolved from public concern over premature discharges of new mothers as part of managed care insurance directives. Longer stays help health care providers identify potential problems in the mother or the baby before discharge, such as difficulty breast-feeding. Continued legislative work on insurance reform may improve family planning services so that couples can plan pregnancies to better meet their sociocultural and financial goals and needs (USDHHS, 2000). Insurance reform, driven by legislative change, may also improve health care coverage for underinsured individuals who lack a consistent source of prenatal care or report difficulties in receiving care because of communication, structural, or personal barriers within their insurance system (Physicians for a National Health Program, 2004).

Economics

When the pregnant woman begins prenatal care, personal financial resources influence the kind of care she receives, whether she works during or after a pregnancy, her acceptance of a pregnancy, her nutritional status, and other choices. The expenses of planning and experiencing a pregnancy may determine whether the woman or her family face a financial crisis. The nurse must understand the financial history and priorities of the couple, because this information will affect access to and use of prenatal care.

The nurse inquires in a sensitive fashion about a woman's or couple's finances to make appropriate referral to resources for care (e.g., Title V or Medicaid programs). Until recently, Medicaid provided no adolescent family planning services, a situation that may have influenced high rates of pregnancy in some sectors of this country (USDHHS, 2000). Many low-income women qualify for the U.S. Department of Agriculture's supplemental feeding program for women, infants, and children (WIC). This program provides essential foods such as milk, cheese, and eggs to pregnant and lactating women. During prenatal visits, the nurse may help a woman or family plan a budget for food and other essential requirements based on individual family needs, cultural values, need for a healthy diet during pregnancy, and income. Local food banks and secondhand clothing and baby supply stores may provide needed items for these families. Occasionally women may access free transportation and child care at the prenatal clinic if the nurse provides information about this program.

Health Care Delivery System

Options for care during pregnancy range from medical-based care by an obstetrician or general practitioner to more health promotion–focused care by a nurse or lay midwife. Geographical availability of options, finances, previous experience, partner's preference, cultural or social acceptability of certain options, and preexisting or newly recognized risk factors will influence a woman's choice of care. Based on her culture and the belief that pregnancy is not an illness, a woman may not seek Western medical prenatal care, but rather may rely on individuals of her culture to provide care until the actual labor, when she will go to a hospital.

A woman generally chooses where she will labor and deliver and the extent of labor and delivery intervention unless complications arise. The movement toward home birth that began during the early 1970s continues to meet some consumer needs for a more family-oriented, natural, health-focused experience. However, most couples choose a hospital birth setting because of availability of emergency equipment and personnel in case of complications. Some insurance companies will cover only deliveries done in hospitals and in birth centers or birthing rooms attached to a hospital. The nurse helps expectant couples become aware of the care and delivery alternatives to make an informed choice for a positive labor and delivery experience. Women who lack resources to access the health care delivery system and teaching by the nurse during regular prenatal visits generally are less able to make informed decisions that affect their childbearing experiences.

Many expectant couples also make an informed choice about the actual process of labor and delivery by developing a birth plan, those components of care and intervention that the couple desires for the birth experience. A pregnant woman and partner may choose natural childbirth or a method of analgesia or anesthesia. The nurse helps the pregnant woman and her partner choose the most appropriate method by providing information about options and encouraging questions about each one. Collaboration between the nurse and woman or couple in meeting their birth plan goals is important, because research shows that women remember their labor and delivery experiences for a long time. A positively viewed birth experience may support a couple's involvement as active health care consumers, thus facilitating their future health.

The nurse may encourage the pregnant couple or woman to attend prenatal classes. These provide valuable information and preparation for birth for many couples. The International Childbirth Education Association, the American Society for Psychoprophylaxis in Obstetrics (ASPO), and many local groups offer a variety of classes for the expectant couple. These classes may include information on early pregnancy, Lamaze-ASPO or Bradley methods, cesarean birth, breast-feeding, infant cardiopulmonary resuscitation, and parenting. Sibling classes for the newborn and involvement of children in the birth experience may also increase sibling bonding.

NURSING INTERVENTIONS

Teaching the pregnant woman and her partner during the prenatal period is the most important role of the nurse. Even the woman who has previously delivered or who has a high degree of education may need or want information from the health care team that will assist her family to adapt effectively to changes of pregnancy to support a healthy birth outcome.

To provide appropriate teaching, the nurse must perform a comprehensive assessment that involves the entire family, such as that presented in **Web Site Resource 16H.** Assessment, the first step in the nursing process, allows the nurse to determine maternal and fetal physical and psychological risks, the woman's informational base for pregnancy and birth, and cultural and family needs. Assessment should also include physical, spiritual, emotional, and sociocultural inspection and recognition of abuse. Battering increases during pregnancy and may be detected by physical, emotional, and history assessment of the woman (see Hot Topics box). Pregnant women at high risk for abuse include adolescents, those with low incomes, and those with a history of alcohol or drug abuse, as well as a partner with a similar history (American College of Obstetricians and Gynecologists, 2002; U.S. Preventive Services Task Force, 2004c). In cases of suspected abuse, the nurse, in consultation with other members of the health care team, provides support and resources for the woman to make an informed decision about protecting herself and her fetus during pregnancy. The nurse may also want to refer the person to a professional counselor for a brief counseling outreach intervention demonstrated to decrease the incidence of family violence (McFarlane, Soeken, & Wiist, 2000).

As discussed in this chapter, assessment may also be made by using Gordon's functional health patterns, a common conceptual framework for clinical assessment (see Box 16-3). Data used in the assessment process will likely be collected during the prenatal visit and may change, based on life occurrences of the pregnant woman. A woman may be defined as high risk during her pregnancy if she experiences heavy bleeding, premature labor, elevated blood pressure, extreme anxiety, if there is fetal distress, or if she shows unexpected behavior or symptoms. After noting these high-risk conditions, the nurse should refer the pregnant woman to an obstetrical specialist or other resources for pregnant women and their families (see Case Study).

After a complete assessment during each prenatal visit, the nurse develops a teaching plan for the individual. Throughout the prenatal course, the nurse collaborates with the woman and her partner to assess their learning and support needs. For example, literature on bottle feeding or breast-feeding may be provided to help a woman decide on a method, and books videos, and Web sites may help couples understand more about birth and, therefore, feel that they have more control during labor and in meeting their birthing goals. If the woman plans to attend group prenatal classes, the nurse should coordinate her teaching

---

| Box **16-5** | Topics for Prenatal Care Teaching |

1. Rationale for and interpretation of physical findings and laboratory results
2. Value of keeping appointments
3. Danger signs that should be reported
4. Breast care
5. Breast-feeding versus bottle feeding
6. Exercise and rest
7. Fetal growth and development
8. Physical and psychological changes during pregnancy and relief measures
9. Effects of smoking, drinking, and drugs on the fetus
10. Nutrition
11. Work and play
12. Body mechanics
13. Personal hygiene
14. Sex during pregnancy
15. Preparation for labor and birth
16. Superstitions and old wives' tales
17. Signs of impending labor
18. Supplies and preparations for the baby
19. Husband's and siblings' responses

---

content and process with those expected in the classes, thereby preventing undue repetition. The nurse teaching prenatal classes should provide a list of topics to participants in the class to share with their health care providers. A woman may be knowledgeable in some areas, and the nurse can use this knowledge as a foundation for further individualized teaching. Box 16-5 covers relevant topics to be covered by the nurse during prenatal care interactions with pregnant women. These topical areas relate to nursing interventions covered earlier in this chapter. Basic handouts detailing information such as danger signs will provide information that a woman can post at home should she experience unexpected complications of her pregnancy.

SUMMARY

Dramatic changes occur during pregnancy; a new life forms and develops and the expectant family members (mother, father, siblings, and other close members) experience major changes in their roles and relationships with each other. Although all fetal development processes, changes in pregnant women's bodies, and role transitions among family members share common elements, each family uniquely experiences pregnancy because of life experience and personal values. The focus is the entire family, although the nurse most often deals directly with the pregnant woman. The nurse provides valuable resources and information that the family may use to meet its specific needs. The overall nursing goal involves assisting each family to have a healthy pregnancy and birth outcome, to lay the foundation for satisfactory parenting and family life.

AL STUDY MATERIAL

ons in the back of the book, see page 663.

WEB SITE MATERIALS

erials are located on the book's Web site at
olve.elsevier.com/Edelman/.

Links
atent Updates
eb Site Resources

16A   Summary of Fetal Growth and Development During Pregnancy
16B   Structure of Placenta
16C   Systematic Adaptation of the Fetus to Extrauterine Life
16D   Effects of Teratogens on Embryo and Fetus
16E   Physical and Diagnostic Tools Used During Pregnancy
16F   Common Birth Injuries
16G   Cultural Context of Childbearing: Questions for the Nurse to Ask the Client
16H   Prenatal Assessment Guide

REFERENCES

Allen, L. (2000). Anemia and iron deficiency: Effects on pregnancy outcome. *American Journal of Clinical Nutrition, 71*(Suppl), 1280S-1284S.

American College of Obstetricians and Gynecologists. (2002). *Guidelines for women's health care* (2nd ed.). Washington, DC: Author.

Askin, D. (1999). The newborn at risk: Acquired and congenital conditions. In D. L. Lowdermilk, S. E. Perry, & I. M. Bobak (Eds.), *Maternity nursing* (pp. 772-806). St. Louis: Mosby.

Association of Women's Health, Obstetrical, and Neonatal Nursing. (1998). *Standards and guidelines for professional nursing practice in the care of women and newborns* (5th ed.). Washington, DC: The Association.

Association of Women's Health, Obstetrical, and Neonatal Nursing. (2000). *Evidence-based clinical practice guidelines. Nursing management of the second stage of labor.* Washington, DC: Author.

Association of Women's Health, Obstetrical, and Neonatal Nursing. (2004). SUCCESS: Nursing care for pregnant women who smoke. Retrieved May 19, 2004, from: *http://www.awhonn.org/awhonn/?pg=874-2190-6070-6080.*

Bennett, A. (1999). Perinatal substance abuse and the drug-exposed neonate. *Advances in Nursing Practice, 7*(5), 32-36.

Brown, H., & Abernathy, M. (1998). Cytomegalovirus infection. *Seminars in Perinatology, 22*(4), 260-266.

Carlson, B. M. (1999). *Developmental disorders: Causes, mechanisms, and patterns. Human embryology and developmental biology.* St. Louis: Mosby.

Carlson, E. J., & Dattel, B. J. (2000). Infectious disease complications. In A. T. Evans & K. R. Niswander (Eds.), *Manual of obstetrics* (pp. 163-198). Philadelphia: Lippincott Williams & Wilkins.

Centers for Disease Control and Prevention. (1998). Guidelines for treatment of sexually transmitted diseases. *Morbidity and Mortality Weekly Report, 47*(RR-1), 1.

Cobb, M. A. (1998). CNS role in women's health promotion and maintenance in a collaborative practice. *Clinical Nurse Specialist, 12,* 112-115.

Cole, J. (1997). What can babies see at birth? *Mother Baby Journal, 2*(4), 45-47.

Cook, A. J., Gilbert, R. E., Buffolano, W., Zufferey, J., Petersen, E., Jenum, P. A., et al. (2000). Sources of *Toxoplasma* infection in pregnant women: European multicentre case-control study. *British Medical Journal, 321*(7254), 142-147.

covertheuninsuredweek.org. (2005). Retrieved April 19, 2005, from *http://www.covertheuninsuredweek.org/factsheets/display.php?FactsheetID=101.*

Creasy, R., & Resnik, J. (1999) *Maternal-fetal medicine: Principles and practices* (4th ed.). Philadelphia: W. B. Saunders

Cunningham, F. G., Gant, N. F., Leveno, K. J., Gilstrap, L. C., Hauth, J. C., & Wenstrom, K. D. (2001a). The placenta and fetal membranes. *Williams obstetrics* (21st ed., pp. 85-108). New York: McGraw-Hill.

Cunningham, F. G., Gant, N. F., Leveno, K. J., Gilstrap, L. C., Hauth, J. C., & Wenstrom, K. D. (2001b). Maternal adaptation to pregnancy. *Williams obstetrics* (21st ed., pp. 167-200). New York: McGraw-Hill.

Cunningham, F. G., Gant, N. F., Leveno, K. J., Gilstrap, L. C., Hauth, J. C., & Wenstrom, K. D. (2001c). Prenatal care. *Williams obstetrics* (21st ed., pp. 221-247). New York: McGraw-Hill.

Cunningham, F. G., Gant, N. F., Leveno, K. J., Gilstrap, L. C., Hauth, J. C., & Wenstrom, K. D. (2001d). Prenatal diagnosis and fetal therapy. *Williams obstetrics* (21st ed., pp. 765-810). New York: McGraw-Hill.

Cunningham, F. G., Gant, N. F., Leveno, K. J., Gilstrap, L. C., Hauth, J. C., & Wenstrom, K. D. (2001e). Multifetal pregnancy. *Williams obstetrics* (21st ed., pp. 1095-1110). New York: McGraw-Hill.

Cunningham, F. G., Gant, N. F., Leveno, K. J., Gilstrap, L. C., Hauth, J. C., & Wenstrom, K. D. (2001f). Antepartum assessment. *Williams obstetrics* (21st ed., pp.). New York: McGraw-Hill.

D'Apolito, K. (1998). Substance abuse: Infant and childhood outcomes. *Journal of Pediatric Nursing, 13,* 307-316.

DeNavas, C., Proctor, B. D., & Mills, R. J. (2004). *Income, poverty, and health insurance coverage in the United States: 2003.* Current population reports, P60-226. Washington, DC: U.S. Census Bureau, U.S. Government Printing Office.

Duff, P. (2002). Maternal and perinatal infection. In S. Gabbe, J. Niebyl, & J. Simpson (Eds.), *Obstetrics: Normal and problem pregnancies* (4th ed.). New York: Churchill Livingstone.

Fanaroff, A., & Martin, R. (1997). *Neonatal-perinatal medicine: Diseases of the fetus and infant* (6th ed.). St. Louis: Mosby.

Frenea, S., Chirossel, C., Rodriquez, R., Baquet, J. P., Racinet, C., & Payen, J. F. (2004). The effects of prolonged ambulation on labor with epidural analgesia. *Anesthesia and Analgesia, 98*(1), 224-229.

Garrett, C. (1999). Assessment for risk factors. In D. L. Lowdermilk, S. E. Perry, & I. M. Bobak (Eds.), *Maternity nursing* (5th ed., pp. 578-600). St. Louis: Mosby.

GeographyIQ (n.d.). *World atlas—rankings—infant mortality rate (all ascending).* Retrieved April 12, 2005, from *http://www.geographyiq.com/ranking/ranking_Infant_Morality_Rate_aa11.htm.*

Georges, J. M. (2000). Female genital and reproductive function. In L. C. Copstead & J. L. Banaski (Eds.), *Pathophysiology: Biological and behavioral perspectives* (2nd ed., pp. 742-781). Philadelphia: W. B. Saunders.

Gordon, M. (1995). *Nursing diagnoses: 1995–96.* St. Louis: Mosby.

Gorrie, T. M., McKinney, E. S., & Murray, S. S. (1994). Effects of drug use during pregnancy and breastfeeding. In *Foundations of maternal newborn nursing* (pp. 973-977). Philadelphia: W. B. Saunders.

Gupta, J., & Nikoderm, V. (2000). Women's position during second stage of labor (Cochrane Review). *The Cochrane Library,* Issue 4. Oxford: Update Software.

Guyton, A. C., & Hall, J. E. (1997). *Human physiology and mechanisms of disease* (6th ed., pp. 670-683). Philadelphia: W. B. Saunders.

Institute of Medicine, Subcommittee on Nutritional Status during Pregnancy and Lactation. (1990). *Nutrition during pregnancy.* Washington, DC: Institute of Medicine, National Academy of Sciences.

Juretschke, L. (2000). Apgar scoring: Its use and meaning for today's newborn. *Neonatal Network, 19*(1), 17-19.

Kost, K., Landry, D., & Darroch, J. (1998a). Predicting maternal behaviors during pregnancy: Does intention status matter? *Family Planning Perspectives, 30*(2), 79-88.

Kost, K., Landry, D., & Darroch, J. (1998b). The effects of pregnancy planning status on birth outcomes and infant care. *Family Planning Perspectives, 30*(5), 223-230.

Lee, M. (1998). Marihuana and tobacco use with pregnancy. *Obstetrics & Gynecology Clinics of North America, 25*(1), 65-83.

Lowdermilk, D. L., & Perry, S. E. (2003a). Genetics, conception, and fetal development. In *Maternity nursing* (6th ed., pp. 140-165). St Louis: Mosby.

Lowdermilk, D. L., & Perry, S. E. (2003b). Anatomy and physiology of pregnancy. In *Maternity nursing* (6th ed., pp. 166-186). St Louis: Mosby.

Lowdermilk, D. L., & Perry, S. E. (2003c). Psychologic and behavioural approaches. In *Maternity nursing* (6th ed., pp. 439-460). St Louis: Mosby.

Lowdermilk, D. L., & Perry, S. E. (2003d). Maternal and fetal nutrition. In *Maternity nursing* (6th ed., pp. 233-255). St Louis: Mosby.

Lowdermilk, D. L., & Perry, S. E. (2003e). Pregnancy at risk: Gestational complications. In *Maternity nursing* (6th ed., pp. 604-647). St Louis: Mosby.

Lowdermilk, D. L., & Perry, S. E. (2003f). The newborn at risk: Acquired and congenital problems. In *Maternity nursing* (6th ed., pp. 748-793). St Louis: Mosby.

Lynfield, R., & Guerina, N. (1997). Toxoplasmosis. *Pediatric Review, 18*(3), 75-83.

Manning, F. (1999). General principles and application of ultrasonography. In R. Creasy & J. Resnik (Eds.), *Maternal-fetal medicine: Principles and practice* (4th ed., pp. 169-206). Philadelphia: W. B. Saunders.

McFarlane, J., Soeken, K., & Wiist, W. (2000). An evaluation of interventions to decrease intimate partner violence to pregnant women. *Public Health Nursing, 17,* 443-451.

O'Leary, J. M., & Thorwick, C. (1997). Impact of pregnancy loss on subsequent pregnancy. In J. R. Woods & J. L. E. Woods (Eds.), *Loss during pregnancy or the newborn period* (pp. 431-451). Pitman, NJ: Jannetti Publications.

O'Toole, M. L., Sawicki, M. A., & Artal, R. (2003). Structured diet and physical activity prevent postpartum weight retention. *Journal of Women's Health, 12,* 991-998.

Pagana, K., & Pagana, T. (2001). *Mosby's diagnostic and laboratory test reference* (5th ed.). St Louis: Mosby.

Perry, S. E. (1999). Conception and fetal development. In D. L. Lowdermilk, S. E. Perry, & I. M. Bobak (Eds.), *Maternity nursing* (5th ed., pp. 158-184). St. Louis: Mosby.

Physicians for a National Health Program. (n.d.). *A national health program for the United States: A physician's proposal.* Retrieved April 12, 2005, from *http://www.pnhp.org/publications/a_national_health_program_for_the_united_states_pnhp.*

Piotrowski, A. (1999). Nursing care during labor and birth. In D. L. Lowdermilk, S. E. Perry, & I. M. Bobak (Eds.), *Maternity nursing* (5th ed., pp. 348-406). St. Louis: Mosby.

Rubin, R. (1967). Attainment of the maternal role. Part I. Processes. *Nursing Research, 16,* 237-245.

Rubin, R. (1972). Fantasy and object constancy in maternal relationships. *Maternal and Child Nursing Journal, 2,* 101-111.

Rubin, R. (1977). Binding in the postpartum period. *Maternal and Child Nursing Journal, 6,* 67-75.

Rubin, R. (1984). *Maternal identity and the maternal experience.* New York: Springer.

Sable, M. R., & Herman, A. A. (1997). The relationship between prenatal health behavior advice and low birth weight. *Public Health Reports, 112,* 332-339.

Santos, I. S., Victora, C. G., Huttly, S., & Carvalhal, J. B. (1998). Caffeine intake and low birth weight: A population-based case-control study. *American Journal of Epidemiology, 147,* 620-627.

Smedley, B. D., Stith, A. Y., & Nelson, A. R. (2003). *Unequal treatment: Confronting racial and ethnic disparities in health care* (pp. 80-198). Washington, DC: National Academies Press.

Spratto, G. R., & Woods, A. L. (2001). *PDR: Nurses' drug handbook.* Montvale, NJ: Medical Economics Company.

Stratton, K., Howe, C., & Battalgia, F. (1996). *Fetal alcohol syndrome: Diagnosis, epidemiology, prevention, and treatment.* Washington, DC: National Academy Press.

U.S. Department of Health and Human Services. (2000). *Healthy people 2010: Vol. 1* (Conference ed.). Washington, DC: U.S. Government Printing Office.

U.S. Preventive Services Task Force (2001). Screening for bacterial vaginosis: Recommendations and rationale, 2001. *American Journal of Preventive Medicine, 20*(3S), 59-61. Retrieved May 11, 2004, from: *http://www.ahrq.gov/clinic/ajpmsuppl/bvrr.htm.*

U.S. Preventive Services Task Force (2003, November). Counseling: Tobacco use. Retrieved April 12, 2005, from: *http://www.ahrq.gov/clinic/uspstr/uspstbac/htm.*

U.S. Preventive Services Task Force. (2004a). Screening for Hepatitis B Virus Infection. Retrieved July 16, 2005, from: *http://www.ahrq.gov/clinic/3rduspstf/hepbscv/hepbrs.htm.*

U.S. Preventive Services Task Force. (2004b). Screening for Rh(D) incompatibility: Recommendation statement, February 2004. Retrieved May 19, 2004, from: *http://www.ahrq.gov/clinic/3rduspstf/rh/rhrs.htm.*

U.S. Preventive Services Task Force. (2004c). Screening children for family violence. Retrieved May 11, 2004, from:*http://www.ahrq.gov/clinic/3rduspstf/famviolence/childrev.htm.*

17

SUSAN SCOTT RICCI

Infant

objectives

After completing this chapter, the reader will be able to:

- Evaluate the infant's health status and give examples of basic growth and developmental principles.

- Analyze the developmental tasks for the infant and the behavior indicating that these tasks are being met.

- Explain the immunization schedule and other safety and health-promotion measures to a parent.

- Identify common parental concerns about infants and describe a model for parent education to allay these concerns.

- Describe accidents that occur during infancy and recommend appropriate counseling for accident prevention and safety.

- Indicate ways in which nurses can be active in making major policies and influencing legislation concerning health.

- Outline governmental strategies to meet the goals of improving infant health.

key terms

Active immunization
Birth defects
Denver Developmental Screening Test II

Failure-to-thrive syndrome
Growth index
Passive immunization
Reflexes

Sensorimotor period
Sudden infant death syndrome
Weaning

THINK About It

Car Safety Seats

Infants are at particular risk from automobile accidents. The proper use of occupant protection systems (infant car safety seats with seat belts) can reduce the risk of death and injury significantly. Although many public service campaigns encourage parents to restrain their infants while riding in automobiles (and all states have laws requiring some type of passenger safety restraint for infants) some parents remain negligent or unaware of the importance of providing safety for their vulnerable infants.

Nurses must have up-to-date knowledge about car occupant protection systems and their proper use to help

parents find new products and obtain the most current information available. Parents often rely on the salesperson of the infant car seat for their information about protection systems and the proper use of car seats. Informational brochures and media campaigns fall short, because they usually fail to provide explanations or demonstrations. As a result, parents may misinterpret the information that they receive.

1   What type of program might you develop to reach and inform parents about the importance of car seat safety?

Continued

Car Safety Seats *cont'd*

THINK About It

2 In what settings might such a program be implemented?

3 How would you modify your teaching plan to meet the needs of illiterate parents?

4 How would you modify your program to ensure that parents who come from cultural backgrounds different than your own would respond well to the information?

Providing a safe and sound source of attachment and contact interaction is paramount to healthy infant development. Caregiving and mothering activities are the primary ingredients of an infant's preparation for life and ultimate independence. Nurses play a vital role in influencing this positive interaction through health promotion and education.

This chapter focuses on the infant and family during the infant's developmental period of 1 to 18 months. Because the infant is completely dependent, this chapter addresses the infant's parents and significant others in terms of health-promotion activities. The relationship initiated at birth between parents and infant is the basis for the interdependence that is required for proper psychological and physical infant development. Health care professionals must focus on parent education as a means of fostering healthy, satisfying relationships within the family unit and promoting the development of healthy future generations.

The principles of normal growth and development are used as a structural framework for this chapter. Understanding these principles helps the nurse identify deviations from the norm and institute appropriate preventive measures.

To promote and maintain health during infancy, a balance between the infant's internal and external environmental forces must be established; any disruption places the infant at risk. Several processes that greatly influence this balance are identified, and appropriate interventions are outlined to assist the nurse in promoting a healthy infant population (*Healthy People 2010* box).

Healthy People 2010

Selected National Health-Promotion and Disease Prevention Objectives for Infants

- Reduce iron deficiency to less than 5% among infants age 1 to 2 years. (Baseline is 9% for children age 1 to 2 years. *Note:* iron deficiency is defined as having abnormal results for two or more of the following tests: serum ferritin concentration, erythrocyte protoporphyrin, or transferrin saturation.)
- Reduce nonfatal poisonings to no more than 292 nonfatal poisonings per 100,000 population. (Baseline is 348.4 nonfatal poisonings per 100,000 population in 1997.)
- Reduce growth retardation among low-income children age 5 and younger to less than 5%. (Baseline is 8% of low-income children under age 5 years were growth retarded in 1997, depending on race and ethnicity. *Note:* growth retardation is defined as height-for-age below the fifth percentile in the age-gender appropriate population using the NCHS-CDC growth charts.)
- Reduce infant deaths to no more than 4.5 per 1000 live births by the year 2010. (Baseline is 7.2 per 1000 live births in 1998.)
- Reduce deaths from SIDS to less than 0.30 deaths per 1000 live births by the year 2010. (Baseline is 0.77 deaths per 1000 live births were from SIDS in 1997.)
- Increase the percentage of healthy full-term infants who were put down to sleep on their backs to 70% by the year 2010. (Baseline is 35% of healthy full-term infants were put down to sleep on their backs in 1996.)

- Reduce or eliminate indigenous cases of vaccine-preventable disease through universal vaccination by the year 2010. (Target: total elimination for congenital rubella syndrome, diphtheria, *Haemophilus influenzae* type b, measles, mumps, polio, rubella, and tetanus; 41% improvement for pertussis; 99% improvement for hepatitis B; and 99% improvement for varicella.)
- Increase the number of infants age 18 months and younger who have a specific source of ongoing primary care to at least 96%. (Baseline is 93% in 1997.)
- Increase the number of mothers who breast-feed their infants during the early postpartum period to at least 75% and the proportion who continue to breast-feed until 6 months of age to at least 50%. (Baseline is 64% were breast-fed during the early postpartum period in 1998; 29% breast-fed infant until 6 months of age in 1998.)
- Eliminate elevated blood lead levels in children age 1 to 5 years by the year 2010. (Baseline is 4.4% of children age 1 to 5 years with blood lead levels exceeding 10 µg/dl during 1991 to 1994.)
- Increase the use of occupant child restraints by the year 2010 to 100%. (Baseline is 92% of motor vehicle occupants aged 4 years and under used child restraints in 1998.)

From U.S. Department of Health and Human Services. (2000). Healthy *People 2010: Vol. 1 and 2* (Conference ed.). Washington, DC: U.S. Government Printing Office.
NCHS-CDC, National Center for Health Statistics, Centers for Disease Control and Prevention; *SIDS*, sudden infant death syndrome.

PHYSICAL CHANGES

...opment begins when a single sperm penetrates ...m. The changes that follow are undeniable and ...Box 17-1).

...this early period of growth and development the ...pends completely on others, primarily the parents, ...all personal needs. To assist the parents in their ...anding of their infant's progress, the nurse must ...what behaviors to expect at certain age levels. These ...opmental landmarks serve as a basis for anticipatory ...ance (Table 17-1). Parents must be aware of age-...propriate behavior to anticipate and facilitate these ...velopmental landmarks. This knowledge, along with the ...urse's anticipatory guidance, can also promote closer ...amily relationships.

In addition to the growth landmarks, the infant must accomplish several developmental tasks for a healthy personality progression.

Developmental Tasks

Everyone faces developmental tasks and must accomplish them individually. Different practices in various societies affect the perception and resolution of the tasks, but all must be faced (Pillitteri, 2003).

The infant's first and most basic task is survival, which includes the physical tasks of breathing, sucking, eating, digesting, eliminating, and sleeping. Because many of these tasks involve the infant's mouth, this stage of life often is referred to as the *oral stage* of development, reflecting the primary importance of the mouth as the center of pleasure. Duvall and Miller (1984) outline several more developmental tasks that must be accomplished during infancy (Box 17-2).

To assist the infant's parents in encouraging achievement of these developmental tasks, the nurse should discuss the importance of stimulation and environmental interactions. Genetic potential, in terms of the development of the anatomical structures of the brain, is not reached at birth; many neurological structures are far from complete (Silberg, 2001). To continue growing, the brain depends not only on internal, embryological, and maturational forces, but also on the interaction of external stimulation with these forces. Stimulation, as provided by the parents, is necessary for a child to develop fully. This external stimulation appears to influence the internal, anatomical, and maturational processes by at least three different mechanisms (Berger, 2004):

1. Stimulation favors progressive complex arborization of dendrites (the connection between nerve cells).
2. Stimulation increases the degree of vascularization of certain anatomical structures of the brain, such as the centers associated with vision.
3. Stimulation increases the process of myelination, which is closely related to the rate of development of a variety of functions. Myelin coats the brain and nerve tissue, which then becomes activated.

When counseling parents, the nurse stresses the importance of a variety of stimuli within the infant's environment. Several auditory and visual stimuli should be available, such as colorful mobiles, television, radio, spoken voice, and toys, to assist the infant in achieving developmental tasks. The sense of touch is an extremely important stimulus, bringing the infant in tune with the external environment, making it a reality. These parenting tasks are vital to the infant's growth and developmental progression (Pillitteri, 2003).

Concepts of Infant Development

The study of how a helpless infant grows and develops into a fully functioning, independent adult has fascinated many researchers. Their theories are descriptions of the development of human behavior as overlapping stages that occur in somewhat predictable patterns in an individual's life (Mandler, 2004). Because these developmental theories are presented in Chapter 15, only their specific application to the infant is discussed here.

Psychosocial Development

Erikson's psychosocial developmental theory is concerned primarily with a series of tasks or crises that each individual must resolve before encountering the next one. The central task during infancy is the development of a sense of trust versus mistrust. Establishing this basic trust or mistrust determines the manner in which the infant approaches all future stages of growth. The infant first develops a sense of trust in the mother (or other caretaker) and then in other significant people. Trust influences the infant's future relationships, allowing for deeper commitment and intimacy. The infant requires maximal gratification and minimal frustration to provide the balance between inner needs and outer satisfaction, which results in the development of trust. If the mother or caretaker is consistently responsive to the infant's care, meeting physical and psychological needs, the infant will likely learn to trust his or her caretaker; view the world as a safe place; and grow up to be secure, self-reliant, trusting, cooperative, and helpful towards others.

Prompt, skillful, and consistent response to the infant's needs helps foster security and trust; the mother is essentially relieving the infant's tension. Part of developing trust depends on the infant's ability to predict what will happen within the environment. When unpredictability and disorganized routines exist, the infant will develop fear, anger, and insecurity, which eventually lead to mistrust. The infant can demonstrate desire by crying but depends on the sensitivity and willingness of others to provide relief. If the most important people fail to do this, the infant has little foundation on which to build faith in others or self in adulthood.

Cognitive Development

Piaget's cognitive developmental theory focuses on intellectual changes that occur in a sequential manner as a result of continual interaction between the infant and the

Box **17-1**   **Growth and Development During Infancy**

ONE MONTH

Follows and fixes on bright object with eyes when it moves within field of vision
Still has head lag when pulled to sitting position
Displays tonic neck, grasp, and Moro reflexes
Turns head when prone, but unable to support
Displays sucking and rooting reflexes
Holds hands in fists
Makes small, throaty sounds
Gains 5 to 7 ounces weekly for 6 months
Grows 1 inch monthly for 6 months
Cries when hungry or uncomfortable
Lifts head momentarily when prone

TWO MONTHS

Has closed posterior fontanel
Listens actively to sounds
Lifts head almost 45 degrees off table when prone
Follows moving object with eyes
Recognizes familiar faces
Pays attention to speaking voice
Assumes less flexed position when prone
Vocalizes; distinct from crying
Turns from side to back
Begins to have social smile

THREE MONTHS

Visually inspects object and stares at own hand with apparent fascination when either appears in field of vision
Has longer periods of wakefulness without crying
Laughs aloud and shows pleasure in vocalization
Holds head erect and steady; raises chest, usually supported on forearms
Smiles in response to mother's face
Begins prelanguage vocalizations (coos, babbles, and chuckles)
Carries hand or object to mouth at will
Actively holds rattle, but will not reach for it
Turns eyes to object placed in field of vision

FOUR MONTHS

Begins drooling, indicating appearance of saliva; does not know how to swallow it
Holds head steady when in sitting position
Recognizes familiar object
Shows almost no head lag when pulled to sitting position
Rolls from back to side and abdomen to back
Inspects and plays with hands; pulls clothing or blanket over face in play
Begins eye-hand coordination
Chews and bites
Enjoys social interaction
Demands attention by fussing
Reaches out to people
Is aware and interested in new environment
Grasps object with two hands
Squeals

FIVE MONTHS

Reaches persistently; grasps with entire hand
Plays with toes

Smiles at mirror image
Begins to postpone gratification
Shows signs of tooth eruption
Sleeps through night without food
Weighs twice the birth weight
Sits with slight support
Vocalizes displeasure when desired object is taken away
Is able to discriminate strangers from family
Makes cooing noises
Squeals with delight
Looks for object that has fallen
Rolls from back to stomach or vice versa

SIX MONTHS

Gains approximately 3 to 5 ounces weekly during the second 6 months
Grows approximately 1 inch monthly for 6 months
Is able to lift cup by handle
Begins to hitch in locomotion
Sits in high chair with straight back
Begins to imitate sounds
Vocalizes to toys and mirror image
Babbles with one-syllable sounds: "ma, ma, da, da"
Has definite likes and dislikes
Likes to be picked up
Plays peek-a-boo
Makes "guh" and "bah" sounds

SEVEN MONTHS

Has eruption of upper central incisors
Bears weight when held in standing position
Sits, leaning forward on both hands
Fixates on one very small object
Produces vowel sounds: "ba-ba" and "da-da"
Shows fear of strangers
Displays emotional instability by easy and quick changes from crying to laughing
Repeats activities that are enjoyed
Bangs objects together
Approaches toy and grasps it with one hand
Imitates simple acts

EIGHT MONTHS

Feeds self with finger foods
Sits well alone
Stretches out arms to be picked up
Greets strangers with bashful behavior
Begins to show regular patterns in bladder and bowel elimination
Responds to "no"
Makes consonant sounds: t, d, and w
Dislikes dressing and diaper change
Releases object at will
Shows nervousness with strangers
Pulls toy toward self

NINE MONTHS

Creeps and crawls (backward at first)
Shows good coordination and sits alone
Responds to adult anger; cries when scolded
Explores object by sucking, chewing, and biting it
Responds to simple verbal requests

Continued

owth and Development During Infancy *cont'd*

cup or glass with assistance
o standing position
show fears of going to bed and being left alone
waving "bye-bye"
s object with flexed wrist
s facial expressions of adults
thumb and index finger in pincer grasp

MONTHS

s by falling down
ys "da-da" and "ma-ma"
Understands "bye-bye"
Looks at and follows pictures in book
Crawls and cruises about well
Pays attention to own name
Picks up object fairly well
Extends toy to another person without releasing
Pulls self to standing position and stands while holding onto
   solid object

11 MONTHS

Is able to push toys and place several objects in container
Attempts to walk without assistance
Begins to hold spoon
Stands erect with help of person's hand
May have lower lateral incisors erupting
Holds crayon to mark on paper
Imitates definite speech sounds
Reacts to restrictions with frustration

12 MONTHS

Loses Babinski sign
Develops evident hand dominance
Weighs triple the birth weight
Has equal circumference head and chest
Walks with help
Knows own name
Has slow vocabulary growth because of increased interest
   in walking
Develops lumbar curve

Uses spoon in feeding, but often puts it upside down in
   mouth
Drops object deliberately for it to be picked up
Shakes head for "no"
Plays pat-a-cake
Recovers balance when falling over
Tries to follow when being read to
Does things to attract attention
Imitates vocalization lead

15 MONTHS

Creeps up stairs
Uses "da-da" and "ma-ma" labels for correct parents
Tolerates some separation
Drinks from cup well, but rotates spoon
Asks for object by pointing
Plays interactive games such as peek-a-boo and pat-a-cake
Expresses emotions; has temper tantrums
Walks without help

18 MONTHS

Has closed anterior fontanel
Has long trunk, short and bowed legs, and protruding
   abdomen
Walks up stairs with help
Turns pages of book
Has short attention span
Begins to test limits
Has bowel movements at appropriate time when placed on
   potty
Indicates wet pants
Gets into everything
Fills and handles spoon without rotating it, but spills
   frequently
Runs clumsily and falls often
Is extremely curious
Places object in hole or slot
Becomes communicative, social being
Imitates behavior of parents, such as mimicking household
   chores

Table **17-1** Parenting Tasks for Developmental Landmarks in Infancy

Age (Months)	Landmark	Parenting Task
1	Lifts head when prone	Place infant in prone position and dangle colorful object above head
2	Has social smile	Promote by talking to infant and allowing opportunity to smile
4	Squeals	Encourage and praise for doing
5	Rolls from back to front	Place infant in protected area (crib or playpen) and encourage to move by placing toy out of reach
8 to 9	Uses pincer grasp to feed self	Make finger foods available
10	Pulls self to standing position	Provide safe environment; place chair or object of appropriate height within reach
11 to 12	Initiates vocalization	Talk to infant frequently and include in family gatherings
12 to 15	Walks	Encourage and provide clutter-free, safe walkway; praise for attempts
15	Drinks from cup	Supply cup with appropriate drink; do not scold for clumsiness in handling cup or spills
18	Mimics household chores	Give rags to help with chores, dusting, allow to fold clothes, and so on

Box **17-2** | Developmental Tasks Accomplished in Infancy

1. Achieves physiological equilibrium after birth
2. Establishes self as a dependent person, but separate from others
3. Becomes aware of animate versus inanimate and familiar versus unfamiliar and develops rudimentary social interaction
4. Develops a feeling of affection for others and the desire for affection from others
5. Manages the changing body and learns new motor skills, develops equilibrium, begins eye-hand coordination, and establishes rest-activity rhythm
6. Learns to understand and control the physical world through exploration
7. Develops a beginning symbol system, conceptual abilities, and preverbal communication
8. Directs emotional expression to indicate needs and wishes

From Duvall, E., & Miller, B. (1984). *Marriage and family development* (6th ed.). New York: Harper & Row.

Table **17-2** | Piaget's Five Stages of Infant Development

Stage	Description
Stage 1: birth to 1 month	Modification of reflexes
	Practices and perfects reflexes present at birth
	Sucking reflex becomes more refined and voluntary
Stage 2: 1 to 4 months	Primary circular reactions
	Repeats behavior that previously led to an interesting event
	Only the infant's own body involved in activities
Stage 3: 4 to 10 months	Secondary circular reactions begins
	Repetitions involve events or objects in the external world
	Appears to perform actions with a purpose
	Hand-eye coordination
Stage 4: 10 to 12 months	Coordination of secondary reactions
	Combines two or more previously acquired strategies to obtain a goal
Stage 5: 12 to 18 months	Tertiary circular reactions
	Uses active experimentation to achieve previously unattainable goals
	Infant purposely varies movements to observe results

environment (Hockenberry, 2005). Piaget's sensorimotor period (up to age 18 months) describes the infant's involvement in mastering simple coordination activities to interact with the environment. The infant solves problems using sensory systems and motor activity rather than symbolic processes that develop later.

Research has shown that fetuses are able to distinguish light from dark and that sight is present at birth. Rod cells in the retina of the eyes, which are responsible for light perception, are functional at birth; the retina (the organ of visual perception) is not fully developed until approximately 4 months of age. However, the infant can perceive color and shape. Infants are startled by loud noises and are soothed by soft voices, which indicates that their sense of hearing is functioning. This can be tested with audio equipment at birth. Babies cry when pricked with a diaper pin and fuss when too hot or too cold; therefore, the senses of pain and temperature are operative, also. Touching, stroking, and rocking typically soothe a fussing infant. Infants will also react to odors and tastes.

In addition to perceiving stimulation, the newborn is capable of reflexive behavior. **Reflexes** are responses that normally are exhibited after a particular type of stimulation (Pillitteri, 2003). Because the response occurs after the stimulus, reflexes are unlearned. Some infant reflexes, such as rooting and sucking, have survival value. The rooting reflex, activated by lightly stroking the angle of the lips or cheek, helps the infant locate the food source. The infant will turn toward the side that is being stroked and will open the lips to suck. The sucking reflex is initiated when an object is placed in the infant's mouth. Together, these reflexes ensure that the infant can obtain food. Infants also have reflexes that result in grasping, yawning, hiccoughing, coughing, and sneezing.

Armed with these reflexes and sensory capabilities, the infant is ready to begin interacting with the environment (seeing, hearing, touching, tasting, and smelling) to acquire valuable information.

The infant progresses in various ways between birth and age 18 months, with early capabilities changing and becoming intentional. Piaget outlines five stages within the sensorimotor period that describe the infant's development, from the early reflexive behavior to differentiation between self and environment (Table 17-2).

The infant in the **sensorimotor period** uses behavioral strategies to manipulate objects, to learn some of their properties, and to reach goals by combining several behaviors. The infant's behavior is tied to the concrete and the immediate; schemes can be applied only to objects that can be perceived directly.

Kohlberg, a leading theorist of moral development, states that it is prefaced by the child's ability to reason and is part of a sequence that corresponds with the development of intellect. The nurse recognizes the interrelationship between the developmental phases in the different dimensions (physical and psychosocial) of each individual.

Knowledge of child developmental theories is extremely valuable to the nurse during interactions with infants. Understanding the infant's level of cognitive thought and emotional and social development helps the nurse decipher a child's communications more meaningfully and interpret behaviors and the processes that motivate the child more accurately. This knowledge can be incorporated in the dance offered to the parents. The nurse ... a variety of sensory and motor stimuli will ... within the infant's environment.

...evelopmental Screening

...r Developmental Screening Test (DDST) is a ...d tool that screens for developmental problems ... from birth to 6 years of age. The original DDST ...ed, restandardized, and renamed the Denver II ..., 2003). Three purposes have been identified ...inistering the Denver II: (1) screening apparently ... infants for developmental problems, (2) validating ...ve concerns about an infant's development with an ...ive test, and (3) monitoring high-risk children for ...opmental problems. The **Denver Developmental ...ening Test II** and directions for administration are pre-...ed in **Web Site Resource 17A.**

...Four areas of development are screened: (1) personal-...cial, (2) fine motor–adaptive, (3) language, and (4) gross ...otor. Unique features of the Denver II are its recent and ...ophisticated standardization and its inclusion of norms for various subgroups based on place of residence, ethnicity, and mother's level of education.

The Denver II includes four test behavior descriptors to rate the infant's behavior, reflecting the administrator's subjective impression of the infant's overall behavior. Behavioral ratings are established for compliance with the examiner's requests for alertness and interest in the sur-roundings, fearfulness, and attention span.

Although administration of the Denver II is not difficult, only nurses or other personnel trained specifically in its pro-cedures and interpretation should make the attempt. This precaution is necessary to ensure the validity of the results.

The nurse tells the parents before the test that the DDST is not an intelligence test but, rather, a test of the child's developmental level. By adding the number of accom-plished and unaccomplished items on the test form, the screener estimates the child's developmental level. By refer-ring to guidelines on the instruction sheet, the child is scored P (passed) or F (failed) on each item. The DDST can be administered with minimal materials and time and, ideally, should be administered to an infant at approxi-mately 3 or 4 months of age, again at 10 months, and again at 3 years (Hockenberry, 2005).

The infant's **growth index,** height and weight measure-ments plotted on a standard growth chart to assess for normal progression, is also important. Physical growth (height and weight) is a valid health status indicator that should be measured during each routine office or clinic visit. During the first year of life, growth is rapid. An infant who is growing properly is at low risk for developing a chronic disease (Lowdermilk & Perry, 2004).

The nurse plots the infant's length and weight measure-ments against exact chronological age on growth grids. In 2000 the National Center for Health Statistics published growth grids that have been standardized to the present growth charts for female and male infants from birth to age 36 months. These growth charts are presented in **Web Site Resources 17B** and **17C.** Body mass index is a feature of the new pediatric growth charts recently released by the Centers for Disease Control and Prevention (CDC). The charts are used by most pediatricians and were developed by the National Center for Health Statistics in collaboration with the National Center for Chronic Disease Prevention and Health Promotion (2000). With the addition of body mass index to the charts, the CDC significantly increased the usefulness of this tool as an early warning signal for potential obesity as early as 2 years of age. Parents have an opportunity to change their children's eating habits before a weight problem develops. The revised pediatric growth charts more accurately reflect the United States' cultural and racial diversity and can track children and young people through age 20. The growth charts indicate that children are heavier today than in the past, but height has remained virtually unchanged.

An infant's growth index, as determined by length and weight, is only one factor in assessing health status. The nurse must have an overall understanding of growth and development principles to counsel parents regarding their infant's progress. **Web Site Resource 17D** presents height and weight measurements for girls and boys.

Gender

The infant's gender is determined at the moment of fertil-ization. Immediately after delivery, the parents usually ask, "Is it a girl or a boy?" The answer has far-reaching implica-tions for many family units. The infant's gender is one of the many important factors that influence the parents' way of relating to the infant.

Studies have revealed many biological and behavioral differences between male and female infants. Boys are, on average, larger and have proportionately more muscle mass at birth. Girls are generally smaller but physiologically more mature at birth and are less vulnerable to stress. Boys show more motor activity, whereas girls display a greater response to tactile stimulation and pain (Kail & Cavanaugh, 2004). As the infant develops, further differences are noted. By 6 months, girls respond to visual stimulation with longer attention spans and are more socially responsive than are boys; girls also tend to sit up, walk, and crawl earlier than do boys. Female infants develop language earlier and respond to speech better than do boys. Therefore female infants learn to communicate with language from an early age, whereas male infants use their bodies (Pillitteri, 2003).

The gender of the infant, a major concern of many expectant parents, may well influence parental relationships and expectations. The infant's gender can evoke disap-pointment; in some cases, a woman may feel disappointed in a girl only because she knows that her husband wanted a boy. Today, the trend is to want one child of each gender. Because of the availability of better forms of contraception and economic factors such as the expense of raising chil-dren, couples are having fewer children today when

Developmental Tasks Accomplished in Infancy

1. Achieves physiological equilibrium after birth
2. Establishes self as a dependent person, but separate from others
3. Becomes aware of animate versus inanimate and familiar versus unfamiliar and develops rudimentary social interaction
4. Develops a feeling of affection for others and the desire for affection from others
5. Manages the changing body and learns new motor skills, develops equilibrium, begins eye-hand coordination, and establishes rest-activity rhythm
6. Learns to understand and control the physical world through exploration
7. Develops a beginning symbol system, conceptual abilities, and preverbal communication
8. Directs emotional expression to indicate needs and wishes

From Duvall, E., & Miller, B. (1984). *Marriage and family development* (6th ed.). New York: Harper & Row.

Table **17-2** **Piaget's Five Stages of Infant Development**

Stage	Description
Stage 1: birth to 1 month	Modification of reflexes
	Practices and perfects reflexes present at birth
	Sucking reflex becomes more refined and voluntary
Stage 2: 1 to 4 months	Primary circular reactions
	Repeats behavior that previously led to an interesting event
	Only the infant's own body involved in activities
Stage 3: 4 to 10 months	Secondary circular reactions begins
	Repetitions involve events or objects in the external world
	Appears to perform actions with a purpose
	Hand-eye coordination
Stage 4: 10 to 12 months	Coordination of secondary reactions
	Combines two or more previously acquired strategies to obtain a goal
Stage 5: 12 to 18 months	Tertiary circular reactions
	Uses active experimentation to achieve previously unattainable goals
	Infant purposely varies movements to observe results

environment (Hockenberry, 2005). Piaget's sensorimotor period (up to age 18 months) describes the infant's involvement in mastering simple coordination activities to interact with the environment. The infant solves problems using sensory systems and motor activity rather than symbolic processes that develop later.

Research has shown that fetuses are able to distinguish light from dark and that sight is present at birth. Rod cells in the retina of the eyes, which are responsible for light perception, are functional at birth; the retina (the organ of visual perception) is not fully developed until approximately 4 months of age. However, the infant can perceive color and shape. Infants are startled by loud noises and are soothed by soft voices, which indicates that their sense of hearing is functioning. This can be tested with audio equipment at birth. Babies cry when pricked with a diaper pin and fuss when too hot or too cold; therefore, the senses of pain and temperature are operative, also. Touching, stroking, and rocking typically soothe a fussing infant. Infants will also react to odors and tastes.

In addition to perceiving stimulation, the newborn is capable of reflexive behavior. **Reflexes** are responses that normally are exhibited after a particular type of stimulation (Pillitteri, 2003). Because the response occurs after the stimulus, reflexes are unlearned. Some infant reflexes, such as rooting and sucking, have survival value. The rooting reflex, activated by lightly stroking the angle of the lips or cheek, helps the infant locate the food source. The infant will turn toward the side that is being stroked and will open the lips to suck. The sucking reflex is initiated when an object is placed in the infant's mouth. Together, these reflexes ensure that the infant can obtain food. Infants also have reflexes that result in grasping, yawning, hiccoughing, coughing, and sneezing.

Armed with these reflexes and sensory capabilities, the infant is ready to begin interacting with the environment (seeing, hearing, touching, tasting, and smelling) to acquire valuable information.

The infant progresses in various ways between birth and age 18 months, with early capabilities changing and becoming intentional. Piaget outlines five stages within the sensorimotor period that describe the infant's development, from the early reflexive behavior to differentiation between self and environment (Table 17-2).

The infant in the **sensorimotor period** uses behavioral strategies to manipulate objects, to learn some of their properties, and to reach goals by combining several behaviors. The infant's behavior is tied to the concrete and the immediate; schemes can be applied only to objects that can be perceived directly.

Kohlberg, a leading theorist of moral development, states that it is prefaced by the child's ability to reason and is part of a sequence that corresponds with the development of intellect. The nurse recognizes the interrelationship between the developmental phases in the different dimensions (physical and psychosocial) of each individual.

Knowledge of child developmental theories is extremely valuable to the nurse during interactions with infants. Understanding the infant's level of cognitive thought and emotional and social development helps the nurse decipher a child's communications more meaningfully and interpret behaviors and the processes that motivate the child more accurately. This knowledge can be incorporated in the anticipatory guidance offered to the parents. The nurse should stress that a variety of sensory and motor stimuli will foster learning within the infant's environment.

Denver Developmental Screening Test II

The Denver Developmental Screening Test (DDST) is a standardized tool that screens for developmental problems in children from birth to 6 years of age. The original DDST was revised, restandardized, and renamed the Denver II (Pillitteri, 2003). Three purposes have been identified for administering the Denver II: (1) screening apparently healthy infants for developmental problems, (2) validating intuitive concerns about an infant's development with an objective test, and (3) monitoring high-risk children for developmental problems. The **Denver Developmental Screening Test II** and directions for administration are presented in **Web Site Resource 17A.**

Four areas of development are screened: (1) personal-social, (2) fine motor–adaptive, (3) language, and (4) gross motor. Unique features of the Denver II are its recent and sophisticated standardization and its inclusion of norms for various subgroups based on place of residence, ethnicity, and mother's level of education.

The Denver II includes four test behavior descriptors to rate the infant's behavior, reflecting the administrator's subjective impression of the infant's overall behavior. Behavioral ratings are established for compliance with the examiner's requests for alertness and interest in the surroundings, fearfulness, and attention span.

Although administration of the Denver II is not difficult, only nurses or other personnel trained specifically in its procedures and interpretation should make the attempt. This precaution is necessary to ensure the validity of the results.

The nurse tells the parents before the test that the DDST is not an intelligence test but, rather, a test of the child's developmental level. By adding the number of accomplished and unaccomplished items on the test form, the screener estimates the child's developmental level. By referring to guidelines on the instruction sheet, the child is scored P (passed) or F (failed) on each item. The DDST can be administered with minimal materials and time and, ideally, should be administered to an infant at approximately 3 or 4 months of age, again at 10 months, and again at 3 years (Hockenberry, 2005).

The infant's **growth index,** height and weight measurements plotted on a standard growth chart to assess for normal progression, is also important. Physical growth (height and weight) is a valid health status indicator that should be measured during each routine office or clinic visit. During the first year of life, growth is rapid. An infant who is growing properly is at low risk for developing a chronic disease (Lowdermilk & Perry, 2004).

The nurse plots the infant's length and weight measurements against exact chronological age on growth grids. In 2000 the National Center for Health Statistics published growth grids that have been standardized to the present

growth charts for female and male infants from birth to age 36 months. These growth charts are presented in **Web Site Resources 17B** and **17C.** Body mass index is a feature of the new pediatric growth charts recently released by the Centers for Disease Control and Prevention (CDC). The charts are used by most pediatricians and were developed by the National Center for Health Statistics in collaboration with the National Center for Chronic Disease Prevention and Health Promotion (2000). With the addition of body mass index to the charts, the CDC significantly increased the usefulness of this tool as an early warning signal for potential obesity as early as 2 years of age. Parents have an opportunity to change their children's eating habits before a weight problem develops. The revised pediatric growth charts more accurately reflect the United States' cultural and racial diversity and can track children and young people through age 20. The growth charts indicate that children are heavier today than in the past, but height has remained virtually unchanged.

An infant's growth index, as determined by length and weight, is only one factor in assessing health status. The nurse must have an overall understanding of growth and development principles to counsel parents regarding their infant's progress. **Web Site Resource 17D** presents height and weight measurements for girls and boys.

Gender

The infant's gender is determined at the moment of fertilization. Immediately after delivery, the parents usually ask, "Is it a girl or a boy?" The answer has far-reaching implications for many family units. The infant's gender is one of the many important factors that influence the parents' way of relating to the infant.

Studies have revealed many biological and behavioral differences between male and female infants. Boys are, on average, larger and have proportionately more muscle mass at birth. Girls are generally smaller but physiologically more mature at birth and are less vulnerable to stress. Boys show more motor activity, whereas girls display a greater response to tactile stimulation and pain (Kail & Cavanaugh, 2004). As the infant develops, further differences are noted. By 6 months, girls respond to visual stimulation with longer attention spans and are more socially responsive than are boys; girls also tend to sit up, walk, and crawl earlier than do boys. Female infants develop language earlier and respond to speech better than do boys. Therefore female infants learn to communicate with language from an early age, whereas male infants use their bodies (Pillitteri, 2003).

The gender of the infant, a major concern of many expectant parents, may well influence parental relationships and expectations. The infant's gender can evoke disappointment; in some cases, a woman may feel disappointed in a girl only because she knows that her husband wanted a boy. Today, the trend is to want one child of each gender. Because of the availability of better forms of contraception and economic factors such as the expense of raising children, couples are having fewer children today when compared with the 1950s. The importance and stress of producing the right-sex infant is evident. Being the wrong sex can be combined with other factors to place the infant at risk for child abuse. The parents may find fault with and place blame on the infant for not meeting this expectation (Olson & DeFrain, 2003).

Health intervention focuses on the identification of high-risk families and the promotion of a positive relationship between infant and parents. The nurse promotes the good health, appearance, and developmental potential of the infant. Increasing the parents' feelings of adequacy and self-esteem will promote their acceptance of the infant. Most importantly, follow-up care for these families is a high priority to ensure that adequate support and help are available.

Race

Race refers to the classification of human beings into groups based on particular physical characteristics, such as skin pigmentation, head form, and stature owing to a common inheritance. Caucasoid, mongoloid, and negroid are the three racial types generally recognized (O'Toole, 2003).

A range of physical variation exists among people of different races with regard to growth rate, dentition, body structure, blood groups, susceptibility to certain diseases, and a great many other variables.

In assessing an infant, the nurse not only collects data, but also compares the data with established norms, such as a standardized growth chart. When the norms chosen are not appropriate for the individual (for example, an Asian infant's growth is assessed based on norms for white children), the assessment will not be accurate.

The nurse who works with families from a variety of racial groups must have an understanding of each background and how it relates to health and health care. To facilitate nursing care for a family from a racial group different from that of the health care provider, effective communication must be established. This communication will help foster an understanding of the other's point of view and frame of reference. Each family member should be viewed as an individual, and there should be no stereotyping of families within a racial group. Despite common language, color, or historical background, not all members of a particular racial group are alike. This diversity presents, without doubt, considerable challenges for nurses who work with families with infants (Schwartz & Scott, 2002). Universal norms by which to measure one's growth and skill capacity do not exist. The nurse must recognize the differences and intervene appropriately. The orientation of health maintenance and disease prevention is basic to good health practices, regardless of racial makeup. This concept should be the main focus of all health care.

Genetics

The desired and expected outcome of any pregnancy is the birth of a healthy, perfect baby. Unfortunately a small, but significant, number of parents experience disappointment when they discover that their baby has been born with a defect or genetic disease. A birth defect is an abnormality of structure, function, or metabolism as a result of a genetic or environmental influence on the fetus, often a combination of both. Couples may refrain from having another child because they have had one with a serious birth defect and do not want to risk another. In these situations, genetic counseling provides information that is needed to understand a hereditary disorder and its associated risks. The main goal of counseling is to explain birth defects to affected families and to allow prospective parents to make informed decisions about childbearing.

Using the basic laws governing heredity and knowing the frequency of specific birth defects in the population, the genetic counselor can often predict the probability of recurrence of a given abnormality in the same family. An important aspect of primary prevention is identifying families at increased risk and referring them for counseling (Burton, 2003). Aspects to be reviewed in the initial interview follow:

1. *Maternal age.* The risk of having a child with Down syndrome increases significantly for the woman older than 35 years of age. In this syndrome, three chromosomes appear in the 21 chromosome group (trisomy 21). Characteristic features include upward slanting eyes; small, malformed ears; large, protruding tongue; broad hands and feet; and some degree of mental retardation.

2. *Ethnic background.* Several genetic disorders occur with higher frequency in certain groups. Eastern European Jews have a 10 times greater chance of carrying the Tay-Sachs gene than does the general U.S. population. Abnormal deposits of lipids (fats) in the cells of the cerebral cortex, spleen, liver, and lymph nodes are characteristics of Tay-Sachs disease. An autosomal recessive gene transmits it. Blacks have a much greater chance of carrying the sickle cell trait than does the general population. Sickle cell anemia is an autosomal recessive condition that occurs in 1 out of every 400 black births and causes severe hemolytic anemia crises.

3. *Family history.* Certain diseases, such as Huntington's chorea, hemophilia, or mental retardation, are often hereditary. Huntington's chorea (an autosomal dominant disease involving the brain) is characterized by deterioration of intellectual functions and involuntary movements of the limbs, face, and trunk. Once manifested, a steady deterioration leads to death after some years. Hemophilia is a sex-linked recessive coagulation disorder caused by a functional deficiency of a clotting factor; bleeding is prolonged. Hemophilia passes from an unaffected carrier mother to her male offspring and occurs in 1 out of every 10,000 births (Burton, 2003).

4. *Reproductive history.* Spontaneous abortions, stillbirths, and previous live-born children with birth defects or slow development may indicate an increased risk.

5. *Maternal disease.* Several maternal disorders are associated with a higher frequency of birth defects, including diabetes mellitus, seizure disorder, mental retardation, and phenylketonuria.

Prenatal diagnosis offers the couple the option of aborting a fetus that is affected with certain genetic disorders. For many people, this option is unacceptable. Chapter 16 discusses the various tests used for prenatal diagnosis.

The nurse's role throughout the genetic counseling process is to provide the vital link between the counseling team and the high-risk couple. The nurse is involved in case finding, referral, and family education. The nurse should have a sound background in the principles of genetics to provide families with appropriate information as part of preventive guidance (Lea, 2002).

GORDON'S FUNCTIONAL HEALTH PATTERNS
Health Perception–Health Management Pattern

Health promotion is aimed at assisting the infant and family to change behavior to produce better physical and emotional health in adulthood. To reach this goal, the nurse encourages child-rearing practices that promote normal growth and development, fosters attitudes and values compatible with health, and teaches appropriate use of health services (Chitty, 2004). The nurse promotes the infant's health through the parents, who determine the care practices for the dependent infant.

Health is largely a subjective judgment; each person's perception of health is related to physical and mental capabilities, self-concept, relationships with others and the environment, and personal goals and values (Jarvis, 2003). With this understanding, the nurse uses every opportunity to convey confidence in the parents' health perception–health management pattern and their ability to act to enhance the infant's health. When parents learn and adopt behaviors that improve their own health, they are more likely to ensure that the health needs of their infant are met. Parental modeling increases the chances that good health practices will be retained throughout the child's life.

The goals of nursing practice with infants and their families are to promote individual motivation for health, to assist the family to identify health needs, and to develop problem-solving skills using the family's own resources. To meet these goals, the nurse must identify the family's perception of good or bad health practices, which greatly influences participation in health-promoting activities. Age, gender, educational level, cultural orientation, financial status, and occupation combine to influence health perception. When parents believe that the infant is more susceptible to a health problem if promotional behavior is not enacted, they become more motivated to adopt the behavior.

The nurse's task is to help the parents recognize the infant's susceptibility and the potential consequences when healthy practices are not instituted. The nurse works within the family's health perception framework to become acquainted with the characteristics that influence the infant's health. Unless caregivers meet their own personal needs, they will be unable to meet their infant's developmental needs (M. J. Clark, 2003).

The nurse supports the parents, strengthening their parental confidence and self-esteem, providing information on meeting their infant's needs, and reinforcing their health perception–health management pattern.

Nutritional-Metabolic Pattern

One of the most important aspects of health promotion in the infant is nutritional status. Many opinions have been expressed about the infant's nutritional needs. As research in this area continues, recommendations and opinions will change; however, some basic facts about nutrition remain fairly consistent. Infant nutritional requirements are based on what is considered necessary to (1) support life, (2) provide for growth, and (3) maintain health.

Essential Nutrients

Water, proteins, fats, carbohydrates, vitamins, and minerals are the essential nutrients in any diet. Because the first year of life is a period of rapid growth, nutritional needs during this period are especially important and always changing.

Water is vital to survival. A person can live for several weeks without food but can survive only a few days without water. Because the infant's body weight is approximately 75% water, the baby must consume large amounts of fluid to maintain water balance. Water requirements average between 125 to 150 ml/kg of body weight per day during the first 6 months of life and 120 to 135 ml/kg per day during the second 6 months (Riordan, 2004). The sources of water are fluids (primarily milk) and food; most strained foods are 75% to 85% water. Most infant diets meet the basic water requirement.

The infant must also consume sufficient high-quality protein to facilitate growth and development. Recommended protein requirements are 2.2 g/kg per day during the first 6 months and 2 g/kg per day during the second 6 months (Cataldo, Debruyne, & Whitney, 2002).

Carbohydrates should supply 30% to 60% of the energy intake during infancy. Approximately 37% of the calories in human milk and 40% to 50% of the calories in commercial formulas are derived from lactose or other carbohydrates (Samour, Helm, & Lang, 2004).

A minimum of 3.8 g/kcal and a maximum of 6 g/kcal of fat (30% to 54% of calories) are recommended for infants (Samour, Helm, & Lang, 2004). This quantity is present in human milk and in all formulas prepared for infants. Significantly lower intakes, such as in skim milk feedings, can result in an inadequate energy intake.

Vitamins are essential nutrients in the infant's diet that regulate metabolism and allow more efficient use of carbohydrates, fats, and proteins within the body. Although most infants receive adequate vitamin intake through formula, breast milk, and food, recent research has raised a concern about a vitamin D deficiency in infants who receive only breast milk. According to researchers Peng and Serwint

(2003), nutritional rickets is on the rise in the United States among American children with certain risk factors: dark-skinned infants, breast-fed for long periods without receiving any vitamin supplementation, and decreased exposure to sun light. Based on their research, they recommend that this population needs vitamin D supplementation at 400 international units/day to be initiated earlier than 3 months of age, and it needs to be continued throughout the time the infant is breast-feeding (Peng & Serwint, 2003).

Minerals are found in relatively small amounts in the infant's body but are vital elements in body structure and control of certain bodily functions. Mineral intake for infants appears to be adequate, except for iron and fluoride.

The full-term infant is born with stores of iron adequate to meet bodily needs for hemoglobin production for up to approximately 4 to 6 months. After this time, body stores may need to be replenished. Although iron in human milk is bioavailable, both breast-fed and formula-fed infants should receive an additional source of iron by 6 months of age. Iron-fortified formula and cereals are the most commonly used food sources.

Fluoride, concentrated in the bones and teeth, helps reduce dental caries. The Committee on Nutrition of the Academy of Pediatrics has recommended that optimal fluoride intake for infants is 0.25 mg per day (Samour, Helm, & Lang, 2004). Supplementation is necessary when the diet contains insufficient fluoridated water.

A review of these requirements shows that milk (breast or formula) meets most of the infant's nutritional needs when consumed in adequate amounts, plus vitamin D supplementation for the high-risk infants. No data support the theory that solid foods are needed to meet these nutritional needs, at least during the first 6 months of life. Nevertheless, many parents introduce semisolid foods to their infants as early as 2 weeks of age.

Breast-Feeding

Research throughout the years has demonstrated unequivocally that exclusive breast-feeding is the preferred method of infant feeding for the first 4 to 6 months of life. Breast milk is often called the *perfect food* for the infant and for the mother, because she does not have to buy it, cook it, store it, or clean up after it. Both the American Dietetic Association and the American Academy of Pediatrics have released position statements in support of breast-feeding. This has influenced a number of health-promotion strategies in the United States. The surgeon general has recommended that by the year 2010, 75% of all postpartum women should be breast-feeding when they leave the hospital, and 50% should still be breast-feeding 6 months later (Research Highlights box). If the nation is to meet the surgeon general's goal by the year 2010, efforts to promote breast-feeding must be strengthened in hospitals, health maintenance organizations, private health care offices, and public health clinics.

The World Health Organization (WHO) and the United Nations Children's Fund (UNICEF) have jointly adopted the Baby-Friendly Hospital Initiative in an attempt to establish a global effort to increase breast-feeding. To become a baby-friendly health care facility, the 10 steps to successful breast-feeding must be implemented, as shown in Box 17-3.

Nurses can be instrumental in working toward the national goal to increase breast-feeding by educating all

---

research highlights

Pacifiers and Breast-Feeding

Improving nutrition is a key area in the government's *Healthy People 2010* initiative, and breast milk is widely acknowledged to be the most complete form of nutrition for infants. There is strong evidence for both short-term and long-term benefits of breast-feeding, including reduced mortality in preterm infants and reduced infant morbidity. Breast-feeding has also been associated with reduced risk of type 1 diabetes, lower blood pressure, and lowered risks of urinary tract and middle ear infections. The benefits appear to increase with longer duration of breast-feeding.

The UNICEF Baby-Friendly Initiative statement recommends that pacifiers should not be given to breast-feeding infants. Shorter breast-feeding duration has been associated with pacifier use by a number of researchers. This research review aimed to answer the question: Does the use of pacifiers shorten breast-feeding duration in infants?

The Cochrane library, Medline, CINAHL, and Embase databases were searched for systematic reviews, randomized controlled trials, and cohort studies examining the effect of pacifier use on breast-feeding duration. This review found evidence to suggest that there is a relationship between pacifier use and shortened breast-feeding duration. Several of the research studies reviewed a classic "dose–response" relationship, with greater pacifier use being associated with earlier cessation of breast-feeding. Most studies confirmed this association between frequency and duration.

Although no study can be 100% accurate, the weight of evidence does suggest that pacifier use may cause a reduction in long-term breast-feeding (beyond 3 months), although in line with the research review there is little evidence of harm associated with occasional pacifier use (e.g., restricted to the period when the infant settles). The recommendation is that nurses should inform breast-feeding mothers of this association and advise them according to the "ten steps to successful breast-feeding" recommended by the Baby-Friendly Initiative.

Data from Ullah, S., & Griffiths, P. (2003). Does the use of pacifiers shorten breastfeeding duration in infants? *British Journal of Community Nursing*, 8(10), 458-463.

Box **17-3** Baby-Friendly Hospital Initiative Breast-Feeding Guidelines

1. Have a written breast-feeding policy that is communicated routinely to all health care staff.
2. Train all health care staff in the skills necessary to implement this policy.
3. Inform all pregnant women about the benefits and management of breast-feeding.
4. Help the mother initiate breast-feeding within 30 minutes after birth.
5. Show mothers how to breast-feed and how to maintain lactation even when they are separated from their infants.
6. Give newborn infants no food or drink other than breast milk unless medically indicated.
7. Practice rooming-in; allow mothers and infants to remain together 24 hours a day.
8. Encourage breast-feeding on demand.
9. Give no pacifiers to breast-feeding infants.
10. Foster the establishment of breast-feeding support groups and refer mothers to these groups when discharged from the hospital or clinic.

From Saadeh R & Akre J: Ten steps to successful breast feeding: a summary of the rationale and scientific evidence, *Birth* 23(3):145, 1996.

Box **17-4** Advantages of Breast-Feeding

BREAST MILK
- Has the correct balance of all essential nutrients for infants
- Is full of immunological agents to protect against disease
- Is easier to digest than is formula
- Contains antiinflammatory properties
- Promotes growth of *Lactobacillus bifidus*

BREAST-FEEDING
- Is cheaper and more convenient than formula
- Provides a unique bonding experience for both infant and mother
- Assists in process of uterine involution for mother
- Promotes weight reduction for new mother

women about the advantages of the practice (Box 17-4). Community nurses who are caring for breast-feeding mothers should stress the following tips to increase the duration of this activity:

- Drink up to eight glasses of fluids daily to produce sufficient quantity of breast milk.
- Consume the proper amount of calories to avoid excessive weight loss.
- Educate nursing mothers about the appropriate interventions for engorged breasts, sore nipples, plugged ducts, infection, and leaking (Health Teaching box).
- Instruct employed nursing mothers about the use of breast pumps and milk storage.
- Encourage participation in breast-feeding support groups for continued help within the community.
- Advise nursing mothers of the effects of drugs, environmental pollutants, alcohol, and nicotine on breast milk.

Introduction of Solid Foods

No scientific evidence is available on the best time to introduce solid foods during infancy. At approximately 4 to 6 months of age, the infant is usually physiologically and developmentally ready to have solid foods, either commercial or home prepared. Some authorities believe that waiting until the child is 4 to 6 months of age to introduce solid food decreases the tendency to develop food allergies. The introduction of various foods was recommended to (1) supply a more appealing, diversified diet for the infant, (2) supply energy, iron, and vitamins, and (3) provide needed trace elements (Burns, 2004). The decision to start solid foods at 4 to 6 months of age is be based more on neuro-

muscular and developmental readiness of the infant rather than on any hard scientific data.

All infants develop according to their own schedules, and some are ready to start eating solid foods before others are. The addition of foods should be governed by an infant's nutritional needs and readiness to handle different forms of foods (Biancuzzo, 2003). The order of food introduction and specific amounts to be given are based on tradition rather than on scientific fact. No scientific studies have been performed to determine whether there is a specific order of infant food introduction necessary or amounts needed for optimal development. The sequence of solids typically recommended by the American Academy of Pediatrics is cereal, fruits, vegetables, and meats. The typical sequence in which foods are introduced is shown in Box 17-5.

A few tips to assist the parents in making the introduction of solid foods to their infant's diet a smooth process are listed in Box 17-6.

Recommendations for food introduction by age and sequence are shown in Table 17-3.

Weaning

Weaning is a gradual, caring process that introduces the infant to a cup, which replaces the bottle or breast. Weaning should be started when the infant is ready. Developmentally, the infant can usually learn to use a cup by age 5 to 6 months; however, many children continue to nurse after they start using a cup. The American Academy of Pediatrics recommends breast-feeding for at least the first year of life. WHO and UNICEF suggest that the health benefits of breast milk are important throughout the second and third years of life. Weaning should be started at this age by periodically offering sips of water or juice. Initially the infant may not be eager to do so but should become accustomed to this new experience fairly quickly.

Some infants accept the cup readily; other infants are extremely reluctant to give up the bottle, especially the bedtime bottle. Allowing infants to sleep with propped

HEALTH TEACHING Breast-Feeding

How to Hold Your Baby for Feedings

- Sit or lie down comfortably with your back supported.
- Make sure your baby has one arm on either side of your breast as you pull the baby close.
- Use firm pillows or folded blankets under the baby as a means of support during the feeding. As your baby gets older, the extra support will likely be unnecessary.
- Support the baby's back and shoulders firmly. Do not push on the back of the baby's head.
- After the baby's mouth is open wide, pull your baby quickly to your breast.

Four Common Breast-Feeding Positions

Football

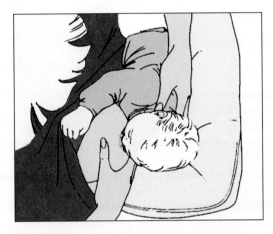

- Hold the baby's back and shoulders in the palm of your hand.
- Tuck the baby up under your arm, keeping the baby's ear, shoulder, and hip in a straight line.
- Support the breast. After the baby's mouth is open wide, pull the baby quickly to you.
- Continue to hold your breast until the baby feeds easily.

Lying Down

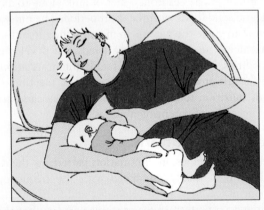

- Lie on your side with a pillow at your back and lay the baby such that you are facing each other.
- To begin, prop yourself up on your elbow and support your breast with that hand.
- Pull the baby close to you, lining up the baby's mouth with your nipple.
- After the baby is feeding well, lie back down. Hold your breast with the opposite hand.

Cradling

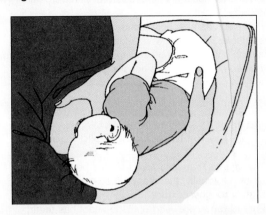

- Cradle the baby in the arm closest to the breast with the baby's head in the crook of your arm.
- Have the baby's body facing you, tummy to tummy.
- Use your opposite hand to support the breast.

Across the Lap

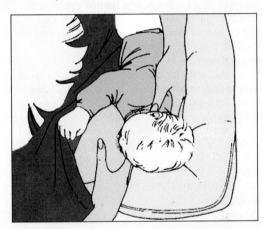

- Lay your baby on firm pillows across your lap.
- Turn the baby, facing you.
- Reach across your lap to support the baby's back and shoulders with the palm of your hand.
- Support your breast from underneath to guide it into the baby's mouth.

Breast-Feeding is Going Well When . . .

- Your newborn is feeding approximately 8 times in 24 hours for 30 to 40 minutes at each feeding. Some newborns need to eat more frequently until they learn to breast-feed efficiently. Other babies gain weight although they feed less often.
- At least one breast softens well at each feeding.
- You feel a tug, but not pain, when the baby sucks.
- The baby's arms and shoulders are relaxed during the feeding.
- The baby has bursts of 10 or more sucks and swallows at the beginning of each feeding.
- As your breast softens, the baby slows down to two to three sucks and swallows at a time.
- Your baby is content when you finish breast-feeding.
- By the time the baby is 4 days old, you should see at least six wet diapers and two bowel movements every 24 hours.

Used with permission of Lactation Consultants of North Carolina. Illustrations from a handset accompanying the video, *Breastfeeding: A special relationship*. Courtesy of Eagle Video Productions.

| Box **17-5** | Solid Food Introduction Sequence |

1. *Cereals,* particularly rice because of nonallergenic property
2. *Fruits* such as peaches, pears, and applesauce
3. *Vegetables,* with yellow vegetables (squash and carrots) given before green vegetables (peas or beans)
4. *Strained meats,* such as nonallergenic lamb or veal

| Box **17-6** | Tips for Introducing Solid Foods |

1. The infant's first solid foods should be smooth and runny. Gradually, the infant will be ready to accept a slightly rougher texture.
2. Puréed foods are used until the infant has teeth; chopped foods are used when the infant can chew.
3. Introduce only one new food at a time and in small amounts. When the new food is not tolerated or the infant is allergic to it, the new food can be identified quickly and discontinued.
4. The infant must learn how to handle solid foods. Because infants use sucking movements, part of the food is ejected from the mouth. With time and practice, the infant learns how to take solid food from a spoon.
5. Do not mix solid foods together; the infant should learn to appreciate different tastes and textures.
6. Do not add solid foods to the infant's formula bottle; do not make a larger hole to allow drinking of foods.
7. Do not start to reduce the milk supply until the infant is taking food successfully from the spoon.
8. Until 1 year of age, feed the baby milk before solid foods.
9. Look at, smile at, and talk to the infant during feeding.
10. Do not give honey to infants less than 12 months of age*

*Honey has been credited throughout the centuries with therapeutic and medicinal uses. However, honey should not be given to infants under 1 year of age. Honey is a known source of bacterial spores that produce a toxin that can cause infant botulism. This rare, but serious, form of food poisoning affects the nervous system of infants and can result in death. Researchers also suspect a link between infant botulism and some cases of SIDS, because breathing is affected in the most severe stages of food poisoning. Botulism spores are quite common, found in dust, soil, and uncooked food. Honey is the only food implicated in infant botulism. Because honey is not essential for the nutrition of infants, parents and caregivers should be reminded not to feed it to infants younger than 1 year. Honey should never be added to baby food or placed on the nipple of a pacifier.
SIDS, sudden infant death syndrome.

bottles can lead to aspiration if the milk flows too rapidly or the infant becomes too sleepy to coordinate sucking and swallowing. Another potential problem is baby bottle tooth decay, of all upper teeth and some of the lower posterior teeth, from direct contact with sugar, syrup, honey-sweetened water, or fruit juice. Tooth decay occurs when the infant falls asleep and stops sucking on the bottle. The sugary solution pools around the infant's teeth and remains

| Table **17-3** | First Foods for the Infant |

Age (Months)	Addition
4 to 6	Iron-fortified rice cereal, followed by other cereals
5 to 7	Strained vegetables and fruits and their juices
6 to 8	Protein foods (cheese, meat, fish, chicken, and yogurt)
9	Finely chopped meat, toast, teething crackers
10 to 12	Whole egg, whole milk (allergies less likely now)

there for long periods. The carbohydrate in the solution is fermented into organic acids that demineralize the teeth until they decay. By not using the bottle as a pacifier, parents can prevent this condition.

Some additional tips for counseling parents are as follows:

1. Keep a calm, relaxed attitude throughout the weaning process.
2. Do not force an infant to use a cup; it is more detrimental to wean sooner than later.
3. Introduce the cup for one feeding per day and progress until the breast or bottle is surrendered.
4. Put only purified tap water into the bottle, and give the infant juice and milk from a cup.
5. Remember that infants enjoy the accomplishment of using a cup; it is one of their first steps toward independence.

Anticipatory Guidance

The infant progresses from a diet of milk alone to a diet of milk and solid foods within a short period. The nurse, in an attempt to guide the parents in meeting their infant's nutritional needs, understands these needs and developmental capabilities, and helps foster family-infant relationships. The health-promotion activity used in meeting proper infant nutrition focuses on parent education and positive reinforcement of parenting abilities.

Elimination Pattern

The infant develops an elimination pattern by the second week of life, usually associated with the frequency and amount of feedings. Both breast-fed and bottle-fed infants progress to a pattern of fewer stools per day after the first few months of life.

A breast-fed infant's stools have an orange-yellow color and a soft, even consistency, with a slightly sour but clean smell, dissimilar to stools passed later in life. A bottle-fed infant's stools are harder, smellier, and resemble those of an infant eating solid food. The breast-fed infant has many daily stools during the first and second months of life, progressing to one stool per day or even every one stool every 4 to 5 days in the later months before solid foods are introduced. The bottle-fed infant has two to four stools per day during the first month, tapering to one a day or even fewer at the end of infancy (Littleton & Engebretson, 2005).

For the first year of life, an infant cannot control the bowels. Bowel evacuation remains under involuntary, reflexive control until myelination of the spinal cord is complete, usually by 14 to 18 months of age (Pillitteri, 2003). Nurses advise overanxious parents to delay toilet training until the infant is developmentally ready.

The stress in American culture on daily bowel movements makes many mothers concerned about their infant's elimination patterns. The breast-fed infant may go for several days without having a bowel movement, which usually is not a problem. When the infant's behavior and feeding and sleeping patterns are normal, no elimination problem exists. A breast-fed infant rarely becomes constipated when consuming adequate amounts of breast milk. Usually the nurse only has to reassure the parents and discuss normal elimination patterns.

Urination increases as fluid intake increases. An infant who voids 6 to 12 times a day during the first few months of life is usually healthy and well hydrated. Voiding is involuntary until sometime during the second year of life, when bladder sensation develops. Irregular patterns of voiding characterize the remaining period of infancy.

Anticipatory Guidance

Anticipatory guidance and health promotion concerning elimination patterns of the infant should consist of parental teaching and reassurance, with special emphasis on good hygienic practices. Reassuring the parents about the infant's inability to control elimination is important so that their expectations are realistic. Despite how it might seem, the infant does not "save it up" until just after a clean diaper was put on.

Activity-Exercise Pattern

Physical activity and exercise contribute to development and coordination throughout the life span; infants receive their exercise through play. Initially infants engage in play with themselves with their hands or feet, with sounds, and by rolling and getting into various positions. By manipulating objects and achieving pleasurable sensations, infants learn about themselves and the objects in the environment.

Activity Through Play

Although the word *play* suggests physical activity, the infant's first play is actually an exercise of the senses. The infant's first toys are visual in nature. Through play, infants learn to hone their senses, to exercise their physical abilities, and to relate to other people. Most of the infant's play is solitary and repetitious. As each discovery is made, self-confidence and pride in the achievement are reinforced (as is the skill) through repetition.

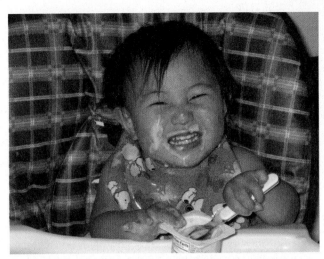

Figure 17-1 The family provides an infant with opportunities for spontaneous play.

As the infant enters the second half of the first year and becomes mobile, the family should provide the infant with increasing opportunities for spontaneous play and exploration. A planned play period in a safe environment should be established. The infant should have unrestrictive clothing so that movement can be free and unhampered. The caregiver should not interfere directly with the play but should be attentive to the infant's needs.

An important nursing role is assisting parents to promote play, stressing the importance of providing opportunities that are appropriate for the infant's age. Buying expensive toys is unnecessary; common household items, such as pots, pans, lids, and spoons, provide excellent objects for play purposes.

Activity Through Stimulation

Parental stimulation of the infant is an important developmental technique; the infant needs stimulation to learn about the world. This activity does not require expensive objects, but rather, it involves experiences in sight, sound, and touch, which are free and can be provided by any parent (Figure 17-1). Examples of stimulating experiences for infants include the following:

- Having lullabies sung to them
- Listening to tape recordings of a heartbeat
- Seeing colorful mobiles in crib
- Being rocked in a rocking chair
- Having a familiar face smiling close by
- Having space to wander when developmentally ready
- Looking at themselves in mirrors
- Listening to music

Anticipatory Guidance

Knowledge of developmental landmarks allows the nurse to guide parents in proper play and stimulation for infants. Handing a 15-month-old child a ball and placing the child in a fenced-in back yard to play is not enough. These

Table **17-4** Normal Sleep Patterns for Infants	
Age (Months)	**Hours in 24-Hour Period**
2 to 3	Low: 10 Average: 16½ High: 23 (2 to 4 naps)
3 to 4	Low: 8 to 10 nightly High: 11 to 12 nightly (2 or 3 naps daily)
6 to 12	11 to 12 nightly (2 or 3 naps daily)
12 to 18	8 to 12 nightly (1 or 2 naps daily)

activities must provide interpersonal contact, activity, and exercise. Activity and exercise through stimulation and play are extremely important for adequate and healthy development (Kelly, 2003).

Sleep-Rest Pattern

The amount of sleep that infants need is closely related to their rate of growth. Initially infants sleep approximately 80% of the time, as demanded by their rapid growth. As growth begins to slow toward the middle of the first year of life, less sleep is needed. The 12-month-old infant sleeps only 12 of 24 hours, a pattern that remains essentially unchanged through the second year (Moore & Persaud, 2003). To assist parents in understanding normal sleep and rest patterns, the nurse should stress that no set schedule exists (Table 17-4).

Nursing Suggestions

Health-promotion activities can also help the parents determine the individual needs of their infant. The nurse should stress that longer sleep patterns are signs of maturation and that sleep and rest are recognized as having a significant influence on the infant's growth and development. The nurse may offer the parents helpful comments for promoting infant sleep patterns, such as the following:

1. Provide a quiet room for the infant that is separate from the parents' room.
2. Learn behavioral clues that signal that the infant is going to sleep and is not interacting socially.
3. Learn to become sensitive to sleep cycles and rest periods that the infant is establishing and base care accordingly.
4. Attempt to schedule feeding times during wakeful rather than drowsy periods.
5. Learn that certain cycles are intrinsic to infants and that each infant is unique.
6. Perform rituals for the infant, such as rocking or reading a bedtime story, to provide comfort and security and let the infant know the expected behavior.

If parents express a sleep concern, the nurse must assess their reactions, consider their definition of the concern, assess the sleep environment, and observe the infant's own unique sleep patterns. Only then can the nurse's health-promotion approach be individualized to assist the family in caring for the infant.

Sudden Infant Death Syndrome

Sudden infant death syndrome (SIDS) is the sudden, unexplained death of an infant younger that 1 year of age that remains unexplained after review of the clinical history, examination of the scene of death, and postmortem examination (Creery & Mikrogianakis, 2003). The incidence of SIDS has varied over time and among nations. By definition, the cause of SIDS is not known. Observational studies have found an association between SIDS and several risk factors, including prone sleeping positions, prenatal or postnatal exposure to tobacco smoke, soft sleeping surfaces, hyperthermia or overwrapping, bed sharing, and lack of breast-feeding (Smith, Pell, & Dobbie, 2003).

Research focuses on sleep pathophysiology, particularly in relation to apneic spells that last longer than 10 seconds. The carotid body network and brainstem reflexes normally control physiological variations in heart and respiratory rates during sleep. For unexplained reasons, in SIDS cases these mechanisms likely fail to work during sleep, and respiration ceases. The mechanism of the relationship between apnea and SIDS is unsubstantiated. It has been proposed that a sleeping infant can become hypoxic with positional narrowing of the airway and respiratory inflammation. Research is ongoing.

SIDS refers to the sudden and unexpected death of an infant who has been healthy, with the cause of death unexplained after a thorough postmortem examination (Hot Topics box). Extensive research, debate, and uncertainty surround this phenomenon; its etiological factors remain a mystery.

The American Academy of Pediatrics Task Force on SIDS recommends the following: (1) healthy infants should be placed to sleep in the supine position in a crib that meets Consumer Product Safety Commission and American Society for Testing and Material standards, (2) avoid allowing infants to sleep on soft bedding (including waterbeds, sofas, and soft mattresses) or with pillows, soft comforters and coverings, loose bedding, or stuffed toys, (3) avoid overheating that occurs, for example, by placing excessive clothing or blankets on infants or by keeping the room temperature too high, (4) stop maternal smoking in the infant's environment, and (5) avoid bed sharing (Scheers, Rutherford, & Kemp, 2003).

Infants who are considered at high risk for SIDS include survivors of near-SIDS, subsequent siblings of SIDS victims, and premature infants with recurrent apneic episodes during sleep. From a preventive perspective, apnea monitors have been used in certain cases. However, controversy remains over this type of respiratory monitoring at home; parents face a heavy psychological responsibility when left in charge of their extraordinarily vulnerable young infant's life and monitoring may increase their anxiety and protectiveness of the infant.

The American Academy of Pediatrics (AAP) (2003a) has issued a policy statement concerning the use of home

INFANT SLEEP POSITION AND SUDDEN INFANT DEATH SYNDROME

HOTtopics

SIDS is the leading cause of infant mortality between 1 month and 1 year of age in the United States, occurring in approximately 4 per 1000 live births. SIDS, defined as the sudden death of an infant less than 1 year of age, remains unexplained after a thorough investigation. SIDS tends to occur at a higher-than-usual rate in the infants of adolescent mothers, infants of closely spaced pregnancies, and underweight male infants. However, even these profiles are inconsistent.

A variety of population characteristics have been explored, such as families with smokers, breast-feeding versus bottle feeding practices, or side or back sleeping positions for the infant. The primary contributor to a 50% decline in SIDS deaths in seven countries, including the United States, over a 12-year period was a decline in the facedown sleeping position of infants. The studies indicate that infants being put down to sleep should be positioned on their sides or backs.

In 1992 the American Academy of Pediatrics published a recommendation that "healthy infants, when being put down to sleep, be positioned on their side or back" in an attempt to decrease the incidence of SIDS. Since that time, the frequency of prone sleeping has decreased from greater than 70% to less than 20% of U.S. infants, and the SIDS rate has decreased by more than 50% (Tighe, 2004). It is therefore imperative that nurses continue to stress "back to sleep."

SIDS Facts

1. Incidence is highest between 1 and 8 months of age, with peak incidence at 2 to 3 months.
2. Infants of families of low socioeconomic status with a history of heavy smoking or drug abuse are at greater risk.
3. Infants with low birth weight are at greater risk of dying from SIDS than are term infants of normal weight.
4. SIDS occurs most often during the infant's sleep cycle.
5. Peak incidence is during the fall and winter seasons.
6. SIDS affects more male infants than it does female infants.
7. SIDS is a specific disease entity.
8. No evidence to date suggests hereditary or contagious causes.
9. SIDS is unexpected and unexplained.
10. No sign of distress, crying, or coughing is apparent at the time of death.
11. A mild upper respiratory infection may be present in some infants, but not all.
12. Autopsy findings are remarkably similar, including pulmonary congestion, intrathoracic petechiae, edema, and inflammatory infiltrates in the upper airway.

American Academy of Pediatrics Task Force on Infant Postioning and SIDS. (1992). Postioning and SIDS. *Pediatrics*, 89: 1120-1126; Tighe, C. M. (2004), Back to sleep. *American Journal of Nursing, 104*(6), 17.
SIDS, sudden infant death syndrome.

monitoring devices as a preventive measure for SIDS. Their recommendations include:

- Home cardiorespiratory monitoring should not be prescribed to prevent SIDS.
- If it is prescribed for premature infants with high-risk respiratory conditions, it should be equipped with an event monitor.
- Parents should be advised that monitors have not been proven to prevent SIDS.
- Pediatricians should continue to promote proven practices that decrease the risk of SIDS:
  Supine sleep position
  Safe sleeping environments
  Breast-feeding
  Elimination of prenatal and postnatal exposure to tobacco smoke (AAP, 2003b)

When an infant dies suddenly, unexpectedly, and for no apparent reason, a crisis occurs. The parents are devastated and completely unprepared for the shock, reacting with intense guilt, blaming themselves and each other, and agonizing over the part they may have played in the infant's death. Because many unanswered questions remain, these feelings are universal. Parents think there is something they could have done to prevent the tragedy. In most cases, nothing could have been done. Too frequently, the first sign that something was wrong is death.

Box 17-7 Parental Grieving Guidelines

1. Allow the parents and other family members to mourn in their own way.
2. Let them know that help is available when needed.
3. Present the factual information available about SIDS to help alleviate guilt.
4. Inform the parents that their reactions to the loss are not abnormal and that many other parents have had similar experiences.
5. Review the autopsy findings with them to substantiate the definite cause of death and to reduce guilt.
6. Reassure the parents that accepting the reality of the loss takes time.
7. Stress that communication is important in the adjustment process that follows a crisis.
8. Give the parents and other family members the opportunity to share the experience of losing an infant to SIDS by being a good listener.

The nurse is in an excellent position to help the family through this crisis. Box 17-7 provides some helpful guidelines.

Dealing with the family's grief is not an easy task. Many families find strength in God to help them through this difficult time. Other family members and close friends can assist the family in their grieving process.

Table **17-5** Visual Development During Infancy	
Age	**Behavior that Indicates Vision**
1 to 3 months	Fixes gaze on object 12 to 24 inches away
	Takes interest in bright colors and faces
	Follows objects in field of vision
3 to 6 months	Begins to show interest in hands
	Follows in range of 90 degrees
	Recognizes familiar objects
	Able to see full color by now
6 to 9 months	Visual scanning becomes more integrated
	Capable of organized depth perception
	Begins to perceive distances accurately
	Both eyes should focus equally now
9 to 12 months	Able to look for concealed items
	Converges on objects in close proximity
	Peripheral vision is well developed
	Judges distances well
12 to 18 months	Eye-hand coordination develops
	Depth perception more refined
	Ability to identify forms and shapes

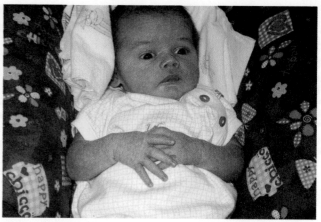

Figure 17-2 Babies respond to startling, loud noises, confirming their sense of hearing.

Many receive solace and support from talking to other parents who have lost an infant to SIDS. Several parent groups are available from local chapters of the SIDS Foundation; the nurse can refer them to their local chapter.

The nurse's main supportive role with families coping with SIDS is listening and offering compassionate guidance through the weeks and months that follow. The nurse encourages parents to talk about their infant. Too soon, family and friends expect the surviving family to get over it. A parent is never over it; it is only put in perspective and not so near the surface (Horchler & Rice, 2003).

Nursing assessment of the infant at risk for SIDS includes observing the infant for apneic episodes. Usually, however, nursing assessment occurs after death and consists of observing for appropriate grief patterns in the family. Nursing diagnoses for sudden infant death might include the following:

• Spiritual distress related to coping with death
• Ineffective family coping related to the loss of an infant
• Dysfunctional grieving related to the parents' inability to cope

Nurses also discuss with the family feelings about caring for future children. Life can appear out of control and parents may believe that they cannot care for another infant. These feelings must be resolved before another pregnancy is contemplated.

When dealing with the families of SIDS victims, nurses can feel uncomfortable and helpless. As health professionals, they might speak in terms of easing the pain or alleviating the guilt of these families, but many times simple

nonverbal human contact is sufficient to express concern and understanding.

Cognitive-Perceptual Pattern

Cognition is the process by which an individual recognizes, accumulates, and organizes the knowledge of the environment, beginning with the perception or recognition of an event within that environment. Cognitive development is concurrent with biological, adaptive, and psychosocial achievement. The infant's biological and cognitive developmental patterns (Piaget's sensorimotor period) are discussed earlier in this chapter. The focus of this section is on the infant's sensory and language development and the importance of stimulation to both developmental areas.

From birth, infants possess sensory capabilities; all sensory organs are well developed and functioning. As the infant is cared for and handled, the special senses become organized neurologically into a pattern of behavior that will greatly influence subsequent development.

Vision

The infant's initial visual impressions are unfocused, bizarre, unfamiliar, and without meaning. Because everything is new and only somewhat significant, visual stimuli must be moving, bright, or flashing to capture the infant's attention. The infant's eyes are well developed at birth, but the muscles that attach the eyes to their sockets are weak. This weakness may be stressful to parents, because the infant's eyes do not appear to function together. Parents can be assured that most infants coordinate their eye movements by the age of 3 months; by 6 months this function is mature. Table 17-5 summarizes visual developmental milestones.

Hearing

After the amniotic fluid drains from the middle ear several days after birth, the infant's hearing becomes acute. Hearing is one of the better-developed senses in the infant; the fetus can even hear in utero and responds to loud sounds (Figure 17-2). The newborn can distinguish sound frequencies and

Table **17-6** Normal Development of Hearing

Age	Behavior That Indicates Hearing
1 to 3 months	Is startled by loud noises
	Stops activity when spoken to
3 to 6 months	Turns eyes and head toward sound
	Responds to mother's voice
	Imitates own noises: "ooh" and "ba-ba"
6 to 9 months	Responds to own name
	Looks toward sounds
	Recognizes familiar sounds
9 to 12 months	Points to familiar objects or people
	Imitates simple words and sounds
	Locates a sound in any direction
12 to 18 months	Follows simple spoken directions
	Distinguishes between sounds
	Spoken words are well on their way

turns toward a voice or another sound. The infant may be familiar with the mother's voice early in life. Sounds gradually gain significance and meaning when they are associated with caregivers, food, and pleasure.

The ability to listen and discriminate among sounds is an important task during infancy. The closer the infant is to the sound, the easier the sound can be discriminated.

The groundwork for verbal ability begins to develop long before words appear, and many believe that infants whose mothers talk to them tend to speak earlier than infants who are not exposed to these sounds (Dacey & Travers, 2004). Table 17-6 summarizes the infant's auditory development.

Smell

The ability to smell is fully developed at birth. The infant has many receptors in the nose, but it lacks the cilia that line the inside of the adult's nose. As a result, the infant has a keen sense of smell, because odors reach the receptor cells easily. Within 2 weeks after birth, an infant can differentiate the odor of the mother's milk from others', an ability developed when the infant is held close (Hockenberry, 2005). At this time the infant begins associating the parents with their body odors, a perception that is important to infant-parent bonding.

Taste

The sense of taste is present at birth and salivation begins at approximately 3 months of age. The four primary sensations are sour, salty, sweet, and bitter. The taste buds for sweet tastes are more abundant during early life than they are in later life, which may account for the preference for sweets that is characteristic of infants and children.

Touch and Motion

Tactile sensation is well developed at birth, particularly on the lips and tongue. Perceptions of motion and touch are

perhaps the most important of all senses. Rocking and other motions are sensations of equilibrium picked up by the middle ear. Skin-to-skin touching should be performed regularly; evidence shows that touch helps relieve the unspent tensions that infants develop and accelerates neuromuscular development (McKinney, James, Murray, & Ashwill, 2005). Infants respond with pleasure to rocking and other motion and to tactile sensations of warmth, closeness, and cuddling.

Language Development

Language development, an important aspect of the infant's cognitive and perceptual pattern, is affected by intellectual development, maturation of the central nervous system, development of the organs of speech, and exposure to human verbalization.

As in other areas of development, language acquisition follows a definite sequence. During the first 2 months, most of the infant's sounds are vowels and are made primarily in the front part of the mouth (Hockenberry, 2005). Crying is the means of communication during this period. Cooing sounds are heard at approximately 2 to 3 months, usually in response to an adult's voice. By 6 months, babbling sounds are heard, and by 9 to 10 months, the infant forms two-syllable sounds. By 12 months, words such as "ma-ma," "bye-bye," and "da-da" are emerging. From 15 to 18 months, an expressive jargon with rhythmic intonations develops, but words are recognized only rarely. The infant uses jargon along with pointing to express wishes.

Nursing Suggestions

The nurse's knowledge and understanding of an infant's cognitive and perceptual behavior facilitates interaction with infants and serves as a guide in parental counseling. The main focus centers on stimulation, because each of the infant's senses is receptive to environmental stimulation. This activity helps the infant learn from the environment. When an infant is exposed to appropriate sensory stimulation, greater curiosity, improved mental capabilities, accelerated neuromuscular growth, enhanced gastrointestinal functioning, quicker weight gain, more rapid language development, and pleasing mother-infant interactions are likely to occur (Mandler, 2004).

Parents are the primary providers of pleasurable and stimulating experiences for the infant. The nurse assists them by offering suggestions about suitable stimuli for each sensory modality.

Self-Perception–Self-Concept Pattern

Self-perception has a pervasive influence on all aspects of life. Self-concept consists of a set of attitudes regarding what each person thinks, believes, and feels about the self. These attitudes form a personal self-belief that is an abstraction referred to as *me*. Many researchers believe that the infant determines self-existence by first noting that actions such as crying or smiling have an effect on others, which depends on receiving feedback (Klaus, Kennell, & Klaus, 2000).

Studies confirm that infants have the ability to identify themselves and therefore form a self-concept. Infants at 4 months of age were found to be particularly fascinated with their images in mirrors and smiled more at themselves than they did at pictures of other infants (Karmiloff & Smith, 2001).

As the infant continues to grow and mature, many circumstances combine to influence self-concept. How others relate to the infant's body and the messages that the infant receives from the body lead to knowledge of a physical self. The ability to use the body to influence others can lead the psychological self to conclude that someone cares about the infant (London, Ladewig, Ball, & Bindler, 2003).

The infant's development of body image is gradual. At birth the infant has diffuse feelings of hunger, pain, anger, and comfort, but no body image. Initially, all the infant knows is the self and regards the external world as an extension of the self. Only when infants begin to experience the environment through sensory modalities are they able to distinguish their bodies from animate and inanimate objects.

Nursing Suggestions

The nurse plays a vital role in assisting parents to foster the development of a positive self-concept and a good body image in their infant. The nurse first identifies personal self-concept and how it influences individuals (Kenner & McGrath, 2004). The nurse stresses that the way in which parents treat the infant influences the infant's self-concept. Basically, infants and young children incorporate their parents' interactions with them (good or bad) into their own view of self. Parents must understand that their infant's self-concept is an important, continuing event. What the infant knows and later believes about the self will affect all interactions with others, and by influencing what the infant will later attempt, the self-concept may have broad effects on the development of new skills (Kopp, 2003).

Roles-Relationships Pattern

Researchers have explored extensively the effect of early bonding between parents and their infants, emphasizing that this initial attraction sets the stage for the later development of love and affiliation (Gerhardt, 2004). The bonding process has many other implications for the infant's future development, as well (Klaus, Kennell, & Klaus, 2000).

Attachment and Bonding

The parent-infant relationship does not begin with the birth of the infant; many aspects have been molded by the life experiences of the parents long before they reached parenthood. The kind of mothering that a woman received as an infant and the concept of mother that she developed as she grew represent early effects that can influence the mother-infant relationship. The mother's overall self-concept will affect her ability to relate to her infant, as will her relationship with the infant's father.

The establishment of this emotional bond between the mother and her infant is known as *attachment*. This emotional bond is considered crucial for the optimal physical and emotional development of the infant. Maternal behaviors such as how the mother holds, feeds, and looks at the infant demonstrate the process of attachment (Brazelton & Sparrow, 2002).

Various theories have attempted to explain the basis for attachment behavior. Freudian psychoanalytical theory emphasizes that the bond between child and mother develops as a result of the mother's satisfying the infant's innate desire to socialize and the physical requirements for survival. Social learning theory contributes the principles of reinforcement to the attachment process; as the mother meets the infant's needs, discomfort is reduced or removed. The infant associates the pleasurable feeling of being satisfied with the mother, who becomes a significant other in the infant's life. The bonding process is the basis for the mother-infant relationship, which, in turn, forms the basis for the interdependence that is necessary for the infant's psychological and physical development (Korones & Bada-Eilzey, 2000).

In their early studies on attachment, Klaus, Kennell, and Klaus (2000) formulated the following seven crucial principles:

1. A sensitive period appears to exist during the first minutes and hours after birth, when it seems necessary for the mother and father to have close contact with their infant for later development to be optimal.
2. Species-specific responses to the infant appear to exist in the human mother and father when the infant is first given to them.
3. The attachment process seems to be structured such that the parents become attached to one infant at a time or in the case of a multiple birth to each infant simultaneously.
4. For attachment to occur appropriately, the infant must respond to the mother and father by some signal, such as body or eye movements. This principle has been called the *you can't love a dishrag phenomenon*.
5. Individuals who witness the birth process become strongly attached to the infant.
6. Some adults find it difficult to go through the processes of attachment and detachment simultaneously. Becoming attached to an infant while mourning the loss or threatened loss of another person is difficult for parents.
7. Some early events may have long-lasting effects. For example, anxiety over an infant with a transient disorder in the child's early days may result in long-term concerns or behavior that will have implications for future development.

Just as the infant's behavior influences attachment, it also continues to influence the evolving maternal-paternal-infant relationship as the infant develops. Studies have shown that if the process of attachment is encumbered, later problems are more likely to occur, such as child abuse, **failure-to-thrive syndrome,** and behavior problems (Tideman, Nilsson, Smith, & Stjernqvist, 2002).

Many factors are present when a relationship is being established and maintained. Most people enter a relationship with unrealistic expectations; parents are no exception—they are going to be wise, patient, and devoted, and they will nurture their infant. Because the parents' self-esteem is associated closely with their infant's interactions and accomplishments, when parents' self-esteem is low, disappointment, anger, and a disturbance in the relationship with their infant can occur. In some instances this disturbed parent-infant relationship is short-lived and nothing harmful develops. When a disturbed parent-infant relationship continues, however, the infant is at risk for abuse and behavior problems. (See Innovative Practice box, p. 412.)

The process of bonding is also important for fathers. Recently, a process called *engrossment* has been used to describe the behavior pattern of fathers when they interact with their infants. The major characteristics of engrossment include: (1) visual awareness of the infant, (2) tactile awareness, often expressed in a desire to hold the infant, (3) awareness of distinct characteristics, with emphasis on the features that resemble the father, (4) perception of the infant as perfect, (5) development of a strong feeling of attraction to the infant that leads to intense focusing of attention, (6) a feeling of extreme elation, and (7) a sense of deep self-esteem and satisfaction (Brazelton & Sparrow 2002).

Child Abuse

Family traditionally has been considered a safe place for its members, but many infants are at risk for maltreatment. Infant and child abuse has always been a part of human history. Acceptable behavior toward infants is largely a learned phenomenon; the art of parenting is not instinctively acquired, as many people believe. Abusing parents are seldom monsters; they are merely individuals who are attempting to cope with the demands of parenthood, for which there is little or no preparation.

The scope of the problem is extensive: estimates indicate that more than 3 million infants and children in the United States are victims of abuse (U.S. Census Bureau, 2000b). Children under 3 years of age are the most frequent victims. Women are more frequent abusers than are men, because they are the primary caregivers. Men abuse more severely and commit sexual abuse more frequently. Child abuse does not discriminate; it occurs in families of every race, creed, and socioeconomic class.

The child-abuse syndrome is a clinical condition in infants who have suffered serious active or passive abuse at the hands of their parents or other caregivers. Physical trauma is not the only facet, but it is the most overt indicator of a dysfunctional family unit and a disturbed parent-infant relationship (Joughin, 2003).

Active manifestations of abuse include the following:
1. Brain injuries, subdural hematomas, and skull fractures
2. Soft-tissue injuries, such as bruises, lacerations, or burns
3. Fractures of the long bones and ribs; multiple fractures in varying stages of healing
4. Sexual abuse manifested by genital tissue injury; sexually transmitted infections

Passive manifestations of abuse include the following:
1. Poor nutrition, failure to thrive, and severe malnutrition
2. Poor physical condition: neglected safeguards against disease, poor skin condition, and lack of medical attention
3. Emotional neglect: rejection, indifference, and deprivation of love
4. Moral neglect: allowing the infant or child to remain in an immoral atmosphere

Abusing parents often have common patterns of behavior. As children, their own parents may have abused them. In this way, child abuse is cycled from generation to generation. The development of the maternal role on which the infant depends for health, progress, and survival begins during the mother's early childhood. Unless she received love and proper mothering, she will have difficulty with a relationship that entails the complete dependency of another person. She may find the relationship with her own infant to be unrewarding, threatening, and frustrating. Feelings of inadequacy and guilt in the mother and father roles compound the problems.

Abusing parents are often socially isolated and have few people to whom they can turn during times of crisis; they also cannot support one another emotionally. These parents may view the infant as the person who can provide the love, support, and nurturing that is lacking in their own lives. When the infant does not fulfill their expectations, the risk of abuse becomes acute (Paavilainen & Astedt-Kurki, 2003).

The abused infant or child is usually singled out as someone who is different. This infant may be chronically ill, may have been premature, may be hyperactive, may have been the product of a difficult and complicated pregnancy, or may have an obvious anomaly. Early bonding disturbances (inadequacies in feeding, holding, and caring for the infant) are characteristic signals.

The long-term effects of child abuse are profound. The victims lack basic trust (a major task of infancy) and confidence and self-worth. These deficits follow the victims into adulthood and parenthood, and the vicious cycle continues. One of the discouraging findings is that infants and children who were abused frequently grow up to be abusing parents (Tomlin & Viehweg, 2003). Infant maltreatment is prevalent, and there is universal agreement about the detrimental effects on their welfare in general, as well as on their development.

Across the United States great interest has been generated in attempts to identify parents in the prenatal and perinatal periods who have significant potential for child abuse. Nurses play a critical role in recognizing infants who have been intentionally harmed, because they are often the first to begin taking a history on the infant. Nurses need to work collaboratively with community agencies to provide

| Box **17-8** | Nursing Interventions to Prevent Abuse of Infants |

- Promote and facilitate early parent-infant bonding.
- Promote a trusting relationship.
- Provide more frequent office visits and be available by phone.
- Provide infant care instructions to enhance mothering ability.
- Provide for community health person to make home visits.

follow-up care for the infant in danger of continued abuse. Nurses must take appropriate action if they suspect an infant is at risk. Doing nothing is not an option. The following measures have been undertaken to help prevent child abuse:

1. Predictive questionnaires to be given to parents on postpartum units
2. Recognition of parents who have difficulty relating to their infants through body language clues or verbalizations
3. Closer follow-up during the postpartum period by the public health nurse
4. Crisis hot lines made available to parents in distress

Before focusing on nursing interventions (Box 17-8), the nurse can make several observations to assist in identifying a high-risk infant by answering the following questions:

- Does the mother hold the infant close and establish eye contact?
- Does the mother speak negatively about the infant?
- Does the mother intensely dislike the duties of motherhood, such as diapering, feeding, and so on?
- Does the mother expect too much of the infant at a particular stage of development?
- Does the mother focus her attention on the infant rather than on her husband?
- Does the mother have a good support system available?
- Does the mother act overly concerned about the infant's gender?

Most communities are seeking ways in which child abuse can be prevented through educational efforts, improved agency coordination, and development of new collaborative efforts and services for parents and infants. Laws for reporting abuse have been enacted in every state. Reporting all cases of suspected abuse and neglect is mandatory. Everyone must assist in this endeavor to prevent continued abuse. It takes a community effort to address the problem.

Homelessness

Along with food, health, and personal safety, probably no greater basic need for human beings exists than shelter. The loss of shelter is detrimental to the health and well-being of all people. Homelessness in the United States is a national disgrace. Most estimates place the number of homeless at 3 million. One of every four homeless people is a child (Anderson, 2003).

To say that the well-being of the next generation is being jeopardized by homelessness is not an exaggeration. Homelessness devastates every aspect of a child's life, doing damage with long-term implications that remain unknown. Homelessness endangers a child's health throughout childhood. Homeless infants are often exposed to unsafe and unsanitary conditions in shelters in which infectious diseases thrive. These dangers are combined with a lack of access to regular health care; common childhood ailments such as ear infections become extremely serious and sometimes life-threatening illnesses before they are treated.

Ear infections are among the most common health problems encountered in children. For a bacterial infection, a course of antibiotics usually relieves the condition. Rarely are long-term complications encountered. For the homeless infant, however, the story is different. Families are cut off from their regular clinics and providers. The struggle for basic life needs is intense. The poverty, isolation, and disorientation of prolonged homelessness can be complicated by drug or alcohol abuse, provoked, at least in part, by situational despair. The fundamental ability of a family to function is hampered or paralyzed.

For the homeless family, the fever caused by an infant's acute ear infection may not have the highest priority. Availability, accessibility, and affordability of medical care are serious concerns. As a result, the infection may never be treated, and the problem becomes prolonged (the infection evolves to a chronic state). Hearing and language development can be impaired.

These children simply do not receive routine, reliable health care. They remain at high risk for many health problems. Their health problems remain undiagnosed and undertreated, if they receive attention at all. Complications and secondary problems abound.

Infants are born onto the streets without cribs and are rarely held. They may find refuge in an overcrowded shelter one night, and the next night their shelter is a doorway hidden in an alley; the following night home is an abandoned car. From the beginning of life these infants encounter an unbeatable cycle of nowhere to go, no place to call home, no safe sanctuary, only the feeling of aloneness and unpredictability (Smolen, 2003).

The pioneering work of Erik Erikson has defined the necessary stages of human development. Each level of maturation must be mastered sequentially, but to do so takes a secure environment, opportunities to succeed, and emotional support. The hidden tragedy for homeless children is the stifling of their personal growth. These losses, dissimilar to the loss of a home, may be irrevocable. Theoretically homelessness can be eliminated. The key factors are increased affordable housing, increased income for low-income families, and strengthened service and support for families at risk of homelessness. Families at risk of homelessness for solely economic reasons can often be helped with short-term loans and grants. Community-based programs can help identify these families before they lose their homes.

CASE STUDY

Homeless Infants

As a community health nurse in an inner-city health center, you are increasingly aware that the homeless population in your city appears to be the forgotten aggregate. Your community health center provides primary care to a culturally diverse and indigent population. As a nurse, you believe that the homeless population within your city has numerous health needs. Beyond the basic requirements, many homeless people have mental and substance abuse problems, lack of life skills, poor family support, and most of all no child health access.

The homeless population has all of the usual health problems you would expect in the general population in addition to other problems resulting from their homeless lifestyle. Although there are several glaring concerns, you plan to focus your attention first on securing immunizations for the homeless infants and, secondly, to obtain formula for them.

Reflective Questions

1. In planning health services for this special population, what facts do you need to know?
2. What barriers to accessing health care for infants confront the homeless family?
3. How can you overcome some of the barriers in developing your plan for health care?

Discussion

1. In planning health services for this special population, what facts do you need to know? Some of the first questions that should be asked are:
   - How many homeless infants are in this aggregate?
   - Where are they?
   - How can they access health care in the city?

To answer these questions, it might be prudent to collaborate and partner with other health and social service agencies, local hospitals, and the state health and human services agency. Collaboration and partnering can bring in additional resources and reduce duplication and gaps in services.

2. What barriers to accessing health care for infants confront the homeless family?
   - Lack of transportation
   - Lack of trust in the medical establishment
   - Judgmental care on the part of health care providers
   - No health insurance to cover medical visits
   - Preventive care, such as immunizations, not a priority when you are hungry
   - No money to get prescriptions filled
   - Waiting until condition is serious before seeking treatment

3. How can you overcome some of the barriers in developing your plan for health care?
   - Provide health care in the city shelters for use by homeless families.
   - Set up a mobile health care team and visit the shelters to provide care.
   - Offer free immunizations for all family members.
   - Set up educational sessions within the shelters to provide information.
   - Stress importance of preventive measures to reduce illness in infants.
   - Obtain free formula from company or hospitals to give to homeless infants.
   - Work closely with other health care interests within the community.

Efforts should be made to link the homeless with all available programs and services, such as the Special Supplemental Nutrition Program for Women, Infants, and Children (WIC), food stamps, Head Start, and housing subsidies. These programs should continue to provide assistance after the family is resettled in permanent housing. These families will need more comprehensive services with special problems such as domestic violence, mental illness, and substance abuse.

Because there is a multitude of needs, a partnership that provides a multitude of resources must be developed. Nurses can take a leadership position in helping the homeless achieve a sense of security and adequate health care. Nursing involvement in community health care for the homeless and providing compassionate care gives the homeless a clear signal of hope and concern about their plight. Bringing attention to this social problem by speaking to community groups to obtain their support is another way that nurses can help. Volunteering time in community shelters and organizing health care days through the local health department is another way to address the problem. Nurses can become active in raising the nation's conscience and helping to call attention to this national disgrace. Housing and support services must be provided to assist the homeless in regaining a foothold in society. With the right support services and health care, many homeless people can be stabilized and reintegrated into the community. These families with infants are not throwaways, but people who have fallen on hard times and need someone to offer a helping hand. Through this help, the nation's health can improve (Case Study and Care Plan boxes).

Sexuality-Reproductive Pattern

An infant's identity begins at birth, when the child is named and caretakers behave a certain way toward the infant because of its gender. The infant's sexuality gives direction to its physical, emotional, social, and intellectual responses throughout life. Infants have a great oral sensitivity, enjoy skin-to-skin contact, and explore their own bodies for pleasure during the first year of life. A healthy, accepting attitude by caretakers is important in an infant's evolving sexual development.

Coping–Stress Tolerance Pattern

The term *stress* implies intense reaction to an experience and changes in usual behavior. Stress is a normal phenomenon that occurs throughout the life span when an individual experiences a developmental or situational crisis.

CARE PLAN

Homelessness

(Related to Homeless Infants Case Study)

Homelessness is a community dilemma and an example of an economic problem that places infants at risk. Families are the fastest growing group of homeless people. Homeless families do not have health insurance; infants within these families are more likely to lack immunizations, proper nutrition, safe environment, and a stable family situation. The community health nurse in this chapter's Case Study wanted to address two aspects of homeless infants: (1) immunizations and (2) nutrition.

Nursing Diagnosis Altered Health Maintenance Related to Nonadherence to Appropriate Immunization Schedule as Manifested by Increased Incidence of Communicable Diseases

DEFINING CHARACTERISTICS

History of lack of health-seeking behavior by caregiver; lack of financial or other resources; reported or observed impairment of personal support systems; lack of knowledge regarding health-promotion practices; inability to access health care; limited basic personal resources

RELATED FACTORS

Ineffective family coping; perceptual-cognitive impairment; lack of material resources; ineffective individual coping

EXPECTED OUTCOMES

Caretaker of infant will:
- Begin health-seeking behavior on behalf of infant
- Increase health-promotion and health maintenance knowledge
- Gain access to available health care resources
- Participate in life change to improve health status; meet goals for health care maintenance

NURSING INTERVENTIONS

- Assess caretaker's feelings, values, and personal situation.
- Assess for family patterns, economic issues, and cultural patterns that influence compliance.
- Assist caretaker and family to access health care resources available to them.
- Refer caretaker and family to community agencies to address social and economic issues.

- Educate caretaker and family on the importance of immunizations and disease prevention.
- Provide for follow-up to increase chance of health status change taking place.

Nursing Diagnosis High Risk for Altered Nutrition—Less than Body Requirements; related factors and socioeconomic factors as manifested by low height and weight measurements for chronological age on growth chart

DEFINING CHARACTERISTICS

Pale conjunctival and mucus membranes; poor muscle development; inadequate food intake to maintain body weight; weight loss, fatigue, frequent irritable, fussy, crying behavior; growth and development milestones not met; frequent illnesses suggesting depressed immunity

RELATED FACTORS

Inability to obtain adequate food or fluid or both to nourish body because of socioeconomic factors

EXPECTED OUTCOMES

Infant will demonstrate the following:
- Progressive weight gains toward desired goal
- Weight within normal range for height and weight
- Infant consuming adequate nourishment
- Infant free of signs of malnutrition

NURSING INTERVENTIONS

- Assess healthy body weight for age and height.
- Observe infant's ability to consume food and fluids.
- Monitor food and fluid intake weekly.
- Access nutritional resources for the caretaker or family.
- Refer to appropriate community agencies to meet needs.
- Assist the caretaker or family to identify area needing change which will make the greatest contribution to improve nutrition.
- Implement instructional dialogue that is appropriate for their level.
- Provide for follow-up care to assist them in changing their health status.

Developmental Crisis

Developmental crises are turning points or periods of great change. Most stressors that the infant experiences are a necessary part of growth and development. For example, learning new skills creates stress. The infant who is unable to move forward while learning to crawl experiences stress. The infant expresses this stress by crying for help. Other stressors are more psychosocial in nature, such as being left with a baby-sitter or in an unfamiliar place.

Situational Crisis

Situational crises are not anticipated easily and do not occur necessarily as part of the normal growth and development

process. One major situational crisis during infancy is separation from the significant other. The following three distinct phases are evident in the reaction to separation (Hockenberry, 2005):

1. *Protest.* Infant cries loudly, screams for the mother, and refuses attention of the substitute caregiver.
2. *Despair.* Infant stops crying and becomes less active, withdraws, and becomes apathetic.
3. *Withdrawal.* Infant takes an interest in surroundings but tends to ignore or reject the mother when she returns, because she failed to meet the infant's needs.

Initially, with no time framework and no understanding of waiting, the infant has little ability to cope with stress.

Nursing Interventions to Assist in Stressful Situations During Infancy

- Attempt to meet the infant's needs promptly.
- Allow favorite toy or item of security to be present during stressful experiences.
- Allow familiar caregiver to be present to calm the infant.
- Attempt to keep the number of strangers interacting with the infant to a minimum.
- Attempt to provide a warm and accepting environment for the infant.
- Allow freedom of expression (crying) to reduce tension in the infant.
- Identify the infant's established daily routine and try to follow through with it.
- Reinforce the infant's need for expression.
- Establish a trusting relationship with the infant.
- Provide opportunity for play so the infant can vent fears.
- Provide emotional support for the parents so they can, in turn, give support to their infant.

As maturity and a sense of security provided by the caregiver increases, the infant begins to wait a short time to have needs met without protest. An infant who experiences stress reacts by crying, the main tool of communication. The infant gradually learns to tolerate greater stress with time.

Nursing Interventions

Nursing suggestions to assist the infant and family in stressful situations are listed in Box 17-9. By allaying anxiety in the infant's caregiver, the nurse facilitates coping behaviors in the infant. The stressful situation and the problem-solving activities can be turned into growth-producing experiences for the family, with coping capacities strengthened for the future.

Values-Beliefs Pattern

A value is a standard or principle that is considered to be good or proper. When people communicate, they send both the content message of the spoken words and the unspoken message of who they are and what they believe. Values are pervasive and important and give a focus to people within a particular culture. Because values are attitudes learned from significant others within the environment, the values-beliefs pattern is undeveloped in the infant. The infant has yet to reach the cognitive level of incorporating the parents' values into the behavioral system. The parents, through parenting behaviors, serve as a model as the infant develops into a boy or girl.

Nursing Interventions

By understanding and respecting the parents' value system, the nurse works within their framework of values in the counseling situation. The nurse communicates personal values to the family. To work successfully within a different value system, the nurse should incorporate the following attitudes concerning the values-beliefs pattern into the nursing process (M. J. Clark, 2003):

1. Believe in the ultimate worth of the infant and the family, regardless of their behavior or situation.
2. Grant families the freedom to make their own informed choices and to experience the responsibilities and consequences of their decisions.
3. Use knowledge of the family's value system in specific ways to reward and reinforce positive health practices.
4. Value the growth potential inherent in developmental and situational crisis situations.
5. Recognize your own value system and its influence on your behavior.
6. Work with families without applying your personal value system in judging their behavior.
7. Broaden your value system by accepting lifestyles different from your own.

The nurse influences the behavior of the parents, who have the greatest influence on their infant's values-beliefs pattern. The nurse accomplishes this task by modeling (living congruently with professed values), acting as a consultant by sharing pertinent information with parents, and modifying one's own values (Betz & Sowden, 2004).

Modeling can be a potent influence on another individual's behavior. In the counseling situation, the family looks to the nurse for guidance and assistance in promoting healthy child-rearing practices. The methods by which the nurse interacts with the infant, listens to the parents' concerns, and demonstrates respect for the family unit are influencing factors in changing behavior.

Second, the nurse acts as a consultant to influence values. Advice on child-rearing practices is overwhelming to parents; everyone has opinions. The nurse listens before giving advice to determine whether parents will accept the advice and to allow them to decide whether the advice can be useful. Repeated attempts to convert parents to the nurse's value system can make them defensive and resistant to the advice.

Third, by expressing values and attitudes, but remaining open to other approaches, the nurse influences the values-beliefs pattern. Parents should realize that they are free to change and are not bound to traditional values that others outside their value system express (Shah, 2004).

The nurse who uses these communication skills can deal with families more effectively. The nurse's open attitude increases the likelihood that the parents will discuss their concerns and adhere to the health-promotion guidelines that the nurse has offered.

PATHOLOGICAL PROCESSES

This section discusses various factors within the environment that can affect the infant's health status. The entire realm of accident prevention and safety promotion is applicable here.

Accidents are always unexpected and, in retrospect, usually could have been prevented. Adults take for granted that they are living in a world designed by adults for adults. They must remind themselves constantly that infants also live in this complex world and, although they learn at a remarkable rate, infants are unaware of most environmental dangers. This inexperience renders them extremely vulnerable to accidents, a major problem and a challenging field for preventive measures.

Accidents occur in many situations: in the home, in the street, on the playground, and in automobiles. The use of safety belts prevent infant injury (Figure 17-3). Most accidents, however, occur in the home. Their number and seriousness are closely linked to the infant's developmental stage. Accidents tend to increase with the mobility of the infant, but even a 2 month old can wiggle or fall from a high place.

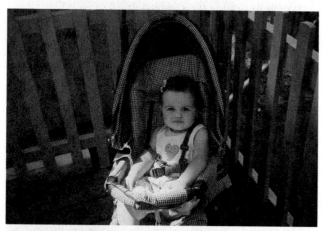

Figure 17-3 Accident prevention for infants in their strollers includes the use of safety belts.

Box **17-10** Safety Tips to Prevent Falls

1. Whenever the infant is in the crib, keep sides up and securely fastened.
2. Place the infant seat in the playpen or on the floor; always strap the infant in securely.
3. Check high chairs, strollers, and carriages for safety, and restrain the infant who is active.
4. Lock windows if the infant is capable of climbing on the windowsill.
5. Clean up food or liquid spills immediately from the floor.
6. Remember that polished floors are hazardous, especially when throw rugs are present.
7. Close off stairways with doors, gates, or some other safety device as the infant becomes mobile.
8. Do not leave items that the infant might use to climb out of the crib.
9. To prevent falls, set the crib mattress at the lowest adjustment level after the infant can pull up and stand.
10. Strap the infant into a shopping cart to prevent falls.

From Wootan, G. (2000). *Take charge of your child's health: A parent's guide to recognizing symptoms and treating minor illnesses at home* (2nd ed.). New York: Marlowe & Co.

Nurses have the opportunity to help parents and caregivers anticipate and understand the common hazards of early life and provide specific guidance for accident prevention.

Unintentional Injuries
Falls

Falls are most common after 4 months of age, when the infant has learned to roll over, but they can occur at any age. The best advice is never to place an infant unattended on a raised surface that has no type of guardrails. When in doubt, the safest place is the floor (Altman, 2004). Safety tips to assist parents in preventing falls are listed in Box 17-10.

Burns

Burns are the most frequent and frightening of all accidents during infancy. Because nearly all burns are preventable, the attendant caregiver can experience severe guilt.

Fire from matches or other sources, hot liquids, ultraviolet light from the sun, electricity or electrical outlets, and heating elements such as radiators, registers, and floor heaters can all cause burns. Box 17-11 lists safety tips to assist parents in preventing burns.

Box **17-11** Burn Prevention Guidelines

1. Keep the infant out of the sun when ultraviolet rays are strongest, generally from 10:00 AM to 3:00 PM.
2. Sunscreen, clothing with long sleeves, pant legs, and a brimmed hat are essential to prevent sun overexposure.
3. Remember that fireplaces can be a serious hazard. Fine-mesh screens attached to a frame are safer than freestanding screens. Never leave an infant alone in a room where a fire is burning; make sure the fire is out before going to bed.
4. Avoid bathing the infant in a sink or adult tub near hot water faucets. Test the bath water temperatures before placing the infant in it; keep one hand on the infant at all times during the bath.
5. Be sure that all infant's clothing is made of nonflammable materials.
6. Avoid handling hot liquids near the infant.
7. Turn the handles of cooking utensils toward the back of the stove.
8. Keep all electrical cords taut, especially those for coffee pots; keep cords out of the infant's sight.
9. Cover electrical outlets with protective plastic caps.
10. Place a barrier in front of any heat-producing element, especially floor heaters.
11. Keep all matches and lighters out of the infant's reach.
12. Teach the older infant the meaning of hot.
13. Close oven doors when the oven is in use or when cooling.
14. If you must smoke, keep the heat of cigarettes or cigars away from the infant.

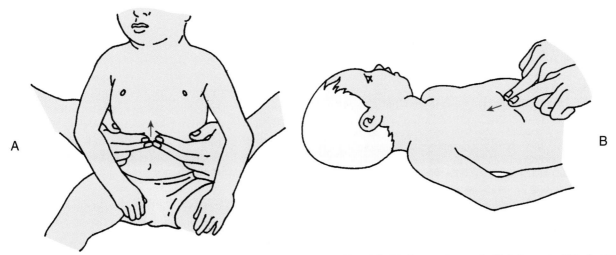

Figure 17-4 The Heimlich maneuver for infants can be performed two ways. **A,** Place infant in lap, reach around with index and middle fingers of both hands placed against abdomen (above navel and below rib cage), and give quick, upward thrust; **B,** Position infant face upward on firm surface, face infant, and deliver upward thrust with index and middle fingers. Repeat either maneuver if necessary.

Swallowing/Choking on Foreign Objects

Any small object that an infant puts in the mouth has the potential to be swallowed and choked on. Parents should be advised that objects such as safety pins, peanuts, beads, coins, hot dogs, paper clips, nuts, corn, buttons, popcorn, chips, apple with peel, and parts of broken toys are frequently swallowed. Many objects can fit into this category and into the infant's mouth. The carelessness of a caregiver, relative, friend, or baby-sitter in leaving small objects available and within reach, or giving toys unsuited to the infant's stage of development, frequently cause these accidents.

When choking occurs, the infant should be placed across the adult's knees (facedown on an incline, with the head at the lower end) and thumped sharply between the shoulder blades (Brenner, 2004).

The nurse gives parents another basic method to prepare them for a choking incident. The Heimlich maneuver should be learned and used in a life-threatening situation caused by swallowing a foreign body (Figure 17-4) (Daly, 2004).

Prevention of swallowing foreign objects is the best treatment. Some safety•measures for parents and caregivers of infants are listed in Box 17-12.

The entire balance of safety for infants rests on allowing them plenty of opportunity to explore and play within the environment while protecting them from harmful physical agents. According to the American Academy of Pediatrics, the greatest threat to the health of infants is not illness, but injuries, many of which can be prevented. The nurse should inform the infant's primary caregivers about ways to child-proof their home (Box 17-13).

Biological Agents

The fetus is protected from biological agents in the environment by the placental barrier and the mother's defense

---

> **Box 17-12** **Nursing Interventions to Reduce Choking Hazards for Infants**
>
> - Keep small objects out of an infant's reach.
> - Avoid propping bottles and making large holes in nipples to prevent aspiration of formula into the infant's lungs.
> - Discourage the use of powder on infants to reduce the risk of pneumonia from inhaling zinc stearate.
> - Burp the infant thoroughly before placing in the crib; place infant in side-lying position.
> - Older children should not give food to the infant, who may choke on it. An adult should be near to supervise children around infants.
> - Adults should not set a bad example by putting pins or other objects in their mouths; older infants like to mimic adults.
> - Inspect toys for loose, removable parts that could end up in the infant's mouth.

---

system. After birth, however, the infant is thrust into an environment that is filled with infectious, disease-causing agents. These bacterial or viral organisms can be found in food, cribs, the air, pets, the parents, and the siblings—literally everywhere. Even the healthiest environment harbors disease-causing agents. Although the infant cannot escape exposure to these pathogens without being completely isolated, immunizations are given to assist the infant's defense against communicable diseases.

Acquired Immunodeficiency Syndrome

Acquired immunodeficiency syndrome (AIDS) is spread by contact with the human immunodeficiency virus (HIV) through blood and bodily secretions. The virus attacks the T cell lymphocytes, affecting formation of T_H4 (T helper or T inducer) cells, which direct the immune response. The

Box **17-13** Home Childproofing Tips

1. Remove any heavy, sharp, or breakable objects from tables and low shelves.
2. Bolt bookcases to the wall and remove heavy books to prevent falls.
3. Test floor and table lamps to make sure they cannot be pulled over.
4. Disconnect unused appliances and wrap up cords.
5. Secure all other cords to prevent appliances from being pulled down.
6. Safely discard unused and unneeded medicines.
7. Avoid referring to medicines as candy.
8. Store potentially toxic substances out of sight and reach.
9. Close reachable outlets with safety covers.
10. Tie drapery and blind cords out of the infant's reach.
11. Choose stair gates with openings too small for an infant's head and child-resistant fasteners such as pressure bars.
12. Avoid accordion or expandable gates with openings that can trap an infant's head.
13. Install smoke detectors and check the batteries at least once a month.
14. Use sturdy screens in front of fireplaces.
15. Place crib, playpen and high chair well away from heaters, fans, and electrical outlets.
16. Install childproof latches on drawers and cupboards. Store all cleaning compounds and detergents in a high, locked cupboard.
17. Buy all medicines in bottles with childproof lids and keep them in their original labeled containers for identification in case of accidental ingestion.
18. Install lids on garbage pails and never leave any harmful materials in them, such as sharp can lids or spoiled food.
19. Check the floor regularly for objects small enough to be swallowed.
20. Cut blinds cord into two pieces.

infant with HIV infection is unable to resist normal infections. Transmission of HIV from mother to infant is the most likely cause of childhood HIV. Transmission can occur during pregnancy, at delivery, or during breast-feeding (Koop, 2003). There is no immunization against HIV infections.

Because infants can retain maternal antibodies for HIV infection for as long as 18 months, the diagnosis of HIV infection in an at-risk infant (one whose mother is infected) is extremely difficult. In the last few years, investigators have demonstrated the utility of highly accurate blood tests in diagnosing HIV infection in infants 6 months of age and younger (Koop, 2003). Although signs and symptoms of illness can occur at any time, they usually begin during the first year of life. In infants the symptoms of the disease include failure to thrive, oral candidiasis, recurrent bacterial infections, persistent pulmonary infiltrates, delays in reaching important milestones in motor skills and mental

development such as crawling, walking and speaking, and chronic diarrhea (Zeichner & Read, 2004). Early diagnosis is essential for effective treatment.

Nursing assessment focuses on a careful and complete history of the infant and mother, signs and symptoms of the disease, growth and development history, and psychosocial concerns. Parents must be assessed carefully to determine their level of anxiety; knowledge of the disease process, including prognosis, treatment, and transmission; and awareness of resources, support systems, coping strategies, and the infant's needs.

No other disease causes as much public awareness and panic as does AIDS. Part of this behavior is ignorance. Nurses play a major role in educating the public about the disease process, its mode of transmission, and most of all, preventive measures. Preventive education should begin with young children. Most school health programs include information on AIDS. School nurses can contribute to the success of these programs, as can nurses working in prenatal clinics, to spread the *prevention word*. Nurses in all settings can engage in research related to AIDS to gather further clarification of this fatal disease.

Although the infant is not an active participant in the spread of HIV, parents should understand the means by which the virus is transmitted and not allow their infant to become a passive participant because of their own high-risk behaviors.

Immunization

Disease prevention by immunization is a public health priority in the *Healthy People 2010* initiative and society as a whole. Progress continues toward the goal of protecting children from serious disease through immunizations. The most recent schedule emphasizes the preference for administering the first dose of the hepatitis B vaccine series at birth before hospital discharge, expands the use of influenza vaccine to healthy children ages 6 months to 23 months, and the change from using oral polio vaccine (OPV) to inactivated poliovirus (IPV) vaccine, because OPV is no longer used routinely in the United States (Centers for Disease Control and Prevention, 2003).

The two types of immunization are active and passive. In **active immunization,** all or part of a disease-causing microorganism or a modified product of that microorganism is injected into the body to make the immune system react defensively. This substance is generally a toxin of the disease organism; depending on the virulence and certain other characteristics of the organism, it is used in the vaccine in a live, killed, or attenuated form (D'Lugoff & Schalla, 2000). The attenuated form is alive, but its virulence has been reduced significantly by treatment with laboratory procedures that use, for example, heat or chemicals, which reduces potency of microorganisms. Examples of active immunization include diphtheria, tetanus, and acellular pertussis (DTaP); inactivated polio vaccine (IPV); and measles, mumps, and rubella (MMR). Active immunization affords lifelong immunity.

Table **17-7** Recommended Immunization Schedule for Infants	
Age (Month)	**Immunization**
Birth	HBV-1
1 month	HBV-2
2 months	DTaP-1, Hib-1, IPV-1, PCV-1
4 months	DTaP-2, Hib-2, IPV-2, PCV-2
6 months	HBV-3, DTaP-3, Hib-3, IPV-3, PCV-3 Influenza (yearly)
12 to 15 months	Hib-4, MMR
15 to 18 months	DTaP-4, varicella

Modified from the American Academy of Pediatrics. (2004). Recommended childhood immunization schedule: United States (Online). Retrieved July 5, 2005, from: http://www.cdc.gov/nip/. *DTaP*, diphtheria, tetanus, acellular pertussis vaccine; *HBV*, hepatitis B vaccine; *Hib*, *Haemophilus influenza* type b conjugate vaccine; *IPV*, inactivated polio vaccine; *PCV*, pneumococcal vaccine; *MMR*, measles, mumps, rubella vaccine.

Passive immunization is accomplished by injecting blood from an actively immunized person or animal. After an individual has been exposed to a disease, a passive immunization is given to prevent the disease from developing. Passive immunizations provide a short immunity, usually 1 to 6 weeks, which will protect the person until the danger of contracting the disease is passed. Passive immunization also helps reduce the severity of the disease when it is contracted. Because of the short duration, active immunization is still needed to remain permanently immune. Passive immunity occurs naturally in newborns when maternal antibodies are passed through the placenta or in breast milk.

The Committee on Infectious Diseases of the American Academy of Pediatrics (2004) recommends immunization schedules that are revised periodically as new information arises. Table 17-7 lists the current recommendations for healthy infants. More detailed immunization information is provided in **Web Site Resource 17E.**

Immunization provides one of the most cost-effective means of preventing infection in infants. Immunizations not only help protect those receiving the vaccinations from developing potentially serious diseases, they also help protect entire communities by preventing and reducing the spread of infectious agents. Immunization is additionally important because currently available antibiotics cannot destroy viruses; therefore, immunization offers the only means of control. Nurses have a special responsibility to keep informed of the recommendations and document all vaccinations given. Emphasis must be placed on educating parents about the importance of immunization. Children need a series of vaccinations, starting at birth, to be fully protected against 12 potentially serious diseases. To motivate parents to have their infants immunized, the nurse can work toward increasing health education to achieve greater health maintenance knowledge, send reminders for upcoming visits and needed immunizations, vigorously advocate for all infants to receive comprehensive health care, including immunizations, provide health services that make immunizations feasible and available, develop a close relationship with the family, and continue the surveillance of the immunization status of every infant in the health care system.

Nutrition Problems

Nutrition problems include undernutrition, in which infants do not receive an adequate supply of an essential nutrient, and overnutrition, in which they receive more of a certain nutrient than is needed for healthy growth and development (Dudek, 2005). For infants in the United States, both of these problems are present.

A parent who wants the infant to have family foods rather than commercial baby food can blenderize a small portion of the table food at each meal. This choice necessitates cooking without salt or sugar as is the practice of baby food manufacturers. Making baby food is easy and economical. Written resources are available on the reference pages for parents who are interested in more details about home food preparation for infants.

Parents should be encouraged to read baby food labels carefully. Nurses can obtain lists of baby foods and their ingredients from the manufacturers. The best overall recommendation that nurses make to parents is to provide their infants with a well-balanced diet and avoid excesses.

Chemical Agents
Drugs

Aspirin is the medicine most commonly ingested, with acetaminophen and vitamins close behind. Ibuprofen and other aspirin substitutes, is becoming increasingly popular with parents as an antipyretic. Vitamins themselves are usually harmless; however, many vitamins contain iron, making them potentially lethal. Infants are attracted to vitamins because of their appealing colors and flavors.

Recent changes in packaging and limits on the number of tablets contained in each bottle have reduced deaths resulting from overdose. Drug manufacturers are using childproof caps increasingly as a safety measure. Despite a concerted effort by manufacturers, childproof bottle caps vary in effectiveness (Carroll, 2004). Frequently the safety caps are adult-proof, although children can readily open them.

This points to the dangers of medications, regardless of the bottle. All medications still must be kept locked away when infants are in the home. Some additional guidelines to help prevent accidents involving drugs include the following:

1. Use a prescription drug only for the purpose and the person for whom it is intended. Do not use medication prescribed for someone else for a similar condition in the infant.
2. Discard unused drugs by flushing them down the toilet; many infants have been poisoned by eating tablets found in the trash.
3. Request safety caps on all prescription drugs.

Table **17-8** Poisonous Parts of Common House and Garden Plants

Plant	Toxic Part	Symptoms
Apple	Seeds	Release cyanide when ingested in large quantities; can be fatal
Azalea	All parts	Nausea, vomiting, dyspnea, paralysis; can be fatal
Buttercup	All parts	Inflammation around mouth, stomach pains, vomiting, diarrhea, and convulsions
Castor bean	Seeds	Burning of mouth and throat, excessive thirst, and convulsions; one or two seeds are near the lethal dose for adults
Croton species	Plant juice	Gastroenteritis
Daffodil	Bulb	Nausea, vomiting, and diarrhea; can be fatal
Dieffenbachia	All parts	Intensive burning and irritation of the mouth and tongue; death can occur when base of tongue swells enough to occlude air passages
English holly	Berries	Nausea, vomiting, diarrhea, central nervous system depression; can be fatal
English ivy	Leaves and berries	Dyspnea, vomiting, diarrhea, coma, and death
Hyacinth	Bulb	Nausea, vomiting, and diarrhea; can be fatal
Iris	Underground stems	Digestive upset
Jasmine	All parts	Hallucinations, elevated temperature, tachycardia, and paralysis
Lily of the valley	All parts	Arrhythmia, mental confusion, weakness, shock, and death
Mistletoe	Berries	Acute stomach and intestinal irritations with diarrhea; can be fatal
Oak tree	Acorns	Kidney failure, gastritis
Oleander	All parts	Digestive upset, bloody diarrhea, respiratory depression, cardiac arrhythmia, blurred vision, coma, and death
Philodendron	All parts	Burning of lips, mouth, and tongue; swelling of tongue; dyspnea, kidney failure; death
Poinsettia	Leaves	Severe irritation to mouth, throat, and stomach; can be fatal
Potato	All green parts	Cardiac depression; can be fatal
Tomato	Green parts	Cardiac depression; can be fatal
Violet	Seeds	Taken in quantity, cathartic effects can be serious to infant
Yew	Foliage, seeds, bark	Nausea, vomiting, diarrhea, dyspnea, and dilated pupils; death is sudden

4. Keep all medicines under lock and key.
5. Have the telephone number of the nearest poison control center readily available.

The main points to be emphasized in giving parents guidance in accident prevention are (1) to eliminate specific environmental hazards, such as drugs, from exploring infants and (2) to supervise infants while they play, gradually replacing supervision with safety training (Shu, 2004).

Plants

Houseplants are another source of poison. Most people fail to think of houseplants as potentially poisonous, because people do not consider eating them. However, infants test almost everything by putting it in their mouths, and a number of plants can be deadly when eaten. As a result, plants are one of the leading sources of poisoning of infants, and amateur foragers frequently learn the hard way that not everything that looks good can be eaten.

Household plants are frequently placed on the floor, where the leaves or flowers are easy to pull off and taste. The best treatment for plant poisoning is prevention which, in this case, means previous knowledge. Table 17-8 identifies several common household and garden plants that are poisonous. The nurse must know which plants are harmful when ingested and must inform parents of the potential dangers to infants.

The National Clearinghouse for Poison Control Centers lists plants as the third most commonly ingested poison, after aspirin and household cleaning agents. Safety education should be stressed at all well-baby conferences beginning in the first 6 months of life. Prevention of plant poisoning and other accidents depends on a reciprocal relationship between protection and education that must be related to age. Safe behavior is a learned behavior, gradually acquired in a progressive process with increasing age. Box 17-14 lists specific safety measures for parents to prevent plant poisoning for infants (Etzel, 2003).

Food Additives

In addition to their questionable nutritional value, additives in commercial baby food can negatively influence an infant's health status. The purposes of food additives vary, including (1) added nutritional value, (2) preservation or extension of shelf life, (3) aid in processing preparation, (4) improvement of flavor, color, and texture, and (5) help in keeping flavors and textures consistent (Samour, Helm, & Lang, 2004).

Commercially prepared baby foods are generally safe, nutritious, and of high quality. In response to consumer demand, baby food manufacturers have removed much of the added salt and sugar that their products once contained and have eliminated most food additives.

Box **17-14** **Nursing Interventions to Prevent Plant Poisoning in Infants**

- Keep plants out of reach of infants and young children.
- Never eat any part of a plant except the parts that are grown or sold as food.
- Keep jewelry made from unknown seeds or beans away from exploring infants.
- Learn to identify poisonous plants around your house and garden.
- Do not use unknown plants as medicines or teas.
- Pay close attention to infants at play inside and outside.
- Seek help whenever anyone chews or swallows a poisonous plant.
- Be aware that infants are more susceptible than are adults to the effects of poisonous plants.
- Keep the poison control center telephone number handy (800-222-1222).

Toxins

Infants are at particular risk from toxic factors in the environment; as dependent, developing organisms, they are inherently vulnerable. Generally the exposure of infants to potential toxins is quite different from that of adults because of differences in physical environment, activities, and diet. Daily activities of infants, such as proximity to the floor or carpet inside the home and the lawn or soil outside, hand-to-mouth behaviors, and smaller body size and composition, place them at great risk for environmental toxins. Infants are exposed to a host of environmental pollutants on a regular basis. These exposures occur through all possible environmental media: air, water, soil, and food. Infants have a unique exposure pattern and unique vulnerabilities. For example, the infant's oral habits and unique diet (ingesting more fruits, vegetables, and water than do adults) magnify their exposure to certain agents. Finally, because infants have a longer life span, toxins that have a long latency or cumulative toxicity (such as certain carcinogens) pose a greater risk to them than to adults (Shannon, 2000).

Some pesticides that are used to control insects that feed on cereal grains, fruits, and vegetables are notorious for their slow accumulation in human tissue. Over sufficient time, exposure to relatively small amounts of pesticides can result in the buildup of toxic quantities and lead to chronic disease in humans.

Lead is another environmental toxin, which has no known physiological role in the human body. Although lead is essentially a contaminant, most people absorb a certain amount daily through air, food, and drink. Studies have revealed a high lead content in dust, dirt, and soil. Lead in the air comes primarily from automobile emissions (Godish, 2004). Absorption of lead is closely related to particle size. Airborne lead of small particle size is readily absorbed through the lungs, whereas larger particles fall to the ground. Lead affects practically all systems within the body.

At high levels, lead can cause convulsions, coma, and even death. Lower levels of lead can adversely affect the brain, central nervous system, blood cells, and kidneys.

Infants are vulnerable to lead exposure for several reasons. In proportion to their weight, infants breathe in more air and more lead than do adults. Additionally, infants breathe closer to the ground, where a higher concentration of lead is located. Their dust-raising play and habit of putting their hands in their mouths add to their lead consumption; they also have a greater rate of gastrointestinal absorption of lead and other chemicals than do adults. Both exercise and blockage of the nasal passages increase mouth breathing, and the mouth is a far less capable filter than the nose. Mouth breathing, coupled with their greater frequency of respiratory tract infections, exposes infants to a greater amount of environmental toxins. The growing prevalence of asthma is also evidence of environmental exposure to lead and other pollutants. Approximately 5 million children have asthma. Statistics show that asthma rates have doubled in the last decade and death rates from asthma have increased in recent years. The reality is that we do not know why asthma is becoming more prevalent, but air pollution is a contributing factor (Godish, 2004).

Human potential and development are clearly important natural resources, and a growing body of evidence now links increased lead exposure to impaired intellectual performance and potential. Clinical lead poisoning affects many children, but it is preventable; excess lead in the infant's environment is made by, and should be eliminated by, human beings. Progress has been made in reducing blood lead levels in infants and young children. The following factors have contributed to these improvements (U.S. Department of Health and Human Services [USDHHS], 2000):

- Decline in lead used in gasoline
- Decline in manufactured food and soft drink cans containing lead solder
- Ban on leaded paint for residential (indoor) use
- Established standard for lead exposure in industry
- Ban on lead-containing solder in household plumbing
- Implementation of lead poisoning prevention programs

Parents need to be educated to take steps to reduce their infant's exposure to lead:

- Keep areas in which infant plays as dust free and clean as possible.
- Do not remove lead paint yourself.
- Do not bring dust into the home.
- If work or a hobby involves lead, change clothes before entering the home.
- Do not burn painted wood in fireplace.
- Eat a balanced diet, rich in calcium, iron, and vitamin C.

Infants do not necessarily escape noxious chemicals when they are indoors. The contaminants that cause air pollution are approximately the same indoors as they are outdoors, with perhaps more indoors from carbon monoxide, nitrogen dioxide, and various hydrocarbons from tobacco

Table **17-9** Major Pollutants and Their Health Effects

Pollutants	Major Sources	Effects
Carbon monoxide	Vehicle exhaust	Replaces oxygen in red blood cells; causes dizziness, coma, or death
Lead	Antiknock agents in some gasoline, old paint chips, metal pieces, pottery, and soil	Accumulates in the bones and soft tissues; affects blood-forming organs, kidneys, and central nervous system
Nitrogen dioxide	Industrial wastes, vehicle exhaust	Causes structural and chemical changes in lungs; lowers resistance against URI
Radon	Earth and rock beneath homes, well water, and building materials	Lung cancer
Ozone	Formed when hydrocarbons and nitrogen dioxide react	Produces smog; irritates mucous membranes, causing coughing, choking, and impaired lung function; contributes to asthma and bronchitis
Sulfur dioxide	Burning coal and oil, industrial processes	Increases colds, coughs, and asthma; contributes to acid rain
Passive smoking	Tobacco products	Causes high incidence of URI, pneumonia, bronchitis, and asthma; linked to cancer

From the Environmental Protection Agency. (2003). Air quality (On-line). Retrieved July 5, 2005, from: *http://www.epa.gov/iaq.*
URI, upper respiratory infection.

smoke, poorly ventilated heating and cooking equipment, and aerosol sprays. Many air pollution aftereffects may not be observed during infancy, but can surface in problems that affect both physical and mental well-being over a lifetime.

Among the acute illnesses of infancy, respiratory disease is ranked number one, representing between 50% and 75% of all childhood diseases (Wootan, 2000). In addition to the inconvenience and incapacity induced by respiratory diseases, medical costs are high. Dirty air aggravates, and in some cases, causes nearly all respiratory problems. Infants with chronic respiratory disease can become adults with respiratory problems.

Water pollution causes gastrointestinal disturbances in the infant. Parents and health care providers are quick to blame food, teething, or a virus for simple diarrhea, when the underlying cause may come from the kitchen tap. Numerous strong chemicals are used today to purify drinking water. These chemicals can irritate the delicate lining and cause disturbances in the infant's gastrointestinal tract. Nurses should encourage parents to boil all water before they give it to their infant to help eliminate any potential problem.

Table 17-9 lists major pollutants and their health effects.

Motor Vehicles

This section refers to the effects of motion or action of forces on the infant; the focus here is on motor vehicle accidents.

Automobiles present a danger to people of all ages, but especially to infants. Usually an infant is injured because of improper restraint inside the automobile. Many parents have been misled by thinking that it is better to be thrown clear of an accident than it is to be restrained. Many also

think that it is safer to hold an infant on the lap in the front seat rather than to have the infant restrained in the back seat. On the contrary, these practices tempt fate and increase the probability of a fatality. A free-moving child not only distracts the driver, but is in a more vulnerable position for being thrown.

Adult seat belts are unsuitable for infants or children under 4 years of age, because their pelvic structure is small; the American Academy of Pediatrics recommends that safety seats for infants be used (USDHHS, 2000). A variety of car seats is available: for infants up to 20 pounds, the recommended type is the rear-facing, molded plastic shell seat, which includes a shoulder restraint and employs the adult seat belt (Wong, Perry, & Hockenberry, 2002). The shield-type car seat offers maximal protection for the child weighing 24 to 48 pounds. All children should be in the back seat because of the potential danger posed by air bags. Infant safety in motor vehicles depends entirely on the responsible adults.

The nurse can also suggest the automobile safety precautions listed in Box 17-15.

Much of automobile safety is common sense, but the nurse must cover all areas in anticipatory preventive teaching. The importance of automobile safety cannot be overemphasized.

Radiation

Radiation, in its broadest sense, means the transfer of electromagnetic waves or energy through space (O'Toole, 2003). Radiation of all types presents a potential hazard in the infant's environment. The risk is proportional to the amount of radiation and the length of exposure and to the particular tissues involved. The infant's rapidly growing and immature cells are especially vulnerable.

Box **17-15** Automobile Safety Precautions

1. Never leave a child unattended in a parked car.
2. Never hold a child in the lap in the front seat.
3. Always use an infant car seat that is properly installed.
4. Keep car doors locked.
5. Use safety restraints for passengers and driver.
6. Do not be distracted by an infant while driving.
7. Continue to use car seats until the child reaches 40 lb and then use adult seat belts. (Some states mandate this precaution and offer resources.)

From Pillitteri, A. (2003). *Maternal and child health nursing: Care of the childbearing and childrearing family* (4th ed.). Philadelphia: Lippincott Williams & Wilkins.

Box **17-16** Nursing Interventions to Prevent Cancer in Infants

- Identify high-risk infants from family history, physical examination, screening programs, and so on.
- Educate parents, caregivers, and day-care personnel about warning signs that may indicate the presence of cancer.
- Refer and provide follow-up care for high-risk infants.
- Update your knowledge concerning cancer and the environment's continuing effect on cancer.
- Be aware of the benefits and risks of radiographic examinations to reduce unnecessary exposure.
- Promote parents' personal habits that are favorable to their own and their infant's health.

The infant is exposed to two basic categories of radiation: (1) natural background radiation, which comes from cosmic rays and radioactive material existing naturally in the soil, water, and air, and (2) human-made radiation, which includes x-rays and radiation from nuclear power plants, microwave ovens, and other electronic devices found in the home (USDHHS, 2000).

Cancer

Most people think of cancer as a disease of adults. Cancer, however, is the leading cause of death from disease in children over 1 year of age. The most common cancers found from infancy to age 5 years are Wilms tumor, retinoblastoma, acute lymphocytic leukemia, neuroblastoma, and rhabdomyosarcoma. Nursing interventions to prevent cancer in infants are listed in Box 17-16.

Nursing intervention to identify risk factors includes taking a careful history, which usually reveals a slow progression of symptoms (e.g., cat's eye reflex, strabismus, painful red eye, and blindness). The nurse who suspects retinoblastoma should ask questions such as the following to identify risk factors:

- Are tumors of the eyes common in your family?
- If so, can you identify which relatives had this and what was done for these tumors?
- Have you noticed your child having any eye problems, such as crossed or lazy eyes, or difficulty seeing?
- Have you noticed any changes in your child's eyes?

Nurses with physical assessment skills can perform screening and ophthalmoscopic examinations on high-risk infants and children. These eye tests include checking for the following:

1. Visual acuity, which can be determined by the fixation test, used to screen vision in infants and children 6 months to 5 years of age
2. Red reflex, which appears whitish in the infant with retinoblastoma (the cat's eye reflex, the most common presenting sign of this cancer)
3. Lid lag, which is found in exophthalmos

Nurses can play a big role in cancer detection, treatment, and prevention through their astute assessment skills, interview techniques, and community education to increase awareness of this disease to parents.

SOCIAL PROCESSES
Community and Work

As infants grow and develop, their boundaries may extend beyond the home environment. Many mothers return to the work force while their infants are still young, placing them in community day-care centers.

Today few young families can escape financial burdens. The two-income family is now a way of life and the trend will continue. With more than one half of all American mothers working outside the home, the need for day-care service is growing.

This situation is usually an emotional issue for families; the separation process can be traumatic for both infant and parent. The comforting realization in this dilemma is that most studies agree that the quality of time spent with an infant is important, not the quantity (London et al., 2003).

Findings from social science research regarding the effects of day care on an infant's development and health can be summarized as: (1) little evidence suggests that day care permanently enhances or slows intellectual development, (2) day care can be used, even from earliest infancy, without damaging the mother-infant relationship, and (3) day care can lead to a slight increase in minor illnesses, but excluding ill infants from the center is not an effective means of reducing the spread of illness (M. J. Clark, 2003).

The question of how old an infant should be before being placed in day care is frequently asked of health professionals. Many experts believe that a mother and infant should have 4 to 6 months together before the mother goes to or returns to work. Brazelton and Sparrow (2002) make a good case for the mother and infant going through four stages of attachment together before the mother goes to work. In the first stage, which takes 10 to 14 days, the infant learns to be attentive to the mother, and the mother learns cues from the infant about being both ready for and tired of attentiveness. The second stage, which lasts 8 weeks, is a stage of playful interaction, when the mother learns how to

| Box **17-17** | Prospective Day-Care Facility Questions |

- Licensed by the state?
- Open all year?
- Number of children present?
- Age range of children?
- Teacher-to-child ratio? (For infants, 1:3 is recommended.)
- Describe day-care program.
- What meals are served?
- What is the cost?
- Are there openings?
- What are the qualifications of caregivers?
- Are the caregivers happy and interacting with the infant?
- Are infants content?
- Are parents welcome to drop in?

recognize the infant's nonverbal cues and helps the infant maintain the alert state. The third stage, from the tenth week to the fourth month, is when the mother and infant learn to play games together. During the fourth stage, which occurs in the fourth month, infants rapidly learn about themselves and their world. Brazelton suggests that a mother, when possible, should spend the first 4 months with her new infant; however, every mother must make her own decision.

A nationwide survey of family day care found that nearly 50% of all infants in day-care centers in the United States are cared for in one of three types of arrangements (M. J. Clark, 2003):

1. Private homes that provide informal day care to infants of relatives, friends, and neighbors
2. Regulated independent care licensed by state agencies
3. Regulated, sponsored care provided by licensed workers operating as part of home networks under umbrella agencies

The nurse has a vital role in assisting families with infants who need day care. Many factors are reviewed when a family is looking for an appropriate day-care program; the nurse can counsel and guide the family in its search. The means by which the nurse counsels and guides the family in selecting a day-care center are as follows:

1. Promote awareness of the three types of day care available in their local communities.
2. Counsel parents on what to ask employees of a prospective day-care facility (Box 17-17).
3. Help parents to deal with the separation behaviors that are manifested by their infant:
    - Remain calm in the situation.
    - Attempt to reduce the number of strange adults who interact with the infant and always introduce them.
    - Encourage the parents to bring an infant's special cuddly toy from home to the day-care facility to promote security.

- Elicit the parent's understanding of the separation and expected behaviors.
- Reassure parents that it takes time for the infant to make the transition from parent to another caregiver and vice versa.
- Emphasize that at certain developmental levels stranger anxiety may be heightened (8 months), and separation behaviors of crying and clinging may be repeated.
- Work toward promoting a good relationship among parents, infant, and caregiver by providing opportunities for open discussions of concerns.

Culture and Ethnicity

The developing infant is subject to the influences of culture from the moment of conception. Partly because of the long dependency period, the family environment is the setting within which the infant experiences overall cultural attitudes. The lives of infants tend to be more under the direct control of parents or other caregivers than the lives of older children, who often are actively involved in selecting their own environments through contacts with peers, teachers, and other adults. The special demands of infancy require extensive and specific caregiving routines across cultures. The parents' perceptions of illness, wellness, roles, child-rearing practices, religious values, language, and health practices are all modeled for the infant. In short, culture helps form the infant's view of the world (Schwartz & Scott, 2002).

The family's ethnicity includes ideas about health, illness, food preferences, moral codes, and family life that persist across generations and survive even the upheaval of coming to a new country. All cultural groups confront repeated challenges as they transfer their families from familiar to unfamiliar surroundings. Infants are exposed to an appropriate mode of behavior that is in accordance with their families' cultural standards. By observing and imitating family members, infants take cues for behavior. These perceptions are then incorporated into their own self-concepts (Olson & DeFrain, 2003).

To assess and plan appropriate interventions for different ethnic groups, nurses must be aware of their own cultural backgrounds. An important consideration is to examine all customs and values in relative terms, seeing none as altogether good or bad. Change is inevitable in family life, whether it is resisted or welcomed. An important function of the nurse is to help families monitor the rate of change that is acceptable to various members and reach a consensus (Box 17-18).

The nurse identifies the power structure within a given cultural group. This knowledge may help dictate which family member to approach with the health teaching. Although the nurse might assume it would be the infant's mother, this may not necessarily be the case. Among some Native American tribes, the grandmother, not the parents, has the authority over the grandchildren. In many Latin cultural groups, the infant's father, not the mother, makes decisions about the infant's welfare (Leininger, 2001). The nurse assesses the cultural groups' practices and beliefs before planning interventions. Approaches to infant care practices vary among cultural groups (Multicultural Awareness box).

In American culture the number of women choosing to breast-feed has steadily increased in recent years. Many factors are involved in the decision-making process, such as cultural beliefs and nurses' attitudes while working with the mother and infant. Nurses who deal with mothers must be aware of the multiplicity of factors influencing feeding choice and should encourage and support parents in their decisions.

The family is the primary health care provider for the infant. The family determines when an infant is ill and decides when to seek help in managing an illness. Many cultural groups choose between the traditional or folk beliefs that they believe to be appropriate to them and Western medical treatment. The Vietnamese use both. For example, to decrease an infant's fever, a basil leaf is tied to the wrist with a piece of cheesecloth. For colic, a silver coin is dipped in wine and rubbed or scratched on the infant's back. Nurses must be cautious in imposing their own values, beliefs, and attitudes on others. Rather than judging people by the nurse's cultural standards, the family should be viewed as a member of a different culture, and the nurse should ascertain how this family's culture influences its health practices and outcomes.

Nurses actively work to reduce culture shock for families raising infants, remembering that American beliefs and behaviors may appear strange to others. The nurse should remember that all behaviors must be evaluated from within the context of the family's cultural background and experiences. Nurses who strive to foster health-promoting attitudes and behaviors must begin at the most basic level: empathic concern and respect for the individual. By incorporating the assessment of cultural beliefs and practices into the infant's plan of care, nurses demonstrate respect, reduce alienation, and take a step toward developing culturally appropriate patterns of health promotion. Respecting another's language and religion is extremely important.

Box 17-18 Factors That Facilitate Multicultural Health Care by Nurses

- Self exploration of own values and beliefs concerning other cultures and their beliefs
- Knowledge of the historical experience, recent and long-term, of ethnic groups that live in the community
- Demographic data that include family size, socioeconomic status, and future expectations that are characteristic of diverse ethnic groups
- Understanding and sensitivity to cultural health care practices different from own
- Recognition of folk beliefs and cultural attitudes toward health and illness
- Awareness of the nature of problems encountered by ethnic group members when they enter the health care system, including fear and distrust of health care professionals, language barriers, and discrimination by caregivers

From Shah, M. A. (2004). *Transcultural aspects of perinatal health care: A resource guide*. Elk Grove Village, IL: American Academy of Pediatrics.

MULTICULTURAL AWARENESS

Quick Guide for Cross-Cultural Nursing Care

The dominant American attitudes about infants and approaches to infant care have undergone many changes in the past several years. With the increased numbers of women in the work force, fathers are becoming more involved in infant care and day care for infants is increasing. Although children are valued, and raising children within the nuclear family remains a priority, an increasing number of American women are focusing on careers, delaying childbirth, and limiting family size.

Members of some cultures view childbearing and childrearing differently. The birth of a child is crucial for many Hispanic, Navajo, black, Middle Eastern, and Mormon women, whose social role and status are attained through reproduction within the marital relationship. Preference for a male child exists among families of many cultures, particularly Middle Eastern and Asian (Shah, 2004).

In the dominant American culture, an infant frequently is wrapped warmly in blankets, placed in an infant seat or stroller, and put to sleep in a crib in a room separate from the parents. Mothers of other cultures may choose to carry or wrap their infants differently; women from some cultures carry their infants with them at all times and sleep with them. Southeast Asian infants may be carried in a hip sling or a blanket carrier; Native American infants often are carried in cradleboards. A cradleboard is a traditional wooden frame into which an infant is bundled and tied. The cradleboard is properly blessed before it is used and can be carried, attached to the mother's back, hung from a tree, or propped up to keep the infant comfortable, safe, and secure (Shah, 2004).

Cultural beliefs and practices are continually evolving and changing. Nurses acknowledge and explore their meanings with all the families with which they meet. Nurses work actively to reduce the experience of culture shock for ethnic minority families, remembering that American medical beliefs and practices may appear strange to others. All behavior must be evaluated from within the context of the family and their cultural background and experience.

Nurses must facilitate health-promoting attitudes and practices and show empathic concern and respect for individuals of all cultural backgrounds. By incorporating the assessment of cultural beliefs and practices into the individual's plan of care, nurses can demonstrate respect and take a step forward in developing culturally appropriate patterns of caring.

Language

Language is an important medium for understanding and working together. The nurse may avoid or tend to mumble a person's name when it is foreign; people hesitate to express themselves when the material is unfamiliar. The nurse must consider how the individual who speaks a different language feels about being unable to express thoughts and feelings or to understand what is being said. Both parties may play the avoidance game.

The nurse must make provisions to remove communication barriers, including the following:

1. Using a professional interpreter to help in the communication process
2. Using pictorial flash cards in the individual's native language to assist in explaining instructions
3. Sending a health care worker to school to learn the basics of the language to help in the interpreting process in the health care facility

Even when a person speaks the nurse's language, understanding and comprehending instructions does not necessarily follow.

Religion

In this pluralistic and democratic society, Americans are confronting the ethical and religious values that impinge on health care services. Interestingly, some providers believe that religion plays no role in individuals' health care practices; therefore, they eschew people's religious or ethical concerns and deal mainly with the physical or psychological problems at hand. The individual's religious and ethical concerns are generally the major source for human values when evaluating health care services.

Religious beliefs as risk factors focus primarily on decisions concerning treatment. An example may be the parents who refuse a blood transfusion, surgery, or other medically indicated treatment required to save their infant's life. A court order is needed in many instances to treat these infants. The decision is the parents' responsibility, based on their customs and beliefs, and should be respected. Deciding not to offer an opinion may be extremely difficult, but usually the opinion is unwanted. Religion is often a powerful force, and when the nurse causes conflict and interferes, a gap can be formed. This gap may force the parents to seek nonprofessional health care to help them with their health-related and religious ideas about birth, death, stress, birth control, and other matters. To work successfully with an individual, the person's religious background should be investigated and understood thoroughly.

Legislation

Health and well-being have become generally accepted rights of everyone, without regard to color, gender, age, economic or social status, or creed. The federal government has pledged to promote the general welfare of the United States in the belief that it belongs to everyone.

To fulfill this pledge, several goals were established. One of these concerns is infant health. The goal, as described by

---

Box **17-19** Low-Birth-Weight Risk Factors

MATERNAL FACTORS

Low socioeconomic status
No prenatal care
Preeclampsia and eclampsia
Hypertension
Chronic renal disease
Advanced diabetes
Malnutrition
Cigarette smoking (10 per day or more)
Drug addiction
Maternal age (under 15 or over 35)
Alcohol abuse
Marital status

FETAL FACTORS

Multiple gestation (twins)
Congenital malformation
Chromosomal abnormality
Chronic intrauterine infection
Placental insufficiency

---

the U.S. Department of Health and Human Services, is to "Improve health and well-being of infants" (USDHHS, 2000, p. 16-10).

The infant mortality rate has been on a steady decline since the turn of the century, a result of better infant nutrition, improved housing, and improved prenatal, obstetrical, and pediatric care (USDHHS, 2000). To meet the goal of improving infant health, major health problems in this age group must be reduced. A major hazard for infants is low birth weight. To address this problem, factors that increase the risk of low birth weight in infants must be identified (Box 17-19).

Many of these factors can be prevented, or risks can be identified early and managed to prevent low birth weight in infants. The major focus for prevention is prenatal care for all women.

Another major threat to infant survival is congenital disorders, such as malformations of the brain and spine (e.g., microcephaly and myelomeningocele), congenital heart defects (e.g., ventricular septal defects), and combinations of malformations, such as Down syndrome or Tay-Sachs disease. Some congenital abnormalities cannot be prevented, but many can be through prenatal screening and research to discover the "why" in the development of these **birth defects.**

Other factors identified by the U.S. Department of Health and Human Services (2000) that contribute to the high infant mortality rate are (1) injuries at birth, (2) SIDS, (3) accidents, (4) respiratory distress syndrome, and (5) inadequate parenting.

The federal government's plans to attain the goal of healthy infants are the following:

1. Promote family planning services such that all pregnancies are planned and all infants are wanted.
2. Provide pregnancy and infant care services through Maternity and Infant Care (MIC) projects to high-risk populations. The WIC program improves the nutritional status of both mother and infant.
3. Encourage educational efforts by schools, health providers, and the media to promote prenatal care.
4. Promote massive immunization efforts such that each infant is protected from communicable disease.

Nursing's Role

The nurse plays a tremendous part in bringing about change in response to a continually expanding knowledge base, consumer health care needs, and governmental legislation. The nurse can play a tremendous part in bringing about change in policies related to health care by actively participating in groups involved with health planning.

The nurse's role in the development of health care policies has three stages: (1) identifying resources for the community to meet its specific need, (2) planning for resources not available to the community, and (3) coordinating the resources available to the community to promote better use of them.

The nurse can become a member of a health planning council, a concerned citizen's group, or an advisory group to a local legislator or to a state health department grant task force. In this capacity, the nurse's responsibility is to inform the other committee members. Because nurses have first-hand experience with many community needs, they are in a good position to speak out and inform others.

The nurse within the community also has several resources available to assist when a need is identified to promote the infant's health, including resources on the federal level (U.S. Department of Health and Human Services), state level (public health department), local level (MIC clinics and well baby clinics), and community groups (Parents Anonymous, hot lines, La Leche League, March of Dimes, and SIDS groups).

Coordinating for resources, the nurse actively participates in assessing the availability of services within the community and makes recommendations to consolidate or expand existing services. To make the public aware of community resources, their services, and existing needs is the basis of the nurse's role in developing policy.

Economics

Even in this society of considerable affluence, many people live below the poverty level. Poor families tend to be characterized as having a lack of education, high unemployment rates, large size and female heads of household, residential crowding, and a lack of adequate bathroom facilities (U.S. Census Bureau, 2000a). Virtually every major health problem is found more frequently in segments of the population with low income than in high-income groups. The infant mortality rates in low-income families remain significantly higher than do rates in high-income families, despite

> ### Box 17-20 Nursing Interventions to Help Economically Deprived Families and Infants
>
> - Contact resource agencies (TANF, WIC programs, MIC programs, and Medicaid) to ascertain available services for the family.
> - Assume the role of advocate for the deprived family to help members interact with the array of health and social welfare agencies.
> - Participate in supporting legislation to reduce the social and economic stresses that affect deprived families.
> - Use the knowledge of healthy infant-parent interactions to foster this relationship within the family unit.
> - Be aware of a different value system when working with low-income families and do not let this difference interfere with developing a trusting relationship.
> - Offer the parents helpful hints as to how they can facilitate their infant's development by using common household items: measuring spoons, plastic cups, and so on.
> - Emphasize the need for protecting the infant's health by fostering safety measures within the home environment and receiving immunizations.

MIC, Maternity and Infant Care; TANF, Temporary Assistance for Needy Families WIC, Special Supplemental Nutrition Program for Women, Infants, and Children.

an overall decrease in infant mortality rate nationally (Clement, 2003).

Studies have demonstrated that parents with low incomes are often unaware of their infant's developmental needs; they frequently are faced with many environmental and social stresses that demand their time, energy, and other resources (Thomlinson, 2002). Many parents have so many unfulfilled needs of their own that they cannot meet their infants' needs.

In many cases infants from families in poverty have delayed language development. Their parents, with limited educational and life experiences, limit the amount of vocalization that the infant will hear. Infants learn early language sounds from their parents, but their attempts at language must be reinforced.

Armed with the knowledge of how economics can affect the infant's growth, development, and health status, the nurse, before deciding interventions (Box 17-20), must assess the family situation by performing the following tasks:

1. Establish a relationship with the family to obtain pertinent information.
2. Evaluate the home environment in which the infant interacts.
3. Elicit the parents' health perceptions about their own health and that of the infant.
4. Complete a thorough physical examination of the infant to identify any problem areas.
5. Identify community resources that are available to the low-income family.

Box **17-21** Infant Health Care Programs

GOVERNMENT AGENCIES

U.S. Department of Health and Human Services, Office of Child Development (responsible for nationally funded health programs)
U.S. Food and Drug Administration (regulates ingested substances)
U.S. Public Health Service (responsible for community's health)
State health departments (establish immunization requirements)

VOLUNTARY AGENCIES (NATIONAL FOUNDATIONS)

March of Dimes (goal is to prevent birth defects)
Sudden Infant Death Syndrome Foundation (information, research, and education regarding SIDS)
Child Abuse Prevention Foundation (promote public awareness of the problem)
Childbirth education associations (provide education to expectant parents)

INTERNATIONAL AGENCIES

World Health Organization
United Nations Children's Fund (goal is to improve children's health worldwide)

LOCAL AGENCIES
Parenting Education

College or school courses
Hospital and clinic classes
Cooperative extension services
Social health department
Childbirth education classes

Financial Assistance (Reduced-Fee Health Care)

City or county health department
WIC program
Well baby clinic
Immunization clinic
Prenatal clinic
Family planning clinic

Ambulatory Care

Pediatrician
Family practice
Pediatric nurse practitioner
Public health nurse

WIC, Special Supplemental Nutrition Program for Women, Infants, and Children.

innovative practice

The Touchpoints Model

The birth of a baby is a life-changing event for a couple and family. Although most infants develop through predictable yet individual patterns of development, parents, especially first-time parents, are usually unaware of these patterns and or have difficulty assessing their infant's progress and problems. All of these processes can be stressful for the parents, the entire family, and the infant.

The Touchpoints Model Program at Children's Hospital in Boston, Massachusetts, delivers a training model for practitioners, emphasizing the building of supportive alliances between parents and professionals around key points in the development of young children. The model is an outgrowth of Dr. T. Berry Brazelton's book, *Touchpoints* (2002), and research at Children's Hospital in Boston. The Touchpoints model provides a form of outreach through which multidisciplinary practitioners can engage parents around important, predictable phases of their baby's development. The Touchpoints model stresses preventive health through development of relationships between parents and providers; acknowledges that developing and maintaining relationships is critical to appreciating cultural, religious, and societal family dynamics; and encourages the practitioner to focus on strengths in individuals and families. Touchpoints is not a stand-alone model; it is intended to be integrated into ongoing pediatric, early childhood, and family intervention programs.

Contact Information:
The Touchpoints Project
Child Development Unit
Children's Hospital
1295 Boylston Street, Boston, MA 02215

Touchpoints has gone on-line. Parents and professionals can get advice and information from Dr. Brazelton at: Brazelton, T. B. (2005). *Brazelton Touch Points Center* (online). Available at *http://www.touchpoints.org.*

Courtesy Carol Lynn Mandle.

The value of preventive health care has been validated; it is cost-effective and is here to stay. As nurses' roles continue to expand within the various parts of the health care system, their duty is to keep pace with the needs, concerns, and available strategies (Lowdermilk & Perry, 2004). Because many conditions that cause morbidity or mortality in infants are preventable when health-promotion practices are employed, nurses have the mission of working within the health care system to promote infant health.

NURSING INTERVENTIONS

Health maintenance, promotion of wellness, and prevention of illness and injury are the goals that have been emphasized throughout this chapter. The federal government has identified areas of concern and made recommendations to promote a healthy infant population. Table 17-10 lists a suggested schedule for health-promotion infant care.

Nurses are the agents of prevention within the health care system (McKinney, James, Murray, & Ashwill, 2005). The opportunities for nurses to share in this major respon-

Health Care Delivery System

The U.S. health care delivery system is diverse and large; many different sectors merge to provide infant care. The nurse within this enormous, multidisciplinary system is a family advocate to facilitate its passage through the many facets of care. Box 17-21 lists health care programs that have been established for the infant and the family for the purpose of disease prevention and health promotion and maintenance.

Table 17-10 Suggested Schedule for Health-Promotion Infant Care

Age (Months)	Promotional Activity	Age (Months)	Promotional Activity
1	Complete physical assessment PKU test Immunizations: HBV-2 Parent discussion includes: Basic infant needs: to be touched, held, fondled, rocked, and talked to Appropriate toy: colorful mobile Nutrition: formula or breast milk		Use of finger foods Playing games with infant: pat-a-cake, peek-a-boo, waving bye-bye, and shaking hands Appropriate toys: blocks, stack toys, and jack-in-the-box Fear of strangers
2	Complete physical assessment Immunizations: DTaP-1, Hib-1, IPV-1, and PCV-1 Parent discussion includes: Placing infant in prone position to allow lifting of head Need of infant to be exposed to a variety of stimuli within environment Need of infant for change of scenery Colic and other common problems	12	Complete physical assessment Immunizations: TB test Laboratory work: CBC Parent discussion includes: Accident prevention Getting into things Infant's need to touch and investigate environment, with supervision Parent's need to read, show pictures, and repeat body parts to infant Infant's need for limited independence Sleeping patterns
4	Complete physical assessment Immunizations: DTaP-2, Hib-2, IPV-2, and PCV-2 Parent discussion includes: Stimulation of infant Providing a mirror in which the infant can see reflection Being talked to and played with Appropriate toy: rattle		Appropriate toy: sets of measuring cups, nesting toys, pots and pans, and wooden spoons
6	Complete physical assessment Immunizations: DTaP-3, Hib-3, HBV-3, IPV-3, PCV-3, and flu vaccine Laboratory work: hematocrit level Parent discussion includes: Accident prevention Teething and use of cool rings Allowing infant to crawl to explore environment Stranger anxiety	15	Complete physical assessment Immunizations: MMR, Hib-4, varicella Parent discussion includes: Negativism as normal aspect of development Age of curiosity in infant Toys appropriate for age: push-pull toys and ball Accident prevention Elimination patterns Discipline: stress positive aspects of behavior, when possible
9	Complete physical assessment Parent discussion includes: Accident prevention Dental caries prevention: cleaning teeth with gauze daily Infant's need for space to crawl about Use cup if weaning	18	Complete physical assessment Immunizations: DTaP-4 Parent discussion includes: Accident prevention Begin toilet training, if child is ready Encourage vocalization Socialization with other small children Importance of reading to child Setting limits on behavior Coping mechanisms of parents

CBC, complete blood count; *DTaP,* diphtheria, tetanus, acellular pertussis vaccine; *HBV,* hepatitis B vaccine; *Hib, Haemophilus influenza* type B conjugate vaccine; *IPV,* inactivated polio vaccine; *MMR,* measles, mumps, rubella vaccine; *PCV,* pneumococcal vaccine; *PKU,* phenylketonuria, *TB,* tuberculin.

sibility are exciting and challenging. If health promotion and disease prevention are to become national realities, then nurses must take the initiative now to preserve the United States' most precious natural resource: its future generations.

SUMMARY

Society is changing, as are people's needs and ideas. Families today want more information and knowledge, and they demand that health care professionals be more responsive to their needs. Their demand has been a catalyst for the nurse's expanded health care role and responsibility for health maintenance.

Health-promotion and disease prevention practices that are applicable during infancy can be used in the nurse's expanded role. A three-pronged approach is stressed:

1. Giving anticipatory guidance to the family unit as the infant grows and develops
2. Teaching and counseling to ensure the infant's optimal development
3. Being a family advocate to ensure the safety and development of the family unit

Anticipating potential health problems during infancy and effectively intervening to avert these problems are nursing processes that are used to promote health. Early detection and reduction of risk factors avoid many health problems, such as abuse. By anticipating problems and helping families to avoid them, the nurse promotes health maintenance.

Using the infant's normal growth and development, psychosocial tasks, common health problems, and health maintenance strategies, the nurse can make an assessment of the infant, the family, and the infant's developmental status to provide anticipatory guidance.

In teaching, an essential component of the nursing process, the nurse transmits knowledge to families to ensure continuity of care and long-term health maintenance. In counseling, the nurse listens to the identified problem, helps the family to recognize the real issues, and allows the family to make its own decisions regarding health care.

Because the infant is in no position to advocate effectively, the nurse assumes this role. The ultimate goal of nursing intervention in maintaining the infant's health is future self-care. As the infant grows and matures, well-established family health maintenance habits can only enhance the lives of healthy future generations. The nurse is challenged to join this effort of investment in the future.

ADDITIONAL STUDY MATERIAL

Study Questions in the back of the book, see page 663.

evolve WEB SITE MATERIALS

These materials are located on the book's Web site at http://evolve.elsevier.com/Edelman/.

- WebLinks
- Content Updates
- Web Site Resources

17A   Denver Developmental Screening Test II and Directions for Administration
17B   Growth Chart for Girls, Birth to 36 Months
17C   Growth Chart for Boys, Birth to 36 Months
17D   Height and Weight Measurements for Girls and Boys
17E   Detailed Immunization Schedules

REFERENCES

Altman, S. J. (2004). *The kidfixer baby book: An easy-to-use guide to your baby's first year.* New York: Ballantine Books.

American Academy of Pediatrics. (2003a). American Academy of Pediatrics Policy Statement: Apnea, Sudden Infant Death Syndrome, and Home Monitoring Committee on Fetus and Newborn. *Pediatrics, 111*(4), 914-917.

American Academy of Pediatrics. (2003b). *Campaign launched to avoid sudden death in childcare settings.* Retrieved April 5, 2005, from *http://www.aap.org/advocacy/archieves/jansids.htm.*

Anderson, L. H. (2003). *Homeless.* Milwaukee, WI: G. Stevens.

Berger, K. S. (2004). *The developing person through the life span* (6th ed.). New York: Worth.

Betz, C. L., & Sowden, L. A. (2004). *Mosby's pediatric nursing reference* (5th ed.). St. Louis: Mosby.

Biancuzzo, M. (2003). *Breastfeeding the newborn: Clinical strategies for nurses* (2nd ed.). St. Louis: Mosby.

Brazelton, T. B., & Sparrow, J. A. (2002). *Touchpoints: Your child's emotional and behavioral development.* Cambridge, MA: Perseus.

Brenner, M. L. (2004). *Pacifiers, blankets, bottles, and thumbs: What parents should know about starting and stopping.* New York: Simon & Schuster.

Burns, C. E. (2004). *Pediatric care: A handbook for nurse practitioners* (3rd ed.). St. Louis: Saunders.

Burton, H. (2003). Genetic education for primary health care nurses. *Primary Health Care, 13*(4), 35-38.

Carroll, P. L. (2004). *Community health nursing: A practical guide.* Clifton, NY: Delmar Learning.

Cataldo, C. B., Debruyne, L. K., & Whitney, E. N. (2002). *Nutrition and diet therapy: Principles and practice* (6th ed.). Bellmont, CA: Wadsworth.

Centers for Disease Control and Prevention. (2003). Recommended childhood and adolescent immunization schedule (Online). *Morbidity and Mortality Weekly Report, 52*(04), Q1-Q4. Retrieved April 5, 2005, from *http:/www.cdc.gov/nip/recs/child-schedule.pdf.*

Chitty, K. K. (2004). *Professional nursing: Concept and challenges* (4th ed.). Philadelphia: W. B. Saunders.

Clark, A. M. (2003). *The ABC's of quality child care.* Clifton Park, NY: Thompson Delmar Learning.

Clark, M. J. (2003). *Community health nursing: Caring for populations* (4th ed.). Upper Saddle River, NJ: Prentice Hall.

Clement, M. S. (2003). *Children at health risk.* Malden, MA: Blackwell Science.

Committee on Infectious Diseases, American Academy of Pediatrics. (2004). Recommended childhood immunization schedule—United States, January-June 2004. Retrieved April 5, 2005, from *http:/www.cdc.gov/nip/recs/child-schedule.pdf.*

Creery, D., & Mikrogianakis, A. (2003). Sudden infant death syndrome. *American Family Physician, 68*(7), 1375-1376.

Dacey, J., & Travers, J. (2004). *Human development across the lifespan* (5th ed.). Boston: McGraw-Hill.

Daly, S. (2004). *Nursing procedures* (4th ed.). Philadelphia: Lippincott Williams & Wilkins.

D'Lugoff, M. I., & Schalla, K. M. (2000). Vaccine guide: Demystifying childhood immunizations for nurses. *Pediatric Nursing, 26*(1), 69-75.

Dudek, S. G. (2006). *Nutritional essentials for nursing practice* (5th ed.). Philadelphia, PA: Lippincott Williams & Wilkins.

Duvall, E., & Miller, B. (1984). *Marriage and family development* (6th ed.). New York: Harper & Row.

Etzel, R. A. (2003). *Handbook of pediatric environmental health* (2nd ed.). Elk Grove Village, IL: American Academy of Pediatrics.

Gerhardt, S. (2004). *Why love matters: How affection shapes a baby's brain.* Hove, East Sussex, New York: Brunner-Routledge.

Godish, T. (2004). *Air quality* (4th ed.). Boca Raton: Lewis.

Hockenberry, M. J. (2005). *Maternal child nursing care* (2nd ed.). St. Louis: Mosby.

Hockenberry, M. J. (2005). *Wong's essentials of pediatric nursing* (7th ed.). St. Louis: Mosby.

Horchler, J. N., & Rice, R. (2003). *SIDS & infant death survival guide: Information and comfort for grieving family & friends and professionals who seek to help them.* Cheverly, MD: SIDS Educational Services.

Jarvis, C. (2003). *Complete physical exam: Health assessment* (4th ed.). St. Louis: Elsevier Health Sciences.

Joughin, V. (2003). Working together for child protection in A & E. *Emergency Nurse, 11*(7), 30-37.

Kail, R. V., & Cavanaugh, J. C. (2004). *Human development: A life-span view* (3rd ed.). Belmont, CA: Thomson/Wadsworth.

Karmiloff, K., & Smith, A. (2001). *Pathways to language from fetus to adolescent.* Cambridge, MA: Harvard University Press.

Kelly, K. (2003). The power of simple play. *US News & World Report, 135*(20), 72.

Kenner, C., & McGrath, J. (2004). *Developmental care of newborns and infants: A guide for health professionals.* St. Louis: Mosby.

Klaus, M. H., Kennell, J. H., & Klaus, P. H. (2000). *Bonding: Building the foundations of secure attachment and independence.* New York: Perseus Book Group.

Koop, C. E. (2003). Pediatric AIDS (On-line). Retrieved April 5, 2005, from: *http://www.drkoop.com/ency/93/000594. htm.*

Kopp, C. B. (2003). *Baby steps: A guide to your child's social, physical, mental, and emotional development in the first two years* (2nd ed.). New York: Henry Holt & Co.

Korones, S. B., & Bada-Eilzey, H. S. (2000). *Neonatal decision making* (2nd ed.). St. Louis: Mosby.

Lea, D. H. (2002). What nurses need to know about genetics. *Dimensions of Critical Care Nursing, 21*(2), 50-62.

Leininger, M. M. (2001). *Culture, care diversity and universality: A theory of nursing.* Sudbury, MA: Jones and Bartlett.

Littleton, L. Y., & Engebretson, J. C. (2005). *Maternity nursing care.* Clifton Park, New York: Thomson Delmar Learning.

London, M. L., Ladewig, P. W., Ball, J. W., & Bindler, R. C. (2003). *Maternal-newborn & child nursing.* Upper Saddle River, NJ: Prentice Hall.

Lowdermilk, D. L., & Perry, S. E. (2004). *Maternity & women's health care* (8th ed.). St. Louis: Mosby.

Mandler, J. M. (2004). *The foundations of mind: Origins of conceptual thought.* Oxford, New York: Oxford University Press.

McKinney, E. S., James, S. R., Murray, S. S., & Ashwill, J. W. (2005). *Maternal-child nursing* (2nd ed.). St. Louis, MO: Saunders.

Moore, K. L., & Persaud, T. V. N. (2003). *Developing human: Clinically oriented embry- ology* (7th ed.). Philadelphia: Elsevier Health Sciences.

National Center for Health Statistics, Health Resources Administration, U.S. Department of Health, Education, and Welfare. (2000). *Height and weight measurement for girls.* Hyattsville, MD: National Center for Health Statistics.

Olson, D. H., & DeFrain, J. D. (2003). *Marriages and families: Intimacy, diversity and strengths* (4th ed.). Boston: McGraw-Hill.

O'Toole, M. T. (2003). *Encyclopedia & dictionary of medicine, nursing, & allied health* (7th ed.). Philadelphia: W. B. Saunders.

Paavilainen, E., & Astedt-Kurki, P. (2003). Functioning of child maltreating families: Lack of resources of caring within the family. *Scandinavian Journal of Caring Science, 17,* 139-147.

Peng, L. F., & Serwint, J. R. (2003). A comparison of breastfed children with nutritional rickets who present during and the first year of life. *Clinical Pediatrics, 42,* 711-717.

Pillitteri, A. (2003). *Maternal and child health nursing: Care of the childbearing and child-rearing family* (4th ed.). Philadelphia: Lippincott Williams & Wilkins.

Riordan, J. (2004). *Breastfeeding and human lactation* (3rd ed.). Sudbury, MA: Jones and Bartlett.

Samour, P. Q., Helm, K. K., & Lang, C. E. (2004). *Handbook of pediatric nutrition* (2nd ed.). Sudbury, MA: Jones and Bartlett.

Scheers, N. J., Rutherford, G. W., & Kemp, J. S. (2003). Where should infants sleep? A comparison of risk for suffocation of infants sleeping in cribs, adult beds, and other sleeping locations. *Pediatrics, 112*(4), 883-889.

Schwartz, M. A., & Scott, B. M. (2002). *Marriages and families: Diversity and change* (4th ed.). Paramus, NJ: Prentice Hall.

Shah, M. A. (2004). *Transcultural aspects of perinatal health care: A resource guide.* Elk Grove Village, IL: American Academy of Pediatrics.

Shannon, M. W. (2000). Risk assessment of children exposed to environmental pollu- tants. *Journal of Toxicology: Clinical Toxicology, 38*(12), 201.

Shu, J. (2004). *Baby and child health.* New York: DK.

Silberg, J. (2001). *125 Brain games for babies: Simple games to promote early brain development.* New York: Fine Communications.

Smith, G. C. S., Pell, J. P., & Dobbie, R. (2003). Risk of sudden infant death syndrome and week of gestation of term birth. *Pediatrics, 111*(6), 1367-1371.

Smolen, A. G. (2003). Children born into loss: Some developmental consequences of homelessness. *Journal for the Psychoanalysis of Culture & Society, 8*(2), 250-257.

Thomlinson, E. H. (2002). The lived experience of families of children who are failing to thrive. *Journal of Advanced Nursing, 39*(6), 537-545.

Tideman, E., Nilsson, A., Smith, G., & Stjernqvist, K. (2002). Longitudinal follow-up of children born preterm: The mother-child relationship in a 19-year perspective. *Journal of Reproductive and Infant Psychology, 20*(1), 43-56.

Tighe, C. M. (2004). Back to sleep. *American Journal of Nursing, 104*(6), 17.

Tomlin, A. M., & Viehweg, S. A. (2003). Infant mental health: Making a difference. *Professional Psychology Research and Practice, 34*(6), 617-625.

U.S. Census Bureau. (2000a). *Characteristics of the population below the poverty level* (pp. 755-757). Washington, DC: U.S. Government Printing Office.

U.S. Census Bureau. (2000b). *Statistical abstract of the United States: 2000. Child abuse* (120th ed., pp. 365-366). Washington, DC: U.S. Government Printing Office.

U.S. Department of Health and Human Services. (2000). *Healthy People 2010: Vol. 1 and 2* (Conference ed.). Washington, DC: U.S. Government Printing Office.

Wootan, G. (2000). *Take charge of your child's health: A parent's guide to recognizing symptoms and treating minor illnesses at home* (2nd ed.). New York: Marlowe & Co.

Zeichner, S. L., & Read, J. S. (2004). *Textbook of pediatric HIV care.* New York, NY: Cambridge University Press.

Chapter 18

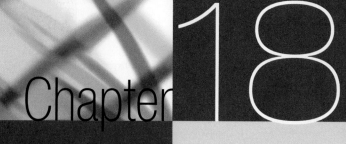

MARTHA DRIESSNACK

Toddler

objectives

After completing this chapter, the reader will be able to:

- Describe the physical growth and developmental changes that occur during the toddler period.

- Outline the recommended schedule of preventive health visits for the toddler and appropriate subjects for the nurse to discuss with parents during each visit.

- Discuss developmentally appropriate approaches to toddlers for both parents and health care providers.

- Describe the factors that contribute to the heightened vulnerability of toddlers to injury and abuse.

key terms

Amblyopia	Object permanence	Sensorimotor stage
Autonomy	Otitis media	Strabismus
Child abuse	Parallel play	Toilet training
Egocentrism	Preoperational stage	
Night terrors	Ritual	

THINK About It

Reframing the Terrible Twos

A young mother tells the nurse that she is convinced that her 22 month old, who used to be the sweetest child around, has entered what must be the terrible twos. She reports that her child's favorite words include "mine" and "no," with "no" being the response to every request the mother makes. In addition, the child is getting increasingly stubborn and just threw her first public temper tantrum. The mother says that she is tired of saying and hearing "no" and turns to the nurse for help.

1. How does the nurse explain the relationship between the child's stage of psychosocial development and meaning behind the child's behaviors?

2. What suggestions can the nurse give to the mother to respond sensitively to her child's evolving need for independence while balancing her own need to provide for and protect her child?

3. If the child doesn't learn she can say "no," ask the mother how she expects her to "Just say no" to drugs, for example, when she is older.

The author acknowledges the work of Marinda Allender as the author of this chapter in the previous edition.

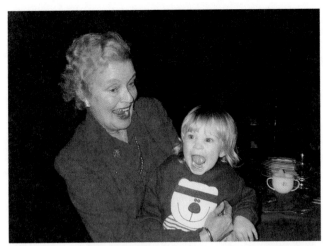

Figure 18-1 A toddler and her grandmother share a happy moment.

Having spent their first year of life getting to know and trust their parents and their immediate environments, toddlers' increasing mobility now allows them to begin to expand their worlds, bringing excitement and challenges to both themselves and their parents. Toddlers are ready to develop a sense of self and separate from their parents, and understanding and respecting this evolving independence is a common parental challenge. Their behaviors can be frustrating, but the toddlers' delight in their own emerging competence and achievements can bring a sense of joy and accomplishment to everyone around them (Figure 18-1).

Nurses need to emphasize the many physical and developmental changes that occur in toddlers and how these changes contribute to their vulnerability to injury, their overall health, and that of the family unit. Unfortunately, the recommended schedule for health-promotion and disease prevention visits for this age group provides for fewer contacts than during infancy. Parents may begin to fall into a pattern of illness care, missing the continued opportunity to receive anticipatory guidance and health-promotion information until preschool or school requirements bring them back in. The nurse plays an integral role in encouraging health-promotion efforts and behaviors.

AGE AND PHYSICAL CHANGES

The toddler period extends from 12 to 18 months to 3 years of age. The overall growth rate slows significantly, and the increasingly active toddlers begin the process of shedding baby fat and straightening their posture. Toddlers have a protuberant abdomen, accentuated by a lumbar lordosis, and a characteristic gait, in which their feet are planted wide apart and appear flat because of an extra fat pad in the instep for stability.

A slow, steady growth in height of 2 to 4 inches per year and in weight of 4 to 6 pounds per year occurs during toddlerhood and remains steady until puberty. Birth weight usually quadruples by 2½ years of age, and the toddler's height at age 2 years is approximately 50% of final adult height (Hockenberry, Wilson, Winkelstein, & Kline, 2003).

The toddler's stature may be measured in a recumbent position for length, as in infancy, or in a standing position for height. Depending on the position, the nurse must select the appropriate Centers for Disease Control and Prevention (CDC) growth chart. The nurse continues to measure head circumference throughout the toddler period. The anterior fontanel usually closes by 18 months, the skull begins to thicken, and by 24 months it is 80% of its adult size (Hockenberry et al., 2003).

The kidneys are well differentiated by the toddler years, and specific gravity and other urine findings are similar to those of adults (Grodner, Anderson, & DeYoung, 2003). The daily excretion of urine for the 2-year-old child is 500 to 600 ml (15 to 18 ounces) and 600 to 750 ml for the 3 year old. The toddler empties the bladder less frequently than does the infant and has more voluntary control of urination because of maturation of the neurological pathways to the bladder and sphincter.

The toddler's gastrointestinal tract also reaches functional maturity, although it continues to grow into adulthood. The toddler tends to need meals and snacks more frequently than an older child or adult. Most toddlers develop sufficient voluntary control of internal and external anal sphincters to accomplish successful bowel training.

No difference exists in lung topography or function after infancy. Lung capacity, however, continues to increase as the toddler grows, and the respiratory rate decreases from a mean of 30 breaths per minute at 1 year of age to 25 breaths per minute at 3 years. The diameter of the toddler's upper respiratory tract is small when compared with that of an older child or adult. This small diameter, coupled with toddler's exploratory nature and lack of judgment in deciding what to place in the mouth, can result in airway obstruction, which demands emergency action.

The anatomy of the ear, eustachian tube, and nasal pharynx continue to resemble those of the infant more closely than those of the adult, continuing the risk for otitis media. The tonsils and adenoids remain proportionately large during the toddler years (Seidel, Ball, Dains, & Benedict, 2002).

With the exception of reproductive functions, most endocrine organs become functionally mature during the toddler and preschool years, although function continues at a minimum. The production of glucagon and insulin can be limited or labile, producing variations in blood glucose levels that can be demonstrated throughout early childhood. The production of cortisol, aldosterone, and deoxycorticosterone by the adrenal cortex remains somewhat limited, but they appear to function effectively in protecting the young child from the hazards of fluid and electrolyte imbalance well known in infancy. Secretion of epinephrine and norepinephrine from the adrenal medulla increases sufficiently to perform homeostatic functions of the autonomic nervous system and to mediate certain aspects of increased emotional components of behavior. Regulation of growth during early childhood remains one of the most important functions of the endocrine system. Growth hormone, thyroid hormone, insulin, and corticoids are probably the most vital hormones for normal growth and development during this period (Guyton & Hall, 2000).

Permanent circulatory pathways are fully established by toddlerhood. Changes in the system's function, including decreases in heart rate, increases in blood pressure, and changes in vascular resistance of various body areas in response to growth in the size of the vessel lumen, continue gradually. The toddler's heart rate ranges from 80 to 120 beats per minute and the mean blood pressure is 90/56 mm Hg. Getting the toddler to sit still for a blood pressure reading can be difficult, but it's worth the effort to obtain several baseline readings for future reference.

The capillary beds gradually increase their capacity to respond to heat and cold in the environment, providing the toddler with more effective thermoregulation. Toddlers can also begin to take voluntary measures to relieve the discomfort of heat or cold. For example, the older toddler can put on clothing or move to warmer or cooler areas, assisting physiological efforts to maintain a constant internal thermal environment.

Some common organisms have been encountered and immune responses have begun to function adequately. When toddlers enter the world of playgrounds, nurseries and day care, exposure to new and different organisms is greatly increased, and they may experience a period during which they appear to succumb to many minor respiratory and gastrointestinal infections. As immunity begins to develop against the organisms of the new environment, their resistance similarly increases.

Passive immunity to communicable disease acquired through transfer of maternal antibodies during fetal life has disappeared, and active immunity through the initial immunization series is usually completed by the age of 18 months. The next scheduled immunizations do not occur until age 4 to 6 years, prior to entering school. If a toddler is behind in the initial immunization series, a separate schedule is available that gives catch-up schedules and minimum intervals between doses. See **Web Site Resource 17E** for detailed immunization schedules. All 20 primary or deciduous teeth erupt by the end of toddlerhood. The sequence is generally as follows: mandibular central incisors, mandibular lateral incisors, maxillary central incisors, maxillary lateral incisors, mandibular first molars, maxillary first molars, mandibular cuspids, maxillary cuspids, mandibular second molars, and the maxillary second molars. Timing of these eruptions can vary widely, but a variation in the sequencing should alert the nurse to inquire about early trauma to the mouth or familial traits for out-of-sequence tooth eruption. Fluoride is an important aspect of preventive dental care and its use should be continued throughout toddlerhood. Other important aspects of dental care at this age that are included in health teaching are listed in Box 18-1.

A mature swallowing pattern, using the tongue rather than the cheeks, has not yet developed, and toddlers continue to be at risk for choking. Toddlers who are mouth,

---

Box 18-1 Nursing Interventions to Promote Dental Health Care for Toddlers

BRUSHING

- Use a soft-bristled brush. The gauze method used during infancy is no longer adequate, because the teeth are too close together to allow a finger wrapped in gauze to reach all surfaces.
- Introduce only a moist toothbrush at first. After the toddler has accepted the toothbrush, begin using toothpaste. A pea-size amount is adequate. If the child does not like the taste of the toothpaste, then use plain water.
- Toothpaste should contain fluoride.
- Toddlers do not have the motor coordination to brush their own teeth. They may enjoy imitating parents and put the toothbrush in their mouths, but an adult should be responsible for the actual brushing.
- Brush daily; for many toddlers, this practice becomes part of the bedtime routine. When the child appears too tired to cooperate in the evening, the parent should choose some other time of day when this important task will not be so difficult.

FOODS

- Limit foods high in sugar.
- When the young toddler still drinks from a bottle, only plain water should be given. Milk and juices should be offered by cup. If milk or juice is given in a bottle, it should never be done at naptime or bedtime.

VISITS TO THE DENTIST

- The first visit to the dentist should occur during the toddler years. Many dentists suggest an inspection-consultation type of visit when the child is approximately 18 months of age. This type of visit provides an early, enjoyable introduction to the dental examination.

---

rather than nose, breathers because of ongoing respiratory illness or allergies may have an underdeveloped palatal arch. With normal breathing, the tongue rests on and naturally widens the palate; however, when the child is forced to breathe through the mouth, the tongue rests in the lower jaw, not on the palate. This resultant narrowing of the palatal arch sets these toddlers up for dental crowding when the permanent teeth erupt.

An increase in the size and strength of muscle fibers continues. During this period, as during infancy, the use of muscle tissues is the primary stimulus for increased size and strength (Figure 18-2). Myelination of the corticospinal tract is functionally sufficient to support most movement, but achievement of full control does not occur until much later in life. Throughout early childhood, voluntary motor movement is often accompanied by involuntary movements on the other side of the body. This mirroring of action is more pronounced in children who suffer some damage of the central nervous system, but the mechanisms by which this occurs are unknown. The toddler generally does not

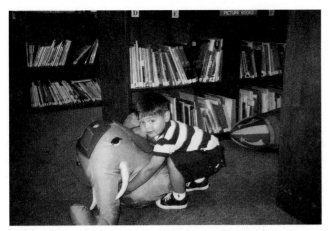

Figure 18-2 Toddlers enjoy learning coordination of large muscle groups.

show complete dominance of one-sided body function and may still switch hands when eating, throwing a ball, or engaging in other-handed activities.

Most genetic syndromes and disease entities are diagnosed either during the prenatal period or during infancy. However, some genetic syndromes and diseases are not detected until the toddler years or even later. The most common initial sign is a failure to thrive or grow or a mild developmental delay. These delays often are not diagnosed during infancy, because the subtle language, motor, or cognitive deficiencies do not interfere with expected performance and behavior.

GORDON'S FUNCTIONAL HEALTH PATTERNS

Health Perception–Health Management Pattern

Toddlers may come to know that being sick means feeling bad or having to stay in bed, but they have little, if any, understanding of the meaning of health. They may perform or request some health-promotion activities, such as brushing teeth, but they do it as part of their bedtime ritual and not because they know this activity will prevent caries. Toddlers depend on their parents for health management, and their overall health will be greatly influenced by their parents' health perceptions and health management priorities (see *Healthy People 2010*).

Toddlers identify with parents, caregivers, and other important role models, internalizing a wide range of lifestyle attributes. Parents' and caregivers' health perceptions and health behaviors should model the perceptions and behaviors desired for health promotion. Toddlers whose parents eat a variety of foods are more likely to try new foods. Such modeling increases the chances that good practices will be retained throughout the toddler's life. The nurse's task is to help parents strengthen their confidence and self-esteem as parents and provide them with the information needed to anticipate and meet the developmental needs of their toddler as they develop as a family.

Healthy People 2010

Selected Health-Promotion and Disease Prevention Objectives for Toddlers

- Reduce iron deficiency to less than 5% among children between ages 1 and 2 (baseline is 9% among children between ages 1 and 2 in 1994).
- Reduce drowning deaths among children ages 4 and younger to no more than 0.9 per 100,000 (adjusted baseline is 1.5 per 100,000 in 1997).
- Increase use of child restraints to 100% of children ages 4 and younger (baseline is 92% in 1998).
- Reduce number of courses of antibiotics for ear infections for young children to 88 antibiotic courses per 100 children under age 5 years (baseline is 108 courses of antibiotics per 100 children in 1996 and 1997).
- Reduce nonfatal poisoning among children ages 4 and younger to no more than 292 per 100,000 (baseline is 348.4 per 100,000 in 1997).
- Achieve total elimination of blood lead levels exceeding 10 mg/dl among children ages 1 to 5 years (baseline is 4.4% of children ages 1 to 5 years had blood level exceeding 10 mg/dl in 1994).

From U.S. Department of Health and Human Services. (2000). *Healthy People 2010*. Washington, DC: U.S. Government Printing Office.

Nutritional-Metabolic Pattern

Weaning from the breast or bottle usually occurs before or during toddlerhood. Adequate iron intake must be ensured as the toddler changes from breast milk or iron-fortified formula and cereal to whole milk, which is low in iron. The continued use of a bottle, rather than the switch to drinking from a cup, has been associated with iron-deficiency anemia. A toddler who continues to ingest whole milk from a bottle tends to drink up to 32 ounces per day. This practice blunts the child's appetite for other foods that contain iron. The use of a bottle with milk or juice, especially at bedtime, has also been associated with dental caries (baby bottle tooth decay). If parents want to give a bottle at bedtime it should contain only water.

The use of prepared toddler foods, as opposed to serving the same foods the rest of the family is eating, presents a special concern, because these products may not provide optimal nutrition or the variety that the toddler requires. Helping parents understand the information labels on prepared foods, especially the high sodium content, is valuable in conveying the principles of nutrition, sound marketing, and consumer protection. Additionally, parents may not realize the expense of these foods, and when convenience in preparation is not a major consideration the child can be fed more economically and nutritionally with the regular family diet. Little extra preparation is needed by the time the child's first molars appear.

PLAN FOR YOUR YOUNG CHILD...The Pyramid Way

Use this chart to get an idea of the foods your child eats over a week. Pencil in the foods eaten each day and pencil in the corresponding triangular shape. (For example, if a slice of toast is eaten at breakfast, write in "toast" and fill in one Grain group pyramid.) The number of pyramids shown for each food group is the number of servings to be eaten each day. At the end of the week, if you see only a few blank pyramids...keep up the good work. If you notice several blank pyramids, offer foods from the missing food groups in the days to come.

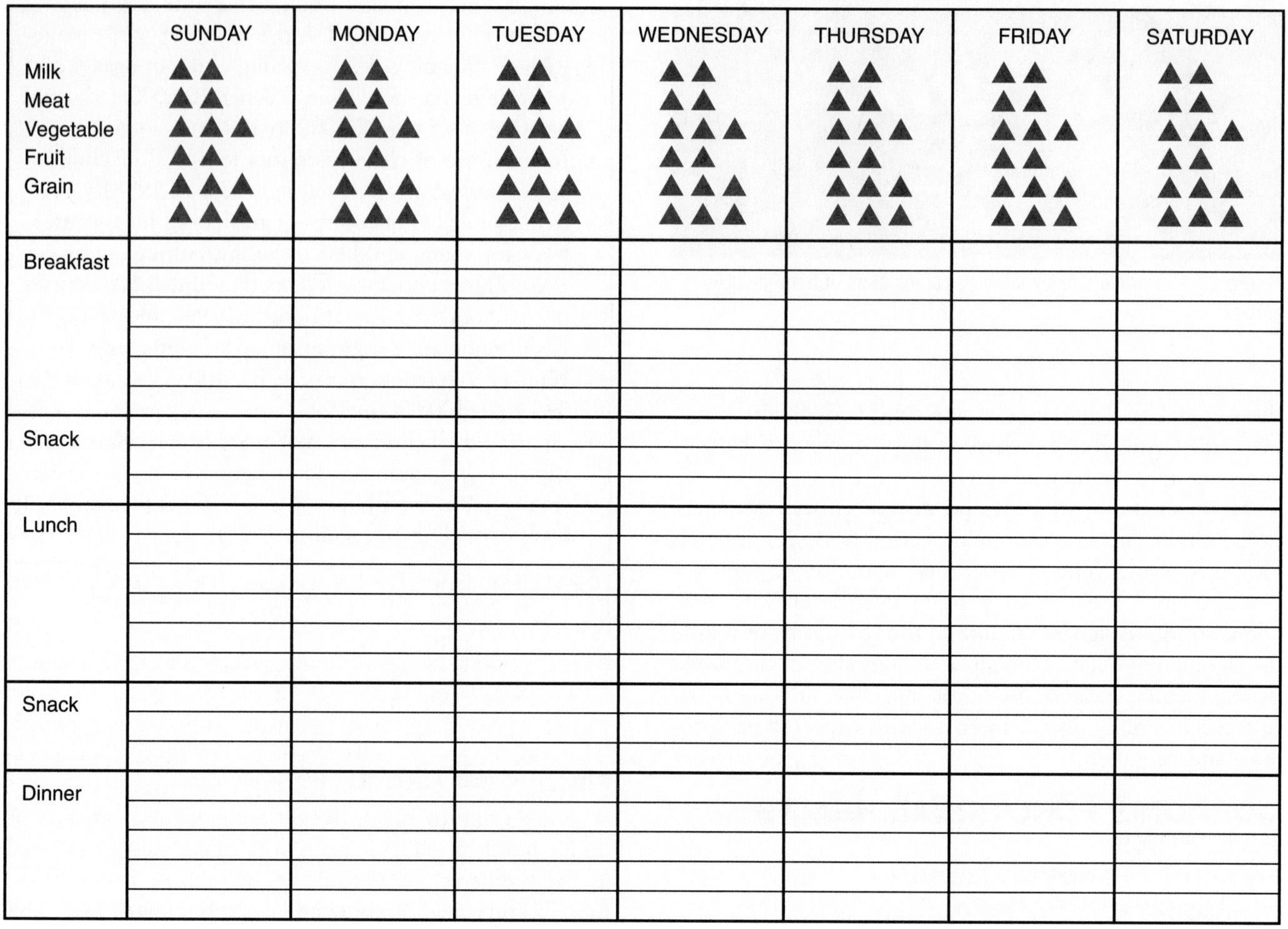

	SUNDAY	MONDAY	TUESDAY	WEDNESDAY	THURSDAY	FRIDAY	SATURDAY
Milk / Meat / Vegetable / Fruit / Grain	▲▲ ▲▲ ▲▲▲ ▲▲ ▲▲▲ ▲▲▲	▲▲ ▲▲ ▲▲▲ ▲▲ ▲▲▲ ▲▲▲	▲▲ ▲▲ ▲▲▲ ▲▲ ▲▲▲ ▲▲▲	▲▲ ▲▲ ▲▲▲ ▲▲ ▲▲▲ ▲▲▲	▲▲ ▲▲ ▲▲▲ ▲▲ ▲▲▲ ▲▲▲	▲▲ ▲▲ ▲▲▲ ▲▲ ▲▲▲ ▲▲▲	▲▲ ▲▲ ▲▲▲ ▲▲ ▲▲▲ ▲▲▲
Breakfast							
Snack							
Lunch							
Snack							
Dinner							

Figure 18-3 Plan for Your Young Child . . . The Pyramid Way. A chart to track the foods a child eats. (From U.S. Department of Agriculture.)

The decreased rate of growth during toddlerhood results in a decrease in required calories and in appetite. Parents should be reminded of this if they begin to worry about their toddler's nutrition. Keeping a record, such as the Plan for Your Young Child . . . The Pyramid Way (Figure 18-3), over 3 to 5 days presents a clear picture of a child's intake and is a useful teaching tool.

Toddlers often use mealtime as an occasion to assert individuality, to control the environment, and for simple exploration of food textures and qualities. Definite food preferences emerge. The nurse uses the lifestyle of the family as a basis for offering counseling and guidance related to feeding; families vary greatly in their expectations of feeding behavior and mealtime routines. For example, when the adults in the family consistently eat a wide variety of foods and enjoy mealtime together, their expectations of the young child will differ greatly from family members who eat meals individually or have a limited variety of foods.

The nurse can ask parents to explore their expectations of the toddler's mealtime behavior and determine which expectations are appropriate at various developmental levels. If the parents want the child to learn to eat the foods served at mealtime, then they may need assistance in anticipating the necessary adjustments for the toddler to acquire these feeding behaviors. If the parents find that the toddler is disruptive of family interactions during mealtime, then they may prefer to continue feeding the toddler separately except for one meal each day.

Within the limits of family resources, the nurse can assist parents by providing specific directions and assistance in the selection of a variety of foods and in their preparation such that their toddler will accept and be able to chew and swallow the foods adequately.

Nursing Interventions

1. Offer simple, single foods, because mixtures of foods are often rejected.
2. Serve your toddler's favorite foods along with new ones. Several introductions may be necessary before the toddler accepts a new food. Make sure you eat it, too.
3. Encourage the use of utensils, but accept that toddlers still often need to use their fingers.
4. Routines are important to toddlers. Serve scheduled meals and snacks. Parents are responsible for what, when, and where the toddler eats. The toddler decides whether to eat and how much.
5. Mealtime should be a relaxed and pleasant time, free of distractions.
6. Do not use food to bribe, reward, or punish your toddler.
7. Schedule meals and sleep periods such that the child is awake and alert during mealtime.
8. Serve small portions and let your toddler ask for more.
9. Avoid foods that may cause choking, such as hard candy, mini-marshmallows, popcorn, pretzels, chips, spoonfuls of peanut butter, nuts, seeds, large chunks of meat, hot dogs, raw carrots, dried fruits, and whole grapes.
10. Drinking more than 2 cups (16 ounces) of milk per day can reduce your child's appetite for other healthy foods. For those under age 2 years, do not use reduced-fat, low-fat, or fat-free (skim) milk.

An important point to discuss with parents is that the toddler may at times refuse a meal altogether. The reasons for this refusal range from the assertion of independence to simple fatigue. Parents should not be concerned or punish the child for this behavior. If a major family crisis follows, the toddler may learn how easily the parents can be controlled by refusing food and may continue this behavior. When the evening meal is considered the main meal and the toddler does not eat it, parents might think their child will be poorly nourished. However, using a record of intake (see Figure 18-3), the nurse can demonstrate the adequacy of the nutrients that the toddler is already receiving during other meals of the day or help the parent work out a plan to offer more of the essential foods during these meals.

The family who has a vegetarian diet may need some assistance, from the nurse or a dietician, in offering a diet adequate in protein, vitamin B_{12}, and vitamin D, especially if they exclude dairy products and eggs. Vegetarian diets vary widely, so it is important to assess precisely what foods are eaten, what foods have been eliminated from the diet, and what supplements are used (Story, Holt, & Sofka, 2002).

Elimination Pattern

Toilet training is often a major parental concern during toddlerhood. The nurse anticipates this developmental stressor and initiates discussion with the parents to determine their understanding of the child's signs of developmental readiness and their attitude and commitment to establishing a toileting pattern for their toddler. Emotional and physical readiness for toilet training rarely develops before 18 months of age. Parents who begin before their child is ready usually experience frustration.

Nursing Interventions

By suggesting the sequence in the Health Teaching box, Initiating a Toileting Program for Toddlers, the nurse can assist parents with toilet training. The parent who can approach toilet training with a relaxed attitude, accepting some delays and frustrations, will have a better chance of success and a more positive outcome for the toddler.

Activity-Exercise Pattern

Toddlers are always busy—emptying wastebaskets and drawers, building and destroying towers, throwing, kicking, chasing after balls, or dressing and undressing. Many of their

---

HEALTH TEACHING Initiating a Toileting Program for Toddlers

- Interest in and awareness of bowel and urinary elimination usually begins by 18 months of age.
- Before beginning toilet training, parents should begin to check their toddlers for the prerequisite skills, which include being able to walk well, stoop and recover, stay dry for at least 2 hours during the day, and communicate sensation before elimination, as well as the discomfort of wet or messy pants and the need for assistance.
- When these prerequisites are present, introduce the child to a potty seat or chair. The potty chair should provide secure seating with the child's feet touching the floor. The potty seat should be used with a small step stool to create the same effect.
- Because of the gastrocolic reflex, bowel elimination is more likely after a meal, so this is a good time to place the toddler on the potty. When a pattern of bowel or urinary elimination is noticed, use this pattern as a guide for placing the child on the potty.
- Encourage the toddler to stay on the chair for 2 to 3 minutes and always explain what to do ("Go potty") rather than what not to do ("Don't wet your pants"). Do not refer to elimination as dirty or yucky. Remember this is your child's first creation.
- Praise the child for desired behavior. Introduce underwear as a badge of success. Ignore undesired behavior and never punish the child by scolding, spanking, or other punitive measures.
- Anticipate that your toddler may want to touch his or her genitals.
- Remember that daytime dryness usually is achieved by 3 years of age and ahead of nighttime dryness.

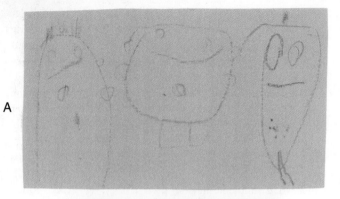

A

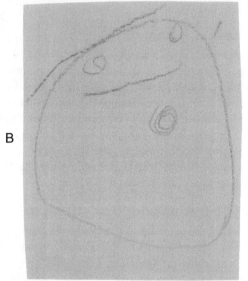

B

Figure 18-4 Tadpolelike drawings created by a toddler. **A,** Family portrait. Everyone looks the same but there are a few distinguishing details. The dad is on the right, with the scratchy face. The toddler is in the center, and the mom is on the left. Both the mom and the toddler (a girl) have bellybuttons. Mom was 8 months pregnant at the time. **B,** The same toddler drawing herself. Note the bellybutton.

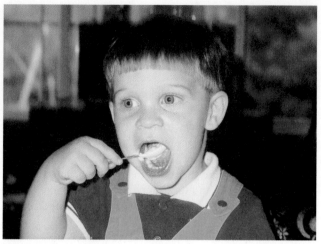

Figure 18-5 Toddlers learn to use a spoon and a fork with fairly good success.

activities are repeated over and over, providing practice opportunities for their newly realized skills.

During the toddler period, they will advance from taking their first step to running, climbing stairs, and even pedaling a tricycle. They enjoy pushing and pulling, whether it is an unsuspecting laundry basket or a push-pull toy made for the job. They scribble spontaneously, usually with vigor, and will emerge from toddlerhood capable of copying a circle and creating tadpolelike figures (Figure 18-4). They learn to use a spoon and a fork with fairly good success and to wash their hands (Figure 18-5). They also advance from being dressed by others to dressing themselves with assistance, although at times they resist it.

Toddlers spend most of their waking hours at play—exploring their expanding environment, imitating others' actions, and creating a safety net of rituals around eating, sleeping, and everything in between. In their enthusiasm to try many activities, toddlers invariably take on tasks that are beyond their abilities, which can result in frustration and an occasional well-known temper tantrum. Their

exploratory nature and limited, but advancing, skills also make them vulnerable to injury.

Most toddlers are interested in other children. However, this interest is limited because toddlers, although ready to be with other children, are not ready to share. Successful social encounters with toddlers are best described as **parallel play,** where children play side by side, doing similar things with similar toys, but each working independently (Berger & Thompson, 2000). Sharing and cooperative play will not develop until well into the preschool age.

Nursing Interventions

When parents inquire about what toys and activities to provide for their toddler, the following are suggested:

1. Provide toys that challenge the child to develop new skills: toys that require skills slightly above the child's present level, but not advanced such that the child cannot achieve some success. For example, the toddler who has mastered a ride-on toy may be ready for a tricycle.
2. Provide opportunities for new learning, which may be as basic as a book with pictures of new animals or a walk through the produce section of the grocery store to point out fruits and vegetables (Figure 18-6).
3. Provide opportunities for social encounters with other children, but do not force playing together. Creating separate, yet parallel space, with the use of small mats or hoola hoops is recommended.
4. Follow the child's lead. Let the toddler choose and explore new toys or objects, within safe limits.

The desire of some parents to raise the smartest, most coordinated, or most musically talented super kids usually has its roots early in the toddler period. Some of these children have indeed shown the ability to learn at a younger age than was ever considered in the past. A big concern among child development specialists is that the time commitment and intensive drill may interfere with the child's need for self-structured play and exploration.

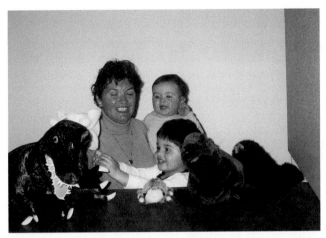

Figure 18-6 Playing with puppets can be a new learning opportunity.

Sleep-Rest Pattern

Toddlers' need for sleep has decreased to 12 hours a day, including 1 or 2 naps of shorter duration. One of the naps usually is replaced by quiet time, a brief period to unwind from a busy or noisy activity. Occasionally the parents or caregivers need these rest breaks as much or more. Sitting together in a rocking chair for a soothing song or quiet music or reading side by side or together can be suggested by the nurse.

The toddler may be highly involved in an activity and not be aware of fatigue, especially when visitors are in the home or some interesting new toys have been discovered. All parents are familiar with the child who is overtired but unable to relax enough to sleep. Parents can avoid this dilemma by scheduling nap and quiet time even when there are houseguests or holidays that preempt the toddler's routine.

Rituals are characteristics of this age, and most toddlers have a nap and bedtime ritual. A typical pattern might be: a snack, followed by bathing, brushing teeth, a story, a kiss, and overhead lights out and night light on. Following this ritual is important, because the toddler gets a sense of security when ending the day. Changing this ritual can be upsetting. The nurse should encourage parents to establish and follow the sleep time ritual as closely as possible, even when visitors, family illness, or travel makes the routine more difficult.

Many toddlers will try to delay sleep by calling for water, another story, another kiss, or by making other requests. Parents should be certain that the toddler has ample opportunity for interaction with them during the day, follow the usual bedtime ritual, and be firm and consistent in resisting any requests for attention after the final good nights have been said. Encouraging toddlers to use transition or security objects, such as stuffed animals or blankets, helps them to self-quiet and console themselves both at bedtime and in new situations.

Night terrors may begin in toddlerhood. Night terrors are different from nightmares, which generally begin at a later age and result in the child awakening and being able to recall the frightening dream. The child who experiences night terrors does not waken completely, but cries out, looks terrified, and cannot be aroused for several minutes. Eventually, usually after 5 to 10 minutes, the child falls back into quiet sleep. Parents need to be reassured that these episodes will become less frequent as the child develops. The parents should talk in a soothing voice but should not try to awaken the child. If the child does waken, then the parents should provide comfort and tuck the child back in bed.

Cognitive-Perceptual Pattern

Toddlers who experienced the security of a nurturing and reliable source of protection and attachment during infancy have a strong base from which to begin to explore and learn about their expanding world. They begin toddlerhood in Piaget's **sensorimotor stage** of cognitive development and begin moving to the **preoperational stage.** Their advancing thought processing skills and abilities to use the language are heralded by the development of **egocentrism,** an inability to put oneself in another's shoes. Toddlers who come running into a room asking their parents "Where is it?" are confused when parents respond "Where is what?" They assume their parents and all others share their same thoughts and cannot understand why they don't.

Toddlers interpret and learn about objects and events, not in terms of general properties, but in terms of their relationship with them or their use to them. Their thoughts are dominated by what they see, hear, or otherwise experience, and they want to experience everything. Their two-word to three-word phrases are most often related to present events, describing an action ("mommy up"), a desire ("more French fries"), or possession ("my kitty").

Both receptive and expressive language skills are developing rapidly in toddlers; however, their receptive language skills far outweigh their expressive language ability, and toddlers often use gestures until words are found to represent the meanings already acquired. Toddlers also learn the use of inflection. "Mommy" may mean "pick me up, I want to see" on one occasion and or "I'm scared" or "Where are you?" on another. Often frustrated by their limited repertoire of expressive language, which usually includes about 400 words, young toddlers default to using "NO" as a method of gaining control over a situation or expressing themselves.

By age 3, children have mastered the basics of language function, form, and content, and these fundamentals will continue to be refined throughout childhood and adolescence. Table 18-1 outlines the landmarks of speech, language, and hearing ability in this age group.

Toddlers have a solid understanding of **object permanence** and are no longer easily distracted when a desired toy, blanket, or parent is not to be found. Many a toddler will sit patiently in front of the washing machine while a favorite blanket is laundered or stare out a front window awaiting a parent's return. They often inadvertently put themselves in harm's way as they pursue an object or person they sense is just out of view.

Table **18-1** Landmarks of Speech, Language, and Hearing Ability During the Toddler Period

Age (Months)	Receptive Language	Expressive Language	Related Hearing Ability
18	Up to 50 words; recognizes between 6 and 12 objects by name, such as *dog, cat, bottle, ball;* identifies three body parts, such as *eyes, nose, mouth;* understands simple one-step commands such as *give me the doll, open your mouth, stick out your tongue*	Up to 20 words; jargon and echolalia are present; uses names of familiar objects and one-word sentences, such as *go* or *eat;* uses gestures; uses words such as *no, mine, eat, good, bad, hot, cold,* and expressions such as *oh-oh, what's that, all gone;* use of words can be quite inconsistent, 25% of speech intelligible	Has begun to develop gross discrimination by learning to distinguish between highly dissimilar noises, such as doorbell and train, barking dog and auto horn, or mother's and father's voices
24	Up to 1200 words; knows *in, on, under;* identifies *dog, ball, engine, bed, doll, scissors, hair, mouth, feet, nose, cup, spoon, car, key;* distinguishes between one and many and formulates a negative judgment (a knife is not a fork); understands simple stories; follows simple two-step directions; is beginning to make distinctions between *you* and *me*	Up to 270 words; jargon and echolalia almost gone; averages 75 words per hour during free play; talks in words, phrases, and two-word to three-word sentences; averages two words per response; first pronouns appear, such as *I, me, mine, it, who, that;* adjectives and adverbs are only beginning to appear; names objects and common pictures; refers to self by name, such as *Katrina go bye-bye;* uses phrases such as *I want, go bye-bye, want cookie, ball all gone;* 60% of speech intelligible	Refinement of gross discriminative skills
30	Up to 2400 words; identifies action in pictures and objects by use; carries out one-part and two-part commands, such as *pick up your shoe and give it to mommy;* knows what is used to drink liquids, what goes on the feet, what is used to buy candy; understands plurals, questions, difference between boy and girl, the concepts *one, up, down, run, walk, throw, fast, more, my*	Up to 425 words; jargon and echolalia no longer exist; averages 140 words per hour; names words such as *chair, can, box, key, door;* repeats two digits from memory; average sentence length is approximately two and one-half words; uses more adjectives and adverbs; demands repetition from others, such as *do it again;* nearly always announces intentions before action; begins to ask questions of adults; 75% of speech intelligible	—
36	Up to 3600 words; understands *both, two, not today,* what to do when thirsty (hungry, sleepy), why people have stoves, understands *wait, later, big, new, different, strong, today, another,* and taking turns at play; carries out two-item and some three-item commands, such as *give me the ball, pick up the doll, and sit down;* identifies several colors; is aware of past and future	Up to 900 words in simple sentences, averaging three to four words per sentence; averages 170 words per hour; uses words such as *when, time, today, not today, new, different, big, strong, surprise, secret;* can repeat three digits, name one color, say name, give simple account of experiences, and tell stories that can be understood; begins to use more pronouns, adjectives, and adverbs; describes at least one element of a picture; is aware of past and future; uses commands such as *you make it* and expressions such as *I can't, I don't want to;* verbalizes toilet needs; expresses desire to take turns; communication includes criticisms, commands, requests, threats, questions, answers; 85% of speech intelligible	Starts to distinguish dissimilar speech sounds, such as the difference between *ee* and *er,* although there may be some difficulty with the concepts of *same* and *different*

Modified from Chinn, P. L. (1976). *Child health maintenance: Concepts in family-centered care* (2nd ed.). St. Louis: Mosby; Gillam, R. B., Marguardt, T. P., & Martin, F. N. (2001). *Communication sciences and disorders: From science to clinical practice.* San Diego: Singular Publishers.

The toddler period is dominated by play, often referred to as a child's *work*, which is repetitive and ritualistic. When toddlers bounce a ball over and over and over again they are not trying to drive their parents crazy. They are trying to learn about balls, and repetition is the best teacher. Toddlers' ritualistic behaviors help them master skills and decrease anxiety, and the addition of a seemingly endless string of questions to these behaviors can test the limits of the most patient parents. These queries, however, must be acknowledged and responded to in a manner that not only provides answers but also validates and reinforces the toddler's burgeoning curiosity (Green & Palfrey, 2000). The nurse can reframe the terrible twos by teaching parents and caregivers that toddlers might better be viewed as "young scientists" in need of a safe "laboratory" in which to conduct their trial and error research (Green & Palfrey, 2000). Better now and in parents' close proximity than in adolescence, a developmental period that mirrors and repeats many of the parent-child challenges of toddlerhood.

Hearing

The ability to hear and listen to others is critical for speech and language development. Listening includes attending to what is heard, discriminating among the various qualities of sound, cognitively associating what is heard with previously learned experiences, and remembering what is heard. The quantity and quality of language that the toddler is exposed to is thought to be more important for the development of listening ability and therefore receptive language skills than it is for the development of expressive language skills. Toddlers often seek repetition of auditory input, as observed in their seemingly endless repetition of sounds, words, and combinations of words. This repetition is their way of practicing and organizing new language (see Table 18-1).

Hearing loss is one of the most common conditions present at birth. If undetected, even mild hearing loss will impede speech, language, cognitive, and emotional development (Green & Palfrey, 2000). Health care providers need to continue to monitor, screen, and refer for formal audiologic evaluation any child with risk indicators or signs of hearing loss. This includes toddlers (1) whose parents or caregivers are concerned about their hearing, speech, or language abilities, (2) with a history of head trauma associated with loss of consciousness or skull fracture, (3) with a family history of sensorineural hearing loss, and (4) with recurrent or persistent otitis media.

Younger toddlers are screened using visual reinforcement audiometry in which stimulus tones and visually animated reinforcers (e.g., a lighted toy) are paired and presented together. After the toddler has been conditioned to expect this relationship, the visual reinforcer is withheld and the sound is presented alone. The toddler looks for the visual reinforcer in response to the sound, and the visual reinforcer is then presented as a reward. Conditioned play audiometry is used for older toddlers and preschool children. The child is first taught to play listening games, using blocks or rings. The child learns to wait and listen for a sound, then performs a motor task (e.g., places a block a bucket or a ring on a stacking stick) in response. The motor task is followed by social reinforcement. Noncalibrated toys or noisemakers and signals that lack frequency specificity are inappropriate screening methods and should be used only as gross indicators for monitoring.

Otitis media, or inner ear infection, is one of the leading causes of visits to health care providers during the toddler years and the number one reason for which antibiotics are prescribed for these children. Discussing the current literature and evidence-based reports and recommendations often helps parents understand the proper use of antibiotics, which is also imperative in preventing antibiotic resistance. When it is deemed necessary to use an antibiotic, nurses need to teach how to administer the medication safely and stress the importance of taking the medication at the prescribed time and for the full duration of the course.

Vision

Toddlers' visual acuity is usually around 20/40, although gaining their cooperation for screening is often difficult and not recommended unless parents, caregivers, or health care providers identify a concern. Depth perception is still immature, although more developed than in infancy.

Amblyopia is one of the major health care concerns of this age group and occurs in 2% to 5% of children. It is defined as diminished, or loss of, vision in an eye that has not received adequate use. The eye looks normal, but it is not being used normally. Because the brain favors the other eye, the term *lazy eye* is often used. The most common cause of amblyopia is strabismus, but it may also occur when one eye is more nearsighted, farsighted, or astigmatic than the other. Occasionally amblyopia is caused by other eye conditions such as a cataract.

Strabismus is a deviation of the line of vision from the midline resulting from extraocular muscle weakness or imbalance and is commonly referred to as *crossed eye*. One or both eyes may turn in, out, up, or down and can be constant or intermittent. Marked or continuous strabismus usually is noticed early by the parents and health care providers and is therefore treated early; the more subtle deviations are often unnoticed until older toddlerhood or the preschool years. Every toddler should be screened for strabismus as part of the routine eye examination that is performed by the physician or nurse practitioner during well-child visits. Best results are obtained when the condition is diagnosed and treated early.

Management of amblyopia depends on the cause and may include surgery or paralytic, autonomic, and centrally acting pharmacological agents. However, no matter what the cause, management will involve making the child use the lazy eye, the eye with reduced vision. There are two ways to do this: (1) atropine eye drops or (2) patching the stronger eye. Researchers have found that atropine eye drops, when placed in the stronger eye once a day, work as well as eye patching and may result in better compliance (The Pediatric Eye Disease Investigator Group, 2002). In

The Eye Patch Club

It is estimated that 2% to 5% of all children suffer from amblyopia. Prevent Blindness America is creating a support group called the Eye Patch Club for families coping with a child's amblyopia treatment. The *Eye Patch Club News* is a newsletter featuring tips and techniques for promoting compliance, stories from and about children whose eyes are patched, and professional advice from optometrists, ophthalmologists, and orthoptists. Each issue also includes a Kid's Page, and there is a classroom guide for teachers with explanations for the classroom, as well as activities for everyone to learn more about their eyes. An Eye Patch Club calendar and stickers that allow children to track their patch-wearing activity, a refrigerator magnet with helpful hints, and pen pal opportunities are also available. To learn more about Prevent Blindness America and The Eye Patch Club, visit their Web site at: http://www.preventblindness.org/children/EyePatchClub.html.

Maternal Limit Setting and Toddler Outcomes

Gail Houck and Elizabeth LeCuyer-Maus are nurse researchers at Oregon Health & Science University. The purpose of their research was to examine maternal limit-setting patterns and toddlers' responses to limits with respect to the outcomes of self-concept and social competence at 36 months of age. One hundred twenty-six mother-toddler dyads were examined over time using videotaped sessions. Mothers were classified according to the control strategies they used and their level of sensitive responsiveness during a limit-setting interaction with their toddlers. Toddlers were classified on the basis of their compliance, autonomy, and engagement. Four types of maternal approaches emerged: indirect, teaching based, power based, and inconsistent.

Mothers whose discipline was teaching based provided more opportunities for their children to practice self-regulatory behaviors, by providing clear limits along with empathy, sensitivity, and assistance with strategies to cope with their distress. Mothers who never clearly asserted a limit and whose primary strategy was to distract the toddler were classified as indirect, while inconsistent classification was assigned to mothers who seemed inattentive or insensitive with a general lack of responsiveness.

Development of a more optimal self-regulatory behavior in the toddler, as embedded in self-concept and social competence over time, was clearly associated with a maternal teaching-based limit-setting pattern. The toddlers who fared the worst had mothers who used indirect or inconsistent approaches to limit setting.

How might this research assist nurses who are counseling parents of toddlers?

Houck, G. M., & LeCuyer-Maus, E. A. (2002). Maternal limit-setting patterns and toddler development of self-concept and social competence. *Issues in Comprehensive Pediatric Nursing, 25*, 21-24.

addition, 2 hours of patching may produce an improvement in visual acuity that is of similar magnitude to the improvement produced by 6 hours of daily patching (The Pediatric Eye Disease Investigator Group, 2003). Shorter patching time should lead to better compliance and improved quality of life (Innovative Practice box).

Other signs of vision problems that the nurse observes or parents report in their toddlers include the following red flags:

1. Rubs eyes excessively
2. Shuts or covers one eye, tilts head, or looks sideways to view an object
3. Has difficulty or is irritable when doing close work
4. Blinks, squints, or frowns when viewing objects
5. Holds books close to eyes
6. Has red, encrusted, or swollen eyelids
7. Has red, inflamed, or watery eyes
8. Develops recurring styes

Taste and Smell

Toddlers are beginning to take control of their world and have the capacity to taste and smell, new skills that are rapidly put to use. Toddlers often refuse to even taste something that looks or smells displeasing to them or eat something that they recall as tasting terrible. They are able to react accurately to a sensation that a taste or smell arouses in them, and they begin to learn conditioned association between certain smells and culturally acceptable values. Foods and smells found in one family or culture become palatable and accepted, and those that are unacceptable become displeasing. Many of our adult eating habits, food likes and dislikes, and visceral responses to odors have their roots in this period.

Self-Perception–Self-Concept Pattern

According to Erikson (1993, 1997), the developmental task of toddlers is to acquire a sense of autonomy while overcoming a sense of doubt and shame. To exert **autonomy,** toddlers must relinquish the dependence on others that was enjoyed during infancy. Continued dependency has the potential to create a sense of doubt in toddlers about their ability to take control of, and ultimately take responsibility for, their own actions. Toddlers seem to thrive when parents can accommodate their increasing autonomy yet maintain a strong parenting presence that includes a full measure of patience, enough parental self-confidence to set appropriate limits, and the ability to realize that their toddler's negative behavior is not directed at them and that their egocentrism is not a reflection on them (see Research Highlights).

The toddler must explore the world, not only the physical aspects but also the interpersonal aspects of relationships, to develop a true sense of autonomy. Exploring the physical world involves poking into, climbing onto, crawling under, tasting, smelling, and taking apart the objects encountered. The child explores relationships with others by searching for the limits of the child's power: if a "no" or a temper tantrum means control of another person's behavior, the child learns that one's own self is more powerful than the other person's self. The toddler continually practices separateness to develop a sense of autonomy.

This process can be trying and confusing for parents. The toddler may say a vehement "no" when offered a drink and then scream and cry when the drink is put away; the parents may wonder if the toddler wants the drink or not. Likely the answer is "yes," but the toddler may also need to express autonomy by refusing it. Occasionally the same toddler who displays a strong need for autonomy spontaneously cuddles or even clings to a parent. These conflicting desires can be confusing to both the parent and the toddler.

The toddler's need for more autonomy may conflict with parental expectations, safety limits, or the rights of other children or adults. Any of these conflicts results in feelings of frustration. A typical toddler response to frustration is the well-known temper tantrum.

Nursing Interventions

The nurse assesses the toddler-parent relationship to determine the following:

1. How is the toddler expressing the need for autonomy?
2. How do the parents perceive these actions?
3. How does the toddler respond to frustration in exploring the environment or controlling personal and others' actions?
4. How do the parents respond to the toddler's display of frustration?
5. What provisions are the parents making to allow safe choices for the toddler?

The nurse's teaching focuses on the aspects that are troublesome for the toddler-parent relationship. Some general concepts to include are:

1. Match the environment to the child's needs and abilities. Childproof the home such that the child can explore safely. Provide toys that the child can master. Give opportunities to play with more challenging toys, but do not make these toys the rule.
2. Give advance notice of a change in activity, such as lunch or nap time. Utilize transition rituals and objects.
3. Do not offer a choice if there isn't one. For example, rather than ask if the toddler wants to take a bath, say it is time to take a bath, do you want to take it upstairs or downstairs, or do you want to start at the face and move down to the toes or start with the toes and wash the face last? This allows for the toddler to be in charge and the task of bathing achieved.
4. Set and enforce consistent limits such that the toddler will come to develop control within these limits.
5. To prevent temper tantrums, keep routines simple and consistent, set reasonable limits and give rationales, avoid head-on clashes, and provide choices.
6. If temper tantrums occur, provide a safe environment for the toddler, identify the tantrum's cause, and help the

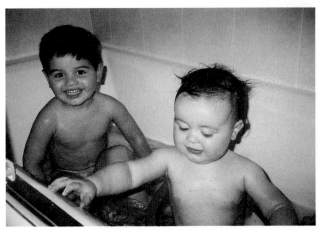

Figure 18-7 Toddlers might have to learn to deal with a new family member.

toddler regain control. Do not reason, threaten, promise, hit, or give in. Respond consistently and follow through on discipline free of anger. Overcriticizing and restricting the toddler may dampen enthusiasm and increase feelings of shame and doubt.
7. Praise the toddler's skills and abilities. Never miss an opportunity to catch your toddler being good. Be positive. Remember to say "yes" once in a while.

Roles-Relationships Pattern

By toddlerhood children typically know their mother, father, and older siblings and have established some form of reciprocal relationship with them. Toddlers' capability for relationships is limited and usually reflects their egocentric approach to everything else. Parents' and siblings' roles are understood, just like everything else in their lives, in terms of how those roles relate to the toddler. One family member may be the fixer of toys or the comforter of bruises, another the troublemaker who takes away toys.

Toddlers are interested in everything, and their parents' and siblings' activities and possessions are often imitated and preferred. Frequently the desire to be like or have something that belongs to a sibling creates sibling rivalry. This happens between toddlers and their older siblings, but even more when a new younger sibling is introduced (Figure 18-7). A new baby who is often loud, unable to play, not to be touched or explored too vigorously, and demands and gets too much parental attention quickly becomes a nuisance to toddlers who have been known to inform their parents that they can "Take the new baby back where it came from now." Realizing the new sibling is here to stay, toddlers often regress, reverting to earlier, previously abandoned infantile behavior such as losing toileting skills, wanting to be fed or dressed, or even talking baby talk. They are usually trying to retain or regain a sense of mastery and once reassured will move on. This process is not the end of sibling rivalry, but only the beginning of what will take on many forms and require ongoing negotiation from all family members.

Box **18-2** Warning Signs of Child Abuse

- Parental delay in seeking help
- Inconsistencies in the history of how the injury occurred
- Injury inconsistent with the history or child's developmental capability
- Old, unexplained fractures evident on radiographs
- Bruises confined to back surface of the body—neck to knees
- Bare spots and broken hair
- Pattern of injury or bruising descriptive of object used to inflict injury (belt or belt buckle, hand, cigarette, hot water)
- Burns with sharply demarcated edges or circumferential patterns
- Perineal injuries of any kind

From Cheung, K. K., & Yetman, R. (1999). Practice guidelines: Identifying and documenting findings of physical child abuse and neglect. *Journal of Pediatric Health Care, 13,* 142-143; Garfunkel, L. C., Kaczorowski, J., & Christy, C. (2002). *Pediatric clinical advisor.* St. Louis: Mosby.

Parents cannot stop sibling fighting by forbidding it, but reasonable limits can be established. One way to tone down fighting is to remove the gain. Generally the desired outcome in the toddler's mind is to see the self rewarded and the sibling punished. When parents do not reward or punish, or when they do not take sides, the gain is missing and fighting becomes less satisfactory. This approach does not mean that all fighting will stop, but the child will look for other ways of getting approval.

Sibling relationships and parent-child relationships can be difficult subjects for parents to discuss. Parents may think that any hint of discord indicates an unhealthy family. The nurse should include normal family development and role relationships as part of the anticipatory guidance given during the toddler years. Toddler behaviors are trying for all parents, and discipline can often be influenced as much by parental emotions as by parenting knowledge and skill. When parental anger, criticism, and restrictions go unchecked, physical and emotional abuse can occur.

Child Abuse

Child abuse is not limited to a particular age or particular families. However, it is more likely to occur with a major change or turmoil in the family and when parental role models were abusive. Toddlerhood is a trying time for the most patient of parents, and nurses need to be alert to family changes and stresses as well as to signs of abuse (Box 18-2). Many injuries are difficult to differentiate from accidental injury and, at times, may even be confused with culturally appropriate healing practices (Multicultural Awareness box).

Typically parental responses to childhood injuries include a spontaneous reporting of the details of the illness or injury accompanied by concern, questions about progress

MULTICULTURAL AWARENESS

Evaluating for Child Abuse With Cultural Sensitivity

Nurses are required by law to report cases of suspected child abuse to Child Protective Services. The nurse who takes a careful health history may discover that what might appear to be characteristic burns or bruises associated with child abuse may instead be the product of a traditional culturally appropriate healing practice. The following are two examples of healing practices found in the Pacific Islander and Asian populations that might create such confusion.

COINING *(CAO GIO)*

Coining is a common healing practice used among Pacific Island and Asian families within the United States. Traditionally, coining is used for conditions associated with "wind" illnesses, as well as a wide variety of febrile illnesses. The lesions seen from coining are produced by rubbing a warm oil or balm on the skin and firmly abrading the skin with a coin or special instrument. The practice produces linear petechiae and ecchymosis on the chest and back that often resemble strap or belt marks. The appearance of the deep red-purple skin color is confirmation that the person had bad wind in the body.

CUPPING *(VENTOUSE)*

Cupping involves creating a vacuum inside a special cup or glass by burning the oxygen out of it and then promptly placing it on a person's skin surface. Cupping draws blood and lymph to the body surface that is under the cup or glass, increasing local circulation. The purpose for doing this is to remove cold and damp "evils" from the body or to assist blood circulation or both. The procedure frequently is used to treat lung congestion. The resulting circular ecchymotic marks are approximately 2 inches in diameter and resemble nonaccidental trauma.

and discharge, difficulty in leaving the child, and an attempt to identify with the child's feelings. These parents may also experience guilt for not protecting the child from the accident and may offer gifts to compensate for these feelings of guilt. In contrast, neglectful or abusive parents are often hesitant to provide information about the illness or injury; they may be evasive or even contradict themselves, irritated by the inconvenience of being asked questions. Abusive parents may not exhibit guilt feelings and often contend that the toddler was solely responsible for the injury.

Although these signs of potential abuse are certainly not present in all abusive parents, their presence should alert the nurse to assess and observe further. The nurse must also remember that some of these signs may be found in nonabusive parents, and their presence serves only as a cue for further assessment, not as a conclusive diagnosis. All nurses are required by law, however, to report suspected child abuse to the local child protective services agency.

Sexuality-Reproductive Pattern

The toileting process, during which attention is focused on the genital area, may precipitate curiosity about the genital organs. The nurse should include this aspect in early teaching about toilet training, giving parents time to consider their feelings and decide on their approach to genital exploratory behavior and masturbation. Some parents accept the child's curiosity, whereas others see this as an opportunity to introduce their own sexual values and taboos.

The nurse can help parents approach this curiosity and exploration, as well as masturbation, as a normal developmental process. These behaviors provide toddlers with an opportunity to become better acquainted with their bodies. Many parents are uncertain about the vocabulary they should use and often create cute, unrelated words rather than provide the correct anatomical terms. The use of cute alternative words often is a reflection of parental discomfort or embarrassment. Using correct terms will help toddlers be better understood, especially if inappropriate touching by others occurs.

Coping-Stress Tolerance Pattern

Perceptions of events and reactions to them are filtered through children's developing cognitive, emotional, and social capacities. The relevance of life events and the child's vulnerability to their impact depend on the given developmental period (see Care Plan). A child's temperament, which is defined as an individual's style of emotional and behavioral response across situations, especially those involving change or stress, serves as a foundation for coping (Burns, Brady, Dunn, & Starr, 2000). Although temperament generally has been accepted as inborn, it is influenced by environmental characteristics and exerts an influence on psychosocial adjustment by way of its effect on parent-child interactions. Nurses need to assist parents in recognizing their toddler's innate behavioral qualities as expressions of temperament and in developing management strategies (Hot Topics box).

Toddlers are developing new ways to cope with the myriad new stresses that come with being a toddler. As is typical of their stage of development, coping is egocentric and reflective of their need for autonomy. Typical stressors include new siblings, baby-sitters, day care, toilet training, parental limit setting, and an endless string of tasks involving skills they have yet to develop.

Toddlers often imitate their parents' behavior and this includes their methods of dealing with stress. They also regress, at times, to earlier infantile behavior when overwhelmed, until they regain some sense of mastery. Parents can help to anticipate and prepare toddlers for stressful experiences before they happen. However, they need to remember that toddlers' sense of time and ability to recall are limited. Preparations should be honest, simple, and focused on what the toddler will experience. Enough time should be allowed for the toddler to rehearse the coping

---

CARE PLAN

Family Situational Crisis

Nursing Diagnosis Altered Parenting Related to Situational Crisis

DEFINING CHARACTERISTICS
- Verbal concerns about changes in parental role, family function, or family communication
- Inattentiveness or inability to attend to child's needs
- Reluctant or inappropriate caretaking behaviors
- Compulsive seeking of role approval from others
- Disruption in caretaking routines

RELATED FACTORS
- Financial difficulties
- Recent move
- Change in marital relationship
- Dysfunctional relationship between parents

EXPECTED OUTCOMES
Goal: Provision of Stability for Child During Family Situational Crisis
- Parent verbalizes increasing confidence in parenting abilities
- Parent demonstrates nurturing behaviors toward child
- Parent identifies effective ways to express negative emotions
- Parent identifies appropriate community and extended family resources

INTERVENTIONS
- Encourage expression of feelings.
- Explore personal, family, and community resources.
- Help parent identify deficits in parenting skills.
- Initiate a plan to assist parent in developing appropriate parenting skills.

---

behavior with the parent, but not so far off from the event that the toddler forgets.

The nurse can help the parents anticipate developmental stressors and can suggest age and temperament–appropriate coping behaviors for toddlers. Early efforts at dealing with stress are an essential step to a more mature coping response as the child grows.

Values-Beliefs Pattern

Healthy behaviors are expressions of positive values and beliefs. These values and beliefs are learned phenomena, and their recognition and acceptance are fundamental to the integrity of every child. Toddlers believe rules are absolute and behave, according to Kohlberg, out of a fear of punishment. However, toddlers' environments should not only help them become aware of right and wrong but also contribute to their sense of security, belonging, and autonomy. Development of moral integrity is enhanced if toddlers believe they are valued.

HOTtopics

COPING WITH A CHILD'S TEMPERAMENT

Temperament is defined as the style of behaviors that a child habitually uses to cope with the demands and expectations of the environment. Chess and Thomas (1986) originally described three common temperament patterns that they believe are innate: (1) the easy child, (2) the difficult child, and (3) the slow-to-warm-up child.

The easy child is cuddly, affectionate, and easy to manage. The way in which a child with an easy temperament elicits positive reactions from adults is obvious.

Children with a difficult temperament, however, are less adaptable, are more intense and active, and have more negative moods. These behaviors can be distressing to parents and caregivers and may cause them to feel ineffective in their roles.

Temperament affects development throughout the life span but is especially significant for toddlers when placed in the context of development. Toddlers are increasingly mobile and are striving for independence at a time when parents become more demanding. Various approaches to parenting, teaching, and providing health care, including the adults' own temperament styles, culture, and gender-related biases, can influence the way in which the child's behavior is viewed.

According to the goodness-of-fit interactive model of temperament, adults can accommodate their demands and expectations in ways that match the child's behaviors, including learning strategies to help toddlers adapt positively to social expectations.

Questions

1. What are some of the consequences of labeling a toddler as *difficult, easy,* or *slow to warm up*?
2. What are common reactions to girls who are extremely active and highly distractible? Boys who are clingy, cry often, and prefer to play with dolls? What influences these reactions in adults? What influence do they have on children?

From Burns, C. E., Brody, M. A., Dunn, A. M., & Starr, N. B. (2000). *Pediatric primary care* (2nd ed.). New York: W. B. Saunders; Chess, S., & Thomas, A. (1986). *Temperament in clinical practice.* New York: Guildford Press.

Because most of toddlers' developing values and beliefs depend on their interactions with parents, the nurse's assessment questions are often directed to or focused on the parent or caregiver.

- What are the family's values and beliefs about what is right and wrong?
- How does the parental approach to limit setting reflect these values and beliefs?
- What religious, spiritual, or cultural traditions and activities does the family have?
- How is the toddler included in these traditions and activities?

Children are exposed to and begin to participate in and imitate their family's religious rituals and practices during toddlerhood. They are often taught prayers and songs with a religious theme that are tied into what the family believes is right and wrong. Toddlers may be able to learn the words to these simple prayers and songs, but parents should be cautioned that knowing the words does not mean that toddlers understand the full meaning of what is said. This early introduction into the family's religious beliefs is important as a socialization factor but should not be assumed to produce a good child.

The creation of values and beliefs in young children is related to their developmental stage and reflected in their behaviors. An important aspect of teaching young children what is right and wrong involves stating what acceptable behavior is and then reinforcing the behavior when it occurs. Parents often attend to toddlers only when they are misbehaving, leaving them alone when they are being good. In this scenario toddlers receive no attention for acceptable behavior but gain their parents' attention when they misbehave. The nurse can remind parents to catch their toddlers being good and give them the same or more attention.

PATHOLOGICAL PROCESSES
Accidents

"If a disease were killing our young children in the proportions that injuries are, people would be outraged and demand that this killer be stopped."
C. Everett Koop, M.D., Former Surgeon General

Toddlers are at high risk for accidental injury, because they lack judgment and experience and have only rudimentary problem-solving skills, limited physical coordination, and a heightened level of curiosity about their environment. Most parents think that it is natural for children to get hurt and that childhood injuries are just a part of growing up. However, most injuries are predictable and preventable and can cause disabilities requiring long-term care. Furthermore, they cause more deaths than all childhood disease combined.

One out of every ten toddlers who comes to the emergency room is treated for accidental injury. Males tend to have more injuries than their female counterparts, but the overall numbers of accidental injuries peak during toddlerhood for both males and females. A second peak occurs for males during adolescence. Major causes of accidental injury in toddlers involve structural hazards, sports, drowning, burns, motor vehicles, and poisoning.

Structural Hazards

Houses and other buildings can be hazardous for toddlers. Their desire to explore lures them to locations to which older children or adults would not consider going. The toddler will climb onto furniture or fixtures, out of windows, or into small spaces. Injuries that result from these explorations can range from minor scrapes and bruises to fatal head injuries. Ideally homes are baby proofed before the infant begins scooting and crawling and toddler proofed

CASE STUDY

Grandparents Provide Care

Mary and John are the parents of 18-month-old Jeremy. They plan to take a week-long vacation while leaving Jeremy with his grandparents at their house. Because Jeremy is the first grandchild, the elderly couple is eager to spend time with him, but they have expressed concern about caring for a toddler.

Reflective Questions
1. What do the parents need to discuss with the grandparents concerning safety issues?
2. What psychosocial issues of a toddler are important for both the parents and the grandparents to consider?

before the toddler becomes increasingly mobile. Parents should reassess the safety of their home as their child acquires new skills. Injuries to toddlers occur most often when they fall from furniture, high chairs, changing tables, stairs, windows, and playground equipment. When the child or family visits the home of a friend or relative, it must be inspected for hazards, or the toddler must be confined to one safe room. Many injuries occur in unfamiliar environments.

Preventive measures for structural hazards include the following:

- Don't leave a toddler unattended.
- Use gates at the top and bottom of stairways and at doors.
- Keep chairs away from countertops and tables to prevent toddlers from climbing.
- Lock doors to dangerous areas and use gates and window guards.

Toys

Toys commonly found in homes are another source of injury. Parents should inspect not only the toys that are in their own homes, but also the toys given to the toddler outside the home by relatives, friends, baby-sitters, or day-care personnel (Case Study). Many toys that are likely to be safe for older children are extremely hazardous for the toddler. Of concern are small removable parts and batteries, toxic paint or stuffing, sharp edges, and flammability.

Sports

Although sports and recreational equipment is recognized as a major source of accidents in older children and adolescents, parents and health care personnel occasionally forget that these items can also be dangerous to toddlers. Improper storage of this equipment is a primary danger. Firearms that are left loaded and unlocked are deadly hazards, and bodybuilding weights and other heavy equipment easily overwhelm toddlers who may pull these objects down on themselves. Toddlers should always be supervised closely, especially in new environments or on playground equipment.

As toddlers becomes more mobile, they are introduced to riding toys, tricycles, and bicycles. Nurses need to remind

parents about the need for, and in most states the requirement of, bicycle helmets that are fitted properly and worn every time the toddler rides or is a passenger on a bicycle.

Drowning

Children between the ages of 1 and 3 years are at highest risk of drowning, because most do not know how to swim and do not have the skills to keep their heads above water or to get out of the water. Toddlers can drown in water just deep enough to cover their noses and mouths. Although swimming pools and other natural bodies of water are a big part of the problem, even pails of water, toilets, bathtubs, and wading pools are dangerous. When toddlers fall into a pail of water or toilet it is hard for them to straighten up because all of their weight is forward. Toddlers should never be left unattended—even for a few seconds—near a bathtub, hot tub, wading or swimming pool, toilet, or pail of water. All swimming pools should be fenced and have self-closing gates and latches. Toddlers must be supervised constantly and competently whenever they are near any body of water and fitted properly with personal flotation devices whenever they are on a boat.

Burns

Each year more than 100,000 children between the ages of 0 and 4 years require emergency room treatment for scalds from hot liquids. Hot tap water, boiling water, coffee, tea, and food are the most common sources of injury. These very painful and often debilitating injuries often happen as toddlers begin to gain mobility and explore their environments, inadvertently touching hot surfaces or spilling hot liquids on themselves. They may also put their mouths on live electrical cords or their fingers into electrical sockets and get serious burns, as well as tip their walkers or themselves into fireplaces or woodstoves.

Nurses need to give parents these reminders:

- Never eat, drink or carry anything hot while holding a child.
- Lower water heater temperature to 120° to 125° Fahrenheit.
- Never leave hot beverages or foods within a child's reach.
- Put children in a playpen while cooking.
- Never leave a toddler unattended in the bathtub. It takes only a moment to turn on the hot water.
- Put screens around fireplaces or woodstoves.
- Do not let children handle food directly from the microwave oven.
- Use burners at the back of the stove and turn pot handles in toward the stove.
- Install and maintain smoke detectors, replacing batteries annually.

Motor Vehicles

Motor vehicle–related injury, which includes both passenger and pedestrian injuries, is one of the leading causes of death in children from 1 to 4 years of age. For the toddler, passenger injury is more frequent and often involves the lack of use or misuse of child safety seats. Child safety seats, when properly installed and used, have reduced the risk of death and serious injury to children by 70%. Unfortunately, improper installation and use of child safety seats are widespread problems, with some experts reporting that over 80% of them are misused in some way. Most health care providers and hospitals are knowledgeable and should provide safety checks or refer families to a nearby child safety center if they have questions.

As children reach 20 pounds, the nurse needs to confirm with parents that they are switched to forward-facing child safety seats. Rear seat position is preferred and safer than the front seat, and a special warning has been issued that no child should be seated in the front passenger seat if the car has airbags. During the toddler years children may progress in size and weight to a transition or booster seat. The nurse can provide a list of approved car seats and local retail outlets or agencies that sell, lend, or rent car seats. The American Academy of Pediatrics has published a comprehensive pamphlet on choosing a car seat (American Academy of Pediatrics, 2000).

Toddlers are also injured or killed when they are hit by motor vehicles in their own driveways and often by members of their family or nearby neighbors. They are too small to be seen by a driver backing up and too quick to run out after a departing parent or relative who thinks they are still safely inside.

Biological Agents

Recent events have heightened concern about bioterrorism, and concerns about agents such as anthrax are becoming more common questions for health care providers. Nurses can provide information that can assist parents in dealing with their toddler's and their own fears. Nurses should encourage parents to:
- Talk about their fears and worries
- Stick to family routines that help toddlers feel comfortable and secure
- Supervise toddlers' television viewing
- Educate themselves, the best protection against unnecessary fear. Toddlers will be less fearful if they see that parents are not afraid.

Many parents feel that toddlers, because of their exploratory nature and limited cognitive competence and understanding, are especially vulnerable to certain agents such as anthrax. This is accentuated by knowing that no anthrax vaccine exists for this age group. Fearful parents might request antibiotics that they can keep on hand, just in case. The nurse can teach parents that giving children antibiotics when they are not needed can do more harm than good. Many antibiotics, especially those identified for anthrax management, have serious side effects and using them when they are not needed can lead to the development of drug-resistant forms of bacteria. If this happens, the antibiotics will not be able to kill the resistant bacteria the next time the child needs the same antibiotic to treat common ear, sinus, or other infections.

| Box **18-3** | Interventions to Prevent Poisoning in Toddlers |

- All household, garden, and car products should be kept out of reach.
- Keep medications out of reach in locked cabinets.
- Use childproof caps on medication.
- Keep all products and medication in their original containers for easy identification.
- No poisonous plants should be kept in the house. A list, which includes poinsettia, amaryllis, aloe vera, English ivy, mistletoe, mums, and spider plants, is available from local poison control centers.
- Avoid outdoor plants and shrubs that are poisonous, including azaleas and mums.
- Supervise toddler's activity at all times.
- Post the poison control center number (800-222-1222) next to every telephone, including your cell phone.

The American Academy of Pediatrics Web site addresses numerous issues related to bioterrorism and children (*http://www.aap.org*), including the development of a teaching toolkit for parents to use with their children.

Poisoning

Studies have shown that poisoning happens 10 times more often among young children between the ages of 1 and 4 years than in their older counterparts. Toddlers between the ages of 1 and 2 years are at the greatest risk. They are becoming more mobile, enabling them to explore and discover poisonous substances in the home. These include prescription and over-the-counter medications, household products, plants, cosmetics, lead-based paint, and cigarettes (Box 18-3). They are also at risk because they still use their mouths as a way of exploring. Although many parents take precautions against poisoning in their own homes, some forget that toddlers can be poisoned away from home, while visiting grandparents or other relatives, for example (see Case Study).

The toddler, because of limited experience and cognitive level, is unaware that these items are harmful. Many emergency room calls and visits are precipitated by a toddler's ingestion of a questionably or actually harmful substance. These incidents are likely to occur in the kitchen, bathroom, bedroom, or work area and usually are discovered by the parent or caretaker who finds an open or empty container or a half-eaten leaf or other substance.

When parents or caregivers suspect that a toddler has ingested a poisonous substance, they should call the poison control center, even if the child appears perfectly healthy. Each center is part of a nationwide effort to provide immediate information about poisonings. Parents should not attempt to induce vomiting without specific instructions from the center. Vomiting can cause further harm if the child is drowsy, unconscious, or convulsing, or if the substance ingested is corrosive, such as lye or a strong acid (Guyton & Hall, 2000). When vomiting is recommended by the poison control center, instructions often are given to use ipecac syrup to stimulate the vomiting rapidly. This medication should be stored as carefully as any other medication or hazardous household product and replaced often because of its short shelf life.

Chronic poisonings, such as lead poisoning, are often undetected until irreversible damage has occurred. Primary prevention involves teaching parents about risk factors and dangers of lead poisoning and the importance of a diet that encourages decreasing fat intake, because lead is retained in fat. Vitamin C, calcium, and iron intake reduce lead levels in the body. Secondary prevention involves doing periodic screening of blood lead levels on all young children identified at risk. See the Multicultural Awareness box in Chapter 15 about childhood lead poisoning.

Consumer protection laws in the United States require that all toys and furniture manufactured for small children be free of lead-based paint products. However, imported toys and furniture or antique and older family furniture may have been painted with a lead-based product.

SOCIAL PROCESSES
Day Care

During the toddler years many parents return to work or decide that an experience in a group setting would be beneficial for their child. The nurse can provide counseling about the decision to place a child in day care and the resulting emotions, as well as guidelines for selecting a child-care or day-care provider.

The U.S. Department of Health and Human Services Administration for Children and Families recommends a four-step approach as a guideline for selecting a child-care provider or day-care center:

Step 1: Interview potential child-care providers and observe the program or setting.

Ask about cost, enrollment, ages served, daily activities, accreditation and licensing regulations, caretaker credentials and experience, and policies about visiting, illness, and nutrition.

Look at provider-child interactions, safety, and the quality of the learning material and toys.

Step 2: Check references.

Talk to parents with children in the center or being cared for by the provider about discipline and responsiveness to parents, and talk to local child care resource or referral agencies and licensing offices.

Step 3: Make a decision based on specific criteria.

Think about safety, values, fit for you and your toddler, and affordability.

Step 4: Get and stay involved.

Talk to the provider regularly about how your child is doing, to your child about what the children are doing each day, and to other parents.

Visit often, announced and unannounced, and at various times of the day.

Many organizations have developed guidelines and checklists on choosing child care. Child Care Aware

(*http://www.childcareaware.org* or 800-424-2246) is a national initiative designed to improve the quality of care and increase the availability of quality child care in local communities. Services include helping to find child care and connecting parents with local child care resource and referral agencies. Their brochure, *Give Your Child Something That Will Last A Lifetime—Quality Child Care*, outlines the steps to finding child care and includes an observation checklist.

Regardless of the reasons for the parents wanting or needing day care for their child, the traditional expectation of caring for the young child at home continues to influence the parents' concept of what they should do for their child. Parents must be reassured that a day-care environment congruent with the family environment is not detrimental to the child. If a child has been placed in a setting that is detrimental to physical or emotional development, then the parent may need assistance in selecting an alternative setting. Changes in caregivers are difficult for toddlers, and regressive behaviors may surface during transition periods.

Culture and Ethnicity

Culture influences everything we do, know, and believe in. Each culture possesses its own values, attitudes, and practices with regard to family and child-rearing. Toddlers continue to be shaped by the cultural values and beliefs of their parents and families, the first of many socializing forces they will encounter. As their world expands, other forces and subcultures, including peers, the media, and their schools, will also be encountered.

Unlike older children, toddlers do not question the cultural practices of the family. The toddler who refuses to do certain expected things usually does so out of a need for autonomy and control rather than a questioning of beliefs. However, the nurse needs to remind parents of this, because parents may be feeling the pressure of cultural norms and expectations. This is especially true for families that have emigrated recently.

Nurses need to be prepared to provide culturally sensitive and competent care. Knowledge and respect for various cultural world views, customs, values, and traditions are needed to negotiate different approaches in developing a health-promotion plan with families. Health care practices are culturally influenced. For example, if a culture views immunizations as dangerous or unnecessary, the toddler may go unprotected from certain communicable diseases. Incorporation of knowledge, respect, and negotiation facilitates the development of a therapeutic relationship grounded in trust, as well as effective, high-quality health care outcomes (Burns et al., 2000).

Legislation

Local and state legislation specific to the toddler is directed primarily toward safety and injury prevention. Many states have passed laws requiring use of child safety seats, bicycle helmets, and temperature limits for household hot water heaters.

Each state has passed laws that provide protection for a child or developmentally disabled adult, define abuse and neglect, require that a report be made to a designated agency in the case of actual or suspected abuse or neglect, and define the responsibility of the protecting agency. These laws also provide for a central registry of reported cases of abuse. Nurses should be aware that they are required by law to report suspected child abuse and should familiarize themselves with the child abuse and neglect laws in their states.

Another key legislative issue for the toddler is the Education of the Handicapped Act amendment of 1986 (Public Law 99-457). This law creates programs that assist states in planning, developing, and implementing systems within states for handicapped children from birth to 3 years of age. Nurses who work with young children with disabilities need to investigate and familiarize themselves with the programs in their states.

Economics

Toddlers are completely incapable of contributing to the economic resources of the family; however, a lack or paucity of economic resources is capable of affecting the toddler's health and well-being. Toddlers who live in poverty have higher mortality rates, poorer health, poorer growth, and more physical morbidity from respiratory infections, gastrointestinal infections, anemia, asthma, dental caries, otitis media, and visual loss, as well as higher rates of accidental injury and psychological and developmental disorders (Burns et al., 2000).

About 25% of all children in the United States are enrolled in Medicaid programs and another 10 million are uninsured. In 1997 the Children's Health Insurance Program was developed to address this need. Other services that are available to low income families with toddlers include Temporary Assistance for Needy Families and the Special Supplemental Nutrition Program for Women, Infants, and Children. The nurse can play a critical role in mobilizing these resources for families.

Health Care Delivery System

The health of toddlers is significantly affected by the health care delivery system in the place where they live (Burns et al., 2000). Private physicians or nurse practitioners and public well-child clinics are the most frequently used resources for ongoing health maintenance or illness care for toddlers. Some public clinics sponsor special immunization days for young children who do not receive routine health care.

Each health care visit should include an interval history, assessment of growth and development, physical assessment, a discussion of age-appropriate developmental concerns, and anticipatory guidance. Immunizations should be given according to the current Recommended Childhood and Adolescent Immunization Schedule, which is published at least once a year in January by the CDC (*http://www.cdc.gov/nip*) (see **Web Site Resource 17E**). The nurse can inform parents that they can anticipate and keep track of their toddler's immunizations with the CDC Childhood Immunization Scheduler available at *http://www.cdc.gov/nip/kidstuff/scheduler.htm*.

Toddlers need to explore their environment to master it, and this is also valid for their health care encounters. They may need to observe and listen as their parents interact with the health care providers, be introduced to and allowed to manipulate examination equipment, and be given simple explanations and choices so that they can maintain some degree of control. Taking the time to enlist the cooperation of a toddler will make the health care visit more productive and conducive to information exchange and health care teaching.

SUMMARY

This period can be an exciting and challenging time for both toddlers and their parents. Parents who have encouraged their toddlers' desire to explore can now delight in their developing sense of adventure as they enter their preschool years. The world is a wonderful place for the toddler who has known and experienced support, affection, and protection.

ADDITIONAL STUDY MATERIAL

Study Questions in the back of the book, see page 663.

🖉evolve WEB SITE MATERIALS

These materials are located on the book's Web site at http://evolve.elsevier.com/Edelman/.

- WebLinks
- Content Updates

REFERENCES

American Academy of Pediatrics. (2005). *Car safety seats: A guide for families.* Elk Grove, IL: The Academy. Available from: AAP, 141 Northwest Point Blvd., P.O. Box 927, Elk Grove, IL 60007-0927. Retrieved April 5, 2005, from *http://www.aap.org*.

Berger, K. S., & Thompson, R. A. (2000). *The developing person through the life span.* New York: Worth.

Burns, C. E., Brady, M. A., Dunn, A. M., & Starr, N. B. (2000). *Pediatric primary care* (2nd ed). New York: W. B. Saunders.

Cheung, K. K., & Yetman, R. (1999). Practice guidelines: Identifying and documenting findings of physical child abuse and neglect. *Journal of Pediatric Health Care, 13,* 142-143.

Chinn, P. L. (1976). *Child health maintenance: Concepts in family-centered care* (2nd ed.). St. Louis: Mosby.

Erikson, E. H. (1993). *The magic years* (35th anniversary ed.). New York: Norton.

Erikson, E. H. (1997). *The life cycle completed.* New York: Norton.

Garfunkel, L. C., Kaczorowski, J., & Christy, C. (2002). *Pediatric clinical advisor.* St. Louis: Mosby.

Gillam, R. B., Marguardt, T. P., & Martin, F. N. (2001). *Communication sciences and disorders: From science to clinical practice.* San Diego: Singular Publishers.

Green, M., & Palfrey, J. S. (2000). *Bright futures; Guidelines for health supervision of infants, children, and adolescents* (2nd ed.). Arlington, VA: National Center for Education in Maternal and Child Health.

Grodner, M., Anderson, S. L., & DeYoung, S. (2003). *Foundations and clinical applications of nutrition: A nursing approach* (3rd ed.). St. Louis: Mosby.

Guyton, A. C., & Hall, J. E. (2000). *Textbook of medical physiology* (10th ed.). Philadelphia: W. B. Saunders.

Hockenberry, M. J., Wilson, D., Winkelstein, M. L., & Kline, N. E. (2003). *Wong's nursing care of infants and children* (7th ed.). St. Louis: Mosby.

Seidel, H. M., Ball, J. W., Dains, J. E., & Benedict, G. W. (2002). *Mosby's guide to physical examination* (5th ed.). St. Louis: Mosby.

Story, M., Holt, K., & Sofka, D. (2002). *Bright futures in practice: Nutrition*. Arlington, VA: National Center for Education in Maternal and Child Health.

The Pediatric Eye Disease Investigator Group. (2002). A randomized trial of atropine vs patching for treatment of moderate amblyopia in children. *Archives of Ophthalmology, 120,* 268-278.

The Pediatric Eye Disease Investigator Group. (2003). A randomized trial of patching regimens for treatment of moderate amblyopia in children. *Archives of Ophthalmology, 121,* 603-611.

Chapter 19

ANNE RATH RENTFRO

Preschool Child

After completing this chapter, the reader will be able to:

- Describe the physical and psychosocial changes that occur during the preschool years as they relate to child and family health needs.

- Discuss the concepts of cognitive development of the preschooler using Piaget's theory.

- Review the *Healthy People 2010* concepts that pertain to the preschool child and the family.

- Describe typical sleep disturbances of the preschooler that are relevant to family teaching and nursing support.

- Discuss appropriate vision and hearing screening tools for the preschooler and the nursing roles regarding their use.

- Compare the coping skills of the preschooler with those of a younger child.

- Outline the immunization requirements of the preschooler that are relevant to primary prevention.

- Identify warning signs of cancer in the preschooler.

- List risk factors for asthma in the preschooler.

- Identify causes of injuries in the preschooler.

key terms

Acquired lactase deficiency
Acute lymphocytic leukemia
Amblyopia
Asthma
Chloroma
Doll or puppet play
Draw-a-Person and Draw-a-Family tests
Early and Periodic Screening, Diagnosis, and Treatment (EPSDT)
Egocentrism
Expressive language
Heterophoria
Heterotropia

Homeostasis
Inductive explanation
Irreversibility
Ishihara's test
Mnemonic techniques
Mutual storytelling
Myopic vision
Neuroblastoma
Nightmares
Night terrors
Otitis media
Parental divorce
Peabody Picture Vocabulary Test
Preoperational stage

Preschool Readiness Experimental Screening Scale (PRESS)
Receptive language
Refractive errors
Retinoblastoma
Snellen E chart
Strabismus
Transductive reasoning
Vineland Social Maturity Scale
Wilms tumor

THINK About It

Aggressive Behavior

Phillip, age 4, started preschool 2 weeks ago after spending his early years at home with his mother and his 18-month-old sister. His mother recently returned to her job as an accountant, works 9 hours a day, and is fatigued when she picks up Phillip at 5:00 PM. Phillip's father travels for his job but is home on weekends to spend time with his family. Although Phillip's mother always believed that he was shy because he was quiet, during the last week at child care he started hitting his peers and becoming loudly vocal at story time. His mother, believing that Phillip's behavior is related to her return to work, feels embarrassed and frustrated by his behavior, especially because she enjoys her new job and the extra income.

1 What factors might be contributing to Phillip's changed behavior?

2 How might you define Phillip's temperament? Why?

3 What discussions might you have with Phillip's parents to help them understand, respond to, and change their son's behavior for the better?

The preschool child (ages 3 to 6 years) has a more mature body structure, the ability to control and use the body, and a facility with language that more closely resembles that of the adult than that of the toddler. The major psychological thrust of this period of development is mastery of self as an independent human being, with a willingness to extend experiences beyond those of the family. With more families being headed by the mother, more reliance has been placed on child-care settings that expose children to learning opportunities beyond the typical family. Although historically the end of early childhood in the Western world was marked by entrance into the formalized educational system, increasing numbers of children are starting formalized schooling during their preschool years. The *Healthy People 2010* box presents objectives related to this developmental stage.

AGE AND PHYSICAL CHANGES

The protuberant abdomen of the toddler disappears during the preschool years as the pelvis begins to straighten and the abdominal muscles develop. The hips gradually rotate inward, replacing out-toeing with straight or slight in-toeing. Mild in-toeing (metatarsus adductus) can remain during the preschool years, but anything beyond a mild level should be investigated and treated.

Growth rate remains relatively steady from ages 3 to 6 years. The average preschooler gains approximately 2 kilograms (4 pounds) of body weight and 7 centimeters (2 inches) of height each year. Head circumference increases less than 2 centimeters during the entire preschool period.

During early childhood, the skin matures in its ability to protect the child from outer invasion and loss of fluids. The skin's capacity to localize infection increases but remains less than mature. Negligible secretion of sebum makes the skin fairly dry. Changes occur both in color and texture of the hair. Hair usually turns darker and becomes straighter. Eccrine sweat gland function, which is the body heat-regulation mechanism, gradually matures, but the quantity of eccrine sweat produced in response to heat or emotion remains minimal. Apocrine sweat glands, located primarily in the axillae, areolas of the breast, and the anal area, remain nonsecretory during this period.

The kidneys have reached full maturity by the end of infancy and early toddlerhood. The only change during the preschool years is in size. By the end of this period, daily excretion of urine is 650 to 1000 milliliters (19 to 30 ounces). Under normal homeostatic conditions, the renal system conserves water and concentrates urine on a level that approximates adult abilities. Under conditions of stress, however, the preschooler's kidneys lack the ability to respond fully and to maintain **homeostasis** when compared with the more rapid response of the adult system.

Growth of the gastrointestinal organs continues through the preschool years, but no basic changes in function occur. Children who did not achieve full voluntary control of elimination during the toddler period generally attain this function by the end of the preschool period. **Acquired lactase deficiency,** intolerance to milk products manifested by diarrhea, often appears during the preschool years. This condition, more common in black, Asian American, and Native American children, can be managed successfully by eliminating lactose from the diet.

Lung capacity continues to increase, with a gradual decrease in respiratory rate. The preschooler makes better decisions than does the toddler about what to put in the mouth; thus, fewer instances of choking and obstruction occur. As ears gradually increase in size and shape the incidence of **otitis media** (inner ear infection) decreases slightly. The tonsils and adenoids become large in relation to the throat, which may contribute to noisy breathing and upper respiratory infection.

The cardiovascular system enlarges in proportion to general body growth. Heart rate for the preschooler is 70 to 40 beats per minute. The mean blood pressure is 100/60 mm Hg. Early hypertension can develop during the preschool years; therefore, blood pressure monitoring becomes important, particularly if there is a strong family history of hypertension (see Chapter 20). The preschool child maintains adequate hemoglobin levels with sufficient dietary intake. The bone marrow of the ribs, sternum, and vertebrae becomes fully established as the primary site for red blood cell formation. The liver and spleen continue to form erythrocytes and granulocytes.

Healthy People 2010

Selected National Health-Promotion and Disease Prevention Objectives for Preschool Children

- Increase the proportion of people who have a specific source of ongoing care to 96% (baseline is 93% for children and youth in 1997).
- Reduce the proportion of families that experience difficulties or delays in obtaining care or do not receive needed care to 7% (baseline is 12% in 1997).
- Establish a single toll-free telephone number for access to poison control centers on a 24-hour basis throughout the United States to 100% (baseline is 15% of poison control centers shared a single toll-free number in 1999).
- Increase the number of tribes, states, and the District of Columbia with trauma care systems that maximize the prevention, survival, and functional outcomes of trauma patients to 100% (baseline is five states in 1998).
- Increase the number of states and the District of Columbia that have statewide pediatric protocols for on-line medical direction to 100% (baseline is 17 states in 1997).
- Eliminate elevated blood lead levels in children (baseline is 4.4% of children age 1 to 5 years had blood lead levels exceeding 10 mcg/dl in 1994).
- Reduce indoor allergen levels to 29 million homes with dust mite allergens exceeding 2 mcg of dust in the bed (baseline is 36.3 million homes in 1999).
- Increase the proportion of people visiting primary health care who receive mental health screening and assessment.
- Reduce the proportion of children and adolescents who have dental caries to 11% (baseline is 18% of children age 2 to 4 years from 1988 to 1994).
- Increase the proportion of children and adolescents who view television two or fewer hours per day.
- Increase the proportion of preschool children age 5 years and under who receive vision screening.
- Increase the proportion of people who have hearing examinations on schedule.
- Reduce otitis media in children and adolescents to 294 per 1000 (baseline is 344.7 per 1000 in 1997).
- Reduce the rate of death for children age 1 to 4 years to 25.0 per 100,000 (baseline is 34.2 per 100,000 in 1998) and for children age 5 to 9 years to 14.3 per 100,000 (baseline is 17.6 per 100,000 in 1998).
- Reduce deaths from asthma to 1 per million children under age 5 (baseline is 1.7 per million in 1998).
- Reduce hospitalization rates for pediatric asthma to 17.3 per 10,000 (baseline is 23 per 10,000 in 1996).

From U.S. Department of Health and Human Services. (2000). *Healthy People 2010*. Washington, DC: U.S. Government Printing Office.

The immune system continues to develop. Preschoolers boost their immune response to common pathogens as exposure occurs. Group activities, such as joining a preschool or play group, increase exposure and subsequently escalate the incidence of common contagious illnesses for a time, regardless of the age of the child. The first encounter with such group activities usually results in some increase in illness. Later these children may be less prone to disease because of their early exposure to infectious illnesses and their consequent immunity.

All primary teeth have erupted by late toddler or early preschool years. The first permanent tooth may erupt toward the end of the preschool period. On average, girls tend to get permanent teeth approximately 6 months earlier than boys. Older preschoolers usually take responsibility for dental hygiene, although they may need gentle guidance about proper brushing and appropriate nutritional intake for healthy teeth. Parents should continue to assist with and supervise flossing. Because this is an age of caries formation, regular dental checkups are essential. The nurse assesses whether the child is receiving preventive dental care. Parents should be encouraged to begin or maintain this care. Suggestions for promoting good oral hygiene as part of general health-promotion teaching can be found in Chapter 20.

Musculoskeletal and neurological development reaches a level that allows for seemingly effortless walking, running, and climbing. Older preschoolers' ability to copy figures and draw recognizable pictures indicates their advancing fine motor abilities, and they are eager to demonstrate these skills to others. Practice, increases in muscle size, continuing associations among existing neural pathways, and the establishment of new pathways for already accomplished tasks are a few of the many complex factors that contribute to the advances in function observed during early childhood. These advances in fine motor and gross motor skills are outlined in Table 19-1.

Gender

Boys tend to experience more childhood illnesses than do girls during ages 3 to 6 (see Chapter 18). Preschoolers are more aware of their sexual identity than are toddlers and may imitate societal stereotypes more closely. Traditionally boys have been encouraged to take more risks than girls have been and they have more accidents than do preschool girls, who may have been encouraged to choose more sedate activities. In today's society boys and girls have opportunities to choose the same activities. Whether this change will reflect accident statistics in the future will be interesting to observe.

Race

Race, with its related economic and cultural issues, can influence health care practices at this age, as is the case during all ages. Race also influences dietary choices because of cultural preferences and economics (Haas et al., 2003).

Table 19-1 Developmental and Behavioral Milestones for Preschool Children

Age	Expectations	Age	Expectations
3 years	At this age, the typical child: Opens doors Kicks a ball; jumps in place; rides on a tricycle Builds a tower of nine cubes; imitates bridge made from three cubes Demonstrates speech that is mostly intelligible. (The child who fails to speak in sentences or whose speech is unintelligible to strangers should be referred for speech, language, and hearing evaluation.) Knows own name, age, and gender May comprehend *cold, tired, hungry;* may understand the prepositions *over* and *under;* differentiates *bigger* and *smaller;* can convey the use of scissors, key, and pencil Copies a circle, may imitate a cross, and begins to visually discriminate colors Describes action in picture books and shows some early imaginative behavior Puts on some clothing and shoes Eats without assistance		Is imaginative and intensely curious Distinguishes between fantasy and reality Has formed gender identification Copies a cross and circle Draws a person with two to three parts Enjoys the companionship of other children, plays cooperatively, and shows interest in other children's bodies Meets the challenges of kindergarten class Rides with training wheels Aware of gender of others
4 years	At this age, the typical child: Alternates feet when descending stairs; jumps forward; hops on one foot, and can stand on 1 foot for up to 5 seconds Climbs a ladder Rides a tricycle or a bicycle with training wheels Can walk on tiptoes Throws a ball overhand Holds and uses a pencil with good control Builds a tower of 10 or more cubes Is able to cut and paste Gives first and last name Engages in conversational give-and-take Asks, *why, when, how,* and inquires about meanings of words Talks about daily experiences and things that are used at home (food, appliances) Can name three or four primary colors Can count from 1 to 5 Enjoys jokes Can sing a song Knows about things used at home (e.g., food, appliances) Washes and dries hands and brushes teeth Dresses and undresses with supervision, except for handling laces and buttons, when allowed sufficient time to dress; begins to be selective about clothes Initiates dramatic make-believe and dress-up play during which the child assumes a specific role	5 years	At this age, the typical child: May be able to skip; can walk on tiptoes; broad jumps Can cut and paste Names four or five colors and can identify coins Tells a simple story and knows several nursery rhymes Defines at least one word (*ball, shoe, chair, table, dog*) Dresses and undresses without supervision Knows address and telephone number Can count on fingers Copies a triangle from an illustration Recognizes many letters of the alphabet Prints some letters Draws a person with a head, body, arms, and legs Begins to understand right and wrong, fair and unfair Engages in dramatic make-believe and dress-up play during which the child assumes a specific role; engages in domestic role playing and dressing up Enjoys the companionship of other children; plays cooperatively Has formed gender identification ("Are you a boy or girl?")
		6 years	At this age, the typical child: Bounces a ball 4 to 6 times; throws and catches Skates Rides a bicycle Ties shoelaces Counts up to 10; prints own first name; prints numbers up to 10 Understands right from left Draws a person with six body parts, with the figure depicted wearing clothing

Modified from Green, M., Palfrey, J. S. (2002). *Bright futures: Guidelines for health supervision of infants, children, and adolescents* (2nd ed.). Arlington, VA: National Center for Education in Maternal and Child Health. Retrieved July 31, 2004, from: *http://www.brightfutures.org/bf2/pdf/pdf/EC.pdf* and *http://www.brightfutures.org/bf2/pdf/pdf/MC.pdf.*

Genetics

Signs and symptoms of most genetic problems appear during infancy or the toddler years, whereas other genetic problems will be noted during adolescence. Those most likely to appear during the preschool years are cystic fibrosis, Duchenne muscular dystrophy, fragile X syndrome, and Williams syndrome (Cunniff et al., 2001; Hockenberry, Winkelstein, & Kline, 2003). Genetic conditions diagnosed early in life affect the child's health, and nursing strategies focus on continuing parent education, screening for complications, and interventions to improve family coping (Hockenberry et al., 2003).

GORDON'S FUNCTIONAL HEALTH PATTERNS

Health Perception–Health Management Pattern

Preschoolers have a fairly accurate perception of the external parts of their own bodies based on what they can see and do; they may be extremely curious about the body of a member of the opposite sex. Their concept of what is inside the body and how its internal functions operate are vague and inaccurate. Preschoolers view the internal part of the body as hollow. Most preschoolers can name one or two items inside the body (blood, bones). Many of their questions involve body functions. Anxiety surrounding the body and fear of mutilation and death pervade the children's concerns. Their size as compared with that of adults produces a sense of vulnerability and fear of loss of control (Popovich, 2000).

By age 4 or 5, children have amassed their beliefs about health from the family. They begin to understand that they play a role in their own health. The preschooler often becomes upset over minor injuries. Pain or illness may be viewed as a punishment. The preschooler's declaration, "If you don't put your seat belt on you will get in an accident" is a statement that reflects the idea of expected immediate and absolute cause and effect. The preschooler cannot conceive that the purpose of the seat belt is to prevent injury in the event of an accident, not prevention of the accident itself.

Although preschoolers are not completely responsible for their own health management, they certainly contribute by brushing their teeth, taking medication, wearing appropriate clothing for inclement weather, and performing other actions. Preschoolers' memory for these activities can be sporadic, but they are at least beginning to be health care agents for themselves (Denham, 2002).

Reinforcement of health-promotion activities, which occur in the home and the child-care environment, helps to instill behaviors that affect self-esteem, safety, and an individual's overall balance with life (Denham, 2002; Dennison, Erb, & Jenkins, 2002; Msall, 2002; Robert & Yogue, 2004). Many community bookstores carry health promotion–focused books appropriate to the preschool population; these references provide information for discussion among parents, caregivers, and children on the importance of healthy behaviors for success in life. See **Web Site Resource 19A** for a detailed list of recommended books.

Nutritional-Metabolic Pattern

Establishing healthful nutritional and physical activity behaviors begins during childhood. The American Dietetic Association Position Statement concludes that most American children do not meet the Food Guide Pyramid recommendations. Children should eat a variety of foods with at least five servings of fruits and vegetables per day. Grains should also be plentiful, but fat consumption should be low, with saturated fat, *trans*-fatty acids, and cholesterol intake as low as possible. Salt and sugar intake should be moderate. The Fitness Pyramid depicts typical situations intended to encourage physical activity among children. (American Dietetic Association [ADA], 2004). The American Dietetic Association position statement also advises adequate consumption of calcium-rich and iron-rich foods. Although iron-deficiency anemia is decreasing generally, it is more prevalent in vulnerable populations (ADA, 2004).

A new food guidance system was announced in April 2005, which replaces the Food Guide Pyramid. The new system, called MyPyramid, remains based on the pyramid approach. It was developed to be a personalized approach to healthy eating and physical activity (USDA/CNPP, 2005). A child-friendly version of MyPyramid is being developed for children 6 to 11 years old.

Preschoolers need approximately 90 kcal/kg of body weight per day for health maintenance, activity, and growth. Table 19-2 lists a typical daily distribution of foods that provides the essential calories and nutrients. As early childhood progresses, intense food preferences emerge. This behavior is a natural outgrowth of the increased physical capacity to react to the taste and textures of foods and the realization that expressing an opinion about food is a way to control the environment. Older preschoolers frequently refuse to try new foods. Favorite foods for this age are meat, cereal grains, baked products, fruits, and sweets. Parents should provide nutritious foods, avoiding salty and sweet foods. Parents should encourage good nutritional habits to help establish healthy eating behaviors (Ruxton, 2004).

Increased consumption of fats and processed foods along with diminished physical activity have contributed to a significant increase in obesity and type 2 diabetes in children and adolescents (Crespo & Arbesman, 2003; Racette, Deusinger, & Deusinger, 2003; Ruxton, 2004; U.S. Department of Health and Human Services [USDHHS], 2000, 2001).

Family tolerance for individual food preferences varies, and children vary in their tendency to develop strong likes and dislikes. When a family and a child reach extreme differences over this matter, major conflicts arise and insightful counseling may be needed to reach a mutually satisfying solution. The nurse determines the nutritional adequacy of the foods that the child prefers and then collaborates with

Table 19-2 Food Pattern for Preschool Children, Ages 4 to 6

Food	Portion Size	Number of Recommended Portions
MILK AND DAIRY PRODUCTS		
Milk[†]	4 oz	*2
Cheese	½ to ¾ oz	May be substituted for 1 portion of liquid milk
Yogurt	¼ to ½ cup	May be substituted for 1 portion of liquid milk
Powdered skim milk	2 tbsp	May be substituted for 1 portion of liquid milk
MEAT AND MEAT EQUIVALENTS		
Meat,[‡] fish,[§] poultry	1 to 2 oz	*2
Egg	1	*1
Peanut butter	1 to 2 tbsp	
Legumes: dried peas and beans	¼ to ⅓ cup cooked	
VEGETABLES AND FRUITS		
Vegetables[‖]		
Cooked	2 to 4 tbsp	*3; includes 1 green leafy or yellow
Raw	Few pieces	
Fruit		
Canned	4 to 8 tbsp	*2 citrus fruit or other food rich in vitamin C
Raw	½ to 1, small	
Fruit juice	3 to 4 oz	
Bread and Cereal Grains		
Whole-grain or enriched white bread	½ to 1 slice	*6
Cooked cereal	¼ to ½ cup	May be substituted for 1 serving of bread
Ready-to-serve dry cereals	½ to 1 cup	May be substituted for 1 serving of bread
Spaghetti, macaroni, noodles, rice	¼ to ½ cup	May be substituted for 1 serving of bread
Crackers	2 to 3	May be substituted for 1 serving of bread
Fat		
Bacon	1 slice	**
Butter	1 tsp	**
Other		
Desserts	¼ to ½ cup	***
Sugars	½ to 1 tsp	***

From the American Dietetic Association. (2004). Dietary guidance for healthy children ages 2 to 11 years. *Journal of the American Dietetic Association*, *104*(4), 660-677.
*Acceptable distribution of macronutrients
Carbohydrates: 45% to 65% of total calories. *Fat:* 30% to 40% of energy for children 1 to 3 years old. *Protein:* 5% to 20% for young children.
**Saturated fat, trans-fatty acids, and cholesterol should be as low as possible
***Added sugars should not exceed 25% of total calories
Adequate intake for total fiber: Children 1 to 3 years: 19 g total fiber/day; 4 to 8 years: 25 g/day
[†]Approximately 2/3 cup can be incorporated easily in the child's food during cooking.
[‡]Liver once a week can be prepared as liver sausage or cooked liver.
[§]Should be served once or twice per week to substitute for meat.
[‖]When child"s preferences are limited, use double portions of preferred vegetables until appetite for other vegetables develops.

the family to discover comfortable approaches to the situation. It is important for both the nurse and the family to maintain a flexible approach and recognize the wide range of possibilities that exist for all families of varying cultures (Ball, Marshall, & McCargar, 2003; Dennis & Small, 2003).

Many preschoolers eat at least one meal a day away from home. Minimal standards require that licensed child-care centers and preschools serve foods that provide recommended dietary allowances of basic nutrients. Parents should communicate regularly with agency personnel about the foods eaten at home and away in order to understand

the child's food habits and to provide a varied diet important for growth. Preschoolers in group settings can learn positive or negative eating skills and food preferences from the teacher and other children; communication of these habits from the child's caregiver to the parents allows reinforcement of the positive or discouragement of the negative habits at home (Innovative Practice box).

Condition of teeth affects nutrition at all ages. Pain from dental caries, infection, and poorly cared-for teeth will affect a child's appetite and ability to chew, and it will also have an impact on future nutritional status. Dental caries

Healthy Start

Risk factors for cardiovascular diseases are prevalent by 3 years of age, the most common of which are hypercholesterolemia and obesity. Healthy Start, a project located in Valhalla, New York, sponsored by the Child Health Foundation and the American Health Foundation, is a 3-year demonstration and research program to evaluate the effectiveness of interventions for reducing cardiovascular risk factors in preschool centers. Two interventions are recommended. The first is the preschool food service, which is designed to reduce the total fat in the preschooler's meals and snacks to less than 30% of calories and to reduce saturated fat to less than 10% of calories. The second intervention is a comprehensive preschool health education curriculum, which focuses on nutrition and exercise.

The effectiveness of this program is evaluated using many components. Changes in the nutritional behaviors (including dietary intake of school snacks and meals of the preschoolers) are being recorded, as are those in snacks and meals consumed at home. Special attention is being given to the intake of total and saturated fat.

Additionally, changes in the health knowledge of preschoolers are being assessed to evaluate the education component. Physical examination data include semiannual assessments of growth and body weight and blood lipid levels.

The specific details of rationale and methods of the randomized controlled trial studies within the Healthy Start project are described in Williams, C. L., Squillace, M. M., Bollella, M. C., Brotanek, J., Campanaro, L., D'Agostino, C., et al. (1998). Healthy start: A comprehensive health education program for preschool children. *Preventive Medicine, 27*(2), 216-223.
Courtesy Carol Lynn Mandle.

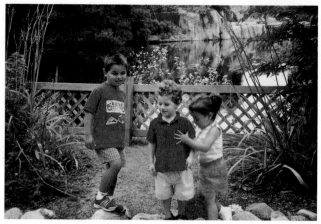

Figure 19-1 The preschool child enjoys playing with other children.

Most researchers agree that the prevalence of food allergy in the United States is increasing (ADA, 2004). Most allergies develop before the age of 2. The foods most likely to cause allergic reactions are milk and milk products, eggs and egg products, peanuts and peanut products, tree nuts and tree nut products, soybeans and soybean products, fish and fish products, shellfish and shellfish products, cereals containing glutens, and seeds. Reactions to milk tend to decrease over time, whereas allergies to peanuts and tree nuts usually remain with the child for life (Wood, 2003). Clear food labeling and education are essential for preventing allergic reactions. Many preschools have banned foods such as peanut products as a precautionary measure. Parents may need help identifying potential hazardous situations and communicating their child's needs to agency personnel (Sheetz et al., 2004).

Elimination Pattern

Older preschool children are capable of and responsible for independent toileting. They may forget to flush the toilet or wash their hands when they are rushed, but they have the physical ability to perform the skills. Preschoolers should not be teased or punished when they are unable to perform independently. If their clothing becomes soiled, they should be responsible for changing their clothes and reminded gently and encouragingly of ways to avoid problems in the future. (Enuresis and encopresis are discussed in Chapter 20.)

Activity-Exercise Pattern

Play continues to be the primary activity of the preschooler and toddler group. Preschoolers explore intently and demonstrate increased coordination and confidence with motor activities. They venture farther from home than toddlers do. Many play activities involve other children (Figure 19-1) and involve modeling the behavior of others. Particularly in group care settings, children should be monitored for safe activities that will enhance their gross and fine motor skills and create fun in movement.

in children have declined dramatically in recent years because of preventive measures such as tooth brushing with fluoride toothpaste, community water fluoridation, sound dietary practices, and dental sealants. Approximately 75% of dental caries today occur in 25% of children, particularly children in low-income families (Amschler, 2003). Oral health promotion involves not only self-care and population-based initiatives, but also professional care. Adequacy of professional dental care varies significantly by age, race, educational level, family income, and dental status (Formicola et al., 2004; Lee, Rozier, Norton, Kotch, & Vann, 2004).

Young preschoolers struggle with the intricacies of using utensils. Older preschoolers have attained skill with spoons, demonstrate fair proficiency with forks, and manage knives for spreading soft foods on bread or crackers. Most children, however, need help cutting meat and pouring from large, heavy containers.

Preschoolers often enjoy helping to prepare family meals and may be capable of making their own sandwiches. Involving young children in meal preparation teaches them about healthy nutrition. Sharing important family functions nurtures self-esteem and a sense of value.

Most 4-year-old children separate easily from their parents, play simple interactive games, dress themselves, copy a number of basic geometric figures well, and draw recognizable people. Preschoolers enjoy using language skills in telling stories and asking questions and they can balance on one foot, jump, and run well (Marston, 2004; Robert & Yogue, 2004; Rudisill & Wall, 2004; Yackel, 2003). Generally, these children appreciate an audience, enjoy practicing new skills, and demonstrate mastered skills to others.

Play constitutes an important role in preschoolers' social and psychological development. Play offers a vehicle for exploring, experimenting with who they are, who they might become, and how they relate to others socially. The drama of play allows preschoolers to view themselves from another perspective. Play often reveals the child's reality and perception of the world.

Children mimic the behavior of people familiar to them, rehearsing what has been demonstrated to them as appropriate behavior. Young children seldom assume the role of a younger child or infant while playing. They usually assume adult roles and use a doll for the younger child. Through play preschoolers learn to exert control over their own behavior. Assuming an adult role in play allows children to consciously adopt more mature behaviors.

Patterns of behavior used in play can be transferred to actual situations. For example, children who express their anger in a play situation aggressively by vocalizing their distress, scolding the offending party, or using withdrawal of attention are likely to respond with aggression or tantrum behavior when facing frustration or anger in real life situations. Observation of play reveals children's physical capacities in a natural setting better than an examination or testing environment and provides further evidence of the child's social and inner development.

Observing imitation play in peer groups helps the nurse assess social competency. At first the new child in a peer group may be expected to stand back and observe other children for a time and then approach before he or she manipulates a toy object. The preschool child engages in more interactive play, particularly dramatic play, than at any other age. Two or more children may become involved in an imaginary plot, especially when toys and equipment support a particular scenario, such as toy kitchen equipment. Much of the preschooler's play involves fantasy. The young child frequently invents an imaginary companion who plays, eats, and sleeps with the child. (The section about cognition and perception addresses more fully the aspects of fantasy during the preschool stage.)

Most preschoolers spend some time in a group setting each week. Ground rules at these facilities govern sharing, quiet times, and group activities. The preschooler regulates bodily activity and copes with limit setting better than the toddler.

Although time orientation remains incompletely developed in preschoolers, they have an idea about past and future. They enjoy planning activities with their parents for the future. Visiting the library to review books about wild animals, packing lunches, and choosing what clothes to wear may preface a trip to the zoo.

Many preschoolers spend long periods each day watching television. Occasionally parents use the television inappropriately to entertain the child. Although some excellent television shows are available for preschoolers, a significant amount of airtime focuses on adult themes and violence. Many experts agree that television disengages the child's mind and supports less learning (see Chapter 20). Parents should remember that preschoolers who watch television (1) do not have enough life experiences to interpret many of the issues presented in adult shows (violence, interpersonal relationships, moral decisions), (2) might be missing opportunities for interacting with other children or adults and other opportunities for active learning, and (3) cannot judge which shows are appropriate for them. In addition, television, a sedentary activity, inhibits children from developing an active healthy lifestyle.

Parents should choose which shows are appropriate for their child and, when possible, watch these shows with the child, which provides an opportunity for discussion and for the child to ask questions (Wertlieb, 2003). Nurses should explain to parents and preschoolers the relationship between watching television and lack of physical activity that leads to health problems such as obesity (Dennison, Erb, & Jenkins, 2002).

Sleep-Rest Pattern

Most preschoolers sleep from 8 to 12 hours during the night, with wide variation from child to child. For many older preschoolers, a nap is not necessary. The preschooler who still naps usually requires only 30 to 60 minutes a day (American Family Physician, 2001; Watamura, Donzella, Alwin, & Gunnar, 2003). Quiet time provides a welcome respite for the parent, along with a chance for the active preschooler to relax before afternoon activities. Many childcare environments routinely provide these rest periods, enhancing rest and relaxation with soft music and a story. An afternoon rest also prepares the young child with energy for the evening routine when family members have other duties beyond work and school.

Bedtime Ritual

Preschoolers usually require a ritual of activities at bedtime to move from playing and being with others to being alone and falling asleep. These children prolong bedtime routines more often than the toddler. They insist on sleeping with the light on, take a treasured object to bed, request parental attention after being told good night, and experience delays falling asleep. The bedtime ritual generally lasts 30 minutes or longer. Parents should honor reasonable rituals, but repeated requests for attention afterward should generally be handled firmly and consistently. Vigorous resistance to bedtime challenges parents more during the preschool period than any other developmental stage. Preschoolers learn to use the behaviors that meet their needs and control the family regardless of the disruption created.

Nursing Interventions

When a demanding bedtime behavior extends beyond one year or one episode persists longer than 1 hour, the nurse explores the family situation. A comprehensive assessment in this case includes the following elements:

1. Description of early episodes
2. The manner in which these early episodes were managed and the progression of events since then
3. Current bedtime behaviors of the child and siblings
4. Identification of parental temperament and the resulting responses of parent and family members
5. Feelings of the parents and child about each other and about the bedtime situation
6. Stressful events and changes that have occurred over the past several years
7. Behavior of the child at other times of the day
8. Parents' thoughts about reasons why these episodes continue
9. Parents' ideas about strategies to use now

The nurse observes interactions within the family. A home visit at mealtime provides an excellent method to observe active interaction. In the office or clinic setting the nurse can ask a parent to teach the child a task or give directions. The nurse remains as unobtrusive as possible while observing the interaction. The first-hand observation of parent-child interaction, along with the detailed history, usually provides the nurse with adequate baseline information to decide whether to manage the situation in the primary care setting or refer the family to a child behavior specialist. Sharing recent literature about management techniques for children with differing temperament characteristics helps families understand more about the behaviors. Research-based strategies should be used to help parents reach their goals related to managing bedtime concerns (Denham, 2002).

Sleep Disturbances

Night terrors and nightmares characterize the nighttime wakening problems that generally occur during the preschool years. **Night terrors** manifest as frightening dreams that cause the child to sit up in bed, scream, stare at an imaginary object, breathe heavily, perspire, and appear in obvious distress (see Chapter 18). The child, not fully awake, may be inconsolable for 10 minutes or more, before he or she relaxes and returns to a deep sleep. The child, in most cases, does not recall the dream and in the morning does not remember the incident. These night terrors can start at approximately age 2 but are more common during the preschool years. Night terrors rarely occur in older children and adults, and only approximately 6% of preschool children have them. Night terrors and nightmares trigger apprehension for the parents.

Nightmares (anxiety dreams) are a more common cause of night wakening. Although infants and toddlers likely have nightmares, their limited verbal skills hinder relating details of the incidents. After age 3 nightmares occur fre-

quently. Approximately 20% of the night is spent dreaming. Dreams frighten preschoolers as they connect to the larger world with their active imaginations and fantastic ideas. These children usually waken fully and feel fearful and helpless. Usually they provide vivid descriptions at the time, and they frequently remember the event the following morning. Consolation can be given by a parent who sits with the child, listens to descriptions and fears about the dream, and reminds the child that dreaming is natural and sleep will soon return.

Helping children appreciate the meaning of the words *pretend* and *real* facilitates growth during this phase of childhood. When the parent reads a story to the child or the child tells a make-believe tale, the parents can specify that these are "pretend" and did not really happen. The parent relating a true event can say, "This is real." Children differentiate between the two concepts as they develop cognitively.

Recommendations

Parents of a preschooler can benefit from knowing the following facts:

1. Bedtime rituals of 30 to 45 minutes are common for preschoolers. These rituals, because of their importance to children, should be respected within reasonable limits.
2. Night-wakening events are common during the preschool years. Children who waken at night should be reassured and encouraged to remain in their own beds.
3. Parents should have clear rules about children sleeping with them if the children will not stay in their own beds.
4. Restricting frightening television shows and stories and discussing "real" versus "pretend" ideas and stories can help lessen the incidence of nightmares.

Cognitive-Perceptual Pattern

During the preschool years children cultivate their conceptual and cognitive capacities. The quality of the child's care environment enhances these gains. The child gradually differentiates today from yesterday and defines tomorrow and the future as concepts of time emerge. The child becomes more oriented in space and develops an awareness of the location of the home within the neighborhood. The child also begins to structure daily activities and to value certain activities, objects, and people above others.

Piaget's Theory

The older toddler enters the first substage of the **preoperational stage** described by Jean Piaget (see Chapter 18). The hallmark of this preconceptual substage includes the ability to function symbolically using language. The preschool child demonstrates increased symbolic functioning during the intuitive substage, from age 4 to 7 years. The predominant feature of this and the following period is the concrete thought process, as compared with adult thinking. As they experience symbolic mental representations, preschoolers process mental symbols as though they were actually participating in the event. An adult analyzes and synthesizes symbolic information without concrete connections between the mental process and the actual event. At this stage, mental abstraction, such as skipping from one part of an operation to another, reversing the operation mentally, or thinking of the whole in relation to the parts is not feasible.

The **egocentrism** that is characteristic of the preschool years exemplifies this concept of concrete thinking. At this stage, children concentrate solely on their own perspective. They consider only their own personal meanings for symbols. The preschooler wonders why another person fails to follow these idiosyncratic communications.

Furthermore, attention focuses solely on one part of an object without shifting. This behavior, termed *centering* by Piaget, illustrates the child's inability to consider more than one factor at a time when solving simple problems. For example, a child can be given two identical cups containing equal amounts of water and asked which cup contains the greater amount of water. During the preoperational stage, the child responds that they contain the same amount of water. The child is then asked to pour the water from each cup into two different containers (one flat and wide, the other tall and narrow). When asked which container has more water, the child always identifies one, usually the taller, narrower container in which the water reaches a higher level. When the water is again transferred to the identical cups and the experiment repeated, the child returns to the original conclusion that the amounts are equal.

This experiment also illustrates the trait of **irreversibility.** The child is unable to connect the reversible operation, the transfer of the water back into the original cup, to reach the logical conclusion that the differently shaped containers may hold the same amount of water. The child cannot mentally associate that the transformation from one state to another relates to the shape of the container, not the amount of the water.

Finally, Piaget describes the preoperative stage of thinking as **transductive reasoning.** The child cannot proceed from general to particular (deduction) or from particular to general (induction); rather, the child moves only from particular to particular in making associations and solving problems. For example, Piaget relates an association made by one of his children between being hunchbacked and being ill. When a hunchbacked neighbor was unable to visit one day because he had a communicable illness, the child understood that the neighbor was ill. However, when the child was told later that the neighbor was better and that she could go see him, her conclusion was that now his hunched back was straight and well. She thought in terms of the man being well or ill, but she placed the man in one or the other category and assumed that he possessed all the attributes and meanings that she linked symbolically with either trait.

The cognitive development of preschoolers is reflected in their symbolic games, which becomes significantly more

---

| Box **19-1** | Play as a Method of Learning: Preschool-Age Child |

Throughout life, play develops cognitive, affective, and psychomotor skills that are important to the effective performance of life skills. For the preschool-age child, the following play activities provide the foundation for later competency and socialization-skill refinement:
- Arts and crafts (jewelry making, painting, drawing, ceramics, printmaking)
- Group sports (softball, volleyball, soccer, swimming)
- Skating, skateboarding
- Bicycling
- Puzzles
- Gymnastics
- Games (board, card, knock-knock jokes, computer)
- Secret clubs
- Imaginary play (being in playhouse productions)
- Horseback riding

---

orderly and representative of reality (Box 19-1). They begin to incorporate the reality of the world, as it exists outside the self. They increasingly seek play objects that represent models of authentic objects in their environment. Preschoolers progressively imitate more social rules in their play. Social interactive play predominates as the young child develops a more secure sense of self.

The preschooler may have one or more imaginary companions who exist for varying periods. These fantasy companions assume the form of another child, an animal, or some other friendly or fearsome creature. The preschooler may save special chairs, insist that an extra place be set at the table, and talk at length to this companion. Imaginary companions serve an important function; they are controlled totally by the child and are not a threat. The preschooler practices social interactions, controls a fearsome beast, or blames someone for naughty behavior without fear of scolding, shame, or attack. Imaginary companions do and say only what the child wills.

Vision

Vision capabilities, which are well developed by 2 years of age, continue to undergo refinement during the early childhood period. By approximately age 6, the child should approach a 20/20 visual acuity level. The possibility of developing **amblyopia** decreases; it appears most frequently during infancy through approximately the fourth year (see Chapter 18). Depth perception and color vision become fully established, and the child recognizes subtle differences in color shading by the sixth year. Maximal visual capability usually is achieved by the end of the preschool years.

Visual capacity throughout the rest of life deteriorates rather than improves. This phenomenon relates partly to changes in the refractive power of the lens and developmental changes that occur in the shape of the eyeball. In the normal sequence of growth, the eyeball becomes increasingly spherical, losing the short shape typical of infancy and progressing to the point at which light converges accurately on the surface of the retina. This change occurs at approximately 6 years of age. When this change occurs before the sixth year, growth continues past the point of ideal light conversion, the eyeball lengthens, and the child may develop early **myopic vision,** which will progress with age. Glasses are always indicated for the child who develops myopia before approximately age 8.

Early detection requires regular screening with standardized tests such as the Denver Eye Screening Test or the Snellen Screening Test. The Denver Eye Screening Test was designed for preschool children and includes detection of the commonly occurring visual problems, such as **refractive errors, strabismus** (crossing of the eyes), and amblyopia.

The Snellen screening test, when administered under standardized procedures, has the advantage of rendering a reliable estimate of actual visual acuity. The child must be able to understand the test requirements of either pointing in the direction of the Es or naming the letters.

The **Snellen E chart** is designed for preschool children; a version for home testing is available from the National Society for Prevention of Blindness. Home testing has been demonstrated to be reliable and offers the advantage of obtaining an estimate for younger children who might not cooperate with this type of testing in a strange environment.

The pupillary light reflex provides a screening approach for **heterotropia,** a condition in which the child's eyes do not focus together to transmit effective, coordinated binocular vision. When the child has heterotropia, the light from a penlight held approximately 20 inches from the eyes reflects off the pupil slightly off center. Consistent and observable strabismus may be noted. The cover test provides further evidence of a tendency for the child's eyes to cross, known as **heterophoria.** The child focuses on a spot 14 inches away, then 20 feet away. As the child gazes at the designated spot, one eye is covered completely for several seconds (the eye and eyelashes must not be touched), and then the cover is removed abruptly. If the covered eye moves from the line of vision of the uncovered eye, that eye has a tendency toward muscle imbalance and must be evaluated further (Bickley & Hoekelman, 2002; Hockenberry, Winkelstein, & Kline, 2003).

Color blindness presents a particular problem for younger children, because many cues encountered at school depend on the child's ability to distinguish colors. With early detection, the child is able to receive assistance to interpret visual cues, thus minimizing the disadvantage of being colorblind. The nurse screens for certain types of color discrimination difficulties by asking the child to respond to various colors in the environment; however, accurate testing for all types of color blindness requires a specialized tool, such as **Ishihara's test,** which uses a series of cards with color-tinted letters and figures.

The preschooler may be aware of some discomfort or limitations with vision. The nurse gathers history from the parents, including the questions listed in the Vision section in Chapter 18 about signs of eye problems. The preschooler is asked questions to elicit information about the following symptoms:
1. Itching, burning, or "scratchy" eyes
2. Poor vision
3. Dizziness, headaches, or nausea after close eye work
4. Blurred or double vision

Hearing

During the preschool years, hearing develops to the level of an adult's, when the ability to attend to and interpret what is heard becomes more refined. The 4-year-old preschooler begins to discriminate among remarkably similar speech sounds, such as the difference between sounds made with "f" and "th" or "f" and "s." It is generally accepted that hearing ability of the preschooler can be hindered by repeated middle ear infections (otitis media). Otitis media with effusion occasionally can result in temporary hearing loss. Parents who notice language delays because of ear infections should be referred to their health care provider for appropriate follow-up (Al-Shehri, 2003; Bush, 2003). Parental reports of difficulty should be taken seriously. One study demonstrated that parents often recognized hearing loss months before the physician did (Cunningham & Cox, 2003).

Audiometric methods most accurately measure the child's ability to hear. Preschool children possess the developmental capability to perform the standard audiometric test. The child can follow directions by this age, and most preschoolers enjoy demonstrating their abilities and cooperate easily during vision and hearing screening (Bush, 2003; Finitzo et al., 2000). The American Academy of Pediatrics on-line resources supply a wealth of information for nurses and families at *http://www.aap.org/healthtopics/visionhearing.cfm*.

To ensure success, the nurse encourages a positive experience by adhering to the following points:
- Use equipment skillfully.
- Use age-appropriate language. Avoid the word *test* to limit anxiety or fear of failure.
- Encourage the child to ask questions and scrutinize the equipment.
- Perform screening before other intrusive or painful procedures.
- Perform screening in a quiet private area without distractions.
- Praise the child for cooperating.
- Allow rest periods when the child becomes distracted or tired.
- Discuss results with the child in age-appropriate language.

Sensory Perception

Sensory abilities contribute to the preschooler's skills in perceiving and interacting with the world. Both sensory acuity and sensory perceptual abilities mature during the preschool years. The nature of the visual stimulus determines the response. Preschoolers respond powerfully to visual illusions and have difficulty discriminating right and left mirror images. Confusion commonly occurs with the letters "b," "d," "p," and "q."

Language

Cognitive and sensory abilities all contribute to the preschooler's language development. Toward the end of the preschool period, **expressive language** rivals that of an adult except for minor deficiencies in refinement, vocabulary, and structure. The child's language ability depends on aptitude, the opportunity for using the language, the quality and quantity of language used at home, and the child's range of experiences. Regardless of the child's expressive capacity, the development of **receptive language** during the preschool years provides a vital foundation for later communication (Roulstone, Peters, Glogowska, & Enderby, 2003). Throughout early childhood, receptive capacity exceeds expressive capacity. Children comprehend meanings of words and phrases not contained in their expressive vocabulary. Associations between concepts materialize, although the child lacks the ability to explain these concepts. Table 19-3 outlines the receptive and expressive language skills of the preschooler.

During the early childhood years, the rhythm develops as an important dimension in speech capacity. Between ages 3 and 5 years, children practice speaking as adults do. This practice expands neuromotor capacities, and the verbal interaction develops their vocabulary and sense of grammatical structure. Hesitations, repetitions, and frequent revisions in speech reflect the children's attempts to expand their capacity. Adults may label such preparation as stuttering, but these inaccuracies actually represent normal speech maturation. Many authorities believe that stuttering originates during this developmental period, arising not from inadequacy of the child, but rather from the adult's response to this normal broken speech pattern. Adult reactions of impatience while waiting for the child to express thoughts decrease the child's opportunities to use language. Insisting that the child correct the speech pattern before the capacity for fluent speech is developed may hinder normal speech development. As many as 60% of expressive language delays resolve during the preschool years (Roulstone, Peters, Glogowska, & Enderby, 2003). Suggestions for the nurse to give parents to facilitate the preschool child's language development are listed in Box 19-2.

Memory

Memory is an important component of language development and of learning in general (Bauer, Wenner, & Kroupina, 2002). At the preschool level children label pictures, group objects, and mimic others as ways to aid memory, performing these tasks with less precision than the older child. The younger child benefits when adults suggest characteristics of an object or action that should be used for grouping items to be remembered. Preschoolers remember pictures better by saying the name of the picture rather than simply hearing the name when the picture is first shown.

Preschoolers do not use rehearsal or other **mnemonic techniques** for remembering spontaneously, but they do use and benefit from rehearsal when it is suggested (Zgaljardic & Benedict, 2001). The nurse tests memory by asking the child to repeat an arbitrary sequence of numbers. By approximately age 5, children should be able to repeat four consecutively named numbers easily (Guskiewicz, 2001; Liben, Bigler, & Krogh, 2002; McKeever & Schatz, 2003).

Testing of Developmental Level

Parents of preschoolers frequently want to determine their child's readiness for school programs. The child's skill level, the child and family's psychosocial status, and the characteristics of the school program under consideration determine readiness. Questions about readiness should be answered considering all three of these components. Developmental testing modalities used during the toddler years appear less accurate as the child approaches school age. Tools designed for this purpose can help identify the child's skill level.

Historically, tools to evaluate skills that might indicate the child's readiness for the school environment have been used. One instrument, called the **Preschool Readiness Experimental Screening Scale (PRESS)** has been used in the past. This reliable tool screens easily for developmental lags or abnormalities that might interfere with academic and social success in school. Constructed for use with 5-year-old children, it may also estimate readiness of slightly older or younger children. The test measures school readiness and addresses specific skills, not intellectual level.

Other components of readiness, family dynamics and school environment, have concerned experts. La Paro and Pianta have developed and tested a 9-point assessment of the environment called the Classroom Assessment Scoring System. The scales assess global classroom quality: positive climate, negative climate, teacher sensitivity, over-control, behavior management, productivity, learning formats, concept development, and quality of feedback (La Paro, Pianta, & Stuhlman, 2004). Evaluating the whole environment using a comprehensive approach contributes important information about readiness. Children who are ready for school demonstrate competencies in areas other than measurable skill performance. The complex home environment with stable adults who care for them, a safe predictable physical environment with regular activities, peers, and materials that stimulate children indicate readiness more than specific skill performance (Allor & McCathren, 2003; Pianta & La Paro, 2003).

To obtain a more specific measure of developmental age, the nurse uses one of several screening tools designed for use with the preschool child. These validated instruments provide rough estimates of ability to identify (Pianta & La Paro, 2003) whether a child needs referral for further evaluation. The **Peabody Picture Vocabulary Test** examines verbal intelligence but also estimates verbal ability. When used with predominantly middle class children who have

Table **19-3** Landmarks of Speech, Language, and Hearing Ability During the Preschool Period

Age (Months)	Receptive Language	Expressive Language	Related Hearing Ability
42	Up to 4200 words; knows words such as *what, where, how, funny, we, surprise, secret;* knows number concepts to 2; knows how to answer some questions accurately, such as, *do you have a dog, which is the girl, what toys do you have?*	Up to 1200 words in mostly complete sentences averaging four to five words per sentence; uses all 50 phonemes; 7% of sentences are compound or complex; averages 203 words per hour; rate of speech is accelerating; relates experiences and tells about activities in sequential order; uses words such as *what, where, how, see, little, funny, they, we, he, she, several;* can recite a nursery rhyme; asks permission; 95% of speech is intelligible	
48	Up to 5600 words; carries out three-item commands consistently; knows why people have houses, books, umbrella, key; knows nearly all colors; knows words such as *somebody, anybody, even, almost, now, something, like, bigger, too,* full name, one or two songs, number concepts to 4; understands most preschool stories; can complete opposite analogies such as *brother is a boy, sister is a girl,* and *in daytime it is light, at night it is dark*	Up to 1500 words in sentences averaging five to six words per sentence; averages 400 words per hour; counts up to 3, repeats four digits, names three objects, repeats nine-word sentences from memory; names the primary colors, some coins; relates fanciful tales; enjoys rhyming nonsense words and using exaggerations; demands reasons why and how; questioning is at a peak, up to 500 a day; passes judgment on own activity; can recite a poem from memory or sing a song; uses words such as *even, almost, something, like, but;* typical expressions might include *I'm so tired, you almost hit me, now I'll make something else*	Begins to make fine discriminations among similar speech sounds, such as the difference between *f* and *th* or *f* and *s*. Child has matured enough to be tested with an audiometer. At this age, formal hearing testing usually can be carried out. Not only has hearing developed to its optimal level, but listening has also become considerably refined.
54	Up to 6500 words; knows what materials a house, window, chair, and dress are made of and what people do with eyes and ears; understands differences in texture and composition, such as *hard, soft, rough, smooth;* begins to name or point to penny, nickel, dime; understands *if, because, why, when*	Up to 1800 words in sentences averaging five to six words; now averages only 230 words per hour—is satisfied with less verbalization; does little commanding or demanding; likes surprises; about 1 in 10 sentences is compound or complex, and only 8% of sentences are incomplete; can define 10 common words and counts up to 20; common expressions are *I don't know, I said, tiny, funny, because;* asks questions for information and learns to manipulate and control people and situations with language	
60	Up to 9600 words; knows number concepts to 5; knows and names colors; defines words in terms of use, such as *a bike is to ride;* defines *wind, ball, hat, stove;* understands qualifiers such as *if, because, when;* knows purpose of *horse, fork,* and *legs;* begins to understand *right* and *left*	Up to 2200 words in sentences averaging six words; can define *ball, hat, stove, policeman, wind, horse, fork;* can count five objects and repeat four or five digits; definitions are in terms of use; can single out a word and ask its meaning; makes serious inquiries—*what is this for, how does this work, who made those, what does it mean;* language is now essentially complete in structure and form; uses all types of sentences, clauses, and parts of speech; reads by way of pictures, and prints simple words	

Modified from Chinn, P. L. (1979). *Child health maintenance: Concepts in family-centered care* (2nd ed.). St. Louis: Mosby.

Box 19-2 Nursing Suggestions to Encourage Language Development in Preschoolers

- Read to the child. Encourage the child to be an active listener. Pause during the story to ask questions, such as "What do you think will happen next?" and "Why do you think the boy said that?" and "What would you do now?" See **Web Site Resource 19A** for a list of suggested books to read aloud to a child.
- Praise the child's storytelling and creativity with stories.
- Always respond to the child's questions. Occasionally a response must be delayed; for example, when the parent is driving in heavy traffic and the child asks a question that requires a complex answer, the parent might say, "That's a very good question; let's talk about that as soon as we get home." The parent should remind the child of the question later and respond if the child still expresses interest.
- Never tease or criticize a child about speaking style. If the child speaks so fast as to be fumbling over words, then the parent might say, "I can't listen that fast. Slow down a little for me." This is much more encouraging than is the statement, "You talk too fast. No one can understand you."
- Play language-focused games, such as naming the colors of houses or kinds of flowers as parent and child walk to the store.

acquired standard English-speaking ability, accuracy is reliable. Insufficient language stimulation or cultural differences may influence scores negatively. Also children sometimes find the process uninteresting and randomly point to options so that they will finish more quickly. The examiner must remain alert to eye movement to identify changes in the child's response behaviors (Bracken & Shaughnessy, 2003).

Draw-a-Person and **Draw-a-Family tests** approximate intelligence and emotional development; however, scoring figure drawings requires standardized test conditions and analysis of findings by a psychometric specialist. Drawings may indicate general developmental level, fine motor control, and evidence of concept formation. Perceptions of family relationships can also be assessed. The 4-year-old child draws a person with at least six body parts in the appropriate locations. Normal children name the parts correctly. The representation may be an approximation, but it should resemble the actual body parts and be drawn with strong, evenly flowing lines. The family drawing may be less sophisticated than a drawing of a single person and may lack some family members. The normal child names the family members readily and describes unique characteristics of each member from a child's perspective. The nurse provides a pencil and plain sheet of paper and asks the child to draw the best picture possible. The nurse explains that the picture will remain with the nurse but that another sketch may be drawn to take home (Allor & McCathren, 2003; Gleason, Jarudi, & Cheek, 2003; Vygotsky, 2004).

Self-Perception–Self-Concept Pattern

During the preschool years the basic concept of self emerges from the child's personal struggle for autonomy. As children develop beyond the toddler years, they refine their sense of self through both task-oriented and socially oriented experiences. By reinforcing skills and successfully accomplishing tasks, the preschooler builds self-esteem, enhancing overall health. Social acceptance helps the child feel successful in the roles of child, sibling, and friend. The preschooler investigates other roles through rich imagination. Pretending to be the parents or the baby allows the preschooler to imagine the experiences and feelings of others and safely experiment with new ideas (Denham et al., 2003; Gleason, Jarudi, & Cheek, 2003; Vygotsky, 2004).

Preschool children learn about their roles in their child-care environments and learn that being dependable within their world is important. When children perceive their value in improving the world in which they live, they experience good feelings about themselves and, ultimately, demonstrate improved mental and physical health. Many simple ways to improve the environment are available, and when children learn ways to contribute to environmental health, they often reinforce these behaviors in their parents (Health Teaching box).

Erikson's Theory

Preschoolers develop a sense of initiative through their vigorous motor activity and active imaginations. Erikson views this growth as the most central developmental task in the emerging self-concept of the preschool years. By praising the preschooler's efforts and providing opportunities for new experiences, parents promote development of initiative. Rather than requiring a particular behavior, parents should provide avenues for experimentation. The preschooler then feels mastery, thus encouraging repetition. With mastery, preschoolers become more confident about trying new actions.

Preschoolers remain sensitive to criticism by others. When ridiculed for ideas or behaviors, they may develop feelings of guilt and inadequacy. Parents, caregivers, and health care professionals should nurture their ideas, while encouraging behaviors to support a positive self-concept.

Roles-Relationships Pattern

Family members continue to play a vital role in the preschooler's life, but peers become increasingly significant as the child develops. Preschoolers receive ideas and information from their peers that they then introduce into family situations. They may question why rules or expectations at home are different from those at friends' houses. Discussion about family values and behaviors that are acceptable one place but not another help them understand these differences.

Preschoolers understand gender expectations regarding jobs, activities, and competencies of people in their lives. Ideas about gender differences in work roles or activities are

HEALTH TEACHING Health Promotion With Preschoolers: Environmental Accountability

Rationale for Teaching Preschoolers About Environmental Protection

- Environmental education at an early age will produce environmental practitioners of the future.
- Preschoolers can learn basic concepts of environmental accountability and gain a sense of empowerment when they perceive that they make a difference to the future world.
- Health care providers, in consultation with child-care providers, can promote environmental education that is based on their knowledge of child growth and development and concerns about overall health.

Basic Ways for Preschoolers to Help the Environment and Promote Overall Societal Health

- Use water wisely.
- Use electricity only when necessary.
- Recycle.
- Avoid using balloons.
- Plant trees, protect plants, and grow a garden.
- Create a compost pile.
- Care for birds.
- Clean up the neighborhood.
- Decrease the amount of trash; say "no" to Styrofoam and plastic garbage bags, and use paper cups and reusable cloth bags for groceries.
- Recycle old toys by giving them to less fortunate people.
- Buy and use only earth-friendly school supplies.
- Walk rather than ride in the car.
- Save Christmas trees and replant.

Box 19-3 Evaluating a Child-Care Setting

Child care that meets the needs and expectations of parents will most likely ensure a happy preschooler, as well. Questions that parents should consider in evaluating and choosing a child-care setting include the following:

- Will my needs and those of my child be best met with a caregiver in a family home, commercial center, or preschool, or by having a person come to my home to care for my child?
- What kinds of backup plans will I need or will be available if the provider becomes ill?
- What are my standards for nutrition, safety, sanitation, and health, and can these standards be met at the chosen child-care facility?
- How important is it to my child to be with other children? How many children would be ideal for my child's socialization needs?
- What personality attributes and educational preparation do I desire in my child's caregivers? What attributes do I dislike and how will I deal with these attributes to maximize the care given to my child? How important is caregiver stability to me? Can I comfortably communicate with the staff to collaborate with my child's learning?

- What educational philosophy do I want in the setting? What involvement do I wish to have in the educational mission of the facility?
- Do the hours of the facility meet my personal and professional needs? Is close access to my job or home important to me?
- How are the children grouped and what is the caregiver-to-child ratio?
- Does the cost of the service meet my financial needs? Can I pay part-time fees during vacation or when my child is ill for a lengthy period?
- Is accreditation of the facility mandatory for me to use it?
- What is my internal response or my general feelings about the setting when I visit it before my child's enrollment? Are the caregivers interacting with and responsive to the children? Are the children happy and interactive? Are the children's individual needs addressed appropriately? Is the environment supportive of my child's care? Is discipline appropriate?

---

based on models in the home, at child-care or preschool centers, and on television. Parents and caregivers should be aware of the powerful influence that these environments have on role perceptions (Box 19-3). When inaccurate portrayals of male and female roles are depicted, parents and caregivers should discuss more accurate ones with the children. The preschooler tries out many roles through play, including family roles. As the mother or father in a play situation, the preschooler can set limits, punish, praise, and make outlandish demands on the invented child. This play represents an important strategy that preschoolers use to alleviate stress and experiment with new roles. By playing different roles, they can safely experience the effects of the

behavior and understand others' roles more clearly. Parents also better understand the effects of their own actions when they observe the behaviors of their child. The nurse can help parents use their observations to improve interactions with their child.

Preschoolers relate to older children in the family on a more equal basis than do toddlers. Although their cognitive, motor, and language skills are less refined, preschoolers are able to participate in some activities with their older siblings. The younger child may admire an older sibling to the point of wanting to imitate the sibling exactly. This behavior may flatter the older child initially, but its persistence may develop into a source of frustration.

Social interaction during this period prepares the preschooler for school. Through experience within the family, with peers, and with other adults, the child acquires readiness to interact in group situations, follow directions, take turns, recognize others' rights, channel energy toward an assigned activity, and demonstrate increasing independence. School readiness can be assessed by using several relevant tests, as discussed in this chapter. The nurse who sees the child repeatedly in an office, clinic, or group care or preschool setting assesses progress as the child develops social competencies. Comparing the child's current, more mature behavior with previous behavior provides insight into the preschooler's readiness for school. This method of evaluation, however, prevents comparison with other children of the same age. For example, school personnel may view a child who reflects a quiet temperament and is introverted or subdued as overly attached to the mother in comparison with other children the same age. However, if the child's earlier social behavior is known, the behavior may be interpreted as a progression toward independence. When the mother is not available, the child may make sufficient adaptations to remain comfortable and secure.

Evidence of social competency can be obtained by discussion and evaluation of the child's drawing of the family. The nurse observes the drawing and responds to any comments or questions volunteered by the child. When asked for advice or assistance, the nurse encourages the child to proceed with drawing. Positive encouragement for the child's efforts may be used, particularly if reluctance is exhibited. After the drawing is finished, the nurse discusses the sketch with the child to identify the people and describe individual characteristics. The nurse writes the names of each family member on the picture and documents the perceptions the child describes. Open-ended questions such as "What do you like best about your brother?" or "When do you get angry with your sister?" can be posed to encourage the child to describe the family interaction patterns. When an adult family member is present, the nurse explains the purpose of the drawing and interview and requests that the adult withhold comments or questions until the activity is completed. Any areas of concern or questions should be discussed and the parent assured of confidentiality. The child's perceptions can be verified with the adult at the conclusion of the interview, or further information can be sought to clarify them.

The **Vineland Social Maturity Scale** provides an objective, standardized estimate of social functioning and social maturity. This tool profiles the child's self-help skills, self-direction, locomotion, communication, and social relations. The scoring system seems to be culturally and socioeconomically neutral. The investigator collects data by observing the child's behavior and interviewing the mother or primary caregiver. Designed to measure progression toward independence, this instrument uses direct observation of the child's behavior whenever possible, using the interview data only if needed to complete the assessment (Denham et al., 2003; Pillay, 2003; Taneja et al., 2002).

These kinds of tools elicit cues indicative of family stress and strain. **Parental divorce** commonly creates disruption in family relationships. Discussion of results of the assessment offers the opportunity to discuss family situations that otherwise might have gone unmentioned. Children's responses to changes in family circumstances depend on their developmental stages and their relationships before the change. Divorce represents a final decision, usually culminating from a period of conflict, stress, and changing relationships, limiting the child's exposure to these issues. Although preschoolers definitely sense stress in the home, they cannot articulate their feelings or determine their origin. Children react to changes in various ways, including regression, confusion, or irritability. Asking the same questions repeatedly, such as, "Is Daddy coming home for supper tonight?" or "Why doesn't Daddy stay here anymore?" can be a child's way of expressing difficulty in coping with or comprehending the situation.

Parents in the midst of marital problems or divorce frequently lack the psychological energy or patience to deal with the preschooler's questions and altered behavior. Nonetheless, these children desperately need closeness, patience, and consistent responses from their parents. The nurse advocates for children by helping parents explore ways to address their children's regression and irritability. As parents develop skills to explain situations, they realize that even when children's behavior is unchanged during times of family disruption, they are nevertheless deeply affected (Cohen, 2002; Rao, Ranga, & Sekhar, 2002). Parents need to learn skills to connect emotionally with their children to demonstrate that their love will continue despite the dissolution of the marriage. In many cases, books that are appropriate to the preschooler's cognitive and emotional level can help parents address the feelings and needs of children involved in a divorce.

Child Abuse

The social processes within the family and community that create child abuse are multifactorial and complex. Research focuses on the complexity of the abuse cycle and the challenges involved in resolution. In some communities, hitting children as a form of discipline remains socially acceptable. Parents and caregivers who experience workplace stressors, financial worries, and other frustrations may project their anger onto their children by abusing them physically, emotionally, or sexually. Effective primary and secondary prevention interventions involve promoting awareness of violence as a social problem, opposing violence to women, and offering community and school programs to teach nonviolent conflict resolution skills to people of all ages. Apparent child abuse, however, must be reported.

Sexuality-Reproductive Pattern

The role of the preschooler as a girl or boy defines self-concept in this age group. Preschoolers recognize the two genders and identify with their own. Appropriate and positive representation of both genders on television and in role models, such as working mothers, allows preschoolers to interpret gender roles broadly and define their own roles more realistically.

Body image, a part of gender identity, also includes perception of sex organs. Preschoolers develop curiosity at this age, including inquisitiveness about other people's bodies and sexual functions. Their questions should be answered simply and factually. Parents and others should avoid teasing the preschooler about this interest or implying that sexual information is unacceptable or naughty. Positive feelings about all aspects of the self (including gender role) create positive self-esteem. Many children's books address self-esteem in young children and provide interesting and informative approaches to nurturing overall health promotion in this age group (Giami, 2002; Popovich, 2000). See **Web Site Resource 19A** for a list of recommended books for preschool children.

Coping-Stress Tolerance Pattern
Play Approaches

Assessing self-concept in preschool children who struggle to articulate their feelings presents a challenge for the nurse. Play approaches can elicit behaviors that indicate the child's sense of self and self-esteem, future success or failure, sense of acceptance, and competence.

Doll or puppet play provides valuable insight into a child's sense of self. Dolls or puppets, including one that represents a young child of the same gender, race, and cultural background as the preschooler, should be the only toy objects available for this kind of play (Cherney, Kelly-Vance, Glover, Ruane, & Ryalls, 2003; Justice & Pullen, 2003; Liben, Bigler, & Krogh, 2002; Rudisill & Wall, 2004; Taneja et al., 2002). If the child spontaneously begins to engage the dolls or puppets in imaginary activity, no further guidance should be given. With a reluctant child, the nurse begins to pretend, using examples for the child, such as going to the store, moving the dolls through the related activities, and then involving the child. Frequently preschoolers continue the scenario to tell their personal stories.

A related technique is **mutual storytelling.** The nurse begins a story for the child to finish. The nurse might begin with a standard line, such as, "Once upon a time there lived a [girl, boy, cow, monkey, etc.] who . . ." The nurse then pauses for the child to continue. If the child hesitates, the nurse resumes the story for another sentence or two and asks what the figure in the story is doing. As the child supplies details, the nurse offers encouragement to continue, asking questions such as "And then what happened?" or "How did the child feel?"

The child's inner nature can be explored along several dimensions. The emotional theme of the story is noted and should be congruent with the child's tone and expression. For example, a child who centers on a theme of aggression and destruction but describes the character's anger in a monotone is demonstrating incongruence between content and expression. The child's emotionless response suggests difficulty with expressing feelings. At the conclusion of the story, possible meanings can be revealed by asking whether the child feels similar to any of the characters or would like to be any of the characters.

Although these dimensions may be explored for meaning, interpretation of a child's behavior in these play situations remains highly speculative. To determine possible themes or estimate the child's self-esteem requires several encounters. Additionally, the nurse's personality and approach influence the child's spontaneity and ability to tell a story. Observed behavior and responses without associated interpretation should be recorded for future reference. Interpretations are avoided until validated by a specialist.

Coping Mechanisms

Preschoolers use coping mechanisms similar to those of the toddler (separation anxiety, regression, denial, repression, and projection). Protest behavior in the form of temper tantrums normally disappears as a stress response in the older preschooler. Temper tantrums that persist through the fifth year indicate a lack of matured coping responses. The child uses tantrums and continues to gain the desired result.

Preschoolers lack the cognitive awareness, social abilities, and motives for communication of adults and older children. They display temperaments and tantrums that appear oppositional to older individuals. Through positive interactions with parents and caregivers, preschoolers frequently learn how to organize their bodies, abilities, and environment to move successfully to the next stage of development (Buckley, Klein, Durbin, Hayden, & Moerk, 2002; Kalpidou, Power, Cherry, & Gottfried, 2004; Mehrabian, 2000; Mendez, Fantuzzo, & Cicchetti, 2002; Orme, 2001; Schor et al., 2003). A positive relationship between the child's temperament and the demands of the environment (also known as *goodness of fit*) can be attained by social interaction which, in turn, prevents the development of problem behaviors later (Hot Topics box).

Preschoolers possess a considerable range of experiences and memories; therefore, they respond more maturely to stress than do toddlers. Positive coping resources are determined by some of the following variables:

1. Availability of emotional comfort and the child's inner resilience
2. Ability to work on task
3. Availability of play materials and toys
4. Opportunity to engage in activities (Kalpidou et al., 2004)

Preschoolers use many of the coping mechanisms developed during their toddler years, but they generally show greater ability to verbalize frustration, fewer temper tantrums, and more patience in experimentation to resolve difficulty than the typical toddler. Preschoolers refine their problem-solving skills. Through fantasy play, they investigate solutions or responses to stressful events and find inner control for challenging situations.

THE CHALLENGE OF TEMPERAMENT AND PRESCHOOLERS

HOT topics

Temperament describes the way in which an individual behaves or responds to new situations and to life occurrences. Most children can be defined as *easy, difficult,* or *hard to warm up to,* based on the way in which they react to their surroundings and to people. For many adults the challenge in parenting is to learn how to work with a child's temperament, which can vary from the parents' or other children's temperaments, in efforts to attain family happiness.

CASE STUDY

Ricky

Ricky, age 4, arrives in the clinic with his mother. Ricky lives with his mother and father, who both work full time, and his infant sister. Their extended family lives in a different state over 100 miles away. Both parents are of average height and in good health. Ricky's mother mentions that Ricky often exhibits a strong will, particularly in regard to food. Conflict over food occurs every day. Mealtime is a battle to get him to eat, unless his mother feeds him. Ricky's baby sister eats no table food and seems to be able to tolerate any food given. Ricky's mother is quite frustrated and concerned that he will become malnourished.

Reflective Questions

1. What additional assessment information would you collect?
2. What questions would you ask and how would you further explore this issue with the mother?
3. In what ways does the distance of the extended family influence this family's approach to health promotion?
4. What factors would you consider to determine whether malnourishment is a factor in this family?

Occasionally projection and fantasy lead parents to consider their child dishonest. When faced with the question, "Did you break this dish?" the preschooler might respond, "No, Teddy did it." The child might even relate a detailed story of the toy bear's mishap. Preschoolers tend to project blame. Active fantasies help tell the story. Parents should not accuse preschoolers of lying, but rather the adult should help the child decide whether the story is pretend or real. The concepts of pretend and real help encourage children to discuss nightmares, television shows, stories, and their own active imaginations (Gleason et al., 2003; Vygotsky, 2004).

Preschoolers perceive their ability to control and manage situations better than does the toddler. Strict adherence to rituals or game rules controls situations. As discussed, the preschooler has a longer and more rigid bedtime ritual than the toddler. The preschooler also dislikes losing games and may structure the rules to ensure winning. Older children and adults may be able to accept these structures, but these controlling behaviors frustrate other preschoolers, because they also need to win. Gentle consistent direction by parents and caregivers about how to play games fairly and how to move toward positive group outcomes assists the preschooler to develop a sense of morality, which is important for later life success and happiness. See the Case Study and Care Plan for an example of ineffective coping in a preschool child.

Values-Beliefs Pattern

Preschoolers, like toddlers, lack fully developed consciences; however, at age 4 to 5 years these children do demonstrate some internal controls on their actions. Immaturity limits the consistency and effectiveness of these internal controls. With the child's concrete perspective, the internal controls may be rigid; therefore, a preschooler may feel overwhelming guilt when behavior and internal controls conflict. Cognitive developmental level determines, for the most part, preschoolers' maturity and their feelings about their behavior fluctuations. Cognitive development continues with dramatic transformation during these years, explaining the differences from child to child and from time

to time in the same child. Modeling and **inductive explanation,** which move from specific to general, by parents and caregivers influence moral behaviors appreciably. Modeling stems from many sources, not all of which leave positive impressions. Parents affect the availability of models by screening television shows, carefully selecting child-care situations, and monitoring play sessions. Responsible parents verify suitability of the models. More detailed inductive explanations, based on the child's cognitive level, generally are comprehended by the preschool population.

Preschoolers control their behavior to retain parental love and approval. From their perspective, parental disapproval represents a decrease in a child's importance from the parent's viewpoint. The child therefore suffers a decline in self-esteem, which motivates a change in behavior. Guilt results from perceived reduction of self-esteem, a critical step in the conscience development.

Moral actions are demonstrated in simple activities, such as taking turns and sharing. These actions stem from the assumption that other people have rights and desires that are as important as the rights and desires of the preschooler.

Preschoolers frequently express their values by stating who or what they like or what they want to be when they become adults. These values can change frequently, even within a few minutes. Preschoolers occasionally use these statements of value as punishment for playmates or family members and display insensitivity to the effect of their remarks on others.

Preschoolers ask endless questions. When they ask these questions about moral actions or feelings, they may simply be asking, "How does this work?" and not questioning the underlying parental value. The same intent exists when the child asks about the spiritual values that the parent may be

---

CARE PLAN

Ineffective Coping in Preschool Child

(Related to Ricky Case Study)

Nursing Diagnosis Ineffective Coping Related to Parental Feedback for Regressive Behaviors and Lack of Consistent Limits and Fulfillment of Appropriate Responsibilities

DEFINING CHARACTERISTICS

- Parent verbalization of need for help
- Changes in the usual behavior patterns

RELATED FACTORS

- Inconsistent methods of parental discipline
- Inadequate impulse control
- Lack of social skills

EXPECTED OUTCOMES

- The child will separate from his parents without incident (tantrum, crying).
- The child will join a community or church peer group activity.
- The child will perform one household task (picking up his toys) before bedtime every evening.
- The child will demonstrate independent self-care behaviors (feed himself).
- The parents will have clear, consistent, and age-appropriate expectations for behavior.
- The parents will explain the rationale for limiting a socially unacceptable or unsafe behavior as soon as it is displayed.

INTERVENTIONS

- Discuss with parents the process of growth and development and the child's need to learn how to compromise, take turns, and channel energy appropriately.
- Use the Prescreening Developmental Questionnaire to validate general assessment data.

- Encourage the parents to leave the child in someone else's care while they go shopping or to see a movie.
- Encourage the mother to formulate a bedtime ritual with the child that does not include her sitting in his room until he falls asleep.
- Discuss with the parents and the child what "jobs" he can do at home and the expectation that they be performed daily.
- Suggest laying out the child's clothes so that he can dress himself. Set a time to be dressed, such as before or after a certain television program.
- Explore with the parents the availability of playgroups or community activities for the child.
- Encourage the parents to take the child to the neighborhood playground so that he can meet and play with other children.
- Have the child help around the house alongside his parents. Specify "work" and "play" times.
- Encourage the parents to praise the child for age-appropriate behaviors, being careful not to bribe him to perform.
- Discuss the principles of discipline consistency, immediacy, realistic expectations, and clear explanations.
- Recognize the parents' frustration and encourage them to try different approaches, such as limited choices, diversion, and incentives ("when you finish your meat, we'll play a game").
- Suggest that the parents keep a diary of how long an approach was tried and how consistently the child responded.
- Discuss the decrease in appetite and reliance of food fads that typify the child's age. Review the principles of nutrition, timing of snacks, and ways of making food attractive to children.
- Refer the parents and the child to a nutritionist for nutrition counseling.

Modified from Carpenito-Moyet, L. J. (2004). *Handbook of nursing diagnosis* (10th ed.). Philadelphia: Lippincott Williams & Wilkins.

---

teaching. Parents may enroll their child in Sunday school or other faith-oriented classes or activities. The preschool child generally enjoys the social aspects of these activities and receives some important modeling of values from the involved adults and from working with peers as they struggle to develop morality.

Life beginnings and death concepts fascinate preschoolers. Because of their limited emotional experiences with death, some ask about dead insects and the process of death with great interest, occasionally with insensitivity. Others become upset with the idea of dying, assuming that when someone becomes angry and wishes them dead, they will cease to exist. Many children worry about who will care for them if their caregivers die, whether pain comes with death, what causes death, and what happens after someone dies. Children who actually lose a loved one to death can experience sleep disturbances and other behavioral changes as

part of the grieving process. Parents, based on their own religious and cultural values, should respond to children in a supportive and open manner to provide an accurate interpretation of death. In some cases, counseling may be needed if the parents are unable to cope with their duties or if the child has significant behavioral problems as a result of the family disruption. Increasingly, books appropriate to the preschooler's level of understanding are available to help deal with this delicate issue (Elkins & Cavendish, 2004).

PATHOLOGICAL PROCESSES

For many children physiological, psychosocial, and environmental factors create health problems that interfere with physical, social, and educational activities of normal development. Major disruptions limit fulfillment of the child's potential in adulthood (Anderson et al., 2002; Bradley & Corwyn, 2002; Denham et al., 2003; Pianta &

Box 19-4 Environmental Safety for Preschoolers

A safe and developmentally stimulating environment allows children of all ages to explore without negative consequences. When teaching parents how to modify their homes for preschoolers, the following requirements for child safety should be considered.

SAFE SLEEP ENVIRONMENT

Provide beds with guardrails (as needed), soft corners, and appropriate bedding to prevent suffocation.

WELL-VENTILATED BUT OPTIMAL TEMPERATURE ENVIRONMENT FOR PLAY

Provide safe play areas by using electrical outlet covers, handrails in stairwells, toy boxes with lids that lock securely, nonslip floor materials, well-anchored furniture, and appropriate soft ground coverings and padding for outdoor play equipment.

BURN PREVENTION

Use only cool mist humidifier for management of upper respiratory infections; dress child only in flame-retardant clothing, particularly at bedtime.

APPROPRIATE INSTALLATION AND USE OF EMERGENCY HOME EQUIPMENT

Discuss the importance of properly operating smoke detectors, fire extinguishers, and practicing an escape plan from the home in case of emergency.

CONNECTION TO EMERGENCY SERVICES

Post 911 on all phones; teach the child how to use 911 and how to report the child's name and address over the phone; parents should be trained in cardiopulmonary resuscitation and the Heimlich maneuver.

PREVENTION OF ASPIRATION

Monitor use of balloons and eating habits of the preschooler.

SAFE DAILY HOME ENVIRONMENT

Close doors of dishwasher, oven, washer, and dryer; mark all glass doors with decals to delineate doors; use gates at the top and bottom of stairs for the younger child; set water heater temperature at a maximum of 120° F to avoid burns; store all poisonous substances out of the reach of children; discourage running in the house; avoid throw rugs on bare floors.

PREVENTION, RECOGNITION, AND MANAGEMENT OF POISON INGESTION OR EXPOSURE

Know how to use syrup of ipecac and have the nearest poison control center phone number within easy access; learn how to evaluate burns or blisters around the mouth, odor of poisons, empty containers around the child, stomach distress, or changes in normal activity level that might indicate poison ingestion.

WATER SAFETY

Monitor bathtub and pool activity; teach preschooler swimming skills (usually by age 4); ensure that all pools are fenced.

BICYCLE SAFETY

Ensure that the child is riding a developmentally appropriate bicycle with a federally approved safety helmet and is schooled in the rules of riding in the street and interacting with strangers.

LEAD CONCERNS

Avoid items with a high lead content in home (paint, wrapping paper, earthenware, colored newspaper); ensure that children are monitored when lead exposure is a concern.

ENVIRONMENTAL CONTAMINANTS HAZARDOUS TO THE CHILD'S HEALTH

Avoid exposure to tobacco smoke, nitrous oxide from wood-burning stoves, asbestos, pesticides, radiation, and factory-produced irritants.

La Paro, 2003; Rosenthal et al., 2004; Yaden & Tardibuono, 2004; Yeung, Linver, & Brooks-Gunn, 2002). Environmental processes that affect toddlers also affect preschoolers (Hambrick-Dixon, 2002). Occurrence rates and outcomes of health problems differ in this age group, likely because of developmental differences (USDHHS, 2000). Preschoolers have more refined problem-solving skills, are more coordinated, and have more experience with a variety of situations than do toddlers. Although preschoolers recognize and avoid some environmental hazards, they remain impulsive and immature. Population-based programs assure that screening takes place at the most developmentally appropriate time (Box 19-4 and Research Highlights box).

Because many preschoolers attend child-care programs, many have been trained to use 911 and can access help in emergencies when this phone code exists. At this age, children need to know their name, address, and how to say "no" to strangers.

Injuries

Approximately 55 American children die every day from injuries; 43% of the deaths of children age 1 through 4 years are a result of injuries, "4 times the number of deaths due to birth defects, the second leading cause of death for this age group" (USDHHS, 2000).

Accidents and injuries are often predictable and preventable (USDHHS, 2000). As preschoolers become more independent, causes of injury change; they may chase a ball into a busy street or suffer from sports-related injuries. Preschoolers continue to need supervision to prevent injury related to their developmental age.

Of all injuries, two thirds occur in children and adolescents. The rate of death from injuries is decreasing in the United States. On the other hand, death rates continue to be higher than in countries with long-term comprehensive preventive approaches that focus on widespread community change (e.g., Great Britain and Scandinavian countries) (Deal, 2000).

research highlights

Screening Preschoolers

The goals of this study were to assess (1) whether preschool children enrolled in a Medicaid managed care clinic received recommended preventive screenings, including blood lead and hematocrit levels, and tuberculosis testing, and (2) the prevalence of positive findings during the screening process.

All children (N = 812) between the ages of 12 and 35 months were included in the study. Records were reviewed for the dates and results of all blood lead, hematocrit, and tuberculosis tests. Of the 812 children, 690 (85.0%) had a documented blood lead test. Of those screened, more than one fourth (190 of 690, or 27.5%) had at least one result greater than or equal to 10 mcg/dl. A hematocrit result was documented for 742 (91.4%) of the study children, and 377 of these children (50.8%) were anemic for at least one testing. Two

thirds of the study children (536) had documentation of a tuberculosis screening, with two thirds of these having a documented reading. None of the 342 children had a positive tuberculosis test result.

Screening rates were excellent in this study group; children not seen regularly in the practice were included in the study. The results provide evidence for the high burden of lead poisoning and anemia in this indigent population. Considering that many populations have a much lower rate of screening, often around 24%, this type of data may not be as available in other populations. The study demonstrates that it is feasible to conduct assessments based on defined primary prevention strategies using a population-based approach to health care.

Vivier, P. M., Flanagan, P., Simon, P., Diana, B. J., Brown, L., & Alario, A. J. (2001). An assessment of selected preventive screenings among children aged 12 to 35 months in a hospital-based, Medicaid managed care practice. *Ambulatory Child Health, 1*(7), 3-10.

Although preschoolers have fewer accidents than toddlers, motor vehicle accidents continue to be a major cause of fatalities in this age group. Although many state laws mandate federally approved car seats for children who are less than 4 feet tall or weigh less than 40 pounds and booster seats for children up to the age of 6, many parents fail to place their children in appropriate restraint systems, or they use them incorrectly. Although parents may know that infants should be placed in the back seat, they do not always know that children in the front seat of a motor vehicle face danger, even if they are using restraint systems. Federal investigations concluded that children under age 13 should ride in the back seat of a motor vehicle, particularly because of potential injury or death from a passenger seat air bag that could inflate in a severe car accident (Deal, 2000; Taft, Mickalide, & Taft, 1999).

Household furniture and fixtures also remain a hazard for preschoolers, as do structural features such as stairs and windows. Nursery and toy injuries decrease during the preschool years. Sports and recreational injuries increase markedly. This elevated incidence likely reflects a change in the preschoolers' involvement in group sports, riding bicycles, and using playground equipment. Preschoolers need a broad range of play areas and experiences. Conscientious parents supply age-appropriate limits and supervision (Deal, 2000).

Preschoolers lack the skill or judgment to ride bicycles in the street. They need instruction about safe use of playground equipment. Adult supervision of most preschooler activities, group sports in particular, is required to prevent injury.

Preschoolers begin to safely handle basic tools, kitchen equipment, and cleaning supplies. The child at this age takes pride in participating in household projects with a supervising parent. They spend much of their time in the home and in the preschool or child-care center. The facil-

ities pose the same potentially harmful environmental conditions as the home, as well as some additional threats to safety (Deal, 2000; USDHHS, 2000).

In a response to concern about firearm safety in homes with small children, several states have passed legislation to encourage safe storage of firearms. Owners in these states take responsibility when a child injures or kills someone with their firearm. Dealers in some of these states must offer locks at the time of purchase (Schuster, Franke, Bastian, Sor, & Halfon, 2000). Among children 5 to 14 years old, firearms remain the fourth leading cause of unintentional injury (USDHHS, 2000). In the United States 35% of children live in homes with guns (Schuster et al., 2000).

Burns

Scalds and direct flame burns are major hazards for the preschooler. In children ages 1 through 9 years the number of burn injuries is second only to the number sustained in motor vehicle accidents. In preschool children the number of deaths in house fires is nearly double that of other ages. Children of this age experiment with matches and fire, and they may be unable to escape from a fire once it starts (Bull et al., 2000; USDHHS, 2000). Home fire deaths occur more often in the African American, Hispanic, and Native American preschool population than in the non-Hispanic white population (USDHHS, 2000). Measures discussed in Chapter 18 to reduce scald burns in the home apply to this age group as well. Preschoolers should be taught about the dangers of matches, open flames, and hot objects. Parents and caregivers should model appropriate use of active and potentially dangerous burning devices.

Drowning

The child over 3 years of age is at lower risk for drowning in the bathtub, but at greater risk for drowning in a swimming pool, than the toddler. In most states preschool children were more likely to drown in swimming pools and older children in natural bodies of water. Over 30% of drowning episodes occur in children aged 1 to 4 years. With this in mind, it is important to supervise young children when they are near a body of water, install fencing to isolate a residential pool from the house, use personal floatation devices while bathing or playing near a natural body of water, and to teach children how to swim and that swimming alone is unsafe. Preschoolers should receive instruction in water safety and swimming and should always be supervised by a trained adult or older person. For children under age 5, drowning represents a major cause of injury death in the United States (Agran et al., 2003; Brenner, Trumble, Smith, Kessler, & Overpeck, 2001; Bull et al., 2000).

Preschoolers have the cognitive ability to learn water survival. They should always wear a personal flotation device (i.e., life jacket) when they are on boats, even when they know how to swim, and they must be supervised when near water, even shallow water (Brenner, Saluja, & Smith, 2003; Hess, 2003).

Mechanical Forces

As mentioned, bicycle accidents become a greater source of injury during the preschool years. Many bicycle accidents involve automobiles, and most of these accidents result from the child's errors. Parents should set reasonable and age-appropriate limits about bicycle use. The transition from tricycle to bicycle provides an excellent time to begin using a helmet. Federally approved bicycle helmets are effective in reducing head trauma, a major cause of death among young children (USDHHS, 2000). In many communities helmets must be worn by all bicyclists and rollerbladers, regardless of age. (Coffman, 2003).

The preschooler, as a passenger or pedestrian, is at great risk for an auto-related accident. At this age pedestrian injury is more likely to occur than is passenger injury. Preschoolers should be taught proper street-crossing techniques and, generally, should be supervised when crossing streets. Approved car seat restraint systems should be used by young children at all times during car travel. Many accidents occur as a result of improper use of restraint devices. It is important for nurses to be informed and to instruct families about how to restrain the child in the car (Taft et al., 1999). The back seat is safer than the front seat, and all car doors should be locked. If the preschooler refuses to use the seat belt or appropriate restraint, then parents must insist that the outing be postponed. Parents who provide a good example by using their seat belts directly influence the child's acceptance, and it meets the child's desire at this age to imitate the parent. The child who uses a car seat from infancy on will generally accept the seat belt quite well.

Biological and Bacterial Agents

Preschoolers seem healthier than toddlers, with fewer respiratory and gastrointestinal illnesses. They have developed antibodies to many common organisms through exposure.

Children usually become ill more often when they enter their first group situation, where they are exposed to organisms new to them. This concerns parents and should be discussed by the nurse before the child begins attending a group setting. Increasingly, child-care settings provide instruction to children about appropriate hand-washing techniques to decrease disease transmission and provide relevant health-promotion teaching (McCutcheon & Fitzgerald, 2001; Roberts, Jorm et al., 2000; Roberts, Smith, et al., 2000).

The child with a full course of immunizations as an infant receives a booster dose of the diphtheria, tetanus, and pertussis vaccine in the fourth year (Paulson & Hammer, 2002). A second injection to protect against measles, mumps, and rubella is recommended between ages 4 and 6 years. Many states require that all children in a school setting be fully immunized. Parents who choose not to immunize their children usually make this choice for religious reasons, but some parents worry about the risk of the immunization itself. Although vaccines provide an extremely safe way to combat communicable disease, issues about safety do arise. Because autism is often diagnosed around the same time a child is vaccinated, some parents have connected the onset of their child's autism with the vaccine (Paulson & Hammer, 2002; Woo et al., 2004). The American Academy of Pediatrics position statement refutes this association as coincidental. The risk of consequences of the disease itself far outweighs any vaccine risk. However, nurses must remain informed about the risks in order to provide accurate information to parents.

Nurses who remain informed about reasons for avoiding immunization will be better able to increase parents' understanding of the possible consequences of omitting a dose. Incomplete immunization may also occur as a result of parental forgetfulness or procrastination. Mandatory immunization for school entry provides an effective incentive for these parents. In addition, community immunization initiatives make administration less expensive and more accessible in many communities (Kempe et al., 2004; Tung et al., 2003).

One of the newer developments in childhood immunizations is the introduction of a conjugate vaccine to prevent pediatric pneumococcal disease, which was added to the recommended schedule in the United States in 2001. Other advances on the horizon are more combination vaccines to decrease cost of administration. Noninjectable vaccines that could be inhaled or eaten would greatly enhance pediatric immunization programs. Administration and storage of these vaccines would be easier (Paulson & Hammer, 2002).

Continued efforts to vaccinate all children are needed, especially children living in poverty, particularly in large cities, where they are traditionally under-vaccinated (Tung et al., 2003). Nurses use immunization registry programs to consolidate records, to remind parents, to evaluate the client's scheduled program, and to analyze issues for a particular population. With registry programs duplication may be avoided in the preschooler whose immunizations are not up to date (Kempe et al., 2004; Tung et al., 2003). The Centers for Disease Control and Prevention (CDC) publishes recommendations for scheduled immunizations and for individuals who have omitted doses for some reason. These schedules are updated regularly and are available online in a variety of formats, in both Spanish and English, at the CDC Web site (*http://www.cdc.gov/nip/recs/child-schedule.htm*). When immunizations have been omitted or delayed, the immunization schedule continues from the dose of the last vaccine. **Web Site Resource 17E** presents several immunization schedules, including a catch-up schedule for children who start late or are more than 1 month behind (Centers for Disease Control and Prevention's Advisory Committee on Immunization Practices, 2004; Rennels et al., 2004). Parents should be fully informed about the potential side effects of immunizations. In most office and clinic settings, parents sign state-developed informed consent documents that describe potential side effects.

Occasionally parents of children with disabilities do not allow them to attend preschool in an effort to protect them from inadvertent harm or scorn from other children. Financially and socially disadvantaged children remain at home because of economic constraints or ignorance about advantages of preschool preparation. Nurses facilitate the exploration of advantages and disadvantages of preschool for these children, helping their families obtain information about local opportunities and sources for assistance with cost.

Chemical Agents

Preschoolers face exposure to environmental pollutants. The young child's skin area is twice that of an adult's, which increases the risk of toxicity. Environmental exposure has been implicated in the increased prevalence of learning disabilities, because of the unique vulnerability of a child's brain to chemicals (Schettler, 2001). Disparities exist among populations with regard to their risk. Ethnicity, socioeconomic status, and geographical location all have an impact on the risk of exposure. Chemical agents of concern for toddlers, such as pesticides, lead poisoning, and passive smoke, continue to merit consideration in the preschool population (Ames, 2002; Rogge & Combs-Orme, 2003; Ross & Birnbaum, 2003). Preschoolers, however, become more independent and understand the concepts of safe and poisonous.

More than one half of all poisonings occur in children under the age of 6. Each year poison control centers receive more than 1.1 million calls about accidental poisonings among children ages 5 and under. Calls to poison control centers peak between 4 PM and 10 PM, which is known by poison centers as the *arsenic hour*. Most poisonings occur in the home (University of Pittsburgh, 2004). Even though companies enclose many children's medications in child-proof packaging, the product may be administered incorrectly by the caregiver, or the child may experiment with another family member's colorful pills. For example, the medication used to treat attention-deficit/hyperactivity disorder, methylphenidate, poisons many children. Klein-Schwartz's analysis (2003) of data from a 7-year period indicates that over 40% of these methylphenidate poisoning were in children under the age of 6 years. About 60% of all poisonings in children, however, involve products other than medicines such as plants, cleaning products, cosmetics, pesticides, paints, and solvents, with the remaining 40% attributed to medications (University of Pittsburgh, 2004). **Web Site Resource 19B** presents recommendations on how to childproof a home from poisons.

Many household products, drugs, carbon monoxide, pesticides, lead, mercury, polychlorinated biphenyls, ethers, and poisonous plants pose hazards to the preschooler. Secondary smoke and lead exposure represent negative chemical influences on the growing child.

Preschoolers should receive verbal explanations about poisonous or dangerous substances, but parents cannot rely on the preschooler to remember instructions. A poison control program from the University of Pittsburgh introduced a character called Mr. Yuk in 1971. The ability to identify warning symbols such as Mr. Yuk helps preschoolers remain safe. Preschools and child-care facilities often incorporate topics about environmental pollutants and dangerous substances into their curricula to promote the health of the preschooler. Information about poison control is widely available on-line (American Association of Poison Control Centers, 2002; Children's Hospital of Pittsburgh, 2004). The national, toll-free poison control center number is 800-222-1212. From that number the caller is directed to the nearest poison control center.

Parents should teach children about the four forms of poison which are (1) solids: air fresheners, pills, vitamins, aspirin, lipstick (2) liquids: cleaning products, fuel, alcohol, (3) sprays: furniture polish, oven cleaner, room deodorizer, and (4) invisibles: carbon monoxide, space heater fumes. Communication with parents about environmental dangers, thus creating a healthier living environment, remains a major role of the child-care provider.

Cancer

With over 8000 children diagnosed with cancer and about 1500 deaths annually in the United States, the disorders represent the leading cause of death from disease in children under age 15. However, with an average of 1 to 2 children (per 10,000) developing some kind of cancer each year, the diseases are considered rare (National Cancer Institute, 2002). Over one half of these cancers are types of leukemia, with brain and central nervous system tumors making up most of the rest. Acute lymphocytic leukemia, the most common childhood cancer, accounts for over one third of the cases of cancer in preschool children. Brain tumors such as gliomas and medulloblastomas are the most common solid tumors, with neuroblastomas, Wilms tumors, and rhabdomyosarcomas occurring less often. Although less common than other solid tumors, retinoblastoma merits attention because of the possible loss of vision. Remarkable advances in long-term survival of children with cancer have occurred. Early detection remains the key to successful treatment; therefore, early aggressive efforts have been put into detection programs. Some of the increases in rates of diagnosis may be attributed to improved imaging techniques and early detection (National Cancer Institute, 2002).

Leukemia

Acute lymphocytic leukemia (ALL), the most common leukemia of childhood, accounts for about 75% of all childhood cancer and one third of the deaths from childhood cancer. The incidence of ALL rises from age 2, peaks at age 5, and diminishes through later childhood and adolescence.

The dominant signs and symptoms of ALL appear suddenly, but often the child demonstrates a prodromal period of weakness, malaise, anorexia, fever, and tachycardia. Bone pain, petechiae, and hemorrhages after minor procedures such as dental extractions are encountered frequently. When an unexplained infection does not respond to management, suspicion should arise. Early detection and treatment of ALL has resulted in a marked increase in 5-year survival rates. Survival is dependent upon age at diagnosis, with the best survival rates occurring when diagnosis occurs during the preschool years (Smith, Gloeckler Ries, Gurney, & Ross, 1999).

With suspected leukemia, the nurse institutes secondary prevention strategies with an assessment that includes the following parameters:

1. Examination of the cervical and peripheral lymph nodes
2. Palpation and percussion of the liver and spleen
3. Inspection of the skin for systemic signs of leukemia, such as pallor, purpura, petechiae, and **chloroma**, a localized tumor mass that has a greenish appearance and may be found in the skin, orbits, or other tissues in granulocytic forms of leukemia
4. Inspection of the mouth for enlarged tonsils, hyperplasia of the gums, and red, friable gingivae
5. Palpation of the sternum, bones, and joints for tenderness and pain

The rate of leukemia is higher in children with Down syndrome; therefore, school nurses and public health nurses should monitor these children for early signs of the disease.

Wilms Tumor

Most cases of **Wilms tumor** occur in children under 5 years of age. A strong correlation exists between Wilms tumor and several congenital malformations. Genetic links may contribute to its occurrence in children with bilateral tumors and those who have family members with the disorder. When Wilms tumor, aniridia (a congenital malformation of the iris of the eye), genitourinary malformations, and mental retardation occur together, the genetic association strengthens. However, survivors of Wilms tumor that is unilateral at diagnosis possess a low risk for producing a child who will develop the disease. Information about the risk factors for Wilms tumor is not definitive. The 5-year survival rates for children with this disease are excellent (Bernstein, Linet, Smith, & Olshan, 1999).

Retinoblastoma

Even as the most common intraocular tumor in younger children, **retinoblastoma** affects only 300 children younger than 20 years of age each year. Most of these children are less than 5 years old. Genetic mutations contribute to the incidence of retinoblastoma, usually causing the bilateral form of the disease. Even though the tumor is uncommon, the scientific work surrounding its diagnosis and management has resulted in many of the methods used for other cancers. Survival rates are excellent (Young, Smith, Roffers, Liff, & Bunin, 1999).

The history usually reveals a slow symptom progression. To reveal risk factors, the following questions should be asked:

- Do tumors of the eye run in your family?
- If tumors of the eye run in your family, which relatives were affected and how were they treated?
- Have you noticed that your child has eye problems (crossed or lazy eyes or difficulty seeing)?
- Have you noticed any changes in your child's eyes?

Screening eye examinations for high-risk children include:

1. Visual acuity
2. Red reflex, which appears whitish with retinoblastoma (cat's eye reflex)
3. Ophthalmoscopic findings
4. Lid lag, which is found with exophthalmos
5. Strabismus, by doing the cover-uncover test

The cat's eye reflex and strabismus are the most common signs of retinoblastoma. Any suspicious findings indicate referral for further evaluation.

Neuroblastoma

Neuroblastoma, a cancer of the sympathetic nervous system, begins in the abdomen, primarily in the adrenal gland, approximately 70% of the time. The remaining 30% originate in cervical, thoracic, or pelvic areas. Approximately one half of these cancers occur in individuals younger than 2 years. More than 90% of diagnoses occur by age 5. Unfortunately, many of the children have metastases when the cancer is identified. Frequently symptoms of secondary spread bring the child to the health professional. The survival rate for children diagnosed during the preschool years is improving, but in other age groups it has remained static. There is little convincing evidence of specific risk factors. Prenatal exposure to pesticides, hormones, and use of certain medications suggest an increased risk (Goodman, Gurney, Smith, & Olshan, 1999).

Secondary prevention strategies include the simple procedure of screening children at risk for catecholamines in the urine and for neurofibromatosis.

Cancer in a child can be frightening to parents, particularly if there is a strong family history of cancers of any kind.

Box 19-5 **Warning Signs That May Indicate Childhood Cancer**

Cancer remains a leading cause of death in children under 15 years of age, second only to injuries.

GENERAL

- Documented weight loss without explanation, failure to thrive
- Persistent poor appetite
- Tires easily or lack of energy

LEUKEMIA OR LYMPHOMAS: "LIQUID TUMORS" (CANCER OF THE BLOOD, BLOOD-MAKING SYSTEM, LYMPH NODES)

- Persistent fever (more than 2 weeks)
- Bruising without injury and purple or red patches appearing on the skin
- Swollen glands (lymph nodes) unrelated to infection
- Persistent bone pain or limping
- Paleness of the lips, skin, nails, or lining of the eyes

BRAIN TUMOR

- Recurrent headaches, especially accompanied by vomiting, particularly in the morning
- Reflection in the pupil of the eye (eye tumor)
- Unexplained, persistent changes in behavior

KIDNEY TUMORS

- Lump in the abdomen or abdominal enlargement
- Blood in the urine
- Bulging of the eyes
- Unexplained, persistent cough or chest pain
- A firm mass in the muscles

MAKE BATH TIME EXAMINATION TIME

- These complaints or physical findings should be interpreted only as warnings of possible serious disease. When these warnings are present, you should consult your physician at once.
- Do not forget that your children must be examined by a physician every year. The earlier that cancer is detected, the better the chances are for a cure. With current treatment methods of surgery, radiation therapy, and chemotherapy (administration of anticancer drugs), the survival rate of children with certain forms of cancer has improved dramatically.

Modified from the Cancer Association of Greater New Orleans, Inc., 211 Camp St., Room 600, New Orleans, LA 70130.

Early detection continues to be associated with increased survival rates. Secondary prevention programs should include the warning signs of cancer in children. Routine procedures, such as a bath, provide opportunities for parents to examine the child for physical symptoms of disease that are outlined in Box 19-5.

Asthma

Thee incidence of **asthma,** a chronic inflammatory disorder of the airways, is rising more rapidly in preschool-age chil-

dren than in any other group (Rogge & Combs-Orme, 2003). The inflammation in this disorder contributes to a hyperresponsive airway, limited airflow, and respiratory symptoms that include breathlessness, wheezing, cough, and chest tightness. Causes include genetic predisposition, allergens such as animal dander or dust mites, and nonspecific precipitants such as infections, exercise, weather, or stress. Rates for boys exceed those for girls, and rates in the black and Hispanic population exceed those in the non-Hispanic white population. Poverty contributes significantly to asthmatic illness, disability, and death (Lara et al., 2002; Van Bever, Desager, & Hagendorens, 2002). Multiple factors contribute to exacerbation of asthma symptoms. High levels of exposure to tobacco smoke, pollutants, and allergens contribute. In addition to the generally known allergens of house mite dust and pet and rodent dander, cockroach particles have been implicated. Access to quality medical care, financial resources, and social support to manage the disease on a long-term basis exist in significantly different proportions from one population to another in the United States (USDHHS, 2000).

SOCIAL PROCESSES
Community and Work

Some preschoolers experience groups outside their families, such as group child-care settings, church groups, or family involvement in other activities, by age 3. Other children of the same age experience little outside contact. A preschool setting introduces the child to a wider social arena. Parents learn to release their child to encourage independent activity in a safe, supervised setting. Preschoolers test their independence, interactive skills, and self-discipline as they learn to function in a group. Preschool provides a transition to kindergarten and first grade, where group interaction skills are expected. Parents often select a preschool based on geographical closeness to their home or a friend's recommendation, using the most practical approach. With many child-care facilities and options now available, parents frequently visit and evaluate a number of settings to determine the most appropriate for their needs (Denham et al., 2003; Mendez, Fantuzzo, & Cicchetti, 2002).

Culture and Ethnicity

Family cultural heritage continues to shape preschoolers. Unlike toddlers, preschoolers frequently ask why the family follows certain practices. These young children notice differences from one family to another. Their playmates may celebrate different holidays or practice family rituals different from their own. As preschoolers experience more activities outside their home, differences become more apparent. Discussion about the strength of cultural differences provides an excellent learning opportunity (Rao, Ranga, & Sekhar, 2002; Xu, Crane, & Ryan, 2002).

Preschoolers also notice ethnic differences in appearance and pronounce skin colors, eyes, and hairstyles as "pretty" or "ugly." The socialization process forms presumptions similar to those of their family or playmates. Parents and caregivers who teach and role model positive behaviors allow children to see differences in others as being positive rather than negative. Mass media influences on physical attractiveness also contribute and become more significant to the adolescent.

Certain cultures apply more pressure for children to assume responsibility for younger siblings or household tasks. Confusion develops in the preschooler when the family's culture varies from that of most playmates. Disciplinary approaches vary from culture to culture. Uncertainty also results when parents integrate their cultural background into the community standards, but the grandparents adhere to traditional cultural practices, rituals, and child-rearing ideas.

Legislation

Many safety-focused legislative bills have affected the preschooler (see Chapter 18). School issues, as discussed in Chapter 20, also affect this age group. With current concern about health care costs, financial programs that focus on children may lose when competing with the whole of health care. If overall funding for vulnerable populations such as the homeless and the poor decrease, child health care in general in this country suffers. In the United States one in every four children under the age of 6 lives in poverty. Over 50% of the occupants of urban homeless shelters at a given time will be children under the age of 6 years (Fields & Smith, 2004; Huebner, 2000; Keogh, 2000; Markos & Lima, 2003; U.S. Census Bureau, 2003).

Economics

Poverty influences the preschooler as it does any child. Unlike toddlers, preschoolers become more aware of family economic status. A preschooler may know that the family lacks money for toys but recognizes less the comprehensive limits to resources that influence the family lifestyle. In some cases the family's financial history prevents attendance at preschool or influences exposure to expanded learning activities. Preschoolers realize money acquires food, toys, and clothes, but they do not yet have a concept of economic values. The child might trade an expensive item for a trinket that looks more interesting. A child who uses the earnings to buy something realizes that more must be earned to buy more things. The child thus begins to learn the concepts of earning and spending.

Health Care Delivery System

Access to health care resources remains the same for preschoolers as toddlers. When preschoolers enter a school setting, admission may require that a health care worker screen them physically and developmentally. For indigent children **Early and Periodic Screening, Diagnosis, and Treatment (EPSDT),** a Medicaid program, may fund the visit. Screening for children under age 21 who meet the economic criteria for Medicaid occurs in private offices, local health departments, and community clinics. Medicaid pro-

vides one screening examination per year, which includes the following elements:

1. Medical history
2. Assessment of physical growth, nutritional status, and mental development
3. Inspection of ears, eyes, nose, mouth, teeth, and throat
4. Vision screening
5. Auditory screening
6. Screening for cardiac abnormalities
7. Screening for anemia
8. Screening for the sickle cell trait
9. Urine sampling
10. Blood pressure reading
11. Assessment and updating of immunizations
12. Tuberculosis screening, when indicated
13. Referral to a dentist for diagnosis and treatment for children 3 years of age and older

Referral for a complete physical examination addresses any health or developmental concerns identified during this screening. Eligible children receive EPSDT as a comprehensive service administered by Medicaid. **Web Site Resource 19C** presents recommendations for preventive pediatric health care from the American Academy of Pediatrics.

NURSING INTERVENTIONS

Preschoolers show much interest in the tools and procedures of a health screening examination (American Academy of Pediatrics, 2000) (Box 19-6). These inquisitive children may play with the stethoscope, otoscope, and other diagnostic instruments. The nurse explains the tests in age-appropriate terminology and expects the child to cooperate for most of the visit. The preschooler may show self-control during injections but definitely needs a parent close by to offer support and encouragement. The nurse includes the preschooler in the history by directing questions about dietary intake and health practices, such as tooth brushing, favorite activities, and friends. At this age children begin taking some interest in health, developing the cognitive maturity to learn many health-promotion skills that they will use for the rest of their lives.

SUMMARY

Schedules for preventive health care during the preschool years include visits at 4 and 5 years of age. Each visit includes an ongoing history; growth, physical, and developmental assessment; and discussion of age-appropriate developmental concerns.

In addition to the office or clinic contact, the nurse may consult with a preschool or a nurse for a primary school and preschool. Early exposure to and reinforcement of health care information as part of preschool education lays a foundation for later healthy lifestyle habits, which influence overall societal health. Health as a curricular subject during the school-age years continues this focus. The school nurse's role in health promotion and prevention of illness is discussed in Chapter 20.

Box **19-6** Health-Promotion Interventions

ANNUALLY

- Health history
- Height and weight
- Blood pressure
- Vision screening (age 3 to 4 years)
- Developmental and behavioral assessment
- Physical examination

PERIODICALLY

- Immunizations based on recommended schedule
  Ensure currency
  Diphtheria, tetanus, pertussis
  Oral poliovirus
  Pneumococcal
  Measles, mumps, rubella
  Haemophilus influenzae type b
  Hepatitis B
  Varicella
- Hematocrit or hemoglobin level at least once after age 9 months
- Urinalysis at 5 years old

SCREENINGS FOR HIGH-RISK CHILDREN

- Lead
- Tuberculosis
- Cholesterol

ANTICIPATORY GUIDANCE

- Injury Prevention
  Child safety car seat (age less than 5 years) or seat belt
  Lap and shoulder belt (age 5 years and older)
  Use helmet and avoid traffic when bicycling
  Smoke detectors, flame-retardant sleepwear
  Hot water temperature less than 125° F
  Window and stair guards, pool fence
  Safe storage of drugs, toxic substances, firearms, matches
  Close availability of syrup of ipecac, poison control phone number
  Parents and caretakers trained in cardiopulmonary resuscitation
- Violence prevention
- Nutrition and exercise
  Limit saturated fats, maintain caloric balance, and emphasize grain, fruit, vegetables intake
  Regular fun physical activity
- Tobacco
  Effects of passive smoking
  Antitobacco messages
- Dental health
  Floss, brush with fluoridated toothpaste at least daily
  Regular visits to dentist

ADDITIONAL STUDY MATERIAL

Study Questions in the back of the book, see page 663.

⟨evolve⟩ **WEB SITE MATERIALS**

These materials are located on the book's Web site at http://evolve.elsevier.com/Edelman/.

- WebLinks
- Content Updates
- Web Site Resources

19A   Recommended Literature for Preschool Children
19B   Childproof Your Home from Poisons
19C   Recommendations for Preventive Pediatric Health Care

REFERENCES

Agran, P. F., Anderson, C., Winn, D., Thayer, S., Trent, R., & Walton-Haynes, L. (2003). Rates of pediatric injuries by 3-month intervals for children 0 to 3 years of age. *Pediatrics, 111*(6), e683-e692.

Allor, J. H., & McCathren, R. B. (2003). Developing emergent literacy skills through storybook reading. *Intervention in School & Clinic, 39*(2), 72-79.

Al-Shehri, A. M. (2003). Speech and language development disorders in the ENT practice. *Journal of Otorhinolaryngology, 2*(1), 37-43.

American Academy of Pediatrics. (2000). Recommendations for preventive pediatric health care (RE9535). *Pediatrics, 105*(3), 645-646.

American Association of Poison Control Centers. (2002). Toxic exposure surveillance system (TESS). Retrieved July 29, 2004, from: *http://www.aapcc.org/poison1. htm.*

American Dietetic Association. (2004). Position of the American Dietetic Association: Dietary guidance for healthy children ages 2 to 11 years. *Journal of the American Dietetic Association, 104*(4), 660-677.

American Family Physician. (2001). Sleep disorders and sleep problems in childhood. *American Family Physician, 63*(2), 277-284.

Ames, R. G. (2002). Pesticide impacts on communities and schools. *International Journal of Toxicology, 21*(5), 397-402.

Amschler, D. H. (2003). A hidden epidemic: Dental disparities among children. *Journal of School Health, 73*(1), 38-40.

Anderson, L. M., Shinn, C., Charles, J. S., Scrimshaw, S. C., Fielding, J. E., Normand, J., et al. (2002). Community interventions to promote healthy social environments: Early childhood development and family housing. *Morbidity & Mortality Weekly Report, 51*(4), 1-12.

Ball, G. D. C., Marshall, J. D., & McCargar, L. J. (2003). Fatness and fitness in obese children at low and high health risk. *Pediatric Exercise Science, 15*(4), 392.

Bauer, P. J., Wenner, J. A., & Kroupina, M. G. (2002). Making the past present: Later verbal accessibility of early memories [memory testing]. *Journal of Cognition & Development, 3*(1), 21-47.

Bernstein, L., Linet, M., Smith, M. A., & Olshan, A. F. (1999). *Cancer incidence and survival among children and adolescents: United States: Renal tumors* (No. 99-4649 ed.). Bethesda, MD: National Cancer Institute. Retrieved July 29, 2004, from: *http://seer.cancer.gov/publications/childhood/.*

Bickley, L., & Hoekelman, R. A. (2002). *Barbara Bates' guide to physical examination and history taking* (9th ed.). Philadelphia: Lippincott Williams & Wilkins.

Bracken, B., & Shaughnessy, M. F. (2003). An interview with Bruce Bracken about the measurement of basic concepts in children. *North American Journal of Psychology*, 5(3), 351-363.

Bradley, R. H., & Corwyn, R. F. (2002). Socioeconomic status and child development. *Annual Review of Psychology*, 53(1), 371-399.

Brenner, R. A., Saluja, G., & Smith, G. S. (2003). Swimming lessons, swimming ability, and the risk of drowning. *Injury Control & Safety Promotion*, 10(4), 211-216.

Brenner, R. A., Trumble, A. C., Smith, G. S., Kessler, E. P., & Overpeck, M. D. (2001). Where children drown, United States. *Pediatrics*, 108(1), 85-89.

Buckley, M. E., Klein, D. N., Durbin, C. E., Hayden, E. P., & Moerk, K. C. (2002). Development and validation of a Q-sort procedure to assess temperament and behavior in preschool-age children. *Journal of Clinical Child & Adolescent Psychology*, 31(4), 525.

Bull, M. J., Agran, P., Laraque, D., Pollack, S. H., Smith, G. A., Spivak, H. R., et al. (2000). Reducing the number of deaths and injuries from residential fires. *American Academy of Pediatrics*, 105(6), 1355-1357.

Bush, J. S. (2003). AAP issues screening recommendations to identify hearing loss in children. *American Family Physician*, 67(11), 2409-2411.

Centers for Disease Control and Prevention's Advisory Committee on Immunization Practices. (2004). Recommended childhood and adolescent immunization schedule—United States, July-December 2004. *Morbidity and Mortality Weekly Report*, 53(16), Q1-Q3.

Cherney, I. D., Kelly-Vance, L., Glover, K. G., Ruane, A., & Ryalls, B. O. (2003). The effects of stereotyped toys and gender on play assessment in children aged 18-47 months. *Educational Psychology*, 23(1), 95-106.

Children's Hospital of Pittsburgh. (2004). Mr. Yuk poison control program. Retrieved July 29, 2004, from: *http://www.chp.edu/mryuk/05a_mryuk.php*.

Coffman, S. (2003). Bicycle injuries and safety helmets in children. *Orthopaedic Nursing*, 22(1), 9-11.

Cohen, G. J. (2002). Helping children and families deal with divorce and separation. *Pediatrics* 110(5), 1019-1023.

Crespo, C. J., & Arbesman, J. (2003). Obesity in the United States. *Physician & Sports Medicine*, 31(11), 23-29.

Cunniff, C., Frias, J. L., Kay, C. I., Moeschler, J., Panny, S. R., & Trotter, T. L. (2001). Health care supervision for children with Williams syndrome. *Pediatrics*, 107(5), 1192.

Cunningham, M., & Cox, E. O. (2003). Hearing assessment in infants and children: Recommendations beyond neonatal screening. *Pediatrics*, 111(2), 436-440.

Deal, L. (2000). Unintentional injuries in childhood: Analysis and recommendations. *The Future of Children*, 10(1), 3-188. Retrieved July 27, 2004, from: *http://www.futureofchildren.org/usr_doc/Unintentional_Injuries.pdf*.

Denham, S. A. (2002). Family routines: A structural perspective for viewing family health. *ANS Advances in Nursing Science*, 24(4), 60-75.

Denham, S. A., Blair, K. A., DeMulder, E., Levitas, J., Sawyer, K., Auerbach-Major, S. (2003). Preschool emotional competence: Pathway to social competence? *Child Development*, 74(1), 238-256.

Dennis, B. P., & Small, E. B. (2003). Incorporating cultural diversity in nursing care: An action plan. *ABNF Journal*, 14(1), 17.

Dennison, B. A., Erb, T. A., & Jenkins, P. L. (2002). Television viewing and television in bedroom associated with overweight risk among low-income preschool children. *Pediatrics*, 109(6), 1028-1035.

Elkins, M., & Cavendish, R. (2004). Developing a plan for pediatric spiritual care. *Holistic Nursing Practice*, 18(4), 179-184.

Fields, J. M., & Smith, K. E. (2004). Poverty, family structure, and child well-being: Indicators for the SIPP. Retrieved May 5, 2004, from: *http://www.census.gov/population/www/documentation/twps0023.html*.

Finitzo, T., Sininger, Y., Brookhouser, P. S., Erenberg, A., Roizen, N., Diefendorf, A. O., et al. (2000). Year 2000 position statement: Principles and guidelines for early hearing detection and intervention programs. *Pediatrics*, 106(4), 798-817.

Formicola, A. J., Ro, M., Marshall, S., Derksen, D., Powell, W., Hartsock, L., et al. (2004). Strengthening the oral health safety net: Delivery models that improve access to oral health care for uninsured and underserved populations. *American Journal of Public Health*, 94(5), 702-704.

Giami, A. (2002). Sexual health: The emergence, development, and diversity of a concept. *Annual Review of Sex Research*, 13, 1-3.

Gleason, T. R., Jarudi, R. N., & Cheek, J. M. (2003). Imagination, personality, and imaginary companions. *Social Behavior & Personality: An International Journal*, 31(7), 721-737.

Goodman, M. T., Gurney, J. G., Smith, M. A., & Olshan, A. F. (1999). *Cancer incidence and survival among children and adolescents: United States: Sympathetic nervous system tumors* (No. 99-4649 ed.). Bethesda, MD: National Cancer Institute. Retrieved July, 29, 2004, from *http://seer.cancer.gov/publications/childhood/*.

Guskiewicz, K. M. (2001). Concussion in sport: The grading-system dilemma. *Athletic Therapy Today*, 6(1), 18-27.

Haas, J. S., Lee, L. B., Kaplan, C. P., Sonneborn, D., Phillips, K. A., & Liang, S. (2003). The association of race, socioeconomic status, and health insurance status with the prevalence of overweight among children and adolescents. *American Journal of Public Health*, 93(12), 2105.

Hambrick-Dixon, P. J. (2002). The effects of exposure to physical environmental stressors on African American children: A review and research agenda. *Journal of Children & Poverty*, 8(1), 23-34.

Hess, P. D. (2003). Summer is prime time for diving injuries. *Nurse Practitioner*, 28(6), 28-32.

Hockenberry, M. J., Winkelstein, M. L., & Kline, N. E. (2003). *Wong's nursing care of infants and children* (7th ed.). St. Louis: Mosby.

Huebner, C. E. (2000). Community-based support for preschool readiness among children in poverty. *Journal of Education for Students Placed at Risk*, 5(3), 291-314.

Justice, L. M., & Pullen, P. C. (2003). Promising interventions for promoting emergent literacy skills: Three evidence-based approaches. *Topics in Early Childhood Special Education*, 23(3), 99-113.

Kalpidou, M. D., Power, T. G., Cherry, K. E., & Gottfried, N. W. (2004). Regulation of emotion and behavior among 3- and 5-year-olds. *Journal of General Psychology*, 159(2), 131-178.

Kempe, A., Beaty, B. L., Steiner, J. F., Pearson, K. A., Lowery, N. E., Daley, M. F., et al. (2004). The regional immunization registry as a public health tool for improving clinical practice and guiding immunization delivery policy. *American Journal of Public Health*, 94(6), 967-972.

Keogh, B. K. (2000). Risk, families, and schools. *Focus on Exceptional Children*, 33(4), 1.

Klein-Schwartz, W. (2003). Pediatric methylphenidate exposures: 7-Year experience of poison centers in the United States. *Clinical Pediatrics*, 42(2), 159-164.

La Paro, K. M., Pianta, R. C., & Stuhlman, M. (2004). The classroom assessment scoring system. *Elementary School Journal*, 104(5), 409-426.

Lara, M., Rosenbaum, S., Rachelefsky, G., Nicholas, W., Morton, S. C., Emont, S., et al. (2002). Improving childhood asthma outcomes in the United States: A blueprint for policy action. *Pediatrics*, 109(5), 919-924.

Lee, J. Y., Rozier, R. G., Norton, E. C., Kotch, J. B., & Vann Jr, W. F. (2004). Effects of WIC participation on children's use of oral health services. *American Journal Public Health*, 94(5), 772-777.

Liben, L. S., Bigler, R. S., & Krogh, H. R. (2002). Language at work: Children's gendered interpretations of occupational titles. *Child Development*, 73(3), 810-828.

Markos, P. A., & Lima, N. R. (2003). Homelessness in the United States and its effect on children. *Guidance & Counseling, 18*(3), 118-124.

Marston, R. (2004). An early childhood laboratory model: Kindergym. *Teaching Elementary Physical Education, 15*(2), 6-8.

McCutcheon, H., & Fitzgerald, M. (2001). The public health problems of acute respiratory illness in childcare. *Journal of Clinical Nursing, 10*(3), 305-310.

McKeever, C. K., & Schatz, P. (2003). Current issues in the identification, assessment, and management of concussions in sports-related injuries. *Applied Neuropsychology, 10*(1), 4-11.

Mehrabian, A. (2000). Beyond IQ: Broad-based measurement of individual success potential or "emotional intelligence". *Genetic, Social & General Psychology Monographs, 126*(2), 133-239.

Mendez, J. L., Fantuzzo, J., & Cicchetti, D. (2002). Profiles of social competence among low-income African American preschool children. *Child Development, 73*(4), 1085-1100.

Msall, M. E. (2002). Tools for measuring daily activities in children: Promoting independence and developing a language for child disability. *Pediatrics, 109*(2), 317-319.

National Cancer Institute. (2002). National Cancer Institute research on childhood cancers: Cancer facts. Retrieved July 29, 2004, from: *http://cis.nci.nih.gov/fact/6_40.htm.*

Orme, J. G. (2001). Foster family characteristics and behavioral and emotional problems of foster children: A narrative review. *Family Relations, 50*(1), 3.

Paulson, P. R., Hammer, A. L. (2002). Pediatric immunization update 2002. *Pediatric Nursing, 28*(2), 173-182.

Pianta, R. C., & La Paro, K. (2003). Improving early school success. *Educational Leadership, 60*(7), 24-29.

Pillay, A. L. (2003). Social competence in rural and urban children with mental retardation: Preliminary findings. *South African Journal of Psychology, 33*(3), 176-181.

Popovich, D. M. (2000). Sexuality in early childhood: Pediatric nurses' attitudes, knowledge, and clinical practice. *Pediatric Nursing, 26*(5), 484.

Racette, S. B., Deusinger, S. S., & Deusinger, R. H. (2003). Obesity: Overview of prevalence, etiology, and treatment. *Physical Therapy, 83*(3), 276.

Rao, A. B., Ranga, S. V., Sekhar, K. (2002). Divorce: Process and correlates: A cross-cultural study. *Journal of Comparative Family Studies, 33*(4), 81.

Rennels, M. B., Baker, C. J., Baltimore, R. S., Bocchini, J. A., Dennehy, P. H., Frenck, R. W., et al. (2004). Recommended childhood and adolescent immunization schedule—United States, July-December 2004. *Pediatrics, 113*(5), 1448.

Robert, D. L., & Yogue, B. (2004). Developing quality preschool movement programs: CHAOS and Kinderplay. *Teaching Elementary Physical Education, 15*(2), 9-12.

Roberts, L., Jorm, L., Patel, M., Smith, W., Douglas, R. M., & McGilchrist, C. (2000). Effect of infection control measures on the frequency of diarrheal episodes in child care: A randomized, controlled trial. *Pediatrics, 105*(4), 743-746.

Roberts, L., Smith, W., Jorm, L., Patel, M., Douglas, R. M., & McGilchrist, C. (2000). Effect of infection control measures on the frequency of upper respiratory infection in child care: A randomized, controlled trial. *Pediatrics, 105*(4), 738-742.

Rogge, M. E., & Combs-Orme, T. (2003). Protecting children from chemical exposure: Social work and U.S. social welfare policy. *Social Work, 48*(4), 439-450.

Rosenthal, J., Rodewald, L., McCauley, M., Berman, S., Irigoyen, M., Sawyer, M., et al. (2004). Immunization coverage levels among 19- to 35-month-old children in 4 diverse, medically underserved areas of the United States. *Pediatrics, 113*(4), e296-e302.

Ross, P. S., & Birnbaum, L. S. (2003). Integrated human and ecological risk assessment: A case study of persistent organic pollutants (POPs) in humans and wildlife. *Human & Ecological Risk Assessment, 9*(1), 303-324.

Roulstone, S., Peters, T. J., Glogowska, M., & Enderby, P. (2003). A 12-month follow-up of preschool children investigating the natural history of speech and language delay. *Child-Care, Health & Development, 29*(4), 245-345.

Rudisill, M. E., & Wall, S. J. (2004). Meeting active start guidelines in the ADC-motion program: Preschool. *Teaching Elementary Physical Education, 15*(2), 25-29.

Ruxton, C. (2004). Obesity in children. *Nursing Standard, 18*(20), 47-52.

Schettler, T. (2001). Toxic threats to neurologic development of children. *Environmental Health Perspectives Supplements, 109*(Suppl. 6), 813-816.

Schor, E. L., Billingsley, M. M., Golden, A. L., McMillan, J. A., Meloy, L. D., Pendarvis Jr., B. C., et al. (2003). Family pediatrics report of the Task Force on the Family. *Pediatrics, 111*(Suppl. 6), 1541-1571.

Schuster, M. A., Franke, T. M., Bastian, A. M., Sor, S., & Halfon, N. (2000). Firearm storage patterns in U.S. homes with children. *American Journal of Public Health, 90*(4), 588-594.

Sheetz, P. G., Goldman, K. M., Franks, J. C., McIntyre, L., Caroll, C. R., Gorak, D., et al. (2004). Guidelines for managing life-threatening food allergies in Massachusetts schools. *Journal of School Health, 74*(5), 155-160.

Smith, M. A., Gloeckler Ries, L. A., Gurney, J. G., & Ross, J. A. (1999). *Cancer incidence and survival among children and adolescents: United States: Leukemia* (No. 99-4649 ed.).

Bethesda, MD: National Cancer Institute. Retrieved July 29, 2004, from: *http://seer.cancer.gov/publications/childhood/.*

Taft, C. H., Mickalide, A. D., & Taft, A. R. (1999). Child passengers at risk in America: A national study of car seat misuse. Retrieved July 27, 2004, from: *http://www.safekids.org/tier3_cd.cfm?folder_id=680&content_item_id=2530.*

Taneja, V., Sriram, S., Beri, R. S., Sreenivas, V., Aggarwal, R., & Kaur, R. (2002). "Not by bread alone": Impact of a structured 90-minute play session on development of children in an orphanage. *Child-Care: Health & Development, 28*(1), 95-100.

Tung, Y., Duffy, L. C., Gyamfi, J. O., Wojtaszczyk, F., Dozier, A., Tempfer, T., et al. (2003). Improvements in immunization compliance using a computerized tracking system for inner city clinics. *Clinical Pediatrics, 42*(7), 603-611.

U.S. Census Bureau. (2003). Current population survey: Poverty: 2002 Highlights. Retrieved May 14, 2004, from: *http://www.census.gov/hhes/poverty/poverty02/pov02hi.html.*

U.S. Department of Agriculture, Center for Nutrition Policy and Promotion. (2005). *MyPyramid.* Retrieved May 31, 2005, from *http://mypyramid.gov.*

U.S. Department of Health and Human Services. (2000). *Healthy people 2010: Understanding and improving health* (Government Rep. No. 017-001-001-00-550-9). Washington, DC: U.S. Government Printing Office, Superintendent of Documents.

U.S. Department of Health and Human Services. (2001). *The surgeon general's call to action to prevent and decrease overweight and obesity* (Government Report No. 02NLM:WD 210 59593 2001). Washington, DC: U.S. Department of Health and Human Services, Public Health Service, Office of the Surgeon General.

University of Pittsburgh. (2004). Child health library: Common childhood injuries and poisonings. Retrieved July 29, 2004, from: *http://www.chp.edu/greystone/poison/chilprof.php.*

Van Bever, H. P., Desager, K. N., & Hagendorens, M. (2002). Critical evaluation of prognostic factors in childhood asthma. *Pediatric Allergy & Immunology, 13*(2), 77-83.

Vygotsky, L. S. (2004). Imagination and creativity in childhood. *Journal of Russian & East European Psychology, 42*(1), 7-97.

Watamura, S. E., Donzella, B., Alwin, J., & Gunnar, M. R. (2003). Morning-to-afternoon increases in cortisol concentrations for infants and toddlers at child care: Age differences and behavioral correlates. *Child Development, 74*(4), 1006-1010.

Wertlieb, D. (2003). Converging trends in family research and pediatrics: Recent findings for the American Academy of Pediatrics Task Force on the Family. *Pediatrics, 111*(6), 1572-1587.

Woo, E. J., Ball, R., Bostrom, A., Shadomy, S. V., Ball, L. K., Evans, G., et al. (2004). Vaccine risk perception among reporters of autism after vaccination: Vaccine adverse event reporting system 1990-2001. *American Journal of Public Health, 94*(6), 990-995.

Wood, R. A. (2003). The natural history of food allergy. *Pediatrics, 111*(6), 1631-1637.

Xu, Y., Crane, P., & Ryan, R. (2002). School nursing in an underserved multiethnic Asian community: Experiences and out-comes. *Journal of Community Health Nursing 19*(3), 187.

Yackel, E. E. (2003). An activity calendar program for children who are overweight. *Pediatric Nursing, 29*(1), 17.

Yaden Jr., D. B., & Tardibuono, J. M. (2004). The emergent writing development of urban Latino preschoolers and instruc-tional environments for second-language learners. *Reading & Writing Quarterly, 20*(1), 29-61.

Yeung, W. J., Linver, M. R., & Brooks-Gunn, J. (2002). How money matters for young children's development: Parental invest-ment and family processes. *Child Develop-ment, 73*(6), 1861-1879.

Young, J. L., Smith, M. A., Roffers, S. D., Liff, J. M., & Bunin, G. R. (1999). *Cancer incidence and survival among children and adolescents: United States: Retinoblastoma* (No. 99-4649 ed.). Bethesda, MD: National Cancer Institute. Retrieved July 29, 2004, from: *http://seer.cancer.gov/publi-cations/childhood/*.

Zgaljardic, D. J., & Benedict, R. H. B. (2001). Evaluation of practice effects in language and spatial processing test performance. *Applied Neuropsychology, 8*(4), 218-223.

Chapter 20

CAROLYN SPENCE CAGLE

School-Age Child

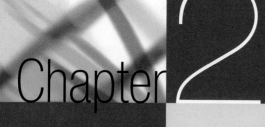

objectives

After completing this chapter, the reader will be able to:

- Discuss expected variation in physical changes occurring in the school-age child.

- Screen the school-age child for health risk factors and relevant health-promotion needs.

- Discuss with families some of the common developmental problems that occur in school-age children.

- Describe the school-age child's cognitive stage of development relative to academic skills.

- Discuss with parents ways to improve child self-concept and decrease stress in the school-age child.

- Analyze the needs for and influence of peer relationships on development of the school-age child.

- Discuss cultural and societal influences, including affluence and poverty, on the school-age child.

key terms

Achievement tests
Astigmatism
Attention-deficit/hyperactivity disorder
Braces
Caries
Chronic serous otitis media
Concrete operations
Conservation
Conventional level
Coping strategies
Depression
Dyslexia
Encopresis
Enuresis
External locus of control
Hyperopic (farsighted)

Industry versus inferiority
Intelligence
Intelligence quotient
Internal locus of control
Learning disabilities
Limit setting
Malocclusion
Menarche
Myopia (nearsightedness)
Ossification
Peabody Picture Vocabulary Test
Pediculosis
Peer group
Phonics
Positive reinforcement
Preconventional level

Puberty
Public Law 94-142
Punishment
Rehearsal
Self-esteem
Semantics
Sexual abuse
Sleep talking
Sleepwalking
Socialization
Somatization
Stanford-Binet Test
Syntax
Tympanograms
Wechsler Series

Homework Procrastination

Sally Paul, 9 years of age, has shown a pattern of homework procrastination since the third grade. She has performed reasonably well in school, primarily because of the pressure from her parents to complete her homework and other projects. This pressure has created an intense home environment that has left Sally and her parents feeling frustrated about her ownership of the problem.

Sally says, on occasion, that she has no homework because she finished it at school. She is active, wants to go outside to play after school when the weather is good, and must be encouraged to finish her homework completely and neatly after dinner. Her parents, both employed full-time outside the home, often help Sally complete a project because she whines that she "can't do it." This collaboration helps Sally, but leaves her parents wondering who did the work, and decreases the time her parents have to finish their own work in the evenings.

1 Is Sally's behavior typical for a 9-year-old child?

2 Discuss the values inherent in Sally's and her parents' behavior and how these might be related to the scenario as described.

3 How might you, as the health care professional, guide this family in finding ways to increase Sally's ownership of the homework duty and the quality of her work and thus decrease family stress? These ways might include structuring the homework environment, timing the homework, defining the value of homework, and supporting parent and child needs.

4 How might a behavior contract be used effectively in improving homework completion?

The school-age years, ages 6 to 12 years, frequently define a period of calm before the storm of adolescence. Dramatic changes occur during this period, when one compares the size and skills of a beginning school-age child with those of one entering adolescence. The former grows more slowly in height and weight than in infancy and adolescence, but growth occurs at a steady pace. The child develops new motor skills and perfects them through practice. Mental abilities grow remarkably as the child learns to read, write, and understand mathematics and other academic subjects. As motor and mental abilities develop through exposure to school and peer relationships, a sense of competence develops. Competency also develops with a child's emotional connections to peers and others outside the family.

For most people, the school-age years are the healthiest time of their lives. Children ages 6 to 12 years recover from injury or infection rapidly and relatively completely. Their energy level is high and appears infinite as they socialize and learn. Nursing interventions in a variety of settings and in collaboration with a variety of groups will facilitate school-age children's eventual attainment of adult health and productivity.

AGE AND PHYSICAL CHANGES

Compared with the preschool child, the school-age child has an overall slimmer shape and longer legs relative to the rest of the body. From age 7 years to **puberty,** a time during which each gender becomes capable of sexual reproduction, the child gradually reaccumulates fat and distributes it throughout the body (Wong, Perry, & Hockenberry, 2002). The child gains an average of 3 kilograms (6 pounds) and 6 centimeters (2 inches) per year. However, many children have "spurts" of growth alternating with periods of minimal growth. During these years, girls and boys are similar in size. Black school-age children tend to be somewhat larger and Asian American children somewhat smaller than white children, as plotted on child growth curves believed reliable for various ethnic backgrounds (Jarvis, 2000; Wong et al., 2002).

Children's growth reflects their genetic inheritance and the sociocultural environment in which they live. Growth changes include lengthening legs, a lower center of gravity, and improved posture, allowing school-age children to effectively ride bikes, climb, and engage in other physical activity (Wong et al., 2002). A preadolescent increase in height and weight tends to occur in girls around age 10 and boys around age 12 (Wong et al., 1999). Many girls tower over their male classmates during this time. However, some late-maturing girls do not begin this growth spurt until ages 12 to 14, and early-maturing boys may enter this growth stage at age 10. Thus a classroom of children 10 to 12 years old has a wide range of sizes of both genders. The average 12-year-old child stands 59 inches tall and weighs about 88 pounds (Wong et al., 2002).

The child's head continues to grow, but at a much slower rate than in the preschooler. After age 5 the head circumference grows only minimally until puberty, when the head and brain reach adult circumference of about 53 or 54 centimeters (21 inches) (Wong et al., 2002). The child's hair often darkens and skin matures and becomes less sensitive, approaching adult appearance and texture. Little sebum and eccrine sweat production occurs throughout childhood.

Most body systems reach an adult level of function during this age if they have not already done so. The gastrointestinal system matures, and the child shows the ability to eat adult foods on a schedule similar to that of an adult, with fewer needs for snacks. By puberty, all endocrine functions, except those regulating reproduction, approach adult capacity. Differences may occur in lung capacity due to a child's size, but most children have slower, more regular, and deeper respirations than when they were preschoolers. The child may have more sinus infections and headaches related to allergies (Schulte, Price, & Gwin, 2001). The heart increases in size, and the heart rate slows to an average rate of 70 to 100 beats per minute, approaching that of an adult. Mean blood pressure, however, is lower in this age group than in adults and ranges from 96 to 107 mm Hg systolic and from 57 to 66 mm Hg diastolic (Schulte et al., 2001).

The long-term effects of hypertension in adults are well known. The realization that adult hypertension begins during childhood has encouraged efforts to screen young children for elevated blood pressure (BP) values. Both the American Academy of Pediatrics (2004) and the American Heart Association (2005) recommend that children have their BP measured and plotted yearly, beginning at 3 years of age, because of increasing concerns about higher BP values in children over the past 15 years that may indicate potential cardiovascular disease. BP values among school-age children may vary greatly. See **Web Site Resource 20A** for detailed tables of BP levels for girls and boys according to height and weight. Black children should be followed closely, because hypertension occurs earlier with more organ damage than in white, Hispanic, or Native American children (American Heart Association, 2005; Saunders, 1995). A family history of elevated BP or identification of elevated BP in a child mandates close monitoring and assessment

of cardiovascular risk factors during well-child checkups during the school-age years (Schulte et al., 2001). If a child is tall and lean or weight is proportional to height, then a higher than average reading can be normal (Sadowski & Faulkner, 1996).

Although the school-age child experiences many physical changes before adolescence, changes in the three physical areas of oral development, lymphoid tissues, and motor skills are particularly noteworthy.

The school-age child appears to be constantly losing or gaining a tooth. The first permanent teeth, the 6-year molars, erupt first, followed by the loss of the deciduous (baby) teeth, usually in the same order in which they erupted. Figure 20-1 shows deciduous teeth and the 32 adult teeth and their average time of appearance. The child between ages 6 and 13 loses and gains approximately four teeth per year. A 13-year-old child should have 28 teeth, having lost 20 deciduous teeth (Wong et al., 2002). When deciduous teeth come out, only the crown is lost; the root has been reabsorbed in the developing permanent tooth. As

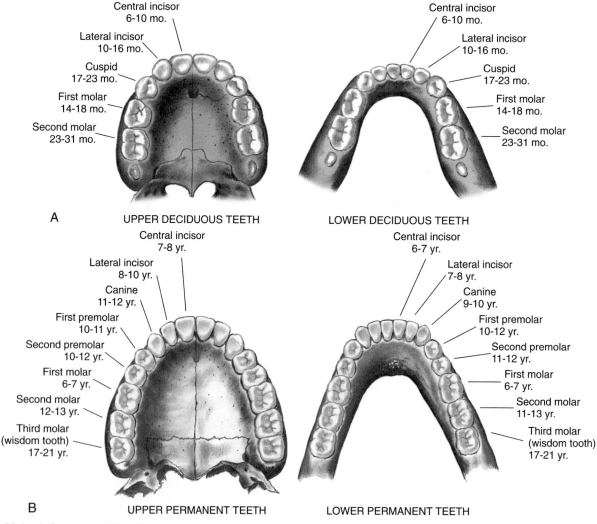

Figure 20-1 **A,** Development of deciduous teeth and their sequence of eruption, **B,** Development of permanent teeth and their sequence of eruption. (From Seidel, H. M., Ball, J. W., Dains, J. E., & Benedict, G. W. [2003]. *Mosby's guide to physical examinations* [5th ed.]. St. Louis: Mosby.)

the child's mouth becomes filled with the larger, permanent teeth, the shape of the jaw and the facial appearance normally change. Girls tend to experience earlier permanent tooth eruption than do boys.

Dental problems, primarily **caries** (cavities), periodontal disease, and malocclusion, are among the most common health problems in school-age children today. Present in over one half of second graders (U.S. Department of Health and Human Services [USDHHS], 2000), caries occur more frequently in poor and ethnically diverse children and those who lack insurance or access to preventive dental care. The rapid change in the number and type of teeth and the uneven growth in the child's jaw may cause **malocclusion,** an unacceptable relationship of the teeth in one jaw to those in the other. A dentist should evaluate children with overbites, gaps between teeth, and other alignment problems that may influence speech and eating. Some children will grow out of these problems, but others may need orthodontic care and appliances (**braces**) to correct problems or improve their appearance. Peer reaction to braces should be addressed as part of the teaching about body changes; this teaching may decrease problems with the child's self-concept or body image as a result of looking different. School dental programs should include education about conscientious tooth care for the child who wears braces, because these frequently make brushing and flossing more difficult, especially for the school-age child who lacks manual dexterity (Box 20-1).

Lymph tissue grows rapidly throughout childhood, reaching maximum size before puberty, after which it begins to decrease in size, most likely due to sex hormones. The amount of lymphoid tissue of a 12-year-old child often exceeds that of an adult (Jarvis, 2000), most often reflected in the size of the tonsils. What appears pathologically enlarged to a parent can be normal for the child's age. Additional lymphoid tissue during the school-age period generally helps this group to have a stronger immune response than do younger and older children (Wilson, Lewis, & Penix, 1996).

Neurological, skeletal, and muscular changes combine to increase the child's overall motor abilities. With maturation of the nervous system by age 7 or 8 years, the brain's two hemispheres articulate to allow the child more control over and coordination with motor tasks (Behrman, Kliegman, & Jenson, 2000; Wong et al., 2002). The child grows taller because of lengthening of the long bones that continues into adolescence. **Ossification,** replacement of cartilage with bone, occurs throughout childhood but is not complete until adulthood. Therefore special attention must be paid to well-fitting shoes, appropriately sized chairs and desks, and backpack loads, to avoid strain on an evolving musculoskeletal system. Children at this age also need protective sports equipment and conditioning exercises before sports to prevent sports fractures. However, the child constantly builds new bony tissue during the entire period of childhood, which generally allows for rapid healing of fractures.

Box 20-1 Dental Health Education

The nurse can implement a school dental educational program by encouraging the following behavior by the school-age child and family:
1. Teach children responsibility for brushing and flossing teeth at least twice a day; use pamphlets from the ADA and state dental societies to teach appropriate brushing and flossing of teeth; utilize local dentists to teach children about dental health and provide brushing resources as part of this teaching.
2. Encourage daily use of fluoride to protect the teeth (e.g., fluoridated toothpaste, rinses, and water).
3. Encourage replacement of personal toothbrushes every 3 months.
4. Use a toothbrush with a straight handle, flat brushing surface, and soft, rounded bristles for teeth and braces; help children less than 8 years to brush teeth; assist children younger than 10 years to brush back teeth (Wong & Hess, 2000; Wong, Perry, & Hockenberry, 2002).
5. Occasionally offer an electric or battery-operated toothbrush to make brushing fun and encourage more frequent and better brushing.
6. Assess children's teeth frequently to ensure successful brushing; parents or health care providers may have children use disclosing tablets to detail areas that need better brushing.
7. Encourage dental visits every 6 months for preventive care (radiographs, sealants).
8. When tooth brushing cannot occur after meals, encourage children to rinse their mouths with water to help clean the teeth.
9. Encourage a low-sugar diet and healthy snacks for dental health; discourage soft drink consumption at home and school.

Wong, D. L., & Hess, C. S. (2000). *Wong and Whaley's clinical manual of pediatric nursing* (5th ed., pp. 132-133). St. Louis: Mosby; Wong, D. L., Perry, S. E., & Hockenberry, M. J. (2002). *Maternal child nursing* (2nd ed.). St. Louis: Mosby.
ADA, American Dental Association.

Muscle mass also increases with muscle strength. During the school-age years, physically active boys are slightly stronger than girls, but this difference is not significant until adolescence. With these changes, the child has the potential to perform more complex fine motor and gross motor functions but must practice to perfect these skills (Table 20-1). Children willingly exercise their newfound skills and feel pride when others see their improved skill level when bike riding, tying shoes, and engaging in team sports.

Gender

Girls tend to mature, enter puberty, and stop growing earlier than do boys. Overall, girls' physical growth is more regular, with fewer spurts and plateaus than boys have. Girls' teeth erupt sooner, and their bones ossify sooner. From birth, girls have more fat than boys, and after puberty they have a greater percentage of body weight devoted to fat. Most physical differences between boys and girls become more evident after puberty. Toward the end of the school-age period for

Table **20-1** Motor Development of the School-Age Child

Age (Years)	Gross Motor	Fine Motor
6 to 7	Balances on one foot for 10 seconds Can perform tandem gait Hops 25 times on one foot, 12 times on the other Pedals a bicycle	Spreads with knife Holds pencil with fingertip Draws a person with 3 to 6 parts Cuts with a knife Aligns letters horizontally Ties a bow Draws a triangle Knows right from left
8 to 9	Has good body balance Enjoys vigorous activities Throws objects farther	Spaces words and letters with writing Draws a diamond Draws a 3-dimensional geometric figure Has good eye-hand coordination Bathes self Sews and builds models
10 to 12	Balances on one foot for 15 seconds Catches a fly ball Has some awkwardness because of prepubertal growth spurt Possesses all basic motor skills	Has skills similar to those of an adult

most children, these physical differences related to maturation involve the development of sexual characteristics.

Discussion of two other areas of difference in the genders appears later in this chapter. First, girls tend to mature faster than do boys in psychological and physical processes. Many psychological processes, such as cognitive abilities and language skills, depend primarily on physical maturation of the nervous system. Second, boys tend to have certain problems, such as enuresis, encopresis, learning disabilities, and other school difficulties, more frequently than girls.

Race

Black and Asian American children mature earlier than do white children in dental development and onset of the **menarche**, the advent of monthly bleeding or menses. As a rule, black children are somewhat heavier and taller than white children during the school-age period. Blacks also have longer and more dense bones than do white and Asian American children (Garn, Pao, & Rihl, 1964; Jarvis, 2000) and tend to have slimmer hips, more muscle, and less fat on their limbs than on their central body as compared with whites (Jarvis, 2000). Most likely, physical differences among white, black, and Asian American children relate to racial characteristics and the socioeconomic climates in which these groups live. Although differences may be attributed primarily to race, poverty probably influences the physical development of black children and an increasing number of Hispanic children. Certainly not all blacks are poor, but the number of poor blacks in proportion to the overall number of blacks is greater than the same ratio in whites (USDHHS, 2000).

Limited data exist in defining factors related to physical differences in Asian American children as compared with white children. Asian American children may be geneti-

cally programmed to be smaller than children of other cultures. However, many Asian American children grow larger than their parents because of better nutrition and resources available in the United States today. However, Asian refugee groups new to the United States often have inadequate socioeconomic resources, exposing these children to malnutrition, overcrowded housing, school challenges, and health problems based on poor access to health care. All of these factors influence their future health and societal productivity.

Genetics

School-age children tend to be concerned about their rate of growth, weight, time of menarche, and final height. They need to understand that the timing and extent of their physical changes usually reflect their genetic inheritance. When assessing a child's height and weight and before referring to standardized growth charts, the nurse should examine the family. For example, the child whose height is in the third percentile may have parents who are shorter than average. Shorter height can be expected because of the family's genetic make-up. Likewise, although the average age of menarche is around 12.8 years, most girls experience their menarche at about the same age their mothers did. With sufficient body fat to stimulate hormones needed for menses, girls can have their first menstrual period between ages 11 and 15 and still be considered normal (Wong et al., 2002). Due to better nutrition and differences in lifestyle, girls appear to experience menarche earlier than did girls of 30 years ago.

Most acute, life-threatening diseases of a hereditary nature become evident before the school-age years. However, some inherited health problems become more difficult to manage during the school-age years (e.g., sickle cell

Physical Activity Among American Indian Children

The purpose of this study was to assess dietary and physical activity behaviors of American Indian children to identify factors that would support interventions for an obesity prevention program. A formative assessment was carried out in nine schools from seven participating tribal groups in three states of the United States. Participants included school-age children in third and fifth grades, child caregivers, and school personnel. Various groups participated in different data collection strategies, including direct observation, child-paired interviews, focus groups, and completion of two quantitative tools. Adherence to human subject requirements occurred in the study. Relevant quantitative and qualitative data analysis produced findings. Participants identified that most schools had a gymnasium or large room for exercise, but inconsistent or infrequent exercise occurred there, because other school activities mandated use of these rooms. Although both parents and students supported the need to increase children's physical exercise to improve their overall health, few parents modeled the behavior due to work and fatigue issues. Most participants identified that unsafe and incompatible environments for exercise prevented outdoor exercise at home. Most students rode a bus to school, so after-school on-campus exercise time was not an option. Assessment of these findings from a variety of stakeholders in the school and community assisted the study authors in defining a strong foundation for an obesity prevention program (Pathways) as part of a health-promotion approach for elementary school students.

Data from Thompson, J. L., Davis, S. M., Gittelsohn, J., Going, S., Becenti, A., Metcalfe, L., et al. (2001). Patterns of physical activity among American Indian children: An assessment of barriers and support. *Journal of Community Health, 26,* 423-445.

disease in African Americans, cystic fibrosis in whites, and lactose intolerance in South Europeans, Arabian and Jewish people, African Americans, and Native Americans) (Wong et al., 2002). Environmental influences may also contribute to diseases believed to have a genetic component. These conditions include obesity, cardiovascular disease, learning problems, and enuresis (Research Highlights box).

GORDON'S FUNCTIONAL HEALTH PATTERNS

Health Perception–Health Management Pattern

The school-age child understands an abstract definition of health and sometimes the factors causing illness, but this understanding differs from that of an adult. Most school-age children perceive symptoms and show an ability to participate in health-promoting behaviors if taught in school and at home ways to prevent illness and stay healthy. Effective health-promotion teaching meets the preschool and school-age child's cognitive level (concrete operations) and moral level (external rules and forces). Teaching strategies using cognitive, psychomotor, and affective senses can help children learn responsibility for their own health. This knowledge may provide an excellent foundation for health-promotion behaviors during the school years.

School-age children, when asked about their ideas on causes of illness, usually state the germ theory, the punishment theory, or the external forces theory. Although many younger school-age children know that germs play a role in illness, they have limited understanding of how germs work. They may believe that a misdeed or misbehavior caused their illnesses. They may also believe that outside elements or people cause illness, such as "the rain gives you a cold." The Haitian culture teaches children that people become ill when they show jealousy, hate, or envy toward another (Schantz, Charron, & Folden, 2003), and black and Native American people may believe a dirty living environment and not eating blackstrap molasses each day will cause illness. Hispanics may believe that illness results when a stranger casts an "evil eye" on a person (Spector, 2004). Thus it is important to consider cultural as well as developmental beliefs of the school-age child in defining strategies for teaching health promotion.

School-age children face challenges in meeting health-promotion goals as defined by *Healthy People 2010*. The *Healthy People 2010* box presents selected objectives related to this age group. However, people in the school-age child's life can facilitate societal attainment of these goals. Parents, caregivers, and teachers teach health-promotion concepts when they spend time monitoring and reinforcing preventive health practices, such as personal hygiene, dental care, and good nutrition. Role playing, reading an age-appropriate book, and modeling of health-promotion behaviors (e.g., washing hands) also may help children make the link between behavior and improved health. Unfortunately, by imitating some caregivers children can become passive health care consumers, asking few questions, doing as they are told, and perpetuating poor choices. This response may also be caused by children's cultural obligation to obey authority figures and partly because many adults who mentor children are not assertive health care consumers. Parents, caregivers, and teachers must make a commitment to demonstrate and teach healthy behaviors at home and in school; this helps children develop health values as part of their educational process toward reaching a healthy adulthood (Cagle & Keen-Payne, 1996; Lozano, 2004).

Counseling the child and family on a broad definition of health, one that includes personal and environmental health and safety, requires an awareness of the school-age child's normal perceptions of health. The nurse, in consultation with teachers, might include the following content areas to support this broader definition: cultural definitions of causes and management of illness as part of regular academic subjects, causes of personal and environmental problems as a foundation for teaching prevention, critical issues affecting children's health (e.g., backpack safety) (Goodgold & Nielsen, 2003), and advocacy skills of assertive health care consumers.

Healthy People 2010
Selected National Health-Promotion and Disease Prevention Objectives for School-Age Children

- Reduce proportion of children and adolescents who experience dental caries in their primary or permanent teeth to 42% for all children in 2010 (baseline is 52% of children ages 6 to 8 from 1988 to 1994).

Special Population Targets

Dental Caries Prevalence	1999 Baseline
Native American–Alaska Native	90%
Asian American–Pacific Islander*	90%
Black	50%
White	51%
Mexican American	68%

*1993 to 1994 baseline.

- Reduce untreated dental caries such that the proportion of children who have them (in permanent or primary teeth) is no more than 21% among all children ages 6 through 8 and no more than 15% among adolescents age 15 (baseline is 29% of children ages 6 to 8 from 1988 to 1994; 20% of adolescents age 15 from 1988 to 1994).

Special Population Targets

Untreated Dental Caries	1988 to 1994
Children ages 6 to 8 whose parents have less than a high school education	44%
Native American–Alaska Native (ages 6 to 8)	69%
Black (ages 6 to 8)	36%
Mexican American (ages 6 to 8)	43%

- Increase the proportion of children who have received protective sealants on surfaces of molar teeth to at least 50% (baseline is 23% of children age 8 and 15% of adolescents age 14 from 1988 to 1994).
- Reduce physician visits for otitis media among children and adolescents to 294 in 1000 visits (baseline is 344.7 in 1000 visits in 1997).
- Reduce the proportion of children and adolescents regularly exposed to tobacco smoke at home to 10% (baseline is 27% of children 6 years and younger in 1994).
- Increase the proportion of people age 2 and older who consume less than 10% of their calories from saturated fat to 75% (baseline is 36% of all children from 1994 to 1996).

Special Population Targets

Saturated Fat Consumption	1994 to 1996
Hispanic-Latino	39%
Mexican American	37%
Black	31%
White	35%

- Reduce the number of asthma deaths among children ages 5 to 14 years to 1% (baseline is 3.3% in 1998) (rate per million).

Special Population Targets

	In 1998
Black	9.7
White	2.0

- Increase the proportion of the nation's public and private schools that require daily physical education for all middle and junior high students to 25% (baseline is 17% in 1994).
- Reduce the proportion of children and adolescents ages 6 to 11 years who are overweight or obese (defined as at or above gender-specific and age-specific 95th percentile) to 5% (baseline is 11% from 1988 to 1994).
- Decrease the incidence of maltreatment of children under age 18 to less than 11.1 per 1000 (baseline is 13.9 per 1000 in 1997).
- Increase the proportion of children and adolescents who view television 2 or fewer hours a day to 75% (baseline is 60% of children ages 8 to 16 years from 1988 to 1994).
- Increase the use of helmets by motorcyclists and passengers to at least 79% (baseline is 67% of motorcyclists and passengers in 1997).
- Reduce deaths caused by motor vehicle crashes to no more than 9.2 per 100,000 people (baseline is 15.6 per 100,000 people (age adjusted) to the year 2000 standard population).

Special Population Targets

Deaths from Motor Vehicle Crashes	1998
Children 14 years and younger	4.4

From U.S. Department of Health and Human Services. (2000). *Healthy People 2010*: Vols. 1 and 2 (Conference ed.). Washington, DC: U.S. Government Printing Office.

Nutritional-Metabolic Pattern

School-age children, like all children, need a well-balanced diet. An average of 2200 to 2400 calories per day meets growth requirements (Consumer Information Center, 2004). Usually these calories are consumed in three daily meals and one or two snacks. School-age children often eat less-than-healthy foods and snacks, foods low in iron and vitamin C, and foods that have a higher fat content than food their parents ate when they were this age. These behaviors place children at risk for poor nutritional habits, iron deficiency anemia, and chronic illnesses such as diabetes and hypertension (USDHHS, 2000).

Factors Influencing Food Intake

Mass media and contemporary busy lifestyles play a role in poor food choices, as well. A multitude of television and billboard messages pressure children to eat certain foods, many of which contain large amounts of salt, sugar, and calories. Frequent and lengthy watching of television has been linked to childhood obesity (Proctor et al., 2003). Working parents spend 40% of their budget on dining outside the home, a behavior that contributes to more "fast food" consumption and food of poor nutritional quality (USDHHS, 2000). Healthy food costs more than unhealthy food, and some cultures value food that has high salt and fat content. These factors also influence poor nutrition among the homeless and children in child-care centers and contribute to the high level of obesity, especially among Hispanic, black, and Native American children. These groups often lack access to safe and nutritious food, causing undernutrition, growth retardation, and iron deficiency anemia (USDHHS, 2000). Thus, successful interventions for school-age obesity must focus on economic, social, and cultural factors that influence access to and use of food (See Research Highlights box).

Although some school-age children willingly try new foods, many continue to dislike vegetables, fruits, casseroles, spicy foods, and iron-rich foods and prefer a small range of foods. Some children may eat only raw vegetables and fruits and go through a phase of eating only one food at lunch, such as a peanut butter sandwich. These practices seldom hurt the child nutritionally. Children frequently make their own after-school snacks and need supervision regarding the content. Foods high in vitamins A and C, fruits, and vegetables should be encouraged daily. With parental, caregiver, or teacher help and positive reinforcement, school-age children can learn to calculate nutrition needs, plan family meals, and eat better for their overall health. These activities also assist school-age children in fostering wise decision-making practices, math skills, feelings of empowerment about health, and healthy food habits for the rest of their lives.

American families have such busy lives that they eat few meals together. Therefore, a positive environment for nutrition and socialization during shared time is important. Parents should encourage positive food habits for each family member, and pressure to eat certain foods should be avoided to prevent power struggles between parent or caregiver and child. A child's nutritional pattern usually reflects family patterns. For example, parents who skip breakfast tend to have trouble convincing their children to eat breakfast. Educating children as a group to eat healthy foods can be successful because of the powerful influence of a **peer group** (people of the same age, experience, and usually gender). The child whose friend is eating a candy bar usually prefers the same rather than an apple for a snack.

Despite evidence that the school can serve as an environment for nutritional health-promotion education (Wong, Perry, & Hockenberry, 2002), not all schools require nutrition education from kindergarten through twelfth grade. Nutrition education, as part of core concepts usually taught in school, could teach students about choices related to weight control and health and help them understand the role of media and culture in nutritional choices. Various Web sites exist to teach children about good nutrition, one of which is KidsHealth at *http://www.kidshealth. org*. Schools that offer nutritious foods that reflect various cultures adhere to principles of the Food Guide Pyramid (Consumer Information Center, 2004; U.S. Department of Agriculture, 1992). The Food Guide Pyramid was replaced in April 2005 by the MyPyramid food guidance system (USDA/CNPP, 2005). These schools may also discourage student use of vending machines that provide "empty calories," foods high in calories and low in nutritional value. Teachers should also serve as role models for optimal eating and exercise habits for children in their charge. Lunch programs exist in most schools and meet guidelines established by the U.S. Department of Agriculture (1992). Many of these programs continue during the summer when school is out of session to support 2 million children's needs for quality food intake (Smith, 2004).

The daily nutritional needs of a child who is 9 to 13 years old include the following (Figure 20-2):

1. Milk group: 2 servings (total of 16 ounces) of unflavored low-fat milk, skim milk, or buttermilk (whole milk or flavored milk may be offered as a substitute, but low-fat milk must be offered)
2. Meat group: 2 servings (total of 4 ounces) of protein-rich canned or cooked meat, fish, tofu, or poultry; 1 egg; 1 cup cooked dry peas or beans; 4 tablespoons of peanut butter; or equivalent combinations of these foods
3. Vegetable and fruit group: 6 to 7 servings (2 cups of vegetables and $1\frac{1}{2}$ cups of fruit)
4. Grain group: 6 to 7 servings (total of 6 to 7 bread slices) of bread or a bread substitute made with enriched flour (Wong & Hess, 2000)

Obesity

Obesity is a major nutrition problem among adults and children in the United States. This problem has increased over the last 40 years, with 11% to 30% of children ages 6 to 19 years estimated as obese (weight above the 95th percentile for height) (Moran, 1999; USDHHS, 2000). Evidence suggests that adult obesity begins in infancy or childhood and

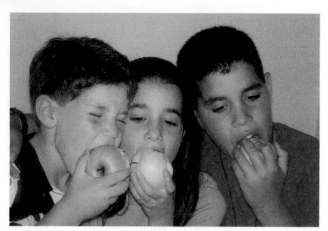

Figure 20-2 Children 9 to 13 years old should eat two or more portions of vegetables and fruit totaling 3 to 4 cups daily.

| Box **20-2** | Nursing Interventions to Prevent Obesity During the School-Age Period |

- Encourage parents to evaluate their cultural nutrition values, patterns, and choices and improve these as needed; encourage parents to consider ways other than food for rewarding child for positive behaviors.
- Discourage eating when watching television.
- Encourage parents to assess snacking habits and change those to improve eating choices and habits for family members.
- Encourage child to engage in daily exercise with family unit and a variety of exercise each week; encourage neighborhood physical activity games to improve neighborhood health and build community relationships.
- Encourage family to assess "fast food" eating habits and develop habits to support a healthier diet as defined by the Food Pyramid (low fat and cholesterol, protein and milk products, whole grains, fruits and vegetables, and fewer sweets and salty foods).
- Encourage parents to balance healthy food intake with ethnic food choices over time.
- Encourage child to occasionally prepare meals of his or her choosing that meet requirements of the Food Pyramid.
- Incorporate discussions of healthy food into daily school life; support lunch choices that meet overall healthy nutritional intake.

results from both genetic and environmental factors. For example, a child whose overweight parents constantly use food as a reward faces a greater risk for obesity than does a child of thin parents who do not reward with food. Excessive food intake and lack of physical activity also cause obesity, and once overweight these children tend to exercise even less. A recent study showed that in an ethnically diverse population, 22% of fourth graders and 16% of eleventh graders in Texas were overweight (Lozano, 2004). Obesity tends to occur more in black and Hispanic children than in white children (15%, 17%, and 11%, respectively) (USDHHS, 2000). Obesity increases the risk of hypertension, diabetes, and heart disease. These higher obesity rates may reflect less physical activity of black and Hispanic children due to living conditions and an inability to purchase higher cost healthy food choices (USDHHS, 2000).

The obese child faces ridicule by peers and discrimination later in life. These responses reinforce an already low self-esteem and poor body image and cause a cycle of personal isolation that influences a child's success, current and future. Helping the obese child change lifestyle patterns requires intensive intervention, including support of parents and teachers. Even with such work, few overweight children achieve or maintain significant weight loss because of the complexity of factors (environmental, cultural, economic, and psychological) involved (Wong et al., 2002). Some success has been achieved by programs that include reasonable caloric restriction, eating a variety of low-fat and low-cholesterol foods, diet support groups, physical exercise, peer counseling groups, and habit changes (American Dietetic Association & HealthLink, n.d.). However, intervention sometimes fails because some school-age children do not show concern about being overweight. Nursing suggestions for parents who are interested in preventing obesity in their school-age children appear in Box 20-2. With more school-age children accessing the Internet, child-friendly sites such as HealthLink (*http://www.healthlink.com*) and keepkidshealthy.com (*http://www.keepkidshealthy.com*) may help children focus on ways to improve their nutrition and avoid obesity.

Elimination Pattern

Most children have full bowel and bladder control by 5 years of age. Control involves the ability to undress and dress and to wipe, flush, and clean hands. The child's elimination patterns are similar to the adult's, with urination occurring 6 to 8 times a day and bowel movements averaging 1 or 2 times a day (Wong et al., 2002). For some school-age children, however, elimination continues to be a problem. White children generally assume earlier control of their elimination habits than do black children, likely based on cultural beliefs about appropriate timing for this type of control.

Enuresis

Involuntary urination at an age when control should be present is called **enuresis**. Children with primary enuresis have never achieved bladder control, and those with secondary enuresis have periods of dryness and recurrent enuresis. Involuntary nocturnal urination (bedwetting) that occurs at least once a month is defined as *nocturnal enuresis*, and wetting during the day has been termed *diurnal enuresis*. Enuresis should not be considered a disease but a variation of normal development. For example, boys and children who were born prematurely experience higher rates of nocturnal enuresis than do girls and children who were born at term (Wong et al., 2002).

Nocturnal enuresis causes disruption for both child and family. The child frequently experiences teasing from classmates and siblings. A night away from home appears impossible because of fear of wetting. Parents may be angry about the frequent bed changes and washes and may try punishments, thinking that the child should be able to control the problem. Parents and caregivers may even become abusive (Wong et al., 2002). Parental stress places additional pressure on the child, who may already have low self-esteem and lack self-confidence due to perceived inability to control the problem.

Often because they lack information, frustrated families seek help. In addition to providing information, the nurse provides active support to facilitate coping. **Web Site Resource 20B** presents helpful information for parents about nocturnal enuresis. If a child does not have a urinary tract infection, various forms of management may be considered. These include wet alarm systems, bladder training and retention control, waking schedules, drug therapy, and hormone therapy. Each method has advantages, disadvantages, and cost considerations, but all require consistency and time from the child and parents, as well as positive reinforcement by the parents, to reach a successful outcome.

Diurnal enuresis is often called *daytime dribbling.* This term describes a urinary pattern most often seen in school-age girls. These children demonstrate "holding on" behaviors, including not voiding first thing in the morning, voiding only 2 or 3 times a day, and voiding exceptionally quickly. It is not clear why children delay urination or empty their bladders only partially, thus promoting overflow incontinence. Evaluation of these children begins with a urine culture to rule out urinary tract infection. If no infection exists or symptoms persist after treatment, then the intervention is focused on increasing fluid intake to prevent "holding" and establishing a voiding routine of every 2 hours, with a conscious effort to empty the bladder completely. The nurse can be instrumental in helping the child and parents understand the problem and its management.

Encopresis

Another elimination problem that may occur in children is **encopresis,** defined as the persistent voluntary or involuntary passing of stool into the child's underpants after age 4 (Wong et al., 2002). In most cases, the problem has no discernable physiological cause and is not related to laxative use. There may be a history of inconsistent toilet training or early life stress in affected children. This problem usually occurs in the late afternoon and af-fects mostly boys of average or above-average intelligence (Wong et al., 2002) who retain stool at least part of the time. This behavior is associated with complaints of recurrent abdominal pain and, for many, enuresis as well. Often these children have emotional difficulties that began before or resulted from encopresis. They experience poor peer relationships and self-esteem, perhaps due to their offensive odor. Nurses should be aware of this childhood problem to identify the affected child, refer the child for treatment, and support the child and family during a bowel management program and counseling.

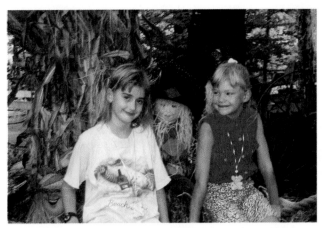

Figure 20-3 Peer play is important during the school-age years.

Activity-Exercise Pattern

Generally, the school-age child is physically active, although Hispanic and black children may be less active than white children (USDHHS, 2000). As previously discussed, impressive changes in motor skills occur between the ages of 6 and 12 years, allowing the child to engage in many activities that develop strength, balance, and coordination. Exercise typically occurs through group activities and organized sports such as Little League baseball and soccer, through individual activities such as gymnastics and ballet, and through unorganized play such as bike riding, sledding, rollerblading, and imaginary play. Typically play provides important learning and health promotion and for this reason should be encouraged consistently during the school-age years. For many children, involvement in physical activities is fun and connects them to their peers and family members, important people in their lives (Figure 20-3).

Play activities also promote social, personal, and cognitive development. School-age children frequently prefer interacting with peers rather than with family. This desire for peer interaction, usually with one of the same gender, extends beyond school and carries over to play and outside activities. A child's skill in motor tasks wins the respect of other children and provides a feeling of self-accomplishment. Organized sports such as baseball teach team cooperation, competition, and other social skills. Concerns that young children have experienced too much physical and psychological pressure to perform in sports has generated a renewed commitment by many parents to focus more on the fun of sports than on the winning of games (Cary, 2004). In addition, organized activities such as scouts and 4H clubs teach children about group functioning, processes involved in carrying out a task, and the power of social relationships to create change. These lessons can prepare them for discipline needed for a job later in life. Overall, children who perform well in these activities, evidenced by prizes or trophies, feel good about themselves, their competence, and their sense of industry. Parents and teachers who compliment children when they perform well enhance self-esteem, as well.

As part of play, school-age children incorporate new cognitive skills, including the ability to count and sort objects. Children of this age express pleasure in their collections of stamps, rocks, or other objects. Understanding the concepts of fair and consistent rules found in games requires cognitive skills of memory, logical reasoning, and the desire to work with others. Many children like to read, which provides ideas about life and cultures that differ from their own, thereby enhancing their acceptance of human diversity.

The nurse helps parents promote healthy play activities for children by encouraging the following:

- Family activities that focus on physical activity and togetherness between parents or caregivers and children, such as daily reading (out loud or silently)
- Use of a library card to encourage reading on a variety of topics and to teach responsibilities involved with borrowing
- Purchase of personal magazines for children's learning and ownership
- Monitoring of daily television and computer use that detract from physical activity and more active mental activities
- Encouragement of both group and solitary activities to support the child's overall development

Sleep-Rest Pattern

Sleep Patterns

Most school-age children have no difficulties with sleep. Generally their sleep requirements and patterns are more similar to those of an adult than those of a younger child. Individual needs vary based on activity, age, and state of health, but most school-age children sleep between 8 and 12 hours a night without naps during the day (Schulte et al., 2001). Unlike younger children, school-age children experience few difficulties with going to bed. Most children and parents can agree on a bedtime with some flexibility on nonschool nights and adhere to that agreement. When problems arise regarding bedtime, children may be testing parents who have not been clear and firm about their expectations for going to bed or have not been willing to discuss the arrangement with their children. Although most Americans accept the idea that school-age children should sleep in their own beds, some African American, Hispanic, or Japanese families may encourage the family or siblings to sleep together (Latz, Wolf, & Lozoff, 1999).

Sleep Disturbances

The most common sleep problems that occur during the preschool and school-age years are night terrors (see Chapter 19), **sleepwalking, sleep talking,** and enuresis. As a group, these disturbances have been called *disorders of arousal* (Rosen, Mahowald, & Ferber, 1995) and share the following characteristics:

- They occur immediately before a REM, or rapid eye movement, state of sleep.
- Most occur 1 to 2 hours after going to sleep.

- There is a family history of sleep problems, and more boys experience sleep problems than girls.
- Problems reflect normal central nervous system (CNS) immaturity of the child.
- Problems may be influenced by fatigue and stress within the child.

Approximately one out of six children between ages 5 and 12 has sleepwalked at least once, but far fewer children walk in their sleep persistently. Sleepwalking often occurs with enuresis (Rosen et al., 1995). Shortly after going to sleep, the child may suddenly sit up in bed, make repetitive finger and hand movements, or walk, usually for a short time. In most cases, however, the child stays in bed. The child may mumble when talking to a parent or other person (sleep talking). The words tend to be simple but unclear to the listener. Often the child falls back to sleep quickly after talking or walking.

Parents who are concerned about sleepwalking or sleep talking need to know that most children outgrow these episodes with CNS maturation. However, parents should protect their child from injury by placing gates at the top of stairs and removing sharp objects from the child's path. Most parents find that the easiest solution is to direct the sleepwalker back to bed, where the child returns to a normal sleep. Occasionally parents can intervene effectively by implementing relaxation techniques for their child before bedtime, avoiding stressful and fatiguing situations, and providing consistency with sleep preparation patterns (Wong et al., 2002). If a child has many episodes of sleepwalking or sleep talking or if parents express particular concern, he or she may need further evaluation and treatment by health care professionals.

Cognitive-Perceptual Pattern

The school-age child spends extensive time in settings that require mastery of new ideas and concepts. The child's basic intelligence, heredity, and environment encourage or discourage learning. Mastery of ideas and learning requires intact senses, such as vision, hearing, and language, and memory capabilities that allow for cognitive development and acquisition of skills needed for later life success. Unfortunately, many children in society lack these capabilities and will have learning problems if not identified early through parental awareness, school observations, or routine health care assessments.

Piaget's Theory

Piaget (1969) refers to the age span of 7 to 11 years as the period of **concrete operations,** a stage when children learn by manipulating concrete objects and lack the ability to perform thinking operations that require abstraction. During this time, the child moves from egocentric interactions to more cooperative interactions and increased understanding of many concepts gained through environmental connections. Children increasingly change their reasoning from intuitive to logical or rational operations (rule-governed actions) and engage in serial ordering, addition, subtraction, and other basic mathematical skills. The operations of this period are termed *concrete,* because the child's mental operations or actions still depend on the ability to perceive specific examples of what has happened. Older school-age children use both concrete and recently acquired abstract operations, which add flexibility and control to their thinking and meet developmental needs of adolescence. Unlike the egocentric preschooler, a school-age child begins to take the other person's point of view into account. This trait does not emerge suddenly and completely. The new skill appears occasionally and then more frequently as the child's mental capacity and experience grow (Piaget, 1969; Wong et al., 2002).

During the school-age period, the child understands a number of expanding concepts regarding objects, including the concept of **conservation** of substance (see Chapter 19). When asked if a difference exists in the amount of liquid poured into two glasses of different shapes, the preschool, preoperational child focuses on the different shapes and says "yes." The concrete operational school-age child realizes that no change has occurred in the substance despite the change in shape. Conservation of numbers, weight, volume, and quantity, required to understand basic mathematics, sequentially develops as the school-age child gains chronological age and experience.

The concept of time also develops during this period. Children begin to learn to tell time and understand the passage of time. By age 8, most children understand the difference between past and present, and history becomes meaningful. The concept of human aging becomes increasingly understandable, and the child can comprehend the difference between an 18-year-old and an 80-year-old person (Wong et al., 2002).

Two major operations of the school-age period are classifying and ordering. The child classifies or groups objects by their common elements and understands the relationship between groups or classes. For example, when given 12 wooden beads, some brown and some white, the child understands that the beads may grouped by their color and by their material. Conversely, the preschool child focuses only on one property of the beads, such as color. The newfound ability to classify shows in the school-age child's interest in collections, such as stamps or coins. Children in school frequently "order" their world; they line up in school according to height, they repeat numbers and letters in their classic order, and they receive numbers in school to reflect an alphabetized surname. These two operations (classifying and ordering) must exist to learn to read, understand the concepts of numbers, and learn subjects based on relations, such as history (the relation of events in time) and geography (the relation of places in space).

Vision

The child's sensory abilities continue to develop during the school-age years. In order to learn satisfactorily, sensory abilities must be intact or accommodations made to improve those abilities (e.g., eye glasses). Visual capacity should reach optimal function by the sixth or seventh year (Wong et al., 2002). Peripheral vision and the ability to discriminate fine color distinctions should be fully developed. Although most 4 year olds have 20/20 vision (Behrman et al., 2000), a school-age child should have a visual acuity of at least 20/30 in each eye, as measured by the Snellen E Chart, an assessment tool for children who can read some letters (Jarvis, 2000). The child coordinates eye movements, sees a single image, and associates incoming visual stimuli with past and present mental images and functions. Throughout childhood, further development of full visual potential occurs through practice during normal activities.

Physiological changes occur in the eye during the school-age years. Eyes in the preschool years are normally **hyperopic (farsighted),** a condition in which the visual image of an object falls behind the retina. However, unlike older individuals, preschool children do not need glasses because their eyes normally accommodate by adjusting their lenses. For most children, vision becomes normal as the shape of the eye changes and lengthens with maturation. However, many school-age children need visual correction to prevent academic difficulties and headaches and dizziness when reading or doing close work. Routine vision screening by a school nurse, as required by many states and as part of a school approach to health promotion, identifies defects early. The nurse encourages parents of children with deficits to seek further optometric care to correct these defects so that these children can learn more effectively.

Two other visual problems are common in the school-age child group. Many school-age children inherit **myopia (nearsightedness),** a condition in which the visual image of an object falls in front of the retina, causing the child to have difficulty seeing distant objects. The other condition, **astigmatism,** causes blurred vision because the image is focused poorly on the retina due to changes in the surface of the cornea or lens. Eyeglasses correct the defects, but the problem must be identified before it can be solved. For example, a child with myopia may not realize that his visual images are impaired. Children with corrective lenses often express delight and surprise when they first see the fully focused and rich detail of the world after experiencing less refined visual acuity for some time.

Hearing

The child's hearing ability (auditory acuity) is nearly complete by 7 years of age, although some maturation continues into adolescence. Hearing deficits occur less frequently than visual deficits, but hearing loss affects over 1 million children from birth to age 21 years in the United States (Berrettini et al., 1999). This deficit compromises learning in school and important socialization with peers. **Chronic serous otitis media,** or long-term fluid in the middle ear, remains a common cause of hearing deficit in both the preschool and the early school-age years. Additionally, at least one author has expressed concern about the potential for long-term hearing loss in children who listen to loud music

(Folmer, 2003). All school-age children, especially those with a history of recurrent ear infections or fluid behind the eardrum, should have periodic hearing evaluations performed as part of a health-promotion program in school and as required by many states. Various treatments exist for acute otitis media, including antibiotics and the recent discovery that Xylitol gum may be of some preventive benefit (Parker-Pope, 2000). Additionally, work continues on a vaccination for otitis media. **Tympanograms,** used to measure the sensitivity of the tympanic membrane to vibrations induced by pressure and sound waves, help detect and monitor this problem as part of well-child and ill-child care (see Chapter 18). The nurse should consider including education on hearing protection for school-age children in order to maintain this important sense for the future.

Sensory Perception

Children learn simultaneously through many senses, and most teaching approaches incorporate this concept. For example, young school-age children see a letter, hear its sound, and feel its shape. With this approach, children learn in a number of ways to interpret an event. For example, some children learn best by listening (auditory learners), others by doing (kinesthetic learners), and others by engaging all sensory modalities (auditory, kinesthetic, and visual learners). Because no two children have exactly the same sensory acuity, sensitivity, or discrimination, all children build slightly different perceptions and conceptions of the world around them and do not follow the same timetable to grasp concepts. Therefore, teaching approaches must be individualized to meet the learning needs of most children.

Of all the senses, visual perception has been studied the most, primarily because of its role in helping children learn to read. Studies have examined children's abilities to discriminate parts of a picture (to see a figure within a picture). Children usually progress from the preschool stage during which they perceive visual stimuli more as a whole, to the school-age stage during which they perceive more details, and finally to the point at which they perceive and integrate both. This process helps children recognize letters, the first step needed for reading. Children may first be able to differentiate between obviously different letters, such as "h" and "o," but may have difficulty with letters similar in appearance, such as "b" and "d," until they can distinguish details more effectively.

Language

Language develops rapidly during the school years. Most school-age children enter this period with an ability to understand and speak a language, but with only a basic knowledge of reading and writing. By the end of the school-age period, most children have acquired at least a functional ability in both areas. Language development mandates that a child have visual perception for reading, auditory acuity and perception for understanding spoken language, and fine motor skills for both articulation and handwriting.

The full capacity to imitate sounds develops during the childhood years. Between 6 and 7 years of age, the child shows the ability to produce proper articulation for most vowel and consonant sounds. However, some have difficulty expressing sounds for "s," "l," "z," "sh," "ch," and "r" (Wong & Hess, 2000). By 7 years of age the child should be able to articulate all sounds for speaking and by age 12 years has a vocabulary of around 4000 words. Understanding of the **syntax** (grammar) and **semantics** (meaning) of language continues to develop. The child uses more complex sentences and understands multiple meanings for the same word and metaphors. The child should be able to recognize and correct spelling and grammatical errors by 8 or 9 years of age. The capacity to learn foreign languages is at an optimal level and provides rationale for foreign language instruction during the school-age years. Foreign language instruction also provides information about other cultures and an opportunity to understand people who are different from themselves.

Much of the child's time in school focuses on learning to read and write. Learning to read is a complex process, beginning with letter and sound recognition. Letters combine to form words that the child must learn to decode. Words combine to form sentences, and so on. Most children need help from teachers, peers, parents, or older children to learn to read effectively. Some researchers believe that children learn best by sounding out the individual letters of a word **(phonics),** whereas others think that learning the word as a whole unit is better. Both processes have value, and likely a combination of both is most effective. Considering the wide range of processes that support development of reading skills (conceptual, perceptual, verbal, and motor), it's not surprising that most children experience some difficulty in learning to read.

Handwriting requires eye-hand coordination, motor control, and perceptual abilities. Primarily a motor skill, handwriting does not reflect mental capacity. Many bright children and adults have poor handwriting, and vice versa. Boys tend to have more problems with legible handwriting than do girls. Writing style does not approach adult-level maturity until the end of late childhood, but the handwriting should reflect the child's handedness. No reversal of letter outlines should occur by age 7 or 8, and the relative size of letters should be uniform. By age 8 or 9, letter strokes should be firm, even, and flow with ease (Wong & Hess, 2000). The individual who has difficulty with handwriting may use a typewriter, computer, or graphics to produce a satisfactory written product. Tutoring by a handwriting specialist can help children with **dyslexia,** a term defining the tendency to reverse the normal appearance of letters and numbers in writing.

Memory

Memory abilities, both short term and long term, improve for school-age children. Strategies such as organizing, classifying, and labeling information help them retain information. **Rehearsal,** repeating an item to be learned, is also a helpful memorization strategy. At age 5 children use rehearsal when someone suggests or models it; at age 10 they rehearse spontaneously. Memory abilities improve with practice and through various strategies, such as placing the words that need to be remembered in a song or by rhyming words.

Intelligence

The concept of **intelligence** usually conveys an ability to think and process information learned earlier in life. Scores on an intelligence test should measure the child's basic abilities as compared with others of the same age and experience level and, ideally, should predict performance in school or society. However, this is not always the case. Intelligence test scores tend to differ because each test, or each form of the same test, measures slightly different samples of abilities and reflects the test author's philosophy on intelligence. **Web Site Resource 20C** contains a list of common developmental and cognitive tests. For example, the **Stanford-Binet Test** places a heavy emphasis on intelligence related to abstract thinking, the **Wechsler Series** emphasizes an aggregate (global) measurement of intelligence, and the **Peabody Picture Vocabulary Test** emphasizes verbal skills. Increases in language ability and mental functioning of later childhood allow the measurement of intellectual capacity to become more reliable and valid. It is important to note that some intelligence tests may be culturally insensitive. For example, the protectionism of the Asian culture may cause lower test scores on self-help skills and socialization among Asian children who demonstrate in other ways that they are good students. Furthermore, words on the test may not be part of an ethnic group's usual vocabulary, causing children to miss these items on an intelligence test.

Children also take **achievement tests** that measure the amount of information learned in a specific area and offer insight into a child's overall intelligence. Although intelligence and achievement tests should measure different issues (basic ability versus learned achievement), their results correlate well. Some researchers believe this correlation exists because both tests actually measure the same thing (achievement, not ability).

Reports from intelligence and achievement testing differ. Intelligence tests usually provide a number that represents **intelligence quotient** (IQ). An IQ of 90 to 110 is considered average. Achievement tests compare the child's performance with that of other children and report scores as percentiles. For example, a score in the twentieth percentile of a test means the child scored better than only 20% of other children of the same age in that skill. Current beliefs accept that people inherit some of their intelligence but that environmental factors also influence opportunities for learning and overall intelligence. Most likely the greatest environmental influence is socioeconomic, reflected in the correlation in scores: children from low-income families tend to score lower on intelligence tests than do children from middle-income or high-income families. The reason for this probably relates to many subfactors, such as nutrition, language, parental reinforcement and encouragement, and sociocultural environmental stimuli. Social programs such as the federal nutrition program for women, infants, and children (WIC) and preschool stimulation programs such as Head Start have attempted to address these subfactors to improve the potential of young children from diverse populations. Many people have suggested less focus on IQ tests, primarily because they label children early in life and influence, often negatively, their self-perception and their performance.

Because of the many interactive elements addressed previously, it is not surprising that some children have problems learning. Learning difficulties may result from a health problem (poor vision or hearing), an emotional problem (anxiety or depression), a cognitive problem (retardation or a learning disability), or a complex mixture of many problems. The child who enters the health care system with a learning problem must undergo a detailed, extensive evaluation by education specialists to identify the cause of the problem and strategies to address the child's needs.

Learning Disabilities

Approximately 20% of children struggle with **learning disabilities** that inhibit school and life success (Goldstein & Mather, 1998). Many terms and definitions have been used to describe the impairments of these children, who have normal or above-normal intelligence and usually do not have visual, hearing, or motor handicaps or emotional problems. One author argues that children have learning differences, not disabilities, and that with knowledge of these differences, effective instructional and life strategies can improve their overall school and life success (Levine, 2002). This author advocates avoiding a label of "learning disabled" for any child. Differences may be found in various systems, including those that influence attention, memory, spatial and sequential ordering, motor or social skills, listening, speaking, and writing, or higher thinking systems. Some children have minor, almost unnoticeable difficulties, whereas other children are so impaired that they appear to be mentally retarded until diagnosed and helped. An individual child may have more than one developmental disorder. Some of these children will develop behavior and self-esteem problems as a response to their inability to function satisfactorily (American Psychiatric Association [APA], 1994; Levine, 2002).

One well-known condition that causes difficulty in the child's adjustment to the school setting is **attention-deficit/hyperactivity disorder** (ADHD), a behavior that reflects developmentally inappropriate degrees of inattention, impulsiveness, and hyperactivity (American Academy of Pediatrics [AAP], 2000; APA, 1994). Frequently these children have high energy, intuitiveness, and creativity, personal characteristics that help them succeed in some facets of their lives (Dumas & Pelletier, 1999). Despite diagnostic criteria for ADHD developed by the American Psychiatric Association (1994) (Box 20-3), the problem has been dif-

Box **20-3**	Diagnostic Criteria for Attention-Deficit/Hyperactivity Disorder

Note: Consider a criterion met only if the behavior occurs more frequently than that noted in most people of the same mental age as the child.

1. A disturbance of at least 6 months exists during which at least six of the criteria for either inattentive behavior or hyperactivity-impulsivity behavior are met.*
2. Some inattentive or hyperactive-impulsive symptoms that caused impairment existed before age 7 years.
3. Some impairment for the symptoms exists in two or more settings (at school or at home).
4. Clear evidence of clinically significant impairment exists in social or academic functioning.
5. The symptoms do not occur only with a pervasive developmental disorder, schizophrenia, or other psychotic disorder and do not support another mental disorder (mood disorder, anxiety disorder, dissociative disorder, and personality disorder).

From American Academy of Pediatrics, Committee on Quality Improvement, Subcommittee on Attention-Deficit/Hyperactivity Disorder. (2000). Clinical practice guideline: Diagnosis and evaluation of the child with attention-deficit/hyperactivity disorders. *Pediatrics, 105,* 1158-1170.
*For specific criteria, refer to American Psychiatric Association. (1994). *Diagnostic and statistical manual of mental disorders.* DSM-IV (4th ed.). Washington, DC: Author.

ficult to assess, primarily because the child manifests symptoms in varying degrees in different settings and with different people. Treatment of children with ADHD has been controversial but includes behavior management, family counseling, classroom management, nutrition therapy, and medication. These interventions may also be successful in management for ADHD-affected adults.

The nurse's role with the child who has a learning disability varies. The nurse may participate in detection of the problem, consultation during evaluations, collaboration with school administration on implementation of a treatment plan, referral to resources, serving as a liaison between school and home environments, and counseling the child and family to improve overall development and the family's adaptation to meet the needs of this unique child.

The nurse plays a vital role in promoting the school-age child's overall cognitive and perceptual health, helping to prevent problems in these areas (see Think About It: Homework Procrastination). The nurse must talk to parents and school administration personnel about any child who has language articulation problems beyond 6 or 7 years, because this child should be evaluated by a professional (Jarvis, 2000). The nurse also helps parents understand their child's level of cognitive and sensory abilities so that learning expectations are realistic. Through educational materials sent home or provided during school meetings, the nurse may address the socialization needs and development of school-age children. The nurse may also need to help parents understand common tests used for child intelligence and achievement screening. See the list of tests in **Web Site**

Resource 20C. In addition, the nurse may help evaluate a child believed to have a learning difference when instead the problem may rest with a health problem, general immaturity, or environmental deficit (poverty or divorce).

Self-Perception–Self-Concept Pattern

Through each of the developmental processes of physiological growth, cognitive development, and social development, children progressively engage in an important process of self-discovery. Through these processes, children actively build and create their own personalities, develop relationships with others, and expose themselves to a wide range of experiences that influence their behavior, attitudes, and values.

Erikson's Theory

The stage of personality development described by Erikson for the school-age child is **industry versus inferiority.** The major task to be accomplished is full mastery of whatever the child is doing (sense of industry). The child focuses on success in personal and social tasks and avoidance of a sense of inferiority. Inferiority occurs with repeated failures at attempted tasks and with little encouragement or trust from people important to the child. With mastery of the tools of the culture in relation to those of the peer group, a sense of worth and understanding of the self develops (Erikson, 1986a, 1986b).

Self-Concept

Self-concept develops over time and through a variety of experiences and relationships. For example, by being responsible for a pet's care and by showing love to this animal, the older school-age child nurtures a positive self-concept. The way in which others, especially peers, view the child influences the sense of self. Increasing cognitive abilities facilitate better understanding of the identifying factors of others (race, ethnicity, disability, or gender) and how those others compare with the child. Self-concept includes self-esteem, sense of control, body concept, and gender role.

Self-Esteem. Self-esteem has been defined as the extent to which an individual believes oneself to be capable, significant, successful, and worthy. The younger school-age child has a limited self-concept, but one that develops with successful completion of the tasks of this period (Erikson's sense of industry). Although engaged in more activities outside of the home, the child still depends on family, as defined by one's culture, to develop high self-esteem. Literature indicates that parents with high self-esteem freely express their affection for each other and their children. In school, teachers or group leaders frequently reward those who have succeeded in a task with badges, stars, or privileges (tangible objects that validate success). People who work with school-age children should communicate the concept that "success breeds success," which can help to build self-esteem early in life (Goldstein & Mather, 1998).

The peer group's influence on the school-age child's self-esteem is unquestionable. Acceptance by a peer group contributes to feelings of self-worth and sense of belonging to a desired group. Competition or collaboration with peers in school, clubs, and activities also influences feelings of adequacy and feelings of success. In one study black children ages 9 to 14 years voiced higher self-esteem than did Asian, Hispanic, or white children because they believed they could make others laugh and others wanted to be like them (Jordan, 2004). Parents must be encouraged to expose their school-age children to interesting activities of their choice, involving peers to nurture their self-esteem and a sense of uniqueness.

Concern has been voiced about school-age girls suffering a decline in self-esteem that affects their school achievements. Some research indicates that boys receive more praise in school than do girls, that girls receive criticism on the content of their work but that boys receive more criticism on the appearance of their work (Jacklin & Martin, 1999). Girls experience greater competition now than in earlier times, and they face pressures about personal appearance, particularly if they are white (Jordan, 2004). Various authors report that these girls need strong adults to support their ways of thinking and behaving in a world often built on male values. Girls tend to have high self-esteem if they perceive parental harmony that supports perceptions of balance within themselves and promotes their emotional health (Bingham & Stryker, 1995; Doswell, 2002; Elium & Elium, 1994). Self-esteem appears to be strong in school-age girls with fathers and teachers who routinely encourage them to take risks, question traditional behaviors, and "listen to their souls" with music and art. Many proponents of education believe that these qualities can best be met with female-only schools, rather than a coeducational approach.

In encouraging development of self-esteem in all school-age children, the nurse remembers that a child needs to experience success with tasks, and completely structured activities may not provide this opportunity for some children. A child who succeeds in some things and receives acceptance by peers gains a sense of competence and worth, is self-confident, and has high self-esteem, which are important qualities for life survival (Cagle & Keen-Payne, 1996).

Sense of Control. As the school-age child matures and makes choices, a sense of control develops about the self and the environment. Children with an **internal locus of control** believe they are responsible for their behavior and accomplishments and tend to have higher levels of achievement than do children who believe in an **external locus of control.** The latter think that fewer reasons exist for them to try hard at a task, because others or fate determines life results. Hispanic and African American cultures may more often support an external locus of control based on a strong belief that God determines one's outcome (Spector, 2004). Older children and girls tend to have a more internalized locus of control than do younger children and boys.

Body Concept. The school-age child's concept of the body and its functioning also changes from the preschool period and adds to overall self-concept. By ages 8 to 11, children know that parts of the body constitute a related whole (Wong et al., 2002). The 11-year-old child can name twice the number and functions of internal body structures as one who is 6 years of age and frequently understands the functions of the cardiovascular, musculoskeletal, and nervous systems. For example, the 7-year-old child knows that the heart is important and that it beats, whereas the 13-year-old child knows that the heart pumps blood. Changes or differences in the body may frighten the school-age child until one understands normal developmental processes such as losing deciduous teeth. Physical differences, such as freckles, can provoke ridicule and isolation. Children in this age group frequently feel threatened by others with deformities (Wong et al., 2002). Children with chronic illness worry that their peer relationships will be negatively influenced if others know about their illness. Children who learn about body differences, through reading and discussion of anxiety about differences, increase their knowledge about the body and ways to maintain health. They also gain an understanding of the value of each person, despite their differences. Ways in which the nurse can help children develop positive self-concepts are listed in Box 20-4.

Box 20-4 — Nursing Interventions to Foster Positive Self-Concept During the School-Age Period

- Remind people working with school-age children that a sense of success is important for all children. Provide a variety of experiences to allow children to identify and use their personal strengths. These approaches help them cope with failure; therefore, they will try for more accomplishments and successes.
- Parents should learn the importance of giving positive feedback to their children, setting realistic goals, spending quality time with them, and helping them to attempt realistic tasks.
- School-age children should be encouraged to make choices to develop their sense of control and decision-making skills and experience consequences of their choices.
- Questions from school-age children about bodily changes, including sexual changes, should be acknowledged and discussed sensitively at home or at school. Open discussions between parents and educators may determine the proper timing and place of teaching. School nurses should play a vital role in developing, teaching, and evaluating sex education programs in the school. They also have a role in collaborating with parents about appropriate teaching in this area.
- School-age children should be encouraged to show pride in their culture and identify with their cultural group by sharing their values and behaviors with peers and others in appropriate forums.

Roles-Relationships Pattern

The family environment provides a sense of security that allows the school-age child to cope with uncertainties in the external environment. Although many live in single, divorced, mixed-race or same-gender parenting households, the family structure generally encourages a child's cognitive growth through exposure to a variety of experiences that bolster the desire to achieve and develop positive self-esteem (Goldstein & Mather, 1998).

Parents, caregivers, and children interact in a variety of ways to show love and companionship for each other. Care-givers, such as grandparents or extended family members (common in the African American culture), protect the dependent child and teach the learning child. The care-giver–child relationship is not equal, primarily because care-givers and parents serve as authority figures that establish the rules needed for the functioning of the family and safe growth of the child. During the school-age years, the child's increasing maturity, independence, and responsibility begin to reduce the amount of parental authority and structure needed. In one study African American parents set higher standards for child independence than did parents of other diverse populations (Jordan, 2004). With increasing independence, the child prioritizes school and peer group relationships to develop socialization skills and understand group social mores. These connections will help prepare the child for future heterosexual relationships.

School-age children also begin to broaden their interests outside the home, often encouraged by parents. Unfortunately, the older ones may become involved in gangs, behavior that causes much stress for both children and their parents. The child's changing world frequently alters family schedules and patterns, supporting studies that have found that parents express the least amount of parental satisfaction when their oldest one is between the ages of 6 and 13. The relationships between siblings vary, depending on birth order, culture, gender, and age differences and perceived power of siblings. Siblings interact with one another in a number of roles, such as playmates, teacher-learner, protector-dependent, and adversaries, based on feelings of jealousy and rivalry that often occur in families (see Chapter 18). School-age children cope with these feelings better than do preschool children because they have outlets outside the family, including school and friends. Parents can minimize conflicts by recognizing each child's needs and level of maturity and by providing guidance and support.

As children mature, they take on more responsibilities within the family and the community. School-age children learn responsibility for money, household chores, self-care, and pets and acquire a sense of empowerment as an integral part of the family. Their health may actually improve with responsibilities associated with pet caregiving (Beck & Myers, 1996). This is the period during which families often give allowances or children earn money through chores or small jobs, such as paper routes. The amount of an allowance may relate to cultural values. In one study Asian children earned higher allowances than did other children from diverse population groups for completing fewer chores and for meeting higher standards of academic performance (Jordan, 2004). School-age children learn valuable life lessons by earning and spending their allowances.

Children learn socially accepted behaviors when their parents engage in **limit setting** (defining expected behavior and consequences when limits are not honored). Some cultures (South Asian) enforce consequences when a child engages in behavior that does not foster the good of the community, a strong cultural value (Maiter & George, 2003). Violent behavior must be discouraged, and nonviolent methods to reach resolutions for personal problems should be encouraged. Parents who express their feelings, explain why things happen, and listen to their children while setting limits encourage the development of self-control and positive self-esteem (Health Teaching box). Some families with school-age children find it helpful to have periodic family meetings during which everyone dis-

---

HEALTH TEACHING The School-Age Child: Points for Effective Discipline

Effective discipline is essential to family harmony and individual child growth and reflects cultural beliefs. The goal of discipline is to encourage and reinforce positive child behaviors, eliminate inappropriate child behaviors, improve parent-child communication, and meet parental needs. The specifics of discipline include:

- Ignoring the misbehavior and acknowledging the appropriate behavior
- Using distraction or substitution to avoid a problem situation
- Offering choices to prevent inappropriate behavior such as whining or emotional outbursts
- Using humor to decrease the intensity of a situation
- Modeling the appropriate behavior

- Setting age-relevant limits
- Giving specific and clear commands for behavior appropriate to the child's age
- Talking calmly, being a good listener, and encouraging negotiation, perhaps in a family meeting, to promote problem resolution
- Limiting a child's environment (distractions such as music and television)
- Setting clear and consistent consequences for misbehavior (withholding privileges, use of contracts)
- Providing one-to-one time, focusing on positive attention
- Taking time for oneself to replenish one's energies as a parent and as an individual

From Lighter, D. (1995). *Gentle discipline*. New York: Meadowbrook Press; Wong, D. L., Perry, S. E., & Hockenberry, M. J. (2002). *Maternal child nursing* (pp. 939-967). St. Louis: Mosby.

cusses family issues, rules, and responsibilities. Behavior contracts between parent and child provide direction and may also encourage improved behavior by delineating favorable consequences when the terms of the contract are followed.

Children frequently model their behavior after that of people they love or admire (parents, friends, and other adults). **Positive reinforcement** (rewards for good behavior) is an effective form of limit setting used often by upper class parents. **Punishment,** a negative reinforcement as reflected in shaming a child in front of his community or family (seen with some Asian cultures, Wong et al., 2002), may stop an undesired behavior, but often only until the child repeats the action and is not caught. Lower class parents tend to use more punishment directed toward misbehavior or failure to adhere to parental values and requirements (Wong et al., 2002).

Recently, spanking has become more popular and several states, including Oklahoma and Nevada, have passed laws that support this form of punishment. However, at least one author warns against child spanking and other punitive approaches, because they cause increased violent and anti-social behavior later in life (Mayer, 2002). Historically, many cultures have invoked discipline through spanking, but further research must be completed to interpret spanking as an abusive behavior within the context of culture (Yerao, Borrego, & Urquiza, 2001). One research study showed that recently acculturated, low-income, ethnically diverse mothers used more aggressive discipline such as spanking and felt less responsible for their child's misbehavior than did white women who were citizens (Ortega, 2001). However, as recently as 1998, the American Academy of Pediatrics did not support any kind of physical punishment directed against children. Despite this stand, many parents believe methods such as "time out" and "living with the consequences of poor choices" have been unsuccessful in "out-of-control" children (Costello, 2000). Recent school shootings by young adolescents have caused concern among many parents who believe that spanking as a disciplinary method might prevent these occurrences in the future.

Child Abuse

Child abuse (physical, sexual, or emotional exploitation of children) and neglect (lack of adequate food, shelter, or emotional support) continue to be significant societal problems. In 1999 an estimated 1100 children died from abuse and neglect, leading causes of mortality for children under 14 years of age (USDHHS, 2001; U.S. Preventive Services Task Force, 2004a). Abused children have an increased likelihood of becoming violent adults and of abusing their own children. Factors that increase the risk of abuse include family poverty, culture, limited maternal education, needy child syndrome, presence of a stepfather, single-parent status, parental drug addiction, and teenage parenthood (U.S. Preventive Services Task Force, 2004a). However, child abuse occurs in families that do not have these risk factors. Cultural factors must be considered in detecting abuse. For example, coin rubbing of the chest (used in the Asian ethnic group for treatment of respiratory infections) leaves abrasions that may be perceived as abuse by a nurse assessing an ill child. Both national governmental agencies and professional organizations recommend that health care providers report suspected abuse and participate in preventing, assessing, and treating victims. Many state nurse practice acts require nurses to report suspected cases of abuse. Ultimately nurses must help interrupt the vicious cycle of abuse by becoming involved in community coalitions and innovative evidence-based programs that prevent and intervene with child and family abuse.

Unfortunately, relationships between children and adults are not always positive. **Sexual abuse,** use of a child for sexual exploitative purposes, has become a more common but often hidden problem for a variety of reasons. The child may be too frightened to talk about the situation, families and society do not want to admit its existence, Internet traffic has supported pornography and pedophilia, and fewer agencies exist to respond to these cases. Many victims know their abusers (many are parents), and people in positions of authority (e.g., doctors or clergy) may be abusers. The child may comply for a variety of reasons, such as a need to be good or a need to keep the family together. Emotions are complex and change as the child grows, but they often lead to adult anxiety, depression, and physical symptoms and illnesses. Males less often report sexual abuse but are more likely than girls to suffer negative emotional effects from incest, a form of sexual abuse (Moody, 1999; Wong et al., 2002).

As in any type of suspected abuse, nurses assist these children by recognizing those at risk and those experiencing abuse and referring them to relevant resources. All people who work with young children must acknowledge the warning signs of abuse (Box 20-5). When sexual abuse is suspected, an in-depth interview and examination must be conducted by a multidisciplinary team that is sensitive to the needs of the child and can validate the abuse. Most authorities believe that children who describe sexual abuse are telling the truth, because the details are usually specific and trauma is evident. Therefore a child's story should be believed unless it is disproved.

Sexuality-Reproductive Pattern

The preschool child learns about gender and begins to model the general societal behaviors expected of a female or male child. The child enters the school-age years with a strong identification with the parent of the same gender. The child continues to learn the concepts and behavior of the gender role and incorporate these into the self-concept. This challenge is significant for all children, but more so for homosexual children. Societal stereotypes related to gender roles continue to influence the school-age child's ideas of male and female roles. Fortunately, most children receive early teaching about gender roles that emphasizes that gender does not determine one's choices, personality, or

| Box **20-5** | Warning Signs of Child Abuse |

- Physical evidence of abuse or neglect, including previous injuries
- Conflicting stories about the "accident" or injury from the parents or others
- Blame placed on sibling or other party for injury to child
- Injury or complaint inconsistent with the child's history or developmental level (e.g., the child received a concussion and broken arm from falling off a bed)
- Signs and symptoms consistent with signs of abuse and inconsistent with history (e.g., chief complaint is a cold when there is evidence of first-degree and second-degree burns)
- Inappropriate response of caregiver, such as an exaggerated or absent emotional response, refusal to sign for additional tests or agree to necessary treatment, excessive delay in seeking treatment, or absence of the parents
- Inappropriate response of child, such as little or no response to pain, fear of being touched, excessive or lack of separation anxiety, or indiscriminate friendliness to strangers
- Child's report of physical or sexual abuse
- Previous reports of abuse in the family
- Repeated visits to emergency facilities with injuries

From Wong, D. L., Hockenberry-Eaton, M., Wilson, D., Winkelstein, M. L., Ahmann, E., DiVito-Thomas, P. A. (1999). *Whaley and Wong's nursing care of infants and children* (6th ed.). St. Louis: Mosby; U.S. Preventive Services Task Force. (2004). Screening for family and intimate partner violence. Retrieved May 11, 2004, from: *http://www.ahrq.gov/clinic/3rduspstf/famviolence/famviolrs.htm*.

behavior. Due to this teaching, children increasingly choose occupations based on their skills and interests, rather than on what appears appropriate because of their gender.

The school-age child's increasing awareness of the body, its functioning, and a need for sexual identity combine to foster a desire for knowledge about the biological aspects of sexual function. Late in the school-age period, when the physical changes of puberty have begun, concern and curiosity about sexual issues frequently grow. A child may become extremely attached to another of the same gender, and they may explore one another's sexual organs. This is common exploratory behavior and does not reflect true homosexuality, even though parents and children may express concerns about it. With the advent of physical changes of puberty, the school-age child desires more privacy in a bedroom shared with no one. As noted earlier, the physical changes of puberty appear gradually over several years.

Children frequently share questions about sexual matters with their peer group. Parents are frequently uncomfortable or unsure of what sexual information to give to their children and when to give it. Many health care agencies sponsor short programs to educate parents and later school-age children about bodily and mental changes during preadolescence and puberty in a supportive environment. An increasing number of age-appropriate books that focus on

emotional and body changes can be used at home and in school to increase children's understanding. Particularly because menstrual cycles start earlier now than they did 50 years ago, education about bodily changes and puberty appears appropriate as part of later school-age education.

The nurse plays an important role in sex education in health care and education settings. This professional should be receptive to answering questions in this area and at each health care visit. The nurse employed in the school is in an ideal position to teach group sex education programs using literature and games. Children at this age appear to respond most favorably with gender-segregated classes, based on their general discomfort with sexual topics and unique needs and questions. Some schools appropriately incorporate these classes into school curricula as part of a health-promotion curriculum. Other schools have special programs focused only on sex education based on parental desires or school board policies. Most school-age children have the cognitive skills to respond to programs on responsible sexuality, including discussions on abstinence and condom use, pregnancy, sexually transmitted diseases, and the human immunodeficiency virus (USDHHS, 2000). The nurse also wants to include program content specific to disabled children who face unique body changes and concerns and need to understand ways others can express affection to them without causing accusations of abuse.

Coping-Stress Tolerance Pattern

The school-age child must learn to cope with stress as part of the developmental process. Through a health-promotion program, children can learn to identify symptoms of stress (pounding heart, stomach "butterflies," and sweaty hands) and ways to cope with these perceived stresses (e.g., deep breathing and walking) before they cause illness. The child actually faces many stressful experiences in life, including competition, homework deadlines, failure at home or school, and decisions whether to cheat, steal, or even join an unpopular peer group. The young school-age child may never have shared his life with other children his age, and cultural values learned earlier in life may not be reflected in school or in peer relationships. Threats to the child's security (e.g., bullying) cause feelings of helplessness and anxiety that may affect the ability to function successfully. Grief over the death of a loved one, parental divorce, loss of a favorite activity because of misbehavior, or expulsion from a favorite peer group may cause negative behavior. Parents need to provide appropriate discipline in responding to this behavior but should also listen and analyze factors related to the problem in order to increase the child's feelings of control and decrease stress for the family (see Health Teaching box, p. 482).

Children use a variety of **coping strategies,** healthy behaviors intended to buffer perceived stressful events (Table 20-2). One study showed that humor helped some school-age children cope with unexpected challenges (Dowling, 2002). However, in a very stressful situation or many stressful situations, a child may be unable to move

Table **20-2** The School-Age Child's Coping Strategies and Nursing Interventions to Promote Coping

Coping Strategies	Nursing Interventions
Use of defense mechanisms (regression, denial, repression, projection, displacement, sublimation)	Accept child's use of defense mechanisms as temporary, healthy coping responses; provide child options for moving to more age-appropriate ways of responding to stressors
Cognitive mastery (problem solving, communication)	Ask children what they know of situation and how they might handle it; encourage questions; use diagrams and models to help explain; encourage child to verbalize feelings and use past successful strategies that might help deal with present stressors; try personalized approaches such as books, puppets, manipulation of equipment, to increase feelings of control when faced with stressful situation; encourage praying and other communications to a chosen deity as appropriate
Controlling, holding behaviors	Encourage child to participate and to make decisions; accept child's need to direct as appropriate; set consistent age-appropriate limits; respond to signals for help; let child be responsible for self-care
Use of repetition	Use books, games, and other communication media to work through feelings; emphasize "ok" for child to continue to ask questions and to receive answers that assist in coping
Use of humor	Be a good listener and participate in riddles and jokes used by child; be a good sport with school-age children's desire to play jokes on each other; share stories and cartoons with child
Motor activity, aggression, protest behavior	Encourage physical activity to deal with stress; accept appropriate behavior; establish limits on behavior for group safety
Withdrawal (resurgence of separation anxiety)	When child is separated from family, may have separation anxiety; encourage close emotional contacts between child and significant others (friends, family, church members); allow favorite objects from home to be brought to hospital or new environment for child

beyond the coping behaviors. In conversations with teachers and parents, the nurse may offer a variety of strategies for coping with a school-age child's problems, enabling the child to cope and learn from others. These strategies may involve role playing or referral to literature on the problem topic to interrupt the child's negative behavior cycle to improve family health. **Web Site Resource 20D** presents a list of books that may be helpful to parents of a school-age child. The nurse may also refer a child to relevant religious and spiritual leaders, based on school-age children's belief that prayer will help them cope with an otherwise uncontrollable situation (Wong et al., 2002).

Parental Divorce

More than one half of all marriages end in divorce, leaving many school-age children to face stress related to their parents' separation. Often children experience a feeling of loss, although they may hope that their parents will reunite at some point. Children's responses vary with their level of development. Factors such as economic security, availability of both of their parents, other family, church, and school supports, and quality of interactions with their parents can influence the child's ability to cope with divorce. Unfortunately, many parents become so immersed in their own feelings that they fail to support their children. Conflicts over custody, child support, and visitation rights add to the child's difficulty in coping. Sometimes the school system must become the child's advocate to encourage the parents

to provide a supportive environment during divorce proceedings. Despite this intervention, some children do not cope well with the divorce and have emotional after-effects that result in juvenile behavior problems or require long-term counseling.

Somatization and Depression

Children, like adults, use defense mechanisms to cope, with varying degrees of success. Two strategies used by the school-age child to respond to uncontrollable situations are somatization and depression.

Some children respond to a stressful situation by transferring their feelings to a physical problem **(somatization).** In this phenomenon, school-age children, unable to discuss their concerns, complain of stomachaches or headaches, symptoms reflective of functional or psychogenic pain. These children may also develop discrete, repetitive movement habits called *tics*. In many cases the child with these problems must be evaluated to determine whether an underlying physiological cause exists. The child and the family will then need assistance in understanding the child's concerns to define successful ways to cope with the behavior.

Depression occurs in 0.8% to 2% of children (U.S. Preventive Services Task Force, 2004b) and more often in boys than girls during the school-age period (Keep Kids Healthy, 1999). **Depression** reflects a disturbance of mood, when a child displays sadness, guilt or worthlessness, and other unusual behaviors that disengage the child from peers and family. In defining depression in children, most authors point out that they refer to a more long-term syndrome in which the child's normal development and functioning become impaired, not a periodic sadness that all children occasionally experience. Factors that place a child at risk for depression include homelessness, death of a parent or significant other, divorce, long-term hospitalization, chronic illness, learning problems, or emotional turmoil at home. Parents and teachers should look for symptoms of depression, including anorexia, sleeplessness, lethargy, changed affect, aggressive behavior, frequent crying, or withdrawal from previously enjoyed activities. The child may also frequently daydream, become more dependent, berate self, or utter words that show low self-esteem (APA, 1994; Goldstein & Mather, 1998).

Although the U.S. Preventive Services Task Force (2004b) has concluded there is insufficient evidence to routinely screen all school-age children for depression, the nurse can serve an important role in identifying any child who appears to be depressed and notifying parents about the need for further assessment. Depending on the child and the situation, varying amounts of counseling and individual child guidance may be required. Although controversial at this time, antidepressant medication may also be prescribed (Mathews, 2004). Nurses in schools and outpatient settings are often the ideal helpers, because they have the skills and time needed to help a child cope with a helpless feeling and its cause.

Values-Beliefs Pattern

Children make decisions related to moral and ethical issues every day. Should they tell the teacher which classmate broke the rule? Should they share their candy with a younger sibling? For these situations, the child makes a decision based on the level of moral development. Moral development involves choosing the most appropriate behavior based on one's values and feelings related to the situation. Environmental factors and culture strongly influence a child's moral development, as do the type of family discipline, role models, people with whom the child identifies, and the child's rehearsal and practice of moral behavior (Wong et al., 2002).

Kohlberg's Theory

Most researchers agree that the younger school-age child is at the **preconventional level,** a level of moral development characterized by self-interest only. The child continues to do many things simply to avoid getting in trouble, does not understand the reason for rules, but also performs actions that will benefit the self (Kohlberg, 1981; Murray, 2001). During later childhood (10 to 13 years) most children progress to the **conventional level,** a stage of moral development defined by concern about group interests and values. The conventional level of moral judgment involves the child looking to others for approval and to societal authority for a definition of rules. Children 10 to 12 years old judge a behavior in terms of the intention of the offender, understand the "golden rule" concept, and engage in behavior that maintains a valued relationship. The conventional level coincides with Piaget's cognitive level of concrete operations and the child's increased social involvement with people outside the home (Kohlberg, 1981; Murray, 2001).

Moral Behavior Problems

Some moral behavior problems, such as lying, stealing, or cheating, are common during the school-age years. Cultural, religious and parental values influence a child's moral development, concept of right and wrong, and consequences of not demonstrating moral behavior. Preschool and younger school-age children frequently lie due to fantasy, exaggerations, or inaccurate understanding. As children grow, they may use the defense mechanism of denial to block upsetting situations and maintain self-esteem. The lie then becomes an unconscious act. Older children often lie because they fear punishment or ridicule. Children may cheat because of a desire to win, do well in competitive society or "look good" for their peers. Children usually steal when they think they will not be caught and they think that there is no other way to get what they want. Although these actions can be quite upsetting for parents, they are common developmental behaviors. Parents frequently need reassurance that the child is normal and probably will outgrow the behavior with parental assistance. They may need help in developing fair rules for behavior and communicating their expectations for a child's behavior to meet parental and cultural values. Therefore the nurse may encourage the parents to warn the child clearly not to steal, lie, or cheat, offer other more socially acceptable ways to cope with the stressor causing the behavior, and then apply appropriate punishment congruent with an understanding of the event.

PATHOLOGICAL PROCESSES

School-age children, similar to those of all other age groups, face daily exposure to environmental agents and factors that may cause injury, illness, or death. Many of these agents and factors are harmless if appropriately used or when exposure is minimal. Examples include physical agents such as fires; mechanical agents such as bicycles, skateboards, and cars; biological agents such as bacteria; chemical agents such as asbestos; and radiological agents such as x-rays. Death rates from these agents vary among ethnic groups because of access to health care and environmental issues. For example, Native Americans and Alaska Natives experience higher death rates from motor vehicle accidents, residential fires, and drowning than do other groups (USDHHS, 2000). Blacks experience higher death rates for unintentional injury than do other ethnic group members (Centers for Disease Control and Prevention, 1999b).

Accidents

Accidents are the leading cause of death in children over age 1 year in the United States and Great Britain (Cole,

SAFETY CONCERNS SPECIFIC TO SCHOOL-AGE CHILDREN

HOTtopics

Because of increased independence, school-age children face significant exposure to situations threatening their health. Consequently, parents of these children must be involved in community and legislative activities that provide safe play environments. Additionally, at appropriate health visits, health care workers should provide anticipatory guidance to parents in the following areas:

Bicycle safety: each child should have a well-maintained bicycle, ride only in safe areas approved by parents, observe rules for vehicle traffic, ride on the side of road with traffic, "bike defensively," and use a federally approved riding helmet

Street safety: children should look right, left, then right again to check safety of crossing a street; cross only at safe and well-monitored intersections, preferably with an adult present; ensure parental supervision when children play close to streets and heavy traffic areas

Motor vehicle safety: children should wear seat belt or be in age-appropriate booster seat as needed; older children should ride with restraint system and in back seat until age 12

Pool safety: all children should have swimming lessons and swim with a buddy or adult who swims well; all pools should have drain covers; children should avoid swimming after a heavy meal and avoid "roughhousing" behavior around the pool; children should be monitored by parents during swimming

Firearm safety: adults need to lock away guns and ensure gun safety locks are intact; parents need to educate children NEVER to touch guns

Playground safety: all playground equipment should meet federally approved standards; children should be trained on how to use equipment safely; equipment should be evaluated for safety and repaired before children use it

Fire safety: working smoke detectors should be in place in home and school; family needs to have a fire evacuation plan and practice it; children need to wear fire-retardant clothing at night; children should not play with matches, open fires, fireworks, or open wires that can cause injury and fire

Toxin safety: children should avoid insecticides, radiation sources, inappropriate use of medications, and pollution sources; parents need to store all known toxins, chemicals, and household cleaning agents in an adequately ventilated location that is inaccessible to children

Stranger safety: children should play with friends, have a plan for returning home, know home phone number and address, play in safe and known area, and report any suspicious activity threatening their safety to an appropriate adult; children should know how to say "no" and how to locate assistance when in an unsafe situation

Sports safety: children need to engage in age-appropriate activities and wear protective equipment relevant to the sport; parents need to ensure safety and maintenance of all sports equipment; parents need to caution children against hazardous sports, such as trampolines

Animal safety: parents should teach children to avoid strange animals, especially sick or injured ones, and ensure that personal pets receive vaccinations; need to teach children not to mistreat pets and not to place their faces close to any animal

Naidoo, & Wills, 1998; USDHHS, 2000). Most accidents do not result in death, but many serious ones cause significant morbidity and disability. Because of this effect, the nurse has a significant role in educating parents and school personnel on ways to prevent dangers to school-age children and to become involved in public initiatives to create a safer society for them (Hot Topics box).

The agent, host, and environment must be considered in developing solutions to decrease the number of accidents. The type of agent varies with the child's age. Most fatal accidents during the school-age period derive from motor vehicle accidents when the child (host) is a passenger or pedestrian (walking or riding a bike). Other fatal accidents occur from fires and burns, bicycles, drowning, and firearm accidents. Most common nonfatal accidents tend to be caused by simple agents that produce simple injuries. Despite helmet laws in several states, many school-age children continue to experience head injuries related to recreational equipment, such as bicycles, swings, skateboards, and trampolines (Wong et al., 2002). Slightly older children have an increased number of accidents from contact sports and cuts, falls, burns, and injuries from firearms.

Specific accident factors relate to the host, the school-age child. Children in this age group tend to become hurt because of their happy-go-lucky attitude, curiosity, love of mimicking older people, and their intense oral tendencies (Wilson, 2001). Typically school-age boys have more accidents than girls, perhaps due to differences in personalities, societal expectations, child-rearing practices, and more risk-taking behaviors. The mechanism varies with the gender of the host. For school-age boys, drowning is the most common fatal accident; for girls, automobile accidents are the most common (Centers for Disease Control and Prevention, 1999a).

The physical environment of the child dictates the type or frequency of accidents, which occur in the home, neighborhood, and school. Most accidents happen outdoors, which means that school-age children face greater risk for automobile or bicycle accidents than for poisoning or falls, indoor accidents that occur predominately in the younger set. More accidents (drowning and pedestrian-vehicle accidents) occur in the summer than in the winter because of children's outside play. Socioeconomic level affects children's physical environments and access to dangers. For example, space heaters place children of low-income families at risk for burns, whereas a private swimming pool places wealthier children at risk for drowning.

The social environment, which includes the family, school, and playmates, also plays a role in accidents. Although little research has focused on the physical trauma caused by heavy backpacks that many school-age children use, appliances such as these exert significant pressure against functionally immature muscles of the back and torso. Daily carrying of bulging backpacks causes muscle strain, headaches, improper posture, shoulder slouch, and other physical problems. At least one study has shown that children will change their backpack carrying behaviors if involved in a school-based program focused on this topic (Goodgold & Nielsen, 2003).

As part of the social environment, the family may influence the rate of accidents in the school-age child. Chronic familial stress (parental unemployment) or a sudden acute stress (parental illness) may contribute to homicide as the third leading cause of death among children ages 5 to 14 years (Osofsky, Cohen, & Drell, 1995; USDHHS, 2000). Homicide is a more common cause of death among black and Hispanic children than white children (Anderson, Kockanck, & Murphey, 1997). Children also face increased risk of accidents when parental supervision is limited, such as during holidays or a move to a new home.

Drowning

Fewer school-age children than infants and adolescents die from drowning. More black children of this age drown than do white children (USDHHS, 2000). Water safety measures can help reduce drowning, along with the many other injuries that occur around water, such as falls in slippery areas. **Web Site Resource 20E** contains a detailed list of safety practices, including water safety. Environment and safety teaching can influence the number of school-age children dying as a result of drowning.

Burns

Each year many children become victims of house fires, many of which occur during the winter months from Christmas tree, space heater, and fireplace malfunctions. Many homes lack working smoke detectors because of incorrect installation or inadequate testing. Most burned children survive, frequently with varying degrees of physical and psychological scars. Children need to learn about fire safety, including the need to avoid situations involving fire and to practice fire drills routinely at school and home. The nurse can encourage parents to understand other practices to prevent fire-related problems, including parental purchase of flame-retardant sleepwear for children. See **Web Site Resource 20E** for fire prevention practices.

Firearms

People in the United States who use firearms frequently cause fatal injury through homicide, suicide, or accidents. Every 2 hours someone's child dies due to a gun accident (Schor, 1998). With many U.S. homes containing a handgun and because of recent shootings by adolescents, concern about children's safety remains well founded. Possibly the best means of preventing accidents with firearms is to ban them from private ownership as seen in England (see Chapter 19). However, because handgun ownership is an important individual right in this country, several states have passed legislation that allows handguns for individual protection. Families with firearms in the home should store guns in a locked area apart from ammunition and consider using nonlethal (wax) bullets. All children should be taught about gun safety.

Sports and Recreation

Accidents from sports and other recreational activities increase during the school-age years and include lacerations, contusions, hematomas, concussions, sprains, and fractures. Some evidence exists that adolescents now have more musculoskeletal injuries due to involvement in repetitive team sports earlier in their lives. This suggests that society needs to examine the current emphasis on initiating young children with musculoskeletal immaturity into team sports such as football, hockey, soccer, and basketball. Intense social pressure for children to participate in these sports means that parents and school systems must ensure that each child has protective body devices to prevent injuries, as well as psychological support to allow a child to benefit from the team sport. There is a further need to increase safety by ensuring that each child fits the sport, has adequate hydration during the game, and engages in conditioning exercises before and after the game for prevention of injuries. Furthermore, literature supports societal need to focus more on the collaborative skills children learn by being part of a team, rather than the winning-despite-the-costs philosophy found in many school-age team sports (Cary, 2004).

Recreation area injuries may be prevented by several measures. The National Bureau of Standards set guidelines in 1976 for home playground equipment, regulating things such as sharp edges, moving parts, and equipment design. Nurses can help prevent accidents by participating in decisions about school playground equipment and counseling families on a variety of issues. See **Web Site Resource 20E** for playground safety practices. Playground safety has become an important issue, because 200,000 children need emergency room assessment each year for related injuries (Reuters Health, 2000). Many of these occur in Hispanic and Pacific Islander students who live in areas where playgrounds fail to meet safety standards (USDHHS, 2000).

Nursing Interventions

Although nurses offer suggestions to parents to improve their children's play safety, studies have shown that few parents follow these suggestions. Reasons for this behavior include parental difficulty in assessing the safety of and age appropriateness of play equipment, the amount of effort involved, and a lack of money to create a safe play area.

Box **20-6**	Nursing Interventions to Prevent Accidents During the School-Age Period

STRATEGIES FOR COUNSELING

- Discuss accident prevention at optimal times, such as during prenatal visits, well-child visits, after the arrival of a new sibling, or after an accident.
- Rather than discussing all topics at once, pick the main concerns for the developmental level of the child at each well-child visit. For the school-age child, these topics include motor vehicle, water, fire, and bicycle safety.
- Repeat information at other visits to emphasize its importance.

COMMUNITY ACTIONS

- Use supplemental materials, such as pamphlets, to reinforce the verbal information.
- Support local and national legislation that sets standards for potentially harmful agents. Mandating standards has been one of the most successful accident preventives, as seen in the Poison Prevention Packaging Act and the Flammable Fabrics Act.
- Encourage children to wear a bicycle helmet and other protective gear when appropriate. Many nurses have been active in lobbying for bicycle helmet requirements in their states.
- Consult with manufacturers on safe designs of materials used by children.
- Report objects that are potentially hazardous.
- Participate in local activities that stress accident prevention, such as those organized by local offices of the National Safety Council.
- Educate groups, such as school children and parent organizations.

Thus the nurse can help them respond to these perceived barriers. With more children using skateboards and rollerblades, the nurse must also encourage child safety helmets and knee, elbow, and wrist guards to prevent muscle sprains and bone fractures. The school offers an on-site opportunity for teaching children, teachers, and parents about accident prevention. In addition to providing this guidance, nurses can participate in legislative and educational actions to increase community consciousness about child safety (Box 20-6).

Mechanical Forces

Motor vehicles and bicycles represent the two most common mechanical agents that cause injury to school-age children.

Motor Vehicles

The leading cause of death in the United States in all groups of children from age 1 to adulthood is motor vehicle accidents (Aetna/U.S. Healthcare, 1998; Durbin, Elliott, & Winston, 2003). Children die as passengers in cars, as pedestrians, and as bicycle riders. In this country, more children die from pedestrian-related accidents than passenger-

related accidents (Wilson, 2001). More than 30% of the people killed in bicycle accidents are children, many of whom did not wear helmets to prevent head injury (Insurance Institute for Highway Safety, 1997). Although not all accidents result in death, children may also sustain injury that causes permanent diability as a result of motor-vehicle accidents.

Automobile passenger injuries can be prevented, or the severity reduced, by altering some aspects of the child's environment. Lower speed limits, alcohol-related laws, better automobile and highway designs, door lock mechanisms, and effective restraint system requirements in all states have reduced the severity and number of accidents and injuries. However, more injuries have been correlated to higher speed limits instituted in the United States several years ago. Furthermore, many children remain at risk for injury, because various school districts and states do not require seat belts in buses used to transport students, despite a recommendation by the American Academy of Pediatrics (1996) to do so.

Studies indicate that proper and consistent use of federally approved belt-positioned booster seats for children ages 4 to 7 years decreases the likelihood of child death by 70% to 95% and decreases serious injury by 50% to 60% (AAP, 1996). However, one study showed that only 19% of such children used these seats (National Highway Traffic Safety Administration, 2004). Less than 10% of children needing the protection of a booster seat ride in one, and younger, smaller school-age children (under 4 feet, 9 inches) often fail to use them correctly (National Highway Traffic Safety Administration, 2004). Reasons given by parents and children for not using seat belts or booster seats include forgetting to use, difficulty reaching and fastening belts, seat belt or seat discomfort, and misinformation about the need for the belt or seat for short trips. Clearly, consistent use of booster seats by young children and seat belts by older children and adults, who model seat belt behavior to their children, will occur only when legal enforcement occurs. Federal government and national professional groups recommend that all children under the age of 12 years ride in the automobile's back seat in an appropriate restraint due to the potential for death from an air bag activated in a motor vehicle accident (Wong & Hess, 2000). Many families have difficulty meeting this recommendation because of long-term acceptance of older children riding in the front seat after they have outgrown booster seats.

Urban children under the age of 15 years experience more than one half of all pedestrian-automobile accidents (Wong et al., 2002). These occur when using rollerblades, skateboards, and skate scooters and tend to be more severe (head injuries) than passenger injuries. Many factors cause pedestrian accidents: children often have difficulty interpreting traffic signs and judging the speed of cars, and they forget to look carefully before crossing the street. Although overcrowding, poverty, high volume of traffic, stress, and unsafe play areas influence children's street safety, various principles can direct interventions to decrease the number of street dangers. Detailed street safety principles are presented in **Web Site Resource 20E.**

Bicycles and Motorized Vehicles

Many accidents occur each year with young children on bicycles, motorized skateboards, and all terrain vehicles (ATVs). Most of these are not serious, but deaths occur among young children who have suffered head trauma or significant bodily injury from inappropriate use of this equipment. The American Academy of Pediatrics (1994) recommends that only people at least age 16 years ride ATVs and then only in rural areas with adult supervision. Bicycle accidents occur most frequently near the child's home and during the day and commonly involve injuries from the spokes when children ride behind the bike seat. More boys than girls experience these injuries from bicycles, motorized skateboards, and ATVs, perhaps based on their greater risk-taking behavior.

In response to children's developmental behavior related to bicycles, motorized skateboards, and ATVs, the nurse needs to address safety issues. See **Web Site Resource 20E** for transportation safety practices for school-age children. Additionally, nurses should encourage parents to teach and reinforce safe bicycling habits to their children and should sponsor helmet and bike programs within the school. At least one school-based intervention involving parental education and mentoring succeeded in increasing from 18% to 66% the numbers of diverse population, low-income school-age children wearing helmets while biking (Hendrickson & Becker, 2000).

Biological Agents

School-age children face constant exposure to bacterial, viral, and other biological agents that pose threats to or improve their overall health (e.g., immunizations). Compared with the preschool child, the school-age child has fewer illnesses. The most frequent illness continues to be upper respiratory infections (URIs), illnesses shared among school children who fail to practice good hand washing and avoidance of ill peers. These illnesses cause children to lose school days and learning opportunities. Most URIs result from viruses, but bacteria can play either a primary or a secondary role. Two problems associated with URIs are streptococcal infection ("strep throat") and otitis media.

Strep throat occurs frequently among school-age children. A child with an infection from Group A streptococcus may have a severe sore throat, fever, and malaise or may have only a minor sore throat. A throat culture confirms the diagnosis, and antibiotic treatment typically cures the infection. Children are noninfectious after 24 hours of treatment and may return to school (AAP, Committee on Infectious Diseases, 2004). If not treated, the affected child may develop rheumatic fever or acute glomerulonephritis as a secondary infection following the sore throat. Greater transmission of streptococcal infection occurs in areas where there is close person-to-person contact during colder weather. The school nurse's preventive efforts focus on teaching the children good hand washing techniques and identifying children who complain of sore throats. Children with throat infections caused by other strains of streptococcus, such as group B, do not usually require treatment, because these infections generally do not cause the same serious complications.

The school-age child may experience other illnesses. The frequency of gastrointestinal infection (gastroenteritis) decreases during the school-age years but is still the second most common acute condition of childhood. Usually caused by a virus, gastrointestinal infection causes vomiting and diarrhea. Older and larger school-age children have little chance of rapid dehydration; they basically react to the illness the same as do adults and need to be treated similarly. Gastroenteritis is contagious and, therefore, the nurse should monitor school children for symptoms of illness and encourage hand washing to prevent transmission of the virus from one child to another.

Scabies and lice (**pediculosis**) are common skin disorders among school-age children. This problem causes extreme itchiness of either the body (scabies) or the head (lice) and is easily spread to other children. The nurse needs to educate parents to visualize or use a lice comb to check their children for scabies and lice when they complain of itchiness or seem to be constantly scratching their heads (Goldsmith, 2003). Previously, children diagnosed with lice could not come to school until they were lice free. This isolated students from their peers and influenced state school funding based on student attendance. The American Academy of Pediatrics now recommends that if children are under treatment for the problem, they should be allowed in school (AAP, Committee on Infectious Diseases, 2004).

A biological agent that many children know about is human immunodeficiency virus, or HIV, which causes acquired immunodeficiency syndrome (AIDS). Of all age groups, the young school-age child is at the lowest risk for contracting the disease, because AIDS acquired by the perinatal route emerges in infancy and toddlerhood, and most young school-age children do not use intravenous drugs or engage in high-risk sexual practices. However, the school-age child may know a person with AIDS or may have heard something about the disease from adults, older children, or the news media. The school-age child and school staff should know basic facts about the disease, its transmission and, most importantly, that it cannot be transmitted through casual contact, such as being in the same classroom with a child who has it. **Web Site Resource 20F** contains resources for AIDS educational materials. Due to widespread misinformation and fear, the United States Surgeon General has called for mandatory, explicit AIDS education beginning with children 8 years of age. The involvement of parents, students, and school personnel in AIDS education programs through age-appropriate materials will increase each group's knowledge and acceptance of people who have the disease. Accepting parents assist their own children in learning to accept others with special needs and in taking better control of their own health.

Children with AIDS may attend school as long as they will not be exposed to illness from other children. Most children with AIDS receive routine immunizations but may need further immunization if exposed to a usual childhood disease (AAP, Committee on Infectious Diseases, 2004). During outbreaks of contagious disease, the chronically ill child may have home tutoring; this approach will need to be evaluated annually to identify the risks versus benefits of school attendance. Certainly, long periods of isolation from peers will contribute to feelings of loneliness in the child with AIDS and may even appear to be a punishment for being ill. The school nurse undoubtedly has an important role in facilitating the multidisciplinary nature of AIDS care while maximizing the learning environment of affected children.

Most states require that the child's immunizations be current before entering kindergarten or the first grade and that additional tetanus immunization be given every 10 years or with an unclean wound. Other immunizations recommended by the American Academy of Pediatrics include a measles, mumps, and rubella (MMR) vaccination at age 11 or 12 years and the series of three injections for hepatitis B during the late school-age and early adolescent years. If the child has no history of chickenpox, a varicella immunization is also recommended (AAP, Committee on Infectious Diseases, 2004; Wong & Hess, 2000). In many states the school nurse has a responsibility to ensure that all students' immunizations are current and, if not, the nurse must inform the parents that the children may not attend school until their immunizations have been brought up to date. Any child lacking age-appropriate immunizations can "catch up" according to a schedule developed by the American Academy of Pediatrics (AAP, Committee on Infectious Diseases, 2004). Although 95% of American children receive immunizations by school entrance time (USDHHS, 2000), increasing numbers of immigrants and transient workers have deepened concern about exposure of Americans to previously conquered diseases (e.g., tuberculosis).

Chemical Agents

A number of potentially toxic chemical agents exist in the environment, and the child is exposed to these through inhalation, ingestion, or direct contact. Children are particularly susceptible to chemical hazards. Food and drugs are two sources of chemicals ingested by children on a regular basis, and some older school-age children ingest tobacco as a result of cigarette smoking. Although normally safe, some foods and drugs can be harmful when used inappropriately. Other environmental hazards include pollution, heavy metals (lead and mercury), and pesticides.

The nutritional needs of the school-age child are discussed earlier in this chapter. As stated, children frequently eat foods with large quantities of sugar, salt, and fat and with chemical additives. The effects of some of these additives have been questioned, and concern has been expressed about the effect of biochemically altered food on children

and future generations. On a short-term basis, some foods may cause allergic reactions; on a long-term basis, some may contribute to the development of coronary disease, hypertension, and cancer. Nurses need to be aware that the child's diet may contribute to future health problems and should assess intake and counsel the child and parents accordingly about ways to improve it.

The incidence of poisoning decreases during the school-age years as children become more aware of the appropriate uses of drugs and other agents. Childproof containers have decreased exposure of children to dangerous poisons and chemicals in the home. However, children continue to face exposure to drugs (alcohol and glue inhalants) due to less monitoring by working parents, and older school-age children face exposure to recreational drugs, primarily through their peers and older children (see Chapter 21). In the school environment the nurse and school personnel need to encourage students to engage in wise decision making about recreational drug use that will affect their future and overall health.

With pressure on older school-age children, particularly African American children, to smoke cigarettes, attention must be paid to effective strategies to prevent these behaviors. Most students who smoke initiate their habit around 12 years of age, and by age 15 years 30% of children smoke. However, more are white than Hispanic or African American (USDHHS, 2000). Attention to smoking as part of a health-promotion program seems merited, because so many begin so young and, because nicotine is highly addictive, many believe that this habit leads people to experiment with more risky drugs (cocaine and methamphetamines). Various governmental efforts (e.g., the tobacco act of 1991), focused on policing businesses selling cigarettes to minors, have so far been ineffective in reducing the number of young smokers (Recer, 2000). Proponents of antismoking campaigns support higher excise taxes and less media support for the activity. Smoking behavior is more common in diverse communities in which billboards advertise its attractiveness, where there is greater access to cigarettes, and where peer pressure and less parental involvement have hindered antismoking efforts (USDHHS, 2000). The federal Tobacco Settlement Project (1998) forbids tobacco advertisements on television. Fewer children may choose to become smokers based on fewer media messages to acquire this habit.

Pollution has become a fact of life for many Americans and, particularly, for the 25% of urban dwelling children who must breathe air that exceeds federal government levels for acceptable ozone (USDHHS, 2000). Air pollution irritates the eyes and the respiratory tract, causing URIs, ear infections, and allergies. More children now experience asthma, and many inner city children face higher rates of this disease due to poor air quality and secondary smoke. Death rates from this illness escalated 67% from 1980 to 1993, and 40% of all activity restrictions of children result from asthma (USDHHS, 2000). Knowing the negative effects of air pollution and smoking to their health, many school-age children participate in school projects to improve their environmental health.

Children also face exposure to toxic materials such as lead (see Chapter 17), cadmium, mercury, arsenic, and asbestos. Mercury is particularly toxic to the developing CNS, and recent recommendations have been made for young children to avoid eating tuna with high mercury levels ("Is the government," 2004). Asbestos may cause breathing difficulties in children, sometimes years after exposure. Children are exposed to lead through parents' clothes, shoes contacting lead-infused soil, lead in older residential water pipes, traditional medications in some cultures, or in school building structures (Wolfe, 2000). Children living in poverty receive high exposure from lead-based paint used on older and cheaper homes. The long-term effects of these metals on children remain unclear, but some evidence indicates children suffer neurotoxic effects from this type of exposure. Moss, Lanphear, and Auinger (1999) also point out that high lead levels in children contribute to dental caries, and other researchers have supported that hearing loss and even criminal behavior can result from early and consistent childhood exposure to lead.

Routine use of chemicals to control insects and undesirable weeds in landscaping has led to increasing concerns about children's exposure to these agents. Animal experiments led to the recent withdrawal of a common pesticide, chlorpyrifos (Dursban), from the marketplace. Each summer, media figures discuss the use of diethylmethyltoluamide (DEET) as an agent protective against mosquitoes and warn parents about using concentrations higher than 10% on their children. With increased interest in more natural substances to control insects and gardening problems, perhaps less reliance will be placed on biological chemicals for these problems in the future.

Radiological Agents
X-ray Exposure

The child receives exposure from both naturally occurring radiation and human-made ionizing radiation. Exposure occurs in varying degrees with radiographic examinations of teeth and bone, from nuclear power plants and explosions, and in the management of many childhood cancers. Children exposed to high levels of radiation risk developing breast or thyroid cancer or leukemia and compromised growth. With little advocacy in this area, nurses and other professionals can improve children's health by becoming active in initiatives that focus on prevention of chemical and radiation hazards as presented in **Web Site Resource 20G.**

Cancer

Leukemia is the most common form of childhood cancer (see Chapter 19). Of those affected, 80% will be cured with current medical treatment (Marcus, 2004). Lymphomas (Hodgkin disease and non-Hodgkin lymphoma) also affect school-age children and adolescents as the third most common group of malignancies. Non-Hodgkin lymphoma

is more common during the school-age years, and boys experience this malignancy 3 times more often than do girls. Mortality rates in the United States tend to be greater in densely populated areas, particularly where the more educated and wealthy live (Wong et al., 2002). The most common symptom is abdominal pain caused by intestinal obstruction and symptoms resulting from organ compression. With effective treatment regimens, children with limited disease may be cured but may experience side effects of treatment later in life (e.g., development of cataracts, dental problems, learning difficulties) (Marcus, 2004). These children present a challenge to the nurse because they are in various stages of recovery, may be developmentally delayed, and may fear a recurrence of their disease. Therefore the nurse must provide psychological and emotional support to affected children and their families, to help children develop peer relationships and meet developmental goals important to them during the school-age years.

SOCIAL PROCESSES

The school-age child interacts daily with other children and adults to become more independent by age 12. Mutual problem solving of child and parents or friends frequently occurs at this age related to a higher level of maturity in social relationships and concerns. Exposure to a variety of social roles and expectations of others strengthens the process of **socialization** so that the child develops social competence, the ability and skills to participate effectively in the social interactions of society (Schor, 1998). Social competence includes both the obvious social behaviors and an inner understanding of the appropriateness of behaviors.

Several elements play a role in the development of the child's social competence. The child's desire for a sense of industry encourages interactions, positive relationships, and accomplishments within society. Cognitive development supports understanding of relationships and effective problem solving. Moral judgment helps the child understand consequences and fairness in relationships. Understanding and obeying authority helps to maintain order in society. Social sensitivity is a result of social interactions and requires the child's ability to perceive the social cues of others, understand the roles of others, and communicate verbally with them. Social behaviors are also a part of social competence; these are learned most frequently through imitation, role modeling, and reinforcement of others' behaviors. The interaction of all these elements produces a level of social competence and simultaneously plays a role in the child's self-perception. Individuals frequently see themselves as others see them.

Community and Work
Peers

The strongest relationships that school-age children develop outside their families are with their peers (other children encountered in the neighborhood and school). The peer group acts as a new social system, becoming increasingly influential in the child's life. All children continue to be influenced significantly by the family, the culture of the family, and many other environmental factors, but the peer group begins to influence lifestyle, habits, and speech patterns and formulate standards of behavior and performance. The standards of the peer group become vitally important, and children attempt to conform to rules. Being accepted by the peer group becomes more important than being accepted by anyone else. Conforming to the pressures of peers becomes an issue, especially when it interferes with the parents' expectations. When children realize that their own goals, desires, and aspirations might be quite different from those held by the peer group or the school, they must find ways to cope and perform according to the new standards if they are to succeed. The degree to which children fit in socially, learn to cope, and receive satisfaction from the group is a powerful determinant of healthy socialization.

A child may have one best friend or several important friends and a mutual understanding and willingness to help each other. Friendship groups that form during this age may change and become goal directed, such as groups composing a sports team. These groups frequently have set rules or rituals that connect the members. During the middle school-age years, friendships often revolve around same-gender relationships, videos, songs, books, and media shared by the group. Later in the school-age years, the development of sexual relationships with the opposite gender occurs during dating and mixed parties.

School-age children also become increasingly involved with adults outside the family, including teachers, coaches, and others who become role models, all of whom influence the child's view of the world and self. Although this influence may not be as significant as that of a child's peers, long-term ideas and beliefs frequently develop from these relationships. Children usually perceive some similarity between themselves and their models, those of the same gender with similar physical or behavior traits. During these years children may not maintain a strong identification with the parent of the same gender, but they tend to adopt other adult models with whom they can identify.

Working Parents

Studies have shown that over one half of mothers with children between ages 6 and 17 work outside the home, and most work full time. Many of these women work out of economic necessity but remain concerned about the welfare of their children during work hours. Both dual-career couples and single-parent families influence their children's safety when no adult is present to monitor the environment after school. Many children who are left alone until their parents return from work follow directions given by their parents. These directions may include beginning dinner in anticipation of their parents' return or completing homework while remaining inside the home with the doors locked.

Parents and school-age children often disagree about how old is "old enough" to be left at home alone or with an older sibling. Although the school-age child might consider being at home alone to be a real mark of maturity, children who look after themselves after school can become more isolated and miss peer relationships important to their development. Nurses can give guidance to families who must cope with the issue of after-school care for school-age children (Box 20-7) to ensure that a relevant and safe decision has been made (see Chapter 19).

Culture and Ethnicity

School-age children focus more on the influences of their culture on their lives than do younger children. Aspects of American culture that the child must confront include poverty and affluence, ethnic and racial differences, acceptance of these differences, and the power of media as a cultural phenomenon in American society.

Ethnic Groups

Preschool children may notice racial and ethnic differences, but school-age children increasingly show evidence of being aware of these differences. This is a time during which attitudes toward race develop based on family and community

---

Box 20-7 After-School Considerations for Latchkey Children

- Each child should be assessed frequently to determine appropriate after-school supervision. One 10-year-old child might be mature enough to be alone for a short time; another might not be ready for this responsibility. The child should play a role in this discussion, but the parents should make the decision.
- Alternatives to a latch-key situation should be considered (after-school day care, neighbors, other family members, or older siblings).
- When the child is alone, a set schedule should be discussed. This schedule might include the time at which the child should be home and whether a parent should be called when the child arrives there. The child should be encouraged not to share that he is home alone after school.
- Rules should be discussed and posted in an accessible place. These rules might define acceptable after-school activities, use of television, homework completion, snacking, play with friends, places that the child may go with others, and need to not enter the home if it looks unsafe.
- Important information (e.g., numbers for police, fire department) should be posted in an accessible place. Have child practice using these numbers before an emergency arises.
- Emergency measures should be planned with the child: plans if the child gets sick, loses the house key, or strangers call on the phone or knock on the door. Plans should include how to reach both a parent and another responsible adult in the neighborhood who has agreed to help as needed. The family should discuss situations defining an emergency and the ways parents can be most easily notified (cellular phone and pager).

MULTICULTURAL AWARENESS

Expectations for Child Behavior Related to Culture

American Indian: expect child to respect elders and take pride in heritage; develop natural talents as child matures; personal independence must balance with accountability to family, community, and tribe; help sought from family members, not outsiders

Mexican American: family environment protects child; child expected to be obedient, respectful, and to work hard to reach goals; "next" generation expected to do better than current generation

Filipino: family raises child in protective environment; expect child to conform to values of culture and child shamed if fails to meet expected behaviors; child taught to avoid direct confrontation and hide emotions and to be respectful and shy; strong emphasis on education for personal and financial gain

African American: child encouraged to walk and to show bowel and bladder control early; child expected to complete family chores, complete schooling, and develop talents such as music or sports to improve self for future; discipline and respectful behavior encouraged

Chinese Americans: child is highly valued, particularly male child; child expected to honor elders and family needs; high value of education to honor family and child

attitudes. Studies of children 5 to 7 years of age show that most identify with and prefer to play with members of their own race. As children get older, they may continue this behavior, as illustrated by one study in which only 19% of a sample of white children interacted with other diverse population children (Jordan, 2004). Although prejudice exists among some school-age children, they may be encouraged to view people from different cultures and ethnic backgrounds in a positive light. Many schools appropriately focus on the importance of other cultures by having multicultural awareness weeks. During these times, children dress, eat, and live as other cultures do, allowing them to recognize the uniqueness of individual cultural beliefs and values (Multicultural Awareness box).

Television, Video, and Computer Games

Television and video and computer games exert a major influence on ideas and behavior in American culture. Unfortunately, many television programs and games pose harm to children because of their messages and because such activities prevent children from engaging in physical activity. Computers connected to the Internet pose danger unless locking devices have been installed to prevent school-age children from accessing inappropriate Web sites. Additional concerns have focused on the violent themes of programming, persuasive television commercials, unrealistic depiction of the world, unhealthy food intake, and the passivity of television viewing.

Violent acts are certainly a part of society. According to Osofsky, Cohen, and Drell (1995), 90% of American elementary school children have witnessed at least one violent or sexually provocative event in their lives. Many times, certain ethnic or racial groups implement the violence in these media sources, leading children to stereotype these groups as the perpetrators of violence. Research has shown that television facilitates negative attitudes and values among children, increases their aggressive behavior, decreases their emotional sensitivity when aggressive acts occur, and leads them to accept aggressive acts (AAP, 2004; Media education, 1999). One positive note is that adults who discuss violence with children by pointing out that these acts are unacceptable and cause pain to others can help inhibit some childhood aggression. Discussion of recent acts of violence committed by young people in such a context also help. Anger control programs, as part of school health-promotion programs, may also help decrease societal violence and produce more collaborative workers needed for the future.

The average child in the culture views an overwhelming number of television commercials by age 18, and these commercials influence daily and future choices and behaviors. Many television commercials focus on sugary foods that cause damage to teeth, diminish overall healthy habits, and lead to increased rates of obesity (Proctor et al., 2003). Young children cannot always separate the program from the commercials and believe that they must purchase products the television says to buy. Many childhood authorities question the ethics of exposing children to any type of advertising. Although concern about the effect of advertising has led to programming changes during children's watching time, more work is needed to send more socially responsible messages.

The world as presented on many television shows does not accurately reflect the real world. Despite an increasingly diverse and aging population, stereotypes of women and minority groups and a predominance of younger actors continue to make money for the media industry. Parents and health care providers should monitor television viewing to ensure age appropriateness of the material, respond to television stations about inaccuracies in the content, and write letters to their newspaper or television networks to express concerns about the material presented. Parents may also participate with their children in responding to media presentations on learning and moral themes. Parents should follow recommendations from the American Academy of Pediatrics (2004) to limit television and media viewing to 2 hours per day, have media-free bedrooms, disallow television viewing while eating, and participate in national Turn Off the Television Week.

Some positive aspects of television viewing exist. A number of children's programs, such as "Mr. Rogers' Neighborhood" and "Reading Rainbow" for younger children and "Call It Macaroni," "Seventh Heaven," and "Full House" for older children, have been deemed developmentally appropriate for children. Likewise, there are excellent Web sites for school-age children that stimulate their learning and promote their health, for example HealthyKids (*http://www.healthykids.com*) and keepkidshealthy.com.

Increasingly, parents engage their school-age children in learning and playing on a home computer. Although this technology serves as a good resource for locating information, writing papers, and organizing information, parents must limit the time students spend on computers. Likewise, limitations must be put on computer games that detract from socialization with peers and family and take time away from school work.

Legislation

Throughout this chapter, laws that support the health and well-being of the school-age child have been discussed. These laws include guidelines for the safe use of products, flame-retardant clothes, mandates against tobacco advertisements, and the nutritional guidelines for federally supported school lunch programs. Another important law is mandatory public education for disabled children.

Public Law 94-142 (Education for All Handicapped Children Act), established in 1977, states that any child with special needs (disabled) ages 5 to 21 years has the right to free appropriate public education in the least restrictive environment and evaluation by school or health professionals to identify learning needs. Disability includes having a limitation in one or more functional areas (USDHHS, 2000) and affects as many as 10% of children ages 5 to 17 years (Hogan, Msall, Rogers, & Avery, 1997). Many states begin educational services for affected children at 3 years of age based on an individualized educational plan (IEP) for that child and as mandated by law (Wong et al., 2002). The school nurse is responsible for collaborating with other school personnel and parents in ensuring that the IEP, including the health care needs of the child and connection to resources addressing the unique learning needs, receives attention. However, some parents have expressed concern that their "normal" or "gifted" child receives less attention in school systems because of the cost and time expenditures associated with implementing IEPs for disabled children. To add further concern, with recent school budgetary shortfalls, lesser trained people than the school nurse often have responsibility for implementing IEPs. Despite these concerns, the value of Public Law 94-142 has been that disabled people have had their problems addressed in the educational arena.

With the recent emphasis on managed care to decrease health care costs in the larger society, costs of implementing Public Law 94-142 will continue to undergo inspection. For the last decade, support has existed for supporting the educational needs of children with special learning needs. Since 1996, the Developmental Assistance and Bill of Rights Act (the Developmental Disabilities Act), as amended by Public Law 104-183, has directed that assistance be given to states and public and private agencies to ensure that all people with disabilities receive services and opportunities to achieve their maximal potential. The act encourages partnerships of groups to help diverse and minority populations in particular to overcome barriers to health care access related to disability.

Economics

Poverty

In the United States more than 18% of children less than 18 years of age live in families whose incomes are below the poverty level (Recer, 2000). Among diverse population groups, 50% of African American, 30% of Hispanic, and an unknown percentage of Native American children live in poor economic conditions that negatively influence their health (Annie E. Casey Foundation, 1999). These conditions include unemployment, inadequate or crowded housing, poor sanitation, poor nutrition, low educational levels, and limited or sporadic access to health and social services perhaps due to lack of health insurance or contextual factors of these persons' lives. The number of uninsured children continues to be high, particularly among Hispanics (30%), and limits the number of children and families receiving primary health care (The Robert Wood Johnson Foundation, 2005; USDHHS, 2000). The lack of primary care among African American, Hispanic, and white children in rural areas prevents needed asthma management, dictating an expanded role for health care providers to connect families to resources for more effective disease control (Horner & Fouladi, 2003; Rose & Garwick, 2003).

Many homeless children face poor living conditions and high rates of depression related to few friends and poor health status (Strehlow & Amos-Jones, 1999). Migrant children face more disease (e.g., tuberculosis, scabies, ear infections), injury, and dental caries and pose treatment challenges due to their transient status (Wong et al., 2002). The effects of few financial resources on children include higher mortality rates at all ages than in those who are not poor or migrant and more lost school days because of illnesses. Numerous problems exist for children of poverty, including developmental delay due to poor nutrition, peer rejection, poor self-concept, increased risk of accidents and drug abuse, abuse or neglect from parents, and overall poor coping.

Nurses interacting with poor families and their children should be familiar with health resources, such as the federal Children's Health Insurance Program (CHIP) (see previous chapters). This program, part of the Balanced Budget Act of 1997 and implemented at the state level, supports comprehensive care to children 0 to 18 years who do not meet Medicaid criteria but live in families too poor to afford private insurance. This program has improved children's health by improving access for many groups, including immigrants; however, recent state budget shortfalls have cut funding for this program (USDHHS, 2000). The nurse can also improve the overall health of poor children by encouraging relationships with appropriate role models and by reinforcing strong family relationships that help children develop strong and positive self-images.

Affluence

The social milieu opposite poverty, affluence, has not been examined with the same frequency as that of poverty. Children of the extremely or moderately rich face risk for health problems. Children who stay at home alone (latchkey children) because both parents work may have a higher risk of injury as a result of inadequate adult monitoring. Family wealth may also have a negative influence on the school-age child if there is frequent substitute caregiving of varying quality due to parental absence, extremely high or unreasonable parental expectations, availability of material possessions but little child awareness of relevant responsibilities, and easy access to drugs and alcohol and similar dangers. The nurse may reinforce the need in wealthy families for consistent demonstration of parental love and support, firm limits on appropriate behavior, and the value of recognizing the child's unique abilities. The nurse may also offer ideas that will help decrease risk-taking behavior (e.g., drugs) and allow parental-child connection until a parent is in the home (Schor, 1998) (see Box 20-7).

When discussing children raised in poverty or affluence, the nurse must remember at least two points. First, many variables affect each child, often in different ways, to influence overall development. Second, although personality and support networks help a child in a socially poor environment to excel later in life, most authorities believe that problems of affluence are easier to overcome than are the all-pervasive problems of poverty.

Health Care Delivery System
Well-Child Care

The American Academy of Pediatrics recommends that children 6 years and older have a well-child examination at least every 2 years by either a physician or a nurse practitioner (Wilson, 2001). In the ideal situation, the child has a primary health care provider, one person or practice from which the child receives wellness and illness care coordinated by members of a health care team. Unfortunately, many American children still do not have this quality of care (see the earlier section on economics). With increasing numbers living in poverty because of family violence, single parenthood, and divorce, many lack a primary care provider for their physical and emotional needs often due to a lack of health insurance. In this situation, they often receive emergency care only when they are very ill or injured.

Table 20-3 provides an example of a health maintenance protocol for this age group. Providers may use this protocol as a guide to the most important age-related issues. Any health history, physical examination, developmental tests, and other observations made by the nurse may be shared with others (teachers and counselors) with parental consent in order to make informed decisions about an individual child's care.

The nurse encourages the school-age child and parents to be active members of any health evaluation. Children may give some of their own history, answer questions, and discuss their health concerns. During the history, the child's privacy should be respected. Some children in this age group want a parent present during the examination; others do not. When possible, the nurse should spend at least some time alone with the child to allow discussions that the child may not feel comfortable with when parents are present. The examinations can also be a time for education on how the body works and ways to keep it healthy. Preventive information on diet and exercise can be offered relevant to

| Table **20-3** | Health Maintenance During the School-Age Period* |

Age (years)	Physiological Processes	Psychological Processes	Emotional-Social Processes
6 to 9	Height, weight	School adjustment, level, and progress	Safety: use of seat belts, water safety, bicycles
	Blood pressure	Developmental level, including speech and cognitive levels	Immunizations reviewed or updated
	Dental: caries, bites, use of fluoride	Stresses in child's life, coping patterns	Responsibilities for household tasks, money, school work
	Diet: snacks	Self-care, hygiene	Relations with parents, siblings, peers, other adults
	Enuresis	Masturbation, homosexual play	Family activities related to culture
	Exercise: motor skills, level of activity, attention		Discipline
	Sleep patterns		After-school work
	Vision and hearing screening		Use of television, computer, video games
9 to 12	Same as ages 6 to 9 plus:	Same as ages 6 to 9 plus:	Same as ages 6 to 9 plus:
	Posture, scoliosis screening	Habits: drugs, alcohol, smoking and other risky behavior	Time and place for privacy
	Menarche, stage of sexual development	Sexual activity	

*Includes areas for which information should be obtained through history, examination, observation, tests, and so on.

prevention of obesity, cardiovascular disease, and diabetes. Information also must be obtained on school adjustment and performance, particularly because this is a major portion of the child's life. School performance can reflect the child's cognitive and general development. If there are any concerns, the nurse should obtain more information through separate testing or discussion with school officials. Health education should be directed to both the child and the parents for the best results. Activities that the child performs alone and with the family can give a picture of relationships and adjustments that relate to the child's health (Care Plan).

NURSING INTERVENTIONS

The challenge for nurses who work with school-age children is to maintain their normal healthy status and prevent illness. This task is accomplished through a variety of health-promotion mechanisms, such as examination, guidance, education, and legislation. The success of this health-promotion approach has been illustrated in at least one study in which African American children improved lifestyle choices when engaged in an intervention focused on cardiovascular health (Fleming, Green, Martin, & Wicks, 2000). Many professionals identify that school-age children guided by the nurse generally seek health and use various resources to attain, maintain, or regain optimal health for their future productivity. Aspects of the nursing process may be implemented when structuring a program to maintain the child's health (such as seen with an assessment of immunization status), promote health habits (seen with teaching bicycle safety), and prevent illness (seen by obtaining throat cultures to detect streptococcal infection).

Nurses have many opportunities and settings to help carry out their interventions as consultants, board members, and active providers of care. For example, nurses and school-age children interact during well-child evaluations and at school. Nurses in other roles, such as in public health and hospitals, also play a role in health promotion, although these nurses must often focus more on helping the child and family respond to an illness or a crisis. Local and national groups influence the health of children through their activities and regulations and include organizations such as Boy Scouts and Girl Scouts, Big Brothers and Big Sisters, charities such as the Red Cross, and government agencies such as the Consumer Product Safety Commission.

CARE PLAN

Child's Isolation From Move to New Neighborhood

Nursing Diagnosis Isolation Related to Placement in New School and Neighborhood and Single-Parent Family

DEFINING CHARACTERISTICS

- Change in quality of schoolwork; 10-year-old child failing classes although has history of doing well in school
- Frequent crying and aggressive behavior at school; visits school nurse complaining of headaches and stomachaches; usually asks to stay at school after dismissal
- Increased daydreaming behavior, according to most teachers
- Aggressive behavior shown at school and on playground
- Mother unavailable for school meetings to discuss child's behavior

RELATED FACTORS

- Child new to area; has attended local school for only 3 months
- Mother works from 8:30 AM to 5:30 PM, 4 days each week; child has to stay at home alone for 2 hours on these days until mother arrives
- Only sibling is 8 years older and works out of home
- Parents recently divorced

EXPECTED OUTCOMES

- Child will decrease number of visits to school nurse for physical complaints.
- Child will display fewer emotional outbursts (crying, aggressive behavior) during school time.
- Grades will improve over next 9-week period.
- Family will become more involved in school setting, to promote effective working relationship between family and school and to focus on child's needs.
- Child will work with student mentor to increase comfort and satisfaction with new school setting.

INTERVENTIONS (SCHOOL NURSE)

- Assess family problems and concerns based on the child's visits to the nurse and visit with family members.
- Over the next 9-week period, document the number of visits the child makes and her physical or other complaints.
- Communicate the child's concerns to her mother and father (if available), encouraging a stronger family-school relationship.
- Work with the parents to develop a plan for meeting academic and emotional needs of the child.
- Offer local resources for child support, latch-key children and, perhaps, for after-school care with the parent of another child in the same grade.
- Offer tutoring support after school for child as desired.
- Seek out a mentor who is a year older to provide friendship and guidance in the child's personal and academic life.
- Involve teachers in identifying ways to improve self-esteem and nurture the child's strengths for improved academic performance.

School and the Nurse

As an integral part of the community, the school system has the responsibility to provide a healthy school environment and a comprehensive health education program. In some areas, nurses, physicians, and other health care workers work as a team in the school health program, which includes health care and maintenance and education. The nurse may advocate and search for resources so that each child has a source of health care, or the nurse may be a nurse practitioner who delivers care. School health programs range from an occasional mention of body care and the changes of puberty to a full program, integrating physical and mental health principles into all aspects of the educational experience as recommended by the Institute of Medicine (1997) and the U.S. Department of Health and Human Services, CDC (2001). **Web Site Resource 20H** presents a list of topics for health education during the school-age period.

Comprehensive school health services require an interdisciplinary, coordinated effort between health care providers and educators. Recommendations state that each school should have an on-site nurse to conduct and mentor students and faculty in health-promotion areas. Nevertheless, many schools share nurses due to budgetary concerns (USDHHS, 2000). However, when available, nurses can offer educational and interpersonal skills to initiate health-promotion teaching that improves the overall health of consumers (students, parents, teachers, community). Nurses have a wide scope of practice, including that of referring parents to relevant resources aimed toward activities that improve the school environment and its inhabitants (Rhodes, 1997). See **Web Site Resource 20I** for parental resources for developmental challenges of childhood.

The nurse's role in planning health maintenance for children of a school varies, depending on the type of health maintenance program. In one system, the school nurse may refer children to resources available to provide a source of health care, whereas in another system, the school nurse may function as a nurse practitioner. Based on scope of practice and state legal requirements, the school nurse monitors and updates children's immunizations and identifies and intervenes with children who have acute or chronic health care problems, such as scoliosis, strep throat, common cold, or child abuse. Increasingly school nurses provide sophisticated care according to evidence-based protocols for chronically ill school-age children who have been integrated into the regular academic environment. Based on state regulations, the nurse also engages in completing vision, hearing, and scoliosis screening at regular intervals. In most schools the nurse works with the school's physician, community physicians, and parents in meeting children's and community health needs.

For all school-age children, the school nurse plays a role in developing a healthy educational environment through promoting a comprehensive and age-appropriate health education program focused on children becoming responsible for their own health (Cagle & Keen-Payne, 1996;

CASE STUDY

Jack

Jack, a 10-year-old fifth grade student, has been caught stealing expensive books from his school library. At first, he denies his involvement in this activity until his best friend, Joey, tells Jack's teacher that Jack hid three of the missing books under his bed. The books cost the library $150.00 when they were purchased 2 years earlier for a new curriculum offering in art. To avoid being caught, Jack throws the books into a river near his home. After several days of questioning, he admits his guilt to the school principal and to his parents. His parents are angry, and his father does not understand why his son is interested in art, a field of study not meant for boys.

Reflective Questions

1. If you were the principal and parents, what disciplinary approaches would you devise to respond to Jack's behavior?
2. Jack's parents do not understand their son's behavior, and his father is so angry that he says he will spank Jack until "he learns his lesson." As a nurse, how might you respond to this statement?
3. Is Jack's behavior appropriate for a 10-year-old boy?
4. What interventions might be effective in preventing further misbehavior by Jack?

USDHHS, CDC, 2001). A program aimed at accident prevention in and around the school should be part of the nurse's role. This should include assessing the school for pedestrian and automobile traffic patterns, broken playground and classroom equipment, ice and snow dangers, poorly maintained toilet facilities, and inappropriately prepared food. Regular practice drills should be held to acquaint teachers and students with emergency procedures (i.e., fire, bomb, or intruder threats or actual events). All people in the school should also be prepared to respond to chemical hazards. The nurse may want to implement existing school-based programs on drug and alcohol abuse. At least one study showed that 19% of children 8 to 12 years old used these substances, particularly if they lived in an urban community and faced family violence (Finke & Williams, 1999). One program (DARE, Drug Awareness Resistance Education) sponsored jointly by schools and local police has successfully prevented school-age children's initiation with drugs. Another program, aimed at cardiovascular health (Heart Healthy) has effectively addressed risk factors and changed lifestyle habits among school-age children (Cowell, Warren, & Montgomery, 1999).

It is also important to consider the role of the nurse in fostering a healthy social environment in the school. The nurse should examine the social interactions of the children and interact with them to promote positive relationships. However, social problems continue to constitute a major concern for many children during this time. Children may experience difficulty in making the initial transition away from family and gaining satisfaction from a group of peers. Children may make the initial adjustment but then have difficulties interacting with others (e.g., bullying). When problems such as these arise, the nurse, parents, and school system may need to determine reasons for this behavior from a child and intervene appropriately.

SUMMARY

Many changes occur in children during the exciting period of the school-age years. The child's development progresses from the immaturity of the preschooler to the beginning of adolescence and eventual adulthood. Cognitive abilities increase dramatically, adding to the desire to master tasks and the ability to develop moral judgment. The child's world expands beyond the family unit as school and peers begin to exert a major influence. Opportunities for nurses during this period occur primarily in ambulatory settings, with the school nurse frequently the most effective and influential health care provider for children of this age group and their families.

ADDITIONAL STUDY MATERIAL

Study Questions in the back of the book, see page 663.

evolve WEB SITE MATERIALS

These materials are located on the book's Web site at http://evolve.elsevier.com/Edelman/.

- WebLinks
- Content Updates
- Web Site Resources

20A   Blood Pressure Levels for Girls and Boys by Age and Height Percentiles
20B   Helpful Information for Parents About Nocturnal Enuresis
20C   Common Developmental and Cognitive Tests
20D   Health-Promotion Literature Related to the School-Age Child
20E   Safety Practices for School-Age Children
20F   Resources for AIDS Educational Materials
20G   Nursing Interventions to Prevent Chemical and Radiation Hazards
20H   Topics for Health Education during the School-Age Period
20I   Parental Resources for Developmental Challenges of Childhood

REFERENCES

Aetna/U.S. Healthcare. (1998). *Caring for your children's health* (Publication No. 12669-8/98). Hartford, CT: Aetna/U.S. Healthcare.

American Academy of Pediatrics. (2004). Policy statements on media. Retrieved April 3, 2004, from: *http://www.aap.org/advocacy/mmpolicy.htm*.

American Academy of Pediatrics, Committee on Infectious Diseases. (2004). *Red Book: Report of the Committee on Infectious Diseases* (26th ed.). Elk Grove Village, IL: Author.

American Academy of Pediatrics, Committee on Injury and Poison Prevention. (1994). Office-based counseling for injury prevention. *Pediatrics, 94,* 566-567.

American Academy of Pediatrics, Committee on Poison Injury and Prevention. (1996). Selecting and using the most appropriate car safety seats for growing children: Guidelines for counseling parents. *Pediatrics, 97,* 761-763.

American Academy of Pediatrics, Committee on Public Education. (1999). Media education. *Pediatrics, 104*(2 Pt 1), 341-343.

American Academy of Pediatrics, Committee on Quality Improvement, Subcommittee on Attention-Deficit/Hyperactivity Disorder. (2000). Clinical practice guideline: Diagnosis and evaluation of the child with attention-deficit/hyperactivity disorder. *Pediatrics, 105,* 1158-1170.

American Dietetic Association & Health-Link. (n.d.). *Healthy habits for healthy kids: A nutrition and activitiy guide for parents.* Retrieved April 28, 2005, from http://www.healthlink.com/healthy_kids/index.html

American Heart Association. (2004). High blood pressure in children. Retrieved June 20, 2004, from: *http://www.americanheart.org/presenter.jhtml?identifier = 4609*.

American Psychiatric Association. (1994). *Diagnostic and statistical manual of mental disorders. DSM-IV* (4th ed.). Washington, DC: The Association.

Anderson, R. N., Kockanck, K. D., & Murphey, S. L. (1997). Report of final mortality statistics, 1995. *Monthly Vital Statistics Report, 45*(Suppl. 2), 11.

Annie E. Casey Foundation. (1999). *Kids count data book: State profiles of child well-being.* Washington, DC: Center for the Study of Social Policy.

Beck, A. M., & Myers, N. M. (1996). Health enhancement and companion animal ownership. *Annuals of Review of Public Health, 17,* 247-257.

Behrman, R., Kliegman, R., & Jenson, H. B. (2000). *Nelson's textbook of pediatrics* (16th ed.). Philadelphia: W. B. Saunders.

Berrettini, S., Ravecca, F., Sellari-Franceschini, S., Matteucci, F., Siciliano, G., & Ursino, F. (1999). Progressive sensorineural hearing loss in childhood. *Pediatric Neurology, 20*(2), 130-136.

Bingham, M., & Stryker, S. (1995). *Things will be different for my daughter.* New York: Penguin Books.

Cagle, C. S., & Keen-Payne, R. (1996). Health promotion teaching in preschoolers. *American Journal of Maternal and Child Nursing, 21,* 96-99.

Cary, P. (2004, June 7). Fixing kids' sports. *US News and World Report, 136*(20), 44-48, 50, 52-53.

Centers for Disease Control and Prevention, National Center for Health Statistics. (1999a, June). Final data for 1997. *National Vital Statistics Report, 47*(10), 1-104.

Centers for Disease Control and Prevention, National Center for Health Statistics. (1999b). Final data for 1997. *National Vital Statistics Reports, 47*(19).

Cole, J., Naidoo, J., & Wills, J. (1998). Reducing accidents. In J. Naidoo & J. Wills (Eds.), *Practicing health promotion: Dilemmas and challenges* (pp. 187-200). London: Bailliere Tindall.

Cowell, J. M., Warren, J. S., & Montgomery, A. C. (1999). Cardiovascular risk prevalence among diverse school-age children: Implications for schools. *Journal of School Nursing, 15*(2), 8-12.

Consumer Information Center. (2004). The food pyramid. Retrieved June 5, 2004, from: *http://www.pueblo.gsa.gov/cic_text/food/food-pyramid/main.htm*.

Costello, D. (2000). Spanking makes a comeback. *Wall Street Journal.* CV(114), W1, W16.

Doswell, W. H. (2002). Overview of female middle childhood in societal context: Implications for research and practice. *Journal of Pediatric Nursing, 17,* 392-401.

Dowling, J. S. (2002). Humor: A coping strategy for pediatric patients. *Pediatric Nursing, 28,* 123-131.

Dumas, D., & Pelletier, L. (1999). Perception in hyperactive children. *Maternal Child Nursing, 24*(1), 12-19.

Durbin, D. R., Elliott, M. R., & Winston, F. K. (2003). Belt-positioning booster seats and reduction in the risk of injury among children in vehicle crashes. *Journal of the American Medical Association, 289,* 2835-2840.

Elium, J., & Elium, D. (1994). *Raising a daughter.* Berkeley, CA: Celestial Arts.

Erikson, E. H. (1986a). *Childhood and society* (2nd ed.). New York: W. W. Norton.

Erikson, E. H. (1986b). *Identity, youth and crisis* (35th ed.). New York: W. W. Norton.

Finke, L., & Williams, J. (1999). Alcohol and drug use of inner-city versus rural school age children. *Journal of Drug Education, 29,* 279-291.

Fleming, T. L., Green, J. L., Martin, J. C., & Wicks, M. W. (2000). Effectiveness of a cardiovascular health promotion education intervention on the attitudes of urban African American school-age children. *Journal of Community Health Nursing, 17,* 49-60.

Folmer, R. L. (2003). The importance of hearing conservation instruction. *Journal of School Nursing, 19,* 140-148.

Garn, S. M., Pao, E. M., & Rihl, M. E. (1964). Compact bone in Chinese and Japanese. *Science, 143*(3613), 1439-1440.

Goldsmith, J. (2003). Nit-picking. *American Journal of Nursing, 103*(9), 22-23.

Goldstein, S., & Mather, N. (1998). *Overcoming underachieving: An action guide to helping your child succeed in school.* New York: John Wiley & Sons.

Goodgold, S. A., & Nielsen, D. (2003). Effectiveness of a school-based backpack health promotion program: Backpack intelligence. *WORK: A Journal of Prevention, Assessment, and Rehabilitation, 21,* 113-123.

Hendrickson, S. G., & Becker, H. (2000). Reducing one source of pediatric head injuries. *Pediatric Nursing, 26,* 159-162.

Hoekelman, R. A., Adams, H. M., Weitzman, M. L., & Wilson, M. A. (2001). *Primary Pediatric care.* St. Jouis: Mosby.

Hogan, D. P., Msall, M. E., Rogers, M. L., & Avery, R. C. (1997). Improved disability population estimates of functional limitations among children 5-17. *Maternal and Child Health Journal, 1*(4), 203-216.

Horner, S. D., & Fouladi, R. T. (2003). Home asthma management for rural families. *Journal of Specialists in Pediatric Nursing, 8*(2), 52-61.

Institute of Medicine. (1997). *Schools and health: Our nation's investment.* Washington, DC: National Academy Press.

Insurance Institute for Highway Safety. (1997). *Facts 1996 fatalities: Bicycles.* Arlington, VA: Author.

Is the government too lax in advice on tuna consumption? (2004). *Consumer Reports, 69*(7), 8.

Jacklin, C., & Martin, L. J. (1999). Effects of gender on behavior and development. In M. Levine, W. Carey, & A. Crocker (Eds.), *Developmental-behavioral perspectives* (3rd ed.). Philadelphia: W. B. Saunders.

Jarvis, C. (2000). *Physical examination and health assessment* (3rd ed.). Philadelphia: W. B. Saunders.

Jordan, M. (2004, June 18). Ethnic diversity doesn't blend in kids' lives. *The Wall Street Journal, CCXLIII*(119), B1, B5.

Keep Kids Healthy. (1999). *Is your child depressed?* Retrieved April 29, 2005, from *http://www.keepkidshealthy.healthology.com/webcast_transcript.asp?b = keepkidshealthy&f = chil*

Kohlberg, L. (1981). *The philosophy of moral development.* San Francisco: Harper & Row.

Latz, S., Wolf, A. W., & Lozoff, B. (1999). Co-sleeping in context: Sleep practices and problems in young children in Japan and the United States. *Archives of Pediatric & Adolescent Medicine, 153,* 339-346.

Levine, M. (2002). *A mind at a time.* New York: Simon & Schuster.

Lozano, J. A. (2004, May 28). Study: Texas kids among the nation's most overweight. *Fort Worth Star-Telegram,* 5B.

Maiter, S., & George, U. (2003). Understanding context and culture in parenting approaches of immigrant South Asian mothers. *Affiliative Journal of Women and Social Work, 18,* 411-428.

Marcus, A. D. (2004, June 9). After leukemia, family struggles to define "normal." *The Wall Street Journal, CCXLIII*(112), A1, A10.

Mathews, A. W. (2004, May 25). In debate over antidepressants, FDA weighed risk of false alarm. *The Wall Street Journal, CCXLIII*(102), A1, A6.

Mayer, G. R. (2002). Behavioral strategies to reduce school violence. *Child Family Behavior Therapy, 24*(1/2), 83-100.

Moody, C. W. (1999). Male child sexual abuse. *Journal of Pediatric Health Care, 13,* 112-119.

Moran, R. (1999). Evaluation and treatment of childhood obesity. *American Family Physician, 59,* 861-868.

Moss, A. J., Lanphear, B. P., & Auinger, P. (1999). Association of dental caries and blood lead levels. *Journal of the American Medical Association, 281*(24), 2294-2298.

Murray, R. B. (2001). Overview: Theories related to human development. In R. B. Murray & J. P. Zentner (Eds.), *Health promotion strategies through the life span* (7th ed., pp. 213-277). Upper Saddle River, NJ: Prentice Hall.

National Highway Traffic Safety Administration. (2004). *Buckle up America Child Passenger Safety Week.* Retrieved June 20, 2004, from: *http://www.nhtsa.dot.gov/people/injury/childps/CPSWeekPlanner/index.html.*

Ortega, D. M. (2001). Parenting efficacy, aggressive parenting and cultural connections. *Child and Family Social Work, 6*(1), 47-57.

Osofsky, J., Cohen, G., & Drell, M. (1995). The effects of trauma among young children: A case of 2-year-old twins. *International Journal of Psychoanalysis, 76,* 595-607.

Parker-Pope, T. (2000). A sugarless gum may help prevent ear infections in kids. *Wall Street Journal, CCXXXV*(129), B1.

Piaget, J. (1969). *The theory of stages in cognitive development.* New York: McGraw-Hill.

Proctor, M. H., Moore, L. L., Gao, D., Cupples, L. A., Hood, M. L., & Ellison, R. C. (2003). Television viewing and changes in body fat from preschool to early adolescence: The Framingham Children's Study. *International Journal of Obesity and Related Metabolic Disorders, 27,* 827-833.

Recer, P. (2000, July 14). Study finds children's status in the U.S. is improving. *Fort Worth Star Telegram,* 8A.

Reuters Health. (2000, June 26). Playground ratings show kids at risk. *Healthweek, 5*(13), 8.

Rhodes, A. M. (1997). Legal issues: Liability for unlicensed assistive personnel. Part I. *Maternal Child Nursing Journal, 22*(5), 269.

The Robert Wood Johnson Foundation. (2005). *Cover the uninsured week.* Retrieved September 1, 2005, from *http:coveretheuninsuredweek.org*

Rose, D., & Garwick, A. (2003). Urban American Indian family caregivers' perceptions of barriers to management of childhood asthma. *Journal of Pediatric Nursing, 18*(1), 2-11.

Rosen, G., Mahowald, R., & Ferber, R. (1995). Sleepwalking, confusional arousals, and sleep terrors in the child. In R. Ferber & M. Kryger (Eds.), *Principles and practices of sleep medicine in the child* (pp. 99-106). Philadelphia: W. B. Saunders.

Sadowski, R. H., & Faulkner, B. (1996). Hypertension in pediatric patients. *American Journal of Kidney Disease, 27,* 305-315.

Saunders, E. (1995). Hypertension in minorities: Blacks. *American Journal of Hypertension, 8*(Suppl. 12), 112S-119S.

Schantz, S., Charron, S. A., & Folden, S. L. (2003). Health screening behaviors of Haitian families for their school aged children. *Journal of Cultural Diversity, 10*(2), 62-68.

Schor, E. L. (1998). Guiding the family of the school age child. *Contemporary Pediatrics, 15*(3), 75-92.

Schulte, E. B., Price, D. L., & Gwin, J. F. (2001). *Thompson's pediatric nursing: An introduction* (8th ed., pp. 252-269). Philadelphia: W. B. Saunders.

Smith, D. (2004, June 5). H-E-B offers free lunches. *Fort Worth Star-Telegram,* B1, B10.

Spector, R. E. (2004). *Cultural diversity in health and illness* (6th ed., pp. 73-89, 253-278). Upper Saddle River, NJ: Pearson Education/Prentice Hall.

State Health Access Data Assistance Center, University of Minnesota. (2004). Characteristics of the uninsured: A view from the states. Retrieved June 18, 2004, from: *http://covertheuninusredweek.org*

Strehlow, A. J., & Amos-Jones, T. (1999). The homeless as a vulnerable population. *Nursing Clinics of North America, 34*(2), 261-274.

U.S. Department of Agriculture. (1992). *The food guide pyramid* (USDA Home and Garden Bulletin, No. 252). Washington, DC: Author.

U.S. Department of Agriculture, Center for Nutrition Policy and Promotion. (2005). *MyPyramid*. Retrieved May 31, 2005, from *http://www.mypyramid.gov*.

U.S. Department of Health and Human Services. (2000). *Healthy people 2010: Vol 1 and 2* (Conference ed.). Washington, DC: U.S. Government Printing Office.

U.S. Department of Health and Human Services. (2001). *Child Maltreatment 1999: Reports from the states to the National Child Abuse and Neglect Data System*. Washington, DC: Author.

U.S. Department of Health and Human Services, Centers for Disease Control. (2001, December 7). School health guidelines to prevent unintentional injuries and violence. *Morbidity and Mortality Weekly Report, RR-22*, 1-73.

U.S. Preventive Services Task Force. (2004a). Recommendation statement: Screening for family and intimate partner violence. Retrieved June 11, 2004, from: *http://www. ahrq.gov/clinic/3rduspstf/famviolence/ famviolrs.htm*.

U.S. Preventive Services Task Force. (2004b). Recommendations and rationale: Screening for depression. Retrieved June 11, 2004, from: *http://www.ahrq.gov/clinic/ 3rduspstf/depression/depressrr.htm*.

Wilson, M. H. (2001). Prevention of injury: Two: Injury control. In R. A. Hoekelman, H. M. Adams, M. L. Weitzman, & M. H. Wilson (Eds.), *Primary pediatric care* pp. 307-311). St. Louis, Mosby.

Wilson, C. B., Lewis, D. B., & Penix, L. A. (1996). Immunodeficiency of immaturity. In E. R. Stiehm, *Immunologic disorders in infants and children* (4th ed., pp. 253-295). Philadelphia: W. B. Saunders.

Wolfe, C. A. (2000). Pediatric alert: Access to lead. *RN, 63*(8), 26-30.

Wong, D. L., & Hess, C. S. (2000). *Wong and Whaley's clinical manual of pediatric nursing* (5th ed., pp. 132-133). St. Louis: Mosby.

Wong, D. L., Hockenberry-Eaton, M., Wilson, D., Winkelstein, M. L., Ahmann, E., & Divito-Thomas, P. A. (1999). *Whaley and Wong's nursing care of infants and children* (6th ed.). St. Louis: Mosby.

Wong, D. L., Perry, S. E., & Hockenberry, M. J. (2002). *Maternal child nursing* (2nd ed.). St. Louis: Mosby.

Yerao, S. Y., Borrego, J., & Urquiza, A. J. (2001). A reporting and response model for culture and child maltreatment. *Child Maltreatment, 6*, 158-168.

Chapter 21

MARTHA DRIESSNACK

Adolescent

objectives

After completing this chapter, the reader will be able to:

- Distinguish between the terms puberty and adolescence.

- Summarize the physical growth and developmental changes that occur during adolescence.

- Outline the recommended schedule of preventive health visits and the appropriate subjects for the nurse to discuss with the adolescent during each visit.

- Analyze the factors that contribute to risk-taking behaviors and situations during adolescence.

- Develop a health teaching plan addressing some of the physical, emotional, and social challenges facing adolescents.

key terms

Acne
Adolescence
Anorexia nervosa
Body image
Bulimia nervosa
Date rape
Depression
Emancipated minor
Formal operations

Gynecomastia
Identity
Klinefelter syndrome
Menarche
Nocturnal emissions
Peer group
Primary sexual
  characteristics
Puberty

Risk-taking behavior
Scoliosis
Secondary sexual
  characteristics
Sexually transmitted disease
Turner syndrome

THINK About It

Risk Behaviors in Adolescents

Increasing numbers of young adolescents are not only becoming sexually active but also are choosing not to use any protection or contraception.

  The mortality rate for adolescents is 3 times higher than it is for school-age children.

  Suicide rates in adolescents are increasing across all ethnic groups.

1 What growth and developmental factors make adolescents susceptible to these risky situations?

2 What anticipatory guidance and strategies might be offered to adolescents and their families to prevent this risky behavior?

The author acknowledges the work of Marinda Allender in the previous edition of the chapter.

The period of adolescence is defined as beginning with the onset of puberty, around age 11 to 13 years, and ending with the achievement of independence from the primary family unit, around 18 to 21 years. The term **adolescence** refers to the psychosocial, emotional, cognitive, and moral transition from childhood to young adulthood, while **puberty** refers to the development and maturation of the reproductive, endocrine, and structural processes that lead to fertility.

Rapid change, in physical, psychosocial, moral, and cognitive growth, is the most characteristic trait of adolescence and creates an extremely tenuous sense of balance. A pivotal developmental period, adolescence offers health care providers unique opportunities for health-promotion and preventive services. Providing knowledge about the changes, challenges, and choices adolescents will encounter, as well as the tools with which to approach them, encourages and reinforces developing competencies and sense of responsibility. The *Healthy People 2010* box presents selected general objectives related to adolescent health.

AGE AND PHYSICAL CHANGES

In contrast to the slow, steady growth of childhood, adolescents experience accelerated growth that dramatically alters their body size and proportions. The most noticeable changes in adolescence involve physical and sexual growth, including the appearance of secondary sexual characteristics. These changes occur in a predictable sequence, but the onset and duration of the sequencing varies from individual to individual. Females usually begin puberty 2 years earlier than males and experience their growth spurt earlier. The appearance and sequence of secondary sexual charac-

teristics and pubertal events are summarized in Table 21-1 and later illustrated in Figure 21-3.

The physical changes experienced during adolescence are mediated primarily by the hormonal regulatory systems in the hypothalamus, pituitary gland, gonads, and adrenal glands (Figure 21-1). The hypothalamus releases gonadotropin-releasing hormone, which stimulates the anterior pituitary to release the gonadotropin hormones (GnRF), luteinizing hormone (LH), and follicle-stimulating hormone. In females, this stimulates ovarian development and estrogen production. Estrogen produces all secondary sex characteristics except axillary and pubic

Healthy People 2010
Selected Health-Promotion and Disease Prevention Objectives for Adolescents

- Reduce the prevalence of overweight and obesity in adolescents ages 12 through 19.
- Reduce the incidence of suicide and injurious suicide attempts among adolescents ages 15 through 19.
- Reduce deaths caused by motor vehicle accidents among youths ages 15 through 24.
- Increase the proportion of high school seniors who associate risk of physical or psychological harm with heavy use of alcohol, regular use of marijuana, and experimentation with cocaine.
- Increase the proportion of adolescents in grades 9 through 12 who abstain from intercourse or use condoms if sexually active.

From U.S. Department of Health and Human Services. (2000). *Healthy People 2010*. Washington, DC: U.S. Government Printing Office.

Table 21-1 Sexual Maturity Rating, Tanner Stages: Developmental Stages of Secondary Sexual Characteristics

Stage	Male Genital Development	Pubic Hair Development	Female Breast Development	Other Changes
1	Prepubertal	No distinction between hair over pubic area and hair over abdomen		
2	Initial enlargement of scrotum and testes; reddening and texture changes of scrotum	Sparse growth of long, straight, downy hair at base of penis or along labia	Enlargement of areolar diameter; small area of elevation around papillae (breast bud)	Usual time of peak height velocity for girls
3	Initial enlargement of penis, mainly in length; further growth of testes and scrotum	Hair becomes dark, coarse, and curly; spreads sparsely over entire pubic area	Further elevation and enlargement of breasts and areolas, with no separation of their contours	Usual time of menarche; facial hair begins to grow on upper lip and voice deepens in boys
4	Further enlargement of penile diameter, testes, scrotum, and glans	Further spread of hair distribution, not extending to thighs	Areolas and papillae project from breast to form secondary mound	Usual time of peak height velocity for boys; axillary hair begins to grow
5	Adult in size and contour	Adult in amount and type; spreads to inner surface of thighs	Adult, with projection of papillae only; recession of areolas into general breast contour	

Modified from Hockenberry, M. J., Wilson, D., Winkelstein, M. L., & Kline, N. E. (2003). *Wong's nursing care of infants and children.* St. Louis: Mosby.

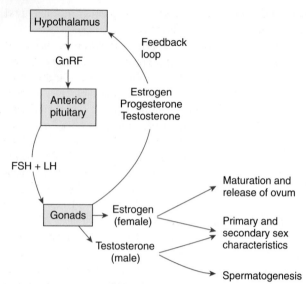

Figure 21-1 Hormonal interaction among hypothalamus, pituitary, and gonads. *FSH*, follicle-stimulating hormone, *GnRF*, gonadotropin-releasing hormone; *LH*, luteinizing hormone. (From Hockenberry, M. J., Wilson, D., Winkelstein, M. L., & Kline, N. E. [2003]. *Wong's nursing care of infants and children* [7th ed.]. St. Louis: Mosby.)

hair, which are controlled by adrenal androgens. In males, luteinizing hormone results in testicular enlargement and the development of Leydig cells in the testes, which produce testosterone. Follicle-stimulating hormone stimulates the development of the seminiferous tubules of the testes, leading to spermatogenesis and fertility. Once sexual maturation is completed, the ongoing release of hormones controls menses, pregnancy, and lactation. **Menarche,** the onset of menses in females, usually occurs late in puberty, as the growth spurt is subsiding. Adolescents who do not follow the normal sequence or who have not begun pubertal development by age 14 years, for males, and age 13 years, for females, should have an endocrine evaluation.

Before the growth spurt, many adolescents experience a transient increase in body fat or adipose tissue. As puberty progresses, the proportion of total body weight composed of fat usually declines, particularly in boys. Body fat begins to accumulate again in both genders after their growth spurt, but at a slightly higher rate in females. In addition the basal metabolic rate is slightly higher in males than in females (Guyton & Hall, 2000).

The heart grows in size and strength. Blood volume and blood pressure increase, and the heart rate decreases to adult levels. These cardiovascular changes occur earlier in females and parallel puberty. Adolescent females also generally have higher pulse rates and slightly lower systolic blood pressure than males. Adolescents are identified as hypertensive when their systolic or diastolic blood pressure is at or above the 95th percentile (based on age, gender, and height) on three separate occasions. Adolescents of African American or Asian–Pacific Islander descent are at higher risk for hypertension (Burns, Brady, Dunn, & Starr, 2000).

Respiratory rate decreases throughout childhood, reaching an average rate of 15 to 20 breaths per minute during

adolescence. Respiratory volume and vital capacity increase, particularly in males. The larynx and vocal cords grow, producing the characteristic voice changes of puberty. Both male and female voices become deeper and laryngeal cartilage enlarges, with both effects more pronounced in males (Guyton & Hall, 2000).

The gastrointestinal and elimination systems enlarge during the growth spurt but have already reached functional maturity during school-age years.

Permanent teeth begin erupting around 6 years of age, and all 32, except the third molars, or wisdom teeth, are in place by 13 to 14 years of age (Burns et al., 2000). Once the permanent teeth have erupted, and sometimes before, necessary orthodontic correction is initiated. Third molars are often pulled during adolescence to make space for the other permanent teeth. However, it is becoming increasingly common for them never to develop.

Both the sweat glands and sebaceous glands become more active during adolescence. The sweat glands are located primarily in the axillary, genital, and periumbilical areas and are the primary source of body odor. The sebaceous glands are located primarily on the face, neck, shoulders, upper back, chest, and genitals. They can become clogged and inflamed, leading to the common teenage condition called **acne.** Acne occurs in up to 80% to 85% of all adolescents and young adults and is more common in females than in males (Burns et al., 2000).

Scoliosis

A common skeletal deformity found in adolescents is **scoliosis,** a lateral S-shaped curvature of the spine (Figure 21-2). The curve is typically convex to the right. Classifications of scoliosis include secondary or functional, congenital, neuromuscular, constitutional, and idiopathic, which has an infantile, juvenile, or adolescent onset. Approximately 10% of all adolescents have a mild truncal asymmetry; however, curves greater than 15 degrees are abnormal and can progress to significant curvature during the growth spurt (Burns et al., 2000). Idiopathic scoliosis is the most common type and is significantly more prevalent in females (Friedman, 1998). Early intervention is important, because untreated scoliosis can result in disfigurement, impaired mobility, and cardiopulmonary complications.

The nurse includes scoliosis screening in the assessment of both prepubertal and pubertal adolescents, paying close attention to the timing of the growth spurt. Most adolescents with scoliosis will require only observation; however, bracing and surgical correction may be necessary and early referral to an orthopedic surgeon is important. Prevention of scoliosis is not possible, but early identification can help avoid more invasive care and prevent the long-term consequences of the disorder.

Acne

Adolescents typically are concerned about their skin changes. The sebaceous glands increase production of sebum, a primary factor in the pathogenesis of acne. The

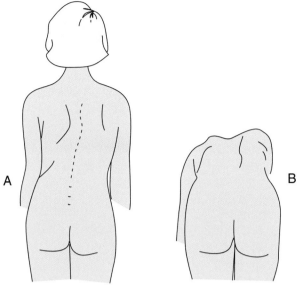

Figure 21-2 Scoliosis screening. So that the entire back can be seen, the adolescent should remove all clothing from the upper body when being assessed for scoliosis. **A,** While the adolescent stands up straight, check for any asymmetry; observe and palpate for differences in shoulder or scapular height, prominence of either scapula or hip, waist asymmetry, and misalignment of the spinous processes. Lateral curvature and thoracic convexity of the spine indicate scoliosis. **B,** With feet together, legs straight, and arms hanging freely, the adolescent bends forward until the back is parallel with the floor. Check for prominence of the ribs, or rib hump, on one side only and hip and leg asymmetry. With scoliosis, the chest wall on the side of convexity is prominent, and the scapula on the side of convexity is elevated.

sebaceous follicles become clogged with sebum and debris, forming open (blackheads) or closed (whiteheads) comedones. The incidence of acne within families suggests that hereditary factors are involved.

Thorough examination of the adolescent's skin and a discussion of its impact on the overall body imagery are necessary to determine appropriate management strategies. Intervention should include teaching the individual about the pathophysiological nature of acne. Knowledge allows the adolescent to become instrumental in its management and helps dispel common myths about acne and its care.

Washing with soap and water 2 or 3 times a day is the best way to remove dirt and oil. Vigorous scrubbing should be discouraged, because the skin can become irritated, leading to follicular rupture. The adolescent should not attempt to remove the pustules and papules that form. Squeezing the lesion can result in further irritation of the gland and permanent injury to the tissue.

Many nonprescription topical medications, such as Oxy-5, Epiclear, and Persadox, contain benzoyl peroxide, which is bacteriostatic and comedolytic. Unfortunately, these agents cause drying and peeling; therefore, therapy is begun with application of 5% strength once a day and after 2 weeks (if tolerated) is increased to twice a day. The nurse

should refer the adolescent with extensive lesions to a nurse practitioner or physician for prescription medication.

Adolescent females should be careful when selecting makeup. Most preparations, when applied extensively over the face, prevent adequate exposure to air and light, especially those that have a fat base. Sunlight can have a beneficial effect on acne; however, prolonged exposure should be avoided. Stress can exacerbate acne in some adolescents. In these cases, stress management techniques should be considered. The effect of diet on acne is a highly controversial issue. Evidence indicates that dietary restrictions specific to acne are unnecessary, and the adolescent is encouraged to adhere to the standard age-specific guidelines.

Adolescents with acne need support and understanding. The nurse can help adolescents and their families understand that management does not result in immediate improvement. In fact, topical agents may make acne appear worse initially, with any improvement occurring slowly over several months.

Gender

During puberty, primary sexual characteristics begin to develop and secondary sexual characteristics emerge. **Primary sexual characteristics** involve the organs necessary for reproduction, such as the penis and testes in boys and the vagina and uterus in girls. **Secondary sexual characteristics** are external features that are not essential for reproduction. Breast development, facial and pubic hair growth, and lowering of the voice are examples of secondary sex characteristics (see Table 21-1). Sexual maturity rating, also referred to as Tanner staging, is used widely to assess and monitor the degree of maturation of an adolescent's primary and secondary sexual characteristics. Each of the characteristics, breast, pubic hair, and genitals, is staged separately (from 1 to 5) and compared with the expected sequencing (Figure 21-3).

Breast development usually is confined to females; however, some degree of unilateral or bilateral breast enlargement, termed **gynecomastia,** may appear early in male puberty, just prior to the growth spurt. Gynecomastia is usually temporary and typically disappears. However, occasionally it persists and leads to body image problems and can be surgically reduced if psychological assessment warrants it.

The first sign of puberty in males is a thinning of the scrotal sac and enlargement of the testicles. Ejaculation is considered a milestone of male puberty and precedes fertility by several months (Guyton & Hall, 2000). **Nocturnal emissions,** or wet dreams, can concern adolescent males, because the event happens beyond their control.

For females the first sign of puberty is the breast buds, followed by the growth spurt. The onset of menstruation, or menarche, occurs approximately 2 years after the appearance of the breast buds and near the end of the growth spurt.

Familiarity with the stages of development of sexual characteristics and their expected sequence helps the nurse

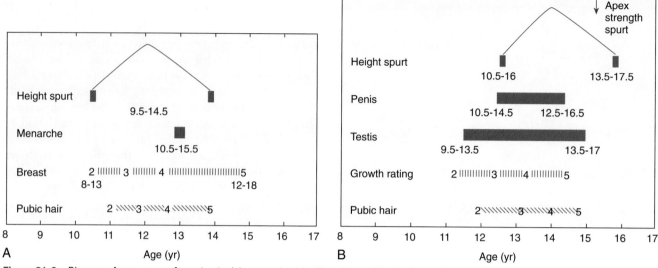

Figure 21-3 Diagram of sequences of events at adolescence in girls **(A)** and boys **(B)**. Single numbers *(2, 3, 4, 5)* indicate stages of development. The average is represented. A range of ages when each event may begin and end is indicated by inclusive numbers listed below each event. (Modified from Marshall, W. A., & Tanner, J. M. [1969]. Variations in pattern of pubertal changes in girls. *Archives of Disease in Childhood, 44,* 291-303; Hockenberry, M. J., Wilson, D., Winkelstein, M. L., & Kline, N. E. [2003]. *Wong's nursing care of infants and children* [7th ed.]. St. Louis: Mosby.)

monitor the adolescent's progression through puberty and detect any variations that might herald an alteration in normal growth and development.

Genetics

Most genetic problems are discovered during infancy and early childhood. Some syndromes, however, may not be diagnosed until adolescence. These genetic disorders frequently are discovered during the assessment of an adolescent with delayed or irregular pubertal development.

Turner syndrome (XO) is a female disorder in which only one X chromosome is present instead of two. Assessment findings include short stature, a webbed neck, a low posterior hairline, low-set ears, a shield-shaped chest with widely spaced nipples, and gonadal-ovarian dysgenesis, resulting in a lack of sexual development and menses during puberty. Cardiac and renal anomalies are often present. Learning disabilities are common. Management consists primarily of growth hormone, to increase height, and estrogen therapy to help develop secondary sexual characteristics and menses. However, the female with Turner syndrome remains sterile. Ongoing emotional support for the adolescent and her family is important (Friedman, 1998).

Klinefelter syndrome (XXY) is seldom diagnosed before puberty. Males have an extra chromosome and typically are tall, initially thin, and do not develop secondary sexual characteristics. They often have gynecomastia. Klinefelter syndrome is associated with learning or behavior problems during childhood. As with Turner syndrome, management typically involves androgen therapy and counseling; however, the adolescent remains sterile.

When the nurse recognizes signs of either of these syndromes during routine screening, the child should be referred to specialists who are qualified to diagnose and manage the physical, social, spiritual, and emotional aspects of these problems.

Most adolescents with delayed development do not have a genetic disorder; their pattern of growth merely falls at the far end of the normal curve and is referred to as a *constitutional delay*. Whatever the cause, delays can have a tremendous effect on psychosocial development, and these adolescents need ongoing assessment and support to promote development of positive self-esteem.

GORDON'S FUNCTIONAL HEALTH PATTERNS
Health Perception–Health Management Pattern

Teens have fewer acute illnesses than do younger children and fewer chronic illnesses than adults. They are seen in health care facilities less frequently than younger children and adults, and they rarely are hospitalized. Yet they need to be monitored, because adolescence is a pivotal developmental period with numerous psychosocial and physical changes. Box 21-1 lists interventions recommended for periodic health examinations for adolescents.

A crucial component for understanding adolescent health is an adolescent's own perceptions of health, illness, and health care services. Too often, their sense of invincibility and "Peter Pan" ideology couples with typical adolescent experimentation and **risk-taking behaviors** to produce deleterious health care choices and outcomes. Caught somewhere between childhood and adulthood, they no longer feel served by pediatricians, pediatric nurse practitioners, and pediatric nurses, yet are often misunderstood by adult health care providers. Health care services for adolescents need to be developed that are available, visible, confidential, and flexible (see Innovative Practice box).

Box **21-1**   **Interventions Recommended for the Periodic Health Examination: 11 to 21 Years of Age**

SCREENING

Height, weight, and BMI
Blood pressure
Scoliosis
Vision and hearing
SMR or Tanner stage
Anemia
Hyperlipidemia
Urinalysis
TB
Eating disorders
Sports injuries
Tattoos and piercings
If sexually active, Pap test and STD screening

COUNSELING
Injury and Violence Prevention

Lap and shoulder belts in car
Bicycle, motorcycle, all-terrain vehicle helmets
Protective gear for sports, work, and other physical activities
Learn first aid and CPR
Skin cancer, sun exposure, sunscreen SPF 15 or higher
Safe storage and use of firearms

Substance Use

Avoid tobacco, alcohol, and drug use
Avoid alcohol or drug use while driving, swimming, boating, riding a bike or motorcycle, or operating farm equipment or other machinery

Sexual Behavior

Abstinence, resisting sexual pressures, saying no
STD prevention and protection
Unintended pregnancy, contraception
Date rape

Diet and Exercise

Choose a variety of healthy foods
Balance caloric intake and energy expenditure
Limit fat and cholesterol; emphasize grains, fruits, vegetables
Adequate calcium, iron, and folic acid

Dental Health

Regular (every 6 months) visits to dental care provider
Brush at least twice a day and floss daily
Avoid tobacco products

IMMUNIZATION

DT vaccine: booster if at least 5 years since last dose of DTP, DTaP, or DT
Hepatitis B virus vaccine (if not given previously)
Hepatitis A virus vaccine (if indicated)
MMR vaccine
VAR vaccine (if not given previously or no reliable history of chickenpox; if 13 or older, two doses 4 to 8 weeks apart)

BMI, body mass index; *SMR,* sexual maturity rating; *TB,* tuberculosis; *Pap,* Papanicolaou; *STD,* sexually transmitted disease; *CPR,* cardiopulmonary resuscitation; *SPF,* sun protection factor; *DT,* diphtheria tetanus; *DTP,* diphtheria, tetanus, pertussis; *DTaP,* diphtheria, tetanus, acellular pertussis; *MMR,* measles, mumps, rubella; *VAR,* varicella.

innovative practice

Boston College Health Fair

A school-based health fair is a combination of intertwining relationships among the students, faculty, and community. When creating a health fair in a university setting, the primary goals are to teach correct and positive health techniques, enhance healthy lifestyle choices, target education toward late adolescent and young adult health care issues and concerns, and conduct age-appropriate health screenings. The Boston College Graduate Nurses Association sponsors the annual Boston College Health Fair with the assistance of faculty, graduate and undergraduate students, and community professionals and agencies.

Each individual who attends the fair completes a five-page health questionnaire. Objective data collected from the questionnaire include general health-related questions, the vendors that were visited by the individual, the reasons for which the person visited those particular vendors, which vendors were most or least helpful, and recommendations for the following year. A comment section is also included to encourage individuals to share health concerns and identify health-related issues they believe need to be addressed within their population.

Booths at the Boston College Health Fair include stress reduction and biofeedback strategies, as well as community safety and awareness, cultural diversity, alternative lifestyles, aromatherapy, domestic and date violence, testicular and breast cancer screening techniques, skin analysis, blood pressure screening, body fat analysis, anemia and blood glucose testing, eating disorder awareness, yoga and Tai Chi, and spinal nerve stress tests.

The Boston College community enthusiastically supports the health fair by donating space, food and beverages, and audiovisual equipment used by various vendors to display their information. Undergraduate nursing students volunteer clinical time to measure blood pressure, faculty members volunteer time to supervise and answer any questions, and members of the Graduate School of Nursing host booths and monitor the efficiency of the health fair.

In summary, an efficient and informative school-based health fair benefits the entire school and surrounding community. Focusing on holistic well-being encourages positive health behaviors for all individuals and a healthy environment.

Courtesy Christine Holborow and Dawnmarie C. Pelrine. Christine Holborow, MS, RN, CS, is a graduate of the Boston College Graduate School of Nursing and is currently practicing as a geriatric nurse practitioner for New England Geriatrics in the Boston area. Dawnmarie C. Pelrine, MS, RN, CS, is a graduate of Boston College Graduate School of Nursing and is currently practicing as an adult nurse practitioner in an acute care cardiology practice at Massachusetts General Hospital in Boston.

Box **21-2** Diagnostic Criteria for Eating Disorders

ANOREXIA NERVOSA

- Refusal to maintain body weight at or above a minimally normal weight for age and height (weight loss leading to maintenance of body weight less than 85% of that expected or failure to make expected weight gain during period of growth, leading to body weight less than 85% of that expected)
- Intense fear of gaining weight or becoming overweight, even when underweight
- Disturbance in the way in which one's body weight or shape is perceived, undue influence of body weight or shape on self-evaluation, or denial of the seriousness of the current low body weight
- Primary or secondary amenorrhea

Specify type:

Restricting type: during the current episode of anorexia nervosa, the person has not regularly engaged in binge eating or purging behavior (self-induced vomiting, the misuse of laxatives, diuretics, and enemas).

Binge eating–purging type: during the current episode of anorexia nervosa, the person has regularly engaged in binge eating or purging behavior (self-induced vomiting, the misuse of laxatives, diuretics, and enemas).

BULIMIA NERVOSA

- Recurrent episodes of binge eating, characterized by both of the following:

1. Eating, in a discrete period of time (within any 2-hour period), an amount of food that is definitely larger than most people would eat during similar period and under similar circumstances
2. A sense of lack of control over eating during the episode (a feeling that one cannot stop eating or control what or how much one is eating)

- Recurrent inappropriate compensatory behavior to prevent weight gain, such as self-induced vomiting; misuse of laxatives, diuretics, enemas, or other medications, such as syrup of ipecac; fasting; or excessive exercise
- Binge eating and inappropriate compensatory behaviors, both occurring, on average, at least twice a week for 3 months
- Self-evaluation unduly influenced by body shape and weight
- Does not occur exclusively during episodes of anorexia nervosa

Specify type:

Purging type: during the current episode of bulimia nervosa, the person has regularly engaged in self-induced vomiting or the misuse of laxatives, diuretics, or enemas.

Nonpurging type: during the current episode of bulimia nervosa, the person has used other inappropriate compensatory behaviors, such as fasting or excessive exercise, but has not regularly engaged in self-induced vomiting or the misuse of laxatives, diuretics, or enemas.

Modified from American Psychiatric Association. (2000). *Diagnostic and statistical manual of mental disorders: Text revision* (4th ed.). Washington, DC: The Association.

Adolescents are in the process of developing health habits and patterns of problem solving that are likely to last a lifetime. The cognitive and psychological changes that they experience can affect their adherence to health-promotion and disease prevention strategies. Teens do not always consider the health risks of their behavior and have an overall sense of insusceptibility to illness or injury. Peer influence is primary, and parental input often is rejected.

Parents, teachers, and health care providers will be more successful in assisting teens to manage their health needs wisely if they treat them as joint partners in planning the care for which the adolescents, themselves, will assume responsibility (Hoffman & Greydanus, 1997). Key components of successful health supervision include a respect for individual differences, support for the adolescent's emerging autonomy, a developmental approach, and a focus on the individual's strengths (Green & Palfrey, 2000).

Nutritional-Metabolic Pattern

Many teens have concerns about their body, proper nutrition, and exercise. The media, and society as a whole, not only portray the ideal body as thin, lean, or muscular, but also promote fast food, soda pop, sweets, and alcohol consumption (Dixon & Stein, 2000). Adolescents may also choose their dietary intake as a mechanism to gain control or independence, or to experiment with a new identity, such as becoming a vegetarian.

The highest nutrient and energy demands occur during the growth spurt, and the addition of sports or other vigorous physical activity can increase these demands. However, the desire to "fit in" prevails and often leads to unhealthy dietary practices. Up to 10% of adolescent females have some form of eating disorder and 62% of female and 20% of male adolescents participate in fad diets (Dixon & Stein, 2000).

Eating Disorders

At one end of the eating disorder spectrum is **anorexia nervosa,** which primarily affects adolescent females, although studies suggest that the incidence among males may be higher than was previously suspected (Neinstein, 2002). Symptoms include self-starving with significant weight loss, amenorrhea, compulsive physical activity, preoccupation with food, and a distorted body image (Box 21-2). Typically the adolescent with anorexia is described as a perfectionist or overachiever who has always performed well academically. The adolescent's family also tends to be achievement oriented, and marital discord is frequently present (Kreipe & Dukarm, 1999).

research highlights

Adolescent Obesity and Depression

Research has shown that both (1) individual eating behaviors, such as binge eating, consumption of fast foods, meal skipping, and excessive consumption of soda pop and snack foods, and (2) inactivity, such as television viewing, which displaces physical activity, increases snacking and caloric consumption, and reduces resting metabolism, place adolescents at increased risk for obesity. However, more researchers are looking at depression as the strongest predictor for obesity in adolescents.

In a prospective study by Goodman and Whitaker (2002), a sample of 9374 adolescents, drawn from the National Longitudinal Study of Adolescent Health, was assessed for depressive symptoms over time. Sociodemographic variables were assessed, as well as self-esteem, delinquent behavior, smoking, and decreased physical activity. After controlling for these factors, depressed mood at baseline predicted follow-up obesity for those not obese at baseline and predicted the persistence of obesity in those already obese at baseline.

This important finding not only emphasizes the need for mental health assessment and services for children and adolescents, but also suggests that individual eating behaviors and inactivity are not the only risk factors for obesity in adolescents and, indeed, may only be the symptoms of underlying depression.

Goodman, E., & Whitaker, R. C. (2002). A prospective study of the role of depression in the development and persistence of adolescent obesity. *Pediatrics, 110*(3), 497-504.

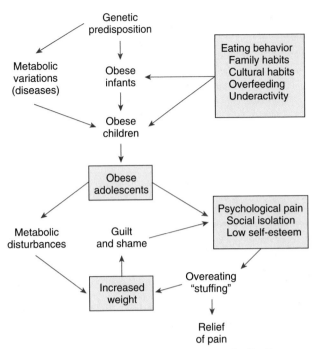

Figure 21-4 Complex relationships in adolescent obesity. (From Hockenberry, M. J., Wilson, D., Winkelstein, M. L., & Kline, N. E. [2003]. *Wong's nursing care of infants and children* [7th ed.]. St. Louis: Mosby.)

The onset of the anorexia is typically in response to real or imagined obesity. With dieting, the adolescent begins to lose weight. Personal pride and positive reinforcement from others lead to continued dieting, which becomes the primary focus of the teen's life. Eventually the adolescent becomes dangerously malnourished. Common complications are fluid and electrolyte imbalance, hypotension, and constipation. Untreated, this disorder can be fatal. Treatment and recovery is an ongoing process that often includes hospitalization and psychotherapy for the teen and the entire family.

Another eating disorder is **bulimia nervosa,** which also affects females more than males. It involves a pattern of binge eating followed by purging, inducing vomiting or using laxatives or both (see Box 21-2). Metabolic acidosis, sometimes fatal electrolyte imbalances, and erosion of dental enamel are secondary to the purging. An adolescent who meets the criteria for an eating disorder should be referred to an interdisciplinary team that is experienced and skilled in working with these disorders (Dixon & Stein, 2000).

At the other end of the eating disorder spectrum is obesity. The obese adolescent consumes too many calories for the amount of energy expended. Studies have shown a strong correlation between inactivity, such as viewing television, playing computer games, and internet surfing, and

the tendency to be overweight (Gortmaker et al., 1996). More recent research is looking at depression as the strongest predictor of adolescent obesity (Research Highlights box).

Obesity can be detrimental to adolescents' self-esteem and social development, and they become trapped in a vicious cycle of social rejection, isolation, inactivity, and continued obesity (Figure 21-4). Adolescent obesity has a poor prognosis, and most obese adolescents become obese adults (Kligh, 1998). In addition, obesity increases the risk of and occurrence of type 2 diabetes mellitus.

More than anything else, adolescents need reassurance about their bodies, even those teens who are "doing well." Parents, teachers, and health care providers will be more successful in assisting teens to manage their health needs if they treat them as partners in planning the care for which the adolescents themselves will assume responsibility (Hoffman & Greydanus, 1997). Nurses need to help every adolescent create an individualized wellness plan that addresses body image, diet, weight concerns, and exercise.

Elimination Pattern

The renal and gastrointestinal systems are functionally mature by adolescence, and elimination patterns are consistent with those found in adults. Abnormal variation can occur in teens with eating disorders. It is important to remember that an adolescent's need for privacy or self-protection may inhibit normal elimination in public places, such as schools.

Box **21-3** Adolescent Preparticipation Sports Examination

AREAS FOR SPECIAL CONCERN
- Previous trauma, including concussion
- Cardiovascular disease
- Hypertension
- Asthma
- Seizure disorder
- Splenomegaly, or enlarged spleen, often seen with infectious mononucleosis
- HIV infection
- Absence of paired organs: eye, kidney, testicle, or ovary

HIV, human immunodeficiency virus.

Activity-Exercise Pattern

During adolescence, the alterations in body composition and growth of lean muscle mass allow the teen to experience increased physical strength and endurance. All adolescents should be taught that regular exercise can improve their endurance, appearance, and general state of health and that these positive effects can extend into adulthood.

Many teens participate in organized sports, and the preparticipation sports examination is one of the most common reasons to seek primary care. This examination offers an opportunity for nurses to identify adolescents at risk, evaluate their general state of health, and promote healthy lifestyle behaviors (Box 21-3). Frequent injuries, stress fracture, secondary amenorrhea, extreme dietary measures to gain or lose weight, exclusion of other activities, deteriorating school work, and chronic pain are a few of the signs of overuse, overexertion, or overinvestment (Dixon & Stein, 2000).

Sleep-Rest Pattern

During adolescence, the amount of time spent each night in sleep declines. Although sleep patterns vary greatly, the average adolescent sleeps 8 hours per night. Working adolescents, or those who have "too much on their plate," are at increased risk for sleep deprivation and daytime sleepiness. Nurses can help these adolescents cope with the challenge of balancing their varied responsibilities and prevent exhaustion or burnout by exploring with them various strategies for daily living.

Cognitive-Perceptual Pattern
Piaget's Theory

Adolescence is characterized by a shift in cognitive abilities to Piaget's stage of **formal operations.** Piaget used the term *formal* to represent the emergence of ability to focus on the "form" of thoughts, objects, and experiences rather than on the exact content which, in turn, lays the groundwork for abstract thinking. These new cognitive abilities are reflected in adolescent behaviors in several ways.

The first change is that, because of their new ability to "think about their thinking," adolescents become highly introspective. As introspection increases, they develop an internalized audience that provides them with a means to evaluate questions such as "Who am I?" "How do others see me?" and "Where am I going?" Introspection also combines with a reemergence of egocentrism, leading to their sense of being the primary focus—special, unique, and exceptional. Being exceptional to the adolescent means being the exception, giving rise to the risk-taking behaviors for which they are well known:
- I can get drunk on weekends and not develop a drinking problem.
- I won't get pregnant; I've had sex for 6 months and haven't gotten pregnant yet.
- I can take those turns at 60 miles per hour and not have a wreck.

Another behavioral manifestation of adolescents' formal operations is an intolerance of things as they are. They are able to conceptualize things as they might or could be, rather than how they are, and can think of elaborate means for achieving these changes—now. With this newfound capability, they constantly challenge the ways things are and challenge themselves to consider the way things can or should be. Teens can be vehement in trying to convince others of their viewpoints and untiring in their support of causes that align with them. This idealism can lead to a rejection of family beliefs, religion, or social causes, which do not appear to the adolescent to be working fast enough to solve the problems of society. Although this idealism appears to most adults to be a flight from reality, it is a necessary stage in formal thinking. Reality is recognized, but only as a subset of many other possibilities that needs to be brought in line with their own thinking. Eventually, their thinking becomes less egocentric and omnipotent, giving way to an appreciation of differences in judgment between themselves and others. This becomes the basis of an adolescent's ability to think about politics, law, and society in terms of abstract principles and benefits rather than focusing only on the punitive aspects (Burns et al., 2000).

When trying to solve the smallest to biggest problems, adolescents are able to try out a variety of solutions in their minds, without having to manipulate anything physical, operating solely through symbolism (Pruitt, 2000). Several relevant variables can be held constant while one variable is manipulated systematically, enabling the them to hypothesize about an outcome under each different condition. This approach is the classic method of experimental science, but adolescents rarely realize that they are using it with such sophistication.

Erikson's Theory

The central task of adolescence according to Erikson's theory of psychosocial development is the establishment of **identity,** with the primary risk being role confusion. Although it may appear that adolescents are involved in a final, rather than a transient or initial, identity formation, adolescence provides a means of moving into and through what might be termed an *identity crisis*.

This crisis involves a restaging of each of the previous stages of psychosocial development. Development of trust in self and others, as emphasized in infancy, is encountered again as the adolescent searches for people and ideologies in which to have faith. Toddlerhood, and its search for autonomy, is also revisited as adolescents search for autonomy from their primary family units. However, searching for autonomy while avoiding shame and doubt leads to an interesting paradox for adolescents. They would rather behave shamelessly in the eyes of their parents than be forced into behavior that would bring ridicule from their peers. The preschooler's challenge, a sense of initiative rather than guilt, resurfaces as the adolescent searches for direction and purpose. The school-ager's developing sense of industry is carried into the adolescent period, also, as teens make choices in social, recreational, volunteer, academic, familial, and occupational activities. The confusion and hesitation in making these choices arise from fears of participating in activities that will not afford them the opportunity to excel or win the approval of their peers.

The extent to which these earlier tasks were accomplished successfully influences an adolescent's resourcefulness and success in experimenting with the new identity. When the threat of identity confusion is exceedingly great, delinquent behavior and alterations in mental health can occur. This threat is enhanced by conditions of poverty, racism, and other social inequities (see the Multicultural Awareness box later in the chapter).

The pursuit for something to which to be devoted and the search for a meaningful ideology frequently create a puzzling combination of shifting devotion and sudden extremes in action (Hot Topics box). Erikson views this behavior as attempts to try on various roles and to search for some stable principle that might last through the testing of extremes and be carried into adulthood.

Time Orientation

Adolescents look at time differently than they did as younger children. They realize that the response to a problem can, and sometimes should, be delayed to think through the possibilities for approaching the problem. Additionally, teens develop a future orientation and are able to delay immediate gratification to gain more satisfaction in the future.

Language

Advances in cognitive skills are reflected in an increased understanding of language. Formal operations and more abstract thought processes require expression in different words than did the more concrete thoughts of younger children. Adolescents give complex definitions, frequently including all possible meanings or uses. Interpretations of pictures or stories are complex and abstract. Older teens are capable of using and understanding complex sentence

---

HOT topics

Body Piercing and Tattooing

Adolescence is a developmental period full of identity experimentation and risk-taking behavior. Body piercing and tattooing have become popular forms of expression of identity, particularly among adolescents. Each carries health risks and potentially fatal complications.

There are very few sites on adolescent bodies that have not been pierced. Ears, nipples, navels, noses, and eyebrows have all succumbed to metallic rings, rods, studs, and barbells. Approximately one in three individuals with a piercing suffers a complication. Most commonly these include localized infection, bleeding, and dermatitis. Intraoral soft tissue piercing of the lips, cheek, uvula, and tongue harbor additional and potentially fatal complications, including a constant risk of aspiration, massive hemorrhage and rapid swelling lending to airway compromise, nerve damage, keloid scar formation, abscess, and tetanus. There is also an increased risk of hepatitis and HIV, as well as tooth injury, gingival recession, and difficulty with speech, taste, and swallowing.

Tattooing carries similar risks of infection, with a heightened concern for the transmission of blood-borne diseases including hepatitis and HIV, especially with colorful tattoos. Color ink is expensive and too often reused to cut costs, increasing exposure risks. Tattoos are also permanent markings and do not age well.

Nurses need to develop health education programs that allow adolescents to make informed decisions about body piercing, tattooing, and other forms of self-expression.

Compiled from Armstrong, M. L., & McConnell, C. (1994). Tattooing in adolescents, more common than you think: The phenomenon and risks. *Journal of School Nursing, 10*, 22-29; Armstrong, M. L., & Murphy, K. P. (1997). Tattooing: Another adolescent risk behavior warranting health education. *Applied Nursing Research, 10*, 181-189; Dyce, O., Bruno, J. R., Hong, D., Silverstein, K., Brown, M. J., & Mirza, N. (2000). Tongue piercing: The new "rusty nail"? *Head & Neck Journal, 22*(7), 728-732; Keogh, I. J. (2001). Serious complication of tongue piercing. *Journal of Laryngology and Otolaryngology, 115*(3), 233-234.
HIV, human immunodeficiency virus.

---

structure, although they, similar to adults, may not use these complex sentences routinely in their speech.

Both receptive and expressive vocabularies increase during adolescence. As with all ages, receptive far exceeds expressive vocabulary. The adolescent's vocabulary frequently includes slang, or argot, words devised and used by participants in a certain subculture. Slang may be centered on topics such as drug use, popular dress, music, and certain peer activities, or it may be more pervasive, in which case adults or "outsiders" may have difficulty following a conversation between two teens.

Self-Perception–Self-Concept Pattern

The term *self-perception*, which often is used interchangeably with the terms *self-concept* and *self-esteem*, refers to both the description of the self and the evaluation of that

---

CARE PLAN

Low Self-Esteem

Nursing Diagnosis Risk for Low Self-Esteem Related to Poor Body Image

DEFINING CHARACTERISTICS
- Verbalizes negative feelings about self
- Self-destructive behavior (alcohol or drug abuse, overeating, promiscuous sexual behavior, and self-mutilation)
- Lack of eye contact
- Rejection of positive feedback
- Excessive passivity

RELATED FACTORS
- Poor body image
- Poor school performance
- Recent changes or stresses in family unit
- Lack of peer group

EXPECTED OUTCOMES
Goal: Increase self-esteem
- Individual acknowledges personal strengths
- Individual decreases verbalization of negative feelings about self
- Individual develops plan for decreasing self-destructive behavior and increasing healthy lifestyle choices
- Individual accepts positive feedback

INTERVENTIONS
- Actively involve the individual in developing a plan of care.
- Assist the individual in identifying personal strengths.
- Give specific feedback regarding positive behaviors.
- Set limits about negative verbalization.
- Identify positive coping behaviors.
- Teach positive behavior skills through role playing, role model, and discussion.
- Provide information about community resources and counseling.

---

description (Burns et al., 2000). **Body image,** on the other hand, specifically refers to the picture of and feelings about one's body (Care Plan). Tied together and brought to the forefront in adolescence, both self-perception and body image dominate, influence, and are influenced by individual, peer, and societal norms and expectations.

Assessment, anticipatory guidance, education, and counseling are strategies the nurse can use to guide the adolescent in developing a healthy self-perception that incorporates a healthy body image. It is important for parents, teachers, and health care providers to remember to praise adolescents for who they are rather than for what they do, value each of them as unique, demonstrate belief in their abilities to grow and develop, and delight in their discoveries of themselves and their unique means of expressing it.

Roles-Relationships Pattern

Until adolescence, the younger child is highly dependent on the parents and other adults. Striving for identity and increased independence, the adolescent begins to spend increased time away from the family. Parents sense a narrowing of their influence as their teen not only begins to prefer the company of peers and other adults but also begins to question familial beliefs and values. Parents may respond by setting unreasonably strict limits and asking intrusive questions about their teen's activities, friends, and ideas or decide to drop all rules and limits and assume that the adolescent can now manage alone. Neither of these approaches works well.

While adolescents are striving for a sense of identity and independence, their parents are learning to let go. Each is temporarily unsure of the relationship with the other, and the family unit may experience more stress than at any previous time.

Some families experience better outcomes than do other families. Families in which parents maintain a willingness to listen, demonstrate an ongoing affection for and acceptance of their adolescent, yet still maintain some consistent limits experience more constructive, positive outcomes during this period. This situation does not mean that parents necessarily agree with their teen's ideas or actions, but rather that they are willing to hear what the adolescent has to say and to negotiate some limits (Pruitt, 2000). Parents may need assistance in determining negotiable versus nonnegotiable rules and in developing ways to voice their concerns in an honest, open way. Even when teens do not want to discuss a topic, they should know the reasons why their parents are concerned.

Peers

Faced with the need to become autonomous, achieve identity, and become productive, the adolescent often turns from family to **peer group** to find safe psychosocial shelter in which to grow. Belonging to an informally organized clique, crowd, gang, or group is the primary means with which to make the transition from primary allegiance as a young child in the family to a member of a group. Identification with a group is proclaimed through conformity to standards of clothing, behavior, language, and values. This feature of the adolescent subculture persists despite the strong inclination in society as a whole toward greater levels of individuality.

The peer group is a vehicle for movement out of and away from the family unit and, as such, provides a means of achieving the goals of independence and individualization (Pruitt, 2000) (Figure 21-5). It provides a sounding board against which young teens can test ideas, as well as a barometer for their own growth and development (Dixon & Stein, 2000).

Adolescents talk a great deal with their peers. Whether on the phone or in person, they can discuss a 10-minute situation for hours on end. This sharing of thoughts and

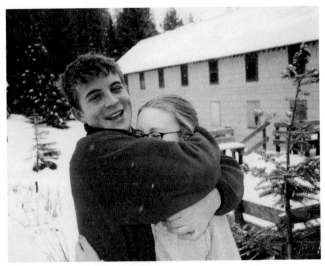

Figure 21-5   Adolescents begin to experiment with peer relationships, preferring them to their families.

impressions is important. The telephone can provide a "safe" mechanism for the young person to interact with members of the opposite sex as they share their most intimate ideas and concerns and begin to experience closeness and caring that will develop into the capacity to form a future intimate relationship.

Sexuality-Reproductive Pattern

The emergence of secondary sexual characteristics increases adolescents' awareness of themselves as sexual human beings. They fantasize about relationships and sex and gradually experiment with dating and a myriad of noncoital physical contacts, as well as coital contacts. Adolescents become sexually active for a variety of reasons. They have sex for affection, peer pressure, as a symbol of maturity, as spontaneous experimentation, to feel close, because it feels good or right, and at times without their consent (Case Study). In the process of establishing a sexual sense of themselves, it is not uncommon for them to question if they are homosexual. Same-sex arousal or experimentation with same-sex physical activity does not necessarily indicate homosexuality or future sexual orientation (Dixon & Stein, 2000).

Knowing adolescents are heavily invested in these and other sexual issues, nurses must be capable and willing to discuss them. Nurses need to be comfortable with their own sexuality, the subject of sex and sexual orientation, and aware of their own limitations and biases. Anticipatory guidance about the decision to become sexually active, contraception, and protection from sexually transmitted diseases (STDs) needs to be provided prior to the situation in which the adolescent needs the information (see Tables 22-2 and 22-3). This is also a good time to introduce the adolescent to breast and testicular self-examination (Health Teaching box).

Adolescent Pregnancy

For health care providers adolescent pregnancy is viewed as a high-risk situation, due to the serious health risks and potential complications for both the mother and the infant (Perrin & Dorman, 2003). For politicians and governmental agencies it is a social problem with an overwhelming use of resources. For adolescents and their families it may be seen as positive and normal or the worst disaster imaginable. No matter what the perspective, adolescent pregnancy represents a myriad of concerns with far-reaching effects.

Although adolescent pregnancy and birth rates are declining, the United States still has the highest rate of adolescent pregnancy in industrialized countries, double that of the United Kingdom (Perrin & Dorman, 2003). Thirty-five percent of adolescent females still become pregnant at least once before the age of 20, resulting in 850,000 adolescent pregnancies each year (National Campaign to Prevent Teen Pregnancy, 2004). The declining rate of adolescent pregnancy has been attributed to a wide range of national, state, and local programs and an increased awareness of STDs, especially human immunodeficiency virus (HIV) and acquired immunodeficiency syndrome (AIDS), and their prevention. However, birth rates for Hispanic and African American adolescents continue to be higher than those of their European and Asian or Pacific Island American counterparts (Perrin & Dorman, 2003).

A review of recent studies identified over 100 precursors to adolescent pregnancy, including economic disadvantage; family structure; family, peer, and partner attitudes and behavior; early menarche and other biophysical changes; detachment from school; and adolescent risk-taking attitudes and behaviors (Perrin & Dorman, 2003). Many of these factors are used to identify at-risk youth and design education and prevention programs.

HEALTH TEACHING Performing Breast and Testicular Self-Examination

BSE or TSE should be performed once a month, so that teens become familiar with the usual appearance and feel of their breasts or testicles. This routine makes noticing any changes from one month to another easier. Finding a change from "normal" is the main idea behind regular self-examination. The best time for females to perform a BSE is 2 or 3 days after their period ends, when breasts are least likely to be tender or swollen. For males, the best time for a TSE is during or right after a warm shower.

Breast Self-Examination

1. Stand in front of a mirror. Inspect both breasts for anything unusual, such as any discharge from the nipples, puckering or dimpling of the skin, or marked asymmetry.
2. While watching closely in the mirror, clasp your hands behind your head and press your hands forward, and inspect again.
3. Next, press your hands firmly on your hips and bow slightly toward the mirror as you pull your shoulders and elbows forward, and inspect again.
4. Next, raise one arm (Figure 1). Use three or four fingers to explore the breast firmly, carefully, and thoroughly. Beginning at the outer edge, press the flat part of your fingers in small circles, moving the circles slowly around the breast. Gradually work toward the nipple. Be sure to cover the entire breast. Pay special attention to the area between the breast and the armpit, including the armpit itself. Feel for any unusual lump or mass under the skin.
5. Gently squeeze the nipple and look for a discharge. Repeat the examination on the other breast.

Steps 4 and 5 should be repeated lying down (Figure 2). This position flattens the breast and makes examination easier. Some women perform BSE in the shower. Fingers gliding over soapy skin make concentrating on the texture underneath easier (Figure 3).

Testicular Self-Examination

1. Cup or support the testicles with one hand and feel with the other.
2. Gently roll each testicle between the thumb and fingers. There should not be any pain. Feel for any swelling or hard lumps on the surface of the testicle. Testicles are normally oval, firm, smooth, and rubbery. One may be slightly larger than the other.
3. A natural tubelike structure, the epididymis, is along the back of the testicle. Learn what it feels like.

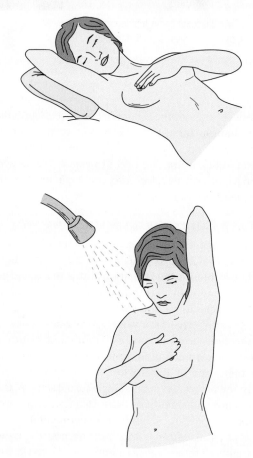

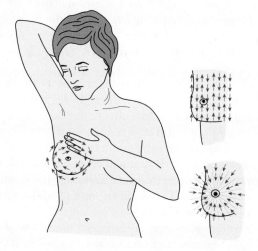

From Lowdermilk, D. L., & Perry, S. E. (2002). *Maternity nursing* (6th ed.). St. Louis: Mosby. *BSE*, breast self-examination; *TSE*, testicular self-examination.

The National Campaign to Prevent Teen Pregnancy (2004) emphasizes the likely negative outcomes of adolescent pregnancy in outreach efforts. For the mother these include a significant decline in her future prospects; serious health risks, including an increased risk of obesity and hypertension; single parenthood; and poverty. For the child born to adolescent mothers there is a higher risk of low birth weight. Low birth weight is associated with infant mortality and other health problems, including cerebral palsy, mental retardation, dyslexia, and hyperactivity. Further, these children often fall victim to abuse and neglect and suffer from poor school performance.

Research also has identified some positive aspects of adolescent pregnancy, identifying mothering as a potential anchor that fosters a sense of purpose and meaning, an ability to reweave connection, and provide a sense of the future

(Smith Battle, 2000). More recently, Perrin and Dorman (2003) conducted a study exploring the personal life stories of now-successful and highly educated women who became mothers as adolescents. Their stories offer insights into formulas for potential success and include the presence of mentors, support, optimism, opportunity, and spirituality.

The hardest thing about being a pregnant adolescent or an adolescent mother is the isolation (Perrin & Dorman, 2003). When pregnancy occurs, adolescents and their families deserve honest and sensitive counseling about all of the options available to them, as well as the support systems available for them throughout the pregnancy, birth, and subsequent parenting (American Academy of Child and Adolescent Psychiatry, 2004). Nurses not only need to reinforce reproductive health education efforts, they also need to encourage adolescents to build on the strengths in their lives and opportunities available to them.

Coping–Stress Tolerance Pattern

When all of the changes that occur in adolescents are aligned with their need to separate from their parents and gain a sense of their own independence, their ability to cope is put to the test. Common coping mechanisms and the strategies the nurse can use to encourage teens to use them in adaptive ways are listed in Box 21-4.

However, too often adolescents are unable to balance the stresses, lacking the appropriate skills and outlets, adequate support systems, or available mental health intervention. Depression, suicide, and substance abuse emerge as life becomes overwhelming and futures unimaginable.

Depression

As with many other diseases, the rate of **depression** increases with age and the incidence continues to increase during adolescence. The term *depression* includes both major depressive and dysthymic disorders. A depressive disorder is defined as a depressed or irritable mood or a diminished interest and pleasure in usual activities, while dysthymia is a depressed or irritable mood that extends over a year-long period with symptom relief for no more than 2 months (Burns et al., 2000).

Depression is suspected when the adolescent uses words such as *down, sad, low, blue, hopeless, worried, bored,* or *discouraged* and exhibits several of the following symptoms:

- Change in weight or appetite
- Insomnia or hypersomnia
- Decreased energy or fatigue
- Loss of interest and pleasure in usual activities
- Out-of-proportion feelings of self-reproach or guilt
- Difficulty concentrating; declining school performance
- Preoccupation with death or suicidal ideation

The nurse needs to refer the adolescent with depression to a mental health specialist.

Suicide

Adolescence is a period of considerable stress, and when coping mechanisms and social supports are inadequate,

---

| Box **21-4** | Coping Mechanisms of Adolescents |

COGNITIVE MASTERY

The adolescent attempts to learn as much as possible about the situation or stressor. This strategy is common for the adolescent with a chronic illness. The nurse can assist by clarifying any misinformation, sharing research findings, and encouraging a discussion of feelings.

CONFORMITY

The adolescent attempts to be a mirror image of peers, which includes dress, language, attitudes, and actions. The nurse must respect this need for sameness and can also encourage discussion of feelings about differences among teens.

CONTROLLING BEHAVIOR

Adolescents must be in charge of some aspects of life and can no longer accept family and school rules without question as they did in the past. This need to control extends to health care. The nurse cannot simply give directions or instructions, but rather should present the options and allow the adolescent to partner with the nurse to work out an acceptable plan.

FANTASY

The adolescent may use fantasy as a way to escape or experiment. The nurse can encourage the teen to use fantasy constructively to develop creative plans to deal with a stressful situation.

MOTOR ACTIVITY

Engaging in sports, dancing, running, or other physical activity can be an effective tension-releasing strategy, as well as provide an instant peer group. The nurse can encourage physical activity and offer information about protective gear and injury prevention.

---

suicide may emerge as an outcome. It is the third leading cause of death in adolescence and has increased 40% over the past 10 years. The dramatic rise was primarily among males (Friedman, 1998).

These figures may not even reflect the full scope of the problem, because many suicides are classified as accidental deaths. Suicide attempts are not included in these statistics, although estimates show that 50 to 200 attempts occur for every successfully completed suicide. Attempts are 3 to 9 times more common in females, but males are 3 times as successful (American Academy of Pediatrics, 2000). Many researchers are convinced that suicide during adolescence is not an impulsive or spontaneous act; it is selected carefully only after other problem-solving methods have failed and suicide is viewed as the only option.

Fortunately, adolescent suicide can be prevented. Distressed adolescents tend to give clues, both verbally and nonverbally. Any single clue may mean nothing, but when several clues are noted, they should be recognized as impor-

Box **21-5** **Warning Signs of Suicide Risk in Adolescents**

BEHAVIORAL CHANGES

- Increased risk taking
- Increased incidence of accidents
- Substance use and abuse
- Physical violence to self, others, or animals
- Decreased appetite
- Alienation from family or peer group
- Giving away personal items
- Writing letters or notes, essays, and poems with suicidal content

COGNITIVE AND MOOD CHANGES

- Expression of hopelessness
- Increasing rage or anger
- Dramatic swings in affect
- Sleep disorders
- Preoccupation with death
- Difficulty concentrating
- Hearing voices, seeing things or people
- Newfound interest in religion or cult

tant warning signs. Box 21-5 outlines warning signs for parents, teachers, health care providers, and peers to be alert to in preventing adolescent suicide.

When the nurse suspects that an adolescent is suicidal, immediate referral should be made to a mental health specialist. A suicide threat should never be ignored, and the adolescent who is in immediate danger of committing suicide should never be left alone.

Values-Beliefs Pattern

Values and beliefs are learned phenomena that serve as guides for adolescent decision making and actions. With the development of abstract thought, adolescents begin to expand their understanding of good and bad or right and wrong, to include autonomous moral principles that have validity apart from the authority of parent or society and instead are based on the individual's beliefs. Their newly discovered maturity in moral reasoning is situational and relational and often is superceded by psychosocial developmental needs and influences. Adolescents may think or feel something is wrong or bad yet may act contrary to that belief because of peer pressure or the need to declare their independence.

Adolescents often align their values and beliefs with a particular religion, philosophical school of thought, social movement or cause, or other formal system, using it to make decisions about what is right or wrong, best or worst, and important or trivial. During adolescence these alignments can change drastically and often, causing strife and concern for parents, yet providing the teen with different ranges of experience from which to base eventual and lasting choices.

According to Kohlberg's theory of moral development (1981), the adolescent begins to make the transition to the

postconventional stage, equating what is right with the idea of justice and basing actions on the recognition of the universal principles underlying laws and social agreements. Gilligan, who developed a parallel theory of moral development for females, proposes that the female adolescent sees "good" as involving self-sacrifice and caring for the relationships in her life (Gilligan, Lyons, & Hammer, 1990). As moral reasoning matures, the female adolescent learns to achieve a balance between what is good for her and what is good for others in her network of relationships.

As adolescents struggle with their journey to discover who they are, parents, teachers, and health care providers need to provide positive role modeling, reinforce positive behaviors, and remember how hard their own journeys were. It is often when we like them the least that they need us the most.

PATHOLOGICAL PROCESSES
Accidents

Accidents, along with suicide and homicide, continue to be the leading cause of death and injury during adolescence. Newly licensed and inexperienced behind the wheel, it is no surprise that adolescents have a motor vehicle fatality rate 20 times higher than that of any other age group (Dixon & Stein, 2000). Whether drivers, passengers, pedestrians, or cyclists, few adolescents take measures to reduce their risk of injury, with 21% rarely or never using a safety belt and 87% rarely or never using a bicycle helmet (Green & Palfrey, 2000).

Nurses should encourage teens to wear their safety belts and avoid driving, or riding with someone, under the influence of drugs or alcohol. The tendency to play loud music and change the tune or disc often, as well as the pressure to answer cell phones, can also be distracting, as can a car full of other teens. Recognizing this and that teens have a much higher nighttime crash fatality rate, many states have enacted new driver restrictions and nighttime curfews.

Sports

Organized sports in and out of school provide adolescents with experiences in competition, team work and effort, and conflict resolution. They also provide a valuable means for adolescents to develop self-esteem. However, adolescents are particularly vulnerable to sports injuries. Their coordination skills are developing, their judgment often immature and inadequate, their epiphyses not yet closed, and their extremities poorly protected by stabilizing musculature. They can also become obsessed or driven to perform beyond their capabilities or to the exclusion of all other activities. The use of performance enhancing substances, such as steroids and creatine, can create another potential extreme scenario that places the adolescent at risk for injury.

The nurse needs to advocate for the proper use of protective gear during all activities and a thorough preparticipation sports examination (see Box 21-3), as well as

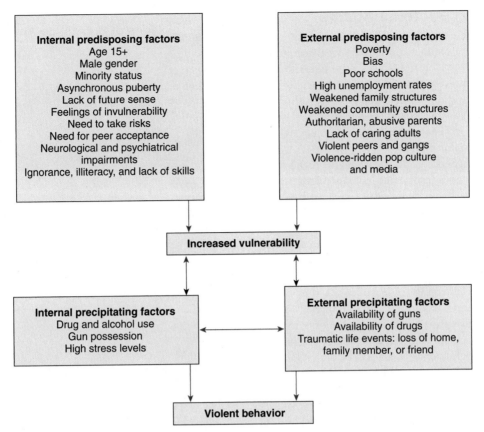

Figure 21-6 Factors contributing to adolescent violence.

monitor for overuse, overexertion, or overinvestment on the part of the adolescent.

Violence

Adolescents today face an unprecedented risk of injury and death from violence in their homes, schools, and communities. Becoming increasingly independent, they test the limits of authority, experiment with a variety of roles, question adult values and authority, and look to peers for affirmation. They may feel pressure to join gangs or feel threatened by them, carrying weapons to either protect themselves or intimidate others. Adolescents often report a fear of violence and try to avoid situations where they might be vulnerable to it, including home or even the bathroom at school.

Many studies suggest that witnessing or observing violence, whether in person or projected on the TV, video, or movie screen, results in a higher incidence of violent behaviors and posttraumatic stress syndrome. The graphic violence in music lyrics and videos has also been implicated.

In his documentary, *Bowling for Columbine*, filmmaker Michael Moore made a compelling case that what endangers America most today is not the act of violence or the crime, but our fear of it. Fear is stoked by a media that trumpets every street murder and bank robbery as an imminent threat and elevates shark attacks and escalator mishaps to

a national crisis. Children and adolescents with fears that go unresolved have been shown to have an increase in violent behaviors, and fear about others often surfaces as racism. Figure 21-6 outlines the interrelationships of internal and external precipitating factors that increase an adolescent's vulnerability to and for violent behaviors.

Nurses need to engage adolescents, examining and discussing the messages in videos, songs, movies, and television shows. Discussing their developing sense of self, their sense of belonging and where that sense is found, and their fears may help to intercept an adolescent who might otherwise turn to violence. Teens who are valued and nurtured by caring adults have the best chance of emerging from adolescence unscathed.

Mechanical Forces
Motor Vehicles

Adolescents become increasingly mobile as they become progressively independent. This increased mobility typically involves the use of motorcycles and motor vehicles. Driver's education certificates and knowledge of traffic rules and regulations unfortunately do not prevent the teen from surrendering to peer pressure or from using driving as an outlet for stress, anger, or to make a statement of independence. The increased numbers of motor vehicle–related injuries and fatalities in adolescence were discussed earlier.

Biological and Bacterial Agents

Infectious mononucleosis is a self-limiting viral infection transmitted by direct contact of oropharyngeal secretions. It is prevalent among adolescents and often referred to as the *kissing disease*; however, it can occur in younger children. It is caused by the Epstein-Barr virus. Typically adolescents complain of a sore throat, lymph node enlargement, and lethargy. Both splenomegaly and hepatomegaly can occur, creating a risk for injury.

Rates of meningococcal disease remain highest for infants, but in the past decade rates have increased among adolescents. Reports have identified an increased risk for meningococcal disease among college freshmen who live in dormitories or residence halls. As adolescents prepare for college, nurses need to review their risk and provide them with information on the available vaccine.

As adolescents experiment with and explore their sexual development and emerging independence, they often become sexually active, exposing them to a myriad of **sexually transmitted diseases.** STDs most commonly include gonorrhea, syphilis, chlamydia, herpes simplex virus, human papilloma virus, trichomonas, hepatitis B, and HIV (see Table 22-3). Considered an epidemic, STDs have the highest rates in adolescents, with minorities, especially African Americans, disproportionately affected (Burns et al., 2000). Inconsistent use of contraceptive and protective devices, increasingly earlier age and frequency of sexual activity, social and peer pressure, and an adolescent's sense of invincibility all contribute to this significant public and adolescent health problem. Although adolescents can be evaluated and treated for STDs, the diseases must be reported and the nurse must be aware of state rules about reporting.

Chemical Agents
Substance Use and Abuse

Society as a whole is increasingly oriented toward using chemicals such as drugs, alcohol, and tobacco to feel better, look better, act more sociable, stay awake, go to sleep, be sexy or erect, or lose weight. Some of the most famous music, movie, and sports stars openly model substance use and abuse. It is no surprise that adolescents are making the choice to experiment with and use substances at earlier and earlier ages.

Substance use is a precursor to abuse, which emphasizes the need for health care providers to be alert and screen for its presence. Identifying an adolescent with substance use or abuse requires a careful nursing assessment that is conducted with an accepting manner.

A brief screening test for adolescent substance abuse developed by Children's Hospital of Boston uses the acronym CRAFFT to guide health care providers when interviewing adolescents about substance abuse:

C—Have you ever ridden in a *car* driven by someone, including yourself, who was "high" or had been using alcohol or drugs?

Box **21-6**	Signs of Substance Abuse

Accidents
Agitation
Appetite loss
Blackouts
Bleeding gums
Chronic cough
Delusions
Depression
Diarrhea
Dyspnea
Eye drops
Headache
Hoarseness
Hyperactivity
Inability to concentrate
Insomnia
Lethargy
Memory loss
Muscle weakness
Paranoia
Rhinorrhea
Seizures
Somnolence
Sore tongue
Stomach pain
Taste loss
Violent outbursts
Vomiting
Withdrawal
Weight loss

From Payne, W. A., & Hahn, D. B. (2002). *Understanding your health* (7th ed.). Boston: McGraw-Hill.

R—Do you ever use alcohol or drugs to *relax*, feel better about yourself, or fit in?

A—Do you ever use alcohol or drugs while you are by yourself, *alone*?

F—Do your family or *friends* ever tell you that you should cut down on your drinking or drug use?

F—Do you ever *forget* things you did while using alcohol or drugs?

T—Have you gotten into *trouble* while you were using alcohol or drugs?

Two or more affirmative answers suggests a significant problem and warrants referral and follow-up.

General signs of substance use and abuse are identified in Box 21-6 and can be used by parents, teachers, and health care providers who assess and monitor adolescent behaviors.

Tobacco Use

Most teens begin smoking during adolescence, especially if a close friend, sibling, or parent also smokes (Burns et al., 2000). The highest rate of smoking is among white females, while "smokeless" tobacco, such as snuff and chewing tobacco, is more popular among males. Adolescents begin using tobacco for a variety of reasons including wanting to appear older, because their friends do, or to imitate adult role models or media images. Advertising by the tobacco industry directed at adolescents has been shown to encourage adolescent smoking.

The nurse's primary prevention focus is on keeping non-smokers from starting and helping smokers to stop. The National Institutes of Health has published guidelines for health care providers to follow, titled The 5 A's for Brief Intervention in Adolescents Who Use Tobacco, which are:

- Ask about tobacco use
- Advise to quit
- Assess willingness to attempt quitting
- Assist in quit attempt
- Arrange for follow-up

By following this brief intervention, which often takes less than 3 minutes, health care providers have doubled the rate of smoking cessation in adolescents (National Library of Medicine, 2000).

Cancer

Adolescents are affected by many of the same cancers as are younger children, such as leukemia, osteogenic sarcoma, lymphomas, and central nervous system tumors. Older adolescents are entering the period of their lives during which cancer of the reproductive and related organs is more common. For females, the focus is on cervical and breast cancer and for males, testicular cancer is of concern.

Peak incidence of breast and cervical cancer is during middle age and is actually rare in the teenage years. Breast self-examination (BSE), which has been highly recommended for over 30 years, has recently been questioned as a routine practice for most adolescents. The extremely small incidence of breast cancer in teens has caused some health care providers to deemphasize this practice for them. However, most still feel that regular examination of the breasts begins a lifelong habit that should begin as soon as the female adolescent develops (see the Health Teaching box).

Cervical cancer is detected with a Papanicolaou (Pap) smear, obtained from the cervix during a pelvic examination. Factors that increase the risk for cervical cancer include sexual intercourse before age 20, multiple sexual partners or a sexual partner who has had many partners, any history of STDs or exposure to exogenous hormones, and smoking. Sexually active adolescents should have a Pap test performed annually and the American College of Obstetricians and Gynecologists recommends annual pelvic examinations by age 18, even when the young woman is not sexually active. The nurse can explain the purpose and the process involved in conducting a pelvic examination and Pap test.

Testicular cancer is the number one cancer in adolescent and young adult males. Adolescent males should learn to do a testicular self-examination and continue this practice monthly (see the Health Teaching box). Nurses should introduce and teach methods of self-examination to adolescents who naturally are interested in their developing bodies.

SOCIAL PROCESSES
School

Junior high and high school are a new social experience, introducing the adolescent to changing classes, multiple teachers and teaching styles, variable class schedules and homework load, and a variety of peer influences. Adolescents must learn to become accustomed to greater anonymity as they navigate the corridors of larger, more impersonal institutions (Dixon & Stein, 2000). Yet despite these challenges, junior high and high school settings also provide meaningful in-school and after-school learning, peer contact, intellectual stimulation, and activities.

Schools and peers, as opposed to home and parents, become the primary setting through which expectations are shared and standards communicated. Adolescent peer groups serve as sounding boards against which teens test their ideas and gauge their physical, intellectual, psychological, and moral growth (Dixon & Stein, 2000). Nurses must remember to ask adolescents about school and their friends, and how they are doing with both. The nurse can also monitor adolescents as they prepare for and make the transition to their next social arena and role whether it is college, vocational training, the military, or another career choice.

Culture and Ethnicity

Cultural and ethnic influences operate throughout childhood and continue into adolescence. The primary difference in adolescence is that teens question, modify, or reject these influences, exchanging them for those of their peers or of the dominant cultural group. First-generation adolescents of immigrant parents have to negotiate two cultures, languages, and sets of expectations. These adolescents live a double life that results in increased stress. Adolescents from minority groups, such as African Americans, Hispanics, Asian Americans, Native Americans, Russian Americans, or Arab Americans, trying to fit in to the dominant adolescent culture may experience discrimination and rejection. Additional stress may also be experienced when their attempts to fit in to the dominant culture are offensive to the values and beliefs of their own.

Young people from minority groups have a particular problem in relation to the culture of adolescence. These teens may desire strongly to fit in to the predominant adolescent culture, which in society is often middle class, white, and Protestant, and they may be able to meet one or two of these criteria but be unable to meet the others because of economics, different appearance, or different education and experiences. Advertising does not emphasize the economically depressed or ethnic-looking model, and the teens' peers are trying every means possible to look and act similar to the dominant culture adolescent. Further pressure comes from their own minority culture when they emulate the majority culture in ways that the family views as offensive to their ideas and beliefs.

Nurses need to recognize and assess for additional stresses experienced by adolescents as they wrestle not only with their own but also with their cultural identities.

Legislation

Many laws and regulations are aimed at adolescents and deal with the minimum age at which they can assume adult responsibilities and decision making. The rationale for these restrictions is that adolescents, although capable, lack the experience, perspective, and judgment to recognize and avoid choices that might be detrimental to them, so they require protection. A question that is raised frequently when considering minimum age is whether strict age criteria are appropriate for any adolescent, particularly because development is variable and experiences are diverse.

The restrictions that have recently been questioned most strongly deal with issues related to sexual activity. The U.S. Supreme Court affirmed the right of all individuals to have equal access to contraceptive service, regardless of age or marital status. However, variations occur from state to state and the nurse must be aware of legal age determinants, as well as variations in definitions of emancipated minors.

The **emancipated minor** provision of certain laws recognizes that some adolescents become independent from their families at an early age and assume adult responsibilities. An emancipated minor is an adolescent who has not reached the standard legal age for certain activities, such as consenting to marriage or seeking certain kinds of health or illness care, but who is permitted to accept full responsibility for these decisions because the individual is economically and emotionally separate from the family.

Most often confidentiality is the more important issue for adolescents. The nurse can assure them that information shared will be kept confidential unless the teens pose a risk to themselves or others or state laws mandate that the information be shared (Burns et al., 2000). For example, abuse must be reported, STDs need to be reported, and some states require report of adolescent sexual activity if an age difference of 3 or more years exists between the sexual partners.

Nurses need to familiarize themselves with the legal rights of adolescents in their state and the resources available in their community.

Economics

Identification with peers, the essence of self-image during adolescence, includes dressing alike, having similar possessions, and doing similar things, all of which require economic resources. This can be a major conflict between parents and adolescents. Parents may think that they should have the power to decide how their adolescent spends money. Adolescents may believe, just as strongly, that they know the best ways to allocate resources and determine the amount of money they need.

Ideally, parents and adolescents should negotiate economic questions, with the parents becoming less controlling as the teen gains more experience and expertise in these matters. However, the family with limited economic resources has fewer choices, and adolescents from these families feel trapped by their circumstance. Poverty is particularly hard on children, and as they become adolescents they often develop a fatalistic view of life (Multicultural Awareness box).

Some adolescents seek employment to earn their own money and have control over it. Others work because their families need the income. It is important for the nurse to assess the economic resources of each adolescent's family and work within them when partnering with the adolescent in health care planning.

Health Care Delivery System

Many health care resources are available to the adolescent. Teens can continue to see their child health care providers in a pediatric center as they did as younger children, but this setting usually is rejected because of the young-child atmosphere.

School-based clinics frequently are available in junior high and high school, and adolescent-focused clinics are available in many communities through both public and private agencies. Each of these clinics serves only adolescents, and the staff is oriented to the needs of this age group. Adolescents frequently have a stronger sense of comfort in these settings than in those in which young children or adults are also served.

Adolescents can also make use of services such as family planning clinics. These settings may designate certain days and hours for teens, whereas other facilities integrate them into the adult-oriented protocols. The pregnant adolescent typically finds prenatal care in an adult-focused setting, although more adolescent-specific programs are being developed. The physical needs of pregnant adolescents may be the same as those of the pregnant adult, but the psychosocial needs are different and should be approached by a professional who has a comprehensive knowledge of their development and responses to stress.

The adolescent is a rapidly changing individual. The nurse who works in an adolescent-focused practice should be well prepared in adolescent health-promotion strategies. The nurse should have a thorough understanding of adolescent physical and psychosocial growth and development and recognize each teen as a person (Box 21-7).

Adolescents not only tend to be fearful about procedures or possible diagnoses but also need to stay in control of the situation. These conflicting feelings can be difficult to manage simultaneously. By establishing the adolescent as a partner with the health care providers in promoting good health and screening for health risks, the nurse can facilitate the adolescent's sense of control.

MULTICULTURAL AWARENESS

African American Youths "Choosing" AIDS

Poor urban African Americans often confront circumstances that the American dream defines as *failures,* and their disproportionate victimization is manifest in the number of violent crimes that target them. Adolescents in this environment rapidly lose their idealism and learn, instead, to hope for little and expect even less.

In a haunting study published in 1998, Sylvie Tourigny provided exquisite documentation of a group of impoverished African American teens in inner city Detroit who deliberately contracted AIDS. Their individual stories of willful seroconversion reveal a world of marginalization, insensitive social policies, and demanding caretaking responsibilities for both themselves and their families.

"I ain't gonna live no 15 years anyway . . . you can't be here in the 'hood' and expect live."

"There is no future to think about anyway."

"There ain't much goin' on for black girls like me, so this be best . . . they'se gonna pay for everything."

"If you got AIDS, you get more."

In a recent editorial entitled "The Complexities of Health Promotion," Morse (2004) asks, "Didn't these teens know that AIDS is terminal?" The answer is yes. However, the attraction of AIDS for these teens was that it would entitle them to much-needed counseling, assistance, and money and yet not cause immediate illness or death. No adolescent should have to choose illness and death for his or her needs to be met.

There is no reason to believe that "choosing" AIDS is only an inner city problem, confined to African Americans, or even to North America. Nurses need to be the leaders in evaluating health promotion and social services support, assessing whether they are truly available to the poorest and youngest of the poor, prior to contracting disease.

Based on Morse, J. (2004). The complexities of health promotion. *Qualitative Health Research,* 14(1), 3-4; and Tourigny, S. C. (1998). Some new dying trick: African American youths "choosing" HIV/AIDS. *Qualitative Health Research,* 8(2), 149-167.
AIDS, acquired immunodeficiency syndrome.

Box 21-7   HEADSSS Assessment

The HEADSSS Assessment provides a mnemonic that guides health care providers through an adolescent's psychosocial assessment. Responses should be interpreted as those that are indicators of strengths or protection from risk and those that are indicators of risky behavior or situations.

Home and health
Education, employment, eating
Activities, affiliations, aspirations
Drugs
Sexuality
Suicide, depression, self-image
Safety

From Reif, C. J., & Elster, A. B. (March 1998). Adolescent preventive services. *Primary Care: Clinics in Office Practice* 25(1). Philadelphia: W. B. Saunders.

The adolescent's questions should be answered thoroughly and honestly. In many instances the adolescent is hesitant to voice concerns, so information should be offered even when questions are not asked. An effective indirect approach to learning about adolescent concerns, especially about potentially embarrassing or stressful topics, is to say, "Many teenagers ask me about [a topic]. Have you ever thought about this?" or "A lot of young people want to know about [a topic]."

Direct questions are also important, even about sensitive topics: "Have you ever thought about suicide?" "Are you depressed?" "Are you sexually active?" "Do you use birth control and/or protection?" However, asking first about friends and the adolescent's feelings about them may be a good lead-in approach: "Are any of your friends doing drugs?" "How do you feel about it?" Vague or circuitous questions may be interpreted as a discomfort or lack of understanding and may cause the adolescent to be equally vague when responding.

Correct anatomical terms and descriptions of laboratory tests, disease processes, and possible outcomes are essential components in treating adolescents as individuals who are capable of being responsible for their own bodies.

SUMMARY

Adolescence is a period of rapid change, when the integration of family, peer, educational, social, cultural, and community experiences begins to take form in teen's sense of self. Many view adolescence as a construction site in its early stages. Onlookers assume that eventually a recognizable structure will emerge but have no idea what that structure will be. Although many parents, teachers, and health care providers feel that hard hats and steel reinforced shoes are needed, each is better equipped with an understanding and respect for the adolescent's developmental struggles with physical and cognitive changes, autonomy, body image, peer relations, and identity. The goal, after all, is for the teen to emerge in young adulthood with a healthy body, mind, and spirit.

ADDITIONAL STUDY MATERIAL

Study Questions in the back of the book, see page 663.

evolve WEB SITE MATERIALS

These materials are located on the book's Web site at http://evolve.elsevier.com/Edelman/.

- WebLinks
- Content Updates

REFERENCES

American Academy of Child and Adolescent Psychiatry. (2004). When children have children. Retrieved August 30, 2004, from: *http://www.aacap.org/publications/factsfam/pregnant.htm.*

American Academy of Pediatrics, Committee on Adolescence. (2000). Suicide and suicide attempts in adolescence. *Pediatrics, 105,* 871-874.

Burns, C. E., Brady, M. A., Dunn, A. M., & Starr, N. B. (2000). *Pediatric primary care* (2nd ed.). New York: W. B. Saunders.

Dixon, S. D., & Stein, M. T. (2000). *Encounters with children* (3rd ed.). St. Louis: Mosby.

Friedman, S. B. (1998). *Comprehensive adolescent health care* (2nd ed.). St. Louis: Quality Medical.

Gilligan, C., Lyons, N., & Hammer, T. (1990). *Making connections: The relational worlds of adolescent girls at Emma Willard school.* Cambridge, MA: Harvard University Press.

Gortmaker, S. L., Must, A., Sobol, A. M., Peterson, K., Colditz, G. A., & Dietz, W. H. (1996). Television viewing as a cause of increasing obesity among children in the United States, 1986-1990. *Archives of Pediatric and Adolescent Medicine, 150,* 356.

Green, M., & Palfrey J. S. (2000). *Bright futures: Guidelines for health supervision of infants, children, and adolescents* (2nd ed.). Washington, DC: National Center for Education in Maternal and Child Health Georgetown University.

Guyton, A. C., & Hall, J. E. (2000). *Textbook of medical physiology* (10th ed.). Philadelphia: W. B. Saunders.

Hoffman, A. D., & Greydanus, D. E. (1997). *Adolescent medicine.* Stamford, CT: Appleton & Lange.

Kligh, W. J. (1998). Childhood obesity. *Pediatrics in Review, 19,* 312-315.

Kohlberg, L. (1981). *The philosophy of moral development.* San Francisco: Harper & Row.

Kreipe, R. E., & Dukarm, C. P. (1999). Eating disorders in adolescents and older children. *Pediatrics in Review, 20,* 410-420.

National Campaign to Prevent Teen Pregnancy. (2004). Teen pregnancy—So what? Retrieved August 30, 2004, from: *http://www.teenpregnancy.org.*

National Library of Medicine. (2000). *AHCRP supported clinical practice guidelines: 18. Treating tobacco use and dependence.* Retrieved May 9, 2005, from *http://www.ncbi.nlm.nih.gov/books/bv.fcgi?rid = hstat2.chapter.7644.*

Neinstein, S. (2002). *Adolescent health care: A practical guide* (4th ed.). Baltimore: Urban & Schwarzenberg.

Perrin, K. M., & Dorman, K. A. (2003). Teen parents and academic success. *The Journal of School Nursing, 19*(5), 288-293.

Pruitt, D. B. (2000). *Your adolescent.* New York: Harper Collins.

Smith Battle, L. (2000). The vulnerabilities of teenage mothers: Challenging prevailing assumptions. *ANS Advances in Nursing Science, 231,* 29-40.

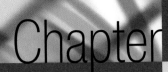

Chapter 22

ELIZABETH C. KUDZMA

Young Adult

objectives

After completing this chapter, the reader will be able to:

- Describe the specific health requirements of the young adult.
- Identify the attitudes, behaviors, and habits that regulate the lifestyles of young adults.
- Identify tasks that are consistent with the adult maturity achieved during this period.
- Differentiate the disease processes that affect the "younger" young adult and the "older" young adult.
- Describe the nurse's role in reducing the rate of unintentional pregnancies in young adult women.
- Describe occupational hazards that infringe on the young adult's welfare.
- Evaluate strategies that the nurse can use to reduce the risks associated with young adult behaviors of smoking, alcohol consumption, and drug use.
- Analyze the cultural and ethnic risk factors that affect young adults.
- Differentiate the nursing roles in preventive intervention for healthy young adults in home and community environments.

key terms

Achievement-oriented stress
Aerobic exercise
Basal metabolic rate
Breast self-examination
Coronary artery disease
Genetic impairments
Genital herpes virus

Hepatitis B
Human immunodeficiency virus (HIV)
Human papilloma virus (HPV)
Hypertension
Infertility
Maternal mortality rate

Metabolic syndrome
Papanicolaou (Pap) smear
Postconventional level of moral reasoning
Rubella
Stress
Testicular self-examination

THINK About It

Assessing Problematic College Drinking Behavior

You are the clinic director and nurse practitioner at a small liberal arts college. Mary, a 19-year-old freshman, has generally been a good student, easily making the adjustment to living away from home during her first 2 months in the dormitory. She comes to you to talk about an episode that occurred the previous weekend and that frightened her.

On Saturday night she was at a party at a private residence in a rural wooded setting away from the campus. She remembers consuming five or six alcoholic drinks; however, any memory after midnight is missing. She woke up in a fellow female student's dormitory room without any memory of leaving the party or returning to the dormitory.

Continued

Assessing Problematic College Drinking Behavior *cont'd*

THINK About It

She was able to piece together information from her friends, who told her that she consumed at least nine alcoholic drinks that night and that she left the party with others who were returning to the dormitory, but they were not the friends with whom she had been seen all evening. She is concerned that she may have been drugged or that she may be having memory lapses. Assessment of her alcohol use in the past reveals that she can recount at least four occasions during which she drank more than seven drinks at a party or family gathering. She describes her family as "social drinkers." Last June, she was involved in a minor car accident that might have been related to her consumption of at least three drinks that afternoon.

1 Do you believe that Mary has a problem with drinking? As what kind of an alcohol user would you classify her? How do you establish appropriate therapeutic communication?

2 What kind of physical symptoms might assist you in making a determination that Mary has a drinking problem?

3 What kinds of monitoring and follow-up mechanisms might assist Mary in keeping her behavior consistent with a treatment plan?

The young adult period encompasses the ages from 18 to 35 years, a time that ranges from the end of adolescence to the beginning of middle adulthood. The major task of this period is preparing for the assumption of adult responsibilities, rights, and privileges.

AGE AND PHYSICAL CHANGES

The young adult period is a time of many physical and emotional changes and is an opportunity for learning by experience and experimentation. All phases of young adult development garner considerable interest. Judging by the increase in books about adult self-development, more adults are exploring topics in holistic healing and spiritual health and development. Health behaviors, safety practices, diet, exercise, sexuality, and addictions are widely discussed topics. Preventive health concerns for young adults can be separated into two basic categories: (1) developing behaviors that promote a healthy lifestyle and (2) decreasing the incidence of accidents, injuries, and acts of violence. *Healthy People 2010* reports that death rates related to traffic and motor vehicle injuries are highest in the age group of 15 to 24 years (U.S. Department of Health and Human Services [USDHHS], 2000).

In 2001, approximately 23.7% of the population was composed of adults ages 18 to 35 (U.S. Census Bureau, 2001). The young adult population is projected to be approximately 22.8% of the general population by the year 2005 and about the same, 22.9%, in 2015. The percentage of young adults ages 20 to 24 years showed a dramatic decline from 9.4% in 1980 to 6.9% in 2001 (U.S. Census Bureau, 2001). A decline in this age group influences birth rates, and the U.S. Census Bureau (2001) reported that the birth rate per 1000 people for women of all ages in 2000 was 14.7; this rate has been dropping since 1990 when it was more than 16.7 live births per 1000. Health-promotion efforts are particularly important for young adults, because health teaching for this age group has the potential to directly influence subsequent generations (*Healthy People 2010* box).

Young adulthood is generally the healthiest time of life. Physical growth is complete by the age of 20; most concerns related to physiological development are focused on ensuring the optimal functioning of body systems. The young adult's physical abilities are in peak condition, and compensatory mechanisms operate optimally during illness to provide minimal disruption in health patterns. Nursing goals for individuals of this age group are oriented toward prolonging this period of optimal physical energy; developing the mental, emotional, and social potential; encouraging proper health habits; anticipating and observing the onset of chronic disease at an early stage; and treating disease when appropriate.

Full adult stature in men is reached at approximately age 21; in women, full growth occurs earlier, typically by age 17. Optimal muscle strength occurs during ages 25 to 30, then gradually declines by approximately 10% from ages 30 to 60. Manual dexterity peaks in young adulthood and declines into the mid-30s.

Women have greater longevity than do men. Women are considered biologically stronger than men, outlive men, and naturally outnumber men. On the average, in the United States women live 5.4 years longer than do men, an increase of 0.1 to 0.2 years within the past decade (Anderson & Arias, 2003). These statistics may be a result in part of female genetic composition or men's greater exposure to environmental and occupational hazards. Men also seek health care services less frequently than do women. The female rate for preventive care is significantly higher than the rate for males (67.1 visits per 100 females versus 37.7 visits per 100 males) and reflects the inclusion of multiple prenatal visits in any 1 year (Cherry, Burt, & Woodwell, 2003).

A classic public health indicator of a nation's health resources and services is the **maternal mortality rate.** Since 1980 maternal mortality has been fairly stable in the United States. In 1980 the rate was 9.2 per 100,000 live births; then mortality dropped to 6.6 in 1987, rose to 8.2 in 1990, and decreased slightly to 7.1 in 1998. In 1999 the maternal mortality rate, calculated using a slightly different formula, was 9.9 (U.S. Census Bureau, 2001). *Healthy People 2010* set a target goal of 3.3 maternal deaths per 100,000 live births, but to reach this goal there is a need for much more early prevention and treatment.

Healthy People 2010
Selected National Health-Promotion and Disease Prevention Objectives for the Young Adult

- Increase the proportion of adults who engage regularly, preferably daily, in moderate physical activity for at least 30 minutes per day. (In 1997 and after, 15% of adults performed the recommended amount of physical activity and 40% of adults engaged in no leisure-time physical activity.)
- Reduce the proportion of adults who are obese. (From 1988 through 1994, 23% of adults age 20 and older were considered obese.)
- Reduce cigarette smoking by adults. (In 1997, 24% of adults were current smokers.)
- Reduce the proportion of adults using any illicit drug during the preceding 30 days. (Illicit drug use in adults age 18 or older has remained fairly stable at the present rate of 6% since 1980; men continue to have higher rates than do women.)
- Reduce the proportion of adults engaging in binge drinking of alcoholic beverages during the preceding month. (Binge drinking remains fairly stable in adults with the highest current rates of 32% among adults ages 18 to 25 years.)
- Increase the proportion of sexually active people who use condoms. (In 1997, 23% of sexually active adults used condoms.)
- Increase the proportion of women 18 years and older who have received a Pap test within the preceding 3 years. (The 1998 baseline was 79%; the 2010 target is 90%.)
- Increase the proportion of adults with recognized depression who receive treatment. (In 1997 and after, 23% of adults who were diagnosed with depression received treatment.)
- Reduce deaths caused by motor vehicle crashes. (Death rates associated with motor vehicle–traffic injuries are highest in the age group 15 to 24 years; the highest intoxication rates in fatal crashes in 1995 were recorded for drivers ages 21 to 24 years.)
- Reduce the number of homicides. (In 1997, 32,436 individuals died from firearm injuries; 42% of these individuals were homicide victims.)
- Reduce the proportion of nonsmokers exposed to environmental tobacco smoke. (Exposure to environmental tobacco smoke among nonsmokers is widespread, with 65% of nonsmokers exposed during the years 1988 through 1994. The overall death rate from asthma increased 52% between 1980 and 1993.)
- Increase the proportion of people who have a specific source of ongoing care. (In 1997, 86% of all individuals had health insurance and a usual source of health care; individuals ages 18 to 24 years were the most likely to lack a usual source of primary care.)
- Increase the proportion of women who begin prenatal care during the first trimester of pregnancy. (In 1997, 83% received prenatal care during the first trimester of pregnancy.)

From U.S. Department of Health and Human Services. (2000). *Healthy People 2010* (Conference ed.). Washington, DC: U.S. Government Printing Office.
Pap, Papanicolaou.

GORDON'S FUNCTIONAL HEALTH PATTERNS
Health Perception–Health Management Pattern

Because excellent physical health frequently is taken for granted, concern about health and well-being is relatively low in individuals in their 20s but begins to increase in individuals in their 30s. Monitoring is both necessary and appropriate to determine health needs and incipient problems. After the mid-30s, an increased sense of the finiteness of life develops with limitations imposed by work choices, well-being, monetary resources, and the deterioration of physical abilities. For more specific health care management, the young adult age span is split into two age groups (18 to 24 and 25 to 35), according to the preventive services that are required.

The assumption that all adults should have an annual physical examination has been supplanted by increased scientifically based information about health screening measures. Screening services provided in a health monitoring program need to meet cost and effectiveness criteria. Evidenced-based practice uses best practices information for clinical decisions instead of intuition and unmethodical clinical experience and, as such, forms the current recommended standard of care. There is, however, considerable debate about what constitutes the best evidence, but there is general agreement that an evidence-based approach will reform clinical practice, particularly through the use of computer resources (Pravikoff, Pierce, & Tanner, 2003). Evidence-based approaches ultimately will determine which screening measures are best supported by scientific data (randomized controlled treatment studies), reduce regional variations in use of diagnostic and therapeutic modalities, and close the gap between practice and research.

Behavioral Health History

A behavioral health history is important for young adults. This tool focuses on risk factors for unintentional injuries, such as alcohol consumption and seat belt use, which are major causes of death and disability in this age group. The safety focus of nursing health promotion for the younger adult takes different forms, from monitoring seat belt use, to air bag use, to concerns about threats such as bioterrorism and globally spreading infections (Nettina, 2002). Figure 22-1 lists questions and content that might be included in a health history for young adults focusing on their age-specific behaviors.

Preventive Care

Basic goals of preventive care are to maximize the period of optimal health status and detect incipient health problems at an early stage. At age 18 (approximately the time of graduation from high school), a full health appraisal is recommended. Table 22-1 illustrates preventive care that is important during the young adult period, along with recommended frequency of screening. As a rule, the recommendation for most procedures is a repeat health history and visit at approximately 2-year intervals. Appropriate intervention in the younger age group is directed toward correcting problems through history assessment and counseling about avoidance of adverse health behaviors. Subsequent counseling sessions focus on rechecking and updating information gathered in earlier meetings.

A physical examination includes a check of height, weight, and blood pressure, with an emphasis on the need to avoid inactivity and obesity and (for women) education about the importance of **breast self-examination** (BSE), including the importance of repeating the technique monthly. Papanicolaou (Pap) smears should be performed within 3 years of the onset of sexual activity or age 21, whichever comes first; the incidence of carcinoma in situ, a precursor of invasive cervical and uterine cancer, is high in this group (1 in 1000 women). **Testicular self-examination** (TSE) should be taught to men. A rectal examination is not recommended unless symptoms are present.

After age 25 the emphasis is on modifying coronary disease risk factors. Recommendations for screening for young adults are undergoing revision as more information becomes available about the interactive risks of high cholesterol, familial high lipid levels, diabetes mellitus, and smoking. The current recommendation is that total cholesterol should be measured at least once during young adulthood. Subsequent recommended screening intervals for young adults with normal cholesterol levels is at least every 5 years starting at age 35 for men and 45 for women (Clinical Preventive Services for Normal-Risk Adults, 2003). Aging is responsible for some degenerative changes in respiratory and cardiac function, but during the young adult years this decline amounts to less than 1% per year and is largely determined by an individual's fitness level (Huether & McCance, 2004). Because cardiovascular disease (along with cancer and cerebrovascular disease) is a primary cause of death accounting for more than one half of all deaths (Anderson & Arias, 2003), cardiovascular assessment of

the young adult includes determining the presence of hyperlipidemia, hypertension, diabetes, chest pain, or heart disease. A *Healthy People 2010* target is to reduce the mean total blood cholesterol levels among adults to 199 mg/dl; the baseline between 1988 and 1994 for adults 20 and older was 206 mg/dl (USDHHS, 2000). A new report suggests that even more watchfulness regarding prevention is indicated, because the number of adults with no known risk factors for heart disease and stroke is decreasing while many individuals with risk factors are living with undiagnosed disease (Declining prevalence, 2004). Health history questions should also elicit pertinent information about hypertension and **coronary artery disease** (CAD) in parents and relatives.

Hypertension results from increases in cardiac output, or increases in peripheral resistance, or a combination of both and is the third leading cause of death worldwide. According to the Seventh Joint National Committee Report, the focus of blood pressure assessment should be on systolic hypertension, and risks from systolic hypertension rise beginning with systolic pressures of 115 mm Hg. The risk from diastolic hypertension starts to rise at 75 mm Hg. The focus of attention should be on lowering blood pressure toward the new normal goal of 120/80 mm Hg or less (Chobanian, 2003). Each increase in blood pressure over this level exerts a consistent rise in risk for heart attack, stroke, and heart failure. Hypertension is a prominent problem for young black adults, especially men. Hypertension can lead to severe complications; more young black people than young white people die as a result of chronic heart disease or stroke (cerebrovascular accident). Although for the entire population, deaths attributable to coronary heart disease and stroke have declined, the mortality rate remains higher for blacks (Anderson & Arias, 2003). A wellness target of *Healthy People 2010* is to increase the proportion of young adults 18 years and older with hypertension whose blood pressure in under control from 18% (in 1988 to 1994) to 50% (USDHHS, 2000). A second target of *Healthy People 2010* is to reduce the proportion of adults with high blood pressure; from 1988 through 1994, 28% of adults age 20 years and older had high blood pressure. The literature also describes a "stroke belt" in the southeastern states, where the incidence of stroke is reported to be above the national average (60 deaths per 100,000 population) (USDHHS, 2000). A target goal of *Healthy People 2010* is to reduce stroke deaths to 48 deaths per 100,000 population (USDHHS, 2000).

A newly recognized cluster of risks is termed the **metabolic syndrome.** This syndrome includes the lethal risks of high lipid levels, insulin resistance, obesity, and hypertension. Metabolic syndrome affects 47 million people in the United States, placing them at increased risk for CAD. A particular feature of this syndrome is central obesity; these individuals are at higher risk for diabetes, CAD, and stroke (Scott, 2003).

Diabetes is seventh on the list of leading causes of death in the United States. Minority populations (blacks,

Well Young Adult Behavioral Health History Content

Sociodemographic content and questions:

What organizations (community, church, lodge, social, professional, etc.) are you involved in?_____

_____

How would you describe your community?_____

_____

Hobbies, skills, interests, and recreational activities?_____

Military service? No_____ Yes_____ From _____to_____

Overseas assignment? No_____ Yes_____

Close friends or immediate family members who have died within the past two years?_____

_____

Names and addresses of relatives or close friends in the area._____

_____

_____

Marital status: S M D W   Length of time _____

Environmental content and questions:

Do you live alone? No_____ Yes_____

When did you last move? _____

Describe your living situation. _____

Number of years of education completed: _____

Elementary?_____ High school?_____ College?_____

Occupation?_____ Employer?_____

How long have you worked for this employer?_____

Are you satisfied with your work situation? No_____ Yes_____

Do you consider your work risky or dangerous? No_____ Yes_____

Is your work stressful? No_____ Yes_____

Biophysical content questions:

Have you smoked cigarettes? No_____ Yes_____

How much? Less than ½ pack per day? About one pack per day? More than 1½ packs per day?

Are you smoking now? No_____ Yes_____ Length of time smoking?_____

Have you ever smoked cigars or a pipe? No_____ Yes_____

If yes, how long?_____ Do you smoke cigars or a pipe now? No_____ Yes_____

Do you drink alcohol (wine, beer, or whiskey)? No_____ Yes_____

If you do, how much each day on the average?_____ Each week?_____

Do you consume large amounts occasionally (binge drinking)? No_____ Yes_____

Have you been drunk on work days? No_____ Yes_____

Have you had alcoholic drinks in the morning sometime in the past year? No_____ Yes_____

How much coffee, tea, or cola do you drink?_____

Do you use seat or lap belts? No_____ Yes_____

What type of exercise do you do each week? Describe type and amount. _____

_____

Are you satisfied with your weight? No_____ Yes_____ Body image? No_____ Yes_____

Do you use a bicycle or motorcycle helmet? No_____ Yes_____ Helmet and pads while roller blading? No_____ Yes_____

How much sleep do you usually get each night?_____

Meals: Do you generally eat: three regular meals per day? two meals per day? irregular meals?

Are you sexually active? No_____ Yes_____

If so, are you aware of the risks of sexually transmitted diseases? No_____ Yes_____

For women: Do you perform breast self-examination (BSE) each month? No_____ Yes_____

For men: Do you perform testicular self-examination (TSE) regularly? No_____ Yes_____

Figure 22-1   Common well young adult behavioral health history content. (Modified from U.S. Preventive Services Task Force. [2003]. *Clinical preventive services for normal-risk adults, January, 2003.* Rockville, MD: Agency for Health Care Research and Quality. Retrieved January 9, 2004, from: *http://www.ahrq.gov/ppip/adulttm.htm*; Somers, A. R., & Breslow, L. [1979]. Lifetime health monitoring program. *Nurse Practitioner, 4*[40], 50, 54.)

Table **22-1** Well Young Adult Health Monitoring

Health Issue	Ages 18 to 24		Ages 25 to 35	
	Intervention	Frequency (Years)	Intervention	Frequency (Years)
Smoking	History and counseling	Each visit	History and counseling	Each visit
Obesity or poor nutrition	History, weight, and counseling	Each visit	History, weight, and counseling	Each visit
Avoid alcohol while driving, swimming, engaging in activities that require mental and physical alertness	History and counseling	At least once	History and counseling	Every 2
Accidental injury, lap and shoulder belts, bicycle or motorcycle helmets, smoke detectors, safe firearm use	History and counseling	At least once	History and counseling	Every 2
Unintended pregnancy	Counseling	At least once	History and counseling	Every 2
Contraception	Counseling	Individually determined	Counseling	Individually determined
Illegal drug use	History and counseling	At least once	History and counseling	Every 2 to 4
Regular physical activity	History and counseling	At least once	History and counseling	Every 2 to 4
Blood pressure, hypertension	Blood pressure measurement	Every 2	Blood pressure measurement	Every 2 to 4
Breast or testicular cancer	BSE or TSE counseling	Every 1 to 2	BSE or TSE counseling	Every 1 to 2
Vision defects	Examination	Once	Examination	Every 4
Tetanus-diphtheria	Booster	Once if 10 yrs since last one	Immunization	Every 10
Hepatitis B	Immunization	If not immunized	Immunization	If not immunized
Cervical dysplasia	Pap smear	Every 1 to 3	Pap smear	Every 1 to 3
Diabetes, proteinuria, bacteriuria	Urinalysis	Once	Urinalysis	Every 4
Coronary artery disease	Serum cholesterol level determination, triglyceride level	Once	Serum cholesterol level determination	Every 5
Dental care	Dental examination and cleaning	Every 1 to 2	Dental examination and cleaning	Every 1 to 2
Tuberculosis	Skin test PPD	Once	Skin test PPD	Every 2 to 3
STD prevention	Counseling	Individually determined	Counseling	Individually determined
Chlamydia	Chlamydia screen	At gynecological examination, if sexually active	Chlamydia screen	At gynecological examination, if sexually active

Modified from U.S. Preventive Services Task Force. (2003). *Clinical preventive services for normal-risk adults, January 2003.* Rockville, MD: Agency for Health Care Research and Quality. Retrieved January 9, 2004, from: *http://www.ahrq.gov/ppip/adulttm.htm*; U.S. Preventive Services Task Force. (1996). An ounce of prevention: Updating clinical practice guidelines. *Advanced Practice Nurse, 5,* 37-40.
BSE, breast self-examination; *TSE,* testicular self-examination; *Pap,* Papanicolaou; *PPD,* purified protein derivative; *STD,* sexually transmitted disease.

Native American–Alaska Natives, and Hispanics) are disproportionately affected. The incidence of diabetes, especially type 2 diabetes (adult onset), and related complications (cardiovascular disease, blindness, and end-stage renal disease) is increasing in the United States (USDHHS, 2000). Only 7% of those diagnosed with diabetes controlled had their blood pressure, glucose levels, and cholesterol levels sufficiently controlled to avoid or delay vascular disease ("Patients With Diabetes Have Poor Control," 2004). Because careful control can delay the beginning and progression of long-term complications, early detection and monitoring of diabetes is important.

Decision Making and Risk Taking

The decision making of a young adult directly affects health and well-being. Peak physical skills stimulate young adults to be venturesome, daring, enterprising, and aggressive. Young adults have less experience with the death of significant others, and they may take inordinate risks. The leading causes of death in individuals ages 15 to 24 years of age are unintentional injuries, homicide, and suicide (USDHHS, 2000). If these trends continue, deaths from firearms will overtake deaths from motor vehicle crashes. The prevalence of adverse behaviors associated with sudden death illustrates a developmental lack of fear in young adults. Underuse of seat belts and helmets by motorcyclists and bicyclists is a cause of many accidental injuries and deaths.

Communicable Disease and Adult Immunization

Communicable (infectious) disease affects young adults with varying degrees of severity. Although the availability of better drug treatments, vaccines, improved hygiene and food handling, and cleaner water supplies have promoted prevention and control of infectious disease, new disease threats are continually emerging. These newer threats include severe acute respiratory syndrome (SARS), Lyme disease, diarrhea caused by *Escherichia coli* O157:H7, and hantavirus pulmonary disease. In 2003, SARS, caused by a respiratory virus harbored by the Chinese civet cat, caused a global threat and the monitoring of individuals traveling to and from Asian countries (Fenwick, 2003). In 1997 approximately 39% of tuberculosis cases in the United States occurred among foreign-born people (USDHHS, 2000), even as the incidence of this disease declined for the fifth consecutive year (to 7.4 cases per 100,000 of the population). An increase in tuberculosis rates, particularly in some minority groups (Asian American–Pacific Islanders, blacks, and Hispanics), illustrates that preventive activities must be reinforced and constant vigilance maintained over monitoring and effectiveness for all communicable diseases.

To reduce **hepatitis B** (HB) transmission in the United States by 2010, vaccination programs are targeted at adolescents and adults in high-risk groups (USDHHS, 2000). A primary way of achieving high levels of vaccination coverage is to identify settings in which individuals can be vaccinated, such as correctional facilities, drug treatment centers, and clinics treating sexually transmitted diseases (STDs) (USDHHS, 2000). HB is a serious infection because of the high incidence of chronic complications; approximately 14% of HB carriers in the United States develop chronic active hepatitis (Tran, 2004).

Rubella in young adults is generally a minor disease; however, when the disease is contracted during the first trimester of pregnancy, miscarriage, stillbirth, or congenital rubella syndrome (CRS) can result. CRS is associated with loss of hearing, ocular defects, developmental delay and growth retardation, and cardiac malformations. Since 1988 the incidence of CRS has increased 15-fold. Most new rubella cases occur in settings in which young adults gather, including colleges, prisons, and religious communities. Large state public health efforts have begun to ensure immunization among these groups, particularly in the college population. All women of childbearing age should be screened (titer monitored) for rubella antibodies and those who are not immune should be immunized. Nurses inform women of childbearing age that antibody testing is recommended before pregnancy and that vaccination is available.

Another target of *Healthy People 2010* is to reduce the incidence of hepatitis C to 1 case in 100,000 population from the 2.4 new cases per 100,000 population occurring now (USDHHS, 2000). Although new infections with hepatitis C dropped during the previous decade, approximately 4 million Americans remain infected (1.8% of the population), making hepatitis C the most common blood-borne infection in the United States. Individuals most at risk are those who have injected illicit drugs, received clotting factors before 1987, are on hemodialysis, are seropositive for **human immunodeficiency virus (HIV),** or have elevated liver function studies (Dieterich, 2000).

Although most outbreaks of meningococcal disease are sporadic, concern is rising among college staff and medical authorities that young adults living in dormitories may be more susceptible than young adults not living in dormitory settings. Between 1994 and 1997, 4 of 42 meningococcal outbreaks occurred in colleges. Although meningococci are sensitive to penicillin and many antibiotics, the case fatality rate is 10% in otherwise healthy adults, and approximately 15% of survivors will have neurological disabilities or loss of hearing (Preventing and controlling, 2000). Most at risk are college freshmen living in dormitories, who have a higher case ratio (4.6 per 100,000) than that of noncollege students 18 to 23 years of age (1.5 per 100,000) or children 2 to 5 years of age (1.7 per 100,000) (Preventing and controlling, 2000).

Other viral agents, such as **genital herpes virus and human papilloma virus (HPV),** commonly affect young adults. Genital herpes virus infections occur frequently in young adults because of the escalation of sexual activity during this period. HPV is spread through sexual contact, and some forms of the virus in combination with smoking are strongly related to the later development of cervical dysplasia and cancer, but at this point routine HPV monitoring is not recommended (U.S. Preventive Services Task Force, 2003).

Nutritional-Metabolic Pattern

Obesity in the United States is attaining epidemic proportions and will shortly be the most pressing public health problem. Young adults value slimness, defined muscle tone, and athletic ability. Regular physical activity increases muscle and bone strength, decreases body fat, aids in weight control, enhances well-being, and reduces depression (USDHHS, 2000). An optimally functioning **basal metabolic rate** in the young adult permits adequate oxygen intake during normal activity and rest periods.

A young man requires approximately 1600 to 1800 calories a day to meet his body's basal metabolic needs, and a young woman only 1200 to 1450 calories a day. As growth stops in the late teens, the basal metabolic rate declines.

During the young adult years, caloric intake increases substantially, particularly in men. Although white men need a higher caloric intake than do black men, the caloric need of all men levels off after age 25. Increased caloric in-

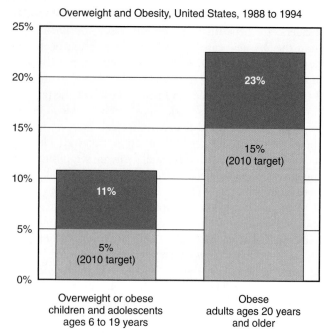

Overweight and Obesity, United States, 1988 to 1994

Figure 22-2 Overweight and obesity, 1988 to 1994. (From U.S. Department of Health and Human Services. [2000]. *Healthy People 2010* [Conference ed.]. Washington, DC: U.S. Government Printing Office.)

CASE STUDY

Kirsten

Kirsten is a healthy 20 year old whose favorite sport is running. Since this spring, Kirsten believes that her breathing capacity is diminishing and her levels of energy are decreasing. During her period these symptoms appear to worsen. Last week, while running up a rather steep course, Kirsten became much more weak, dizzy, and fatigued than usual, and her best friend and running partner recommended that she make a doctor's appointment for a physical examination. Kirsten's running partner also noted that she has appeared pale lately.

In the physician's office, Kirsten is noted to have a normal temperature, an elevated heart and respiratory rate, and a blood pressure of 90/60. Kirsten's description of her period is that it tends to be heavy and has been this way for 5 years. For muscle aches and pains caused by running, she usually takes two aspirin tablets every 3 to 4 hours for as long as 7 days. When her running increases during the summer, she takes aspirin continually for 2 to 3 months. Diagnostic testing indicates that her hemoglobin is 7 g/dl, and her red blood cells are pale and small.

Reflective Questions
1. What common health alteration in young adult women is most likely for Kirsten?
2. What contributing factors place Kirsten at risk?
3. What lifestyle modifications can Kristen implement to decrease her risk?

---

take without a corresponding energy requirement can lead to obesity, which is a precursor to hypertension, coronary disease, and diabetes.

According to data shown in Figure 22-2, 11% of children and adolescents ages 6 to 19 years are overweight or obese and 23% of adults age 20 and older are obese (USDHHS, 2000). According to a 1999 to 2000 study by the Centers for Disease Control (CDC), an estimated 64% of adults are overweight (33%) or obese (31%); obesity prevalence in Medicaid recipients is higher ("Overweight and obesity," 2005). Obesity is frequent in certain ethnic and racial groups; approximately one half of black women and Mexican American women are defined as overweight. Some reports suggest that intellectually challenged individuals have 10% more obesity than individuals with normal intelligence (Marshall, McConkey, & Moore, 2003). To stop or decrease the trend, new behaviors must be learned for nutrition and physical activity. Specifically, decreasing fat intake, increasing fruit and vegetable intake, and increasing physical activity must be emphasized. Food labeling information (particularly for calories, fat, and cholesterol) is now required for processed and packaged foods. Young adults should be counselled to read package labels. Another challenge is the increasing consumption of food prepared and eaten away from home, which is generally higher in fats, cholesterol, and sodium, and lower in fiber and calcium than that prepared at home (USDHHS, 2000).

Health professionals are counseled to investigate weight problems by monitoring waist circumference, blood pressure, cholesterol levels, and activity levels rather than solely monitoring weight, to the frustration of many clients. Assessments should be made of weight and height to calculate body mass index (BMI). Those with a BMI of 25 or less (male waist size of 40 inches or less, women 35 inches or less) should have weight maintenance teaching. Clients with a BMI of 30 or greater who have tried diets and exercise may be considered for weight-reducing drugs (Manson, Skerrett, Greenland, & Vanltallie, 2004). A BMI of 40 or more meets the criteria for bariatric surgery in psychologically stable clients. In clients with comorbidity, bariatric surgery may be suggested with a BMI of 35 or greater (Manson et al., 2004). The focus of professional advice should be conservative at first, recommending careful diet appraisal and increase in exercise patterns. Several repetitions will probably be necessary, because long-term weight management is a frustrating process.

Proper nutrition is particularly necessary during the childbearing years. Prospective mothers should be concerned about high-quality nutrition and avoidance of food additives. Iron deficiency anemia is common in young adult women (Case Study). Contributing factors in this age group are regular loss of blood (during menses) and pregnancy. A blood loss of 2 to 4 milliliters per day (1 to 2 mg of iron) can cause iron deficiency anemia; young women who don't eat a healthy diet and have heavy periods or use nonsteroidal anti-imflammatory drugs are specifically at risk for iron deficncy anemia. Iron supplementation is recommended during pregnancy for optimal growth of the fetus and supporting structures (Lowdermilk & Perry, 2004). The CDC recommends that all women of childbearing age consume 0.4 mg of folic acid daily to reduce the risk of fetal neural tube defects, including spina bifida. Supplementation should include the month before pregnancy and the first trimester during pregnancy. The Association of Women's Health, Obstetric and Neonatal Nurses (AWHONN) further recommends fortification of oral contraceptive preparations with folic acid supplementation to provide additional protection to women of childbearing age (Association of Women's Health, Obstetric and Neonatal Nurses [AWHONN], 2004b).

Most adolescents and adult women fail to meet their calcium requirements, placing them at risk for osteoporosis and bone fractures in later life. Low calcium intake is a direct result of low milk consumption related to soft drink ingestion. Between 1994 and 1996, the amount of soft drinks consumed was twice that used in the 1970s (USDHHS, 2000). An increase in calcium-containing foods is therefore recommended, particularly for teens and young women.

Elimination Pattern

Patterns of elimination are generally well established by young adulthood; although eating disorders (anorexia and bulimia) typically begin at an earlier stage of development, they can persist during young adulthood. The fashion industry is widely criticized for using underweight women as young female models, thereby emphasizing excessive thinness as the ideal female standard.

Activity-Exercise Pattern

Inactivity is a predisposing factor to cardiovascular disease and obesity. A *Healthy People 2010* goal is to reduce the proportion of adults who engage in no leisure-time physical activity to 20% from approximately 40% in 1997, and to increase the proportion of adults who engage in moderate physical activity for 30 minutes a day to 30% from 15% in 1997 (USDHHS, 2000).

Aerobic exercise, in which oxygen is metabolized to produce energy, develops an optimally functioning cardiorespiratory system. Aerobic conditioning achieves cardiovascular fitness through 3 periods of intense exercise weekly, for 30 minutes or more at a heart rate of approximately 220 minus the age of the person multiplied by 65% to 85%. Young adults are encouraged to engage in fitness activities that increase the heart rate to approximately 150 or more beats per minute. After 5 minutes of activity at this rate, the body is required to make adjustments in cardiovascular capacity by enlarging the lungs and the capillaries in the muscles and the heart. Repeated aerobic exercise, such as swimming (Figure 22-3), cycling, running, skipping rope, and walking produces physical fitness and decreases the likelihood of problems caused by inactivity. The major barriers to increasing physical activity seem to be lack of time, access to exercise facilities, and safe environments in which to exercise (USDHHS, 2000).

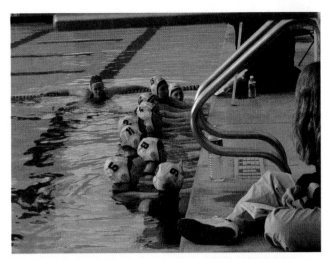

Figure 22-3 Swimming and other sports activities provide young adults with needed exercise.

Radiation and Excessive Sun Exposure

Nurses educate young adults about the risks of sun exposure and tanning, the preventive use of sun-blocking agents, and skin symptoms that might indicate cancer. The use of sun-blocking agents, such as paraaminobenzoic acid, is recommended, particularly because it is rated based on skin type and sensitivity to burning. Many lotions and creams are available with differing radiation protection levels. Women's makeup preparations now include sun-blocking agents. Young adults should avoid sunbathing during the 2-hour period before and after noon, because two thirds of the day's ultraviolet light comes through the earth's atmosphere during this time. A goal of *Healthy People 2010* is to increase the proportion of people who use sun-protective measures such as sunscreen, sun-protective clothing, and avoidance of ultraviolet light. The target is to induce 75% of adults 18 and older to use at least one protective measure (USDHHS, 2000).

Sports

Bicycling and motorcycling are encouraged by environmentalists to decrease automobile pollution; however, this trend is also promoted to relieve traffic congestion, avoid the high costs of fuel and car maintenance, and increase interest in healthy exercise. Cyclists are likely to be involved in accidents with automobiles. Head injury is responsible for approximately 62% of bicycle-related fatalities. In 1997 only 11 states had mandatory helmet requirements for riders under 15 years of age (USDHHS, 2000). Bicycle helmets are believed to be the single most effective preventive measure available to decrease the incidence of brain and head injury. They reduce the risk of bicycle-related head injury by 85% (USDHHS, 2000).

Motorcycles have less occupant protection than do automobiles but are appealing to young adults, primarily because they have high-performance capabilities. Using a motorcycle helmet reduces the chance of dying in an accident by 29% (USDHHS, 2000). A target of *Healthy People 2010* is to increase the proportion of motorcyclists using helmets from 67% in 1997 to 79% (USDHHS, 2000).

Accidental deaths from drowning are also common in young adults. Swimming, boating, and scuba diving are associated with the high number of water-related fatalities. Hang gliding, parachuting, and flying small aircraft are responsible for a large number of outdoor fatalities. Mountain climbing, hiking in poor weather conditions, downhill ski racing, and bobsledding are other hazardous activities. Most so-called *accidents* are not random, uncontrollable events, but predictable and preventable if precautions and risks are analyzed (USDHHS, 2000).

Amateur and professional sports activities generally pose few hazards when rules and safety precautions are observed. Relatively few fatalities are associated with the professionally organized contact sports, such as football, hockey, or boxing, but chronic injuries frequently cause discomfort. A study of football hits and accelerations indicates that some of the blows players endure are similar to those experienced in automobile accidents ("American Footballers," 2004).

A comprehensive history of recreational activities will alert the nurse to specific needs about safety education. Young adults are encouraged to learn and abide by the rules of the sport in which they are engaged. Rules in many sports have evolved from health and safety concerns, enabling the individual to learn the sport well with appropriate instruction.

Sleep-Rest Pattern

Young adults are subject to fatigue induced by work, stress, or inactivity. Changes in activity or stressors can help reduce fatigue. Trying out new and challenging tasks can help reduce mental stress. New physical activities, such as learning a new sport or form of exercise, can also provide stimulation.

Cognitive-Perceptual Pattern
Physical and Mental Patterns

Visual acuity is highest at approximately age 20 and begins to decline at approximately age 40, when farsightedness frequently develops. Hearing is also best at age 20; the ability to distinguish high-pitched tones decreases with age. The other senses, taste, smell, touch, and awareness of temperature and pain, remain stable until age 45 to 50.

Maturation requires young adults to learn skills and behaviors that improve the performance abilities gained as adolescents. Factors that an individual young adult will perceive as essential to learn will depend on specific goals, values, attitudes, and practices as influenced by intrinsic (constitutional) and extrinsic (environmental or community) factors. The development of intellectual maturity influences the selection of behaviors and attitudes that affect health and well-being practices.

Piaget's Theory

Jean Piaget's stage of formal operational thought evolves from concrete operational thought in adolescence and extends through the reasoning process of young adults (Piaget, 1972). Achievement of formal operational thinking allows a person to analyze all combinations of possibilities and construct hypotheses that can be tested. Young adult thought becomes more perceptive and insightful; issues can therefore be evaluated realistically and objectively. Young adults are energetic and can therefore contribute substantially to social and occupational decision making. Although they tend to take greater risks, young adults typically demonstrate the use of appropriate reasoning and analytical approaches.

Intellectual Growth

Organization of information influences memory. Evidence shows that recall performance diminishes with age; at its peak in the twenties, memory starts to diminish during the thirties. Improved strategies for organization of information, however, can enhance recall, and limitation of memory with increasing age is likely a result of retrieval rather than storage mechanisms.

Erikson's Theory

A major goal for young adults is the development of an increased sense of competency and self-esteem (Erikson, 1993). In developing self-esteem, the individual learns to be truly open and capable of trust through the formation of intimate relationships that are characteristic of this period. Erikson (1993) has described this stage of psychosocial development as intimacy versus isolation and loneliness.

Erikson's concept of genuine intimacy extends beyond sexual relations to a broader view of mutual psychosocial intimacy with a spouse or lover, parents, children, and friends. Characterized by the reciprocal expression of affection, intimacy requires mutual trust. These interchanges are spontaneous for the young adult; relationships should be free and allow for self-disclosure. Young adults who are unsure of their identity may avoid intimate contact or engage in promiscuous behavior lacking in true intimacy, which can result in isolation and consequent self-absorption. Healthy adults search for continuity, regularity, or unity of meaningful relationships, while avoiding situations of little commitment.

Moral Development

Young adults who have successfully mastered the previous cognitive, social, and moral stages are usually able to recognize or use principled reasoning. Lawrence Kohlberg identifies this ability as the **postconventional level of moral reasoning** (Kohlberg & Lickons, 1986). During this phase, the individual is able to differentiate the self from the rules and expectations of others and to define principles regarding rights in terms of self-chosen principles. The interests of individuals can be weighed against the needs of society and the state, and violations of law can be justified when individual interests are in accord with principles. Gilligan (1982, 2002), who studied the development of moral reasoning in women and girls, asserts that their moral judgments reflect less of a "rights" perspective and more of an emphasis on relationships.

Although development of principled moral reasoning is possible during young adulthood, it may never occur if the cognitive and social factors that stimulate higher reasoning are not present. Acts of personal violence representative of lower moral reasoning should not be present; however, such acts do occur during this period, illustrating the need for addressing moral development concerns at earlier stages of education and socialization.

Self-Perception–Self-Concept Pattern

In non-Western cultures the entrance to adulthood generally is defined and marked by social events such as marriage. In Western societies, maturation is defined through the individual's achievement of financial and residential independence, and is a more drawn-out, gradual process. Two emotional themes regarding the value of work become evident during young adulthood. During their twenties, young adults yearn to explore and experiment, keeping structures temporary and reversible. These individuals may move from job to job and relationship to relationship, remaining in a transient state. At the opposite extreme is the urge to prepare for the future by making firm commitments. During this period, both men and women question their value to society, the merit of their accomplishments, their success as sexual beings, and the probability of attaining their unfulfilled goals.

The U.S. Census Bureau (2001) reports that more than 70% of women ages 25 to 35 are employed; this percentage is rising and expected to be over 80% by 2010. As more mothers enter the labor force, the need for child care increases. The gap in earnings, or pay differential, between men and women is also significant. Access to insurance and pension benefits is not always available, especially to high-risk groups such as minorities or people receiving the minimum wage. Even when there is sufficient access to health care, some types of employment expose individuals to occupational risks and hazards.

Many young adults are high achievers and seek opportunities to be challenged. Employment problems can be stressful and traumatic to an individual's self-esteem and self-worth. The failure to receive a promotion or a pay raise can accelerate the degree of stress. Employment is more than a source of income; it provides self-esteem and social interaction. Because the adjustment to the job market influences many other aspects of daily living, young adults frequently require assistance in developing coping mechanisms to manage stress. Properly managing the initial stress prevents further complications that can arise if the young adult uses unhealthy stress relievers such as alcohol or drugs.

Young women have many of the same concerns about employment and success as do young men. Many young women postpone childbearing until they have established their careers; many are absent from the job for only a standard maternity leave. Women who return to work when their children are very young frequently risk the emotional strain caused by guilt feelings. In addition to helping parents cope with the stress of being absent from their children, nurses can help them identify ways to provide quality supervision in their absence, either through private baby-sitters, day-care programs, or through neighbors, friends, and relatives.

The U.S. workforce is changing dramatically as companies restructure, downsize, "right size," and shift employees around to meet changing market conditions. There is increasing concern about the global economy and jobs, especially in the computer industry, moving overseas. Job stress can lead to increased absenteeism, which is more common in young adults. Nursing interventions in industrial settings are directed toward improving both working conditions and employer-employee relationships. Healthy work sites increase the chance that young adults will have access to comprehensive health-promotion programs (USDHHS, 2000).

Roles-Relationships Pattern

Young adult friendships are more enduring than are earlier relationships. The focus of the relationship is the sharing of feelings or confidences. True friendship is characteristic of a person who wants to give rather than receive. Friendships are necessary in a constantly changing society; they provide a source of emotional support and a basis of stability for developing the self-concept.

Establishing interpersonal relationships involves agreeable and purposeful interactions with others. Interpersonal relationships can be created with people of the same or the opposite sex; age is typically a less important factor than it was during adolescence. The formation of intimate relationships develops within or outside a family context and occasionally in the work environment. Cell phone and Internet access facilitates relationships through text messaging, e-mail, and instant messaging. For some the significant other is a person of the same sex, and there are current legislative proposals that would legitimize the legal rights of same-sex couples through same-sex marriage or civil union statutes. See the Innovative Practice box about the Gay and Lesbian Wellness Series.

In addition to achieving intimacy, the young adult must accomplish other developmental tasks to achieve true psychosocial maturation. Decision making about life and career directions is the developmental milestone that heralds the transition from adolescence to adulthood. Decisions usually entail establishing independence from the family of origin. This transition may involve an actual physical move from the parent's home (going away to college, joining the military, or getting an apartment); however, movement away is not the sole indicator of independence. Young adults frequently remain in their parent's home for economic reasons, particularly when life choices involve continued schooling or remaining unmarried. In some cultures, unmarried adults live with their parents until they are married, and newly married young adults share the home of their parents until they begin having their own children.

Gay and Lesbian Wellness Series

The Gay and Lesbian Wellness Series is a multidisciplinary educational program offered through the collaborative efforts of the Be Well! programs of the Tanger Center for Health Management and the Lesbian and Gay Advisory Committee at Beth Israel Deaconess Medical Center in Boston, Massachusetts.

The clinician-teachers encourage clients and employees of the hospital and ambulatory care centers and members of the community, whether gay, straight, or bisexual, to participate in these free educational programs. Massachusetts, in 2004, was the first state to implement legislation allowing marriage between individuals of the same sex. The following examples are indicative of educational topics offered at Beth Israel Deaconess Medical Center:

1. Sexual Orientation and the Workplace: Creating an Open Environment. Understanding the dynamics of the work environment, whether as a clinician, manager, or support staff, can be challenging when issues of sexual orientation in the workplace are examined. As a gay or lesbian employee, how comfortable do you feel being "out" at work? Alternatively, as a manager of gay and lesbian employees, how successful are you in creating an environment in which staff members feel safe, comfortable, and valued? This class is a discussion of this topic aimed at creating an open environment for all.

2. A Welcoming Place for All: Improving Access and Quality for Gay and Lesbian Patients. Underestimating the power of a simple word or gesture in providing care for individuals is easy. Sensitivity to the wording of materials and forms, and the way in which questions are asked, can help gay and lesbian clients feel safe and comfortable. This class offers the opportunity to learn more about steps you can take to make your department, unit, or practice a welcoming place for all.

3. Selecting and Communicating with Your Health Care Provider. Asking the right questions and developing a comfortable and trusting relationship with a primary care provider are challenges for everyone. For gay and lesbian clients, the task can be especially difficult. Tips are available for enhancing the lines of communication between the client and health care providers.

4. Supporting and Communicating with Your Gay or Lesbian Child: Understanding Gay and Lesbian Issues in the Family. Parents of gay and lesbian children frequently have few places to turn for support and information. Struggling with love for one's child and the challenges of accepting the child's sexual orientation can be an overwhelming dilemma.
   Contact Information:
   Tanger Center for Health Management
   Lesbian and Gay Advisory Committee
   Beth Israel Deaconess Medical Center
   Boston, MA
   Telephone: 617-667-4695

Courtesy Carol Lynn Mandle, PhD, RN.

Individuals in this age group typically choose life partners and begin families; they make decisions about childbearing and the number and education of children. Additional consideration must be given to decisions related to childbearing, such as finances, safety, family support, housing, the relationship with extended family members, and the roles and responsibilities within the nuclear family unit. Young adults who are establishing a family must have open communication about self-development, which includes issues of dual careers, child-rearing practices, and domestic duties.

Family harmony and development are major goals for many young adults. Although family size and structure have undergone dramatic changes in previous decades, concern about each member's health and safety continues to be a primary focus. Family life is influenced by the qualities of individual family members. Typically, economic security, status, place in the community, and healthy patterns of living, such as good nutrition, personal hygiene, and physical fitness, are associated with healthy family adjustment.

Separation and Divorce

About one half of first marriages and 60% of second marriages terminate in divorce (Golden & Hopkins, 2003). About one quarter of all children in the United States are living in single parent families, and one half of the children affected by divorce never see their fathers again. Many stressors contribute to divorce. It is a difficult process, and lingering anger and hostility may remain for years. Socioeconomic factors often place unreasonable stress on marriages. Age at the time of marriage is correlated with duration of marriage, and young adults whose parents have divorced have an increased rate of divorce (Bramlett & Mosher, 2002). Unmarried cohabitations are even more unstable, with higher breakup rates than marriages (Bramlett & Mosher, 2002). Employment has enabled women to leave unhappy marriages that they formerly would have been forced to tolerate.

Although dissatisfaction and unhappiness are frequent precursors to separation and divorce, the decision to dissolve a marriage is not easy. Considerable emotional strain exists for both partners, their children, their families, and close friends. Divorce requires that young adults reevaluate their basic values, individual personality and ego strength, job potential, and socioeconomic factors to ensure future security for themselves and their children. Divorced young adults frequently suffer severe emotional strain and depression. Some young adults are unable to adjust to role and status changes and to threats to self-concept. For these reasons, support systems in the form of groups, individual counseling, or special social activities are critical. As a result of divorce, many women and their young children are forced to seek emergency shelter in publicly operated homes, including welfare hotels and group shelters.

Many people need support from the nurse to help them work through this difficult period. Nurses help to identify the feelings of guilt, grief, and loss that young adults experience during a separation or divorce. Suggesting that young adults read articles or books on issues related to divorce is helpful, because they provide a reference point for their experiences. The nurse recommends marital counseling by a qualified professional; this may be the most beneficial source of support.

Male and Female Risk of Violence

Violence is becoming more prevalent and a global health problem. Although most cite the World Trade Center incident in 2001 and fighting in the Middle East as examples of organized terrorism, worldwide only one fifth of violent acts are related to organized events. Over one half are suicides and another one third are homicides ("Violence," 2004). Youth are involved as both the perpetrators and the victims of violence. In the United States their targets tend to be elderly, children, and women with whom they are familiar (USDHHS, 2000). Homicide (assault) is the second leading cause of death in the 15-year-old to 24-year-old age group and the leading cause of death for black men in the same age category (U.S. Census Bureau, 2001). Firearms are involved in approximately two thirds of these deaths, and men have twice the risk of dying than do women. When compared with the general population, mortality statistics are higher for men of poorer populations, in urban areas, and with less formal education. Homicide is closely associated with alcohol and drug abuse and frequently is related to other violent acts, such as robbery. Other risk factors include history of detention or prison experience, access to firearms, abuse in the home, mental illness, social isolation, and homelessness. The presence of firearms in the home is associated with the increased risk of

unintentional and intentional injury to children (Health Teaching box). A target of *Healthy People 2010* is to reduce firearm-related deaths from 11 per 100,000 population in 1998 to 4.9 per 100,000 population and to reduce the proportion of people living in homes with firearms loaded and unlocked from 19% to 16% (USDHHS, 2000). The firearm-related death rate for young black men and boys was nearly 5 times the rate for young white men and boys, although there was a substantial decline of 10% per year in the death rate between 1993 and 1997 for young black men and boys 15 to 24 years of age (USDHHS, 2000).

Abuse of women is one of the nation's most common health problems; however, because of social and legal factors, it is probably the most underreported (Hot Topics box). Abuse crosses all socioeconomic, racial, ethnic, religious, and age boundaries. Approximately one half of the women who knew their assailant were murdered by a husband, boyfriend, or former husband (USDHHS, 2000). Nurses and other primary health care providers often fail to assess, detect, or treat violence or abuse in an optimal manner, and more efforts must be made to recognize the scope of the problem and to provide appropriate counseling. A target of *Healthy People 2010* is to reduce the rate of physical assault by current or former intimate partners by 20% (USDHHS, 2000).

Sexuality-Reproductive Pattern

By young adulthood the menstrual cycle generally is well established in the woman. Cyclical hormonal function is responsible for regularity of the cycle and normal functioning of the ovaries and uterus. The normal duration of menses is 5 days; irregularities such as painful menstrua-

---

HEALTH TEACHING   Assessment and Education Regarding Firearm Safety

Nurses are taught to perform community and environmental assessments; however, most fail to incorporate assessment of the presence of firearms in the home. Firearm accidents are the second leading cause of death for individuals ages 10 to 24 years. More than 100 firearm-related deaths occur in the United States each day. The risk of suicide is increased nearly 5 times in homes with firearms. Approximately 38% of families keep at least one firearm in the home, and approximately 55% of those families report that they normally keep the gun loaded. Firearm presence in the home is a risk for violence against women. Between July 1, 1992, and June 30, 1999, 323 school-associated violent death events occurred in the United States.

The presence of firearms in the home continues to be an increasing concern. The American Academy of Pediatrics has published a position paper on gun safety and urges physicians to ask questions about guns when taking client histories. A widely publicized program called *ASK* requests that parents inquire if guns are present in any home where their child will stay or play: "Is there a gun where my children play?"

(Ahmann, 2001). This question should be posed with other questions aimed at ascertaining the adequacy of child supervision in any other site. If there is a gun in the home, the parent can check to see if the gun is stored unloaded in a locked or secure closet, or offer to have the children play in a monitored setting at another location.

Physicians and nurses have unique opportunities to counsel clients about gun safety and recommend removing guns from the home. Becher, Cassel, and Nelson (2000) indicate that many physicians (75% to 90%) do not counsel their clients about gun safety. About one third (29%) of this physician study population were gun owners, and physician gun owners were less likely to express support for counseling but more likely to report actual counseling with their clients. This contradiction about supporting counseling versus actually doing it may be attributed to physician conflicts about endorsing regulations on firearm ownership but also having more actual knowledge about firearm safety precautions (Becher, Cassel, & Nelson 2000).

From Source of firearms used by students in school-associated violent death—United States, 1992-1999. (2003.) *Morbidity and Mortality Weekly Report,* 52(7), 169-172; Ahmann, E. (2001). Guns in the home: Nurses' role. *Pediatric Nursing, 27*(6), 587-590, 605; Becher, E. C., Cassel, C. K., & Nelson, E. A. (2000). Physician firearm ownership as a predictor of firearm injury prevention practice. *American Journal of Public Health, 90*(10), 1626-1628.

VIOLENCE AGAINST WOMEN

HOTtopics

Assessing the Problem

Epidemiological researchers have attempted to determine the risks for intimate partner violence. Understanding the roots of partner violence has been more difficult than ascertaining determinants of physical disease. The unequal position of women in a relationship and the manner in which conflict is managed, as well as differences in education and prestige associated with the partners' occupations, are related to risk of violence (Jewkes, 2002). In the United States more than one third of women who are murdered are killed by their male partners, and approximately 6% of emergency room visits are a result of domestic violence. Domestic violence is a problem in all age, ethnic, and religious groups; in some cultures attitudes toward women even legitimize the practice. Women who have gained positions of respect and power outside the home through activities in their neighborhood or community are less likely to be abused.

Are Nurses Willing to Take Action?

Some studies indicate that nurses have been reluctant to take action regarding violence against women. Some of the traditional reasons for not taking action are based on paternalistic attitudes, in which the victim is blamed for her part in the social situation that becomes violent. Campbell, Harris, and Lee (1995) noted that nurses should take a stronger role in identifying violence against women.

Nursing's strong advocacy stance and emphasis on the communication of nonjudgmental, genuine concern should provide a strong foundation to avoid blaming the victim and to focus on pathological factors that have been identified by much of the health profession's research in this area.

How Can Nurses Recognize Abuse of Women?

Some research demonstrates that nurses should be more aware of indicators of partner violence (Jewkes, 2002). These include the presence, as revealed by a health history, of separation or divorce, alcoholism, frequent verbal disagreements, and high levels of conflict. Other warning signs include repeated visits to the emergency room, complaints of headaches or backaches, psychiatric illness, and incidents of bruises, sprains, and lacerations. Another risk is unemployment in the male partner combined with higher education in the female (Jewkes, 2002).

What Do You Think?

1. Are nurses less than helpful in their detection and management of violence against women? Why do you think this occurs?
2. Are nurses, because of their education and sensitization to people with mental problems, more or less likely than others to experience violence in their own domestic settings? Explain.

From Jewkes, R. (2002). Intimate partner violence: Causes and prevention. *Lancet, 359*(9315), 1423-1430; Campbell, J. C., Harris, M. J., & Lee, R. K. (1995). Violence research: An overview. *Scholarly Inquiry for Nursing Practice, 9*(2), 105-126.

tion, premenstrual syndrome, and prolonged or heavy bleeding can occur. Although these problems are not always abnormal, the symptoms and the individual's reaction to them can signal functional disorders and the need for further investigation.

Reproductive Problems

Infertility is defined as the lack of conception in the presence of unprotected sexual intercourse for at least 12 months. Approximately 10% to 15% of couples in the United States are believed to be infertile (Lowdermilk & Perry, 2004). Infertility has become more of a public issue since the advance of assistive reproductive technologies, such as in vitro fertilization and gamete intrafallopian transfer, which can enable couples with known reproductive problems to conceive children. These technologies frequently create great stress for the couple and often result in marital conflicts and distress. Generally, infertility is not an issue for those 18 to 25 years old; however, after the age of 25 the diagnosis is more frequent. At the other end of this spectrum are those young adult women who choose to be surgically sterilized. In 1995 approximately 1.8% of the 15-year-old to 24-year-old age group were surgically sterile; by the age of 25 to 35 this number had jumped to 23.6% (U.S. Census Bureau, 2001).

Common problems of the male reproductive system include mumps, orchitis, epididymitis, and varicoceles and hydroceles. External conditions such as fungal infections, contact dermatitis, and eczema; parasites such as scabies and lice; and nonvenereal diseases such as erysipelas, abscesses, and fistulas can occur in the scrotum.

Unintended Pregnancy

According to the CDC, the teen birth rate in the United States has dropped 30% during the past decade; this includes an even steeper decline in pregnancy rates for black teens ("Michigan teens," 2004). However, unwanted or unplanned pregnancies can be a considerable source of stress to young adults. Unintended pregnancy is an important public health issue related to increased infant mortality and morbidity, and increased risk of parental neglect, child and wife abuse, and emotional deprivation. Despite the advent of modern contraceptives, unintended pregnancy remains a persistent problem. Approximately one half of all pregnancies are unintended (USDHHS, 2000); from 1987 to 1994 the proportion of unintended pregnancies declined from 57% to 49%. Other industrialized countries report smaller figures, suggesting that more education is needed in the United States. Unwanted pregnancies lead to most of the abortions induced each year; in the United

Contraceptive Method	Risks of Use	Noncontraceptive Health Benefits
OCs (combined and progestin only)	Thromboembolic disorder, CVA, coronary artery disease, especially in presence of smoking, hypertension, diabetes, breast cancer	Reduced risk of functional pelvic inflammation, endometriosis, uterine fibroids, endometrial cancer, ovarian cancer, iron deficiency anemia, ectopic pregnancy, irregular cycles
Transdermal (contraceptive patch)	Similar to OCs	Similar to OCs
Diaphragm	Toxic shock syndrome, allergy to latex or spermicide, urinary tract infection	Reduced risk of vaginitis, cervicitis
Condom	Must be used consistently, allergy to rubber or latex or spermicide	Reduced risk of sexual transmission of HIV and other STDs
Spermicides*	Spermicide sensitivity	Antiviral activity against HPV, decreased activity of other STD organisms, reduced risk of PID
Intrauterine contraceptive device	Bleeding, anemia, difficult removal, PID ectopic pregnancy, cramping	
Injectable progestin (Depo-Provera)	Prolonged amenorrhea, venous thrombosis, thromboembolism	Limited data indicate reduced risk of anemia, PID, cancer of endometrium and ovary
Implants (rods or capsules) (Norplant)	Data limited, but possibly similar to OCs	Limited data indicate reduced risk of PID and endometrial cancer
Sponge	Toxic shock syndrome	Decreased activity of STD organisms
Female sterilization (tubal ligation)	Anesthesia, infection, hemorrhage	
Male sterilization (vasectomy)	Complication rates low, reversal may be difficult	

Modified from Hatcher, R. A., Trussell, J., & Stewart, F. H. (2004). *Contraceptive technology* (18th ed.). New York: Ardent Media; Wallach, M., & Grimes, D. (2000). *Modern contraception: Updates from the contraceptive report.* Totowa, NJ: Emron.
*Often used in combination with other methods.
OCs, oral contraceptives; CVA, cerebrovascular accident; HIV, human immunodeficiency virus; STD, sexually transmitted disease; HPV, human papilloma virus; PID, pelvic inflammatory disease.

States one abortion occurs for every three live births, a ratio 2 to 4 times higher than that of other developed countries (USDHHS, 2000). Although many young adults would consider family planning services as an essential basic health service, health insurance plans traditionally have excluded payment for family planning services (USDHHS, 2000). A target of *Healthy People 2010* is to increase the proportion of intended pregnancies from 51% in 1995 to 70% (USDHHS, 2000). The current lower pregnancy rates among teens probably results from more involvement in school activities, effective birth control and pregnancy prevention programs, and expanding job opportunities ("Michigan teens," 2004).

Approximately one half of unintended pregnancies are the result of contraceptive failure. Both married and unmarried young adults need information about contraceptives to decrease the number of unwanted pregnancies and the need for abortions (Table 22-2). The nurse's role in contraceptive counseling involves helping individuals to choose the method most appropriate to their needs (Hatcher, Trussell, & Stewart, 2004). Laws in some settings restrict nurses and other health care providers from engaging in certain types of counseling, including abortion counseling. Emergency contraception can reduce the number of unintended pregnancies by 50% (Morris & Young, 2000). Several hormonal and nonhormonal methods of emergency contraception are

available in the United States (Morris & Young, 2000). Currently there is discussion about allowing over-the-counter purchase of emergency contraception (AWHONN, 2004a).

Prenatal Care

Access to prenatal care and financing of sufficient care are critical concerns. High-risk and minority women do not receive sufficient prenatal care. A lack of insurance coverage and less-than-adequate referral mechanisms exist. Between 1990 and 1997 the proportion of mothers receiving care during the first trimester of pregnancy increased from 76% to 83%; the largest changes were seen in mothers of racial and ethnic groups with traditionally low levels of use. However, in 1997 a wide variation in receipt of care remained, ranging from 68% for Native American mothers to 90% for Cuban American mothers (USDHHS, 2000).

Another trend affecting young adults is the increasing mean age of mothers. Over the last 3 decades the average age has risen, with mothers having their first and second live births showing the largest increase (Mathews & Hamilton, 2002). In 2000 Massachusetts had the highest mean age and Mississippi the lowest. Education and career have been reported as important factors in the decision to delay childbearing (Mathews & Hamilton, 2002).

Sexually Transmitted Disease

STDs are a leading cause of infection and reproductive dysfunction in adults between ages 15 and 80. Women ages 15 to 19 and men ages 20 to 24 have the highest reported rates of chlamydia and gonorrhea (USDHHS, 2000). The list of STDs (Table 22-3) now includes HIV, *Chlamydia trachomatis* infections, genital herpes, HPV, chancroid (*Haemophilus ducreyi*), genital mycoplasma infections, cytomegalovirus infections, HB, and bacterial vaginitis, in addition to the more widely known diseases of syphilis and gonorrhea. The presence of other STDs increases the risk of HIV infection (USDHHS, 2000). HPV is the most commonly occurring STD (5.5 million cases per year in 1996) followed by trichomoniasis, chlamydia, herpes, gonorrhea, HB, syphilis, and HIV. STDs cost millions of dollars in screening, treatment, and reporting. In addition to creating a substantial problem for young adults, STDs impose tremendous demands on health care facilities. Many cases are unreported and untreated for lack of screening or failure to recognize symptoms.

Human Immunodeficiency Virus

Estimates of the number of people in the United States infected with HIV range from 650,000 to 900,000 (USDHHS, 2000). HIV is transmitted by sexual intercourse, shared needles, and infected blood. Another less common source of transmission is from mother to baby across the placental barrier or through breast milk. The higher level of worry about contracting an STD in young adults is correlated with the implementation of risk-reduction behaviors (Research Highlights box). Nurses are aware that the incidence of STDs is greatly reduced with proper use of condoms. In 1997 only 23% of sexually active adults reported using condoms (USDHHS, 2000). The *Healthy People 2010* target for condom use is 50%. Therefore, all sexually active individuals should be counseled on the hazards of unprotected sexual activity and on the effective use and limitations of condoms, stressing that they must be used properly and can fail. Condom failures occur at an estimated rate of 10% to 15%; therefore, counseling should stress that condom use is not foolproof.

Another AIDS-prevention success is the 66% decline between 1992 and 1997 in perinatal transmission. Rates of HIV transmission are greatly reduced by zidovudine therapy during pregnancy. Therefore the U.S. Public Health Service recommends voluntary testing for HIV and counseling as a part of basic prenatal care (USDHHS, 2000).

The nurse's role in intervening for STDs includes providing treatment and education, and early diagnosis and treatment are essential. When an individual is suspected of having an STD, the nurse obtains a complete history, including sexual history, sexual contacts, previous treatment and test results, any signs or symptoms of a current infection, recent use of antibiotics, and allergic reactions to antibiotics. When treatment is required, the nurse ensures that the person understands the goals of treatment in an attempt to gain cooperation and adherence to the plan of care.

research highlights

Safer Sexual Behaviors

This descriptive study examined predictors of safer sexual practices, in particular the differences between risky and safer sexual encounters (Sadovszky et al., 2002). Young adults are at serious risk for contracting sexually transmitted diseases. A convenience sample of 84 student volunteers was recruited from the psychology classes of a large university. A research questionnaire to examine contextual factors around the sexual encounter was constructed from current research findings. Participants' sexual experiences were separated into "safer" and "risky" categories through the use of the Risky Sexual Intercourse Measure.

Safer sexual encounters were more likely to occur in situations in which the place, partner, and communication with the partner were perceived in a negative fashion. Risky encounters tended to take place in situations where their was a perception of cozy ambiance, more partner attractiveness, when the partner directly asked for the encounter, and in situations associated with parties or celebrations.

In another study the annual college spring break provided an attractive "contranormative" setting for an unhealthy interaction among binge drinking, drugs, and sexual risk taking. Although level of knowledge regarding safer sex is increasing, knowledge alone continues to be necessary, but not sufficient, for the practice of safer sexual behaviors. Because knowledge alone is insufficient, programs to prevent HIV transmission through sexual behavior must be specific and relevant to the intended population. Psychological factors that influence the practice of safer sexual behaviors must be targeted.

Sadovszky, V., Keller, M. L., Vahey, D., McKinney, K., Powwattana, A., & Pornchiakate, A. (2002). Situational factors involved in college students' safer and risky sexual encounters. *Journal of Obstetric, Gynecologic, and Neonatal Nursing, 32*(5), 612-622; Apostolopoulos, Y., Sonmez, S., &Yu, C. H. (2002). HIV-risk behaviors of American spring break vacationers: A case of situational disinhibition? *International Journal of STD & AIDS, 13*(11), 733-743.
HIV, human immunodeficiency virus.

The nurse is an educator not only of the individual, but also of the general public. Appropriate health education for the individual with an STD includes mode of transmission, incubation periods, signs and symptoms, methods of treatment, complications resulting from lack of treatment, and signs of recurrent infections.

Coping-Stress Tolerance Pattern
Assessment of Stress Levels

Stress, the result of forces operating on the individual that disrupt physiological or psychological equilibrium, is an integral part of young adulthood; therefore, a comprehensive health assessment should include questions to determine stress levels. Anxiety, nervousness, depression, or somatic complaints are indicators of stress, such as divorce, loss of employment, failure to be promoted, or financial difficulties. The role of the nurse is to listen, offer support, and

Table 22-3 Summary of Selected Sexually Transmitted Diseases

Disease	Causative Agent	Diagnostic Methods	Treatment	Risks or Complications	Focus of Nursing Teaching
Vulvovaginal candidiasis	Candida albicans, non-C. albicans	Wet mount: evidence of hyphae and spores	Antifungal medication (miconazole [Monistat], clotrimazole [Gyne-Lotrimin])	Recurrence of disease	Recheck for evidence of disease in 14 days, reduce moisture and heat in genital area
Trichomoniasis	Trichomonas vaginalis	Wet mount: observation of protozoa, Pap smear	Metronidazole (Flagyl)	Recurrence, excoriation of genital area	Understand medication regimen, use condoms to prevent new infection
Bacterial vaginosis	Gardnerella vaginalis	Wet mount: presence of "clue cells"	Metronidazole (Flagyl)	Asymptomatic infection	Sexual transmission not proven
Chlamydia	Chlamydia trachomatis	Chlamydia monoclonal antibody test, culture	Doxycycline, azithromycin	Infertility, urethral scarring, PID, endocervicitis, neonatal infection	Understand medication regimen, refer partners for evaluation, use condoms to prevent future infections
Genital herpes	Herpes simplex virus	Herpes (lesion) culture	Acyclovir at first diagnosis or first episode	Urethral stricture, lymph node enlargement	Examine partners, abstain from sex while symptomatic, annual Pap smears
Genital warts	Human papilloma virus	Pap smear, observation of warts, colposcopy, biopsy	Podophyllin, trichloroacetic acid, cryotherapy/laser, valacyclovir, tamiciclovir	Cervical dysplasia	Return for treatment, examine partner, Pap smears
AIDS	HIV	Enzyme immune assay and Western blot	Current recommendations	Opportunistic infections	Monitor lymphocyte count, educate for current treatment recommendations
Gonorrhea	Neisseria gonorrhoeae	Culture	Ceftriaxone, cefixime	PID, infertility, ectopic pregnancy	Monitor antibiotic treatment, examine partner, repeat culture
Syphilis	Treponema pallidum	Venereal Disease Research Laboratory test, rapid plasma reagin test, fluorescent treponemal antibody absorbtion assay	Penicillin G benzathine	Secondary or late syphilis	Monitor antibiotic treatment, test and monitor partners

Based on data from Hatcher, R. A., Trussell, J. & Stewart, F. H. (2004). *Contraceptive technology* (18th ed.). New York: Ardent Media; Lowdermilk, D. L., & Perry, S. E. (2004). *Maternity & women's care.* St. Louis: Mosby.

Pap, Papanicolaou; *PID,* pelvic inflammatory disease; *AIDS,* acquired immunodeficiency syndrome; *HIV,* human immunodeficiency virus.

demonstrate concern. The nurse also suggests referrals to appropriate health providers and support groups.

Achievement Stress

Achievement-oriented stress differs from the stress of situational crises in that the stress of an overachiever is derived from internal pressures to succeed as measured by self-defined goals. Achievement-oriented stress frequently causes workaholic habits, including loss of sleep and omission of meals. When this behavior becomes extreme, serious physical and emotional consequences can occur, such as nutrition problems or burnout which, in turn, leads to severe emotional and physical exhaustion. Workaholic behaviors may not be perceived by the individual and may not be apparent until changes in bodily functions or behavior occur. Young adults are generally health conscious and willing to alter personal lifestyles and behavior patterns to reduce stress and become healthier. Many people have responded to campaigns for physical fitness, exercise, and nutritional adjustment, which should increase their well-being and life expectancy.

Suicide

Suicide is a leading cause of death in the young adult age group. Suicide occurs because many young adults are unable to cope with the pressures of adulthood. For some people, pressure arises when dealing with interpersonal conflicts: marital problems, family discord, or the loss of a close relationship; for others, the precipitating event is a lack of personal resources, unemployment, or dissatisfaction with work or school. Many young adults try to solve their problems before the fatal incident but see no positive solutions; in many cases, a prior suicide attempt was a signal for help.

Suicide rates are higher for men than for women; approximately 4 to 5 times as many men than women take their own lives (U.S. Census Bureau, 2001). However, more women are known to suffer from depressive disorders and to unsuccessfully attempt suicide. Suicide is more common among single or widowed individuals and divorced people. Young adults are more likely as a group to attempt suicide than are older individuals, and professionals are more likely to attempt suicide than are nonprofessionals.

A quick method of screening young adults who may be depressed requires the nurse to ask two questions. First the nurse asks whether in the last month, the young adult has been bothered by (1) little interest or pleasure in doing things and (2) feeling down, depressed, or hopeless (U.S. Preventive Services Task Force, 2002). A "no" answer to both questions indicates a negative screening result. In 1999 approximately 10.3% of all deaths in those ages 15 to 24 were classified as suicides (U.S. Census Bureau, 2001). When the health care provider is concerned that the young adult may be at risk for suicide, the following two questions should be asked: (1) "Have these symptoms or feelings that you have been talking about led you to think that you might be better off dead?" and (2) "What thoughts have you had about hurting yourself or even killing yourself?" To question

further the nurse can ask, "Have you actually done anything to hurt yourself?" (Depression Management Tool Kit, 2001). Suicide continues as a major health problem for young adults; annual rates, especially for men, remain high.

Nursing interventions are directed toward identifying behaviors in individuals who may be contemplating suicide. Physical clues include self-neglect, depression, slowed gait, slumped shoulders, and droopy faces. Presuicidal individuals also tend to exhibit impaired reality testing; feelings of hopelessness, helplessness, and rejection; impaired judgment and decision making; anxiety; weight loss; insomnia; or a radically changed affect. In addition to identifying presuicidal behaviors, the nurse also investigates relationship patterns to determine behaviors that are complicated by feelings of worthlessness and defeat. When the nurse identifies a young adult at risk for a suicide attempt, referrals to other professionals are indicated.

Values-Beliefs Pattern

Young adults enter their twenties with habits, values, and beliefs acquired during childhood and adolescence. Many acquired habits foster continuance of practices that are hazardous to health and well-being in later life. Prevention is directed toward altering value and belief patterns that encourage poor health practices, reorienting them toward those that support optimal health behaviors. Nursing interventions are more effective when the nurse can describe, discriminate, identify, and align value and belief patterns consistent with practices known to maximize health.

Values Involved in Parenting

Parenthood is envisioned by most young adults; therefore, health-promotion and health protection activities to ensure healthy offspring are crucial (Care Plan). **Genetic impairments,** or congenital defects caused by abnormal chromosomes, are responsible for 4% to 6% of perinatal deaths (Lowdermilk & Perry, 2004). Tests are available for about 200 genetic diseases (Lowdermilk & Perry, 2004). Most of the offered genetic testing is for single-gene impairment to mothers who have a history of genetic disease. Young adults with a genetic disease must make many important decisions; predicting the transmission of the disease to potential offspring is key.

Values Regarding Prenatal Diagnosis and Genetic Impairment

Prenatal diagnostic procedures have been available since the mid-1960s. This capability has enabled the identification of high-risk pregnancies and requires the cooperation and education of childbearing women and their partners, both of whom must provide accurate family health and obstetrical histories and comply with suggested screening and follow-up measures. Decisions about the advisability of reproduction are based on current information on genetics and known deleterious genetic factors.

The finding of a malformed or genetically impaired fetus may result in a parental decision to terminate the

CARE PLAN

Preparation for Childbearing

Nursing Diagnosis Health-Seeking Behaviors Related to Preconceptual Assessment and Preparation for Childbearing

DEFINING CHARACTERISTICS

- Expressed desire to improve overall health to prepare for childbearing
- Expressed thoughts about planning for pregnancy in the near future
- Desire to improve nutritional status before childbearing
- Desire to improve nutritional intake of essential vitamins and minerals (iron and calcium)
- Plan to take multivitamin each day
- Plan to limit foods high in sodium and fat
- Plan to limit alcohol consumption
- Plan for exercise program to increase stamina and flexibility
- Seeks physical examination to rule out problems that might negatively affect pregnancy
- Seeks information on pregnancy risk factors (biophysical, psychosocial, sociodemographic, and environmental)

RELATED FACTORS

- Expressed desire to improve the quality of relationship with husband or partner
- Desire to attend education classes to improve knowledge of childbearing and positive health practices
- Plan for room or housing to accommodate children
- Plan for employment arrangements that accommodate child care

EXPECTED OUTCOMES

- Increase in indices of well-being in client
- Healthy pregnancy and future child
- Increase in self-confidence and awareness preparation for childbearing

- Management of pregnancy risk factors before becoming pregnant
- Making the person aware of resources available for pregnancy and child care

INTERVENTIONS

- Assess current level of wellness regarding preparation for childbearing.
- Identify community resources that provide information regarding preconceptual planning and preparation.
- Identify primary health provider, midwife or obstetrician, and hospitals with delivery services.
- Assess biophysical risk factors (genetic disorders, nutrition problems, and current medical problems).
- Assess for history of pregnancy loss.
- Test for blood type and Rh factor.
- Screen for sexually transmitted disease, tuberculosis, rubella titer, sickle cell trait.
- Review immunization history, including hepatitis B.
- Assess need to augment diet, particularly to increase intake of calcium and iron.
- Take a multivitamin daily.
- Assess for psychosocial risk factors (mental problems, use of drugs, alcohol, caffeine, and smoking).
- Counsel to avoid alcohol consumption.
- Assess for possible sociodemographic risk factors (poverty, first pregnancy risks of dystocia or PIH, residence [rural or urban], and ethnicity).
- Assess for environmental risks (exposures to chemicals, drugs, pesticides, pollution, smoke, stress, and radiation).
- Assess current employment situation.
- Identify child-care arrangements.

PIH, pregnancy-induced hypertension.

pregnancy. Theological and political debates in addition to legislative mandates have greatly influenced family control over many of these decisions. Genetic counseling is an important nursing intervention for young adults. A genetic specialist gives technical explanations of genetic disorders; however, nurses have a supportive role in helping young adults decide whether to have children or to carry through a pregnancy that is at risk.

Ethnicity, Race, and Culture

The young adult whose ethnic background is different from that of the dominant culture may encounter prejudice and discrimination, which can occur because of differences in race, creed, language, attitudes, values, preferences, or behaviors. The young adult is susceptible to these prejudices at work, at school, in health care delivery systems, and in the community. Young adults must meet not only personal needs, but also the needs of children or elders; therefore,

nurses must consider the values that are common to specific cultures and ethnic backgrounds.

Race and ethnicity are important influencers of health for young adults. Longevity for nonwhite men and women has increased recently, the result of a decrease in birth-related fatalities and in deaths caused by systemic disabilities. Blacks remain at risk for specific health problems, and the life expectancy of the average black person is shorter than that of the average white person. Race and ethnicity can also influence the clinical response of an individual to drug therapy; unfortunately, many drug investigations underrepresent minority subjects in their samples, so drug recommendations may be incompletely studied for some minority groups (Kudzma, 1999).

Race and ethnicity are closely connected to educational and work-related decisions, which subsequently affect choice of residence. Many minority families live in substandard housing or crowded living spaces. A lifestyle of this type, when combined with insufficient economic resources, frequently affects health. Compared with the general population, divorce rates are proportionally higher among white women than Hispanic and black women; remarriage occurs less frequently for black or Hispanic women than it does for white women in the same age ranges (Bramlett & Mosher, 2002). Poverty is more common among black families, which often leads to unmet basic needs of food, clothing, and housing and, in turn, leads to decreased regard for health needs.

PATHOLOGICAL PROCESSES
Accidents

The largest percentage of accidents occurs before age 35; from 15 to 24 years, deaths from injury exceed deaths from all other causes (USDHHS, 2000). Motor vehicle accidents cause more fatalities than all other causes of death combined. Reducing speed limits contributes to lower fatality rates. Approximately 48 states have seat belt laws, and all states have seat belt requirements for children. All individuals in the car need to use seat belts, because an unrestrained occupant can cause harm to another passenger in a crash (Cummings & Rivara, 2004). The continued high incidence of vehicle accidents in the young adult age group is related to accessibility of cars to young adults and peer pressure on driving behavior; reckless driving and driving under the influence of alcohol and drugs is now viewed as closely connected to violent and abusive behavior (USDHHS, 2000).

Accident-prevention education, long considered appropriate for young children, is an important part of young adult instruction. Most young licensed drivers have participated in driver education courses, and a number of states have adopted progressive licensing programs. The young adult must understand the potentially fatal consequences of aggressive tendencies or thoughtless risk taking. When young adults are encouraged to reflect on the consequences of their actions, they tend to be more willing to control and change unsafe driving behaviors.

Pollution
Noise

Young adults are exposed to high levels of noise in occupational and recreational settings. Long-term exposure to loud noise is directly related to impaired hearing and can increase irritability and stress. Young adults can be exposed to noises in the work setting from industrial machinery and equipment. Although industrial exposure can be difficult to mitigate, many young adults worsen the situation through recreational exposure, by listening to music or videos at excessively high-decibel levels. Ear protection is necessary in some situations to prevent hearing disability. Recognition of hazards and corresponding appropriate preventive education are early nursing strategies for decreasing excessive noise exposure.

Air

Motor vehicles are the largest source of air pollution; vehicles release over 90 million tons of particles and noxious gases each year, most of which is either carbon monoxide or hydrocarbons. Carbon monoxide in high concentrations is deadly; in lower concentrations it causes headaches, dizziness, and heart palpitations. In sunlight and low-lying areas, automobile exhaust becomes photochemical smog that contains ozone, which irritates the eyes and the respiratory tract. Although air pollution is not a problem only for young adults, they frequently work in dirty, entry-level jobs in industrial settings and may be among the age group that is most affected.

Occupational Hazards and Stressors

Occupational hazards pose a threat of illness, injury, or death in all age groups, and occupational safety standards have contributed greatly to the reduction of work-related accidents. Legislation, including the Occupational Safety and Health Act (1970), has resulted in the improvement of work conditions, along with the provision of health care facilities, in many companies.

Young adults should not be allowed to work in certain industrial settings without vocational training to reduce hazards. Young adults frequently want a challenge and high wages; therefore, they work at hazardous jobs, for example, on offshore drilling rigs, on high bridges, or in nuclear plants. Because of their age, physical stamina, and agility, young adults are suitable candidates for positions that require physical ability. Occupational training should include education about personal exposure risks, identification of work-related hazards, and identification of situations in which the severity of accidents is connected to personal behaviors or habits. For example, drivers of heavy construction machinery should be particularly observant and avoid reckless behaviors and fast driving. Working women who are pregnant can expose their fetuses to industrial substances. Proper evaluation and temporary reassignment may be necessary.

Occupational preventive intervention requires that known work hazards and risks be identified early. Health histories should include questions about the place of work, type of work, and young adults' understanding of the risks associated with their occupations. Occupational risk and health are closely related; stress associated with work, the use of alcohol or drugs, and a negative attitude toward work are predictive of occupational injuries. Job counseling aimed at changing the nature of employment can be an appropriate referral for some people with health conditions. Employees in industrial settings should visit a health care provider on a periodic basis for health assessment, update of the health history, and counseling.

Chemical Agents
Drug Use

Misuse of drugs, a major risk for young adults, is associated with injury, disability, violence, homicide, and suicide and

MULTICULTURAL AWARENESS

Racial and Ethnic Variations in Drug Response

Various studies, although limited, indicate that race and ethnicity may be important factors to consider when prescribing certain drugs. Different genetic types tend to metabolize drugs differently, have different binding receptors, or have different environmental influences that change the utilization and uptake.

Gene selection favored chances of survival; for example, sickle cell trait developed through selection factors which favored resistance to malaria. Similarly, gene selection factors also favored the prevalence of glucose-6-phosphate dehydrogenase deficiency, which also provides resistance to malaria but causes drug-related red blood cell hemolysis. In a related study of warfarin response, ethnic differences were shown to affect bioavailability and distribution which were controlled through careful clinical management and dosage regulation (El Rouby, Mestres, LaDuca, & Zucker, 2004).

In studies of people with hypertension, black individuals responded with a greater decrease in systolic pressure in response to thiazide diuretics (hydrochlorothiazide) and calcium channel blockers. Black clients have a blunted response to β-blockers, which can be improved by adding a diuretic.

The situation in Asian clients appears to be the exact opposite. In a study of the effectiveness of propranolol in Chinese and white men, the Chinese men had at least a twice as much sensitivity as did the white men to propranolol administered at several dosage levels. Compared with the white men, the Chinese men experienced a 20% greater reduction in heart rate and a 10% greater reduction in blood pressure.

Studies indicate that Asians are more sensitive to alcohol and its drug effects than are whites. The most outstanding difference is in the amount of facial flushing, which was experienced by a substantial percentage of Asians compared with the white sample. The Asians also experienced other undesirable discomforts, including palpitations, tachycardia, head pounding, and muscle weakness, to a greater degree than did the white subjects. The alcohol dehydrogenase enzyme is reported to be absent in about one half of Asians.

These examples suggest that nurses should be aware of racial and ethnic issues in drug metabolism and effectiveness. In individuals who do not respond to certain drugs as expected, the nurse may consider whether this might be related to constitutional factors within the person's genetic makeup. This research also invites rethinking of managed care practices that restrict diversity of drug use with prescribed drug formulary listings.

This topic is discussed in more detail in Kudzma, E. (2001). Cultural competence: Cardiovascular medications. *Progress in Cardiovascular Nursing, 16*(4), 152-160, 169; El Rouby, S., Mestres, C. A., LaDuca, F. M., & Zucker, M. L. (2004). Racial and ethnic differences in warfarin response. *Journal of Heart Valve Disease, 13*(1), 15-21; Hall, W. D. (1999). A rational approach to the treatment of hypertension in special populations. *American Family Physician, 60*(1), 156-162; Wood, A. J. (1998). Ethnic differences in drug disposition and response. *Therapeutic Drug Monitoring, 20*(5), 525-526; Zhou, H., Kosharji, B., Silverstein, D., Wilkinson, G., & Wood, A. (1989). Racial differences in drug response: Altered sensitivity to and clearance of propranolol in men of Chinese descent as compared with American whites. *New England Journal of Medicine, 320*(9), 565-570.

is related to social problems (criminal behaviors and maladjustment to accepted norms). Drug abuse may be closely related to an inability to cope appropriately with adult responsibilities. Physical health problems associated with drug misuse account for more than 50% of the major acute and chronic problems of young adults. Heroin users have increased mortality rates because of overdosage or chronic disability associated with hepatitis infections. Drug use is an independent risk factor involved in approximately one quarter of HIV infections (USDHHS, 2000).

Use of drugs, such as anabolic steroids, to improve athletic performance is increasing. The risks of using steroids are enormous, and preventive education should focus on healthier sports and exercise values.

Nursing activities include preventive strategies to curb the problem of drug misuse. Distribution of information on drugs, early treatment of complications, and drug treatment centers are only part of the answer. Nursing efforts aimed at increasing individual awareness and altering drug-taking attitudes and behaviors are of critical importance (Multicultural Awareness box).

Alcohol Use

Alcohol-related accidents among individuals ages 15 to 24 continue to be a leading cause of preventable morbidity, disability, and death. Heavy alcohol use, that is, consuming five or more drinks on at least one occasion within a month, is more common in 18 to 25 year olds than it is for younger or older people (USDHHS, 2000). Raising the legal drinking age to 21 reduces not only deaths and injuries connected to motor vehicle accidents, but also homicides and other violent death. Alcohol abuse is directly related to chronic conditions such as cirrhosis of the liver. Modifying alcohol consumption in young adults can decrease the frequency of chronic and disabling conditions in later life.

Alcohol consumption is increasing in the young adult population. Young adults between the ages of 18 and 25 are more likely (27%) to report that they have engaged in binge drinking in the last 30 days (USDHHS, 2000). Although young adults drink less regularly than do older adults, they tend to consume larger amounts of alcohol at one time; the tendency is toward binge drinking, which causes increased loss of control and is related to an additional risk of automobile accidents. Teens with work schedules of more than 10 hours per week are more often involved in heavy or binge drinking or both. Working more time increases the money available to purchase alcohol and exposes the teen to older adults who drink (Paschall, Flewelling & Russell, 2004).

Tobacco Use

Smoking is a leading cause of preventable death in the United States; therefore, smoking cessation is the single most important counseling topic for all people because of its potential to lower the risk of contracting many preventable diseases. Smoking was most prevalent among adults aged 18 to 24 years (28.3%) and 25 to 44 years (28.0%) and declined with age (Schoenborn, Vickerie, & Barnes, 2003). More than one third of current smokers aged 18 to 24 years (37.6%) started smoking before the age of 16. In later adulthood, the incidence of smoking declined: 28% for people 18 to 24 years of age, but only 12% for those over age 65 (USDHHS, 2000).

Individuals employed in high-risk occupations should be informed of the synergistic relationship between smoking and asbestos and radiation exposure. Fear tactics, nagging, preaching, and threats are generally ineffective in convincing people to stop smoking. Major barriers to smoking cessation are the presence of other smokers, particularly in situations where alcohol is also being used. Antismoking strategies tend to focus on the hazards of smoking rather than basic causes such as lack of confidence in stressful social situations and weight control (Kelley, Thomas, & Friedmann, 2000).

State enforcement of no smoking policies is important, as Jemal, Cokkinides, Shafey, and Thun (2003) have reported. Lung cancer death rates declined in states with strong tobacco control enforcement and increased in states where tobacco control was weak. Measures of tobacco control are strongly correlated with smoking cessation rates of young adults ages 30 to 39. Nurses are familiar with the antismoking resources in their communities, enabling them to make the appropriate referrals.

Cancer
Environmental Carcinogens

Young adults can be exposed to environmental carcinogens in their work settings or through unhealthy practices such as having multiple sexual partners. In the work setting, environmental regulations have limited exposure to some hazardous chemicals, but long-term effects on health of exposure to many industrial chemicals remains unknown. In health care, latex, long considered inert and safe, has now been shown to cause long-term immune system disease in some nurses exposed to the agent (or the chemicals that bind it) in surgical gloves.

The risk for developing cervical cancer is related to environmental exposures such as smoking and HPV infection. Cervical cancer has decreased steadily over the years, likely because of the effective use of screening methods, such as **Papanicolaou (Pap) smear** testing. Rates for cervical dysplasia and cancer peak in both white and black women between ages 20 and 30. The rate for black women increases faster than it does for white women over the age of 25. Known risk factors for environmental exposure include smoking, early age of first intercourse, multiple sexual partners, and infection with HPV (USDHHS, 2000).

SOCIAL PROCESSES
Community and Work
Neighborhood Resources

The environment of the community strongly influences the well-being of the young adult and sets the standard for the health of people and families living within a neighborhood. Neighbors can be an excellent source of support, which can be especially important to a young mother who does not have immediate family nearby. Nurses working in the community facilitate the contact of individuals with common interests through community and religious activities and support groups.

Community resources for exercise and recreation can make important contributions to the young adult's physical and emotional health (Figure 22-4). When these resources are available, the young adult can have the opportunity to exercise and release stress in a positive fashion.

Schools within the community are a concern for parents; dissatisfaction with the public school system can cause additional stress. When economic resources are available, private schooling becomes an option. This approach can

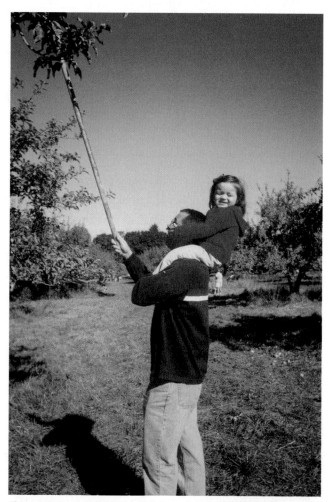

Figure 22-4 Young adults' need for recreation with their family members can make important contributions to their physical and emotional health.

add burdens to the young family that is already financially troubled. When there are inadequate resources, the family can feel frustration and despair.

Health Service Availability

Availability of health services is important. Economic realities, however, influence the effectiveness of resources, particularly for the young adult who lives in an economically depressed area. In some communities health services are lacking or, when available, are not culturally sensitive or adapted to the customs and beliefs of the people who are served. In other communities access to public transportation can be a critical problem, affecting the ability of the young adult to keep appointments. Young adults ages 18 to 24 years are the least likely of any age group to have a usual source of care; thus, a target of *Healthy People 2010* is to increase the proportion of young adults with a usual primary care provider (USDHHS, 2000).

Culture and Ethnicity

Health delivery methods in the United States are based on Western belief systems, which tend to be rigid in their applications. For example, women seeking birth control information and prescriptions are expected to use health clinics and keep to their schedule of return visits. Because health care provider systems have removed many traditional barriers once assumed to be responsible for poor utilization of services by low-income or minority groups (location and scheduling), nonattendance at scheduled clinic visits frequently is interpreted as noncompliance. Among Native Americans, contraceptive education has gained little acceptance, and fertility rates remain high, primarily because conception control may be viewed as both culturally and religiously objectionable.

Appropriate health strategies and interventions require that nurses identify cultural beliefs and health care practices that are harmful to people. Many cultural practices may be allowed because they do not affect appropriate health care. For example, food cravings are common among many pregnant women. In moderation, following dietary patterns directed by these cravings is not harmful. However, when the craving leads to an unbalanced diet or to pica (eating nonfood substances), the pregnancy can be affected (e.g., the incidence of anemia is higher in women with pica) (Lowdermilk & Perry, 2004).

Legislation

Young adults are one of the major political constituencies in the United States; they support many causes and have the time and energy to publicize issues related to the common good. Some of these issues involve the environment, nuclear energy, war, and pollution. Relative to health, predominant issues have involved housing and health care in neighborhoods and rural areas and health, agricultural, and sanitation concerns in foreign countries. Through these efforts, young adults can influence and improve living conditions for future generations.

Economics

One of the young adult's age-related tasks is to choose and develop a lifelong career. This choice is directly related to economic factors; young adults want satisfying occupations that also yield adequate economic returns. To manage financially and maintain a lifestyle in which personal needs can be met, young adults may elect to have fewer children. Caring for aging parents can also cause physical, psychosocial, spiritual, and economic stress.

Although goals vary greatly among young adult couples, they generally are concerned with acquiring material comforts; the desire for housing, transportation, clothing, or recreation generally necessitate that both partners work to meet financial obligations. This desire necessitates the changing of roles and the sharing of responsibilities, and open communication becomes a crucial component. For single parents these challenges can appear insurmountable.

New career opportunities and the economic expansion in the United States during the 1990s have allowed young adults more career choices. During the latter part of the 1990s, college graduates had the best choice of employment opportunities in decades. The booming technology industry provided employment in a wide variety of occupations and start-up companies. Work styles within these companies tend to be different from that in the traditional workplace, including an expectation of longer and more fluid workdays. "Dot.com" or Internet-based companies provide young adults with jobs that have the potential to give them rapid financial rewards at the cost of long-term job stability. From 2000 on there has been contraction in the computer industry combined with the movement of some jobs overseas, especially in areas in which developing countries could provide a skilled, technically proficient inexpensive workforce. Young adults are becoming accustomed to the vision that long-term employment will be less available in the economies of the future.

Homelessness

Homeless people were, at one time, primarily single men; today entire families account for approximately one third of the homeless population. More families are seeking subsidized housing, although homelessness is not only a housing issue but results from poor education, lack of employment skills, substandard health care, domestic violence and abuse, and inadequate child and foster care. Poverty is a key factor; welfare benefits are too low to cover high rents, and long waits for public housing are common. Housing may be located away from transportation and health care facilities, hindering access to health care (Nunez & Caruso, 2003).

Single men tend to use shelters only for night residence, but families tend to use shelter settings longer, an average of 2 to 11 months, before locating housing. Today's shelters are very different from the temporary places of the past; many provide on-site services and programs to eradicate the causes of homelessness. About 26% of those living in shelters are employed, and many shelters provide child care, after-school programs, and job preparedness training (Nunez & Caruso, 2003). Minorities are significantly and disproportionately represented among the homeless in larger cities, reflecting the large number who live below or near the poverty level.

Dual Careers

For many young adult couples, different careers, friends, and varying maturity levels place additional strains on their relationship. These circumstances can provide a basis for domestic difficulty. Domestic quarreling tends to precede family disruption, leading to marital separation or divorce. In addition to the emotional strain placed on family members, domestic arguments can result in aggressive acts of abuse and personal injury. Young adults can also be faced with decisions about day-care facilities; the couple or mother may need support to resolve guilt feelings related to the separation from the child.

Alternative lifestyles include living arrangements with individuals of the same gender or the opposite gender. Although these lifestyles are becoming more acceptable in today's society, attitudes toward alternative lifestyles contribute pressures that lead to further stress and uncertainty.

SUMMARY

Nurses promote health care measures and behaviors at all places where young adults come into contact with the health care delivery system. In community colleges and uni-versity settings, efforts can be directed toward health education curricula with emphasis on positive health behaviors, establishment of peer counseling groups, and better utilization of sports and exercise facilities. Workshops on alcoholism, drug abuse, sports or exercise, mental health and self-expression, relationships, and various aspects of sexual care have been effective in college populations. At the work site, programs of employee counseling, blood pressure monitoring and treatment, exercise, smoking reduction, cafeteria nutrition management, and stress reduction have also been effective. Employee insurance programs should undergo continual review to determine an appropriate level of integrated care and coverage. Preventive care, mental health, dental health, and maternity benefits should be analyzed and increased when necessary. Young adults are generally healthy, which challenges the nurse to be even more sensitive, insightful, and creative in implementing care for individuals within this age group.

ADDITIONAL STUDY MATERIAL

Study Questions in the back of the book, see page 663.

evolve WEB SITE MATERIALS

These materials are located on the book's Web site at http://evolve.elsevier.com/Edelman/.

- WebLinks
- Content Updates

REFERENCES

American footballers endure "car crash" blows. (January, 2004). *New Scientist.* Retrieved May 2, 2005, from *www.newscientist.com/article.ns?id=dn4534*

Anderson, R. N., & Arias, E. (2003). *The effect of revised populations on mortality statistics for the United States, 2000. National vital statistics reports* (Vol. 51, No. 9). Hyattsville, MD: National Center for Health Statistics.

Association of Women's Health, Obstetric and Neonatal Nurses. (2004a). AWHONN urges approval of OTC emergency contraception. *AWHONN Lifelines, 8*(1), 65-66.

Association of Women's Health, Obstetric and Neonatal Nurses. (2004b). Fortifying oral contraceptives with folic acid. *AWHONN Lifelines, 8*(1), 12-13.

Bramlett, M. D., & Mosher, W. D. (2002). Cohabitation, marriage, divorce, and remarriage in the United States. *Vital Health Statistics, 22*, 1-93.

Cherry, D. K., Burt, C. W., & Woodwell, D. A. (2003). *National ambulatory medical care survey: 2001 Summary. Advance data from vital and health statistics* (No. 331). Hyattsville, MD: National Center for Health Statistics.

Chobanian, A. V. (2003). The Seventh Report of the Joint National Committee on Prevention, Detection, Evaluation, and Treatment of High Blood Pressure: The JNC 7 report. *Journal of the American Medical Association, 289*(19), 2560-2572.

Clinical preventive services for normal-risk adults recommended by the U.S. Preventive Services Task Force. (2003, Jan.). Rockville, MD: Agency for Health Care Research and Quality. Retrieved April 29, 2005,, from: *http://www.ahrq.gove/ppip/adulttm.htm.*

Cummings, P., & Rivara, F. P. (2004). Car occupant death according to the restraint use of other occupants: A matched cohort study. *Journal of the American Medical Association, 291*(3), 342-349.

Declining prevalence of no known major risk factors for heart disease and stroke among adults—United States, 1991-2001. (2004). *Morbidity and Mortality Weekly Report, 53*(1), 4-7.

Depression Management Tool Kit. (2001). MacArthur initiative on depression and primary care. Retrieved March 12, 2004, from: *http://www.depression-primarycare.org.*

Dieterich, D. (2000). Chronic hepatitis C: Update on diagnosis and treatment. *Consultant, 40*(9), 1590-1596.

Erikson, E. H. (1993). *Childhood and society.* New York: W. W. Norton.

Fenwick, A. (2003). On the front line of SARS. *American Journal of Nursing, 103*(9), 118-119.

Gilligan, C. (1982). New maps of development: New visions of maturity. *American Journal of Orthopsychiatry, 52*(2), 199-212.

Gilligan, C. (2002). *The birth of pleasure.* New York: Alfred A. Knopf.

Golden, W. E., & Hopkins, R. H. (2003). Divorce. *Internal Medicine News, 36*(17), 22.

Hatcher, R. A., Trussell. J., & Stewart, F. H. (2004). *Contraceptive technology* (18th ed.). New York: Ardent Media.

Huether, S. E., & McCance, K. L. (2004). *Understanding pathophysiology.* St. Louis: Mosby.

Jemal, M., Cokkinides, V., Shafey, O., & Thun, M. (2003). Lung cancer trends in young adults: An early indicator of progress in tobacco control (United States). *Cancer Causes and Control, 14*, 579-585.

Kelley, F. J., Thomas, S. A., & Friedmann, E. (2000). Smoking patterns, health behaviors, and health-risk behaviors of college women. *Clinical Excellence for Nurse Practitioners, 4*(5), 302-308.

Kohlberg, L., & Lickons, T. (1986). *The stages of ethical development: From childhood through old age*. San Francisco: Harper.

Kudzma, E. C. (1999). Culturally competent drug administration. *American Journal of Nursing, 99*(8), 46-51.

Kudzma, E. C. (2001). Cultural competence: Cardiovascular medications. *Progress in Cardiovascular Nursing, 16*(4), 152-160, 169.

Lowdermilk, D. L., & Perry, S. E. (2004). *Maternity & women's care*. St. Louis: Mosby.

Manson, J. E., Skerrett, P. J., Greenland, P., & Vanltallie, T. B. (2004). The escalating pandemics of obesity and sedentary lifestyle: A call to action for clinicians. *Archives of Internal Medicine, 164*, 249-258.

Marshall, D., McConkey, R., & Moore, G. (2003). Obesity in people with intellectual disabilities: The impact of nurse-led health screenings and health promotion activities. *Journal of Advanced Nursing, 41*(2), 147-153.

Mathews, T. J., & Hamilton, B. E. (2002). *Mean age of mother, 1970-2000. National vital statistics reports, 51(1)*. Hyattsville, MD: National Center for Health Statistics.

Michigan teens still having sex, but pregnancy rates are falling. (2004, Feb. 5). *Women's Health Weekly*, 12. Retrieved July 14, 2005, from: *http://www.obgyn.net/newsheadlines/womens_health-Adolescent_Health-20040205-4.asp*

Morris, B., & Young, C. (2000). Emergency contraception. *American Journal of Nursing, 100*(9), 46-48.

Nettina, S. M. (2002). Health promotion: More than just cardiovascular risk reduction. *Topics in Advanced Practice Nursing eJournal, 2*(1). Retrieved March 10, 2004, from: *http://www.medscape.com/viewarticle421467*

Nunez, R., & Caruso, L. (2003, Jan.). Are shelters the answer to family homelessness? *USA Today, 131*, 46.

Overweight and obesity: Economic consequences. (2005). Retrieved May 2, 2005, from *http://www.cdc.gov/nccdphp/dnpa/obesity/economic_consequences.htm*

Paschall, M. J., Flewelling, R. L., & Russell, T. (2004). Why is work intensity associated with heavy alcohol use among adolescents? *Journal of Adolescent Health, 34*(1), 79-87.

Patients with diabetes have poor control of complication risks. (2004, Feb. 4). *Biotech Week*, 81. Retrieved March 18, 2004, from: *http://infotrac.galegroup.com*.

Piaget, J. (1972). Intellectual evolution from adolescence to adulthood. *Human Development, 15*, 1-12.

Pravikoff, D. S., Pierce, S., & Tanner, A. (2003). Nursing resources: Are nurses ready for evidence-based practice? *American Journal of Nursing, 103*(5), 95-96.

Preventing and controlling meningococcal disease: Latest guidelines. (2000). *Consultant, 40*(9), 1654-1657.

Schoenborn, C.A., Vickerie, J. L., & Barnes, P. M. (2003). *Cigarette smoking behavior of adults: United States, 1997-98. Advance data from vital and health statistics* (No. 331).

Hyattsville, MD: National Center for Health Statistics.

Scott, C. L. (2003). Diagnosis, prevention, and intervention for the metabolic syndrome. *American Journal of Cardiology, 92*(1A), 35i-42i.

Tran, T. T. (2004). Current issues in hepatitis B. *Advances in viral hepatitis, CME*. Retrieved July 14, 2005, from: *http://bmj.bmjjournals.com/medscape/gastroenterology/ddw1/a11.shtml*

U.S. Census Bureau. (2001). *Statistical abstracts of the United States: 2002* (122nd ed.). Washington, DC: U.S. Government Printing Office.

U.S. Department of Health and Human Services. (2000). *Healthy people 2010: Vol. 1 and 2* (Conference ed.). Washington, DC: U.S. Government Printing Office.

U.S. Preventive Services Task Force. (2002). Screening for depression: Recommendations and rational. *Annals of Internal Medicine, 136*(10), 760-764.

U.S. Preventive Services Task Force. (2003). Clinical Preventive Services for Normal-Risk Adults, January, 2003. Rockville, MD: Agency for Health Care Research and Quality. Retrieved January 9, 2004, from: *http://www.ahrq.gov/ppip/adulttm.htm*.

Violence a growing public health problem in the Americas. (2004, Feb. 8). *Medical letter on the CDC and FDA, 47*.

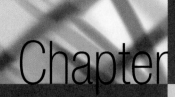

Chapter 23

SHEILA GROSSMAN
CAROL LYNN MANDLE

Middle-Age Adult

objectives

After completing this chapter, the reader will be able to:

- Name three psychosocial and spiritual changes that frequently occur during middle age.
- Explain two normal biological changes that occur as a result of the aging process.
- Identify the major causes of mortality in the middle-age adult.
- Describe the health patterns of middle-age adults.
- Discuss the unique health problems related to the occupations of the adult between ages 35 and 65.
- Discuss the influence of psychosocial stressors on the middle-age adult and the ways the individual's culture and occupation can affect these stressors.

key terms

Advance directive	Generativity	Osteoporosis
Calcium	Gingivitis	Periodontitis
Cardiac output	Glaucoma	Presbycusis
Constipation	Kyphosis	Presbyopia
Degenerative joint disease	Menopause	Stagnation
Durable power of attorney	Midlife crisis	
Functional aerobic capacity	Obesity	

THINK About It

Terminal Illness

Charlie Shelton is dying of lung cancer. His wife, Sarah, finds that she must manage a household and provide for their two children (ages 15 and 18) on her own. The elder child plans to enter college next fall, but the Sheltons wonder whether they will be able to afford this. Although Charlie and Sarah worked hard and saved money all their lives, Charlie's long illness continues to deplete their savings. Their parents are helping as best they can, but they live on limited incomes themselves. The hospital bills continue to come, and the Sheltons are overwhelmed.

1. What can health providers do to help the Sheltons during this stressful time?
2. What health-promotion strategies might be suggested and implemented to help them?
3. What community organizations might the health care provider recommend to meet the needs of this family?
4. What responsibilities do health providers and policy makers have to provide health promotion to middle-age adults?

Middle adulthood is defined as the period between 35 and 65 years of age. During this dynamic time the adult experiences biological, physiological, social, psychological, and spiritual changes (Cottrell, Girvan, & McKenzie, 2001). The middle years represent a stage of development set within major economic productivity and family responsibility. This significant group makes up nearly one half the population of the United States (U.S. Department of Health and Human Services [USDHHS], 1998).

AGE AND PHYSICAL CHANGES

Although their onset is insidious, biological changes come to the forefront during the middle years, affecting most bodily systems. The hair of the adult begins to thin and turn gray. The skin's moisture and turgor decreases, and with the loss of subcutaneous fat, wrinkling occurs. Excessive sun exposure through the years makes this process more pronounced. The result can be a coarsening of the facial features.

Fat deposition increases during these years, with increases in weight. The body contour changes as "love handles" and "saddlebags" appear. Sedentary lifestyles and unchanged dietary habits contribute a great deal to these changes. The inactive lifestyle is further compromised by a decrease in energy; "I'm not as young as I used to be" is a common remark. This proclamation is legitimate, because the capacity for physical work actually decreases. The **functional aerobic capacity** decreases, with a resulting decrease in **cardiac output.**

In the musculoskeletal system, bone density and mass progressively decrease. When 55-year-old adults say that they were an inch taller when they were 18, the observation is likely to be true. A 1-inch to 4-inch (2.5-cm to 10-cm) loss in height occurs as a person ages; thinning of the intervertebral disks accounts for approximately 1 inch. However, dramatic losses in height (as much as 4 inches) can occur with thoracic **kyphosis,** an angulation of the posterior spine (commonly known as *hunchback*). The wear and tear on joints predispose the adult to **degenerative joint disease,** deterioration of the joint(s), with more frequent annoying backaches. The general decrease in muscle tone is categorized by many as *flab,* which reduces physical agility. Degenerative joint disease, specifically osteoarthritis, has its peak onset in middle age. Most frequently the knees and hands, followed by hips, spine, shoulders, and ankles, are involved.

The functional capacity of all organ systems generally decreases. For example, in the gastrointestinal tract, the following chain of events occurs: decreased metabolism leads to less enzyme production, resulting in lower hydrochloric acid levels, decreasing tone in the large intestine. As a result, the middle-age adult may complain of acid indigestion with increased belching.

When the adult leads a sedentary lifestyle as well, the effects of the diminished motility through the gastrointestinal tract can be more pronounced. That Americans eat more refined foods (foods that are low in bulk) than residents of third-world nations is well known. A low-bulk diet can contribute to the problem of **constipation,** a change in bowel habits characterized by decreased frequency or passage of hard, drier stools and difficult defecation, and is believed to be a primary contributor to the increased incidence of colon cancer in the United States.

Between ages 25 and 85, a 35% loss of nephron units occurs. The remaining nephrons increase in size and undergo degenerative changes. The entire weight of the kidneys decreases. Because blood supply is also diminished, the glomerular filtration rate is decreased by nearly one half.

Significant changes occur in the cardiovascular system as the blood vessels lose elasticity and become thicker. This process predisposes middle-age adults to coronary artery disease, hypertension, myocardial infarctions, and strokes. Heart disease is the leading cause of death in middle-age adults (USDHHS, 2000).

When a previously menstruating woman does not have a period for 1 year, she has reached **menopause.** Menopause usually occurs between ages 45 and 55. A great deal more must be learned about what exactly causes many of the symptoms that women frequently report. Sheehy (1993) conducted interviews of 100 women from their midforties to sixties and also interviewed 75 physicians and other experts. Her analysis showed that many of these people felt there was a renewed sexual vitality and surge of mental energy for menopausal women. She characterized menopause as a gateway to a second adulthood and found that most frequently only 15% of women have unrelenting menopausal symptoms, 15% have no concerns, and the other 70% experience some symptoms but not to the extent that they affect their lives negatively. Northrup (2001) and Sheehy (1993) reiterate the importance of taking time to rethink and reprioritize one's life once menopause is in process.

During this time, production of ovarian estrogen and progesterone ceases; the remaining estrogen is produced by the adrenal glands. As a result of the diminished estrogen level, a woman's secondary sex characteristics regress, such as loss of pubic hair and decrease in breast size. The female reproductive organs shrink in size, and vaginal secretions decrease.

Men experience changes in their sexual response cycle as testosterone levels plateau, then decrease, as they approach the end of the middle years. The testes undergo degenerative changes, the viable spermatozoa diminish, and the volume and viscosity of semen decrease. In men, sexual energy gradually declines; achieving an erection takes longer, but it is sustained longer. Stress, however, can significantly diminish function (Rice, 2000).

Mortality Rates

The leading causes of death during middle adulthood are heart disease, lung cancer, cerebrovascular disease, breast

AGES 25 TO 44 YEARS
Unintentional injuries 27,129
Cancer 21,706
Heart disease 16,513

AGES 45 TO 64 YEARS
Cancer 131,743
Heart disease 101,235
Unintentional injuries 17,521

AGE 65 YEARS AND OLDER
Heart disease 606,913
Cancer 382,913
Stroke 140,366

From Centers for Disease Control and Prevention, National Center for Health Statistics, National Vital Statistics Systems. (1999). Washington, DC: Centers for Disease Control and Prevention, U.S. Government Printing Office; U.S. Department of Health and Human Services. (2000). *Healthy People 2010* (p. 23). Washington, DC: U.S. Government Printing Office.

cancer, and colorectal cancer (Box 23-1). Reducing disabilities and deaths from these chronic conditions are national health-promotion and disease prevention objectives (USDHHS, 2000) (*Healthy People 2010* box).

Many of these diseases are preventable, entirely or in part, through behavior changes. Middle adults can influence their own health and that of their children through a healthier lifestyle and primary care (Buttaro, Trybulski, Bailey, & Sandberg-Cook, 2003).

Gender and Marital Status

Male mortality rates have always been higher than female rates for the leading causes of death, with the exception of diabetes. Women live approximately 6 years longer on average than do men. White women have the greatest life expectancy, and black women's life expectancy is now longer than that of white men. Adults in households with annual incomes greater than $25,000 live 3 to 7 years longer on average than do those in households with less than $10,000 income (USDHHS, 2000). The death rate of middle-age men from cardiovascular diseases plays a major part in this disparity. The incidence of lung cancer, however, continues to decrease slowly for men (81.6 per 100,000) and increase for women (41.4 per 100,000), primarily because of the changing smoking and work patterns of women.

Mortality rates also vary with gender. Death rates are lowest among married men and highest in divorced men. Single, widowed, and divorced middle-age men generally demonstrate a higher mortality rate than do those who are married.

Chronic and degenerative diseases are less pronounced in women. The primary cause of death for both genders over age 45 is heart disease. Women are more likely than men to have arthritis, colitis, and gallbladder disease. Men, conversely, have an increased likelihood of developing ulcers, hernias, and emphysema. Injuries are also more common in men.

Race and Gender

Black Americans are the largest minority race (12.8 %) in the nation. The real risk for many diseases is higher in black adults. Between ages 25 and 64, for instance, they have a cerebrovascular accident (stroke) rate nearly 2.5 times that of white adults (USDHHS, 2000). Race is also considered to be one of the risk factors in hypertension (Joint National Committee, 2003; USDHHS, 2000). Black men have an increased incidence of and mortality rates from cancers of the lung, colon and rectum, prostate, and esophagus. Black women are more likely to die of breast and colon cancer than are any other group. Hispanics have higher rates of cervical, esophageal, gallbladder, and stomach cancers (USDHHS, 2000). The differences between the cancer rates in blacks and whites have been related partly to blacks residing in lower socioeconomic areas, which tends to increase their exposure to industrial carcinogens. The educational opportunities available to blacks in urban areas may also be limited, contributing to a lack of knowledge of risk factors, significant signs and symptoms of disease, preventive self-care, and the location of health care resources (Research Highlights box).

In looking at the major causes of death in middle-age adults, the three leading causes in both white and black populations are the same: heart disease, cancer, and cerebrovascular accidents. Although the primary cause of death for both genders over age 44 continues to be heart disease, the death rate is declining. Women continue to have poorer outcomes than do men. The rate of women who die within a year after a myocardial infarction (heart attack) is 44%, whereas only 27% of men die. The heart disease death rate is higher in black Americans than it is in white Americans (USDHHS, 2000). Blacks have the highest rate of stroke among all population groups, with a death rate approximately 80% higher than that of white Americans (USDHHS, 2000) (Figure 23-1).

Genetics

The middle-age adult is at greater risk than is the young adult for diseases known to be associated with genetics (familial characteristics), including diabetes, hypertension, Huntington chorea, arteriosclerosis, gout, obesity, heart disease, and alcoholism.

Some malignancies tend to be hereditary; for example, women with a personal or family history of breast cancer have an increased risk. Additionally, individuals with a family history of colorectal cancer, rectal or colon polyps, or ulcerative colitis are at high risk for colorectal cancer.

Healthy People 2010

Selected National Health-Promotion and Disease Prevention Objectives for the Middle-Age Adult

Overall Goals

1. Increase the quality of life and years of healthy life.
2. Eliminate health disparities.

Objectives

1. Improve access to quality health services.
   - Increase the proportion of people with health insurance to 100% (baseline* is 86% of adults).
   - Increase the proportion of adults who have a specific source of ongoing care (baseline is 84% of adults).
2. Reduce the overall cancer death rate to 158.7 per 100,000 population (baseline is 201.4 per 100,000 population).
3. Reduce new cases of diabetes to 2.5 per 1000 people (baseline is 2.1 new cases per 1000 people).
4. Increase the proportion of adults with disabilities reporting satisfaction with life to 96% (baseline is 87%).
5. Increase the quality, availability, and effectiveness of educational and community-based programs designed to prevent disease and improve health and quality of life.
6. Promote health for all through a healthy environment.
7. Increase the proportion of pregnancies that are intended to 70% (baseline is 51% of pregnancies were unintended).
8. Reduce increases in food-borne illness.
9. Use communication strategically to improve health.
10. Reduce coronary heart deaths to 166 per 100,000 population (baseline is 208 deaths per 100,000 population).
11. Reduce new cases of AIDS among adolescents and adults to 1 per 100,000 population (baseline is 19.5 new cases per 100,000 population).
12. Reduce indigenous cases of vaccine-preventable diseases.
13. Reduce injuries, disabilities, and deaths from accidents and violence.
14. Improve the health and well-being of women, infants, children, and families.
15. Improve mental health and ensure access to appropriate, quality mental health care.
16. Increase the proportion of adults who are at a healthy weight to 60% (baseline is 42% of all adults).
17. Reduce work-related injuries for full-time workers to 4.6 per 100 (baseline is 6.6 injuries per 100 workers) and deaths to 3.2 per 100,000 workers (baseline is 4.5 deaths per 100,000 workers).
18. Increase the proportion of adults who engage regularly, preferably daily, in moderate physical activity for at least 30 minutes per day to 30% (baseline is 15%).
19. Reduce asthma deaths of adults ages 35 to 64 years to 9 per 1 million (baseline is 17 asthma deaths per 1 million).
20. Promote responsible sexual behaviors, including preventing sexually transmitted diseases.
21. Reduce substance abuse to protect the health, safety, and quality of life for all people.
22. Reduce tobacco use by adults to 12% (baseline is 24% of adults).
23. Increase the proportion of people who have a dilated eye examination at appropriate intervals.

From U.S. Department of Health and Human Services. (2000). *Healthy People 2010*. Washington, DC: U.S. Government Printing Office.
*Baseline year for all objectives is 2000.
Note: Target and baseline data identified when available.
AIDS, acquired immunodeficiency syndrome.

Health Care of Women in Rural Areas

Over 14,000 Australian women ages 45 to 50 are participating in the Australian Longitudinal Study on Women's Health. The purpose of this study is to track their health for 20 years. Women from rural and remote areas are deliberately overrepresented in the sample.

To date the women living in the rural and remote areas rate their health as similar to that of women in urban areas, but they have (1) significantly fewer visits to general practitioners, (2) significantly more visits to alternative health care providers, (3) lower levels of stress, (4) higher frequency of being overweight, and (5) fewer gynecological surgeries compared with women from urban areas.

Future follow-up studies will continue to explore the health and health care of these women.

Data from Brown, W. J., Young, A. F., & Byles, J. E., (1999). Journey of distance? The health of mid-age women living in five geographical areas of Australia. *Australian Journal of Rural Health, 7*(3), 148-154.

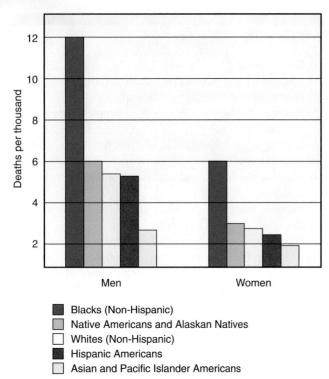

Figure 23-1 U.S. death rates in 1992, ages 45 to 55, by ethnic group, per 1000. (From U.S. Department of Health and Human Services. [2000]. *Healthy people 2010.* Washington, DC: U.S. Government Printing Office.)

GORDON'S FUNCTIONAL HEALTH PATTERNS

Health Perception–Health Management Pattern

To promote health in the middle-age adult, the nurse performs a health assessment that includes the person's values and beliefs, lifestyle patterns, general perceptions of health, and health practices.

Habits

The self-destructive habits of the middle-age adult that have been practiced for years (cigarette smoking, excessive alcohol use, and overeating) begin to have visible consequences. As pressures increase, adults are tempted to turn to substances such as these as a crutch for coping with stress. Prevention is extremely important, primarily because withdrawal from any of these substances is a difficult process.

Risk Factors

The major risk factors for adults in the middle years are environmental and behavioral; they can be changed through teaching, counseling, and other nursing interventions (USDHHS, 2000). Helping adults to take care of themselves and to change, when indicated, can be accomplished on an individual or group basis.

Some of the health-promotion needs of the middle-age adult include acceptance of aging, the need to exercise, and weight control. Decreasing or stopping cigarette smoking and alcohol consumption can also be identified needs. Preventive health screening is vital. The adult needs input into and control of as many of these behaviors as possible.

Total health risks of middle-age adults are composed of group risks (age, gender, race) and personal risks (Flowers & McLean, 1996; Pender, 1996a, 1996b). Precritical secondary prevention includes periodic selective screening for the detection of disease before it becomes clinically apparent, such as performing breast self-examination. A suggested screening examination appears in Box 23-2.

Chronic conditions are defined as those that last for more than 3 months. Approximately 20% of the population age 45 to 64 reports limitations caused by chronic conditions (Lubkin & Larsen, 2002). A significant increase is seen between the ages of 45 and 64. Chronic conditions found in the middle-age adult include heart conditions, arthritis, impairments of the back and spine, chronic obstructive lung disease, diabetes, mental and nervous conditions, and dental disease (Lubkin & Larsen, 2002). Diseases and behaviors for which screening is recommended in the middle-age adult are listed in **Web Site Resource 23A.**

Nutritional-Metabolic Pattern

Dietary factors are correlated with 5 of the 10 leading causes of death in the United States: coronary heart disease, some cancers, stroke, non–insulin-dependent diabetes mellitus, and atherosclerosis (USDHHS, 2000).

Physical activities and nutritional patterns frequently are correlated. The middle-age adult typically leads a more sedentary lifestyle than does the young adult, primarily because of increased responsibilities at work and home and the many convenience devices that infiltrate homes and workplaces. Obesity tends to occur in women (30% to 40%) more than in men (20% to 30%) (Dunphy, 2004). Unfortunately, the less active adult usually fails to alter any dietary habits to compensate, so one of the major health problems of the middle years is obesity.

Obesity

Obesity is defined as a body mass index (BMI) of 30 kg/m^2 or more, and being overweight is a BMI over 27.8 kg/m^2 for adult males and 27.3 kg/m^2 for adult females. At least 127 million American adults are overweight, 60 million are obese; and 9 million are severely obese (American Obesity Association, 2004; Centers for Disease Control and Prevention, 2002; Flegal, Carroll, Ogden, & Johnson, 2002). The proposed target for obesity for 2010 is 15% of American adults (USDHHS, 2000).

"Overweight and obesity substantially raise the risk of illness from high blood pressure, high cholesterol, type 2 (non–insulin-dependent) diabetes, heart disease and stroke, gallbladder disease, arthritis, sleep disturbances and problems breathing, and endometrial, breast, prostate and colon cancers. Obese individuals may also suffer from social

Box **23-2** Screening Examination: Ages 35 to 65

DATABASE

Health history: initial update with nurse or PE
Health hazard appraisal: initial screening
Psychological inventories as needed

PHYSICAL EXAMINATION (EVERY 3 TO 5 YEARS UNTIL AGE 40, THEN ANNUALLY) EMPHASIZING

Weight and height
Blood pressure, pulse
Breasts
Pelvis
Prostate
Testicles
Eyes
Mouth
Skin

LABORATORY PROCEDURES

Pap smear
Hemoccult: three stools for Hemoccult with PE after age 50
Colonoscopy or sigmoidoscopy every 3 to 5 years after age 50 as indicated
Mammography screening at age 35 every 2 years, then yearly after age 50
Urinalysis: examined at the time of PE
Lipid profile (men ages 35 to 65; women ages 45 to 65)
Chest radiograph with PE if heavy smoker

Tetanus and diphtheria booster every 10 years
Influenza vaccine: follow current recommendations
Counseling and testing for HIV as indicated
Rubella serology (women of childbearing age)

SELF-CARE EDUCATION AND COUNSELING

With physical examination; individualized according to individual's risk factors
Injury prevention: seat-belts, helmets, firearms, smoke detectors
Stress reduction
Exercise
Diet: cholesterol, fat, sodium, fiber, multivitamins with folic acid (women of childbearing age)
Calcium
Breast self-examination
Testicular self-examination
Dental care
Mouth care
Sexually transmitted diseases
Contraception
Skin protection from ultraviolet light
Alcohol and other substance abuse
Smoking cessation
Possible hormone prophylaxis (perimenopausal and postmenopausal women)

Data from American Cancer Society (Massachusetts Division); U.S. Department of Health and Human Services. (2000). *Healthy people 2010.* Washington, DC: U.S. Government Printing Office.
PE, physician examination; *Pap,* Papanicolaou; *HIV,* human immunodeficiency virus.

stigmatization, discrimination, and lowered self-esteem" (USDHHS, 2000, p. 29). A study including approximately 7000 middle-age people (conducted 26 years ago) revealed that those who had a BMI between 18 and 25 felt better and had a better quality of life than people who were overweight (Davighis et al., 2003).

Women with less education and low incomes and black and Hispanic women are at an increased risk for being overweight. In addition to gender, race, and socioeconomic status, genetics may be a contributing factor. The most significant variables, however, are health behaviors, particularly food intake and exercise and activity patterns. Although an abundance of health information is available, these challenges persist.

As much as 40% of a typical American family's food budget is spent on food in restaurants or for take-out foods, both of which are usually higher in fat than foods prepared at home (USDHHS, 2000). Losing and maintaining weight may require an individual to change eating and activity behaviors, but the social and food preparation and consumption behaviors of the family must change, as well.

Prevention of obesity is the goal of weight management during the middle years. When the adult is obese, a clear-cut history of the onset is imperative. A lifelong history of obesity is significantly more arduous to alter than that of adult-onset obesity. A decrease in calories should be accompanied by at least 30 minutes of exercise 3 to 5 times a week. When calories are reduced and exercise is increased, weight loss is achieved and maintained.

Weight-management resources available to the adult are plentiful. Weight-management programs using behavior modification can be found in varied settings, such as universities and work sites, Weight Watchers, Overeaters Anonymous, and Take Off Pounds Sensibly. If the nurse identifies a need for weight management and no program is available, a self-help group can be initiated. Input should be solicited from concerned individuals regarding time and location of meetings. A suggested list of topics generated by the group can be assembled. A discussion of basic nutrition with appropriate handouts is a good place to start. Having adults write down their individual goals and keep a 1-week diet log is nonthreatening and helpful for future planning and also gives them some responsibility in the program.

High Saturated Fat Diet

Lipid levels and ratios have a significant influence on cardiovascular and cerebrovascular morbidity and mortality rates. The National Heart, Lung, and Blood Institute regards a blood cholesterol level below 200 mg/dl as desirable. However, the mean cholesterol level for American adults is 206 mg/dl, and approximately 50 million adults in this country are estimated to have blood cholesterol levels that place them at high risk for coronary heart disease and cerebrovascular disease. The Coronary Primary Prevention Trial demonstrates that men at high risk are able to reduce coronary heart disease by approximately 2% for every 1% lower blood cholesterol level. By reducing their intake of saturated fat, total fat, and dietary cholesterol and by normalizing their weight and increasing physical activity, some people can lower their high blood cholesterol levels. Medications are available for those whose blood cholesterol levels remain significantly elevated despite diet modification (USDHHS, 2000).

Calcium

Adequate calcium intake is essential for developing and maintaining bone mass. Additionally, **calcium** is needed for other physiological processes, including muscle contraction and blood pressure regulation. Men and women need a minimal daily intake of 1000 milligrams of calcium. Pregnant and nursing women need 1200 milligrams, and postmenopausal women need either 1000 milligrams (when taking estrogen) or 1500 milligrams (when not taking estrogen). Vitamin D enhances the absorption of calcium (Karch, 2003). When the daily intake of calcium is less than 400 milligrams per day, an adequate serum calcium level will be maintained by leaching calcium from bone, resulting in **osteoporosis.** Exercise also contributes to bone mass by increasing mechanical stress on the bones.

Food Additives

A great deal of controversy surrounds food additives and their relationships to disease, specifically cancer. Sodium nitrate, for example, is used in the preservation of bacon, ham, and smoked meats; butylated hydroxytoluene is found in cereal and potato chips. Saccharin, used in low-calorie foodstuffs, carries a warning label and has been determined to cause cancer in laboratory animals. Studies thus far have been conducted only on laboratory animals and are inconclusive. Importantly, malignancies can take years to develop; many additives have been in use for short periods, so long-term outcomes are unknown (USDHHS, 2000).

Caffeine

Caffeine is a popular stimulant found in coffee, tea, and some soft drinks, such as colas. Caffeine prolongs the amount of time that physical work can be performed and appears to decrease boredom and increase attention span. On the negative side, coffee has come under significant scrutiny from the media recently, with reports of a link between cancer of the pancreas and coffee consumption. There is controversy as to whether daily moderate intake of caffeine has any detrimental effects.

Like alcohol and nicotine, caffeine is readily available and has become an accepted part of daily living. Because caffeine is a strong stimulant with effects that typically are taken for granted, its importance as an addictive substance must be emphasized. Ingestion of 0.5 grams of caffeine (3 to 4 cups of coffee) can increase the basal metabolic rate an average of 10%, and possibly as much as 25% for some people.

Long-term stimulation of the central nervous system results in restlessness, sleep disturbances, cardiac stimulation, and withdrawal effects. Nurses' assessment should screen for stimulating and addicting substances that may be producing these symptoms.

High-Sodium Diet

High-sodium diets play a significant role in hypertension, especially when consumed over many years. The result may be an increase in total body fluids, which increases peripheral vascular resistance. Salt contains approximately 40% sodium and is a contributing factor for hypertension in the 10% to 20% of Americans who are at risk. On average, Americans consume 4 to 5 grams of sodium per day. A major contributor of dietary sodium is the salt found in processed foods.

Over the past 3 decades, many clinical studies have demonstrated the effectiveness of lowering blood pressure by lowering dietary sodium. Other studies have described the relationships between urinary and sodium excretion and the change of blood pressure with age (Joint National Committee, 2003).

Alcohol Abuse

Substance abuse can be a devastating habit. Many adults abuse prescription and illicit drugs and, especially, alcohol.

Initially alcohol appears to be a stimulant, but actually it is a central nervous system depressant and anesthetic. Chronic alcohol use produces tolerance, thereby necessitating gradually increasing doses to achieve the same effect. Alcohol contributes to problems with safety because of decreased reaction time and depression of the central nervous system.

Alcohol is frequently treated as a nondrug, but alcohol addiction is second only to nicotine addiction. Alcohol is readily available, reasonably inexpensive, and considered a part of social exchange; its long-range physiological and psychological effects are well documented. In the United States, two thirds of adults consume alcohol, and 18 million are problem drinkers. Presently men outnumber women as alcohol abusers by approximately 5 : 1, but this ratio is decreasing. Alcohol abuse is associated with motor vehicle accidents, homicides, suicides, drowning, heart disease, cancer, liver disease, pancreatitis, and fetal alcohol syndrome, a major cause of mental retardation in children (USDHHS, 2000). The alcoholic person is at greater risk for cancer of the larynx, oral cavity, and liver.

Since World War II, the number of female alcoholics has increased. Women drink primarily in relation to life crises to relieve loneliness, feelings of inferiority, and gender role conflicts at home and at work. This situation occurs in all social classes and crosses all lifestyles. Interestingly, 9 of 10 husbands leave alcoholic wives, whereas 9 in 10 wives remain with their alcoholic husbands. The alcoholic woman is likely to abuse other substances, as well; her family is likely to protect her and themselves from public exposure, delaying necessary treatment.

The alcoholic may complain of symptoms such as heartburn and gas, stomach distention, poor eating habits, nausea and vomiting, gastric pain, irritation of the mouth, throat, and esophagus, and right upper quadrant pain. Two additional subtle findings are spider angiomata and palmar erythema.

Primary prevention for substance and alcohol abuse is complex, especially because adults consume these agents for many reasons, including peer pressure, loneliness, alienation, frustration, anxiety, and low self-esteem. Heavy drinkers may also be following the example established by influential people in their lives. Merely telling people about the potential physical, emotional, and legal hazards appears to have little effect as a preventive measure. Promoting more realistic portrayals of substance abuse through the media is difficult to implement. Although techniques such as assertiveness training and teaching adults to resist persuasion are helpful, more useful approaches might include helping them learn to manage anxiety and increase their self-esteem. Less anxious and more confident people have greater skills in resisting peer influences to participate in substance abuse; they also are more likely to have fewer episodes of isolation and loneliness.

Early detection and intervention can decrease ongoing and future physical and psychosocial problems resulting from alcohol abuse. Nurses use a variety of screening strategies to identify individuals' perceptions and consequences of drinking. The CAGE questionnaire is the most popular screening tool used in primary care (Dunphy, 2004). The Michigan alcohol screening test (*http://www.ncadd-sfvorg/symptoms/mast_test.html*) and alcohol use disorders identification test (*http://www.niaaa.nih.gov/publications/audit.htm*) are examples of other screening instruments.

Abnormal laboratory test results, including elevations in aspartate aminotransferase, erythrocyte mean corpuscular volume, and serum glutamyltransferase, are not adequately sensitive and specific and may be a result of other causes including trauma, disease, and medications.

A variety of treatments are known to be effective, but no single "best" intervention has been identified. Effective treatments may be to address other problems using tools such as stress management, individual and family therapy, and supportive environments.

Although alcohol consumption per person has gradually decreased since 1981, 72% of adult women and 74% of adult men continue to exceed the recommended guidelines for low-risk drinking, with the 2010 target at 50% (USDHHS, 2000).

Gingivitis

Gingivitis is common among adults who fail to brush their teeth and use dental floss regularly. Redness and swelling develop around the teeth. Bleeding of the gums while brushing the teeth is an early sign of gingivitis. The gums may or may not be tender. When inflammation is not adequately treated and controlled, **periodontitis** involving bone destruction can develop, in addition to tooth loss.

Regular oral hygiene and care are major factors in maintaining oral health. However, less than one half of Americans receive regular oral health care. Middle-age adults have responsibility not only for their own care, but also for the care of their children and elderly parents. Low income is a risk factor (USDHHS, 2000). Untreated dental decay and tooth loss are higher in blacks, Hispanics, and Native American–Alaska Natives compared with the total American adult population (USDHHS, 2000). Regularly scheduled dental care with a dentist and dental hygienist is highly recommended.

Elimination Pattern

Aging brings a gradual decrease of tone in the large intestine. As mentioned, this change, accompanied by a sedentary lifestyle and lack of bulk in the diet, predisposes the adult to constipation. Mass media advertising strongly encourage the population to rely on external controls rather than on exercise and dietary means to solve this problem. Consequently, many adults are dependent on taking fiber products as well as laxatives for regular bowel movements.

As discussed, degenerative changes in the nephron units occur during the middle-age years. Usually, however, the middle-age adult does not have any appreciable kidney malfunction. When a woman has had multiple births and little exercise, she may begin experiencing stress incontinence during this time, which can be socially embarrassing (Newman & Giovannini, 2002).

Activity-Exercise Pattern

Regular physical activity increases life expectancy and quality of life. It can help prevent and manage coronary heart disease, hypertension (American Obesity Association, 2004), diabetes, osteoporosis, and depression. Physical exercise has been correlated with lower rates of osteoporosis (National Osteoporosis Foundation, 1998), back injury, stroke, and colon cancer. Effective weight loss programs that incorporate physical activities also make significant contributions to increased life expectancy and quality of life (Kriketos, Sharp, Seagle, Peters, & Hill, 2000; USDHHS, 2000).

Despite these benefits, few American adults engage in regular physical activity for 30 minutes, 3 to 5 times a week, as recommended. Only a fraction of adults perform the recommended level, and slightly more report no leisure-time physical activities. By age 75, one in three men and one in two women engage in none. Sedentary behavior increases with age (USDHHS, 2000). Continuous, rhythmic exercise maintained for a sufficient period to stress the cardiac system is desirable (Dunn et al., 1999). Some suggested activities include brisk walking, jogging, swimming, bicycling, and skipping rope. Activities that focus on skill and coordination should be attempted by the adult over age 40 rather than activities necessitating speed and strength. Moderation is the key, along with increased caution as the adult approaches age 65. Overexertion, evidenced by symptoms of dizziness, tightness in the chest, and unresolving breathlessness, should be avoided.

The nurse initiates an exercise program with the middle-age adult by asking what activities have been enjoyed in the past. When these activities are realistic today, the nurse encourages the individual to rediscover them; when they appear unrealistic, new options should be explored. Additionally, activities are selected with consideration of potential for injury. Anyone at risk for heart disease (heavy smoking, high blood pressure, family history, diabetes, or prolonged lack of exercise) should have a complete history and physical examination before developing a rigorous activity program. For some of these individuals, an exercise test is recommended. Proper equipment, including supportive shoes and thermally appropriate clothing, is also important.

To be health promoting, physical exercise involves as many muscles as is possible, performed on a regular basis. Adults should do 30 minutes or more of moderate-intensity (brisk) physical activity on most (or all) days of the week, for a total of 3 to 4 hours. The appropriate level of performance for aerobic exercise is determined by achieving a pulse rate that is established for each individual: taking the number 220, subtracting the person's age, and then computing 75% of that number (WebMD, n.d.). A 50-year-old person, for example, should not exceed a pulse rate of 128 ($[220 - 50] \times 0.75 = 128$).

Despite all these considerations, the kind of activity and style should be an individual choice and approached as something done for oneself and for fun, not as another chore or responsibility of middle age (Brownson et al., 2000).

Sleep-Rest Pattern

Rest is a frequently omitted consideration for middle-age adults, who spend less time in deep sleep and need less sleep overall than do young adults. This change may be interpreted as insomnia; therefore, middle-age adults may need reassurance that this is common. Regularly scheduled, quality sleep and occasional napping, when fatigued, are healthful guidelines (Jacobs, 1998; National Sleep Foundation, 1998).

Cognitive-Perceptual Pattern

The notion that at age 21 adults reach their peak and that "it is all downhill after that" is a myth. Continued learning is found throughout adulthood in such areas as reasoning, vocabulary, and spatial perception. Decreases can be observed, however, in reaction time and cognitive flexibility.

Box **23-3**	Developmental Tasks of Middle Age

1. Helping children become responsible, happy adults
2. Rediscovering or developing new satisfaction in the relationship with one's spouse (for the single adult, this can occur in a relationship with a sibling or significant other)
3. Developing an affectionate, but independent, relationship with aging parents
4. Reaching the peak in one's career
5. Achieving mature social and civic responsibility
6. Accepting and adapting to biological changes
7. Maintaining or developing friendships
8. Developing leisure-time activities

Intellectual Ability

"Learning" intelligence accumulates through education and life experiences and continues to increase throughout life, as evidenced by the many scholars and artists who are more productive in their middle years than they were as young adults.

The theories of Havighurst, Piaget, and Bloom are relevant to the middle-age adult. These theorists conclude that the prime time to be in the learner role is when the developmental task for that role is to be accomplished. The adult in the middle years as the learner-performer is a case in point. For example, to balance the responsibilities of caring for children and parents and working, the adult may explore new career options or creative endeavors.

Havighurst defines developmental tasks as the basic tasks of living that must be achieved if the adult is to live successfully. These tasks are dictated by the expectations of society, the physiological changes of the body throughout life, and the individual's own value system and goals. Although initially described in the 1950s, Havighurst and Orr's developmental tasks of middle age remain timely (Havighurst & Orr, 1956) (Box 23-3).

If career goals have been previously identified, then reaching them can be highly rewarding, both psychologically and financially. In addition to career activities, the mature adult has an increased social awareness and assumes more civic responsibility.

In Piaget's theory of cognitive development, formal operations is the final period. This stage begins at approximately age 12 and continues throughout life. Piaget describes the thoughts of adults as being both flexible and effective. The adult can deal efficiently with complex problems of reasoning, including hypothesis testing (Piaget, 1970).

Bloom (1984) developed a hierarchy of cognitive levels in the adult learner. Knowledge is the simplest cognitive level; the adult learner understands and can recall specifics. For example, the individual defines high blood pressure in lay terms.

Comprehension is the second level, as indicated by the learner grasping the meaning of the communicated message and relating it to other material. For example, the individual can state one way that obesity influences high blood pressure.

The third level is application. At this level the learner applies knowledge in the form of abstractions and ideas to concrete situations. For example, the hypertensive person begins a weight reduction and exercise program.

In analysis, the fourth level, the adult breaks down material into its constituent parts while noting their relationships. For example, the individual identifies values and life goals in determining actions to be taken for meeting health care needs.

The final levels, synthesis and evaluation, are at times difficult to achieve. The person is able to combine various elements to form a plan and then judge the extent to which the ideas, materials, and so on satisfy the established criteria. For example, people may develop plans to improve their health care and increase their self-care responsibilities. In turn, they may validate their ongoing health care programs in relation to the expected outcomes that they formulated. Genetic, environmental, and personality factors in early and middle adulthood account for the large difference in the ways in which individuals maintain mental abilities. Schaie (1994) has identified seven of these factors that maintain cognitive function in later life:

1. Absence of chronic diseases
2. Living with favorable socioeconomic factors, including maximal occupational complexity, a low degree of routine, and an intact family
3. Involvement in complex social activities
4. Flexible personality style
5. Marriage to a spouse with high cognitive function
6. Maintaining high levels of performance speed
7. Personal satisfaction with accomplishments in midlife and early old age

Perceptual Changes

Presbyopia (farsightedness) is common in middle-age adults, even in individuals who have had no previous vision problems. This condition is corrected easily with lenses, which may be needed only for reading or close work. Other visual conditions that may not allow for ready correction include decreased peripheral vision and decreased visual sensitivity in the dark. Both conditions are a result of the cornea becoming less transparent, and both are slow and subtle in development. Because all of these conditions are not readily detected by the individual, middle-age adults should undergo a routine professional eye examination every year. **Glaucoma** is a result of increased intraocular pressure, which can damage the optic nerve. Damage to the optic nerve is irreversible, but vision loss can be prevented if damage is identified early. Peripheral vision is affected. Cataracts, opacity of the lens, can develop and cloud the vision in later years of middle age, especially in people who have diabetes. Diabetic retinopathy gradually causes rupture

of vessels in the retina, which leak into the eye, causing lack of color differentiation and central vision changes.

Another common perceptual change in middle age is **presbycusis** (impaired auditory acuity). The first sounds to be lost are higher frequencies, such as a woman's voice. This is important in the work environment and social interaction. Because this process is subtle, middle age is a time for auditory evaluations as a part of routine examinations.

Beginning in the middle years, the sense of taste also diminishes. A progressive loss of taste buds occurs, first affecting those located more anteriorly, which detect sweet and salt, and then the posterior taste buds, which detect bitter and sour. Consequently this change can alter a person's food preferences and present problems for people who insist on adding salt to make up for the deficit. Nurses can suggest using various herbs and spices to enhance flavor.

Self-Perception–Self-Concept Pattern
Levinson's Theory

In Levinson's research on men (1986a, 1986b) and women (1996), a theory on "individual life structures" is posed. Levinson describes age-associated *seasons* or *eras*. The midlife transition, beginning at ages 38 to 40 years, appears to include reappraising one's life, integrating the polarities, and modifying one's life structure toward being who one wants to be. Middle-age adults struggle with meaning, value, and direction of their lives.

Erikson's Theory

In Erikson's eight stages of the life cycle (1986), the last three stages are related to adulthood. Stage 7, generativity versus stagnation or self-absorption, most frequently is associated with the middle-age years.

Erikson identifies **generativity** as the primary task during this stage. Generativity includes a sense of productivity and creativity, as evidenced by reaching previously established goals (Hornstein, 1986; Reifman, Biernat, & Lang, 1991; Thomas, 1995). Generativity also encompasses a desire to care for others and is the opposite of **stagnation,** which is the result of a lack of accomplishment during middle-age's developmental tasks, and self-absorption, the tendency to direct most of one's interest and attention to oneself, thereby excluding others.

Middle age is a time of critical self-review, and some people are sad and disappointed in themselves and their accomplishments. Both women and men question their value to society, the merit of their accomplishments, their success as sexual beings, and the probability of attaining unfilled life goals. Women generally make this life assessment between ages 35 and 50, whereas men do not usually begin until approximately age 40. Because the male life assessment tends to come late, there is a potential problem for couples of approximately the same age. Women begin looking at changes they may want to make in their lives, whereas men remain content with the status quo. This type of self-evaluation and lack of effective communication

Skin Health Care for Middle-Age Adults

Wrinkling, xerosis (dry skin), and lentigines (sun spots, liver spots, age spots) begin to be more evident during the forties and fifties, sometimes being manifested even earlier depending on individual amounts of sun exposure, skin irritation, and genetics. Sloughing of the stratum corneum with aging has been projected to happen about twice as quickly as one reaches middle age. There also are changes occurring in the fat and dermis layers that begin around age 40. This causes sagging as the layers separate from each other.

Some middle-age individuals have one or more benign lesions called *seborrheic keratoses,* which are brown or black wartlike papules. Precancerous lesions such as actinic keratoses begin to manifest during the forties, and skin malignancies are more common with aging. There are about 400,000 new cases of basal cell carcinoma each year. These lesions typically occur on sun-exposed areas and have a 99% cure rate with treatment. There are 100,000 new cases of squamous cell carcinoma diagnosed every year. These lesions also have a high cure rate if treated.

Many people use over-the-counter antiaging creams, lotions, sprays, and pills to moisturize and revitalize their skin. For these products to be effective, they must contain at least 5% to 10% α-hydroxy acids (Kucera, 2004). Eye cream should not contain oil but must have antioxidants such as coenzyme Q10 and an antiinflammatory agent such as vitamin C (Kucera, 2004). Creams containing collagen are not effective, because collagen cannot penetrate the skin. People need to be educated on these over-the-counter products.

Botox (botulism toxin A), a neurotoxin, is effective in managing wrinkles for 4 to 6 months. Another prescriptive treatment is tretinoin (Retin-A), which will decrease pigmented areas such as age spots and hyperkeratosis.

Kucera, K. (2004). Managing common skin problems in the elderly. *The Clinical Advisor, 7*(6), 23-30.

of personal needs to the spouse is a threat to marriage stability (Erikson, 1986; Vaillant & Vaillant, 1990).

Physiological Changes

The effect of physiological changes on mental health is nearly as critical during middle age as it is during adolescence. Some of the most obvious changes that influence self-esteem are graying hair, wrinkles, decreased visual and auditory acuity, and changes in body shape (Hot Topics box). The extent to which these changes are tolerated depends largely on the person's level of self-satisfaction and acceptance. Some people try to "hold on" to youth by dressing as more youthful counterparts dress, whereas others adapt their attire to their age and position in life (Erikson, 1986; Lancaster & King, 1985; Schiff & Parson, 1996).

Although controversial, some researchers believe that hormonal changes during middle age lead to behaviors in

men that represent what menopause does to women. In women, estrogen supplies begin to decrease; the loss of estrogen is thought to be responsible for the hot flashes and the mood changes that often occur (Northrup, 2001). The concomitant emotional aspect of menopause appears to be related to the personality of the individual. Women who have a positive self-concept and have coped effectively in the past are less prone to experience the full range of psychological symptoms that are often associated with menopause (Boston Women's Health Book Collective, 1999). The most common changes include emotional lability (excess or frequently changing emotions), nervousness and anxiety, insomnia, fatigue, and depression. Women need information in making decisions about estrogen supplements, including research on cardiac health, osteoporosis, and breast cancer (Northrup, 2001). Many feel that any estrogen supplementation is risky due to the findings of the Prempro arm of the Women's Health Initiative. This was a study of 16,608 women that ended in 2002 after data showed those who took estrogen replacement therapy were experiencing a higher incidence of breast cancer, heart attacks, strokes, and other thromboembolic events than those who took a placebo. Data further revealed that the women on estrogen experienced less colorectal cancer and osteoporosis (Seaman, 2003).

Similarly, men frequently experience physical and psychological reactions to middle age. The hormonal changes in men are gradual, typically beginning between ages 40 and 55. The symptoms are similar to those experienced by women, with the emotional effects related to other life events, past coping patterns, and general feelings of self-esteem.

Roles-Relationships Pattern

Craig (1989) notes that middle age is frequently a time of reassessment, turmoil, and change. This time has been called **midlife crisis.** The turning point occurs for several reasons. Middle-age adults recognize that their physical agility is decreasing; the inevitability of one's own death is recognized, perhaps for the first time. Lifestyle choices have been made and are less flexible than are those made at age 25. The adult identifies mistakes made in the past.

Family

Duvall and Miller (1984) delineate eight stages of the family life cycle, with stages 5, 6, and 7 in the middle years (see Chapter 7):

Stage 5: families with children, with the oldest child age 13 to 20; lasts approximately 7 years

Stage 6: families launching young adults, from the first leaving until the last; lasts approximately 8 years

Stage 7: families from empty nest to retirement; lasts approximately 15 years

The developmental tasks identified for the families in stages 6 and 7 are similar to those of Havighurst; they focus on changes from a nuclear family to a marital couple with other responsibilities. For example, in stage 6, the parents who are helping their children become independent may also be caring for their aging parents. Additionally, middle-age adults fulfill multiple complex responsibilities within a variety of career, social, and civic positions.

These transitions can be even more challenging for the family headed by a single parent (most typically the mother), which is true of over 10 million American households (out of a total of 35 million). The single most significant health risk in families headed by a single mother is poverty. Nearly one half of all of these families live in poverty, and the median family income for families with two parents is 3 times that of a family headed by a single mother. These inadequate resources make it extremely difficult for middle-age mothers, who are frequently raising grandchildren as well, to fulfill their responsibilities.

Families with young adolescent or young adult children have been described in research studies as both *postparental* and *launching families*. In contrast, criticism of this emphasis on the separation of children (regardless of age) from their families is increasing. Gilligan (1982) criticizes the work of many human development theorists who identify human development in terms of separation from the family. Apter (1991) also challenges the conventional view that adolescent girls must reject their mothers as part of a healthy development. Middle-age parents are encouraged to continue to care for and nurture their adolescent and adult children while recognizing the increasing interdependence of their relationships.

Although many adolescent and young adult children move out of their homes of origin to complete educational or career training, create their own living arrangement, or pursue a career, almost 16 million families had at least one child older than 18 years living at home in 2003, an increase of 7% since 1995 and of 14% since 1985 (USA Today, 2005). Many children of families in these age groups remain dependent on parental help for many more years.

By supporting their children's efforts, parents can increase the self-esteem of their children while being effective role models. The parent assumes less of a parent-child relationship, interacting more on an adult-to-adult level. As the children are "launched," the parents may have uninterrupted time alone and time to share activities. Parents who remove too much care too quickly place their children at risk for depression, substance abuse, violence, and suicide (Silverstein & Rashbaum, 1995).

Family life may also be threatened by older children living at home, opposition to a child's partner, or the inability to establish satisfactory relationships with potential or actual partners or sons-in-law and daughters-in-law. For many parents, the idea of their children leaving home is anticipated with relief that the heavy care responsibilities of parenting are over or with dread over having to fill the void of time and inactivity. The empty nest syndrome may be exacerbated if the husband and wife have never learned to communicate effectively and to enjoy each other's company without the children.

At the other end of the family spectrum, aging parents can place demands on the adult child, primarily because elderly adults frequently are beset with health problems. A caring relationship is in order, in which the aging parent's need for independence is recognized.

Because of the society's emphasis on youth, the adult must associate feelings of self-worth with personal integrity rather than with bodily appearance or physical prowess. Friends of both genders can provide invaluable support systems. With the newly found free time after children have left home, the middle-age adult can share favorite activities and learn new ones. Middle-age adults should remind themselves how much and how well they are doing, especially considering the complexity of the demands placed on them. Never before in history have families pursued such varied and individual-oriented goals as they do today.

Although for many Americans the concept of family remains of major importance, the perceptions are different from those held by previous generations. Parents and children in most families are involved in numerous activities, as evidenced by a "let's-hurry-or-we'll-be-late" orientation. Even younger children frequently have schedules that must be met if they are to get to their dance, drama, play, or enrichment classes. None of these activities necessarily has a negative effect, but the cumulative influence places heavy demands on all family members. Additionally, many activities in which both children and adults are involved have a certain degree of competitiveness. For example, parents frequently get emotionally involved in the athletic activities of their children to the extent that the failure of a 6 year old to play a winning softball game causes a great deal of parental anguish. One only has to listen to the cheering of parents at a Little League baseball game to note whose self-esteem is at stake. Shouts of "Kill her," "Grab the third baseman," and so on do not tend to engender feelings of team spirit or a notion of playing for the sake of having a good time (Erikson, 1986).

Work

Perhaps the most common role that middle-age adults share is that of a worker. Much of their pride and sense of satisfaction is derived from their work. Work is equated with being "grown up"; one can easily recall the "What do you want to be when you grow up?" questioning of youth. Success and achievement are evaluated in terms of careers and family life. The work ethic still persists, especially with individuals born during the Great Depression and many of their offspring. Much of their conversation evolves from what they do, such as, "My name is Leslie Smith. I am a real estate agent." To be mature is to be a responsible, hardworking individual (Erikson, 1986). Research has shown that older adults are more satisfied with their jobs than are younger adults (Mottaz, 1987; Zeitz, 1990).

Middle-age adults make up most of the work force of 110 million people. Vocations play a major role in their levels of wellness. Approximately 10 million work-related injuries occur every year; 3 million of these are severe, including

HEALTH TEACHING Workplace Violence Plan

- Establish a workplace violence policy.
- Define conflict resolution methods.
- Establish and maintain communication between management and staff.
- Establish a threat-reporting process.

- Manage specific cases.
- Analyze the environment for the potential for violence.
- Debrief after incidents.
- Take corrective actions as soon as possible.

From Hinojosa, I. (1996). Taking control of violence in the workplace. *Advances in Nursing Practice, 11,* 36.

3400 to 11,000 deaths and 1.8 million totally disabling injuries (USDHHS, 2000).

More than 22% of fatal occupational injuries involve motor vehicles; other injuries include falls, nonvehicular injuries, blows, and electrocutions. Although the number of fatal injuries appears to be decreasing, work-related illness and injuries appear to be increasing (USDHHS, 2000). Workers in mining, agriculture, fire fighting, transportation, and construction are at an increased risk of dying from a work-related injury. Poor housekeeping and poor design predispose the worker to falls and other illnesses (USDHHS, 2000).

Many injuries that contribute significantly to the morbidity and mortality of adults can be prevented. Fixing faulty steps, repairing faulty electrical wires, and securing carpets are only a few of the many preventive measures.

Accidents are twice as high among smokers than among nonsmokers. Possible explanations include the loss of attention, the use of one hand for smoking, and irritation of the eyes. Other work-related problems include exposure to harmful substances resulting in lung diseases, cancers, and workplace violence (Health Teaching box).

The effect of life events on mental health depends on the personal strength of the individual, availability of supports, and the nature and number of events and their significance for the person. Three common examples of life events with potential disruptive effects are divorce, two or more jobs, and caring for aging parents. Their negative effects may be alleviated if assistance is provided early in the process of a change.

Two-or-More-Job Family: Family and Work Responsibilities

More and more women are in the workforce; many feel the necessity for financial gain, especially with the increased cost of living and college expenses. Other women, who are postmenopausal and have been separated from their last child, have a newfound freedom and begin or rediscover a career. The husband may be a support person in this venture or he may feel threatened by his wife's new pursuit. These role changes can be stressors to the family.

The relationship between marital status, with or without children at home, and employment status determines the psychological well-being of the woman in her middle years. The educated woman who is married, has children at home, and has not worked since her marriage is at an increased risk for psychological disturbances (McKinlay & McKinlay, 1988).

Historically women worked with their husbands within the family farm or business. Only in the few decades immediately after World War II did many middle-class white women stay at home while their husbands went to work. Currently women make up a significant portion of the workforce. Additionally, many women are able to become highly educated and motivated to pursue careers. Both men and women are increasingly taking jobs that do not end at 5:00 PM. The problems and challenges of the workplace are experienced at home as adults bring projects and problems home with them.

Job-related travel has also increased during the last few years for both men and women. Travel by either partner means additional responsibilities for the one who remains at home. Additionally, if one spouse travels far more than the other travels, feelings of resentment may develop, or the common ground for discussion of work events may be altered. The one who stays at home may feel "put upon" when the spouse is perceived as having fun. In contrast, travel is tiring and is not usually as exciting as it appears to observers. The traveling spouse can come home tired and irritable and desire peace and quiet, which may conflict with the expectations of other family members.

Men may feel threatened by highly successful and visible women. For some families, the post-World War II prototype was for the husband to support the family financially and gain status through achievements of work outside the home. As women gain recognition and acclaim for their career accomplishments, even the most "enlightened" man may experience twinges of envy and discomfort. Men have few role models in learning the ways to be a participant in a successful two-career family. Men may need as much, if not more, support than do women in adapting to contemporary family styles. Opportunities to discuss what it means to be a man in today's society can be helpful, such as in support groups with volunteers or professionals who provide services to various agencies and community resources.

In addition to the changes in women and the effect on families of each adult working at one more jobs, the nature of the parental work environment is critical to family coping ability. Work that is emotionally draining, particularly when it is filled with conflict, poses special threats to family stability. When parents come home tired, angry, or frustrated from their experiences at work, they likely have limited emotional support to share with other family members.

When people gain self-esteem from their jobs and generally enjoy going to work, they tend to experience less frustration and dissatisfaction with themselves and their positions, enabling them to give more of themselves to other members of the family (Reifman et al., 1991).

Middle age is important when looking at the career clock. Issues that need to be considered include midcareer changes and preretirement planning. Retirement is a major turning point; to many people, it is the transition from middle age to old age and the period of work to the period of leisure or different work.

Adults are working up to and beyond the age of retirement, and many are entering new careers later in life. As adults progress through the middle years, they become increasingly aware of the time remaining until retirement: "Can I readjust my goals?" "Is there disparity between where I am in my career and where I would like to be?" An example might be the 60-year-old veteran nightclub singer whose goal to cut a solo album remains to be achieved. The heightened awareness of age and the decreased likelihood of finding another suitable job can precipitate increased anxiety or depression in this singer.

Comprehensive health-promotion programs at the work site contain these elements: "(1) health education that focuses on skill development and lifestyle behavior change in addition to information dissemination and awareness building, preferably tailored to employees' interests and needs; (2) supportive social and physical work environments, including established norms for healthy behavior and policies that promote health and reduce the risk of disease, such as work site smoking policies, healthy nutrition alternatives in the cafeteria and vending services, and opportunities for obtaining regular physical activity; (3) integration of the work site program into the organization's administrative structure; (4) related programs, such as employee assistance programs; and (5) screening programs, preferably linked to medical care service delivery to ensure follow-up and appropriate treatment as necessary and to encourage adherence. Optimally, these efforts should be part of a comprehensive occupational health and safety program" (USDHHS, 2000, pp. 7-28). The efficacy of these programs is beginning to be documented (Van der Hek & Plomp, 1997).

Caring for Aging Parents

The needs of aging parents and of the adult's own children can create additional demands during the middle years. The middle-age adult can feel caught between one's children and one's parents. Both children and older parents can present unrealistic, excessive demands and be difficult to please.

Middle-age adults may be faced with having frail and ill parents live within their own family unit or placing them in a nursing home. These dilemmas are complicated by the reality that their parents are growing older and may not have long to live. The recognition of the parents' impend-

ing death heightens middle-age adults' awareness of their own aging and mortality.

Difficulties in caring for elderly parents can be somewhat lessened when potential situations are discussed before a crisis arises. This is particularly true when all members of the middle-adult family are working, space in their home is limited, and the community has few resources for the well or ill elderly adults. Although institutionalization is undesirable to many families, the care of ill, elderly parents may eventually require it. By anticipating these needs and preparing for them, middle-age children and their elderly parents can develop further meaningful relationships with one another.

Divorce

Divorce is a major disruption to the marriage and family and to each individual's short-term and long-term health. As the divorce rate has risen in recent years, individuals and families have been faced with new and multiple problems. When a divorce occurs, each family member must confront the necessity to examine and, in many cases, modify an accustomed style of living and adapting. In a 5-year study of 60 families with 131 children ranging from ages 3 to 18, Wallerstein and Kelly (1977) found the first year after a divorce to be the most difficult, and money constituted a major source of stress. The researchers initially thought that divorce is a time-limited crisis for all involved that taxes the usual coping mechanisms to the extent it does particularly because adults have diminished abilities to parent effectively during the acute stage of adjustment. Wallerstein and her colleagues have subsequently described long-term consequences of divorce (Wallerstein, 1991; Wallerstein & Johnston, 1990; Wallerstein, Lewis, & Blakeslee, 2000).

Death

Similar to divorce, death of a spouse can result in grieving for the loss of companionship and the lost planned-for future, free from the responsibilities of work and children. The surviving spouse may be unprepared to be single again and to live alone. The loneliness may be exacerbated by ill or dying peers or parents. Middle-age adults become increasingly aware of the finite nature of life, thinking not only of the number of years since birth, but also of the number of years left to live. The midlife review is a common outcome of this recognition.

Sexuality-Reproductive Pattern

Men and women can continue to have a satisfactory pattern of sexual functioning throughout the middle and older adult years. As they would in any other developmental phase, middle-age adults may need counseling to make health-promoting decisions about their sexual behaviors.

Unintended pregnancies are high in all ages of American women, but are the highest (77% of all pregnancies) in middle-age women. In contrast, women planning to have children during the fourth and fifth decades of life should know that fertility rates decrease and infant mortality rates increase, especially when mothers are age 44 years and older (USDHHS, 2000). Additionally, the maternal death rate in women 35 years and older is higher (16.1 per 100,000 live births) than for younger women (USDHHS, 2000).

Changes in the reproductive systems of men and women result in changes in sexual function throughout adulthood. During middle adulthood, sexual arousal is slower, orgasms are less intense, and a return to prearousal levels is more rapid, with men having longer refractory periods between erection and ejaculation. When a person continues to be sexually active, these functional changes occur over decades and are minimally noticeable until later in adulthood, unless external factors are present, such as the negative effects of some antihypertensive and antidepressant agents.

After menopause, many women enjoy sex more, especially because no risk of pregnancy exists. Conversely, menopause can bring many challenges to a woman. American culture values women largely for their youth, beauty, and childbearing ability. Middle-age women may confront their own aging for the first time and may be perplexed as to the symptomatic factors and possibly changing roles (Nachtigall, Nachtigall, & Heilman, 1999). Women can experience vaginal dryness, difficulty finding a partner, less interest in initiating sex, and longer times to reach orgasm. No data exist that report decreases in postmenopausal women's interest in and physical capacity for sex.

Although men and women frequently enjoy satisfactory sexual relationships throughout the middle adult years, men in their middle age are more vulnerable to sexual dysfunction than are women. Frequently, men first experience problems with premature ejaculation, impotence, and retrograde ejaculation between ages 40 and 50 (Dunphy, 2004).

Abnormal genital bleeding and secondary amenorrhea are common gynecological complaints that indicate serious physical problems. Abnormal genital bleeding is the most common reason for gynecological office visits by adult women. Although pregnancy and menopause are the most common causes of secondary amenorrhea, other conditions related to abnormal pregnancy, functional disorders, physiological changes, and pathological factors must be considered (Buttaro et al., 2003).

As in adolescents and young adults, sexually transmitted diseases continue to be major public health problems in the middle-age adult. Women and children bear an inordinate share of the burden: sterility, ectopic pregnancy, fetal and infant deaths, birth defects, and mental retardation. Cancer of the cervix can be linked to the sexually transmitted herpes 2 virus and human papillomavirus (HPV). As with many other health behaviors and diseases, the full effect on the life of an individual and family may not be realized until middle age. "Americans 50 years of age and older are a forgotten population at risk for HIV [human immunodeficiency virus] infection and AIDS and presently comprise 10% of reported cases of AIDS in the United States" (Johnson, Haight, & Benedict, 1998, p. 8). As a result, nurses are increasingly aware of the importance of taking a comprehensive sexual history and not missing the diagnosis of HIV infection. Nurses must practice universal precautions when caring for older adults in all settings, including offices, nursing homes, and home care. Each nurse should develop appropriate strategies to enhance communication about sexuality throughout the adult years. Adults need accurate information about sexual health promotion, including developmental changes, sexually transmitted diseases, and related treatment strategies to promote satisfying, responsible health behaviors (Flaskerud & Calvillo, 1991).

Coping-Stress Tolerance Pattern

Long-held myths about women during and after menopause were dispelled in a 5-year study of 2500 middle-age Massachusetts women. The following percentages of these women reported stress from children away from home (8.5%), children living at home (20.3%), children recently returned home (23.6%), husbands away from home (3.6%), husbands living at home (6.3%), and parents or in-laws receiving no care (13%), being cared for outside the woman's home (49.1%), and being cared for in the woman's home (52.7%). This study also found that stress was reduced by one half when the woman had someone close who provided emotional support and practical help (Carpenito-Moyet, 2004, McKinlay & McKinlay, 1988) (Case Study and Care Plan).

Kobasa (1979) studied the concept of hardiness that she identified as including control, commitment, and challenge. Her studies have strong clinical relevance, because they strive to answer the question, "Why do some people's illness progress while others improve despite both groups having similar level of stress?"

In a 45-year longitudinal study of 173 men, Vaillant and Vaillant (1990) found that the extent of tranquilizer use before age 50 was the most powerful negative predictor of both mental and physical health outcomes at age 65. Another important predictor for health outcomes was the maturity of defenses against stress (sublimation, anticipation, altruism, and humor).

Stress and Heart Disease

As reiterated throughout this chapter, heart disease is the leading cause of death in the middle-age adult. In landmark studies, Haynes, Levine, Scotch, Feinleib, and Kannel (1978) describe the relationship of psychosocial factors to coronary heart disease using the Framingham study (Haynes et al., 1978; Haynes, Feinleib, & Kannel, 1980). In the study, 24 measures of psychosocial stress were used. In men, aging worries correlated significantly with systolic and diastolic blood pressure values. Marital disagreement and personal worries correlated significantly with diastolic blood pressure. Both diastolic and systolic pressures correlated significantly with work changes and anxiety in employed women between 45 and 64 years of age. Anger

CASE STUDY

Graham A.

Graham A., a 47-year-old divorced woman, was diagnosed with stage 3 ovarian cancer 4 years ago, for which she had a total hysterectomy, bilateral salpingo-oophorectomy, omentectomy, lymphadenectomy, and tumor debulking followed by chemotherapy, consisting of cisplatin (Platinol), paclitaxel (Taxol), and doxorubicin (Adriamycin). She did well for 2 years and then moved back to her hometown near family and underwent three more rounds of second-line chemotherapy. She took on a less taxing job, bought a house, renewed old friendships, and became more involved with her two sisters and their families.

She developed several complications, including metastasis to the lungs. Then she could no longer work, drive, or care for herself. She had been told by her oncologist that there was nothing else that could be done and that she should consider entering a hospice. She met with her attorney and drew up an advance directive and completed her will. She decided to have hospice care at home and, with the help of her family, set up her first floor as a living and sleeping area. She was cared for by family members around the clock for about 3 days. Graham A. observed that she was tiring everyone out so much that they could not really enjoy each other's company. At this time she contacted the VNA to seek assistance. Her plan was to try to enjoy her family and friend's visits. After assessment the VNA nurse prioritized her problems to include fatigue and caregiver role strain. Other potential problem areas that may need to be incorporated into the care plan include anticipatory grieving and impaired comfort.

Reflective Questions

1. What are some of the stresses on her middle-age sisters and their families?
2. What resources are available to manage these stresses and support the sisters in caring for their dying sister?
3. Describe Graham A.'s feelings about dependency and loss of autonomy because she is unable to do her own activities of daily living any longer.

VNA, visiting nurse agency.

CARE PLAN

Caregiver Role Strain

(Related to Graham A. Case Study)

Nursing Diagnosis Risk for Caregiver Role Strain Related to Sister's Terminal Cancer

DEFINING CHARACTERISTICS

- Ms. A. and sisters are tired doing all of the daily care for Ms. A.
- Ms. A. and family are at a point where they are accepting Ms. A.'s terminal status.
- Ms. A. and family want to prepare for a death at home.

RELATED FACTORS

- Sisters are missing work and neglecting their own families.
- Sisters need assistance with Ms. A.

EXPECTED OUTCOMES

- Ms. A. and sisters will contact the VNA to assist in planning daily hospice care at home.

- VNA and family will plan realistic care.
- Ms. A. will have enjoyable time with sisters and friends.
- Sisters will have quality time to spend with Ms. A.
- Sisters will be able to voice their grief and anger about their sister's upcoming death.

INTERVENTIONS

- Home health aides are scheduled for 24 hours a day.
- Psychiatric nurse practitioner will meet with Ms. A. and family to schedule therapy time for anticipatory grieving.
- The sisters will meet with a support group for families involved in hospice care at home.
- A schedule will be made to allow each sister time at home, time with Ms. A., and rest.

VNA, visiting nurse association.

suppressed, anger discussed, tension, and anger symptoms correlated significantly with diastolic blood pressure in this age group.

Among white collar men in this age group, the Framingham type A and ambitiousness scales also correlated significantly with elevated diastolic blood pressure. The correlation of anger symptoms and anger discussed with diastolic pressures was significant for white collar women between ages 45 and 64. The initial findings by Haynes and her colleagues have been supported by many other studies, including those of Spielberger, Jacobs, Russell, and Crane

(1983), Kawachi, Sparrow, Spiro, Vokonas, and Weiss (1996), and Williams, Paton, Siegler, Eigenbrodt, Nieto, and Tyroler (2000).

The death of a parent enhances awareness of one's vulnerability to illness and death. The more opportunities and time people have to prepare for these stressful events, the more likely they will be to feel more in control and less anxious and helpless. When an individual takes on more responsibility for one's own life, decisions lead to concrete behaviors, such as drafting a will or advance directive, appointing a durable power of attorney, and making funeral arrangements (Scharlach & Fredriksen, 1993). An **advance directive** is a legal document prepared when an individual is alive, competent, and able to make decisions to provide guidelines for health care providers in the future, when the individual is not able to make decisions because of physical disability (being unconscious) or mental incompetence. By appointing a **durable power of attorney,** the individual designates another person (spouse, son, daughter, or friend) to make health care decisions (especially about how aggressive treatment should be in forestalling death) when an individual becomes unable to make such decisions. The nurse helps middle-age adults anticipate stressors so that they are better prepared to cope and to prevent additional physical, psychosocial, and spiritual stressors, thereby optimizing their health.

Values-Beliefs Pattern

When adults make decisions affecting their lives, it is usually the result of a personal, complex pattern of values and beliefs (Amaro, 1988; McFadden & Gerl, 1990; Robertson & Robertson, 1985; Smith, 1995). Much of what people value or believe to be true is formed early in life and

can be the most difficult to alter (Rippe, 1996). Normally people do not spend a great deal of conscious thought on abstract explanations of the meaning of life and why certain things are valued. During times of illness or crisis, however, they frequently take time to review their value systems and seek meaning about what is important (Spector, 2000; Stuart, Deckro, & Mandle, 1989) (Innovative Practice box).

A crisis at any age can be a turning point during which both increased vulnerability and increased potential are present. When the crisis is managed successfully, a virtue or strength will evolve. Erikson names *caring* as a middle-age adult virtue that can be developed.

Committed responsibilities for the care and welfare of others promotes moral development. When middle age is lived with generativity, many opportunities are afforded to live life by one's higher principles. The middle adult can differentiate among personal wants and needs, duties demanded by society, and principles by which to live. Kohlberg's work on moral development delineated these phases as conventional and postconventional. His studies of men described stage 3 as an interpersonal definition of

---

innovative practice

Mind/Body Medical Clinic Symptom Reduction Programs

Research demonstrates that 60% to 90% of health care visits are for symptoms such as headaches, insomnia, weakness or fatigue, and gastrointestinal symptoms, all of which are frequently stress related. The Mind/Body Medical Clinic Symptom Reduction Programs are designed to help clients who have chronic illnesses (including life-threatening illnesses) or stress-related symptoms to better manage their health problems and optimize their quality of life. The interventions combine conventional medical care with knowledge about the effects of behaviors and attitudes on health.

The biopsychosocial-spiritual approach of the assessment and treatment plans with clients includes:
- Eliciting the relaxation response, a state of deep rest that changes responses to stress (decreases vital signs, and muscle tenseness, increased mindfulness)
- Enhancing coping skills through cognitive behavioral strategies
- Encouraging exercise or physical activity
- Providing nutritional counseling
- Monitoring and adjusting medication, when necessary, in consultation with the physician

Insurance claims for these outpatient visits are submitted directly to clients' insurance carriers. Because health insurance policies differ, coverage and reimbursement vary. A client advocate helps clients research their specific health insurance coverage and billing requirements.

Research demonstrates that after these interventions:
- Clients with pain reduced their physician visits by 36%.
- Visits to an HMO were reduced by approximately 50% after a relaxation response–based intervention, resulting in significant cost savings.

- Blood pressure was lowered and use of medications decreased in 80% of hypertensive clients; 16% were able to discontinue all of their medications.
- Sleep patterns were improved for 100% of clients with insomnia; 90% reduced or eliminated the use of sleep medication.
- Infertile women reported decreased levels of depression, anxiety, and anger, and a 35% conception rate.
- Women with severe premenstrual syndrome experienced a 57% reduction in physical and psychological symptoms.
- Health-promoting behaviors, such as nutrition, social supports, self-esteem, health responsibility, and exercise, increased after the program and were maintained until a 6-month follow-up.
- Six months after the program, 80% of clients continued to experience improvement of their physical symptoms.
- Anxiety and depression normalized for most participants and were maintained 6 months following the program.
- Women with menopause reported fewer hot flashes, lower blood pressure, improved sleep, and decreased depression, anxiety, and anger.

Contact Information:
Harvard Medical School
Beth Israel Deaconess Medical Center
Division of Behavior Medicine
Mind/Body Medical Clinic
Symptom Reduction Programs
Telehone: 617-632-9530

Courtesy Carol Lynn Mandle, PhD, RN, CS-FNP.
HMO, health maintenance organization.

morality, whereas stage 4 is a societal definition based on law and order. Kohlberg concludes that most American adults are in these phases of moral development. In contrast, stage 5 is the concern and willingness to sacrifice for the well-being of others (Kohlberg & Lickona, 1986). Subsequent studies by Gilligan on moral development in women and men demonstrate gender differences in describing high morality. Women discussed issues of selfishness versus responsibility, of exercising care with decision making and avoiding hurting others. Men described terms of *justice, fairness,* and *rights of individuals.* Gilligan (1982, 1990) concludes that women possess a process of moral development different from that of men.

Valuing others, having relationships, and being responsible to others enables middle-age adults to make the transitions of moral development. This process is accomplished through raising children, developing more junior employees, and serving the community. As people fulfill these commitments, they increasingly treat others as equals and gradually develop a sensitivity and desire to change barriers to human worth and equality, such as racial prejudice, homelessness, inadequate access to health care, and weapons stockpiles.

ENVIRONMENTAL FACTORS

Environmental factors are significant variables in health promotion. Placing the emphasis on sanitation and preventing pollution must continue. The complex interactions between physical, biological, and chemical agents threaten health. Additionally, "the monitoring of public exposure to increasing numbers of toxins and research into the relationship of toxic exposure to disease are important, but are confounded due to the complexities of measuring the level of toxins in the environment, the relative exposure of the population, and individual characteristics that mitigate the effects of the exposure" (USDHHS, 1999, p. 116).

Because there are approximately 100 million workers in the United States, occupational hazards are a serious threat to national health. Exposures to toxic chemicals, asbestos, coal dust, cotton fiber, ionizing radiation, physical hazards, excessive noise, and stress can precipitate numerous health problems. For the middle-age worker, these problems include cancers, lung and heart diseases, decreased hearing, bodily injuries, and mental health problems (USDHHS, 2000).

Physical Agents

Ionizing radiation is a prime example of a physical agent that can cause cancer. Among the best-known examples is cancer caused by medical procedures that include the use of diagnostic radiography and therapeutic radiation.

Water pollution has become another major concern. Many industrial and agricultural wastes, such as benzene and chlordane, have been recovered in rivers and lakes from which drinking water is obtained. These substances can lead to potential carcinomas and other health problems.

Air pollution from auto emissions, burning fuels, and industrial incineration have warranted smog alerts and air pollution indexes. This issue is especially important to the individual with chronic respiratory or cardiovascular disease (USDHHS, 2000).

Noise pollution in industry is a potential problem for the middle-age adult worker. Hearing loss can be prevented if federal guidelines are followed with regard to noise exposure levels and hearing conservation programs.

Exposure to excessive noise, radiation, sunlight, and vibration can produce problems such as chronic obstructive lung disease, cancer, and degenerative diseases.

Biological Agents

As noted throughout this text, health and disease are influenced by the interactions among the agent, host, and environment. Agent factors can be biological, physical, chemical, or psychological. Many of these agents are transmitted through the air or by contact with certain media, such as water or food. These agents enter through the respiratory or gastrointestinal tracts. The size of the agent is important; if it is extremely small, the portal of entry can be the respiratory tract. Several of the categories merit special discussion in relation to middle adulthood.

Hepatitis A is caused by viral infection, with transmission occurring primarily through the fecal-oral route. This host-agent interaction typically occurs in the middle-age adult living in an environment with poor sanitation and having close contact with an infected person. The person may also be exposed through contaminated food and water. Hepatitis B is transmitted primarily in the blood or plasma of the infected individuals, which is particularly significant for the adult who is employed in a health care setting.

Hepatitis B is an occupational hazard among medical and dental personnel, with surgeons, oral surgeons, and pathologists at the highest risk, 6 times higher than that of the general population.

The biological causes of diseases include bacteria, viruses, rickettsiae, fungi, parasites, and food poisoning. Because these causes are often limited to identifiable occupations, they can be readily diagnosed, treated, and prevented (Table 23-1).

Chemical Agents

Chemicals include a wide variety of substances that increase the risk of morbidity and mortality in the middle-age adult. When a home is located near an industry, there is the risk of exposure to toxic chemicals that pollute the air. Contaminants can also be carried home on the clothing from the workplace.

Workers at increased risk include coal miners, wood handlers, and those who work with asbestos and coke. Pneumoconiosis is found in approximately 15% of coal miners, with "black lung disease" implicated in thousands of deaths per year. Wood handlers have increased risk of certain cancers. The asbestos worker has an increased risk of mesothelioma and asbestosis. Approximately 2 million

Table **23-1**   Examples of Occupational Biological Hazards and Preventive Measures

Disease	Target Organ	Occupational Source	Exposed Occupations	Preventive Measures
Fever (rickettsiae)	Systemic	Placental tissue, excreta from infected cattle, sheep	Laboratory workers, farmers, slaughterhouse workers	Hygiene, immunization
Histoplasmosis (fungus)	Lung	Fowl droppings	Farmers, poultry workers, demolition workers	Dust control, environmental sanitation
Hookworm (parasite)	Small intestine	Larvae in human feces penetrating skin	Farmers, sewer workers, recreation workers	Environmental sanitation, use of shoes, boots, gloves
Tetanus (bacterium)	Nervous system	Soil	Construction workers, farmers	Immunization
Rabies (virus)	Central nervous system	Wild animals, cows	Laboratory workers, veterinarians, hunters	Immunization of humans in contact with dogs, cats, skunks, foxes, bats, raccoons

Modified from Cohen, R. (1990). Occupational biologic hazards. *Occupational Health Nursing, 28*(8), 20-24.

workers each year have been exposed to benzene and vinyl chloride, which may be carcinogens (USDHHS, 2000).

Nine out of ten American industrial workers may be inadequately protected from exposure to at least 10 of the 163 most common hazardous chemicals. More than 2000 of the 50,000 chemicals found in the workplace are suspected human carcinogens (USDHHS, 2000).

Tobacco

Many 50-year-old adults have a 30-plus-year history of cigarette smoking. Cigarette smokers have nearly twice the heart disease death rates of nonsmokers, with the risk being proportional to the amount of smoke inhaled and the number of cigarettes smoked. Smokers are at increased risks for colds, chronic bronchitis, emphysema, and cancers of the mouth, lungs, esophagus, pancreas, and bladder. More blue collar workers smoke than do white collar workers (Centers for Disease Control and Prevention, 1999; Pierce, Fiore, Novotny, Hatziandreu, & Davis, 1989). A study of 2092 urban adults found that knowledge about the health effects of smoking was generally low among women, older adults, blacks, those of lower education levels, and current smokers (Brownson, Alavanja, Hock, & Loy, 1992).

Few smokers realize that cigarettes contain 2000 known chemicals, including tar, nicotine, hydrogen cyanide, formaldehyde, and ammonia. Cigarette smoking is, for most smokers, an addiction to nicotine, which is absorbed into the bloodstream. Nicotine acts on the two divisions of the nervous system: central (brain and the spinal cord) and peripheral (autonomic nervous system and motor and sensory fibers to the arms and legs). Effects of nicotine stimulation can be observed in both electroencephalographic changes and in hand tremors. Nicotine also stimulates the heart, leading to an increased pulse and elevated blood pressure. Although smokers frequently believe that cigarettes have a calming effect, this notion is misleading. Nicotine stimulates the body, whereas carbon monoxide causes lethargy. Smokers may feel calm, although they are actually having their sensations dulled by carbon monoxide. Additive effects such as those from chlorine, cotton dust, and β-radiation can lower midexpiratory flow values. Profound effects can also be observed with asbestos interaction.

SOCIAL PROCESSES
Culture and Ethnicity

Spector (2000) describes culture as the "sum of beliefs, practices, habits, likes, dislikes, norms, customs, rituals . . . we have learned from our families during the years of socialization" (p. 1). Spector further relates the ways in which one's cultural background is a component of one's ethnic background. The major ethnic groups of the United States are Asians, blacks, Native Americans, and Hispanics.

Nurses must understand their own ethnic cultures and those of others, largely because differences in beliefs, practices, and rituals can exist. The middle-age adult may not interpret dizziness as a possible symptom of hypertension, for example; it may be described simply as a *spell*. What the black adult defines as *health* may be completely different from that of the white health care provider or the Asian person. The obese adult who has received positive reinforcement throughout life for being pleasingly plump is less motivated to lose weight than is the adult who defines health as being *svelte* (Smith, 1995).

The health problems of middle-age adults, even within major ethnic groups, are varied. Recent immigrants who live in crowded urban areas have higher mortality rates than do earlier immigrants of the same cultural group who live in healthier environments. Immigrants' working conditions continue to be poor, with long hours and minimal wages. Modern preventive health care is difficult, if not impossible, to obtain.

Hispanic subgroups combined make up the largest minority group in the United States. The Hispanic American adult's primary health care problems, as identified by Spector (2000), are the barriers faced when they seek health care. These barriers include language, poverty, and time orientation. Few health care providers speak Spanish. The problem is compounded by the Hispanic tendency to place little value on the exact time of day, which makes appointment keeping frustrating for both the individual and the nurse. Poverty can predispose the middle-age Hispanic adult, and any other group, to tuberculosis, malnutrition, and delayed screening (e.g., mammography).

Poverty is reported in approximately one third of Native Americans. The middle-age adult Native American is faced with a high rate of tuberculosis, alcohol abuse, inadequate immunization, mental health problems such as depression, and dental problems (Spector, 2000; USDHHS, 2000).

For many women in society, the cessation of menses is associated with aging; the role of the middle-age woman may be shaped by her culture. Nurses who have attained cultural competency can ensure that appropriate health promotion is provided, especially for vulnerable populations and those individuals, families, and communities who have special health care needs.

Economics

Adults in the middle years are frequently at the peak of their careers. Although their net income may be greater than it was during early adulthood, they frequently have significant additional financial obligations. Children may be in college and need financial support, and preretirement planning can stress the budget. The care of an aging parent can be an additional financial burden and can be costly in terms of present lifestyle. When the adult or family members have ongoing health problems, the economic status of the family can be compromised further (Multicultural Awareness box).

The individual's economic status plays a role in the incidence of mental illness. Mental illness is increased in adults at the lower socioeconomic level, with higher rates of anxiety, depression, and phobias.

Health Care Delivery System

The nurse can contact numerous agencies that are geared to middle adulthood. These can be categorized as official, voluntary, and service agencies. Councils of community services frequently publish a directory. Official agencies include those that are state and federally funded, such as public health departments and drug treatment centers. Voluntary agencies include the American Cancer Society, the American Lung Association, and Alcoholics Anonymous. Many educational and self-help programs are sponsored by these organizations. The American Lung Association sponsors a "Stop Smoking" program, which can be conducted on a group basis in a work or community setting. Service agencies include professional organizations, such state nurses'

MULTICULTURAL AWARENESS

Health Care for Middle-Age Gypsies

Culturally competent and effective health care is imperative for all, especially people with several comorbid conditions who do not have a consistent primary care provider or clinic. Middle-age gypsies, or Roma, are in need of consistent health care but, because they tend to travel from one place to another and do not put down roots, health providers need to have understanding of their beliefs so the episodic interactions will be most productive. It is important to realize the Roma prefer to involve their family when it comes to their health. Hence a family member should be allowed to participate in each interaction with a health provider. This involvement with family will increase the client's compliance with the health regimen. Vivian and Dundes (2004) found that health care providers should be aware that the following variables may affect the Roma's health care: pollution, cleanliness, ideal weight, views on death, and medical procedures.

From Vivian, C., & Dundes, L. (2004). The crossroads of culture and health among the Roma (gypsies). *Image: The Journal of Nursing Scholarship*, 36(1), 86-91.

---

associations, the American Medical Association (sponsor of the Tel-Med program), bar associations, Young Men's Christian Association (YMCA), hospice programs, and the Women's Occupational Health Resource Center. **Web Site Resource 23B** presents a detailed list of these agencies.

NURSING INTERVENTIONS

The nurse must first understand the hazards to which the individual is exposed by listening, conferring with other individuals in the same environment, and reviewing health and safety data.

As a health educator, the nurse then initiates programs that emphasize helping adults to accept more responsibility for their own health. This effort can be provided on a one-to-one basis or in a seminar fashion. For example, with the goal of early detection of high blood pressure, the nurse in the community or industry might increase consumers' knowledge of hypertension, screen people who have sought health care for any reason, set up mechanisms to screen people outside the health care system, and refer and follow up on all people with elevated blood pressure.

The target groups identified by the nurse should have common needs, such as individuals exposed to a particular chemical, smokers, substance abusers, women entering the workplace for the first time, or men nearing retirement. In a work environment, the occupational health nurse can assess absenteeism rates for trends. In gathering data, the nurse can initiate research projects with multidisciplinary input.

The preemployment physical examination not only provides the employer with information about proper placement, but also provides a baseline health assessment. Frequently this examination is the only assessment that the individual has had in years.

The Occupational Safety and Health Administration (OSHA) mandates that the employee have a healthy and safe work environment. Therefore a complete health history is essential. Is there a history of hypertension, arthritis, cancer, or hernia? Is there significant family history? Is the person a smoker? How many packs per day? Does the person take medications? Medical limitations must be addressed; for example, decreased visual acuity means no driving, and dermatitis means no oils, chemicals, or solvents. Removing a worker from a particular job may be indicated if the worker might endanger coworkers, has a disease condition that might be aggravated by the job, or if the worker is taking prescribed medications with potentially harmful side effects.

The nurse in the community and in industry should reiterate some key safety issues to the adult, such as wearing seat belts and observing speed limits. With a decrease in visual acuity, driving at night can be hazardous. The middle-age adult's reaction time is also decreasing, which reinforces the need for periodic driving testing as recommended by the National Highway Traffic Safety Administration.

With an increase in leisure time, the middle-age adult is at greater risk for recreational accidents. As noted, moderation should be stressed. Alcohol is a depressant and should be avoided in activities that require attentiveness.

Protection from burns is essential; 56% of fatal residential fires are cigarette related, such as from smoking in bed. Falls can occur at any age, and safety measures should be considered for the entire family, with preparatory planning for aging parents. A few suggestions to the adult might be to avoid highly waxed floors, poor lighting, high beds, and bathtubs without nonslip bottoms.

Handgun availability is controversial at best; however, approximately 20% of American households have them. When the person believes strongly about having a firearm, safety measures to avoid accidental injury should be discussed, such as security locks and proper storage.

The Occupational Safety and Health Act (1970) was designed to ensure that workers are employed under safe and healthy working conditions. The act is applicable to every employer who is engaged in a business that affects commerce. The employer must ascertain that the workplace is free from recognized hazards and must comply with the act. OSHA has offices in most major cities and can provide recommended standards for occupational agents.

Nurses can participate actively in the safety committee of the industry in which they are employed. When no such committee exists, many protection measures will fall on the nurse. Suggestions include:

1. Tour the facilities on a regular basis. Be familiar with resource books, laws, and codes.
2. Develop a toxicology chart with symptoms of overexposure and recommended treatment. Update this chart frequently.
3. Be a role model in safety issues; wear safety glasses, protective footwear, and gloves, and do not smoke.
4. Discuss the preemployment physical with the employee, with an emphasis on risk factors. Monitor health problems and exposure levels in the work setting.

The worker must be aware of the protective clothing that should be worn, sanitation measures for the work environment, general hygiene measures, and proper immunization. The food handler, for instance, should have an annual tuberculosis skin test, wear clean clothing and appropriate hair protection, and use good hand-washing techniques. The nurse should not assume that workers know how to protect themselves and others.

A major challenge for the nurse is to encourage workers to assume responsibility for protecting their own health. Increasingly, organizations are interested in promoting the health of their employees for many reasons, including enhancing their recruiting efforts and minimizing lateness, absenteeism, turnover, physical and emotional inability to work, disability costs, and health and life insurance costs. Health-promotion programs are increasingly recognized for their vital contributions to the financial viability of organizations. It has been validated that providing health care to middle-age adults in homeless centers, showing health-promotion videos during meals, and giving incentives for participating in wellness programs improve health outcomes (Clark, 2002).

Health-promotion programs within an organizational setting can be categorized in one of three levels: (1) awareness, (2) lifestyle change, and (3) supportive environment. The goal of a health program at the level of awareness is to increase the individual's knowledge or interest in a particular health issue, such as smoking cessation. Examples of awareness programs include special events, flyers, lunch seminars, meetings, and newsletters. Changing health behaviors or status are not the goals of awareness programs, but are goals of lifestyle change programs.

Lifestyle change programs last at least 8 to 12 weeks and include assessment, education, and evaluation components to help individuals implement long-term changes in health behavior and status. To maintain these long-term changes and to develop a healthy lifestyle, a supportive organizational environment is needed. This type of environment includes health-promoting physical settings, corporate policies and culture, ongoing programs, and employee ownership of programs (USDHHS, 2000).

Five models of nurse-managed primary health care delivery at the work site have been proposed as part of the American Nurses Association's program for reform of this nation's health care system, known as Nursing's Agenda for Health Care Reform. Each model is developed to enable employers to fulfill the goal of providing accessible, quality, and affordable care at locations that are familiar and convenient for employees. These designs assist employers in introducing or expanding health care services at the work site, controlling health care costs, and meeting the health care needs of their employees (*Nursing facts: Nursing's agenda for health care reform*, 2005).

SUMMARY

Nurses are in a position to help the middle-age adult improve the quality of life, both for the present and for the future, through the identification of risk factors, health promotion, and other nursing interventions. Nurses work in a variety of health care settings available to healthy middle-age adults: outpatient clinics, occupational health clinics, and private practice.

Health promotion and disease prevention are aimed at the personal habits and lifestyles of adults to improve their biological, spiritual, and psychosocial development. Strategies to help an adult achieve a higher level of health include individual or group counseling based on identified risk factors, providing self-help information that is most relevant to the middle-age adult, and describing available resources.

Using these strategies, the nurse can motivate middle-age adults to assume more responsibility for their health behaviors. Changes may be effected after years of poor health practices, decreasing the adult's risk of disability from chronic disease.

ADDITIONAL STUDY MATERIAL

Study Questions in the back of the book, see page 663.

evolve WEB SITE MATERIALS

These materials are located on the book's Web site at http://evolve.elsevier.com/Edelman/.

- WebLinks
- Content Updates
- Web Site Resources

23A   Screening Requirements for Middle-Age Adults
23B   Community Resources for Health Promotion During Middle Adulthood

REFERENCES

Amaro, H. (1988). Women in the Mexican-American community: Religion, culture, and reproductive attitudes and experiences. *Journal of Community Psychology, 16,* 6-20.

American Obesity Association. (2004). Retrieved June 21, 2004, from: *http://www.obesity.org/subs/fastfacts/aoafactsheets.shtml*

Apter, T. (1991). *Altered loves: Mothers and daughters during adolescence.* New York: Ballantine.

Bloom, B. S. (1984). *Taxonomy of educational objectives: Handbook I, cognitive domain.* New York: Longman.

Boston Women's Health Book Collective. (1999). *Our bodies, ourselves for the new century.* New York: Touchstone.

Brownson, R. C., Alvanja, M. C., Hoch, E. T., & Loy, T. S. (1992). Passive smoking and lung cancer in non-smoking women. *American Journal of Public Health, 82*(11), 1525-1530.

Brownson, R. C., Houseman, R. A., Brown, D. R., Jackson-Thompson, J., King, A. C., Malone, B. R., et al. (2000). Promoting physical activity in rural communities: Walking trail access, use and effects. *American Journal of Preventive Medicine, 18*(3), 235-241.

Buttaro, T. M., Trybulski, J., Bailey, P. P., & Sandburg-Cook, J. S. (2003). *Primary care: A collaborative practice.* St. Louis: Mosby.

Carpenito-Moyet, L. (2004). *Nursing diagnosis: Application to clinical practice* (10th ed.). Philadelphia: Lippincott Williams & Wilkins.

Centers for Disease Control and Prevention. (1999). Prevalence of current cigarette and cigar smoking adults—United States, 1998. *Morbidity and Mortality Weekly Report, 48*(45), 1034-1039.

Centers for Disease Control and Prevention. (2002). *National Center for Health Statistics, National Health and Nutrition Examination Survey, Health, United States, 2002.* Retrieved July 31, 2005, from *http://www.cdc.gov/nchs/nhanes.htm*

Clark, C. (2002). *Health promotion in communities: Holistic and wellness approaches.* New York: Springer.

Craig, C. J. (1989). *Human development* (5th ed.). Englewood Cliffs, NJ: Prentice Hall.

Cottrell, R., Girvan, J., & McKenzie, J. (2001). *Principles and foundations of health promotion and education* (2nd ed.). San Francisco: Benjamin Cummings.

Davighis, M., Liu, K., Amber, P., Yan, L., Garside, D., Feinglass, J., et al. (2003). Favorable cardiovascular risk profile in middle age and health relationship of quality of life in older age. *Archives of Internal Medicine, 163,* 2460-2468.

Dunn, A. L., Marcus, B. H., Kampert, J. B., Garcia, M. E., Kohl, H. W., & Blair, S. N. (1999). Comparisons of lifestyle and structured interventions to increase physical activity and cardiorespiratory fitness: A randomized trial. *Journal of the American Medical Association, 281,* 327-334.

Dunphy, L. (2004). *Management guidelines for nurse practitioners working with adults* (2nd ed.). Philadelphia: F. A. Davis.

Duvall, E. M., & Miller, B. (1984). *Marriage and family development* (6th ed.). New York: Harper Collins.

Erikson, E. H. (1986). *Childhood and society* (35th ed.). New York: W. W. Norton.

Flaskerud, J. H., & Calvillo, E. R. (1991). Beliefs about AIDS, health and illness among low income Latino women. *Research in Nursing & Health, 14,* 431-438.

Flegal, K. M., Carroll, M. D., Ogden, C. L., & Johnson, C. L. (2002). *Prevalence and trends in obesity among US adults, 1999-2000. Journal of American Medical Association, 288:* 1723-1727.

Flowers, J. S., & McLean, J. E. (1996). Psychometric studies of the Flowers Midlife Health Questionnaire. *Journal of Nursing Science, 1*(3,4), 115-126.

Gilligan, C. (1982). *In a different voice: Psychological theory and women's development.* Cambridge, MA: Harvard University Press.

Gilligan, C. (1990). *Mapping the moral domain.* Cambridge, MA: Harvard University Press.

Havighurst, R. I., & Orr, B. (1956). *Adult education and adult needs.* Chicago: Center for Study of Liberal Education for Adults.

Haynes, S. G., Feinleib, M., & Kannel, W. B. (1980). The relationship of psychosocial factors to coronary heart disease in the Framingham Study. III. Eight-year incidence of coronary heart disease. *American Journal of Epidemiology, 111*(1), 37-58.

Haynes, S. G., Levine, S., Scotch, N., Feinleib, M., & Kannel, W. B. (1978). The relationship of psychosocial factors to coronary heart disease in the Framingham Study. *American Journal of Epidemiology, 107*(5), 362-383.

Hornstein, G. (1986). The structuring of identity among mid-life women as a function of their degree of involvement in employment. *Journal of Personality, 54,* 551-575.

Jacobs, G. D. (1998). *Say goodnight to insomnia.* New York: Henry Holt.

Johnson, M., Haight, B. K., & Benedict, S. (1998). AIDS in older people. A literature review for clinical nursing research and practice. *Journal of Gerontological Nursing, 24,* 8-13.

Joint National Committee. (2003). The seventh report of the Joint National

Committee on detection, evaluation and treatment of high blood pressure. The 7th Joint National Committee on Prevention, Detection, Evaluation, and Treatment of High Blood Pressure. Journal of Amercian Medical Association, 289. Retrieved April 21, 2005, from *http://jama.ama-assn.org/cgi/content/full/289,19.2560V/*

Karch, A. (2003). *Focus on nursing pharmacology* (2nd ed.). Philadelphia: Lippincott.

Kawachi, I., Sparrow, D., Spiro, A., Vokonas, P., & Weiss, S. T. (1996). A prospective study of anger and coronary heart disease: The Normative Aging Study. *Circulation, 94,* 2090-2095.

Kobasa, S. (1979). Stressful life events, personality and health: An inquiry into hardiness. *Journal of Personality and Social Psychology, 37,* 1-11.

Kohlberg, L., & Lickona, T. (1986). *The stages of ethical development: From childhood through old age.* New York: Harper Collins.

Kriketos, A. D., Sharp, T. A., Seagle, H. M., Peters, J. C., & Hill, J. O. (2000). Effects of aerobic fitness on fat oxidation and body fitness. *Medicine and Science in Sports & Exercise, 32*(4), 805-811.

Kucera, K. (2004). Managing common skin problems in the elderly. *The Clinical Advisor, 7*(6), 23-30.

Lancaster, J. B., & King, B. J. (1985). *An evolutionary perspective. In her prime: A new view of middle-aged women.* South Hadley, MA: Bergin & Garvey.

Levinson, D. (1986a). A conception of adult development. *American Psychologist, 41,* 3-13.

Levinson, D. (1986b). *The seasons of a man's life.* New York: Ballantine.

Levinson, D. (1996). *The seasons of a woman's life.* New York: Knopf.

Lubkin, I. M., & Larsen, P. D. (2002). *Chronic illness: Impact and interventions* (5th ed.). Boston: Jones and Bartlett.

McFadden, S., & Gerl, R. (1990). Approaches to understanding spirituality in the second half of life. *Generations, 14,* 35-38.

McKinlay, J., & McKinlay, S. (1988). *Massachusetts women's health study: 9th Annual scientific sessions.* Boston: Society of Behavioral Medicine.

Mottaz, C. J. (1987). Age and work satisfaction. *Work and Occupations, 14,* 387-409.

Nachtigall, L. E., Nachtigall, R. D., & Heilman, J. R. (1999). *What every woman should know: Staying healthy after 40.* New York: Warner Books.

National Osteoporosis Foundation. (1998). *Boning up on osteoporosis: A guide to prevention and treatment.* Washington, DC: The Foundation.

National Sleep Foundation. (1998). *Women and sleep.* Washington, DC: The Foundation.

Newman, D. K., & Giovannini, D. (2002). The overactive bladder: A nursing per-

spective. *American Journal of Nursing, 102*(6), 36-46.

Northrup, C. (2001). *The wisdom of menopause.* New York: Bantam Books.

Nursing facts: Nursing's agenda for health care reform. (2005). Washington, DC: American Nurses Publishing. Retrieved July 31, 2005, from *http://www.nursingworld.org/readroom/rnagenda.htm*.

Pender, N. (1996a). *Health promotion in nursing practice.* Stamford, CT: Appleton & Lange.

Pender, N. (1996b). *Health promotion.* Norwalk, CT: Appleton & Lange.

Piaget, J. (1970). *Structuralism.* New York: Basic Books.

Pierce, J. P., Fiore, M. C., Novotny, T. E., Hatziandreu, E. J., & Davis, R. M. (1989). Trends in cigarette smoking in the United States: Projections to the year 2000. *Journal of the American Medical Association, 261,* 56-60.

Reifman, A., Biernat, M., & Lang, E. (1991). Stress, social support, and health in married professional women with small children. *Psychology of Women Quarterly, 15,* 431-445.

Rice, V. (2000). *Handbook of stress, coping, and health: Implications for nursing research, theory, and practice.* London: Sage.

Rippe, J. M. (1996). *Fit over forty: A revolutionary plan to achieve lifelong physical and spiritual health and well-being.* New York: William Morrow.

Robertson, V. L., & Robertson, J. F. (1985). *Grandparenthood.* Beverley Hills, CA. Sage.

Schaie, K. (1994). The course of adult intellectual development. *American Psychologist, 49,* 304-343.

Scharlach, A., & Fredriksen, R. (1993). Reactions to the death of a parent during midlife. *Omega Journal of Death and Dying, 27,* 307-319.

Schiff, I., & Parson, A. B. (1996). *Menopause.* New York: Times Books.

Seaman, B. (2003). *The greatest experiment ever performed on women: Exploding the estrogen myth.* New York: Hyperion.

Sheehy, G. (1993). *Menopause: The silent passage.* New York: Random House.

Silverstein, O., & Rashbaum, B. (1995). *The courage to raise good men.* New York: Penguin.

Smith, C. A. (1995). The lived experience of staying healthy in rural African American families. *Nursing Science Quarterly, 8,* 17-21.

Spector, R. E. (2000). *Cultural diversity in health and illness* (5th ed.). East Norwalk, CT: Appleton & Lange.

Spielberger, C. D., Jacobs, G., Russell, S., & Crane, R. S. (1983). Assessment of anger: The state-trait anger scale. In J. N. Butcher & C. D. Spielberger (Eds.), *Advances in personality assessment: Vol. 2.* Hillsdale, NJ: Lawrence Erlbaum Associates.

Stuart, E., Deckro, J., & Mandle, C. L. (1989). Spirituality in health and healing:

A clinical program. *Holistic Nursing Practice, 3,* 35-46.

Thomas, S. P. (1995). Psychosocial correlates of women's health in middle adulthood. *Issues in Mental Health Nursing, 16,* 285-314.

U.S. Department of Health and Human Services. (1999). *Healthy people 2000 review.* Washington, DC: U.S. Government Printing Office.

U.S. Department of Health and Human Services. (2000). *Healthy people 2010.* Washington, DC: U.S. Government Printing Office.

U.S. Department of Health and Human Services, Centers for Disease Control and Prevention, National Center for Health Statistics. (1998). *Health, United States.* Hyattsville, MD: The Author.

USA Today. (January 11, 2005). *Why grown kids come home.* Retrieved from *http://www.usatoday.com/educate/college/careers/news4.htm*

Vaillant, G., & Vaillant, C. (1990). Natural history of male psychological health: A 45-year study of predictors of successful aging at age 65. *American Journal of Psychology, 147*(1), 31-37.

Van der Hek, H., & Plomp, H. N. (1997). Occupational stress management programs: A practical overview of published effect studies. *Occupational Medicine, 47*(3), 133-141.

Vivian, C., & Dundes, L. (2004). The crossroads of culture and health among the Roma (gypsies). *Image: The Journal of Nursing Scholarship, 36*(1), 86-91.

Wallerstein, J. S. (1991). The long-term effects of divorce on children: A review. *Journal of the American Academy of Child and Adolescent Psychiatry, 30,* 349-360.

Wallerstein, J. S., & Johnston, J. R. (1990). Children of divorce: Recent findings regarding long-term effects and recent studies of joint and sole custody. *Pediatric Reviews, 11,* 197-204.

Wallerstein, J. S., & Kelly, J. B. (1977). Divorce counseling: A community service for families in the midst of divorce. *American Journal of Orthopsychiatry, 47,* 4-22.

Wallerstein, J. S., Lewis, J., & Blakeslee, S. (2000). *The unexpected legacy of divorce: A 25 year landmark study.* New York: Hyperion.

WebMD. (n.d.). Pulse measurement. Retrieved April 20, 2005, from *http://my.webmd.com/hw/heart_disease/hw233473.asp*

Williams, J., Paton, C., Siegler, I. C., Eigenbrodt, M. L., Nieto, F. J., & Tyroler, H. A. (2000). Anger proneness predicts coronary heart disease risk: Prospective analysis from the Atherosclerosis Risk in Communities (ARIC) Study. *Circulation, 101*(17), 2034-2039.

Zeitz, G. (1990). Age and work satisfaction. *Human Relations, 43,* 419-438.

Chapter 24

MEREDITH WALLACE

Older Adult

objectives

After completing this chapter the reader will be able to:

- Identify normal aging changes in the older adult.
- Evaluate morbidity data according to age, gender, and race.
- Discuss nutritional factors that affect the health promotion of the older adult.
- Analyze environmental factors that have an effect on older adults.
- Recognize risk factors that could lead to health problems in older adulthood.
- Enumerate the five most prevalent health conditions and the five leading causes of mortality among older people.
- Discuss environmental, biological, physical, and mechanical agents that contribute to disability, morbidity, and mortality in later adulthood.
- Analyze political and social issues that influence the well-being of the older adult.
- List the leading causes of injury among older adults and suggest preventive measures.
- Identify major resources that are available for older adults.

key terms

Alzheimer's disease
Cognition
Constipation
Decubitus ulcer
Dementia
Depression
Euthanasia

Physician-assisted suicide
Mild cognitive impairment (MCI)
Mini-Mental State Examination
Multiinfarct dementia
Osteoporosis

Overflow incontinence
Stress incontinence
Urge incontinence
Urinary incontinence

THINK About It

Older Adult Smokers

You are the director of a senior center in which 10 of your 40 members smoke. Several of the smoking individuals currently experience health problems. One older woman has chronic obstructive pulmonary disease and avoids using her oxygen because she is not supposed to smoke while the oxygen tank is in the room. One older gentleman has high blood pressure; another one of the smokers has been diagnosed with lung cancer. As director of the center, you would like to help these older adults to stop smoking. You have referred them to their physicians to obtain

Continued

THINK About It

Older Adult Smokers *cont'd*

assistance with smoking cessation. However, all of the participants are Medicare recipients and Medicare does not provide coverage for smoking-cessation programs and/or nicotine-replacement therapy. All involved are on limited incomes and cannot afford to pay the charge of either a behavior management class or nicotine-replacement therapy.

1 What types of resources are available to help you obtain the necessary assistance for these smokers?

2 What policy changes might be instituted within the senior center to prevent secondhand smoke from harming the residents in the center's care?

As a result of health promotion and technological advances, health care professionals now enjoy the gift of caring for an older population. To be caring for a group of human beings that was virtually nonexistent 100 years ago is truly extraordinary. The current standard of living, nutrition, prevention and treatment of infectious diseases, and progress in medical care have increased sharply the survival rate for people living in the United States. Once these individuals reach adulthood, they are likely to survive to old age. In 1990 the number of Americans age 65 and older was approximately 28 million, or 12% of the population. By the year 2030 the percentage is projected to increase to more than 18% of the population. The fastest growing age group in the country is that of adults age 75 and older. The fastest growing group within the older adult population is 85 years and older. According to *Healthy People 2010*, individuals age 65 years can be expected to live an average of 18 more years than they did 100 years ago, for a total of 83 years. Individuals age 75 years can be expected to live an average of 11 more years, for a total of 86 years (U.S. Department of Health and Human Services [USDHHS], 2000).

The dominant, white population of adults 65 and older is expected to decrease over the next 30 years, while the percentage of African American, Hispanic, and Asian older adults will continue to rise. Considering this shift in population characteristics, it is imperative that health care providers develop an awareness of the cultural diversity of the population and identify the cultural beliefs that influence health care decisions of older adults (Multicultural Awareness box).

During the past few decades, mostly tertiary care has been provided for older adults. Health care providers waited until they became sick before providing nursing care. Insurance reimbursement and introduction into the health care system has come late for many, resulting in a high prevalence of illness and limited health-promotion interventions. The misconceptions surrounding health promotion for older adults impedes the ability of nurses to provide the best possible care. It is time to overcome these misconceptions and begin to promote their health rather than wait until

MULTICULTURAL AWARENESS

How Different Cultures Care for Older Adults

How fortunate is today's society to enjoy the variety of many cultures? Individuals and families who immigrated to the United States in the early 1900s are now spending their later years as citizens of this country. Although many older adults have lived in the United States for many years, remembering the countries from where they came is of great importance. An understanding of the individual cultural backgrounds of older adults allows nurses to provide care that is respectful of the whole individual.

Schmall (1996) indicates that five major cultural groups in the United States display differing attitudes toward older adults. Most white Anglo-Saxon Protestants show less respect for older adults and their role in the family than do other cultures, in which older men and women tend to share in the family structure more equally. Parents are expected to live away from and not be overly dependent on their adult children. Although this view represents the mainstream American culture, other distinct and important cultures within the United States should be recognized and respected.

The black culture generally has a greater respect for older adults and their family role than do white cultures. Black people also place a value on kinship and the extended family that is no longer present in white cultures. East Asians have an especially high level of respect for older adults: the older an individual is, the more respect that individual is given. Additionally, the oldest son in East Asian cultures assumes responsibility for the care of the aging parents. Hispanic cultures give more overt respect to older adults than do white cultures. In many families aging parents live in households that consist of numerous extended family members. Finally, Native American cultures have a high level of respect for older adults because of their years of accumulated wisdom and knowledge, and they are frequently sought out for advice.

Knowledge of the different cultures in the United States provides the nurse with a broader understanding of the psychosocial mechanics underlying an individual's illness. Understanding the older adult's role within the family gives the nurse the information that is needed to develop an appropriate plan of care. Many of them will be well cared for by family members, and others do not expect or value care from their families. Additionally, the role that older adults are expected to fulfill within their culture, such as grandparent, primary caregiver, or family decision maker, must be considered when nurses are attempting to understand the value of health and illness to the older adult. Although nurses generally believe that the health of the individual should come first, an understanding of the culture can help in planning; for example, an aging Hispanic grandfather prefers to be home when his grandchildren return from school rather than at the clinic receiving dialysis treatments in the afternoon. Enhanced cultural competency among nurses has great potential for improving health care and quality of life for older adults.

Data from Schmall, V. L. (1996). Family influences. In A. G. Lueckenotte (Ed.), *Gerontologic nursing* (pp. 136-166). St. Louis: Mosby.

they are ill to effect the highest quality of life possible. Health promotion is as important in later adulthood as it is in childhood. Older adults can derive the same benefits from health-promotion activity as do their younger counterparts; they are not "too old" to stop smoking, start exercising, change their diet, or relinquish other bad health habits. The potential for improvement is great, and nurses have a key role in changing common societal misconceptions and in creating new fields of knowledge surrounding health promotion and older adults.

The many physical, emotional, and role changes of aging that will be discussed in this chapter are complicated by the great diversity of cultural backgrounds in this country. Older adults who have immigrated to the United States have brought with them different languages, spiritual patterns, eating habits, views toward modern medicine, and other customs foreign to U.S. culture. Furthermore, in other cultures older adults are more highly respected than they are in the United States. Throughout this chapter, cultural norms and behaviors will be discussed within each functional health pattern.

AGE AND PHYSICAL CHANGES

Although the need to promote the health of the older population is great, numerous challenges are presented in fulfilling this need. As stated, one of the great challenges to health promotion among older adults lies in the misconceptions about its benefits. Another challenge concerns separating the normal changes of aging from pathological processes and illness. Normal age-related changes frequently are regarded as inevitable and irreversible. An extraordinary amount of variability exists in the age-related changes that occur in each individual. Exposure to environmental injury, illness, genetics, stress, cultural influences, and many other factors combine to influence the aging process. Most researchers agree that biological changes show that growth and development peak during the thirties, with subsequent linear decline until death. These normal changes must be distinguished from pathological changes to focus health-promotion interventions on behaviors that can and should be changed. For example, older adults experience a decline in their respiratory vital capacity. Therefore when recommending exercise programs, these people must start gradually, allowing them to experience the exercise free from respiratory distress. These changes will be discussed specifically under each section of the physiological and psychological processes.

Another challenge to promoting the health of older adults lies in the large prevalence of chronic illness. Although chronic illness is not a normal change of aging, years of environmental assault, poor health behaviors, and stress have placed older adults at a high risk for developing these illnesses. Generally health deteriorates with aging through an accumulation of chronic disorders and disabilities. According to the Centers for Disease Control and Prevention (CDC), chronic conditions significantly limit daily activity for 39% of people over 65 years of age. Although

Table 24-1 Percentage of Older Adults With Chronic Conditions By Gender

Chronic Condition	Men	Women
Arthritis	49.5	63.8
High blood pressure	40.5	48
Heart disease	24.7	19.2
Cancer	23.4	16.7
Diabetes	12.9	11.5
Stroke	10.4	7.5

From Centers for Disease Control. (2003). Healthy aging: Preventing disease and improving quality of life among older Americans at a glance. Retrieved April 12, 2005, from: *http://www.cdc.gov/nccdphp/aag/aag_aging.htm*.

older Americans make up 12% of the population, they account for nearly 36% of health care costs (Centers for Disease Control and Prevention [CDC], 2001a). Table 24-1 lists the percentage of older adults with chronic conditions. Illness impairs the individual's capacity and motivation to learn new health-promoting behaviors. This prevalence of illness clearly indicates that this population has a great need for health promotion, although it is one of the most difficult in which to effect change.

It is important to note that health-promotion practices among older adults vary by cultural background. In a study of 110 older Korean immigrants in the United States, nutrition practices were considered among the healthiest behaviors, although the mean score on exercise was very low. Self-efficacy and health status were significantly related to health-promotion behaviors. The researchers concluded that elderly Korean immigrants did not practice healthy lifestyles (Sohng, Sohng, & Yeom, 2002). In order to improve the health-promotion practices of Korean immigrants and other cultural groups, cultural norms and behaviors must be taken into consideration. In a study of Chinese Americans, older adults began to shift dependence for health needs from traditional family caregivers to friends and neighbors (Pang, Jordan-Marsh, Silverstein, & Cody, 2003).

GOALS OF HEALTH PROMOTION

The U.S. Department of Health and Human Services (2000) has developed *Healthy People 2010: National Health-Promotion and Disease Prevention Objectives* for health-promotion programs for the older population (*Healthy People 2010* box). These goals focus on increasing health-promotion programs and decreasing morbidity and mortality related to various disease states.

As the population of older adults continues to rise, the number of cultural backgrounds within this population will increase and diversify. Cultural background and race have an effect on the prevalence of disease in the United States. The CDC reports that although the five major cultural groups share eight leading causes of death, heart disease and cancer are the first and second leading causes, respectively, among white, black, Hispanic, and Native American pop-

Healthy People 2010

Selected National Health-Promotion and Disease Prevention Objectives for the Older Adult

- 1-9. Reduce hospitalization rates for three ambulatory care–sensitive conditions (pediatric asthma, uncontrolled diabetes, and immunization-preventable pneumonia and influenza in older adults).
- 2-9. Reduce the overall number of cases of osteoporosis.
- 6-3. Reduce the proportion of adults with disabilities who report feelings such as sadness, unhappiness, or depression that prevent them from being active.
- 6-4. Increase the proportion of adults with disabilities who participate in social activities.
- 6-5. Increase the proportion of adults with disabilities reporting sufficient emotional support.
- 6-6. Increase the proportion of adults with disabilities who report satisfaction with life.
- 6-7. Reduce the number of people with disabilities in congregate care facilities, consistent with permanency planning principles.
- 6-8. Eliminate disparities in employment rates between working-age adults with and without disabilities.
- 7-12. Increase the proportion of older adults who have participated during the preceding year in at least one organized health-promotion activity.
- 8-22. Increase the proportion of people living in pre-1950s housing that have tested for the presence of lead-based paint.
- 10-1. Reduce infections caused by key food-borne pathogens.
- 12-6. Reduce hospitalizations of older adults with heart failure as the principal diagnosis.
- 14-5. Reduce invasive pneumococcal infections.
- 14-28. Increase hepatitis B vaccine coverage in high-risk groups.
- 14-29. Increase the proportion of adults who are vaccinated annually against influenza and were ever vaccinated against pneumococcal disease.
- 15-1. Reduce hospitalization for nonfatal head injuries.
- 15-15. Reduce deaths caused by motor vehicle crashes.

- 15-27. Reduce deaths from falls.
- 15-28. Reduce hip fractures among older adults.
- 17-3. Increase the proportion of primary care providers, pharmacists, and other health care professionals who routinely review with their clients aged 65 years and older and those with chronic illnesses or disabilities all newly prescribed and over-the-counter medicines.
- 19-1. Increase the proportion of adults who are at a healthy weight.
- 19-2. Reduce the proportion of adults who are obese.
- 19-17. Increase the proportion of physician office visits made by clients with a diagnosis of cardiovascular disease, diabetes, or hyperlipidemia that includes counseling or education related to diet and nutrition.
- 19-18. Increase food security among U.S. households and, in so doing, reduce hunger.
- 21-4. Reduce the proportion of older adults who have had all their natural teeth extracted.
- 22-1. Reduce the proportion of adults who engage in no leisure-time physical activity.
- 22-2. Increase the proportion of adults who engage regularly, preferably daily, in moderate physical activity for at least 30 minutes per day.
- 22-3. Increase the proportion of adults who engage in vigorous physical activity that promotes the development and maintenance of cardiorespiratory fitness 3 or more days per week for 20 or more minutes per occasion.
- 22-4. Increase the proportion of adults who perform physical activities that enhance and maintain muscular strength and endurance.
- 24-9. Reduce the proportion of adults whose activity is limited because of chronic lung and breathing problems.
- 24-10. Reduce deaths from chronic obstructive pulmonary disease among adults.
- 27-10. Reduce the proportion of nonsmokers exposed to environmental tobacco smoke.

Modified from U.S. Department of Health and Human Services. (2000). *Healthy people 2010: National health promotion and disease prevention objectives*. Washington, DC: U.S. Government Printing Office. Retrieved April 12, 2005, from: *http://www.health.gov/healthypeople*.

ulations, while cancer is the first and heart disease the second highest among Asian American–Pacific Islanders (CDC, 2002).

THEORIES OF AGING

The study of how and why people age has continued over many years and has been the source of a great deal of debate. Until fairly recently the cause of death on many older adults' death certificates was listed simply as "old age." As the study of gerontology has progressed, researchers have begun to question the physiological, social, and psychological reasons why people die. At the 55th annual meeting

of the Gerontological Society of America, Butler and Olshansky (2002) explored these questions in a presentation entitled, "Has Anyone Ever Died of Old Age?"

Despite this attention, the debates among those studying biogerontological, psychogerontological, and sociogerontological theories of aging continue. There is no formula to predict how a person will age or how long that individual will live. Many theories continue to be tested today. Included in the most prevalent research are the roles of both genetics and diet in aging. Genetic markers to predict the development of disease will play a large role in determining how a person will age and longevity. In addi-

- Growth hormone secretion theory
- Waste product theory
- Cross-linkage theory
- Rate of living theory
- Wear and tear theory
- Social theories of aging
- Gene regulation theory
- Somatic mutation theory
- DNA damage theory
- Free radical theory
- Error theory
- Programmed cell loss theory
- Neuroendocrine theory
- Immunological theory
- Autoimmune theory

DNA, deoxyribonucleic acid.

tion, researchers report that calorie-restricted diets have shown an increase in longevity in animals (Allison et al., 2001). The role of antioxidants in binding free radicals is also being researched as an important influence on increasing longevity (Ness & Smith, 1999). Although no consensus has yet been reached that describes the entire aging process, theories continue to be forthcoming and are very exciting. Explanations of each of these theories is extremely interesting but beyond the scope of this book. Some of the theories used to explain aging are listed in Box 24-1.

GORDON'S FUNCTIONAL HEALTH PATTERNS
Health Perception–Health Management Pattern

The most important factor in maintaining health is the older adult's motivation. Nurses who care for older adults know that all the best nursing in the world cannot make an individual do something believed to be unnecessary. A primary factor in the older adult's motivation to promote personal health is the perception of health and its subsequent management.

The *Harvard Women's Health Watch* (Forestalling frailty, 2003) reports five major activities older adults should engage in to promote health and prevent frailty. These include: (1) maintaining healthy weight and diet, (2) staying active, (3) practicing fall prevention, (4) maintaining relationships, and (5) keeping regular medical appointments. Helping an older adult to understand the importance of these factors for maintaining health is an essential nursing role needed to form positive health perceptions and effective health management patterns.

Ideal health maintenance behaviors include exercise, good nutrition, sexual safety, and appropriate sleep-rest patterns. Health maintenance practices should also include regular health care checkups, which will provide early detection and management of disease. Although these behaviors are important for all older adults, the perception of these activities and the ability to practice good health behaviors varies by cultural groups. It is essential that nurses are culturally competent and understand the cultural values that guide behavior. In so doing, the nurse will be most effective in helping the older adult to form a positive health perception and practice good health behaviors.

Nutritional-Metabolic Pattern

Guthrie and Lin (2002) found that 6.3% of older adult households did not have sufficient access to food to allow a healthy, active lifestyle. Two to three percent of these people admitted to being hungry. The number who did not have access to adequate food increased to 18.2% among lower income older adults. These statistics underscore the problems of maintaining good nutrition. Access to food is compounded by the effect of normal changes of aging. Declines in gastrointestinal organ function can lead to changes in digestive metabolism and the absorption and elimination of nutrients. Additionally, a deterioration of the smell, vision, and taste senses and the high frequency of dental problems makes maintaining adequate daily nutrition even more difficult. Cultural food preferences and lifelong eating habits, such as diets high in fat and cholesterol, are other obstacles to maintaining optimal nutrition.

Living environment further affects nutritional status. Community-dwelling seniors are at high risk for nutritional disorders, because access to food may be limited. Institutionalized older adults do not have a problem with availability of food, but the meals served in institutions frequently contain excessive fat, cholesterol, or salt and a lack of fiber. Additionally, fresh fruit and vegetables are less available, and the nutritional value of produce is reduced significantly when the food is canned or cooked. Finally, institutional food tends to be unappealing, and most institutions are not able to adapt their meals to the cultural diversity of their residents.

Anorexia, or lack of appetite, can accompany disease. Medications or a lack of dentures can also cause older people to eat less than is optimal. Those in acute care hospitals or long-term care facilities may experience a lack of appetite as a result of illness. The hospital stay is a time during which good nutrition is most important to heal wounds and to restore energy; however, a lack of interest in or energy for eating during these stays places the older adult at a high risk of developing nutritional disorders.

Sahyoun and Basiotis (2000), using data from the National Health and Nutrition Examination Survey III, found that poor food intake and nutritional status decreases self-rated health. Good nutrition helps prevent cancer, obesity, and gastrointestinal disorders and provides older adults with the energy required to function in all activities of daily life. Good nutrition can be measured by ascertaining whether the individual is meeting the recommended daily allowance (RDA) for caloric intake established by the National Academy of Sciences and the National Research Council. The RDA is 2000 to 2800 calories for men ages

Geriatric Assessment

The health care system, with its emphasis on acute care, busy office schedules, and fragmented delivery systems, often frustrates older people and their families. The very old or frail person's health problems frequently are overlooked, ignored, or only partially treated. Many communities have a health care service that uses a team approach to meet the special needs of older adults. This service is known as *geriatric assessment*.

GOALS OF GERIATRIC ASSESSMENT

- Maintain health and health maintenance practices
- Minimize hospitalizations
- Establish complete diagnoses that are frequently overlooked, including hearing impairment, vision deficits, early dementia, depression, poor nutrition, and falls
- Decrease overprescription of medications

Geriatric assessment uses an interdisciplinary team consisting of a geriatric nurse practitioner, physical therapist, and a social worker. Each member of the team evaluates the person from a health care, functional, cognitive, or psychosocial point of view. Additional members of the team might include a geriatric psychiatrist, geriatrician, nutritionist, pharmacist, dentist, or podiatrist. The program team evaluates the home environment, advance directives, falls, incontinence, vision and hearing impairments, memory loss, depression and anxiety, functional decline, deconditioning, caregiver stress, economic resources, and quality-of-life issues. The team is coordinated by the geriatric nurse practitioner.

Geriatric assessment is not meant for all older people. The people who benefit are the frail ones. A typical person who might benefit from geriatric assessment would be:

- Over age 80
- Falls frequently
- Is losing weight because of poor nutrition
- Is depressed because of loss of spouse and friends
- Has mild memory loss
- Has been hospitalized 3 times in 2 months
- Takes more than five medications regularly and frequently gets them confused
- Has no close family in the community
- Is in need of health teaching

Geriatric assessment usually identifies the strengths and weaknesses of these people. Following the assessment, the geriatric nurse practitioner begins developing a plan of care to address usable strengths and assist with weaknesses.

The primary care physician, family physician, or internist is a key link between the geriatric assessment team and the individual, primarily because this provider carries out the team's recommendation and monitors the person's progress. In most cases the nurse practitioner coordinates between the team and the person's primary physician and family.

Geriatric assessment clinics are available in many larger cities. As the U.S. health care system changes from its costly system of treating acute health problems with frequent office and hospital visits to a more cost-controlled, coordinated, comprehensive health management system, geriatric assessment will play a key role in identifying individual strengths, correcting problems, and maintaining the health and quality of life of older citizens.

Courtesy Carole Lium Edelman.

---

51 to 75 years and 1650 to 2450 for men 76 years and older. The range for women 51 to 75 years of age is between 1400 and 2200 calories; for women 76 years and older, 1200 to 2000 calories are recommended.

The nurse assists the older adult in maintaining the highest possible nutritional level. Teaching about the food needed to maintain optimal nutritional status is of utmost importance. In the community setting, Guthrie and Lin (2002) note that there are several federally supported nutrition assistance programs available to the older adult, including food stamps, commodity supplemental food program, child and adult food program, elderly nutrition program (Meals on Wheels), and the emergency food assistance program. The nurse may assist the older adult in acquiring transportation to obtain food and applying for these programs. Nurses who work in institutional settings are charged with the difficult task of encouraging good nutrition on the resident and administrative level. Residents who frequently do not want to eat institutional food should be encouraged to eat the types of food that they enjoy. Encouraging family members to bring in food that the resident enjoys is helpful. A pleasant setting with socialization can also enhance the desire to eat.

Elimination Pattern

Bowel and bladder functions in the older adult are altered by the normal changes of age. The bladder retains its tonus, but its capacity decreases. Large bowel motility also decreases as people age. In addition to some of the normal changes of aging, diet plays a significant role in problems with intestinal motility and constipation. Increased incidence of nutritional disorders, particularly decreased intake of fluids and fiber, contributes in large part to elimination problems. Many medications frequently taken by older adults cause elimination concerns. Lack of physical activity and changes in environment that decrease privacy also contribute. To maintain healthy bowel hygiene, the nurse encourages the older adult to have adequate fluids, roughage, and exercise.

Constipation is a major problem for older adults and has far-reaching effects on their quality of life. Researchers report that constipation requires excessive nurse staffing costs (Pekmezaris, Aversa, Wolf-Klein, Cedarbaum, & Reid-Durant, 2002). By encouraging older adults to exercise and change their fluid and dietary intake, nurses can help reduce their incidence of constipation. Exercise has a

Box **24-2** Causes of Urinary Incontinence Among Older Adults

DELIRIUM

New onset of UI may be associated with delirium from acute underlying conditions requiring diagnosis and treatment.

RESTRICTED MOBILITY

Acute conditions causing immobility may precipitate UI; environmental manipulation and scheduled toileting are appropriate while rehabilitative efforts are undertaken.

INFECTION

Acute cystitis may precipitate urge UI. Asymptomatic bacteriuria, with or without pyuria, should not be treated in the absence of symptoms of acute UTI.

INFLAMMATION

Atrophic vaginitis and urethritis can cause irritative voiding symptoms, including UI.

IMPACTION

Fecal impaction may be associated with UI and fecal incontinence.

POLYURIA

Poorly controlled diabetes with glucosuria can contribute to urinary frequency and UI.
Excess intake of caffeinated beverages may exacerbate symptoms.
Edema from congestive heart failure or venous insufficiency can cause nocturia and exacerbate nocturnal UI.

PHARMACEUTICALS

Rapid-acting diuretics (urge UI)
Psychotropic drugs (sedation, immobility)
Anticholinergic agents, α-antagonists, calcium channel blockers, narcotics (urinary retention)
α-Antagonists (stress UI)
Alcohol (sedation, immobility, polyuria)

Modified from Ouslander, J. G. (June, 2000). Incontinence management in LTC. *Annals of Long-Term Care,* 8(6), 35-41.
UI, urinary incontinence; *UTI,* urinary tract infection.

rapid and favorable effect on constipation. Dietary modifications, such as the increase of fiber and fluid, can stimulate the colon and resolve constipation.

Urinary incontinence affects approximately 30% of community-dwelling older adults and half of nursing home patients (Vinsnes, Harkless, Haltbakk, Bohm, & Hunskaar, 2001), with costs estimated at $16.3 billion per year (Wilson, Brown, Shin, Luc, & Subak, 2001). The causes of urinary incontinence are summarized in Box 24-2. The three major types of incontinence among older adults include **stress incontinence,** which is most common and occurs during exercise, laughing, coughing, or sneezing; **urge incontinence,** or the inability to delay voiding after the bladder is full; and **overflow incontinence** caused by an obstruction in the elimination system, such as an enlarged prostate gland or urethral stricture.

Incontinence results in threats to both psychological and physical health, including depression, urinary tract infections, pressure ulcers, and falls (Wyman, 2003). Despite the high prevalence of the problem, older adults frequently fail to report incontinence to their health care providers because of its embarrassing nature. Accepting incontinence as a manageable problem and seeking appropriate treatment is important for continued health and self-esteem.

Incontinent older adults in all cultural groups tend to avoid physical and social activities because of this problem.

Wyman (2003) describes several treatment categories. The first method includes lifestyle modifications and health-promotion behaviors to decrease incontinence, such as weight loss, exercise, and diet. Voiding schedules are most effective when the person can select specific times during the day for urination. After developing a schedule, the individual is instructed to use the toilet 30 minutes before this time each day. This technique may prevent incontinence.

Prompted voiding is another method to decrease incontinent episodes. The individual is reminded or asked about voiding. A structured bladder training program allows older individuals to develop a voiding schedule that is progressive by increasing the time between voids and ensuring that adequate fluids are taken from 7:00 AM to 7:00 PM. Postponing voids by using relaxation, imagery, or distraction is essential to the success of this management strategy. This type of training is difficult, however, and relies on a good working relationship between the individual and the nurse.

Antiincontinence devices, such as pessaries, are often helpful. In addition, pelvic floor or Kegel exercises may be taught to improve the musculature of the urinary system. To perform Kegel or pelvic floor exercises, the first step is to locate the muscle that requires strengthening. The individual is instructed to squeeze around the finger for 10 seconds. Repetitions of 10 cycles of 10 seconds each 6 times a day will result in fewer accidents in a period of approximately 2 weeks. Supportive interventions such as disposable pads may be used to avoid embarrassment, as well.

Activity-Exercise Pattern

The benefits of regular exercise in promoting health and preventing disease are widely accepted. The overwhelming evidence of the positive effects of exercise has led the U.S. Department of Health and Human Services to develop within its program, *Healthy People 2010,* national objectives for increasing the numbers of adults who exercise regularly. Binder, Schechtman, Ehsani, Steger-May, Brown, Sinacore, et al (2002) reported that exercise reduced frailty even in the oldest old. Despite the many benefits of exercise, Friis, Nomura, Ma, and Swan (2003) report that older adults do not often participate in exercise programs. Although exercise is not popular among this age group, no physiological or psychological explanation has been found to explain this decline. Normal changes of aging, pathological conditions, and environmental deterrents do not prevent them from exercising (Figure 24-1).

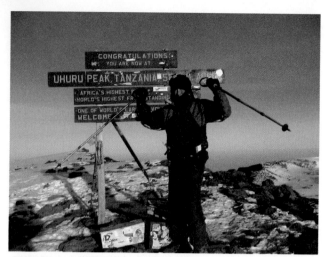

Figure 24-1   Older adults practice health promotion by continuing to achieve new heights through exercise.

Teaching the many benefits of exercise is the first lesson in motivating older adults to participate. With respect to the role that culture plays on the value of exercise, individual counseling is needed to identify exercises that can be enjoyed and continued (Figure 24-2). The nurse assists in designing an appropriate exercise program that will maintain strength, flexibility, and balance. Walking is broadly reported as the most widely accepted form of exercise among older adults. Friis, Nomura, Ma, and Swan (2003) found that 38% of men and 26% of women in their study walked for exercise. Walking is an exercise that can be done in both community settings and health care facilities.

Other popular activities for older adults include weight-bearing and aquatic exercises. Weight-bearing and muscle-building exercises help to maintain functional mobility, promote independence, and prevent falls. Weight-bearing exercises are shown to be highly effective in reducing bone

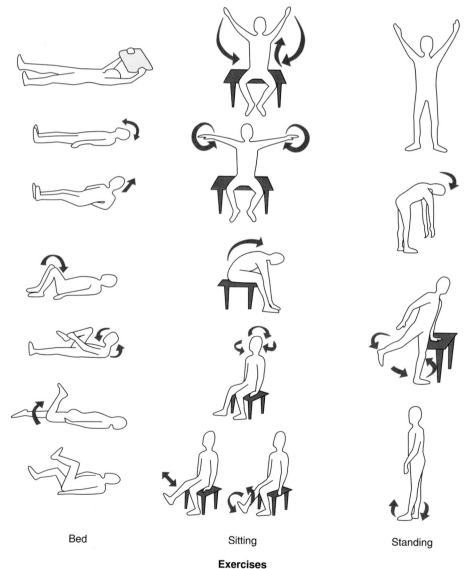

Bed   Sitting   Standing

Exercises

Figure 24-2   Bed-lying, sitting, and standing exercises. (From Ebersole, P., & Hess, P. [1998]. *Toward healthy aging: Human need and nursing response* [3rd ed.]. St. Louis: Mosby).

Box **24-3** Benefits of Exercise in the Older Adult
• Better sleep • Reduced constipation • Lower cholesterol level • Lower blood pressure • Better digestion • Weight loss • Socializing opportunities

wasting common to osteoporosis. Recent research shows that regular exercise promotes bone mineral density among older adults (Florindo et al., 2002). Older individuals who suffer from arthritis find aquatic exercise a pain-free way to promote their health and increase their functional ability. Exercising in the water is also an effective and enjoyable activity for those without arthritis. The effects of exercise on the older adult are extensive. Box 24-3 lists many benefits that can be derived from participating in an exercise program.

Before beginning any exercise program, an older person who has not been exercising should consult a physician or nurse practitioner. After the program begins, activity levels should be increased gradually. Adherence to exercise is a major problem for all populations. The best tools available to encourage continued exercise among older adults are to communicate the role of exercise in maintaining their quality of life, to help them choose an exercise that they enjoy with others, and to choose one that is easily accessible.

Sleep-Rest Pattern

Inability to sleep well is one of the most frequent complaints of older adults (Ramesh & Roberts, 2002). The high prevalence of sleep disorders in this population indicates that they experience a great need for assistance in getting to sleep and staying asleep. Zizi, Jean-Louis, Magai, Greenidge, Wolintz, and Heath-Phillip (2002) state that 25% of the sample in their study of 1118 reported difficulty falling asleep and 52% had difficulty remaining asleep; 28% reported early awakening and 12% reported daytime sleepiness. Sleep complaints result from several normal aging changes that occur among older adults of all cultural backgrounds. The changes result in a decrease in the total hours of sleep that are required, an increase in nocturnal awakenings, shorter periods of sleep, and a decrease in slow-wave activity.

The benefits of a good night's sleep are numerous. Overall increases in energy, motivation to continue a high quality of life, and improved immune function are only a few. Nurses assist older adults in achieving a good night's sleep through assessment that might reveal possible causes of sleep disturbances. Teaching about the normal changes in the aging sleep system can provide reassurance that their sleep patterns have changed but are not necessarily harmful.

Having this information may decrease anxiety. Increasing physical activity can also help them fall asleep more readily in the evening or night hours. Increased pain medication or alternative pain-relief methods can help those who suffer from painful conditions obtain better rest at night.

Residents of nursing facilities or people in acute care facilities may have difficulty adjusting to the environment at night. Adjustments in noise and lighting can help these individuals sleep better. Emotional disorders frequently can be identified, and therapy and medication can be administered during the day to help them sleep peacefully at night. Finally, daytime napping has been viewed as inhibiting a good night's sleep in this population.

Sleep medications may be helpful for short-term use. However, Ramesh and Roberts (2002) report that benzodiazepines should be used cautiously because of the possibility of rebound and morning insomnia, as well as hangover effect and daytime sedation.

Cognitive-Perceptual Pattern
Cognition

Thinking processes (**cognition**) in old age have been the subject of intensive study over the past few decades. Brain weight decreases with aging, and a shift occurs in the proportion of gray matter to white matter. The ways in which these changes are manifested in individuals varies because of culture, heredity, lifestyle, environmental exposures, and many other factors. No consensus has been reached as to the ways in which these changes translate into human behavior.

There is a common belief that most older adults will eventually develop dementia; however, cognitive problems are not a normal change of aging. **Mild cognitive impairment (MCI)** is a pathological collection of symptoms that results in memory loss, language difficulties, and impairments in judgment and reasoning. It is estimated that 10% to 15% of older adults will develop Alzheimer's disease (Rapp, Brenes, & Marsh, 2002).

Dementia is an illness of the cognitive system and is not accepted as a normal change of aging. Dementia is defined by the Alzheimer's Association as a "loss of mental function in two or more areas such as language, memory, visual and spatial abilities, or judgment severe enough to interfere with daily life" (Alzheimer's Association, 1999). It is important to note that most older adults live without cognitive difficulties. Shelkey (2000) reports that approximately 15% of people over age 65 have cognitive impairment. Cognitive alterations are key symptoms indicating changes in physiological function among the aged.

Two main types of dementia exist. The first type is **multiinfarct dementia,** which is caused by the death of brain tissue and diagnosed through brain imaging. Tissue death may be caused by of a lack of blood flow to the brain from a cerebral vascular accident (CVA) or from another cause. The other main type of dementia is **Alzheimer's disease,** the most common type, which makes up about 50% of all dementia diagnoses. The Alzheimer's Association estimates

---

Mini Mental Status Examination Sample Items

Orientation to Time

"What is the date?"

Registration

"Listen carefully,

I am going to say three words.

You say them back after I stop.

Ready? Here they are...

HOUSE (pause), CAR (pause), LAKE (pause).

Now repeat those words back to me."

[Repeat up to 5 times, but score only the first trial.]

Naming

"What is this?"

[Point to a pencil or pen.]

Reading

"Please read this and do what it says."

[Show examinee the words on the stimulus form.]

CLOSE YOUR EYES

Figure 24-3 Mini Mental State Examination sample items. (Reproduced by special permission of the Publisher, Psychological Assessment Resources, Inc., 16204 North Florida Avenue, Lutz, Florida 33549, from the Mini Mental State Examination, by Marshal Folstein and Susan Folstein, Copyright 1975, 1998 by Mini Mental LLC, Inc. Published 2001 by Psychological Assessment Resources, Inc. Further reproduction is prohibited without permission of PAR, Inc. The MMSE can be purchased from PAR, Inc., by calling 800-331-8378 or 813-968-3003.)

that approximately 4.5 million U.S. adults have Alzheimer's disease. Other dementias include Parkinson-related dementia, Huntington disease, Creutzfeldt-Jakob disease, Pick disease, and Lewy body dementia. Each one involves cognitive processes as defined above, although cognitive symptoms may vary depending on the area(s) of the brain affected by the disease.

The symptoms of dementia include forgetfulness, inattentiveness, disorganized thinking, altered levels of consciousness, perceptual disturbances, sleep-wake disorders, psychomotor disturbances, and disorientation. All older adults should be assessed for dementia regularly and again if these symptoms arise. One tool that has been used successfully to screen for cognitive impairments among older adults is the **Mini-Mental State Examination** (MMSE) (Folstein, Folstein, & McHugh, 1975) (Figure 24-3). This instrument was developed to assess the baseline mental status of older adults and to evaluate change or decline in mental functioning. The MMSE is based on a 30-point scale that measures level of awareness and orientation, appearance and behavior, speech and communication, mood and affect, disturbances in thinking, problems with perception, and abstract thinking and judgment. The higher the older adult scores on the examination, the more intact the mental

status is presumed to be. When the scale is 23 or lower, the individual is determined to have a problem with cognition. It is important to note that this instrument has been criticized for its cultural insensitivity, and it is difficult to use among individuals who speak languages other than English and among those with visual impairments and low literacy. Mulgrew, Morgenstern, Shetterly, Baxter, Baron, and Hamman (1999) found that the performance of Hispanic people on the MMSE was lower than that of non-Hispanic white people.

The MMSE is relatively easy to perform after a little practice and has been used for initial and subsequent evaluation of older adults in a variety of settings. The most effective way to perform the assessment is to make the person comfortable and establish a rapport. Eliminating noise and promoting attention and concentration will allow individuals to answer questions to the best of their ability. After the examination, the score can be computed and used as a basis for care planning.

Nonpharmacological techniques for managing the problems associated with dementia include developing and keeping routines, working in a calm, gentle, and unhurried manner, encouraging self-care activity, and reducing sensory overload. Interventions to keep the older adult safe include curtailing wandering behavior and preventing falls, cuts, and bruises. Medications to treat Alzheimer's disease are known as *cholinesterase inhibitors*. These medications are most effective during the early stages of the disease and act by increasing the levels of acetylcholine in the brain to prevent further loss and improve cognitive status.

Researchers are testing the effectiveness of an Alzheimer's vaccine. Preliminary studies suggest that older adults who developed antibodies to β-amyloid plaques (the product that composes the plaques associated with Alzheimer's disease) had less cognitive decline, as measured by the MMSE, when compared with those who did not develop antibodies (Alzheimer's Disease Education & Referral Center, 2001-2002). Brain swelling in the study participants, however, has slowed testing on this vaccine.

Another medication that has shown some promise in treating Alzheimer's disease is Namenda, or memantine. The action of memantine differs from that of cholinesterase inhibitors but works well in combination with this class of drugs and appears to be well tolerated. Lithium is also being suggested as a possible medication to suppress the development of β-amyloid plaque formation among people who already have the disease. However, the cardiovascular and central nervous system side effects of this medication make it difficult for the elderly to tolerate.

Stereotypes suggest that older people are less capable of learning and lose their intellectual capacity, but research has not supported this notion. Although studies indicate that older people do not show a decrease in intellect (Shelkey, 2000), nurses are advised to allow them more time to process information. Nurses should encourage older individuals to take classes, read, engage in stimulating conversation and entertainment, keep their minds active, and continue learning throughout their lives. They should be encouraged to continue with self-care activities rather than to relinquish them to caregivers. Because some memory impairment may be present in cognitively healthy older adults, memory aids and familiar environments should be encouraged (Research Highlights box).

Sensory Factors

Older adults experience several age-related changes in the five senses. Because of the normal and pathological changes associated with their senses, individuals of all cultural backgrounds and in all settings can benefit from nursing interventions. A variety of structural changes cause visual acuity to decrease, color discrimination to become less acute, pupil size and constriction ability to decrease, and peripheral vision to diminish. The lens of the eye becomes yellow and predisposes them to cataracts. The older adult is at increased risk for glaucoma, a group of eye disorders characterized by increased intraocular pressure. Because of the normal changes in the aging eye and the high risk for disease, a baseline eye assessment should be done early in this stage of life. Based on the normal changes and any disease processes assessed, follow-up eye appointments should be scheduled at least annually. Safety, particularly while

---

research highlights

Assisted Living Facilities for Older Adults

The number of assisted living facilities has increased greatly over the past decade because of their philosophical emphasis on maintaining independence and privacy. A study by Hawes, Phillips, Rose, Holan, and Sherman (2003) examined the extent to which these facilities are meeting the philosophical ideals of older adults that they aim to serve. The data revealed that only 11% of the 11,459 facilities offered a high level of services and privacy. Aging in place, or the ability of the older adult to live in the facility when health conditions decreased functional ability, was limited by the policies in these facilities. The authors concluded that the practice of assisted living facilities does not always live up to their philosophy.

Data from Hawes, C., Phillips, C. D., Rose, M., Holan, S., & Sherman, M. (2003). A national survey of assisted living facilities. *The Gerontologist, 43*, 875-882.

---

driving, is a concern for older adults and society. Nurses should encourage them to take driving classes that will help them deal with the diminishment of certain senses and learn how to become safer drivers as these changes occur.

Hearing deficits are common in old age, resulting from inner ear atrophy or sclerosis of the tympanic membrane. The inner ear can also undergo a number of changes, including those that are cell degenerative and nerve related. Sound threshold changes, with an associated difficulty in understanding what others are saying. Similar to the changes of the eye, changes in hearing and high risk for pathology indicate that older adults should begin regular ear and hearing screening early in this stage of life. On the recommendation of the audiologist, audiological testing should be conducted at least annually. Hearing aids can assist those with hearing loss to communicate more effectively. Wallhagen and Strawbridge (2003) report that there is a relationship between hearing impairment and cognitive impairment in this population. The nurse assesses, on an ongoing basis, for the buildup of wax to ensure optimal hearing (Case Study and Care Plan).

Taste changes with aging because of a loss of taste buds. The flavors of sweet, sour, salty, and bitter become blurred with this loss. The sensations brought about by touch may also diminish with sensory nerve losses, especially in the presence of debilitating diseases such as diabetes, stroke, or Parkinson's disease. The ability to smell and the acuity of the olfactory nerve also decrease with age. Because of the loss of smell and taste sensations, older adults have the tendency to use large, perhaps unsafe, amounts of salt and sugar in their food. Teaching about safe cooking and seasoning of food may be appropriate. Additionally, cognition related to common danger signals such as smoke or rotten food is impaired. Older adults should be taught to check the dates on their food packages frequently and be attentive when cooking and preparing meals. A recent issue of the Tufts University Health & Nutrition Letter ("Greater food

CASE STUDY

Larry Johnson

Larry Johnson, a healthy 75-year-old man, lives in his own apartment and is completely independent in ADLs and IADLs. Last Friday morning, Larry left his apartment complex at 8:09 AM to go to the store. While backing out of his driveway, he failed see a school bus passing on the intersecting street, and his car struck the bus. Although no one was injured, this incident indicated the need for a sensory and neurological assessment. The assessment revealed both hearing and visual deficits.

ADLs, activities of daily living; *IADL,* instrumental activities of daily living.

CARE PLAN

Unsafe Driving

(Related to Larry Johnson Case Study)

Nursing Diagnosis Risk for Injury Related to Unsafe Driving

Defining Characteristics
- Altered response time
- Change in vision or hearing

Related Factors
- Past accident
- Stressful life events
- Receipt of traffic tickets
- Witnessed poor driving

Expected Outcomes
- Client will have realistic expectations of ability to drive.
- Client and nurse will set appropriate limitations on driving.
- Client will take a driver refresher course.
- Client will have no further accidents.

Interventions
- Assist Larry in registering for a renewal driving program.
- Assist Larry in finding alternative modes of transportation until visual and hearing alterations are corrected and instead of driving in the evening.
- Schedule hearing and vision appointments for Larry and assist in transportation to appointments.

safety," 2002) advises older adults to avoid the following foods because of the risk of bacteria: deli meats and other ready-to-eat meat and poultry products; smoked fish; refrigerated pâtés and meat spreads; soft cheeses such as feta, brie, Camembert, blue-veined, and Mexican cheeses; unprocessed (homemade) Caesar salad dressing, hollandaise sauce, eggnog, and Key lime pie; cookie or cake batter; raw mollusks, including oysters, clams, and mussels; alfalfa sprouts; and fresh, unpasteurized juice.

The loss of taste and smell sensations, combined with the many other problems of obtaining appropriate nutrition, makes dental care of vital importance to this population. Lack of fluoridated water and preventive dentistry during the developmental years have caused tooth and gum problems to prevail in the older population. Tooth loss among adults is a common contributor to decreased taste sensation. In fact, *Healthy People 2010* has established goal #21-4 to decrease the number of older adults who have had all of their natural teeth extracted (USDHHS, 2000). The inability to chew and swallow food in a comfortable manner works synergistically with decreased smell and taste sensations and other problems to inhibit proper nutrition. The American Dental Association recommends that adults be seen for oral hygiene and counseling at least twice a year. During the initial evaluation, follow-up visits should be scheduled to ensure that teeth and gums remain in good condition or that appropriate dental devices are being used.

Skin changes occur, becoming thinner, wrinkled, and more fragile. Although sweating decreases and injuries take longer to heal, the skin remains capable of sensing and carrying out its protective role. However, chronic disease can place an individual at risk for decreased sensation throughout the body. CVAs or neuropathies resulting from diabetes are two examples of diseases that disrupt the ability to feel pain and pressure through the skin. This lack of sensation can threaten safety. When older adults are homebound, information about cooking on a hot stove and bathing and showering should be provided to prevent burns. The nurse should perform frequent skin assessments to detect alterations in skin integrity at an early stage.

The potential for skin impairment is common for those who suffer sensory deprivation from physical disease or

dementia. A pressure sore **(decubitus ulcer)** is a localized area of tissue necrosis that develops when soft tissue is compressed between two bony prominences or between a bony prominence and an external surface for a prolonged period. In addition to prolonged pressure on the skin, friction, moisture, shearing, and lack of nutrition place the older adult at risk of developing a decubitus ulcer, which is difficult to treat. Preventing the ulcer is the best method for maintaining intact skin. People at risk for decubitus ulcers should shift their position at least every 2 hours to distribute pressure appropriately throughout all areas of the skin. Elevating the lower extremities and maintaining proper body alignment are imperative to prevent decubitus ulcers. Specialty beds are readily available in most care settings to decrease pressure and assist in positioning individuals who are at risk. Positioning pillows and other orthopedic devices provide ways to help maintain the proper support of body parts and body alignment. Proper nutrition, including zinc and vitamins C and E, will help prevent this skin problem.

Self-Perception–Self-Concept Pattern

The variability of self-concept in the older adult is similar to the variability that is seen in the general population. As in all aspects of health, culture, environment, family, lifestyle factors, and heredity combine to form self-concept. Self-concept includes an individual's attitudes, perception of abilities (cognitive, affective, or physical), body image, identity, general sense of worth, and general emotional pattern. Personality traits tend to remain constant throughout life.

Erikson's Theory

The prevailing belief holds that adults no longer grow either emotionally or physically in their later years. Although the rate of physical decline exceeds the rate of physical growth, no evidence was found that emotional growth declines in any way. One needs only to view the classic film *Driving Miss Daisy* to understand that older adults go through many developmental changes in the 30 to 40 years that often make up older adulthood. Erikson's theory of development (1982) asserts that older adults must pass through developmental stages as do infants, children, and younger adults. As in all stages of psychosocial development, unsuccessful passage through a stage yields psychological illness, and successful passage through the stage promotes health (Erikson, 1982).

Ego integrity versus despair is the developmental stage of older adults (Erikson, 1982). The quality associated with successful passage of this stage is integrity, defined as an honest acceptance of the life that has passed and the stage of life that is currently being lived. Individuals who have reached this stage are said to be at peace with themselves. The inability to reach this stage leads to fear of death and despair that life has been lived in vain. Based on the expanding life span, this stage of development was expanded into three additional stages: (1) ego differentiation versus work role preoccupation, which involves achieving identity apart from work, (2) body transcendence versus body preoccupation, which focuses on adjusting to normal and aging changes, and (3) ego transcendence versus ego preoccupation, which involves accepting death (Erikson, 1997).

Nurses working in all settings are charged with helping older adults successfully pass through Erikson's psychosocial stages, enabling them to reach ego integrity. Two successful methods of assistance for older adults at all cognitive levels are reminiscence and life review. Haight (2005) defines these as, "Reminiscence is a multifaceted, multipurpose, naturally occurring mental phenomenon manifested across the life span in a variety of forms and contexts. Life review is one of those forms of reminiscence but it differs in that it is more intense and has more depth." Haight, Michel, and Hendrix (2000) found a positive effect of reminiscence on reducing depression. Puentes (2002) states that reminiscence usually is directed by a listener using questions or topics. The typical reminiscence session takes the form of a semistructured 45-minute to 1-hour meeting focusing on positive memories and the process, rather than product.

Roles-Relationships Pattern

Although the general framework of self-perception remains constant throughout the life span, the source of an individ-

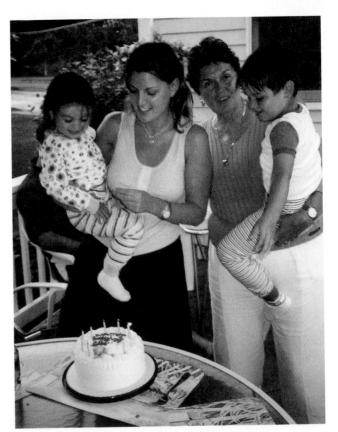

Figure 24-4 Passing on traditions by spending time with grandchildren fulfills a developmental task for older adults.

ual's self-perception often changes with older adulthood. The formation of the self that has focused on a person's role in the family changes when the children become independent or a spouse passes away. Roles such as daughter, son, sister, brother, wife, or husband may be lost because of death or illness. The loss of these roles can bring a great deal of sadness and possibly depression to the older adult. On the other hand, with the loss of these roles, a new role, such as grandparenting, frequently evolves (Figure 24-4). In the United States, 5.8 million, or 3.6%, of grandparents are raising grandchildren (Simmons & Dye, 2003) The role of grandparent frequently brings great joy and happiness at a time when the older adult feels loss; however, grandparents who rear grandchildren encounter several issues. Research suggests that grandparents who rear grandchildren are at increased risk for poor health and increased psychological distress (Kelly, 2000). Encouraging and supporting older adults in this role is necessary to help them fill the void left by the loss of their job or spousal roles, and to prevent the stress and strain of this caregiver role.

With the average life span increasing, older adults can spend many more years in retirement than did previous generations. There were approximately 47 million social security beneficiaries at the end of 2003 (Social Security Administration, 2003), up from an estimated 27.2 million retirees reported in December 1997. Rosenkoetter (2000) offers several theories to help understand retirement. For people who are healthy and view retirement in a positive light, it is a time that is peaceful and less stressful than the work years were. For individuals who have an adequate amount of money, retirement can be a time for travel, golf, painting lessons, or other favorite hobbies and leisure activities for which time was previously unavailable. For other older adults, retirement can be a long void at the end of life that is full of ill health and financial difficulty. Further assaults on the individual's self-concept may include a lowered income, loss of friends, disease, and disability. Volunteering can be an effective method for older adults to continue to feel engaged in the working environment as a productive, contributing member of society. Older adults who volunteer have an external incentive for getting dressed in the morning; they take a great amount of pride in their work. Filling a volunteer position can remedy negative feelings about retirement and other role changes.

Federal and state funding has created a number of subsidized work programs for older adults. With the assistance of this funding through private agencies and local Area Agencies on Aging, they are given the opportunity to work for pay. Although the pay may not be comparable with that earned before retirement, the earnings can be a necessary supplement, after the age of 70, to Social Security benefits. These programs allow older adults to work with children in day care centers, with disabled and ill older adults at home, and in administrative positions. Nurses should provide interested individuals with information about these programs.

Leaving home, widowhood, retirement, and relocation can elicit profound feelings of loss. Older adults who remain engaged in a variety of activities and relationships are happier and healthier. Personality, and its expression over time, is considered as a major determinant of how engaged or active a person will be late in life. Other variables such as culture, health, bereavement, and habit affect activity, as well.

Health-promotion activities center on an understanding of the individual's usual behavior and any unexpected or unexplained deviation in that behavior. Nurses help older adults identify the meaning of their lost roles and the results of those losses, and to work through reactions to the loss. In more traumatic cases, support groups, such as bereavement groups, can be helpful. The nurse supports those going through role changes by eliciting reactions and facilitating communication about these reactions. Significant others, such as children, neighbors, and friends, can provide important ongoing support. The nurse is integral in helping older adults develop and explore their new role as grandparents.

Sexuality-Reproductive Pattern

Pangman and Seguire (2000) define sexuality as "a fundamental and natural need within everyone's life, regardless of age and physical state" (p. 51). A great deal of debate has taken place over the presence or absence of sexual desire among older adults. Society generally believes that older adults do not participate in sexual relationships. The myths regarding sexual activity among older adults include the following:

- Older adults are no longer interested in sex.
- Medical illnesses common to older adults prevent them from having sex.
- Impotence is a normal aging change (Wallace, 2000).

The most accurate predictor of sexual interest in older adulthood is the enjoyment and frequency of sex at a younger age. No data were found to show that men or women lose interest in sexual activity as they age. Older adults must also fulfill the human need to touch and be touched. Touch is an overt expression of closeness and an integral part of sexuality. Although the need to express sexuality continues, older adults are susceptible to many disabling medical conditions, such as cardiac problems, arthritis, and normal aging changes, and these can make the expression of sexuality difficult. In both genders, reduced availability of sex hormones results in less rapid and less extreme vascular responses to sexual arousal. The lack of circulating hormones in both men and women results in changes in four areas of the sexual system: arousal, orgasm, postorgasm, and extragenital changes. Management of a medical condition can hinder sexual response.

Nurses are in an ideal position to help older adults fulfill their sexual desires by helping them to compensate for normal aging changes and disabling medical conditions and medications. Knowledge is essential to the successful fulfillment of sexuality. In a study of 68 older adults living in the community, Walker and Ephross (1999) found that the group was able to answer only 67% of sexual knowledge questions correctly.

After making a sexual assessment, nurses can intervene at an early point to prevent or correct problems, but they frequently choose not to consider sexuality when planning care. One of the reasons for this refusal is that nurses believe the societal myths about older adults' sexuality. Without proper training and experience, they are not sufficiently confident to venture into this delicate area.

One method in which they may gain knowledge is through a game aimed at educating nursing staff about sexual dysfunction in older adults. In a pilot study of five nurses who completed both pretests and posttests, knowledge regarding sexual assessment and treatment increased after playing the sexual dysfunction trivia game (Skinner, 2000). Bauer (1999) concluded that the use of humor was often an effective method for addressing sexual needs.

The expression of sexuality among older adults results in a higher quality of life achieved through fulfilling a natural desire. In long-term care facilities, the need to address sexual needs of the residents is great because of their many disabilities. In the community setting nurses have access to the entire family unit in their natural surroundings. The information that is necessary to make a sexual assessment is readily accessible.

Many nurses believe that acquired immunodeficiency syndrome (AIDS) and other sexually transmitted diseases are not problems for older adults. However, the number of older adults who have contracted the human immunodeficiency virus (HIV) has risen sharply over the past decade. Eleven to fifteen percent of all AIDS cases are among people aged 50 and older; 25% of these are over age 60 (Capozza, 2002). Older adults should use proper precautions, such as a barrier method, to prevent the spread of disease. Nurses use universal precautions to protect themselves from HIV and other blood-borne pathogens. Older adults should follow the safer sex guidelines recommended by the CDC.

Coping–Stress Tolerance Pattern

An individual's ability to cope with the common stresses of older adulthood is a key factor in maintaining self-concept and subsequent integrity. As people age, they tend to encounter many losses, such as the loss of a home, physical functioning, spouses, friends, and siblings. The nurse who cares for the older adult can be extremely helpful in the coping process. In a sample of 99 older adults, it was found that continually thinking about a loss or bad event was not as effective as trying to find the positive and developmental benefits of losses. In this study acceptance of the loss or event resulted in less depression (Kraaij, Pruymboom, & Garnefski, 2002). Cultural background has a profound effect on the manner in which coping with stresses occurs. After assessing the most appropriate way in which the individual desires to cope with a situation, the nurse may help create an appropriate environment for coping.

Depression

The rate of **depression,** symptoms of sadness, decreased ability to experience pleasure, pessimism, inhibition, retardation of action, and physical complaints (Wykle & Zauszniewski, 2000), rises sharply with age. According to *Healthy People 2010* (USDHHS, 2000), adults and older adults have the highest rates of depression. Rates are especially high among those with coexisting medical conditions. Research further reports that 12% of older people hospitalized for problems such as hip fracture or heart disease are diagnosed with depression. Rates of depression in nursing home residents range from 15% to 25%. The cause of this increase is not completely understood. The numerous losses experienced by older people may be partly to blame. Depression is also caused by physiological changes in the aging body. As a manifestation of an individual's self-concept, this disease has been the subject of detailed study. Although it appears to affect older adults in much the same way that it affects younger individuals, certain patterns of symptoms and older adults' overall susceptibility are different from those of younger counterparts.

Nurses are integral in helping to diagnose and manage depression in older adults. Depression can be found in all care environments. Some common behaviors include sullen affect, lack of appetite and weight loss, sleeplessness, fatigue, decreased ability to think or concentrate, psychomotor agitation, decreased participation in daily living activities and social activities, and suicidal ideation. Many instruments are available to assist nurses in assessing for this commonly occurring disorder. The Geriatric Depression Scale (Yesavage et al., 1983) is available in several formats, with 30, 15, 5, and 1 question, and is easily administered. This scale is presented in **Web Site Resource 24A.** Positive results on the screening examinations require referral to social services for a diagnostic workup. After depression is diagnosed, successful management may include antidepressant medications and psychosocial therapy.

Suicide

According to the CDC and unpublished mortality data from the National Center for Health Statistics, suicide rates increase with age and are highest among Americans age 65 years and older (CDC, 2001b). Men accounted for 83% of suicides among people age 65 years and older in 1997. From 1980 to 1997, the largest relative increases in suicide rates occurred among people 80 to 84 years of age. The rate for men in this age group increased 8% (from 43.5 to 47.0 per 100,000). Firearms were the most common method of suicide by both men and women age 65 years and older in 1997, accounting for 77.1% of male and 32.7% female suicides in this age group (CDC, 2001b). The reason for the high number of suicides in the older adult population continues to be explored. The elevated rate of depression helps the medical community understand the motive of many older adults. Many older adults have serious medical illnesses that provide an explanation for wanting to die. Risk factors for suicide include social isolation, alcohol abuse, psychosis, bereavement, and serious medical illness. Lynch, Compton, Mendelson, Robins, and Krishnan (2000) found that other variables related to suicide included feeling sinful, guilty, or worthless, and early depressive onset. The importance of different aspects of life also varies by culture. Some older adults may visit a health care provider with a somatic complaint before the suicide attempt as, perhaps, a final call for help. Nurses working with the older population are aware of their high rate of suicide and are alert for the risk factors. Suicide threats are taken seriously and interventions are implemented to keep the older adult safe.

The chronic illness that frequently accompanies old age raises a concern for ethical care. Many members of society believe that with the increased life span, individuals can be subjected to more suffering. A solution to ending the suffering of those with chronic illness has been **euthanasia,** or **physician-assisted suicide.** In many states people are lobbying to legalize physician-assisted suicide. The American Nurses Association maintained in their 1994 position statement that nurses should refuse to participate in assisted suicide. Nurses are subsequently charged with helping society to understand the many benefits of older adulthood and celebrating the extended life span rather than deeming it wasteful. Nurses caring for chronically ill older adults have the added burden of determining which ones are at risk for wanting physician-assisted suicide and helping them to live free of pain and discomfort. Nurses are instrumental in ensuring that the older person experiences a pain-free

HOTtopics

Herbal and Nutritional Supplement Use in Older Adults

Kales (2002) in a study of 82 older adults with depression or dementia, or both, and 56 of their caregivers, reports that approximately 20% of older adults use herbal medications without discussing them with their health care providers. Among participants in the study, 33.3% used ginkgo biloba, 26.7% used St. John's wort, 6.7 used ginseng, and 20% took other herbal preparations. The author states that herbal medication use among older adults requires further study. However, the findings of this study are important and should alert health care providers to the large use of herbal medications among the older population.

1. Why do older adults use herbs?
2. Are the alternatives used more for health-promotion reasons or for chronic condition relief?

Modified from the work of Kales, H. C. (2002). Retrieved April 12, 2005, from: *http://www.med.umich.edu/opm/newspage/2002/elderlydep. htm.*

death by advocating for an appropriate pain-management program and working with other health care professionals toward this end (Hot Topics box).

Values-Beliefs Pattern

Every older adult for whom nurses have the opportunity to care will have a different sense of spirituality, which will have a profound influence on the person's motivation and ability to live a healthy lifestyle. The individual sense of spirituality is influenced by culture, gender, experiences, religion, economic status, ethnic background, and other beliefs (Brush, 2000). Although no universal sense of spirituality exists among older adults, many researchers report that spiritual resources are related to mental health.

Nurses may find themselves in a difficult position in attempting to promote the spiritual health of individuals. One reason for this perceived difficulty may be the nurse's discomfort with the person's belief system. Bickerstaff, Graser, and McCabe (2003) report that spirituality provides older adults with purpose and meaning in life, as well as guidance regarding personal values and concerns. There may be as many different spiritual values and beliefs as there are individuals. For example, Shih and Shih (1999) report that spirituality was listed as one of the met needs of elderly Chinese men. However, other cultural groups may need more assistance from health care providers in meeting spiritual needs.

Varying spiritual values make helping older adults actualize their spirituality, and thus acquire a high quality of life, difficult for nurses. Because of the highly personal quality of spirituality, an unobtrusive and sensitive presence by the nurse is needed to allow the person in any setting to achieve spiritual health. Additionally, spiritual assessment tools are available to guide nurses with the right questions to help

get to the root of the person's spirituality. Open-ended questions, such as, "What is your perception of God and spirituality?" can encourage discussions about the person's innermost spirituality.

PATHOLOGICAL PROCESSES
Accidents

Falls are a leading cause of morbidity and mortality among older adults. In 2001 more than 1.6 million older adults were treated in emergency departments for fall-related injuries and approximately 383,000 were hospitalized (CDC, 2002). White men have the highest fall-related mortality, followed by white women, black men, and black women (CDC, 2002), and women sustain about 80% of all hip fractures (Stevens & Olson, 2000). Rates increased with advancing age for both sexes but were consistently higher for women in all age categories. Hospitalization rates for hip fracture increased for women from 1988 through 1996, and the rates for men remained stable (Stevens et al., 1999).

Some of the causes of falls in older adults are neuromuscular dysfunction, osteoporosis, stroke, and sensory impairment. Although a fall in a younger individual may not be problematic, a fall in an older adult can have devastating consequences. Because of the higher risk of osteoporosis in the older population, a fall can result in a fracture. **Osteoporosis** is a disease of bone loss common to women age 70 and older and men age 80 and older. The disease occurs 6 times more frequently in women than it does in men. The rapid decline in estrogen secretion at the onset of menopause signals the calcium in the bones to move into the bloodstream, which allows the bones to become weak and brittle. Because of this weakness, falls in older adults with osteoporosis frequently result in fractures, which places these individuals in a spiral of iatrogenic risk, beginning with weeks of immobilization and possibly resulting in decubitus ulcers, psychological trauma, pneumonia, and even death.

Risk factors for osteoporosis include a small, thin frame; white or Asian ancestry; family history; excessive thyroid medication or high doses of cortisone-like drugs for asthma, arthritis, or cancer; a diet low in dairy products and other sources of calcium; physical inactivity; smoking cigarettes; and drinking alcohol. Osteoporosis typically is diagnosed after an older adult sustains a fracture. However, bone density testing is readily available to diagnose individuals at risk before a fracture occurs. Sufficient calcium intake remains vitally important and will continue to reduce the normal bone loss of aging. Most women need 1000 mg a day before menopause and 1500 mg a day after menopause. Consuming this amount of calcium from today's average diet is nearly impossible; therefore, a calcium supplement is essential. For the prevention of osteoporosis and the optimal health maintenance of both psychological and physical well-being in the older adult, physical activity is necessary.

A program to prevent falls is essential in the care of older adults. Because many factors contribute to falls, risk assessment is essential. Recommendations for prevention are abundant in the literature. The American Geriatrics Society (2001) collaborated with the British Geriatrics Society and the American Academy of Orthopedic Surgeons to recommend that all older adults should be screened for falls and that if a prior fall was sustained, the older adult remains at high risk. By identifying the risks and assessing an older adult's vision, hearing, medication usage, blood pressure, mobility, and other factors, falls can be predicted and prevented.

Several fall risk assessments have been developed. These instruments are easy to use and can be employed in acute or long-term care or in home settings. After completing the assessment, scores can assist in preventive care planning. Nurses in all settings will then be prepared to implement environmental, physiological, and psychological interventions.

Table 24-2 lists frequent causes of accidents that occur in the home and nursing interventions to prevent them. Home care nurses are in an ideal position to prevent injuries. During the initial and subsequent assessments, the nurse can evaluate individuals' homes for common factors leading to poisoning, fires, and falls, such as frayed wires on electrical appliances that can produce sparks and start fires or improperly labeled cleaning products that can be accidentally ingested. Health teaching should incorporate the concept of accident prevention for all older adults living not only in the community, but also in acute care and long-term care facilities.

The older adult's ability to feel changes in heat and cold may be impaired due to normal and pathological changes of aging. This process can cause older adults to die from the effects of heat waves or cold spells. During periods of heat and humidity, older people should increase fluid and salt intake; they should stay in cool quarters, remain quiet, have more rest periods, and refrain from going outdoors when the temperature goes above 90° F. Sweating, which tends to be delayed and reduced in older adults, can be facilitated by wearing light-colored, lightweight cotton clothing. If sweating ceases or is inadequate, the older person can be at risk for heat stroke. Heat stroke can contribute to sepsis, myocardial infarction, and CVAs, particularly in people with diabetes. Reduced body heat can also present problems in the older adult. Symptoms of and interventions for hypothermia are listed in Table 24-3.

Preventing Injury

Many causes of death by injury exist for older adults. Some of these causes are motor vehicle accidents, falls, suffocation, fires, and poisoning. Because of normal age-related changes and the increased incidence of illness, older adults can experience a decrease in muscle strength and reaction time and may subsequently become more vulnerable to environmental hazards. Decreased sensory acuity and impaired balance further diminish their ability to interpret the environment.

Table **24-2** Safety Risk Areas and Related Interventions	
Area of Attention	**Intervention**
Stairways	Secure handrails
	Stairways illuminated with light switches at both top and bottom
	Nonskid treads for steps
Bedroom	Night lights
	Tacked-down carpet
	Discourage use of throw rugs
	Furniture securely placed that will not obstruct clear pathways
	Extension cords and telephone wires secured and not in walking areas
Bathroom	Handrails used near tub and toilet
	Nonskid mats in tub area
	Bath thermometer for tub hot water
Kitchen	Nonflammable, lightweight, clothing when cooking
	Dishes and cooking devices at reasonable heights
	Use stepstools according to specifications and only when not alone
	Keep off wet floor and refrain from using slippery wax
	Never climb on chairs
	Keep emergency numbers near the telephone
	Locks should to be easy to open in times of emergency
	Cook at front of the stove rather than at the back
Living room	Furniture that is easy to get in and out of
	Fire detectors installed at appropriate places
Outdoors	Stairs free of breaks and cracks, clear of snow and ice
	Safe handrails
	Good lighting for stairs and walkways

As the percentage of older adults living in the United States increases, the number of older drivers also increases. If current trends in the number of drivers remains consistent, this number could exceed 2.5 times the 1996 levels within 30 years. In addition, it is estimated that between 1990 and 2020, the total annual mileage driven will increase by 465% for male older drivers and 500% for female older drivers (Burkhardt, Berger, Creedon, & McGavock, 1998). Older individuals are at a high risk for hospitalization and death from motor vehicle injuries because of the many changes in their neuromuscular and sensory abilities, which slow response time in emergency situations. According to Burkhardt et al. (1998), the number of elderly traffic fatalities will more than triple by the year 2030, exceeding the number of alcohol-related fatalities in 1995 by 35%. A

| Table **24-3** | Nursing Interventions for Hypothermia |

SYMPTOMS

Cold to touch
Slow respirations
Bradycardia
Low blood pressure
Slurred speech
Drowsiness
Temperature 95° F rectally

INTERVENTIONS

Warm hands and feet
Cover with blanket
Set room temperature to 70° F
Wear cap to bed at night
Wear several layers of clothing
Increase activity
Decrease alcohol intake

survey of 2046 older adults showed that older adults limited or stopped driving because of medical problems or problems with eyesight (Ragland, Satariano, & Macleod, 2004). Some were concerned about getting in an accident or stopped driving because they didn't have anywhere to go.

Older adults are encouraged to relearn how to drive so as to adapt to their neuromuscular and sensory changes. Nurses working in the community may encourage older drivers to contact AARP for driving classes designed to meet their needs. Attending these classes frequently allows savings on car insurance.

Biological Agents

A large emphasis is placed on immunizing young children against disease. However, older adults can require commonly available vaccines that have been shown to lower both morbidity and mortality. In many cases older adults have not received primary immunization against diphtheria and tetanus. Lack of immunity leaves them vulnerable to illness and death from these two diseases. **Website Resource 24B** lists immunization schedules for older adults.

Influenza

Influenza is a major cause of morbidity and mortality in older adults. The 80-and-older population experiences an estimated 42.7 million annual hospitalizations and deaths due to influenza and its complications (Menec, MacWilliam, & Aoki, 2002). Despite the increase in immunization rates and Medicare reimbursement for the vaccine, rates among older adults in senior housing is only 30% to 60%, with the number of institutionalized older adults receiving the vaccine being closer to 80% (McElhaney, 2002). The influenza vaccine can markedly reduce the incidence of complications, hospitalizations, and death (McElhaney, 2002). The vaccine, composed of inactivated whole virus or virus subunits grown in chick embryo cells, is given annually to older adults, especially those with chronic conditions such as pulmonary or cardiac problems and those in long-term care facilities. Vaccination is contraindicated in people who have experienced a reaction to it, and caution should be exercised in administering it to people who have allergies to eggs. A *Healthy People 2010* goal (#14-29 a-b) is to increase the number of older adults who are vaccinated annually against influenza and ever vaccinated against pneumococcal disease (USDHHS, 2000).

Pneumococcal Infections

Estimates indicate that pneumococcal infections were responsible for approximately 90,000 deaths in 1999 (National Institute of Allergy and Infectious Diseases, 2004). Nevertheless, many older adults remain unvaccinated. The CDC recommends that older adults should receive the pneumococcal vaccination every 10 years. However, many barriers, such as the prevailing myth that receiving the vaccination will result in the disease, prevent older adults from receiving immunization.

Tuberculosis

Commonly referred to as *consumption,* tuberculosis (TB) was the leading killer among infectious diseases from the nineteenth century into the mid-twentieth century. The TB organism usually is inhaled and deposited in the lung, where it replicates and causes morbidity and mortality in all populations, especially older adults. The TB epidemic was virtually wiped out with the introduction and appropriate use of various medications. In 1984, however, TB rates began to rise again. The increase in poverty, homelessness, drug and alcohol abuse, and AIDS has produced multiple strains of drug-resistant TB. The CDC estimates that there are 17,528 active cases of TB the United States (CDC, 1999).

The chances of acquiring TB in public areas with adequate ventilation are not significant. Ultraviolet rays from the sun kill the virus. The major risk comes from close contact with individuals who are carrying the TB organism. Nurses who suspect TB infection in older adults should look for these signs and symptoms: cough, fatigue, anorexia, nausea, fever, night sweats, and weight loss. However, atypical symptoms, such as delirium, frequently occur in older adults. A tuberculin skin test will indicate exposure to the TB organism, and a chest radiograph can confirm the presence of the disease in the person's lungs.

Therapy for TB includes isoniazid (300 mg a day) and rifampin (600 mg a day) orally for 9 months. Unfortunately, because of the possibility of concomitant altered liver function in older adults, side effects are possible. People must be instructed to take the medications exactly as ordered and not to skip a dose, because undertreatment leads to drug-resistant strains.

Drug Use

Normal changes of aging have a significant influence on drug use in the older adult. The way in which medications are absorbed, distributed, metabolized, and cleared from the body is affected by changes in organ systems and illness. Even when medications are taken as prescribed, age-related changes and disease can increase the risk of undesirable side effects. In addition to problems caused by the processing of drugs, prescription and non-prescription drug use is much higher in the older adult population than it is in the general population. Morley (2003) reports that the use of excessive and often inappropriate medication among older adults remains a significant problem.

One problem in this population is drug-drug interactions. Evidence suggests that as a person ages, the chance of experiencing a drug reaction is increased, and each prescribed or over-the-counter preparation that is taken multiplies the possibility of an adverse reaction. The Beers criteria, developed from the Health Care Financing Administration Guidelines for Potentially Inappropriate Medications in the Elderly, present medications known to place older adults at risk for adverse reactions. The Beers criteria are presented in **Website Resource 24C.** Federal government regulations (Omnibus Reconciliation Act) developed in 1987, implemented in 1990, and revised in 1997, have attempted to curtail the large use of unnecessary medications by older adults in long-term care facilities. As a rule, nurses should take a medication history to assess for past drug reactions. Medications should be started at their lowest effective dose and slowly increased as needed.

Many older adults who reside at home take their medications independently. Although self-medication with prescription and over-the-counter medications is an effective method of disease management, little is known about the process of taking medications after the person leaves the health care practice or facility. Although it is often assumed that medications are taken as ordered, sensory disturbances, lack of knowledge, and alternative drug, alcohol, and nutrition practices may present challenges to medication self-administration that interfere with medical management of health problems. Amoako, Richardson-Campbell, and Kennedy-Malone (2003) conducted a study of 39 older adults who lived independently to determine their over-the-counter self-medication practices. The researchers concluded that people may not be aware of risks associated with interactions between medications, as well as concomitant alcohol and caffeine use. Moreover, Neafsey and Shellman (2001) conducted a study of 168 older adults and found that 86% of the sample participated in self-medication practices resulting in high risk for adverse drug interactions.

One of the major barriers to drug adherence in the elderly surrounds affordability. Prescription drug costs continue to rise annually and Medicare does not usually pay for medications. Recently the Medicare Prescription Drug Improvement and Modernization act of 2003 approved prescription discount drug cards for Medicare recipients. These cards are available to over 7 million of Medicare's 41 million participants. To be eligible for the discount cards, older adults must apply and, depending on their income, a fee of $30 may be charged. The cards provide discounts on some drugs, but not all. The *American Journal of Nursing* (AJN reports, 2004) reports that older adults with higher incomes may save more by using other prescription drug plans or by shopping around.

The use of illegal drugs among older adults is a problem that has been around since the beginning of time, but it remains widely unrecognized by health care professionals. Because of this lack of acknowledgment, drug abuse frequently is overlooked. In fact, some of the problems of older adults, such as accidents, neglected personal hygiene, malnutrition, noncompliance, and memory loss, may actually be signs of substance abuse. New tools designed to detect the problems of substance abuse are being developed that will help nurses assess this problem and make referrals to treatment programs.

Alcohol Use

Alcohol problems among older adults have been underestimated and hidden. The National Institute on Alcohol and Alcoholism reports that for women of all ages and for men over 65, more than 7 drinks per week or more than 3 drinks per occasion is considered a risk. It is estimated that the number of adults over age 50 who abuse or are dependent on alcohol will increase from 1.7 million to 4.4 million by 2020 (Robert Wood Johnson Foundation, 2001).

Blow, Walton, Chermack, Mudd, and Brower (2000) demonstrated that older adults with alcohol problems who received treatment specific to their needs could achieve positive health outcomes. However, a major barrier to treatment is lack of detection. Alcohol abuse in seniors frequently goes unnoticed, because the symptoms can be similar to those of other common problems of aging, and the affected individuals are no longer in the work force where they could be observed. The longer the problem remains undetected, the greater it becomes.

The elderly are more vulnerable to the effects of alcohol, because their systems do not detoxify and excrete as efficiently as do those of younger people. Alcoholism predisposes them to accidents, nutritional deficiencies, disease, and decreased function. Interestingly, when older adults seek treatment for their alcoholism, their prognosis is many times better than it is for their younger counterparts. When alcohol abuse is suspected, referral to a treatment program will help the person conquer the problem and return to a higher level of functioning.

Tobacco Use

Cigarette smoking causes cardiovascular disease, several kinds of cancer (lung, larynx, esophagus, pharynx, mouth, and bladder), and chronic lung disease. Cigarette smoking also contributes to cancer of the pancreas, kidney, and cervix (USDHHS, 2000). Aging men of today are perhaps the first generation to smoke practically throughout their adult lives. The results of smoking occur slowly over time, and problems usually are not experienced until lung damage has occurred. Research demonstrates that because smoking can initiate and promote disease processes, it is one of the

Table 24-4	Three Leading Cancer Sites in the Elderly in Order of Incidence
Gender	**Cancer**
Men	Prostate
	Lung
	Colon
Women	Breast
	Lung
	Colon

From U.S. Cancer Statistics Working Group. (2003). *United States cancer statistics: 2000 Incidence.* Atlanta, GA: Department of Health and Human Services, Centers for Disease Control and Prevention and National Cancer Institute.

most important negative predictors of longevity. Other diseases common to smokers are chronic obstructive pulmonary diseases, including bronchitis, asthma, emphysema, and bronchiectasis. Smoking is a particular problem for older adults because of the large number of medications they take and the potential for drug interactions. Nicotine-drug interactions can cause many problems.

Older adults can experience the benefits of smoking cessation even after the age of 65. These people may be more motivated to quit smoking than when they were younger, because they are likely to see some of the damage that smoking has caused and anticipate that smoking cessation will restore their health. Nurses in acute care settings are in an ideal position to assist them in making the commitment to quit smoking while recovering from an acute illness. Nurses in long-term care and community settings also have the opportunity and access to resources to help motivate individuals to quit. Behavioral management classes are available to community-dwelling older adults, who may also be candidates for other nonmedical interventions and nicotine-replacement therapy.

Cancer

Cancer rates for older adults are disproportionately high in the United States. Although only 12% of the population is considered as older adults, more than 50% of all diagnosed cancers are found in this population. The reason for the large proportion of cancer in this country is unknown. Theories include longer exposure to carcinogens, increased susceptibility to cancer in the older body, decreased cellular healing ability, loss of tumor-suppressing genes, and decreased immune function. Although the exact cause cannot be determined, cancer is a significant problem for older adults in the United States.

The types of cancer common to older adults are listed by gender in Table 24-4. Prostate cancer is the leading cancer among men of all races and ages and is clearly the most common male cancer and the second leading cause of death from cancer in men in the United States. Estimates are that 8% of all men in the United States will be diagnosed with prostate cancer during their lifetime. Early detection of prostate cancer allows treatment while it is still localized in the prostate gland and highly curable. Evidence suggests that by using a combination of screening techniques, more cases of prostate cancer can be detected earlier. A review of the literature identified the three key components of an appropriate prostate screen: (1) symptomatology, (2) prostate specific antigen, and (3) a digital rectal examination (Lee, 2002). The four major treatment options for prostate cancer are surgery, radiation therapy, watchful waiting, and hormone therapy.

Breast cancer is the most common cancer in older women of all ages and races in the United States. It is surpassed only by lung cancer as the cause of mortality in women. Reports suggest that one in nine women will develop breast cancer in her lifetime. Three quarters of all breast cancers occur in women over 50. The risk is increased in women whose close female relatives (mothers or sisters) have had the disease. Women who have never had children or had their first child after age 30 appear to have an increased risk. The causes of breast cancer remain unclear. The best protection is early detection and prompt treatment. The American Cancer Society recommends that women have annual mammograms and breast examinations beginning at age 40 and practice monthly breast self-examination.

Nurses help older adults change the habits that place them at high risk for developing cancer. Following nutritional guidelines (as suggested earlier in this chapter), reducing stress, adopting a program of regular exercise, and smoking cessation are a few of the approaches that nurses can advise to promote individual wellness. Periodic monitoring and screening in the form of regular visits with a primary health care provider or community screening can alert older adults to early signs and symptoms of cancers that occur during the later years.

SOCIAL PROCESSES
Environments of Care

The incidence of chronic and acute illnesses, the subsequent decline in functional status, changes in economic status, and changes in family structure frequently place older adults in situations for which they are admitted to acute care facilities or must make a temporary or permanent move into another housing situation or a long-term care facility. When providing health-promotion services to older adults, nurses must take into account that they might live in a number of different settings.

When older adults leave their homes, they enter a continuum of care extending from the acute care facility to the long-term care or community setting (Figure 24-5). Nurses who work in each of the settings on the continuum can promote health to this population in many ways. From the acute care setting through each stage of the continuum until they return home, opportunities are available for nurses to introduce older adults and their families to community resources (Table 24-5). The acute care nurse has the opportunity to present health-promotion strategies at a time

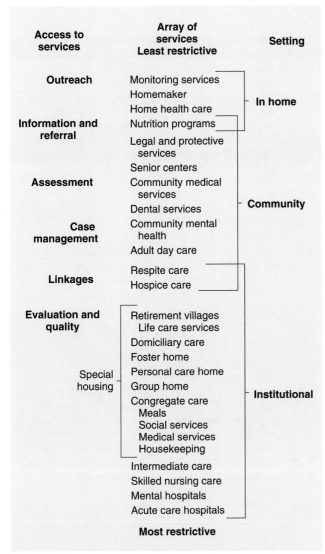

Access to services	Array of services **Least restrictive**	Setting
Outreach	Monitoring services / Homemaker / Home health care / Nutrition programs	In home
Information and referral	Legal and protective services / Senior centers	
Assessment	Community medical services / Dental services	Community
Case management	Community mental health / Adult day care	
Linkages	Respite care / Hospice care	
Evaluation and quality	Retirement villages / Life care services / Domiciliary care / Foster home	
Special housing	Personal care home / Group home / Congregate care / Meals / Social services / Medical services / Housekeeping	Institutional
	Intermediate care / Skilled nursing care / Mental hospitals / Acute care hospitals	
	Most restrictive	

Figure 24-5 Continuum of care for older adults. (From Wetle, T. [1982]. *Handbook of geriatric care.* East Hanover, NJ: Sandoz.)

during which clients perceive the greatest need to change their lifestyle to return to a healthy status. In most cases an acute care admission is a perfect opportunity to introduce health-promotion teaching. However, the acute care nurse may feel frustrated by the inability to see the results of this teaching and may therefore give it a low priority in the plan of care.

Some older adults will rapidly grasp material that they believe will prevent future hospital admissions and restore their health. Visiting nurse appointments, transportation, homemaking and chore services, adult day care, and assistance with grocery shopping or home-delivered meals will help them return to the home care environment better prepared to recover from the illness. Helping older adults to locate adult day-care programs, smoking-cessation programs, stress-management workshops, or weight-loss and exercise programs before leaving the hospital will encour-

HEALTH TEACHING   Sleep and the Older Adult

When you believe that you suffer from poor sleep, ask your health care provider about what is considered normal for adults your age. Follow these suggestions to improve your sleep:

- Plan a regular bedtime and wake-up schedule.
- Pursue activities and hobbies.
- Avoid daytime napping; consider any nap you take as part of your sleep total for the day.
- Exercise will help you fall asleep easily, but avoid exercise immediately before bedtime.
- Avoid caffeine after 10:00 AM.
- Avoid drinking too much alcohol.
- Avoid some over-the-counter medications, such as cough syrup and allergy medicine.
- Avoid sleeping medications.
- Avoid tobacco products.

To further your getting a good night's sleep, your bedroom should include the following:

- Quiet surroundings
- Darkness
- Coolness and comfort
- A firm and comfortable mattress

Contact your health care provider if you are experiencing any of the following:

- Sleepiness while driving
- Depression, anxiety, or severe personal stress
- Trouble doing your usual daily activities

How will my health care provider find the cause of my sleep problem?

To find the cause of your sleep problem, your health care provider may:

- Ask you many questions about your health and your family's health
- Ask your sleep companion questions about your sleeping habits
- Ask you to complete a sleep log; in the sleep log, you record whether you were tired during the day, when you fell asleep, how well you slept, and when you woke up
- Perform tests, which may include a blood test or having you fall asleep in a laboratory so that your sleep can be observed
- Refer you to a sleep specialist

What usually causes sleep problems in older adults?

Sleep problems can be caused by many things, including medications; medical conditions, such as angina, asthma, or anxiety; poor sleeping habits; and sleep disorders.

Modified from Grand Jean, C. K., & Gibbons, S. W. (2000). Assessing ambulatory geriatric sleep complaints. *Nurse Practitioner, 25*(9), 29-32, 35-36.

age them to enter these programs immediately after discharge, while they are motivated.

Long-term care nurses are able to locate and plan community resources during the resident's stay. Some of the community services discussed will allow a return home to an environment in which health promotion can continue.

Table **24-5** Long-Term Care Housing and Assessment Continuum

	Independent Living	Retirement Community	Assisted Living	Nursing Facility
Description	Covers a broad range of housing options (residential houses, apartments, condominiums, townhouses, subsidized senior housing) for older persons who are functionally and socially independent	Provides a living arrangement that integrates shelter and services for older people who do not need 24-hour protective oversight	Provides a living arrangement that integrates shelter and services for frail older people who are functionally or socially impaired and require 24-hour protective oversight	Provides a living arrangement that integrates shelter with medical, nursing, psychosocial, and rehabilitation services for older people who require 24-hour nursing supervision
Primary Services	-A- • Environmental security • Possibly coordination of resident services (transportation, activities, housekeeping) • Or no services are available	-B- "A" plus: • Meals (1 to 3 per day) • Transportation • Activities • Housekeeping assistance • Assistance with coordination of community-based services	-C- "A & B" plus: • Assistance with activities of daily living • Medication monitoring • 24-Hour protective oversight	-D- "A, B, & C" plus: • Medication administration • 24-Hour nursing supervision
Mobility	Capable of moving about independently OR ambulatory with cane or walker Independent with wheelchair, but needs help in an emergency	Capable of moving about independently Able to seek and follow directions Able to evacuate independently in emergency OR ambulatory with cane or walker Independent with wheelchair, but needs help in an emergency	Mobile, but may require escort or assistance resulting from confusion, poor vision, weakness, or poor motivation OR requires occasional assistance to move about, but is usually independent	May require assistance with transfers from bed, chair, toilet OR requires transfer and transport assistance Requires turning and positioning in bed and wheelchair
Nutrition	Able to prepare own meals; eats without assistance	Able to prepare own meals; eats without assistance. Generally a minimum of one meal a day is available	All meals and snacks provided. May require assistance getting to dining room or requires minimal assistance (opening cartons or other packages, cutting food, or preparing trays)	May be unable or unwilling to go to dining room. May be dependent on staff for eating or feeding needs OR fully dependent on staff for nourishment (includes reminders to eat or feeding)
Hygiene	Independent in all care, including bathing	Independent in all care, including bathing and personal laundry	May require assistance with bathing or hygiene OR may require assistance, initiation, structure, or reminders. Resident may be able to complete tasks	May be dependent on staff for all personal hygiene
Housekeeping	Independent in performing housekeeping functions (includes making bed, vacuuming, cleaning, and laundry)	Independent in performing housekeeping functions (includes making bed, vacuuming, cleaning, and laundry) OR may	Housekeeping and laundry services provided	Housekeeping and laundry services provided

Continued

Table 24-5 Long-Term Care Housing and Assessment Continuum *cont'd*

	Independent Living	Retirement Community	Assisted Living	Nursing Facility
		need assistance with heavy housekeeping, vacuuming, laundry, and linens		
Dressing	Independent and dresses appropriately	Independent and dresses appropriately	May require occasional assistance with shoelaces, zippers, or medical appliances or garments OR may require reminders, initiation, or motivation	May be dependent on staff for dressing
Toileting	Independent and continent	Independent and completely continent OR may have incontinence, colostomy, or catheter, but independent in caring for self through proper use of supplies	Same as "retirement community" OR may have occasional problem with incontinence, colostomy, or catheter and may require assistance in caring for self through proper use of supplies	May have problem with incontinence, colostomy, or catheter and requires assistance OR may be dependent and unable to communicate needs
Medications	Responsible for self-administration of all medications	Responsible for self-administration of all medications OR may arrange for family or home health agency to establish a medication administration system	Able to self-administer medications OR facility staff may remind or monitor the actual process OR facility staffed by RN or LPN who administers medications	Medications administered by staff personnel or self if assessed as capable
Mental Status	Oriented to person, place, and time Memory intact, but has occasional forgetfulness AND able to reason, plan, and organize daily events. Mentally capable of identifying needs and meeting them	Oriented to person, place, and time AND memory is intact, but has occasional forgetfulness without consistent pattern of memory loss AND able to reason, plan, and organize daily events. Mentally capable of identifying environment needs and meeting them	May require occasional direction or guidance in getting from place to place OR may have difficulty with occasional confusion that may result in anxiety, social withdrawal, or depression OR orientation to time or place or person may be impaired	Judgment can be poor and may attempt tasks that are not within capabilities OR may require strong orientation and reminder program May need guidance in getting from place to place OR disoriented to time, place, and person OR memory is severely impaired
Behavioral Status	Deals appropriately with emotions and uses available resources to cope with inner stress	Deals appropriately with emotions and uses available resources to cope with inner stress AND deals appropriately with other residents and staff OR may require periodic intervention from staff to resolve conflicts with others to cope with situational stress	May require periodic intervention from staff to facilitate expression of feelings to cope with inner stress OR may require periodic intervention from staff to resolve conflicts with others to cope with situational stress	May require regular intervention from staff to facilitate expression of feelings and to deal with periodic outbursts of anxiety or agitation OR maximal staff intervention is required to manage behavior

Modified from Steven Bender (geriatric social worker), Colorado Springs, CO.
RN, registered nurse; *LPN,* licensed practical nurse.

Community resources that may help older adults who are discharged from long-term care facilities include adult day-care programs, support groups and medical resources, telephone information, and referral services. In addition to their role in individual care planning, long-term care nurses can be more involved in institutional policy changes. Recommendations about smoking policies and healthy diets may prompt interdisciplinary changes that will result in improved health for the entire institution.

The geriatric care manager who sees people in their original residences or in housing complexes may be charged with individual health-promotion planning. Home care nurses provide health care information and services to both individuals and their families. The resources available to community health nurses frequently are rich and enable the nurses to draw on a variety of sources to assist them in promoting the health of community-dwelling older adults. Transportation, home-delivered meals, assistance with housekeeping, socialization, exercise programs, and self-help groups are only a few of the health-promotion resources available within the community. Nurses in all settings may take the opportunity to call the town or city older adult services office for information on the many resources available.

The AARP provides many services to people over age 50, including excellent educational materials and community program packages. The topics reflect a broad range of concerns and generally are presented in a self-help manner. Among the topics covered are smoking, exercise, nutrition, and wellness. Each program serves as a guide to negotiate a system or learn more about a health problem. These topics are written in lay terms, are easily understandable, and are printed in large letters to accommodate vision changes. This self-help method is especially important for those who feel uncomfortable addressing questions on finances or sexuality to nurses and physicians.

Two additional environments of care have emerged over the last half of the twentieth century in the United States: (1) continuing care retirement communities (CCRCs) and (2) assisted living facilities (ALFs). CCRCs are full-service communities offering long-term contracts that provide older adults with a continuum of care, extending from retirement services through assisted living to skilled nursing, all in one location. The mission behind CCRCs is "aging in place." CCRCs are very expensive and require an entrance fee ranging from $60,000 to $700,000, and a monthly payment ranging from $2500 to $4000. Residence in a CCRC requires commitment to a long-term contract that specifies the housing, services, and nursing care provided. ALFs are defined as homelike settings that promote resident autonomy, privacy, independence, dignity and respect while providing necessary support. Wallace (2003) reports that the lower cost of ALFs in comparison with that of skilled nursing facilities and the greater emphasis on functional autonomy makes these facilities appealing to older consumers and their families. Although ALF residents have many long-term health care needs, it is important to realize that the role and availability of nurses in these facilities varies greatly by state guidelines.

Cultural Diversity

The percentage of white older adults is expected to decrease from 1990 to 2030, while the percentage of black, Asian, and Hispanic members of the population is expected to rise. These changes in cultural background bring unprecedented challenges to the Western health care delivery system. Challenges continue to present in the way that each culture perceives disease origin and management, and the traditional manner in which health is maintained or improved will be changed.

Nurses must be aware of the cultural diversity of older adults for whom they care and the cultural beliefs that influence health care decisions of older adults. Cultural competence refers to the ability of nurses to understand and accept the cultural backgrounds of clients and provide care that best meets the clients' needs—not the nurses' needs. In order to develop cultural competence the first step is to examine personal beliefs and the effect of these beliefs on professional behavior. This may best be accomplished by conducting personal cultural assessments. After identifying personal cultural biases that influence care, nurses must bracket these beliefs to make sure they do not affect delivery of care. After this step is accomplished, it is important to increase understanding about population-specific health-related cultural values, beliefs, and behaviors. It is important to remember that although an older person may be part of a cultural group, the individual may have become acculturated while living in the United States. A cultural history is therefore an essential first step in determining the client's health care beliefs and practices. When conducting cultural assessments, it is necessary to remember that some of the standardized assessment tools, such as the Geriatric Depression Scale and the MMSE are available in languages other than English. Caution should be taken in interpreting a tool that has not been formally translated, because the meanings of many words change with cultural background.

The final stage in attaining cultural competence is to develop skills for working with culturally diverse populations. This entails the development of knowledge in working with culturally diverse populations and consistently using those skills with older adults. Conducting cultural assessments, using translation services, and providing culturally competent care are integral components to developing culturally competent institutions and improving care.

Health Care Delivery System

This chapter has brought the need for health-promotion services for older adults into the limelight. Few health care plans pay for health-promotion services. Medicare (the primary health insurance coverage for older adult) offers little coverage for preventive services. Although these people require a wide range of services that ideally exist on a continuum, not all services on this continuum are available regardless of care setting.

Medicare and other federal expenditures for older adults (direct or indirect) constitute a large part of the federal budget. Most goes to old age and retirement programs, disability, and Medicaid. Because of the large percentage of the federal budget consumed by Medicare, this insurance program is undergoing much scrutiny. Legislation to cut the Medicare budget is under review. Lawmakers anticipate that approximately $49 billion in savings could come from more effective use of health maintenance organizations and prospective payment systems instituted in the home. Regardless of the nature of funding cuts, illness prevention contributes to financial stability of the older adult. Nurses will play a key role during the years of Medicare reform in promoting health not only to prevent illness, but also to prevent older adults from losing all their savings and becoming impoverished.

Medigap policies have been promoted to pay for the health care coverage not afforded by Medicare, including prescription drugs (see Drug Use section for discussion of Medicare prescription discount cards). There are approximately nine Medigap policies. Each one provides varying levels of coverage. Choices about whether to purchase coverage for durable health care supplies, prescription medications, and other medical charges must be made to select the most appropriate policy. The charge for the policy varies according to the level of coverage selected. Federal legislation is being explored to improve coverage for prescription medications by Medicare.

Unfortunately, many people are not financially prepared for older adulthood. Although some individuals receive supplemental income from pensions or individual retirement accounts, this situation is rare. Most live on limited incomes. Several resources are available to help those with limited finances live quality lives. Medicaid, authorized by Title 19 of the Social Security Act, is designed to help older adults who are receiving public assistance to pay for medical expenses. Both federal and state governments fund the Medicaid program. To qualify for Medicaid, an individual must have limited income and assets. The coverage afforded by Medicaid is more extensive than that of Medicare. For example, Medicaid covers stays in long-term care facilities, transportation, and prescription drug services. Medicare covers these services only in limited and medically acute situations. Frequently older adults and their caretakers desire the more extensive coverage provided by Medicaid. These individuals are required to "spend down" their assets to be eligible.

Other resources are available to help older adults live this last stage of life in a high-quality manner. Food stamps are available to those who meet certain economic criteria. Food stamps can help them obtain nutritious food at participating markets without depleting their limited budgets. Supplemental medication payment programs assist some in purchasing their prescription medications. When income criteria are met, older adults may be entitled to purchase medications by paying only small co-payments rather than the large amount of money that frequently is charged.

Careful financial planning before the onset of illness is ideal to avoid the need to spend down assets and to help the older adult live at a desirable income level. This task can be accomplished through meeting with lawyers and financial planners as early in life as 30 years of age. Completing advance directives, including naming a conservator in advance of illness, assists caregivers, physicians, clergy, and the family in making difficult decisions at the end of life, when the affected person is no longer able to make them. The better prepared the older adult is, the easier it is to receive appropriate care and treatment during times of illness. Reverse annuity mortgages are one option for increased income during the later years. A reverse annuity mortgage is obtained when a bank or private business purchases the home of an older adult. The bank pays the person a set amount of money each month until the house is paid for in its entirety. The senior continues to live in the home. This approach provides the person with necessary funds and negates the need to move and sell the house if an illness arises.

Long-term care insurance is a newer option for those planning for the possibility of long-term care. As with other insurance programs, younger adults can purchase a policy, now widely available from reputable insurance agents. A premium is paid each month that entitles the beneficiary to receive long-term care benefits at home, in assisted living, in day care, or in a long-term care facility. Older individuals are cautioned to explore the many options available for this type of insurance. The benefits and coverage vary, and exclusions frequently are written into the contract to prevent care in certain situations. An important feature of these policies is the option to hire a personal caregiver if the need should arise.

Because population shifts have created a large number of older adults in the United States, political movements toward protecting older adults' rights are abundant and strong. Nowhere is there more political activity than among the groups responsible for social policy and aging. However, this large number has created problems of consistency, equity, and authority. Several large programs, including those directed by the Social Security Administration, the Health Care Financing Administration, and the Department of Veterans Affairs, have coordination problems because of their size and the large number of cases they handle.

The nurse who specializes in the care of older adults can do a great deal to promote their health and well-being through education, research, and practice. Educational curricula should be evaluated continually to ensure that content is appropriate and accurate with respect to aging. The quality of care depends on the clinician's knowledge base. Education for the older person is equally important and begins with an assessment of the individual's level of understanding of health-promotion activities.

Health-promotion research for this population is only beginning. A great deal more remains to be done in exploring the concepts of health promotion, relating these concepts, and developing and testing hypotheses. Research may best begin with an attempt to debunk commonly held beliefs. Defining some of the concepts of health promotion, such as quality of life and functional ability, will yield immeasurable amounts of information that can be tested. Eventually, with the commitment of qualified nurses, health promotion will be respected for the integral role it plays in the quality of life of these people.

SUMMARY

Life expectancy is now beyond 75 years for both men and women, with the fastest growing age group being those older than 85. This phenomenon is indeed wonderful. However, aging causes physiological changes in many bodily functions. Although some of these changes are benign, older adults have a higher frequency of illness than the younger population. The many physical, emotional, and role changes of aging are complicated by the great diversity in cultural backgrounds. Older adults who have immigrated to the United States have brought with them different languages, spiritual patterns, eating habits, views toward modern medicine, and other customs foreign to U.S. culture. Culturally competent health-promotion services are integral to helping them lead high-quality lives throughout their extended life spans.

Many problems of old age are related to lifestyle. Changes in nutritional needs, sleep patterns, and activity level are required to adapt to normal and pathological processes. Psychological health depends on reassessing spirituality, self-concept, and role functions. Change and adaptation are possible. With the assistance of nurses and other health care professionals, older adults can be empowered to live their final years with integrity.

Some of the dysfunctional aspects of aging have extrinsic causes, such as environmental pollution. Older adults are as susceptible as any age group is to society's problems, such as homelessness, mistreatment, and drug and alcohol abuse. In conjunction with physiological and pathological changes, cancer, TB, and other disorders can result. Internal and public policy changes will continue to help older adults live in a world in which old age can be the most rewarding stage of life.

ADDITIONAL STUDY MATERIAL

Study Questions in the back of the book, see page 663.

evolve WEB SITE MATERIALS

These materials are located on the book's Web site at http://evolve.elsevier.com/Edelman/.

- WebLinks
- Content Updates
- Web Site Resources

24A   Yesavage Geriatric Depression Scale: Short Form
24B   Recommended Adult Immunization Schedule, United States, 2004-2005
24C   Beers Criteria for Inappropriate Medication Usage Among Older Adults

REFERENCES

AJN reports: Pick a card—Any card? (2004). *American Journal of Nursing, 104,* 24-26.

Allison, D. B., Miller, R. A., Austad, S. N., Bouchard, C., Leibel, R., Klebanov, S., et al. (2001). Genetic variability in responses to caloric restriction in animals and in regulation of metabolism and obesity in humans. *The Journals of Gerontology. Series A, Biological Sciences and Medical Sciences, 56A*(Special Issue I), 55-65.

Alzheimer's Association. (1999). *Alzheimer's disease and related dementias fact sheet.* Silver Springs, MD: Author.

Alzheimer's Disease Education and Referral Center. (2001-2002). *Alzheimer's disease: Unraveling the mystery.* Retrieved October 11, 2001, from *http://www.Alzheimers.org/unraveling/11.htm.*

American Geriatrics Society, British Geriatrics Society, & American Academy of Orthopedic Surgeons Panel on Falls Prevention. (2001). Guidelines for prevention of falls in older persons. *Journal of the American Geriatrics Society, 49,* 664-672.

Amoako, E. P., Richardson-Campbell, L., & Kennedy-Malone, L. (2003). Self-medication with over-the-counter drugs among elderly adults. *Journal of Gerontological Nursing, 29*(8), 10-15.

Bauer, M. (1999). The use of humor in addressing the sexuality of elderly nursing home residents. *Sexuality and Disability, 2,* 147-155.

Bickerstaff, K. A., Graser, C. M., & McCabe, B. (2003). How elderly nursing home residents transcend losses of later life. *Holistic Nursing Practice, 17,* 159-165.

Binder, E. F., Schechtman, K. B., Ehsani, A. A., Steger-May, K., Brown, M., Sinacore, et al. (2002). Effects of exercise training on frailty in community-dwelling older adults: Results of a randomized, controlled trial. *Journal of the American Geriatrics Society, 50,* 1921-1980.

Blow, F. C., Walton, M. A., Chermack, S. T., Mudd, S. A., & Brower, K. J. (2000). Older adult treatment outcome following elder-specific inpatient alcoholism treatment. *Journal of Substance Abuse Treatment, 19*(1), 67-75.

Brush, B. (2000). Spirituality. In J. Fitzpatrick, T. Fulmer, M. Wallace, & E. Flaherty (Eds.), *Geriatric nursing research digest* (pp. 91-93). New York: Springer.

Burkhardt, J. E., Berger, A. M., Creedon, M., & McGavock, A. T. (1998). *Mobility and independence: Changes and challenges for older drivers.* Washington, DC: U.S. Department of Health and Human Services and the National Highway Traffic Safety Administration.

Butler, R., & Olshansky, S. J. (2002). Has anybody ever died of old age? *The Gerontologist, 42*(Special Issue 1), 285-286.

Capozza, K. (2002). *HIV in the elderly presents unique challenges.* Retrieved May 9, 2005, from *http://www.aegis.com.*

Centers for Disease Control and Prevention. (1999). *Reported tuberculosis in the United States.* Atlanta: U.S. Department of Health and Human Services.

Centers for Disease Control and Prevention. (2001a). Healthy aging: Preventing disease and improving quality of life among older Americans: At a glance (On-line). Retrieved May 9, 2005, from: *http://www.cdc.gov/aging*

Centers for Disease Control and Prevention. (2001b). Suicide in the United States (On-line). Retrieved May 9, 2005, from: *http://www.cdc.gov/ncipc/factsheets/suifacts.htm.*

Centers for Disease Control and Prevention. (2002). *National Vital Statistics Report*, 50(16).

Centers for Disease Control and Prevention. (2003) *Web-based injury statistics query and reporting system (WISQARS)*. Retrieved May 9, 2005 from *www.cdc.gov/ncipc/wisqars*.

Erikson, E. H. (1982). *Life cycle completed: A review*. New York: W. W. Norton.

Erikson, E. H. (1997). *The life cycle completed*. New York: W. W. Norton.

Florindo, A. A., Latore, M. D. O., Jaime, P. C., Tanaka, T., Pippa, M. G. B., & Zerbini, C. A. F. (2002). Past and present habitual physical activity and its relationship with bone mineral density in men aged 50 years and older in Brazil. *Journals of Gerontology, 57A(10)*, m654-m657.

Folstein, M. E., Folstein, S. E., & McHugh, P. (1975). Mini mental state: A practical method for grading the cognitive state of patients for the clinician. *Journal of Psychiatric Research, 12*, 189-198.

Forestalling frailty. (2003, March 1). *Harvard Women's Health Watch*, 27.

Friis, R. H., Nomura, W. L., Ma, C. X., & Swan, J. H. (2003). Socioepidemiologic and health-related correlates of walking for exercise among the elderly: Results from the longitudinal study of aging. *Journal of Aging & Physical Activity, 11*, 27-31.

Greater food safety precautions needed by the elderly—But what's "old"? (2002, Oct.). *Tufts University Health & Nutrition Letter*.

Guthrie, J. F. & Lin, B. (2002) Overview of the diets of lower- and higher-income elderly and their food assistance options. *Journal of Nutrition Education and Behavior, 34* (Suppl 1), S31–S41.

Haight, B. K, Michel, Y., Hendrix, S. (2000). The extended effects of the life review in nursing home residents. *International Journal of Aging & Human Development, 50(2)*, 151-168.

Haight, B. K. (2005). Reminiscence. In J. Fitzpatrick & M. Wallace (Eds.), *Encyclopedia of nursing research*. New York: Springer.

Kelly, S. (2000). Grandparents raising grandchildren. In J. Fitzpatrick, T. Fulmer, M. Wallace, & E. Flaherty (Eds.), *Geriatric nursing research digest* (pp. 20-24). New York: Springer.

Kraaij, H., Pruymboom, E., & Garnefski, N. (2002). Cognitive coping and depressive symptoms in the elderly: A longitudinal study. *Aging & Mental Health, 6(3)*, 275-281.

Lee, E. H. (2002). Assessment, screening and diagnosis of prostate cancer. In M. Wallace & L. Powell (Eds.), *Prostate cancer: Nursing assessment, management & care*. New York: Springer.

Lynch, T. R., Compton, J. S., Mendelson, T., Robins, C. J., & Krishnan, K. R. R. (2000). Anxious depression among the elderly:

Clinical and phenomenological correlates. *Aging & Mental Health, 4*, 268-274.

McElhaney, J. E. (2002). Influenza: A preventable lethal disease [Guest editorial]. *Journal of Gerontology. Biological Science Medical Science, 57*, M627-M628.

Menec, V. H., MacWilliam, L., Aoki, F. Y. (2002). Hospitalization and deaths due to respiratory illnesses during influenza seasons: A comparison of community residents, senior housing residents, and nursing home residents. *Journals of Gerontology, 57A(10)*, M627-M628.

Morley, J. (2003). Hot topics in geriatrics (Editorial). *Journal of Gerontology Medical Sciences, 58A*, 30-36.

Mulgrew, C. S., Morgenstern, N., Shetterly, S. M., Baxter, J., Baron, A. E., & Hamman, R. F. (1999). Cognitive functioning and impairment among rural elderly Hispanics and non-Hispanic whites as assessed by the Mini-Mental State Examination. *Journals of Gerontology Series B. Psychological Sciences and Social Sciences, 54B*, P223-P230.

National Institute of Allergy and Infectious Diseases. (2004). Pneumococcal pneumonia. Retrieved May 10, 2005, from *http://www.niaid.nih.gov/factsheets/pneumonia.htm*.

Neafsey, P. J., & Shellman, J. (2001). Adverse self-medication practices of older adults with hypertension attending blood pressure clinics: Adverse self-medication practices. *Internet Journal of Advanced Nursing Practice, 5(1)*, 15.

Ness, A., & Smith, G. D. (1999). Mortality in the CHAOS trial. Cambridge Heart Antioxidant Study. *Lancet, 353*, 1017-1018.

Pang, E. C., Jordan-Marsh, M., Silverstein, M., & Cody, M. (2003). Health-seeking behaviors of elderly Chinese Americans: Shift in expectations. *The Gerontologist, 43*, 864-874.

Pangman, V. C., & Seguire, M. (2000). Sexuality and the chronically ill older adult: A social justice issue. *Sexuality and Disability, 18*, 49-59.

Pekmezaris, R., Aversa, L., Wolf-Klein, G., Cedarbaum, J., & Reid-Durant, M. (2002). The cost of chronic constipation. *Journal of the American Medical Directors Association, 3*, 224-228.

Puentes, W. J. (2002). Simple reminiscence: A stress-adaptation model of the phenomenon. *Issues in Mental Health Nursing, 23*, 497-511.

Ragland, D. R., Satariano, W. A., & Macleod, K. E. (2004). Reasons given by older people for limitation or avoidance of driving. *The Gerontologist, 44*, 237-244.

Ramesh, M., & Roberts, G. (2002). Use of night-time benzodiazepines in an elderly inpatient population. *Journal of Clinical Pharmacy and Therapeutics, 27*, 93-97.

Rapp, G., Brenes, S., & Marsh, A. P. (2002). Memory enhancement training for older adults with mild cognitive impairment: A

preliminary study. *Aging & Mental Health, 6*, 5-11.

Robert Wood Johnson Foundation. (2001). Substance abuse: The nation's number one health problem (prepared by the Schneider Institute for Health Policy, Brandeis University). Princeton, NJ: Author.

Rosenkoetter, M. (2000). Retirement. In J. Fitzpatrick, T. Fulmer, M. Wallace, & E. Flaherty (Eds.), *Geriatric nursing research digest* (pp. 34-37). New York: Springer.

Sahyoun, N., & Basiotis, P. P. (2000). Food insufficiency and the nutritional status of the elderly population. Washington, DC: U.S. Department of Agriculture, Center for Nutrition Policy and Promotion.

Shelkey, M. (2000). Cognitive impairment. In J. Fitzpatrick, T. Fulmer, M. Wallace, & E. Flaherty (Eds.), *Geriatric nursing research digest* (pp. 325-333). New York: Springer.

Shih, S. W., & Shih, J. A. (1999). Health needs of lone elderly Chinese men with heart disease during their hospitalization. *Nursing Ethics, 6*, 58-72.

Simmons, T. & Dye, J. L. (2003). Grandparents living with grandchildren: 2000. Retrieved May 6, 2005, from http://www.census.gov/population/www/cen2000/briefs.html. May 6.

Skinner, K. D. (2000). Creating a game for sexuality and aging: The sexual dysfunction trivia game. *Journal of Continuing Education in Nursing, 31*, 185-189.

Social Security Administration. (2003). *Social Security basic fact*. Retrieved May 9, 2005, from: *http://www.ssa.gov/pressoffice/basicfact.htm*.

Sohng, K., Sohng, S., & Yeom, H. (2002). Health-promoting behaviors of elderly Korean immigrants in the United States. *Public Health Nursing, 19*, 294-300.

Stevens, J. A., & Olson, S. (2000). Reducing falls and resulting hip fractures among older women. In CDC recommendations regarding selected conditions affecting women's health. *Morbidity and Mortality Weekly Report, 49*(RR-2), 3-12.

Stevens, J. A., Hasbrouck, L. M., Durant, T. M., Dellinger, A. M., Batabyal, P. K., Crosby, A. E., et al. (1999). Surveillance for injuries and violence among older adults (On-line). Retrieved April 12, 2005, from: *http://www.cdc.gov/epo/mmwr/preview/mmwrhtml/ss4808a3.htm*.

U.S. Department of Health and Human Services. (2000). *Healthy people 2010: National health promotion and disease prevention objectives*. Washington, DC: U.S. Government Printing Office. Retrieved April 12, 2005, from: *http://www.health.gov/healthypeople*.

Vinsnes, A. G., Harkless, G. E., Haltbakk, J., Bohm, J., & Hunskaar, S. (2001). Healthcare personnel's attitudes towards patients with urinary incontinence. *Journal of Clinical Nursing, 10*, 455-462.

Walker, B. L., & Ephross, P. H. (1999). Knowledge and attitudes toward sexuality of a group of elderly. *Journal of Gerontological Social Work, 31,* 85-107.

Wallace, M. (2000). Sexuality and intimacy. In A. G. Lueckenotte (Ed.), *Gerontologic nursing* (pp. 244-256). St. Louis: Mosby.

Wallace, M. (2003). Is there a nurse in the house? The role of nurses in assisted living facilities, past, present and future. *Geriatric Nursing, 24*(4), 218-221, 235.

Wallhagen, M., & Strawbridge, S. S. (2003). Hearing impairment and cognitive frailty: A five year longitudinal study. *The Gerontologist, 43*(Special Issue 1), 20-21.

Wilson, L., Brown, J. S., Shin, G. P., Luc, K. O., & Subak, L. L. (2001). Annual direct cost of urinary incontinence. *Obstetrics and Gynecology, 98,* 398-406.

Wykle, M. L., & Zauszniewski, J. (2000). Depression. In J. Fitzpatrick, T. Fulmer, M. Wallace, & E. Flaherty (Eds.), *Geriatric nursing research digest* (pp. 199-204). New York: Springer.

Wyman, J. F. (2003, Mar.). Treatment of urinary incontinence in men and older women. *American Journal of Nursing,* (Suppl.), 26-35.

Yesavage, J., Brink, T., Rose, T., Lum, O., Huang, V., Adey, M., et al. (1983). Development and validation of a geriatric depression screening scale: A preliminary report. *Journal of Psychiatric Research, 17,* 37-49.

Zizi, F., Jean-Louis, G., Magai, C., Greenidge, K. C., Wolintz, A. H., & Heath-Phillip, O. (2002). Sleep complaints and visual impairment among older Americans: A community-based study. *Journals of Gerontology, 57A*(10), m691-m694.

Unit

Challenges in the Twenty-First Century

25 Health Promotion in the Twenty-First Century: Throughout the Life Span and Throughout the World

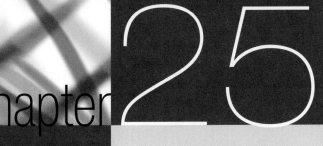

Chapter 25

RATCHNEEWAN ROSS
KATHLEEN HUTTLINGER

Health Promotion in the Twenty-First Century: Throughout the Life Span and Throughout the World

objectives

After completing this chapter, the reader will be able to:

- Discuss global trends and directions for health promotion and disease prevention.

- Discuss the values, goals, and targets of *Health for All in the 21st Century.*

- Analyze major health-promotion priorities for 2000 through 2010 that influence nursing practice, research, and health care policy.

- Evaluate activities across public and private sectors that reflect the *Healthy People 2010* objectives.

key terms

Advocate
Health for All
Healthy People 2010
Human immunodeficiency virus/acquired

immunodeficiency syndrome (HIV/AIDS)
Ottawa Charter
Severe acute respiratory syndrome (SARS)

Socioecological model
Vulnerable populations
World Health Organization

THINK About It

Health Challenges in a Developing Country

Rosa lives in Mombasa, Kenya, with her three children, ages 14, 11, and 4 years. She has been a widow for 10 years and has no family members to help her support her family. Her husband's brothers all succumbed to AIDS several years ago, and Rosa has no way to return to what family she has left in the interior of Kenya. Rosa and her children share a room in the harbor with Huwayda, another widow with no children and no family. There are no cooking facilities or running water in the room so Rosa, Huwayda, and the children must cook on a charcoal fire outside in the street. Water must be hauled from a public well four blocks away. Everyone sleeps on mats on the floor, and it is the oldest child's responsibility each morning to sweep the floor. Rosa can earn a little money by sweeping out local shops before they open in the morning. Huwayda works at the fish market and brings home what leftovers she can from the fish, fruit, and vegetable stalls. None of the children attends school and none has ever been to a clinic or doctor for immunizations or preventive care. Local missionaries provide what food they can to Rosa and Huwayda.

1 What kind of developmental problems would you anticipate that the children might encounter?

Continued

Health Challenges in a Developing Country *cont'd*

2 Visit the World Health Organization Web site *(http://www.who.org)* to identify the incidence and prevalence of HIV and AIDS in Kenya.

3 Who in this family is most at risk for contact with an HIV carrier?

4 What other kinds of health problems do you see not only for the children but for Rosa and Huwayda as well?

Scenario courtesy Doug and Laura Krefting, Maryknoll Missionaries in Mombasa, Kenya. July, 2004.
AIDS, acquired immunodeficiency syndrome; *HIV,* human immunodeficiency virus.

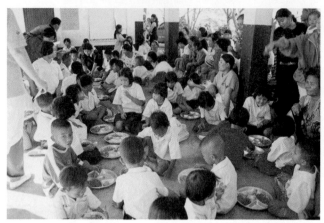

Figure 25-1 Lunchtime for school children in a remote area of Thailand. The food was made possible through donations from health care providers.

Within the past 30 years, a number of changes around the world have alarmed health professionals enough to make them look at their approaches to health promotion and disease prevention more closely, globally, and comprehensively. For example, an outbreak of **severe acute respiratory syndrome (SARS)** that affected over 8000 people worldwide and killed at least 700 people (Centers for Disease Control and Prevention [CDC], 2004) and shocking increasing rates of human immunodeficiency virus (HIV) infection in several regions are raising red flags (Joint United Nations Programme on HIV/AIDS & World Health Organization [UNAIDS &WHO], 2003).

According to the World Health Organization (WHO) (2003), average life expectancy at birth has increased by 20 years around the world, particularly in developed countries, due to advances in medical technology. Nevertheless there were 57 million deaths in 2002 worldwide: over 10 million deaths were among children younger than 5 years, and around 98% of these deaths happened in developing countries. The leading causes are related to pregnancy, labor, and postpartum conditions, lower respiratory tract infections, diarrhea, and malaria. Malnutrition contributes to all causes. Globally children who are poor and malnourished are more likely to die than are those who are not poor and are well-nourished (Figure 25-1). Approximately 332,000 children died in 2002 from **human immunodeficiency virus/acquired immunodeficiency syndrome (HIV/AIDS)** in sub-Saharan Africa (WHO, 2003).

As to adult health worldwide, in sub-Saharan Africa life expectancy has been reduced by more than 20 years due to HIV/AIDS. Despite the fact that antiretroviral medicines have been used in Africa to decrease mother-to-child transmission (Research Highlights box), Botswana, Lesotho, Swaziland, and Zimbabwe are being hit hard by the disease (WHO, 2003). The estimated number of people living with HIV/AIDS at the end of the year 2001 was 40 million people worldwide, with 28.5 million exclusively in sub-Saharan Africa, 5.6 million in South and Southeast Asia, 1.5 million in Latin America, 1 million in Eastern Europe and Central Asia, 1 million in East Asia and the

research highlights

Prevention of Mother-to-Baby (Vertical) Transmission Through the Use of Nevirapine

A randomized trial study was conducted from November 1997 to April 1999 to compare vertical transmission rates among 645 mother-baby pairs in Uganda. One group of 313 HIV-infected pregnant women was randomly assigned regimen A, a single dose of 200 mg NVP, an inexpensive antiretroviral drug, at the onset of labor. Their babies also received NVP (2 mg/kg) within 72 hours after birth. For regimen B, another 313 pregnant women received ZDV 600 mg orally at the onset of labor and 300 mg every 3 hours until delivery. Their babies received ZDV 4 mg/kg orally twice a day for 7 days. Nineteen mother-baby pairs received placebo. Most babies (99%) in the total sample were breastfed for a median of 9 months' duration. HIV testing for infants was performed 5 times. The first testing was done at birth, and subsequently at 6 to 8 weeks, 14 to 16 weeks, 12 months, and 18 months after birth.

Results revealed that single-dose NVP prophylaxis for the mothers and their babies significantly decreased vertical transmission at 14 to 16 weeks compared with those who received ZDV. At 18 months, the infants who received NVP maintained a significantly lower rate of transmission than those given ZDV (15.7% versus 25.8%). However, infant mortality rates between the two groups were about the same at 18 months of age (12%). The results of this study have shed new light for developing countries in terms of using affordable short-course NVP prophylaxis to prevent mother-to-baby transmission. It is projected that this regimen could prevent 246,000 infants (out of 800,000) a year from getting the virus from their mothers.

Data from Jackson, J. B., Musoke, P., Fleming, T., Guay, L. A., Bagenda, D., Allen, M., et al. (2003). Intrapartum and neonatal single-dose nevirapine compared with zidovudine for prevention of mother-to-child transmission of HIV-1 in Kampala, Uganda: 18-month follow-up of the HIVNET 012 randomized trial. *The Lancet, 362*(9387), 859-867.
HIV, human immunodeficiency virus; *NVP,* nevirapine; *ZDV,* zidovudine.

Pacific, 950,000 in North America (900,000 in America and 50,000 in Canada), 550,000 in Western Europe, 500,000 in North Africa and the Middle East, and 15,000 in Australia and New Zealand (WHO, 2003).

Many of these issues require health professionals to focus on and assist individuals and local communities throughout the world in identifying their health care needs. Dealing directly with people by providing information and technical assistance, at personal, community, national, and global levels, is a necessary approach to establishing good health and is vital to health promotion and all forms of prevention activities. The challenge that faces the health care community around the world in the new millennium is for health care professionals, consumers, and communities to develop collaborative skills that foster partnerships, which will allow all people and community levels to make informed decisions about health and health care.

Since World War II people throughout the world have experienced globalization-complex; that is, interrelated economic, political, social, and cultural processes. A variety of workers initiating changes at national and international levels have proposed, encouraged, and supported more comprehensive and global approaches to health promotion (Beukens, Keusch, Belizan, & Bhutta, 2004; Lee, 2000; Waters, 2001).

As discussed earlier, the most significant health-promotion development in the second half of the twentieth century was the creation of the **World Health Organization,** an international agency founded immediately following World War II. In defining health as a state of complete physical, mental, and social well-being and not merely the absence of disease or infirmity, the founders of the constitution of the World Health Organization transformed the definitions for health throughout the world. Furthermore, the writers stated, "The health of all people is fundamental to the attainment of peace and security and is dependent upon the fullest cooperation of individuals and states" (WHO, 1998b, p. 4). This effort has been the world's challenge for over 50 years and continues as the twenty-first century begins (Lee, 2004).

This challenge requires individuals, families, groups, health care professionals, communities, and nations to develop collaborative skills that foster partnerships with each other, which will allow all people to make informed decisions about health and health care, including the many related processes.

Many examples of national and worldwide achievements illustrate this effort, such as women's health programs for disease prevention and health care, issues involving social health, networking projects that facilitate early detection and intervention of AIDS, and child immunization projects (WHO, 2000). One example is "100% condom use program" in Thailand, which decreased the national HIV prevalence from 4% in the mid-1990s to less than 1% in 2002 (UNAIDS & WHO, 2003). However, many government-sponsored programs throughout the world have experienced setbacks, economic shortfalls, and disappointments because of economic rationing, lack of technology, and marketing schemes that fall short of delivery.

In reshaping the national and the world's health care systems, questions arise, such as, "Can health outcomes be purchased from competing providers?" "Can communities combine their resources to act as providers of health promotion?" "Can the economic and technological environments mix community interest with an individualized customer approach in delivering health care as a commodity?" "How can future health care practitioners combine holistic views with the health marketplace to improve health?"

As a profession, nursing has enjoyed a long-standing interest and focus on health-promotion activities throughout the life span and has the reputation of advocating for individuals, families, and communities. Recognition as an **advocate,** a person who supports and pleads for another, has served nursing well by providing opportunities for giving educational guidance and counseling in both institutional and community settings. Education and teaching are considered an integral part of nursing's role (American Association of Colleges of Nursing, 1998), and so is research supported through the efforts of the National Institute of Nursing Research. One goal of this organization is to support and advance the goals of *Healthy People 2010,* which is reflected by its publication of annual initiatives (National Institute of Nursing Research, 2004).

The increased need for health-promotion and disease prevention activities nationally and worldwide has generated many employment opportunities in the public and private sectors for a variety of health care workers, including nurses worldwide. Opportunities exist for teaching personal wellness at workplaces; advising national and local governments; consulting with hospitals, schools, and health insurers; and as client advocates in a variety of settings (Henry & Royer, 2004; Whitehead, 2004). In this way, health promotion and disease prevention has moved from the single realm of health education to modern health policy–driven programs.

Nurses are in a unique position among all health care professionals to act on the opportunities for promoting health care activities. With an enduring emphasis on health promotion and disease prevention, nurses function in a variety of roles, including primary health care practitioner, health advocate and enabler, educator, and researcher. Therefore nurses are critical links in the health care delivery system and function as change agents in the achievement of health for all in the new millennium (WHO, 2000).

This chapter provides a description of national and international trends in health promotion and revisits the philosophies, goals, and strategies of the World Health Organization's *Health for All* and the *Healthy People 2010* initiatives from the U.S. Department of Health and Human Services. Examples of health problems and national health-promotion programs developed by many other countries around the world are also described. Examples of the many roles of nurses in health promotion in the next millennium are discussed from the dimensions of policy development and the advancement of practice, education, and research at both national and international levels. Nurses are challenged to provide experiences, vision, and leadership to fulfill the goals of *Health for All*.

HEALTH PROMOTION: PAST DEVELOPMENTS AND FUTURE DIRECTIONS

Although the world aspires to achieve health for all through health-advancing strategies, many challenges lie ahead. For example, although health promotion and disease prevention are now considered global terms, they are frequently misused, with the inherent values distorted (Lamarche, 1995; Lefebvre, 1996).

When considering future directions in health promotion and disease prevention, reviewing past achievements can be useful. During the 1950s, 1960s, and into the early 1970s, the focus of many health-promotion activities was on the control and prevention of communicable diseases. This goal was achieved though mass immunization and education programs that emphasized major preventive and health-protection strategies. In the 1970s tackling preventable diseases and reducing premature death and risky health behaviors through early identification and education formed key strategies in many countries. Most noteworthy was the initiation of *Health for All in the 21st Century*, the health-promotion goal of the World Health Organization's strategies around the world (1978).

The decade of the 1980s saw the first U.S. Surgeon General's Report on Health Promotion and Disease Prevention (U.S. Department of Health and Human Services [USDHHS], 1981). Subsequently the World Health Organization's European regional office published *Targets for Health for All* in 1985 and reissued this document in 1991 following input from representatives from many European countries. In 1988 Australia published its first set of national health goals and targets, also based on the U.S. model. In addition to national objectives, countries such as Australia and the United States have encouraged their states and communities to develop objectives that are compatible with the national goals but more specific to regional needs (USDHHS, 2000).

Another worldwide event occurred in the 1980s that set the agenda for health promotion. A meeting was held in Ottawa, Canada, in 1986 (WHO, 1986) that was attended by health leaders from around the world. The outcome of this meeting was a set of health-promotion guidelines that can be used worldwide, known as the **Ottawa Charter**. A new health paradigm emerged with an increased focus on determinants and prerequisites outside the health care realm, such as adequate income, employment, housing, food, education, and a safe social and physical environment for health development. One example of the worldwide influence of this conference and charter was the International Conference for Health Promotion in Colombia in 1992 and the adoption of the 1993 Caribbean Charter for

Health Promotion (Pommier, Deschamps, Romero, & Zubarew, 1997).

During the 1990s the importance of reaching people through various settings and sectors, such as schools, families, temples, rural areas, cities, hospitals, and workplaces, and the development of needs-based programs, was initiated in many countries, including Canada, Australia, Thailand, India, and the United States (Tsouros, 1996) and by the World Health Organization (Modawal, 2003). For example, a collaborative project in India between nongovernmental organizations and government sectors created community housing and medical programs, giving pension discounts to older people, especially for traveling in different modes (train, air, bus). These projects have helped a lot of the elderly to have a better quality of life (Modawal, 2003).

The new millennium, which has welcomed contrasting life expectancies between developed and developing countries, brings a need to sustain the momentum and add another dimension to health promotion and disease prevention. In many developed countries, such as Japan, France, and America, people have a life expectancy at birth ranging from 72.5 to 82.9 years (UNAIDS & WHO, 2003). Countries in Africa, such as Botswana and Mozambique, are homes for those whose life expectancy can be as low as 27 years due to HIV infection (Henry J. Kaiser Family Foundation, 2002). These contrasting life expectancies demonstrate the shift from infectious diseases to chronic diseases among developed countries, while more urgent interventions are needed to prevent HIV transmission in developing countries, especially in Africa.

These result in intergenerational, social, economic, cultural, health, and ethical challenges, to name only a few (Cohen, 2000; Howson, 2000; Kalache & Keller, 2000). In the wake of massive demographic and social changes in global trade, emerging diseases, migration, urbanization, transportation, and collaboration between countries in sharing and redistributing knowledge, a new health perspective must certainly be part of the vision (Huttlinger, 2004).

GLOBAL STRATEGY OF *HEALTH FOR ALL*
Health for All

As discussed, the World Health Organization (2004) has developed a series of global health initiatives to fulfill the goal of *Health for All* and these remain a priority today. These initiatives continue to include "the right of all people to a standard of living adequate for health and well-being, including the right to adequate food, water, clothing, housing, health care, education, reproductive health, and social services; and the right to security in the event of unemployment, sickness, disability, old age, or lack of livelihood in circumstances beyond an individual's control. Respect for human rights and the achievement of public health goals are complementary" (WHO, 1998a, p. 3). *Health for All* continues to be a call for social justice, enabling all individuals to live economically and socially productive lives. The World Health Organization along with the United Nations adopted Millennium Development Goals (MDGs). The MDGs call for a dramatic reduction in poverty and marked improvements in the health of the poor. Meeting these goals is feasible but far from assured. Success in achieving the MDGs requires a seriousness of purpose, a political resolve in countries, and an adequate flow of resources from high-income to low-income countries on a sustained and well-targeted basis (WHO, 2004). In addition, supporters of the World Bank agree with the WHO and the United Nations and recommend that governments invest in the health of the socially weak, because decreases in the differences of income and the strengthening of various forms of social cohesion, civic solidarity, legitimate equality, and ethical justice, can substantially improve the health status of populations and social conciliation (Zacek, 2000, p. 163).

More specifically, the World Health Organization proposes in its new program for Europe (*21 Goals for the 21st Century*) that "health status differences among the European states should diminish by one third by 2020" (Zacek, 2000, p. 163). "Furthermore *Health for All* acknowledges the uniqueness of each person and the need to respond to each individual's spiritual quest for meaning, purpose and belonging" (WHO, 1998b, p. 4).

Based on these values, *Health for All* proposes these goals: (1) to provide the highest attainable standard of health as a fundamental right, (2) to strengthen the application of ethics to health policy, research, and service provision, (3) to implement equity-oriented policies and strategies that emphasize solidarity, and (4) to incorporate a gender perspective into health policies and strategies (WHO, 2004). From these goals, 10 global health targets have been prioritized (Box 25-1).

On May 16, 1998, the *World Health Declaration* was annexed to the constitution of the World Health Organization. The major components are described in Box 25-2.

Health Care Systems

Although a variety of health care strategies have been established and progress has been made in improving health and quality of life (decreased maternal and infant mortality rates, improved sanitation and drinking water, increased immunizations) (Brundtland, 2000; Lee, 2004; WHO, 1995), great disparities and inequities continue to exist. More poignant are the injustices within the allocations of resources in industrialized countries. For example, although a wide variety of health-promotion strategies have been instituted in most industrialized countries, technology and expensive health care modalities appear to be the dominant and prevailing paradigm. Despite the evidence that health status cannot be determined by increasing health care

---

Box **25-1**   **Health for All: Global Health**

A new global health policy, *Health for All in the 21st Century*, aimed at meeting the major challenges in health during the next decades has been developed by WHO in consultation with all its national and international partners. This involved member countries, the regional WHO offices, the academic and research community, and a wide variety of nongovernmental organizations. During its session in May 1998, the World Health Assembly endorsed the new *World Health Declaration* and the new global health policy. This policy evolves from the health-for-all approach, which has been a common goal since its inception in 1979. Targets include:

- Health equity: childhood stunting
- Survival: maternal mortality rates, childhood mortality rates, life expectancy
- Reverse global trends of five major pandemics: malaria, AIDS, tuberculosis, hepatitis, and influenza
- Eradicate and eliminate certain diseases (those related to malnutrition)
- Improve access to water, sanitation, food, and shelter
- Measures to promote health
- Develop, implement, and monitor national *Health for All in the 21st Century* policies
- Improve access to comprehensive, essential, quality health care
- Implement global and national health information and surveillance systems
- Support research for health

From World Health Organization. (2004). *Health for all in the 21st century.* Geneva, Switzerland: The Organization.
AIDS, acquired immunodeficiency syndrome.

Box **25-2**   **Major Components of the World Health Declaration Annexed to the World Health Organization Constitution**

The fifty-first World Health Assembly reaffirmed the major components of the *World Health Declaration* that was annexed to the World Health Organization Constitution, May 16, 1998 (WHA 48.16). According to the assembly, this document serves as the basic framework for the development of future policy. These affirmations are:

I. Affirmation (1) of the dignity and worth of every person, (2) that health is a fundamental right of every person, and (3) the equal rights, equal duties, and shared responsibilities of all for health
II. Improvement of health, the ultimate aim of social and economic development, by reducing social and economic inequities through commitment to equity, solidarity, and social justice and incorporation of a gender perspective
III. Strengthening, adapting, and reforming health systems, including the essentials of primary health care
IV. In all nations, communities, families, and individuals are interdependent
V. Full participation and partnership by all member states

resources (infrastructure and work force), a large part of the U.S. health care budget has been used to provide expensive health care services and, in many cases, for only a few people. In this approach, emphasis is not given to other influences such as poverty, education, environment, and social well-being. Additionally, a recent trend is the increasing privatization of health care with profit as the goal (Coburn, 2004; Maskovsky, 2000). In contrast to the industrialized countries, health-promotion initiatives throughout the world have emphasized the importance of ensuring financial and geographical access to health-promotion services and has become the preferred way to improve a population's health (Hassmiller, 2000).

Unfortunately, even in countries with universal access to health care such as Canada, the following is evident:

- Health care expenditure has grown 4 to 5 times faster than the country's collective wealth. In contrast, in the United States, which does not have universal access, spending on health care reached 13.9% of the gross national product in 2000 (Maurer, 2000).
- Social health problems such as AIDS, single-parent families, and the growing number of elderly and minority population groups lead to increasing health care management problems.
- The diminishing effect of health care on health has been clear, because major indexes, such as life expectancy at birth, are not related to investment in health care.

In addition to actual costs of health care delivery services, the value of services being offered at cost is being questioned in many countries. Historically the nursing profession has helped lower the cost of delivery by serving as primary care providers for the urban poor and rural dwellers. In doing so nurses have rendered a prevention-focused and individualized sickness-care service at low cost. The same initiative must now be taken in improving the health status of economically disadvantaged populations by promoting cooperation with other disciplines and encouraging them to be active participants in the provision of health care services for the more inaccessible populations.

New Public Health Movement

The *Ottawa Charter* was published in 1986 and remains an important document and one that emphasizes health promotion activities around the world. The *Ottawa Charter* still influences public health policy and health-related initiatives in many countries and its purpose redefines and resurrects ideas that once formed the basic traditions of public health, but were often lost. The *Ottawa Charter* stresses the importance of health for the continued prosperity and development of countries and maintains that the elements of public health, including health promotion and disease prevention, serve as the framework for health as a human right, an investment in society, and a resource for everyday living (Deschamps, 2003; O'Byrne, 2000).

Legge (1991), a well-known critic of the old or pre–*Ottawa Charter* version of public health, asserted that a

knowledge–action gap existed in most countries. Given this, Legge maintained that knowledge of health promotion and disease prevention is a precondition that must be met before a behavior change can be made. In addition, according to Legge, the pre–*Ottawa Charter* public health system failed to provide guiding frameworks for health care interventions that addressed inequalities in health care. Therefore, the public health effort that was initiated with the *Ottawa Charter* shifted the focus from behavior change to healthy public policy and community empowerment.

Socioecological Foundations of Health Promotion

One conceptual framework or model that can be used to understand health promotion and disease prevention is the socioecological model (Heiss & Walden, 2000; Riley, Taylor, & Elliot, 2001; Sword, 1999). A socioecological perspective has been one of the approaches used in public health theory, and many believe that this approach is central to understanding public health issues and concerns, including health promotion and disease prevention. The **socioecological model** describes health as a product of the interdependence between individuals and the subsystems of ecosystems, and it assumes a connectedness among human beings, their physical and social environment, and their health (Heiss & Walden, 2000; Riley, Taylor, & Elliot, 2001; Sword, 1999). Therefore the thrust of health promotion is on population-based approaches, such as healthy public policies and the integration of environment and health through interdisciplinary collaboration. Brown (1992) along with Riley, Taylor, and Elliot (2001) identified four major areas within the model that have health-promotion implications: equity, sustainability, conviviality, and preservation of the global environment. Socioecological health promotion points to the role of various determinants of health, including economic and social conditions that assist people who engage in healthy behaviors.

Goals and Targets for Health Promotion

Health for All by Year 2010 has been a major focus for the World Health Organization (2000) and has been the impetus for many of their policies and programs. Many nations have used the program to address health disparities and to improve access to health services, and many have refocused their efforts to improve performance measures for all health systems (Musich, Adams, & Edington, 2000; WHO, 2000). Health goals and targets for nations have included statements of direction and intent, including such goals as reducing deaths due cardiovascular disease or change in the social, economic, and physical environment by a certain year.

The United States, in a document entitled *Promoting Health, Preventing Disease: Objectives for the Nation* (USDHHS, 1990), was one of the first countries to develop goals and objectives that were aimed at health-promotion and disease prevention activities. This document, which stressed a health-for-all strategy focused on setting goals and targets and eventually became the framework for all World Health Organization member nations to follow. The document is still in use today and is modified as needed by a task force that operates within the Agency for Healthcare Research and Quality (AHRQ).

Although the *Promoting Health, Preventing Disease: Objectives for the Nation* served the United States well, it was adapted by other countries to meet their own specific needs. For example, European countries initiated an approach to health policy and grouped targets around four major issues: (1) lifestyle and health, (2) risk factors affecting health and the environment, (3) reorientation of the health care system, and (4) infrastructure support to implement changes (Dekker, 2000; Samiel, 2000; Zacek, 2000).

The Australian Report, *Health for All Australians* (Health Targets and Implementation Committee, 1988), was compiled to improve health and reduce inequalities in health status. This document was the result of an analysis of the Better Health Commission (1986) and contained a series of recommendations on priorities for national action. This effort led to the development of better health programs, with funding to establish programs focused on five priority areas: (1) preventable cancers, (2) hypertension, (3) nutrition, (4) injury prevention, and (5) the health of elderly adults (Better Health Commission, 1986). These programs were reevaluated during the 1990s and again in 2000 (Walker, 2003). Continuing reviews indicated a need for greater understanding of the social and environmental determinants of health that are required to achieve greater equity (Commonwealth Department of Health, Housing, and Community Services, 1993; Walker, 2003). Four groups of health targets were selected after a review in 1994 and remain important considerations today: (1) preventable mortality and morbidity, (2) healthy lifestyles and risk factors, (3) health literacy and health skills, and (4) healthy environments. Principles of health promotion have been built into major national health strategies and programs in Australia, such as mental health, rural health, and the divisions of general practice (Smith, 2000; Walker, 2003).

Other countries, such as New Zealand, England, and Wales, have also developed targets to raise the overall status of health. To evaluate progress, monitoring systems and accountability measures in these countries have been established for the use of health-related resources and for achieving health care outcomes. On the other hand, Canada has developed a collaborative strategy in a partnership with interdisciplinary and intersectoral groups of health professionals, including the Canadian Nurses Association. The strategy, known as enhancing prevention practices of health professionals, involves a partnership-building process that uses networks to stimulate change to promote the concepts of participation, empowerment, and ownership of programs by the communities, thereby encouraging local action around health programs. Many other approaches to assessment and planning have occurred in other countries, such

as Brazil (Li & Sander, 2003) and Norway (Mittelmark, 2003).

In addition to its *Healthy People 2010* document, the United States has adopted a "life stage" approach to analyzing the health status of Americans. In this approach, 15 priority issues were identified by using a management-by-objectives approach (USDHHS, 1990). Continual reviews by the U.S. Preventive Services Task Force indicate that a significant improvement has taken place, particularly with regard to infants and children (Agency for Healthcare Research and Quality [AHRQ], 2004). Although there are positive reviews for HIV and AIDS control, there are still gaps in health for minority groups (AHRQ, 2004).

The American Public Health Association has continued to support their criteria for the development of health promotion and education that offer five standards for program design and implementation, which remain a major focus for the organization today as well (Lissi, 2000). These standards indicated that public health programs should do the following:

1. Address one or more risk factors that are carefully defined, measurable, modifiable, and prevalent among the members of the target group
2. Address special characteristics, needs, and preferences of the target group
3. Include interventions that will effectively reduce a targeted risk factor
4. Select interventions that make optimal use of resources
5. Select a program design that ensures continued operation and the ability to evaluate it

Higgins and Green (1994) used these criteria for case analysis of four *Healthy Communities* projects in British Columbia, Canada, concluding that the American Public Health Association criteria would disqualify most of the *Healthy Communities* projects as worthy, because most of these projects lack modifiable risk factor targets of known epidemiological importance to health outcomes or interventions.

Health Rather than Health Care as a Starting Point

In 1974 the Canadian *Lalonde Report* (Department of National Health and Welfare, 1974) promoted the concepts of lifestyle and environment as two major determinants of health, and stated that these determinants were important criteria for any national health-promotion program. Although many countries recognized the importance of the *Lalonde Report* and the *Ottawa Charter*, they developed their own initiatives that were more focused on the nature of funding disparities and service reimbursement (Smith, 2000). For example, answers about social environment, human biology, and health care spending may influence balanced spending on health and health care policy and programs. Some industrialized countries, such as Denmark and Sweden, have changed "the mix" by balancing health care spending and health-promotion and disease prevention spending (Musich, Adams, & Edington, 2000). However, the United States has continued to focus on health care alone, with an emphasis on health risks and disease prevention strategies (Catford & St. Leger, 1996; USDHHS, 2003).

Nursing's focus on disease prevention and health promotion is based on a tradition of providing holistic care to people in a variety of health care settings. The nursing profession prides itself on considering all aspects of the social, physical, and spiritual domains rather than focusing on simply an individual's health status within the prevalent health care paradigm. This view is consistent and in step with a rapidly changing health care environment that is not confined to health care agencies and institutions. Although most nurses still are employed in institutional care settings, many are seeking less traditional roles in various community settings, such as in schools, parish nursing programs, nurse-run clinics, and so on (Croghan, Johnson, & Aveyard, 2004; Smith & Maurer, 2000).

Healthy lifestyles and risk factors, quality-of-life indicators, healthy environments, development of health literacy, and life skills must be linked with target groups and related to specific determinants and health-promotion strategies. Addressing the social perspective within the community and considering individual approaches in the achievement of optimal health are also important for the new millennium.

REFORM OF HEALTH PROMOTION AND HEALTH CARE
Clinical Effectiveness of Preventive Health Care

The U.S. Preventive Services Task Force (1989) was the first to identify the clinical benefits of preventive health care. Their report provided age, gender, and risk factor recommendations for the prevention of more than 60 causes of morbidity and mortality. Methodology involved a thorough examination of the quality of scientific evidence for the effectiveness of screening tests, immunizations, and counseling interventions. *Healthy People 2010* builds on the U.S. Preventive Services Task Force document and focuses on ways to increase the years of healthy life and eliminate health disparities for population groups in the United States (USDHHS, 2000). Relevant implications of these publications for professional nursing indicate the need for education and interventions that are aimed at changing personal health behaviors before the onset of clinical disease. The task stresses the importance of involving all health care providers and individuals in taking responsibility for health promotion. This premise, naturally, assumes that an individual will become self-empowered or highly motivated to make needed health-related behavior changes. This effort requires a constant update on a variety of skills through education (Hot Topics box).

At the state and national levels there is a gradual realization that the current system is costly and still is based on acute hospital care rather than on primary and preventive health care, which may be delivered through community

and public health agencies. Policy makers and the American public have come to realize that the ultimate solution to the current health care dilemma lies in a more comprehensive approach to financing, organization, and the provision of health care services within a more integrated and coordinated system (Coburn, 2004). The concept of equitable access to preventive care for all Americans has been nourished during recent years by the demonstrated effectiveness of preventive services in reducing premature morbidity and mortality (U.S. Preventive Services Task Force, 1996). Despite these efforts, however, an equal opportunity for health promotion and disease preventive care remains unreachable and unrealized for many people (Lissi, 2000).

It is estimated that at least 41 million Americans are without health care coverage (U.S. Department of Commerce, U.S. Census Bureau, 2002). The United States spends more annually on health care costs than any other industrialized nation, with approximately $1.4 trillion having been spent in 2001. Annual costs are expected to exceed $2.2 trillion by 2008 (USDHHS, Center for Medicare and Medicaid Services, 2003). U.S. legislators continue to investigate cost-controlling measures while maintaining quality of services provided (Guico-Pabia & Endsley, 2000). Legislators also are examining ways to improve access to underserved populations (Lissi, 2000) and to add protections for U.S. citizens. The Patient's Bill of Rights of 2002, the Health Insurance Portability and Accountability Act enacted in 2003, and the prescription drug benefits legislation for senior citizens that was passed in 2003 are three examples of recent legislative efforts (Haugh, 2004; USDHHS, 2003).

The clinical approach to health promotion has served its purpose for primary and secondary disease prevention efforts but has been of greatest value to educated middle class populations. The approach has fallen short in meeting the needs of medically underserved and less well-educated groups. For many people in need of health care, responding to the immediate needs of their everyday lives comes before making adaptations to a healthy lifestyle. Nursing's long-standing support of health promotion for underserved groups can play a major role in achieving equitable access to preventive health services for all Americans (Stanhope & Lancaster, 2004).

Cost-Effectiveness of Preventive Health Care

Some believe that prevention should be judged by whether the gains in health are a reasonable return for the costs incurred, primarily because the nation continues to endure the economic burden of preventable illness and death. The portion of the gross national product in the United States spent on health care rose from 5.3% in 1960 to 13.9% in 1999 (National Center for Health Statistics, 2000). The diagnosis and management of diseases, including heart disease, cancer, injuries, and HIV and AIDS, have outstripped society's ability to pay for what are essentially pre-

Severe Acute Respiratory Syndrome

HOTtopics

SARS is a viral respiratory illness caused by SARS-CoV. It is an infectious, flulike disease that emerged in south Guangdong, China, in November 2002 and infected people globally by the spring of 2003. WHO alerted the world regarding international travel warnings when a number of SARS cases were reported from China, Hong Kong, Taiwan, Vietnam, Singapore, and Canada (CDC, 2004; Lingappa, McDonald, Simone, & Parashar, 2004; Weingartl Copps, J., Drebot, M. A., Marszal, P., Smith, G., Gren, J., et al., 2004). So far more than 8200 people have been infected and 700 have died from the disease according to WHO (CDC, 2004). In America, eight people had a positive test result for the virus, and the disease has not spread more widely in the U.S. community. Based on the sequence analysis of SARS-CoV, it is suggested that the virus is different from any other coronavirus and might have evolved and lived in a domesticated animal host. However, a research study that inoculated pigs and chickens intravenously, intranasally, ocularly, and orally with SARS-CoV failed to show that these animals are amplifying hosts for the virus (Weingartl et al., 2004). The origins of SARS-CoV remain unclear (Lingappa et al., 2004). Nevertheless, animal traders carry antibodies to SARS-CoV and indigenous animals in Guangdong province are hosts for a SARS-like coronavirus (CDC, 2004).

It is believed that SARS is spread by close person-to-person contact, especially by respiratory droplets. "Close contact means having cared for or lived with someone with SARS or having direct contact with respiratory secretions or body fluids of people with SARS. Examples of close contact include kissing or hugging, sharing eating or drinking utensils, talking to someone within 3 feet, and touching someone directly. Close contact does not include activities like walking by a person or briefly sitting across a waiting room or office" (CDC, 2004, p. 1). The virus can be deposited on

the mucous membranes of the mouth, nose, or eyes of a person who is within 3 feet when an infected person coughs or sneezes. Also, a person who touches infectious droplets on a surface of an object and then touches the mouth, nose, or eye(s) can become sick (CDC, 2004).

SARS Symptoms

Normally when a person is infected by the SARS virus, early symptoms include a fever with a temperature greater than 100.4° F (38.0° C), headache, malaise and body aches, diarrhea (10% to 20% of SARS patients), and mild respiratory symptoms (for some people). Dry cough develops 2 to 7 days later. Most people end up experiencing pneumonia (CDC, 2004). CDC responded to the 2003 SARS outbreak by working closely with WHO and other international sectors in order to:

- Provide 24-hour coordination and response
- Deploy health professionals to help with on-site investigations around the world
- Provide help and support for health departments locally and nationally in identifying and investigating possible SARS cases and causes
- Initiate a new system in order to alert travelers who may have been exposed to SARS (CDC, 2004)

Although WHO announced that the last chain of human transmission of SARS-CoV was broken on July 5, 2003, all countries should be vigilant for its reemergence. There have been reports of SARS-CoV cases due to (1) laboratory accidents in Taiwan, China, and Singapore and (2) contacts with animal hosts and environmental contamination in China. Therefore, every country in the world should be prepared for a recurrence and prompt detection and response to the reemergence of SARS-CoV transmissions in humans (WHO, 2004).

Centers for Disease Control and Prevention. (2004). Fact sheet: Basic information about SARS. *http://www.cdc.gov/ncidod/SARS/factsheet.htm*; Lingappa, J. R., McDonald, L. C., Simone, P., & Parashar, U. D. (2004). Wrestling SARS from uncertainty. *Emerging Infectious Diseases, 10*(2), 167-170; Weingartl, H. M. Copps, J., Drebot, M. A., Marszal, P., Smith, G. Gren, J., et al. (2004). Susceptibility of pigs and chickens to SARS coronavirus. *Emerging Infectious Diseases, 10*, 179-184.; World Health Organization. (2004). WHO SARS international reference and verification laboratory network: Policy and procedures in the inter-epidemic period. Retrieved April 13, 2005, from: *http://www.who.int/csr/resources/publications/en/SARSReferenceLab.pdf*.
CDC, Centers for Disease Control; *SARS,* severe acute respiratory syndrome; *SARS-CoV,* SARS-associated coronavirus; *WHO,* World Health Organization.

ventable conditions. Although compiling the cost of preventable illness and premature death is certainly possible, determining the value of health-promotion programs and dollar savings is difficult. During the 1990s, attempts have been made to develop health-promotion indicators, standards, and health outcomes (National Center for Health Statistics, 2000).

Reported outcomes generally have been limited to aggregates of changes in health behavior or attitudes for which the cost can be estimated for professional time, materials, and so on, but that underestimates the gains made by the communities from interventions such as empowerment or capacity building to exercise health-related decision making (Smith & Maurer, 2000).

The reality of skyrocketing health care expenditures has ushered in cost-effectiveness analysis as a method for determining the way in which financial resources are being used and the way in which they should be used in health care. The purpose is to help clinicians and policy makers focus on investments that provide the most health for the required expenditure, with outcomes reported either as a single measure (years of life saved) or as several measures combined on a single scale (quality-adjusted life years) (Feldstein, 1999). Cost-effectiveness analyses of preventive services have included screenings for lead, cholesterol, breast cancer, and cervical cancer. Most counseling interventions have not been analyzed for cost-effectiveness, which is consistent with the finding that primary care physicians spend less than 15% of their time counseling individuals on weight reduction, cholesterol reduction, smoking cessation, and breast self-examination (Woodwell, 1989). A primary care provider survey, sponsored by the U.S. Public Health Service to track provider-related *Healthy People 2010* objectives, should help determine the nature and amount of preventive health care delivered by primary health care providers, including nurse practitioners (Health Teaching box).

Estimates indicate that providing coverage for preventive services is likely to increase costs in the short term (Maurer, 2000). Furthermore, preventive services vary in clinical effectiveness and cost-effectiveness when performed by health care providers using different guidelines and methods. Another consideration involves the differential costs per year for services that have undergone cost-effectiveness analysis, suggesting that personal and social values may influence whether a preventive intervention is judged to be cost-effective.

Because the U.S. health care delivery system has evolved with a bias toward coverage for acute illness, providing coverage for preventive services in most public and private insurance plans has been difficult. At a time of heightened attention to health care reform, preventive services of known effectiveness must be incorporated into a comprehensive benefits package for all Americans. A core set of clinical preventive services, including immunizations, screening, and counseling, was prepared by a task for on preventive health care for inclusion in an overall benefits package (Agency for Healthcare Research and Quality, 2004). These services are defined according to age-specific and gender-specific periodic health examinations to ensure their economic efficiency in primary care settings (Kulbok, Laffrey, & Goeppinger, 2000).

Health Promotion and Vulnerable Populations

In 1996 approximately 40 million Americans who might have been classified as medically indigent were without health insurance. Among the people most likely to be uninsured were blacks (21%), people with incomes below the poverty line (42%), the unemployed (36%), and people with less than 12 years of education (30%). Many of these uninsured individuals and families received care as needed at local emergency rooms, and people with higher incomes were more likely to receive their care through ambulatory clinical and private physicians' offices. In 1999 less than 1% of Medicaid funding was directed to early and periodic screening, rural health clinics, and family planning services (National Center for Health Statistics, 2000). Little has changed since the publication of a report by the National Medical Expenditure Survey (Agency for Health Care Policy and Research, 1994) in 1987 that indicated that people who are uninsured or who have inadequate coverage usually forego primary and preventive health care. Additional evidence of this primary care underservice is reflected in several reports by the Robert Wood Johnson Foundation's National Access to Care surveys beginning in 1978, which still identify factors associated with utilization of health care services (Robert Wood Johnson Foundation, 2001). One survey indicated that 40 million Americans had no health care provider, clinic, or hospital as a regular source of health care, representing a 7% increase over an earlier survey. Concurrently the percentage of people who

---

HEALTH TEACHING Smoking Cessation

Tobacco use is a risk factor for over 25 diseases, including lung cancer, which is one of the leading causes of cancer-related mortality throughout the world. In 2002 tobacco was the number 1 leading actual cause of death in America, with 435,000 deaths (CDC, 2004). According to WHO (2002), worldwide one third of male adults and one fifth of teenagers aged 13 to 15 years old smoke. Although smoking is on the decline in developed countries, rates in developing countries are rising at alarming rates, especially among youths.

- In Cambodia, in the male population, 67% in urban areas and 86% in rural areas smoke. Most smokers are older (50 to 70 years) and monks.
- In China, among the whole population, 67% of men and 4% of women smoke. Among teenagers, smoking rates are 30% for males and 8% for females. One third of cigarettes worldwide are smoked by Chinese, and about 3000 people die daily in China from smoking-related illness.
- In Japan 51% of the male population smoke. The number of female smokers has increased dramatically during the

past 10 years to about 10%. There are very few smoke-free public areas in Japan due to weak laws against tobacco consumption.

- In Malaysia about 50% of the men smoke. There are approximately 50 teenage (younger than 18) new smokers each day. Among teenage boys (12 to 18 years), 30% smoke. Smoking among teenage girls is rapidly rising, from 4.8% to 8% between 1996 and 1999.
- In the Philippines approximately 60% of the men smoke, and 40% of teenage boys are smokers. There are no laws in the Philippines to prevent children from buying cigarettes.
- In South Korea 67% of the men smoke. The smoking rate among female adults rose nearly twofold from 3.9% in 1989 to 6.7% in 1997. Throughout the world, South Korea is the eighth largest tobacco market.

School-based interventions and personal contact with teenage groups by nurses can assist in preventing this harmful activity. A thorough assessment of tobacco use is a necessary part of the health intake.

Centers for Disease Control and Prevention. (2004). *Factsheet: Actual causes of death in the United States, 2000.* Retrieved March 11, 2004, from http://www.cdc.gov/nccdphd/factsheets/death_causes2000.htm; World Health Organization. (2002). Smoking statistics: Factsheet. Retrieved March 11, 2004, from: *http://www.cdc.dov/tobacco/research_data/adults_prev/mmwr5253_highlights.htm.*

reported having no ambulatory visits during the previous 12 months rose significantly, from 19% to 33%. Underserved populations were affected disproportionately, with a significantly higher percentage of poor, uninsured, and ethnic minority individuals reporting no regular source of care, no ambulatory visits within the preceding 12 months, and fair or poor health status. Other indicators, such as high infant mortality rate, illnesses related to poor diet, inadequate housing, and lack of other basic necessities of life, are evident among the vulnerable groups (Agency for Health Care Policy and Research, 1994; USDHHS, 2000) (Case Study).

Groups referred to as disadvantaged, at-risk, or as **vulnerable populations** are those with socioeconomic vulnerability factors that may include poverty, lack of education, and homelessness. They are at risk for adverse health outcomes, including premature mortality, comparative morbidity, and low functional status and quality of life (Leight, 2003). Other vulnerable groups include people who have age-related vulnerability and include youth, pregnant adolescents, and frail elderly (Kidd & Scrimenti, 2004). Providing a "band-aid" service when the needs are much greater constantly frustrates nurses. Questions may be raised as to whether the needs are addressed adequately and whether greater health risks, limited control, disenfranchisement, victimization, disadvantaged status, and powerlessness are ever understood when dealing with people's vulnerability.

CASE STUDY

Derek

Derek is a 4-year-old Haitian American boy who was brought to a rural health department clinic by his grandmother. Derek and his family are recent immigrants from Haiti, having lived in this area for less than 2 years. Derek has received all of his care since coming to the United States at the clinic, and his immunizations are up to date. His last visit to the clinic was 6 months ago when his grandmother brought him in with a low-grade fever and diarrhea. The problems were resolved, and the clinic nurse discussed basic child care and health-promotion activities with his grandmother, including nutrition. For the past month Derek has been attending preschool for the first time. Derek lives with his grandmother, a 14-year-old cousin, his 19-year-old mother, and his 2-year-old brother. Derek's grandmother is concerned that Derek has been wetting the bed 2 out of 7 nights a week for the last 3 weeks and appears less interested in food than he was at the time of his last visit.

Reflective Questions
1. Given Derek's age and social situation, what types of health-promotion information might you want to make certain to discuss with Derek's grandmother?
2. What type of nutritional guidance should be shared with his grandmother?
3. What are some possible explanations for the bed wetting?

Among all age groups, older adults and homeless people represent those who are most in need of clinical preventive services to offset disabling and life-threatening conditions (Kidd & Scrimenti, 2004). Examples of these conditions, which frequently are overlooked by clinicians, include numerous types of chronic infections, skin conditions, trauma, and malnutrition (Nabors et al., 2004).

For some vulnerable populations, unstable or dangerous physical environments, isolation, and the lack of adequate and available health services exacerbate the already high rates of preventable illness and death. Perhaps for no other group is the convergence of economic hardship, social isolation, and physical and mental disability more apparent than for homeless individuals and families. For example, a report from the Institute of Medicine (1988) entitled *Homelessness, Health, and Human Needs* revealed that families with young children were one of the fastest growing groups among the American homeless. Since this publication, more recent data state that families with children make up 36.5% of the homeless population, single men 46%, single women 14%, and adolescents 3.5% (Nabors et al., 2004; Waxman & Henderliter, 1996).

IMPLICATIONS FOR NURSING LEADERSHIP IN HEALTH PROMOTION
Implications for Policy Development

The health-promotion priorities that have been presented in this chapter pose an interesting challenge for all nurses. This is an opportune time for nurses, as individuals and as a profession, to play a key role in a health system that must emphasize health promotion and disease prevention. Because nurses have long believed in and practiced the principles of primary prevention, their leadership and participation in health-promotion policy development is critical during an era that might bring dramatic changes in health care reform (Gullotta, 2000). Through a perspective on the development of community-based, health-promotion programs, nurses can bring a balance to decisions that will be made about the appropriate use of health care resources. In 1981 the World Health Organization presented a challenge of *Health for All by the Year 2000* to nurses throughout the world through its proposal that nurses consolidate their resources and become a powerful influence in the world's health (WHO, 1981). The report asserts that responses by nurses have been fragmented, sporadic, planned, and inadequate, involving relatively few nurses practicing beyond their limited clinical paradigms. Since that time, new directions for nurses have been established at the World Health Organization (2000) that involve nurses in roles that incorporate the ability to effect social differences in terms of poverty, population displacement from rural to urban areas, and epidemiological and demographic transitions resulting in a growing number of elderly people (Multicultural Awareness box).

With rapidly advancing health technology, developing an international declaration on nursing, human rights, human genetics, and public health policy is of great signif-

MULTICULTURAL AWARENESS

Health and Health Promotion in a Native American Tribe: The Navajo

The Navajo people of the *Dine' Bike'yah* live on a vast land on which the four states of Arizona, Utah, New Mexico, and Colorado intersect. The *Dine'* hold this land as sacred and as an integral part of their lives. The Navajo believe that health is a part of the *Hozho'*, which is a personal sense of well-being and rightness with the world and is all inclusive. For the Navajo, health is not separate from the overall state of balance among the body, mind, spirit, and the surrounding environment. When one of these is out of balance, *Hozho'* is not achieved. *Hozho'* is everything that a Navajo thinks of as being good, in terms of good and evil or favorable and unfavorable. The Navajo strive to maintain *Hozho'* and to live in harmony with all things that surround them. The goal of Navajo life in this world is to live to attain maturity with *Hozho'* and to die of old age, the result of which incorporates beauty, harmony, and happiness or *sa'ah naagh"ii bik'eh hozho'*. When the body, spirit, or mind fall out of *Hozho'*, a traditional healer or medicine man is sought. In many instances, the medicine man recommends that the individual seek both Western medicine and the traditional ways to cure the problem.

Since 1955 trends in Navajo health have demonstrated a progressive improvement, particularly in the areas of maternal and infant mortality. However, on the increase are lifestyle-related diseases and premature deaths for which health-promotion activities can have an effect. Among these lifestyle-related diseases are adult-onset diabetes, AIDS, and alcohol and substance abuse. Health care providers who work with the Navajo must address all health-promotion and disease prevention activities in terms of an appreciation for the cultural and economic realities and the needs of this community.

Discover Navajo People of the fourth world. Retrieved May 13, 2004, from http://www.discovernavajo.com/culture.html; *Native American tribes interesting facts & legends from the . . . Navajo or Dine.* Retrieved from http://www.geocities.com.willow1d/factnava.html
AIDS, acquired immunodeficiency syndrome.

---

icance (Anderson & Rorty, 2001). The United Nations Educational, Scientific and Cultural Organization, the Council of Europe, and the Human Genome Organization have drafted and proposed legislation regarding applications of human genetic science to countries that wish to adopt or apply such legislation. It is crucial that the international nursing community develops its own legislation, philosophy, and practice-based services dovetailing with those at the international level, yet yielding practices applicable to uniquely cultural communities at a grass roots level (Anderson & Rorty, 2001)

Implications for Practice

Nurses have been challenged to use their capacity to bring about health gains. The preventive services delivered by nurses, including efforts such as health assessment, screening, and counseling, are necessary tools to empower individuals to promote and maintain optimal health and

well-being. Achieving the *Health People 2010* objectives is possible only by a comprehensive implementation of health-promotion activities at the community level, including work sites, schools, homes, and neighborhood settings. In collaboration with other professional and business groups, nurses can educate and empower individuals, families, and communities to become active participants in defining their health needs, in making informed decisions to meet these needs, and ultimately in bringing about improvements in health status and quality of life. New models must be generated (Gebre-Medhin & Wekell, 1999; Howson, 2000), such as with creative inventions (telemedicine), to meet these complex needs (Eminovic, Wyatt, Tarpey, Murray, & Ingrams, 2004).

Furthermore, because individuals will be increasingly responsible for their own health, they will need access to quality information that has not been readily available in the past. For example, Marine and others (1998) have developed Net Wellness, an electronic consumer health information service to provide the best possible health information to the broadest possible populations.

Implications for Education

The demand for primary health care providers will continue to spur the need for more advanced practice nurses, including nurse practitioners and clinical nurse specialists. The demand can be met if undergraduate students, indeed, pre-undergraduate students without specific career goals, are introduced to a global perspective and to the concepts of health promotion and disease prevention early in their education and in their personal lives. Then health promotion, quality of life, and socioeconomic justice will become increasingly valued in cultures throughout the world.

Although some baccalaureate nursing programs in America focus on cultural diversity and international health, nursing programs in other countries, such as Australia, Japan, South Korea, and Thailand, do not (Lambert et al., 2004). Curricula with cultural diversity global frameworks (Brown, 1999; Pomrehn, Davis, Chen, & Barker, 2000) that develop concepts and experiences directed toward maximizing *Health for All* will enable nurses to fulfill innovative roles in reformed health care systems around the world. Faculty and students will work increasingly together in interdisciplinary teams with and in communities, using an expanding variety of health-promotion services. The team will be guided by national and international standards. For example, in 1997 the Bureau of Health Professions of the Health Resources and Services Administration and the Association of Teachers of Preventive Medicine convened a task force to update the 1984 *Inventory of Knowledge and Skills Relating to Disease Prevention and Health Promotion*. In addition to completing this objective, the task force created a list of competencies that are essential to all disciplines, which are described by Pomrehn and coauthors (2000).

Nursing faculty will bring the strength of tested nursing theories to their teaching, practice, and research with nursing students, faculty, and students in other disciplines throughout the university, not simply within health care. Nursing practice and literature will continue to demonstrate the limitations of the biomedical model in promoting health for all. Curricula that provide experiences directed toward maximizing health will enable nurses to fulfill innovative roles in a reformed health care system. Given the increasing focus on self-care in disease prevention and health promotion, nurses can respond directly to the health needs of individuals, families, communities, and groups by focusing on health promotion and by supporting new ways to work and live.

Implications for Research

In the area of research, a heightened need for nurses exists to test individual, family, community, and group interventions that optimize health and well-being of both healthy and ill populations. An example of action research conducted in Thailand during 2000 and 2001 to promote self-reliance and self-esteem among HIV-positive pregnant women was found to be successful. With a combination of counseling, advocacy, education, and services that the nurse researchers provided to the participants at both the hospital and home, most women from the study felt that they could move on and had higher self-esteem than they did before participating in the project (Sawatphanit, Ross, & Suwansujarid, 2004). A support group inspired them to have hope and release tension from the disease. Education and counseling provided by the nurses helped them to use condoms with their partners to prevent them from getting more HIV virus and enabled the women to solve problems more effectively (Sawatphanit et al., 2004). One woman stayed happy throughout her pregnancy, and part of the success was derived from support of the nurse team who advocated her religious practices (e.g., meditation, reading religious stories) according to her beliefs (Ross, Sawatphanit, & Suwansujarid, 2004). Because of the evidence that maximal effectiveness in lifestyle modification occurs through a combination of educational and environmental interventions, future research will identify the most effective combinations of these interventions under different conditions. Nurse researchers will be testing these theories to examine the relationships between the delivery of health promotion interventions and cost, access, utilization, and health outcomes associated with this type of care (Badalik, Hegyi, Farkas, & Honza, 2000).

Given the acknowledged importance of health-promotion and disease preventive care in health care reform deliberations, articulating an agenda that will ensure the nursing profession's role of leadership and active participation is critical. The American Nurses Association (1991) issued a report entitled *Nursing's Agenda for Health Care Reform*, which offers a broad-based strategy that calls for a nationally defined standard package of primary and preventive health services. The American Nurses Association has continued this effort by promoting the development of relationships in health care that are targeted at activities that will improve health outcomes in a cost-effective manner of

an individual, family, group, or community (American Nurses Association, 2000). By acting on this agenda, nursing can assume a position of leadership in promoting the health of all. Nurses need to consider the following three principal goals:

1. *Participate in health-promotion policy development.* Cultivating nursing leadership in health policy development involves time, funds, expertise, authority, and education (American Nurses Association, 2000). Although nurses continue to focus on the care of individuals in acute settings, equal support for altering the contexts that result in preventable illness and disability should be afforded. Professional attention to health-promoting environments and behaviors provides an entry point to the development of community-based models of primary care that emphasize health promotion and disease prevention.

2. *Influence public expectations about health promotion.* Presentations and other forms of public dialogue and education will help raise awareness of the value of individual and community health promotion. Nurses have the collective capacity to change the philosophy of the system from selling health care in the marketplace to creating a milieu for changing health behavior. Encouraging meaningful community participation in addressing health issues provides a significant opportunity to narrow the gap between what is possible in terms of health promotion in this country and what is reality. Increasing consumer demand for preventive health care and provider willingness to offer such care is influenced largely by the coverage of preventive services in health insurance plans. Nurses should participate in a broad range of activities that evaluate options for expanding coverage of preventive health care. Nurses should also lobby for equitable reimbursement of preventive services delivery. One approach might be to advocate a periodic preventive health visit fee, which would specify a package of preventive services for different population groups.

3. *Promote equitable access to preventive health care.* Given the higher rates of preventable conditions among underserved populations, a justified need to promote the distribution and utilization of preventive health services is apparent. Community-based efforts that combine public and private resources should be targeted to people most in need of preventive health care. Delivery models that focus on integrating preventive and primary care should be expanded into more areas.

Preventive health care delivery should be based on a broad research agenda that encompasses multiple health and social science perspectives. Nurses should participate in areas of research that will influence both personal and community health in a cost-effective manner. Service delivery can also benefit from an expanded health services research agenda that fosters collaboration with other disciplines, such as nutrition and education. Most importantly, preventive health care should be adapted to the health and social problems of specific groups and supplemented as needed by innovative practice

Haitian Health Foundation: A Charitable Outreach to Neighbors in Need

A volunteer effort of health professionals initiated in Haiti in 1982 by Dr. Jeremiah Lowney and his wife, Virginia, has grown into an outpatient health care facility supported by a nondenominational foundation called the Haitian Health Foundation, Inc. (HHF). In 1985, after working for 4 years in Port au Prince, HHF moved its outreach to Jeremie, Haiti, at the suggestion of Mother Teresa of Calcutta, to bring health care, hope, and opportunity to this especially poor and remote area. The clinic at Jeremie employs 105 people, including 2 full-time physicians, 1 full-time dentist, 10 registered nurses, 2 licensed professional nurses, a medical technician, a dental assistant, and 70 to 80 auxiliary personnel (all Haitians). The clinic provides health care to 350 to 400 Haitians daily.

The Haitian *Agents de Sante* program currently employs villagers in 936 villages surrounding Jeremie. This program was initiated by a nurse, who enlisted an individual who had a seventh grade education in each village. After being educated in health promotion, the person became the Health Agent of that village. These Health Agents are trained by HHF to provide preventive and basic health care and education. Many villages have also begun mothers' groups, by which women can share experiences and knowledge relating to nutrition, health care, and other topics that have an effect on their quality of life. Breast-feeding classes and immunization programs are available.

Another program was begun by building a food distribution pavilion. This building will be used to store and distribute food to over 1000 children and pregnant women 3 times a week. The pavilion will also be used to educate participants in nutrition and preventive health care. Much of the education in these programs is accomplished through song, primarily because this approach appears to enable the Haitians to remember what is being taught.

For over 8 years, another education program has provided access to schools for poor children in a country in which education is neither free nor mandatory. As of 2004, 1250 students were attending school through this program. Tuition, uniforms, books, and shoes are provided by HHF funds or through the Save-a-Family Program.

The HHF relies heavily on the generosity of donors and the many volunteers who donate their time and talents to supplement the staff in Haiti. Volunteers travel to Jeremie, at their own expense from America, Canada, and Europe, to share their skills and resources with the poor. These volunteers include health care providers, electricians, plumbers, teachers, clergy, and students.

These programs are only a few examples of the health-promotion programs sponsored by the HHF. These efforts show the way in which dedicated professionals can make a difference, even in third world countries in which health care resources are rare.

Courtesy Jeremiah Lowney, MD, MPH.

- Do you believe that a paradigm shift toward health promotion has actually been realized by health care professionals?
- What are the political implications of health promotion for the country of your residence?
- What does "determinants of health status" mean to you? How would you propose to serve as an advocate for them?
- What are some of the positive attributes of collaboration with other health care professionals that you have implemented, or might easily implement, in your practice? Which ones are most important to you?
- As a nurse working in acute care hospital services, what does health promotion mean to you? Does an acceptance of being "doers" to "enablers" cause professional conflict with your values or belief system?
- What outcomes have been achieved by the implementation of *Healthy People 2010* or parallel policies that grab your attention?

PROFESSIONAL PERSPECTIVE

- What lessons are to be learned from past approaches or the over-reliance on health care delivery to solve all health-promotion and disease prevention problems?
- Have national or international public policy developments influenced any negative and positive views of health of people?
- If you have been involved in influencing contemporary policy at the local or national level, what implications does this have for your work as a health-promotion practitioner?
- What are some of the obstacles that nurses must overcome with regard to their involvement in policy debate for social and health policies?
- To what extent have health rights and consumer perspectives been realized by health care professionals? Provide three examples from your practice.
- Do you believe that in the current economic climate, introduction of health-promotion principles is not a cost-effective exercise?
- Do you believe that clinical effectiveness through risk factor identification is a cost-effective, population-oriented approach?
- Would you participate in encouraging community action for public awareness and lobbying against political issues, such as tobacco advertising in sports, the proposed development of a casino in your area, the development of an industry that will emit toxic wastes, and proposed discriminatory laws against certain minority groups?

the services of social workers, nutritionists, translators, and outreach workers. Alternative forms of health-promotion approaches and preventive service delivery should also be examined, including mobile vans, school and worksite clinics, and other community-based, intersectorial collaboration to reorient the health system beyond health care (Innovative Practice box).

SUMMARY

This chapter has described selected past developments and future directions in health promotion and disease prevention throughout the life span and throughout the world. This chapter makes it quite apparent that health promotion as a field of practice is quite complex. For some people the concept of health promotion dwells on idealism, and in the current climate of economic realities health promotion requires a considerable shift of philosophy and resources. Jargon such as healthy public policy, healthy communities, and healthy people have been politicized and interpreted in different ways by different professionals and countries depending on their power base. Most countries have adopted some of the core concepts as a health-for-all strategy.

In this chapter, priority issues and future directions for nursing in the area of health promotion have been pre-

sented. Current health care reform efforts pose significant opportunities and challenges for nurses, educators, and researchers. With an enduring emphasis on (1) individuals, families, communities, and the environments in which people live, work, and play and (2) health promotion and disease prevention, nurses are critical links for promoting the nation's health. As the twenty-first century begins, nurses have the vision, expertise, and experience to truly make a difference in the health of all women, men, and children. This chapter has demonstrated that the nursing profession can make a greater difference if a commitment can be made to realizing an equal opportunity for the improved health status of populations using a variety of investigated strategies. Through a combination of leadership, creativity, and determination, nurses can and will establish a healthier future for all people around the globe (Box 25-3).

ADDITIONAL STUDY MATERIAL

Study Questions in the back of the book, see page 663.

evolve WEB SITE MATERIALS

These materials are located on the book's Web site at http://evolve.elsevier.com/Edelman/.

- WebLinks
- Content Updates

REFERENCES

Agency for Health Care Policy and Research. (1994). *National medical expenditure survey: Health insurance, use of health services and health care expenditures.* Rockville, MD: Public Health Service.

Agency for Healthcare Research and Quality. (2004). U.S. Prevention Task Force reports. *http://www.ahrq.gov.*

American Association of Colleges of Nursing. (1998). *Essentials of baccalaureate education in professional practice.* Washington, DC: The Association.

American Nurses Association. (1991). *Nursing's agenda for health care reform.* Kansas City, MO: The Association.

American Nurses Association. (2000). *Achieving access for all Americans.* New York: The Association.

Anderson, G., & Rorty, M. V. (2001). Key points for developing an international declaration on nursing, human rights, human genetics and public health policy. *Nursing Ethics, 8,* 259-271.

Badalik, L., Hegyi, L., Farkas, D., & Honza, Z. (2000). Research and knowledge for health-important part of the strategy: Health for all in the 21st century. *Eurorehab, 4,* 210-211.

Better Health Commission. (1986). *Looking forward to better health.* Canberra, Australia: Australian Government Publishing Service.

Beukens, P., Keusch, G., Belizan, J., & Bhutta, Z. A. (2004). Evidenced-based global health. *Journal of the American Medical Association, 291*(21), 2639-2641.

Brown, G. (1999). A visit to the Republic of South Africa and Botswana: A modern country with a relic from the past. *Association of Black Nursing Faculty Journal, 10*(5), 116-118.

Brown, V. (1992). Health care policies, health policies or policies for health. In H. Gardiner (Ed.), *Health policy development, implementation, and evaluation in Australia.* Melbourne, Australia: Churchill Livingstone.

Brundtland, G. H. (2000). *Fifth global conference on health promotion* (On-line). Retrieved June 5, 2000, from: *http://www.who.int/directorgeneralspeeches/2000/200000605_mexico.html.*

Catford, J., & St. Leger, L. (1996). Moving into a new decade and a new dimension. *Health Promotion International, 11*(1), 1-7.

Centers for Disease Control and Prevention. (2004). Fact sheet: Basic information about SARS. *http://www.cdc.gov/ncidod/SARS/factsheet.htm.*

Coburn, D. (2004). Beyond the income inequality hypothesis: Class, neoliberalism, and health inequalities. *Social Science & Medicine, 58,* 41-56.

Cohen, G. D. (2000). Aging at a turning point in the 21st century. *American Journal of Geriatric Psychiatry, 8*(1), 1-3.

Commonwealth Department of Health, Housing, and Community Services. (1993). *Towards health for all and health promotion.* Canberra, Australia: Australian Government Publishing Service.

Croghan, E., Johnson, C., & Aveyard, P. (2004). School nurses: Policies, working practices, roles and value perceptions. *Journal of Advanced Nursing, 47*(4), 377-385.

Dekker, E. (2000). Health policy in the Netherlands: Description and analysis of 10 years of national health policy development emphasizing the health of all strategy. *World Health Organization Regional Publications—European Series, 86,* 110-129.

Department of National Health and Welfare. (1974). *A new perspective on the health of Canadians (The Lalonde Report).* Ottawa: Department of National Health and Welfare.

Deschamps, J. P. (2003). A rereading and examination of the Ottawa charter. *Sante Publique, 15*(3), 313-325.

Eminovic, N., Wyatt, J. C., Tarpey, A. M., Murray, G., & Ingrams, G. J. (2004). First evaluation of the NHS direct online clinical inquiry service: A nurse-led Web chat triage service for the public. *Journal of*

Medical Internet Research, 6(2), E17. Retrieved March 20, 2005, from *http://www.jmir.org/2004/2/e17/.*

Feldstein, P. J. (1999). *Health care economics* (5th ed.). West Albany, NY: Delmar.

Gebre-Medhin, M., & Wekell, P. (1999). Focus on children! A model for international development cooperation. *Lakartidningen, 96*(3), 188-193.

Guico-Pabia, C. J., & Endsley, D. (2000). Lessons from a health promotion victory. *Business Health, 18*(8), 43-44.

Gullotta, T. P. (2000). How will we understand prevention in the 21st century? *Journal of Primary Prevention, 21*(2), 145-146.

Hassmiller, S. B. (2000). Public health and primary health care systems and health care transformations. In M. Stanhope & J. Lancaster (Eds.), *Community and public health nursing* (pp. 42-59). New York: Mosby.

Haugh, R. (2004). Banking on privacy: Hospitals must protect patient information and their own liability—As banks balk at HIPAA. *Hospital Health Network, 78*(2), 50-54.

Health Targets and Implementation Committee. (1988). *Health for all Australians: Report to the Australian Minister's Advisory Council and the Australian Health Ministers Conference.* Canberra, Australia: Australian Government Publishing Service.

Heiss, G., & Walden, L. S. (2000). Health promotion and risk reduction in the community. In C. M. Smith & F. A. Maurer (Eds.), *Community health nursing* (pp. 447-476). Philadelphia: W. B. Saunders.

Henry J. Kaiser Family Foundation. (July, 2002). *HIV/AIDS policy fact sheet: The global HIV/AIDS Epidemic.* Washington, DC: Author.

Henry, L. L., & Royer, L. (2004). Community-based strategies for pediatric nurses to combat the escalating childhood obesity epidemic. *Pediatric Nursing, 30*(2), 162-164.

Higgins, W. H., & Green, L. W. (1994). The APHA criteria for development of health promotion programs applied to four healthy community projects in British Columbia. *Health Promotion International, 9*(4), 311-316.

Howson, C. P. (2000). Perspectives and needs for health in the 21st century: 20th century paradigms in 21st century science. *Journal of Human Virology, 3*(2), 94-103.

Huttlinger, K. (2004). Perspectives on international health. In M. Stanhope & J. Lancaster (Eds.), *Community and public health nursing* (5th ed.). St. Louis: Mosby.

Institute of Medicine. (1988). *Homelessness, health and human needs.* Washington, DC: National Academy Press.

Joint United Nations Programme on HIV/AIDS & World Health Organization. (2003). *AIDS epidemic update.* Geneva: UNAIDS.

Kalache, A., & Keller, L. (2000). The graying world: A challenge for the twenty-first century. *Science Progress, 83*(Pt. 1), 33-54.

Kidd, S. A., & Scrimenti, K. (2004). Evaluating child and youth homelessness. *Evaluation Review, 28*(4), 325-341.

Kulbok, P., Laffrey, S. C., & Goeppinger, J. (2000). Community health promotion: An integrative model for practice. In M. Stanhope & J. Lancaster (Eds.), *Community and public health nursing* (pp. 284-303). St. Louis: Mosby.

Lamarche, P. A. (1995). Our health paradigm in peril. *Public Health Reports, 110*(5), 556-562.

Lambert, V. A., Lambert, C. E., Daly, J., Davidson, P. M., Kunaviktikul, W., & Shin, K. R. (2004). Nursing education on women's health care in Australia, Japan, South Korea, and Thailand. *Journal of Transcultural Nursing, 15*, 44-53.

Lee, J. W. (2004). *The world health report 2004: Changing history.* Geneva: World Health Organization.

Lee, K. (2000). For debate. The impact of globalization on public health: Implications for the UK Faculty of Public Health Medicine. *Journal of Public Health Medicine, 22*, 253-262.

Lefebvre, C. (1996). Health reform in the United States: A marketing perspective. *Health Promotion International, 9*(4), 229-234.

Legge, D. (1991). Towards a politics of health. In H. Gardiner (Ed.), *The politics of health: The Australian experience.* Melbourne, Australia: Churchill Livingstone.

Leight, S. B. (2003). The application of a vulnerable populations conceptual model to rural health. *Public Health Nursing, 20,* 440-448.

Li, L. M., & Sander, J. W. (2003). National demonstration project in epilepsy in Brazil. *Arquivos de Neuro-psiquiatria, 61*(1), 153-156.

Lingappa, J. R., McDonald, L. C., Simone, P., & Parashar, U. D. (2004). Wrestling SARS from uncertainty. *Emerging Infectious Diseases, 10*(2), 167-170.

Lissi, P. E. (2000). Setting goals in health promotion: A conceptual and ethical platform. *Medical Healthcare Philosophy, 3*(20), 169-173.

Marine, S., Guard, R., Morris, T., Haag, D., Kaya, B., Riep, J., et al. (1998). A model for enhancing worldwide personal health and wellness. *Medinfo, 9*(2), 1265-1268.

Maskovsky, J. (2000). Managing the poor: Neoliberalism, Medicaid, HMOs and the triumph of consumerism among the poor. *Medical Anthropologist, 19*(2), 121-146.

Maurer, F. (2000). The U.S. health care system. In F. Maurer & C. Smith (Eds.), *Community health nursing* (pp. 107-139). Philadelphia: W. B. Saunders.

Mittelmark, M. B. (2003). The role of professional education in building capacity for health promotion in the global south: A case study from Norway. *Ethnic Disease, 13*(2, Suppl. 2), S35-39.

Modawal, A. (2003). Letter from India: Caring for the elderly. *Annals of Long-Term Care, 11,* 48-50.

Musich, S. A., Adams, L., & Edington, D. W. (2000). Effectiveness of health promotion programs in moderating medical costs in the U.S.A. *Health Promotion International, 15*(1), 5-15.

Nabors, L. A., Weist, M. D., Shugarman, R., Woeste, M. J., Mullet, E., & Rosner, L. (2004). Assessment, prevention and intervention activities in a school-based program for children experiencing homelessness. *Behavior Modification, 28*(4), 565-578.

National Center for Health Statistics, Centers for Disease Control and Prevention. (2000). *Health United States, 2000.* Hyattsville, MD: U.S. Public Health Service.

National Institute of Nursing Research. (2004). *Research themes for the future.* Washington, DC: National Institutes of Health.

O'Byrne, D. (2000). Global conference on health promotion: Mexico 2000. *Promotion & Education, 7*(3), 15-16.

Pommier, J., Deschamps, J. P., Romero, M. I., & Zubarew, T. (1997). Health promotion in adolescents in Latin America. *Promotion & Education, 4*(4), 29-31.

Pomrehn, P. R., Davis, M. V., Chen, D. W., & Barker, W. (2000). Prevention for the 21st century: Setting the context through undergraduate medical education. *Academic Medicine, 75*(Suppl. 7), S5-S13.

Riley, B. L., Taylor, S. M., & Elliot, S. J. (2001). Determinants of implementing heart health: Promotion activities in Ontario public health units: A socio-ecological approach. *Health Education Research, 16*(4), 425-441.

Robert Wood Johnson Foundation. (2001). *Public-private collaboration to expand access to care for the underserved.* Princeton, NJ: The Foundation.

Ross, R., Sawatphanit, W., & Suwansujarid, T. (2004, Mar. 1). *Two contrasting cases of HIV-positive, pregnant women in Thailand.* Paper presented at the meeting of the 28th Midwest Nursing Research Society in St. Louis, MO.

Samiel, S. (2000). Health promotion and health for all. *Caribbean Health, 2*(4), 10-11.

Sawatphanit, W., Ross, R., & Suwansujarid, T. (2004). Development of self-esteem among HIV-positive pregnant Thai women: Action research. *Journal of Science, Technologies, and Humanities, 2*(2), 55-69.

Smith, C. M., & Maurer, F. A. (2000). *Community health nursing: Theory and practice* (2nd ed.). Philadelphia: W. B. Saunders.

Smith, R. D. (2000). Promoting the health of people with physical disabilities: A discussion of public health services in Australia. *Health Promotion International, 15*(1), 79-86.

Stanhope, M., & Lancaster, M. (2004). *Community and public health nursing* (6th ed.). St. Louis: Mosby.

Sword, W. (1999). A socio-ecological approach to understanding barriers to prenatal care for women of low income. *Journal of Advanced Nursing, 29*(5), 1170-1177.

Tsouros, A. D. (1996). World Health organization Healthy Cities Project: State of the art and future plans. *Health Promotion International, 10*(2), 133.

U.S. Department of Commerce, U.S. Census Bureau. (2002). 2002 Data profiles. Retrieved March 16, 2004, from: *http://www.census.gov.*

U.S. Department of Health and Human Services. (1990). *Healthy people 2000: National health promotion and disease prevention objectives.* Washington, DC: U.S. Government Printing Office.

U.S. Department of Health and Human Services. (2000). *Healthy people 2010: Understanding and improving health.* Washington, DC: U.S. Government Printing Office.

U.S. Department of Health and Human Services. (2003). *Administrative simplification under HIPAA: National standards for transactions, privacy and security.* Washington, DC: U.S. Government Printing Office.

U.S. Department of Health and Human Services, Center for Medicare and Medicaid Services. (2003). *Projected costs for health care in the United States 2001-2008.*

Washington, DC: U.S. Government Printing Office.

U.S. Department of Health and Human Services, U.S. Public Health Service, Office of the Surgeon General. (1981). *Report on health promotion and disease prevention.* Washington, DC: U.S. Government Printing Office.

U.S. Preventive Services Task Force. (1989). *Guide to clinical preventive services: An assessment of the effectiveness of 169 interventions.* Baltimore: Williams & Wilkins.

U.S. Preventive Services Task Force. (1996). *Guide to clinical preventive services: An assessment of the effectiveness of medical interventions.* Baltimore: Williams & Wilkins.

Walker, J. (2003). The future of primary care in Australia. *Australian Journal of Rural Health, 11*(6), 257-258.

Waters, W. F. (2001). Globalization, socioeconomic restructuring, and community health. *Journal of Community Health, 26,* 79-92.

Waxman, L., & Henderliter, S. (1996). *Status report on hunger and homelessness in America's cities.* Washington, DC: U.S. Conference of Mayors.

Weingartl, H. M., Copps, J., Drebot, M. A., Marszal, P., Smith, G. Gren, J. et al. (2004). Emerging infectious diseases: Susceptibility of pigs and chickens to SARS coronavirus. *Emerging Infectious Diseases, 10,* 179-184.

Whitehead, D. (2004). Health promotion and health education: Advancing the concepts. *Journal of Advanced Nursing, 47*(3), 311-320.

Woodwell, D. A. (1989). *Office visits to internists: Advance data, vital and health statistics.* Washington, DC: National Center for Health Statistics.

World Health Organization. (1978). *Primary health care. Report of the International Conference on Primary Health Care.* Alma Ata, USSR; Geneva: The Organization.

World Health Organization. (1981). *Global strategy for health for all by the year 2000.* Geneva: The Organization.

World Health Organization. (1986). *Ottawa charter for health promotion.* Copenhagen: The Organization, Regional Office for Europe.

World Health Organization. (1995). *The world health report 1999: Bridging the gaps.* Geneva: The Organization.

World Health Organization. (1998a). *Health for all in the twenty-first century.* Geneva: The Organization.

World Health Organization. (1998b). *World health report 1998: Life in the 21st century— A vision for all.* Geneva: The Organization.

World Health Organization. (2000). *World health report 2000.* Geneva: The Organization.

World Health Organization. (2003). *The world health report.* Geneva: The Organization.

World Health Organization. (2004). *Health for all in the 21st century.* Geneva: The Organization.

Zacek, A. (2000). Determinants of health and health policy (Part 3): From intervention of quality of life. *Časopis lékařů českých, 139*(6), 163-165.

Glossary

A

achievement-oriented stress (Ch. 22) The stress of an overachiever, deriving from internal pressures to succeed as measured by self-defined goals.

achievement tests (Ch. 20) Tests that measure the amount of information learned in a specific area.

acne (Ch. 21) The result of sebaceous follicles becoming clogged with sebum and debris, forming comedones (blackheads or whiteheads).

acquired immunodeficiency syndrome (Ch. 16, 25) A syndrome involving a defect in cell-mediating immunity that has a long incubation period followed by a protracted and debilitating course, and has a poor prognosis.

acquired lactase deficiency (Ch. 19) Intolerance to milk products, manifested by diarrhea.

active immunization (Ch. 17) A substance is introduced into the body that stimulates the production of antibodies to a specific antigen.

acupuncture (Ch. 14) A therapy that manipulates life energy by stimulating precisely mapped points on the skin surface.

acute lymphocytic leukemia (Ch. 19) The most common cancer in children from infancy to 5 years of age.

adolescence (Ch. 21) The period characterized by the psychological, emotional, social, and spiritual changes that result in the transition from child to young adult.

advance directive (Ch. 23) A legal document prepared when an individual is alive, competent, and able to make decisions to provide guidelines for health care providers in the future when the individual is not able to make decisions because of physical disability (being unconscious) or mental incompetence.

advocate (Ch. 3, 25) One who pleads the cause of another.

aerobic exercise (Ch. 12, 22) Activity that uses large muscle groups over an extended time to improve the efficiency of the oxidative energy-producing system and to improve cardiorespiratory endurance; uses stored adipose tissue as the major fuel source.

affirmation (Ch. 13) A positive thought, in the form of a short phrase, which has meaning for the individual.

Alzheimer's disease (Ch. 24) A type of dementia or progressive mental deterioration thought to result from plaque formation in the brain. Its ultimate cause remains unknown.

amblyopia (Ch. 18, 19) The loss of vision or diminished vision caused by the disuse of an eye.

amenorrhea (Ch. 21) The absence of an expected menstrual period.

amniocentesis (Ch. 16) Diagnostic procedure involving removal of amniotic fluid from the uterus to determine chromosomal abnormality or fetal sex.

anaerobic exercise (Ch. 12) High-intensity, short-duration activity that improves the efficiency of the phosphocreatine and glycolytic energy-producing systems and increases muscle strength, power, and speed of reactivity; uses phosphagens, glucose, and glycogen as major fuel sources.

anorexia nervosa (Ch. 21) A disorder of self-starvation characterized by significant weight loss, amenorrhea, compulsive physical activity, preoccupation with food, and a distorted body image.

Apgar scoring system (Ch. 16) The measure evaluating an infant's general condition at birth. The scoring, made at 1 minute and 5 minutes of age, may be repeated until the infant's condition has stabilized. The total score is determined by adding the values allotted to observations of heart rate, respiratory effort, muscle tone, reflex irritability, and color. The highest possible score is 10. A score of 8 to 10 indicates that the baby is adapting well to the extrauterine environment.

applied research (Ch. 1) Research that is done to directly affect clinical practice.

aromatherapy (Ch. 14) The use of aromatic plant materials and essential oils in a therapeutic manner.

assertive communication (Ch. 13) Using nonjudgmental statements that express one's feelings and opinions and reaffirm one's rights.

asset planning (Ch. 1) A planning approach that focuses the family and the providers on the building blocks for their future, given the realities of the present.

asthma (Ch. 19) A chronic inflammatory disorder of the airways.

astigmatism (Ch. 20) Blurred vision caused by a poorly focused image on the retina.

attention-deficit/hyperactivity disorder (Ch. 20) A behavior disorder characterized by developmentally inappropriate degrees of inattention, impulsiveness, and hyperactivity.

autonomy (Ch. 18) The quality of being independent, self-reliant, and self-directing.

B

bacterial vaginosis (Ch. 16) A condition in which there is a change in the normal bacteria that are found in the vagina, in which they are replaced by an overgrowth of harmful bacteria. The cause of bacterial vaginosis remains unknown, but symptoms may include increased vaginal discharge that has an unpleasant odor (which may worsen after sex), itchiness, and burning; however, most women suffer no symptoms at all.

basal metabolic rate (Ch. 22) Rate of oxygen utilization of an individual during minimal physiological activity while awake.

birth defect (Ch. 17) An abnormality of structure, function, or metabolism. It may result from a genetic or environmental influence on the fetus but is usually a combination of both.

body image (Ch. 21) The mental picture of and feelings about one's body.

braces (Ch. 20) Short-term orthodontic appliances.

bradycardia (Ch. 16) Heart rate below 120 beats per minute in a fetus at term or below 60 beats per minute in an adult.

breast self-examination (Ch. 22) A procedure in which a woman examines her breasts and their accessory structures for evidence of change that could indicate a malignant process.

bulimia nervosa (Ch. 21) A disorder characterized by a pattern of binge eating followed by forced vomiting or laxative use, or both, accompanied by a general feeling of lack of control over eating.

C

calcium (Ch. 23) A mineral essential in developing and maintaining bone mass.

cancer (Ch. 11) A neoplasm characterized by the uncontrolled growth of anaplastic cells that tend to invade the surrounding tissue and metastasize to distant body sites.

Candida albicans (Ch. 16) Yeast present in a woman's vagina or cervix.

capitation system (Ch. 3) A system in which each provider, such as a health maintenance organization (HMO), receives a flat annual fee for each individual, regardless of how often services are used.

cardiac output (Ch. 23) The volume of blood expelled by the ventricles of the heart.

cardiorespiratory fitness (Ch. 12) The ability to deliver and use oxygen throughout the body to allow physical activity over an extended period without excessive fatigue.

cardiovascular disease (Ch. 11) Any abnormal condition characterized by dysfunction of the heart and blood vessels.

care management (Ch. 3) This is when an experienced health care professional monitors client care, determines what care is necessary, and arranges for clients to receive the care they need for the most appropriate cost and in the most effective setting.

caries (Ch. 20) Dental cavities.

centering (Ch. 14, 19) The process of becoming calm, fully present in the moment, and connected to another individual.

cervix (Ch. 16) The lower portion of the uterus that protrudes into the vagina.

chi (qi) (Ch. 14) The energy that flows through the body, nourishing organs and promoting optimal functioning.

child abuse (Ch. 18) Intentional injury to a child.

chlamydia (Ch. 16) One of the most common sexually transmitted organisms in North America and a frequent cause of sterility.

chloasma (Ch. 16) Darkening of the skin across the forehead and nose that develops slowly and fades over time.

chloroma (Ch. 19) A localized tumor mass that has a greenish appearance.

cholesterol (Ch. 11) A waxy lipid found only in animal tissues. It facilitates the absorption and transport of fatty acids.

chorionic and amniotic membranes (Ch. 16) The membranes that surround the fetus throughout gestation, supporting the developing infant and protecting it from injury.

chorionic villi (Ch. 16) Placental passages though which fetal circulation flows.

chronic serous otitis media (Ch. 20) Long-term fluid accumulation in the middle ear causing inflammation or infection.

codes of ethics (Ch. 5) Moral standards that provide a normative framework for professional actions. There is implicit acceptance of these codes upon acquiring membership in a discipline. A code of ethics outlines the primary goals, values, and obligations of the profession.

cognition (Ch. 24) Thinking processes.

cognitive restructuring (Ch. 13) A technique or series of strategies that help people evaluate their thoughts, challenge them, and replace them with responses that are more rational. It teaches people to recognize that negative thinking often causes emotional distress. This recognition, in turn, reduces the negative consequences of stress and enhances health.

colostrum (Ch. 16) Breast milk that precedes mature breast milk.

communication process (Ch. 4) A process by which information is exchanged between individuals through a common system of symbols, signs, or behaviors.

community (Ch. 8) A group of people, often living in a defined geographical area, who share common culture, values, and norms and are arranged in a social structure according to relationships that have developed over time.

community-based care (Ch. 1) Care that is provided in health care settings in the community.

community diagnosis (Ch. 8) Description of a community health problem that serves as the basis for planning and implementing interventions and nursing actions and making evaluative judgments about health concerns.

community evaluation (Ch. 8) Identification of a specific or potential health concern and planned actions to achieve the desired community outcome.

community health promotion (Ch. 8) A process including community participation, with representatives from at least three of the following sectors: government, education, business, faith organizations, health care, media, voluntary agencies, and the public; assessment guided by a community assessment and planning model to determine community health problems, resources, perceptions, and priorities for action; targeted and measurable objectives to address any of the following: health outcomes, risk factors, public awareness, services, and protection; comprehensive, multifaceted, culturally relevant interventions that have multiple targets for change; and monitoring and evaluation of the processes to determine whether the objectives are reached.

community nursing intervention (Ch. 8) An action or behavior implemented by the nurse to fulfill a health goal of the community.

community outcome (Ch. 8) A goal that is projected before the implementation of planned actions and is stated in terms of the individual behaviors that are expected to result from nursing actions.

community pattern (Ch. 8) A clustering of information about a community obtained from assessment data.

community risk factors (Ch. 8) Characteristics that contribute to identified potential and existing health-related concerns.

concrete operations (Ch. 20) The stage within Piaget's stages of cognitive development in which a child is able to move from egocentric interactions to more cooperative interactions.

congenital defect (Ch. 16) An abnormality in structure and function occurring in the fetus when cells do not develop adequately at the necessary time and sequence.

conservation (Ch. 20) The concept that certain characteristics of objects remain constant.

constipation (Ch. 23, 24) A change in bowel habits characterized by decreased frequency or passage of hard, drier stools and difficult defecation.

conventional level (Ch. 20) The level of moral judgment in which a child looks to others for approval and to society to define rules.

cool-down period (Ch. 12) A period that allows the body to readjust gradually from the demands of exercise to baseline; it follows the endurance phase.

coping (Ch. 13) The ability to deal with difficulties by finding a balance between acceptance and action and between letting go and taking control.

coping strategies (Ch. 20) Behaviors intended to buffer perceived stressful events.

coronary artery disease (Ch. 22) Any one of the abnormal conditions that may affect the heart's arteries and produce various pathological effects.

coronary heart disease (Ch. 11) A term formerly used for coronary artery disease.

cost-benefit ratio analysis (Ch. 9) An analysis that compares various outcomes in monetary terms.

cost-effectiveness analysis (Ch. 9) An analysis that determines the optimal use of resources to reach a predetermined, constant end point—the desired health outcome.

cost-efficiency analysis (Ch. 9) An analysis used to promote efficiency and budget a limited amount of money toward achieving as much of the preselected desired outcome as possible; the funds are the central issue, not the health benefit.

cultural competence (Ch. 6, 7) The ability to give care to an individual that demonstrates awareness of and sensitivity to the underlying personal and cultural reality of the individual by identifying and using cultural norms, values, and communication and time patterns in collecting and interpreting assessment information.

cultural focus (Ch. 6) One of the five areas of focus that characterize functional health patterns. It includes culturally-based age, developmental, and gender norms.

culture (Ch. 2) An element in ethnicity, consisting of shared patterns of values and behaviors that characterize a particular group.

cytomegalovirus (Ch. 16) A member of a group of large species-specific herpes-type viruses with a wide variety of disease effects. It is the most common infection that can cause serious complications for the fetus.

D

date rape (Ch. 21) Sexual assault occurring between two people who already know each other. Certain drugs are sometimes used to facilitate a sexual assault. Because of the effects of these drugs, victims may be physically helpless, unable to refuse sex, and unable to remember what happened.

decidua (Ch. 16) Fetal-nourishing cells in the uterus.

decubitus ulcer (Ch. 24) A localized area of tissue necrosis that develops when soft tissue is compressed between two bony prominences or between a bony prominence and an external surface for a prolonged period.

degenerative joint disease (Ch. 23) Deterioration of the joint(s) often caused by arthritis and may result in pain and loss of function; mainly affects weight-bearing joints; more common in older adults.

dementia (Ch. 24) A pathological condition that affects cognition in old age. Symptoms include forgetfulness, inattentiveness, disorganized thinking, altered levels of consciousness, perceptual disturbances, sleep-wake disorders, psychomotor disturbances, and disorientation.

demography (Ch. 8) The study of a population. It provides information on population characteristics, such as size, age distribution, gender ratio, racial composition, marital status ratio, nationality, language, religious grouping, and educational and occupational distributions.

Denver Development Screening Test and Denver II (Ch. 15, 17) A standardized tool that screens for developmental problems in children from birth to 6 years of age.

depression (Ch. 20, 21, 24) A disorder characterized by an all-pervasive sadness that is present much of the time.

descriptive theories (Ch. 5) Ethics based on observations of human behavior over time and in a variety of settings. They are not directive—they merely tell us how people act toward each other and their environment, what they seem to believe are "good" or moral actions.

development (Ch. 15) Changes in skill and capacity to function. Qualitative in nature, development evolves from the maturation of physical and mental capacities and learning.

developmental pattern (Ch. 15) A pattern of development of physical and mental abilities showing certain common and predictable characteristics.

developmental theory (Ch. 7, 8) An explanation of the phases of human development—physical, psychosocial, cognitive, and spiritual dimensions—based on descriptive research studies.

Dietary Guidelines (Ch. 11) Federal government nutrition guidelines that form the foundation of the federal nutrition policy in the United States. They were first issued in 1980 in response to the public's desire for authoritative, consistent guidance on diet and health and are reviewed every 5 years.

dilation (Ch. 16) Opening of the cervix during labor and delivery.

dilemmas (Ch. 5) Questions of what is right or what should be done.

disease (Ch. 1) The failure of a person's adaptive mechanisms to counteract stimuli and stresses adequately, resulting in functional or structural disturbances.

disease prevention (Ch. 10) Efforts used to prevent disease and disability.

distress (Ch. 13) Stress that is chronic or excessive, resulting in the body being unable to adapt and maintain homeostasis, producing negative results.

divergent family structures (Ch. 7) Nontraditional family structures. Three predominant types have been described: adolescent unwed mothers whose developmental needs and lack of parenting skills pose particular challenges; couples who, after widowhood or divorce, have remarried and merged two families; and older couples or older individuals (mostly women) living alone.

doll or puppet play (Ch. 19) Use of toy objects to tell a personal story; it provides valuable insight into a child's sense of self.

Down syndrome (Ch. 16) A chromosomal dysgenesis syndrome that results from the presence of an extra chromosome.

draw-a-person and draw-a-family tests (Ch. 19) Psychological tests used to give estimates of intelligence and interpretations of a child's emotional development.

durable power of attorney (Ch. 23) A document in which an individual designates another person (spouse, son, daughter, or friend) to make health care decisions (especially about how aggressive treatment should be in forestalling death) when that individual becomes unable to make such decisions.

dyslexia (Ch. 20) A disturbance in the ability to use language, particularly to read, with the tendency to reverse the normal appearance of letters and numbers.

E

Early and Periodic Screening, Diagnosis, and Treatment (Ch. 19) A health-screening program for children provided by Medicaid.

ecomap (Ch. 7) A form of documentation diagramming a family's social environment.

effacement (Ch. 16) Thinning of the cervix prior to or during labor.

egocentricism (Ch. 18, 19) The outlook of an individual characterized by seeing everything through his or her perspective only and not realizing that other ways of viewing things may exist.

emancipated minor (Ch. 21) An adolescent who has not reached the standard legal age for certain activities, but who is permitted to take on full responsibility for decisions because of being economically separate from the family.

embryo (Ch. 16) The growing baby from 2 to 8 weeks of gestation.

empathy (Ch. 4, 13) The ability to understand another's feelings without losing personal identity and perspective.

encopresis (Ch. 20) A condition in which a child over the age of 4 persistently passes stool in his or her underpants.

endometrium (Ch. 16) The inner lining of the uterus.

energy (Ch. 14) A life force present in all living and nonliving elements of the universe.

enuresis (Ch. 20) The involuntary passing of urine at an age when control should be present; term used in reference to children.

epidemiology (Ch. 1) The study of health and disease in society.

episiotomy (Ch. 16) A surgical incision into the perineum to assist in delivering a baby.

Erikson's theory of psychosocial development (Ch. 15) The theory based on the need of each person to develop a sense of trust in self and others and a sense of personal worth.

estrogen (Ch. 16) A hormone that stimulates the development of female secondary sexual characteristics and promotes growth and maintenance of the female reproductive system.

ethic of care (Ch. 5) Also referred to as the "care ethic," a responsibility to attend to the individual as individual in all of his or her complexities.

ethical issue (Ch. 9) A situation that presents a dilemma involving right and wrong.

ethics (Ch. 5) A search for what shapes the human being and contributes to the growth and development of the person. It is an attempt to discover all the elements required to make and keep life human so a person may achieve the goals of the humanization process and live as properly and well as possible.

ethnic group (Ch. 2) A collectivity within a larger society; a group whose markedly contrasting values, rituals, and maintenance of separate institutions differentiate it from the larger society. A group of people who identify themselves and/or are identified by others as belonging to the same group.

ethnicity (Ch. 2) Kinship patterns, physical contiguity, religious affiliation, language or dialect forms, tribal affiliations, nationality, phenotypic features, or a combination of these that characterize an ethnic group.

ethnocentric perspective (Ch. 2) A perspective that sees other ways as inferior, unnatural, or even barbaric.

eustress (Ch. 13) Stress that can be challenging and useful.

euthanasia or physician-assisted suicide (PAS) (Ch. 24) The painless ending of a person's life with the person's consent.

evidence-based practice (Ch. 1) The conscientious, explicit, and judicious use of current best evidence in making decisions about the care of individual people.

exercise (Ch. 12, 13) Planned, structured, and repetitive bodily movement done to improve or maintain one or more components of physical fitness.

expected outcomes (Ch. 6) Goals set for a person's behavior that, if achieved, reflect positive results from nursing interventions.

expressive language (Ch. 19) Language that is used to coherently express ideas and feelings.

external locus of control (Ch. 20) The view that an outside force in the environment is the source of control over behavior, actions, or the results of a task.

F

failure-to-thrive syndrome (Ch. 17) The term used to describe infants who fail to gain weight, resulting from the failure to obtain or use necessary calories.

false-negative results (Ch. 9) Reports of a test that indicate that individuals do not have a condition when they actually do have it.

false-positive results (Ch. 9) Reports of a test that indicate that individuals do have a condition when they actually do not have it.

family developmental tasks (Ch. 7) Tasks for establishing a mutually satisfying adult relationship that fits into the kinship network.

family function (Ch. 7) The process of continual change in the system as information and energy are exchanged between the family and the environment.

family health status (Ch. 7) The family health pattern that is considered functional, potentially dysfunctional (potential problem), or dysfunctional (actual problem).

family nursing diagnosis (Ch. 7) A concise summary statement of a problem or potential problem. The diagnosis provides direction for outcomes and interventions by identifying the negative health state and the factors that must be changed to alleviate or prevent it.

family nursing interventions (Ch. 7) Actions aimed at assisting the family in carrying out health-related functions that the members cannot perform for themselves.

family pattern (Ch. 7) Family developmental norms and age-specific risk factors.

family resilience (Ch. 7) A framework for studying families that generally addresses three domains: family belief systems, organizational patterns, and communication and problem solving.

family risk factors (Ch. 7) Factors that put the health of a family at risk. They can be inferred from lifestyle, biological factors, environmental factors, social and psychological dimensions, and the health care system.

family strengths (Ch. 7) Factors or forces that contribute to family unity and solidarity and foster the development of inherent family potential.

family structure (Ch. 7) The family's roles and relationships.

fat (Ch. 11) A substance composed of lipids or fatty acids occurring in various forms or consistencies ranging from oil to tallow.

feedback (Ch. 4) A monitoring system through which a person (or group) controls the internal and external responses to behavior (output) and accommodates the responses appropriately.

fee-for-service plan (Ch. 3) Individual health care payment arrangement in which the person pays for each visit.

feminist ethics Feminist thoughts and philosophies that present a viewpoint on moral problems in health care and other areas of life that has been neglected historically.

fertilization (Ch. 16) The union of sperm and egg.

fetal heart monitor (Ch. 16) A machine monitoring fetal heart rate and activity during labor.

fetus (Ch. 16) An unborn offspring that has attained the particular form of the species.

fiber (Ch. 11) A generic term for nondigestible carbohydrate substances found in plant cell walls and surrounding cellular material.

first stage of labor (Ch. 16) The stage that begins with regular uterine contractions and ends with complete dilation and effacement of the cervix.

flexibility (Ch. 12) Adequate muscle length and joint mobility to allow free and painless movement through a wide range of motion.

folk healing system (Ch. 2) A system of healing that embodies the beliefs, values, and treatment approaches of a particular cultural group that is a product of cultural development.

Food Guide Pyramid (Ch. 11) A graphic representation of dietary balance and variety that classifies foods into six groups, each of which contains a variety of nutritionally similar foods. It was replaced in 2005 by MyPyramid.

formal operations (Ch. 21) Piaget's stage of cognitive development in which thought processes develop into mature, adultlike patterns with specific traits that allow for adult accomplishments in thinking.

fourth stage of labor (Ch. 16) The first 2 hours after delivery when the mother faces the greatest danger of postpartum hemorrhage.

function of a community (Ch. 8) The process of dynamic change or adaptation in the community system's parts and the way the community system and its subsystems interact.

functional aerobic capacity (Ch. 23) Oxygen consumption capacity needed to maintain normal physical functioning.

functional focus (Ch. 6) One of the areas of focus characterizing patterns, which refers to an individual's functional level.

functional health (Ch. 1) The ability to function cognitively and physically.

functional health patterns (Ch. 6, 7, 8) An assessment framework of 11 health-related behaviors developed by Gordon; these patterns interact to make up an individual's lifestyle.

fundus (Ch. 16) The upper segment of the uterus.

G

generativity (Ch. 23) A feeling of productivity and creativity as evidenced by reaching previously established goals.

genetic counseling (Ch. 5) Counseling with a person or couple related to genetic screening. It can include assisting people to determine the risks and benefits of screening, to prepare for their future needs, and to help them with procreative planning.

genetic impairment (Ch. 22) Congenital defect caused by abnormal genes.

genital herpes virus infection (Ch. 22) A chronic infection caused by type 2 herpes simplex virus, occurring in the genital area and usually transmitted by sexual contact.

genogram (Ch. 7) A family diagram that depicts each member of the family and shows connections between the generations.

gentrification (Ch. 2) The transformation of a neighborhood from a lower income area to a higher income area, through the displacement of lower-end tenants, renovation of buildings, and opening of higher-priced businesses.

Gilligan's theory of moral development (Ch. 15) The theory suggesting that there is a different process of moral development in women than in men.

gingivitis (Ch. 23) Inflammation of the gums. Redness and swelling develops around the teeth. Bleeding of the gums while brushing the teeth is an early sign.

glaucoma (Ch. 23) A condition that occurs as a result of increased intraocular pressure, which can damage the optic nerve. Damage is irreversible, but vision loss can be prevented when it is identified early. Peripheral vision is affected.

goal setting (Ch. 13) A dynamic process that includes an action plan for change to work toward a more balanced health-promoting lifestyle consistent with an individual's values and beliefs.

gonococcus (Ch. 16) A microorganism that causes gonorrhea. It causes an infection that can infect a newborn's eyes which has been commonly prevented by treating all newborns with silver nitrate or erythromycin eye drops at birth.

group B streptococcus (Ch. 16) A group B streptococcal infection.

group or mass screening (Ch. 9) A screening in which a target population is selected on the basis of an increased incidence of a condition or a recognized element of high risk within the group.

growth (Ch. 15) Changes in structure and size.

growth charts (Ch. 15) Charts that provide measurements of height and weight corresponding to age. They are used to identify children and adolescents as underweight, overweight, or at risk of overweight.

growth index (Ch. 17) Height and weight measurements plotted on a standard growth chart to assess for normal progression.

growth patterns (Ch. 15) Patterns of development for different age periods. Different parts of the body increase in size at different rates. There is rapid growth in the prenatal period through infancy and adolescence, with the head growing the fastest during infancy. From age 1 to adolescence, the legs grow the fastest. There is also growth in the body organs and systems.

gynecomastia (Ch. 21) Some degree of unilateral or bilateral breast enlargement that may appear early in male puberty, just prior to the growth spurt. It is usually temporary and typically disappears.

H

health (Ch. 1) A state of physical, mental, and social functioning that realizes the potential of which a person is capable.

health behaviors (Ch. 10) Any activities that an individual undertakes to enhance health, prevent disease, and detect and control the symptomatic stage of a disease.

health belief model (Ch. 10) A paradigm used to predict and explain health behavior that is based on value-expectancy theory.

health counseling (Ch. 10) Referring people to health education resources or assisting them in acquiring health information pertinent to solving a health problem.

health disparities (Ch. 1) Refers to the wide variations in health services and health status among certain population groups. Examples are the growing problems of access to medical care; differences in treatment based on race, gender, and ability to pay; and related issues such as urban versus rural health, insurance coverage, Medicare and Medicaid reimbursement for care, and satisfaction with service delivery.

health education (Ch. 10) The process of assisting individuals, acting separately or collectively, to make informed decisions on matters affecting individuals, family, and community health.

Health for All (Ch. 25) The health-promotion initiative of the World Health Organization, established in the late 1970s.

health literacy (Ch. 4) The capacity to read, comprehend, and follow through on health information.

health maintenance organization (Ch. 3) The prototypical managed care structure that encompasses two possibilities: (1) a health plan in which providers assume some of the financial risk and (2) a health plan that uses primary care providers as gatekeepers.

health promotion (Ch. 1, 10) The science and art of helping people change their lifestyle to move toward a state of optimal health. The process of advocating health to enhance the probability that person (individual, family, and community), private (professional and business), and public (federal, state, and local government) support of positive health practices will become a societal norm.

health status (Ch. 6) The condition of an individual's physiological state and his or her interaction with the environment.

healthy diet (Ch. 13) Balanced food choices from the five food groups.

Healthy People 2010 (Ch. 1, 25) The latest edition of the *Healthy People* documents, the U.S. federal government's health-promotion initiative, sets out 28 specific areas for health improvement in 467 objectives.

healthy pleasures (Ch. 13) Activities that bring feelings of peace, joy, and happiness.

helping or therapeutic relationship (Ch. 4) A process in which one person promotes the development of another by fostering the latter's maturation, adaptation, integration, openness, and ability to find meaning in a situation.

hepatitis B (Ch. 16, 22) An inflammatory condition of the liver caused by the hepatitis B virus.

herpes simplex (Ch. 16) A virus that causes small, transient, irritating, and sometimes painful, fluid-filled blisters on the skin and mucous membranes.

heterophoria (Ch. 19) A tendency for a child's eyes to deviate from their normal position for visual alignment.

heterotropia (Ch. 19) A condition in which the child's eyes do not focus together to transmit good, coordinated binocular vision.

high-level wellness (Ch. 1) A sense of well-being, life satisfaction, and quality of life.

holism (Ch. 14) The theory that people have an existence other than the mere sum of their parts and must be perceived or studied as a whole.

homeostasis (Ch. 19) A relative constancy in the internal environment of the body, naturally maintained by adaptive responses that promote healthy survival.

human chorionic gonadotropin (Ch. 16) A hormone of pregnancy produced by the placenta.

human immunodeficiency virus (Ch. 11, 22, 25) A retrovirus that causes acquired immunodeficiency syndrome.

human papilloma virus (Ch. 22) A virus that is the cause of common warts of the hands and feet and lesions of the mucous membranes of the oral, anal, and genital cavities. Human papilloma virus is spread through sexual contact and some forms of the virus, in combination with smoking, are strongly related to development of cervical dysplasia and cancer.

humor (Ch. 13) Something comical or amusing.

hyperopia (Ch. 20) The condition in which an image falls behind the retina. Also known as farsightedness.

hypertension (Ch. 11, 22) High blood pressure.

I

identity (Ch. 21) A component of self-concept characterized by persisting consciousness of being an individual, separate and distinct from others.

illness (Ch. 1) A social construct in which people are in an imbalanced, unsustainable relationship with their environment and are failing in the ability to survive and to create a higher quality of life.

imagery (Ch. 14) A practice in which a person relaxes and focuses attention on images chosen or presented.

individual screening (Ch. 9) A screening in which one person is tested by a health professional who has designated the individual as high risk.

inductive explanation (Ch. 19) Answer arrived at by examining specific data to determine a general concept.

industry versus inferiority (Ch. 20) The stage of personality development described by Erikson for the school-age child.

infant mortality rate (Ch. 16) A statistical reflection of the number of infants dying before their first year of life and the leading indicator of a nation's health.

infertility (Ch. 22) The lack of conception in the presence of unprotected sexual intercourse for a period of at least 12 months.

input (Ch. 4) The act of taking in information from outside the individual or group.

insurance (Ch. 3) Individual payment to a fund to provide protection for each contributor against financial losses resulting from an unlikely, but possible, occurrence.

intelligence (Ch. 20) The quantity of information that people possess, their ability to think, and how they compare with others at the same time, chronological age, and experience level.

intelligence quotient (IQ) (Ch. 20) The ratio of a person's performance compared with other individuals, calculated by dividing maturational age (MA) by chronological age (CA) and multiplying by 100 (MA $\div$ CA $\times$ 100 = IQ).

internal locus of control (Ch. 20) The view that a person is the source of control over his or her behavior, actions, or the results of a task.

interobserver reliability (Ch. 9) The occurrence of the same result emerging from a test performed by two individuals.

interview (Ch. 8) Person-to-person meeting to collect information.

interview data (Ch. 8) Verbal statements gathered during an interview.

intraobserver reliability (Ch. 9) The occurrence in which an individual is able to reproduce a result several times in a test.

involuntary migration (Ch. 2) Involuntary movement of people to other lands.

irreversibility (Ch. 19) The inability to correct a reversible situation.

Ishihara's test (Ch. 19) A test for color blindness using a series of cards with color-tinted letters and figures.

J

journal writing (Ch. 13) Self-confessional writing.

K

Klinefelter syndrome (Ch. 21) A condition in which males have an extra chromosome (XXY) and typically are tall, initially thin, and do not develop secondary sexual characteristics. They often have gynecomastia.

Kohlberg's theory of moral development (Ch. 15) The theory that responses to moral dilemmas indicate distinct sequential stages of moral thinking.

kyphosis (Ch. 23) A curvature or angulation of the posterior spine (commonly known as *hunchback*).

L

Lamaze (Ch. 16) A method of childbirth preparation developed in the 1950s. It requires classes, practice at home, and coaching during labor and delivery. The physiology of pregnancy and childbirth and exercises and techniques are taught to promote control and relaxation during labor.

learning (Ch. 15) The process of gaining knowledge or skills that results from exposure, experience, education, and evaluation.

learning disabilities (Ch. 20) Learning impairments of individuals who have normal or above-normal intelligence and do not have emotional problems or visual, hearing, or motor handicaps.

levels of prevention (Ch. 1) Primary, secondary, and tertiary means to avert the development of disease in the future.

limit setting (Ch. 20) Teaching children what behaviors are acceptable in society.

linea nigra (Ch. 16) A darkened line from the symphysis pubis to the umbilicus.

lobbying (Ch. 3) The process of trying to persuade legislators to vote for or against measures important to the represented interest group.

lobbyist (Ch. 3) A registered representative of a special interest group.

M

malocclusion (Ch. 20) An unacceptable relationship of the teeth in one jaw to those in the other.

managed care (Ch. 3) A system that seeks to manage the cost of health care, the quality of that health care, and access to care. It is based on the belief that health care costs can be controlled by "managing" the way in which health care is delivered.

maternal mortality rate (Ch. 22) All deaths related to pregnancy, delivery, and the postpartum period.

maturation (Ch. 15) An increase in competence and adaptability that is reflective of changes in the complexity of a structure that make it possible for that structure to begin to function or to function at a higher level.

measurement (Ch. 8) A method of data collection using instruments to quantify data in information collection.

meconium (Ch. 16) Fetal fecal matter.

meditation (Ch. 14) A self-directed practice for relaxing the body and calming the mind that involves the focusing of concentration on a single point. When the mind wanders, the individual consciously brings the mind back to the point of concentration. The focus of concentration can be a burning candle, a word, a phrase, the breath, or simply a quiet awareness of what is happening in the present moment.

menarche (Ch. 20, 21) The advent of monthly bleeding or menses.

menopause (Ch. 23) The time during which production of ovarian estrogen and progesterone ceases; the remaining estrogen is produced by the adrenal glands, usually occurring between ages 45 and 55. As a result of the diminished estrogen

level, a woman's secondary sexual characteristics regress, such as loss of pubic hair and decrease in breast size. The female reproductive organs shrink, and vaginal secretions decrease.

metabolic syndrome (Ch. 22) A cluster of health risks that includes the lethal risks of high lipid levels, insulin resistance, obesity, and hypertension. A particular feature of this syndrome is central obesity; these individuals are at higher risk for diabetes, coronary artery disease, and stroke.

metacommunication (Ch. 4) A phenomenon that refers to a message about a message. Metacommunication is the relationship aspect of communication. It involves reading between the lines or going past the surface content of the message to glean nuances of meaning.

metaethics (Ch. 5) The philosophical approach that evaluates value theories or ethical perspectives for their congruence and usefulness in human decision making across environments.

midlife crisis (Ch. 23) A time during middle age of reassessment, turmoil, and change.

mild cognitive impairment (Ch. 24) A pathological collection of symptoms that result in memory loss, language difficulties, and difficulty with judgment and reasoning among older adults.

Mini-Mental State Examination (Ch. 24) An instrument developed by Folstein, Folstein, and McHugh to accurately assess the baseline mental status of older adults and monitor progress or decline in mental function.

mini-relaxation (Ch. 13) Response that can be used to help develop awareness and to counter the negative effects of stress on mind, body, and spirit. It can be anything from a few conscious, deep, diaphragmatic breaths to several minutes of sitting quietly.

minority group (Ch. 2) A group that consists of people who receive less than their share of wealth, power, or social status. The identity of the minority group is tied in with the dominant group that is perceived to possess the authority to control the value system and the allocation of resources. A minority may consist of a particular racial, religious, or occupational group.

mnemonic techniques (Ch. 19) Techniques for remembering things.

moral philosophy (Ch. 5) The branch of philosophy concerned with discovering or proposing what is right or wrong, or good or bad, in human action toward other humans and other entities such as animals and the environment.

multiinfarct dementia (Ch. 24) Dementia that is caused by the death of brain tissue, diagnosed through a computerized axial tomography scan of the brain. The death of the tissue may be caused by of a lack of blood flow to the brain from a cerebral vascular accident or from another cause.

multiple test screening (Ch. 9) The administration of two or more tests to detect more than one disease.

muscular fitness (Ch. 12) The strength and endurance of muscles that allows for participation in daily activities with low risk of musculoskeletal injury.

mutual storytelling (Ch. 19) A technique in which a nurse begins a story and the child finishes it.

myopia (nearsightedness) (Ch. 20) The condition in which an image falls in front of the retina, causing difficulty in seeing distant objects.

myopic vision (Ch. 19) The condition of having myopia (nearsightedness).

MyPyramid (Ch. 11) New food guidance system instituted in April 2005 to replace the Food Guide Pyramid.

N

natural history (Ch. 9) The progression of a disease from prepathogenesis to pathogenesis.

neuroblastoma (Ch. 19) A tumor in the sympathetic nervous system.

night terrors (Ch. 18, 19) Sleep disturbances in which a child does not waken completely but cries out, looks terrified, and cannot be aroused for several minutes.

nightmares (Ch. 19) Anxiety dreams.

nocturnal emission (Ch. 21) Wet dream.

nonverbal communication (Ch. 4) Any type of communication that is not verbal, including gestures, facial expressions, movements, body messages or signals, and artistic symbols.

nursing center (Ch. 3) An organization that gives the individual access to professional nursing services. The key components of a community nursing center include a nurse as chief manager, nursing staff who are accountable and responsible for care and professional practice, and nurses as the primary providers of care.

nursing diagnosis (Ch. 6) The identification and naming of an individual's response to actual or potential health problems or life processes.

nursing intervention (Ch. 6) Action taken by the nurse to promote the health of an individual.

nutrition screening (Ch. 11) The process of discovering characteristics or risk factors that are known to be associated with dietary or nutrition problems.

O

obesity (Ch. 11, 23) A body mass index of 30 kg/m^2 or more, or weight about 20% or more over what is considered a healthy weight for that individual.

object permanence (Ch. 18) The realization that an object exists, has permanence, and can be made visible once again.

observation data (Ch. 8) Data obtained by using sight, hearing, touch, smell, or taste.

one-test specific screening (Ch. 9) The administration of a single test that searches for a specific characteristic indicating a high risk of developing a disorder.

ossification (Ch. 20) Replacement of cartilage with bone.

osteoporosis (Ch. 11, 23, 24) Decreased bone mass, resulting in weak and brittle bones.

otitis media (Ch. 18, 19) Inflammation or infection in the middle ear resulting from a buildup of secretions in the middle ear chamber.

Ottawa Charter (Ch. 25) A set of health-promotion guidelines to be used worldwide. It was the outcome of a meeting of health leaders from around the world held in Ottawa, Canada, in 1986. These guidelines put forth a new health paradigm with an increased focus on determinants and prerequisites outside the health care realm, such as adequate income, employment, housing, food, education, and a safe social and physical environment for health development.

output (Ch. 4) The outcome of information processing.

overflow incontinence (Ch. 24) Incontinence caused by an obstruction in the elimination system, such as an enlarged prostate gland or urethral stricture.

overweight (Ch. 11) About 10% to 20% over healthy weight.

P

Papanicolaou (Pap) smear (Ch. 22) Screening test for cervical cancer.

parallel play (Ch. 18) Successful social encounters among toddlers, in which children play side by side, doing similar things with similar toys, but each working independently.

parental divorce (Ch. 19) A final decision of parents to dissolve their marriage, usually culminating from a period of conflict, stress, and changing relationships.

passive immunization (Ch. 17) The injection or ingestion of already-formed antibodies. After an individual has been exposed to a disease, passive immunization is given to prevent contracting the disease or to make the disease less serious if contracted. Passive immunizations provide a short immunity, usually 1 to 6 weeks, which will protect the person until the danger of contracting the disease from exposure is passed. Passive immunity occurs naturally in newborns by ingesting maternal antibodies passed through the placenta or breast milk.

pattern focus (Ch. 6) One area that characterizes functional health patterns. This focus explores patterns or sequences of behavior. The recognition of a pattern is a cognitive process that occurs during information collection. As information is collected, a pattern emerges that represents historical and current behavior. This pattern is easiest to recognize when behavior or information is quantifiable.

Peabody Picture Vocabulary Test (Ch. 19, 20) A test examining verbal intelligence.

pediculosis (Ch. 20) Infestation with scabies or lice.

peer group (Chs. 20, 21) Persons of the same age, experience, and usually gender.

periodontitis (Ch. 23) A gum disease involving tooth loss and bone destruction.

phonics (Ch. 20) A method of teaching beginners to read by sounding out the letters of a word.

physical activity (Ch. 12) Bodily movement that is produced by the contraction of skeletal muscle that substantially increases energy expenditure.

physical fitness (Ch. 12) A set of attributes that people have or achieve that relates to the ability to perform physical activity without undue fatigue or risk of injury.

Piaget's theory of cognitive development (Ch. 15) The theory of mental processes that is concerned primarily with structure rather than content; that is, how the mind works rather than what it does.

pica (Ch. 16) The eating of nonfood substances.

placenta (Ch. 16) The vascular fetal organ that mediates metabolic exchanges with maternal circulation. It provides the primary nourishment to the fetus and protects the fetus throughout the pregnancy.

point-of-service plan (Ch. 3) A health care plan in which members decide how to receive services at the time of service; it combines HMO and indemnity features. As with HMOs, providers are paid through a capitation or risk-based system and, as with preferred provider organizations, individuals can choose a non–plan provider by paying extra.

policy decision making (Ch. 3) Making decisions about health care policy.

politics (Ch. 3) The art or science concerned with guiding or influencing governmental policy; the use of power to promote a change. The political process determines the decision makers who negotiate a desired outcome.

positive reinforcement (Ch. 20) A reward for good or positive behavior.

positive signs of pregnancy (Ch. 16) The signs that indicate fetal existence.

postconventional level of moral reasoning (Ch. 22) The phase during which an individual is able to differentiate the self from the rules and expectations of others and to define principles regarding rights in terms of self-chosen principles.

prana (Ch. 14) The Hindu term for the energy that flows through the body, nourishing organs and promoting optimal functioning.

prayer (Ch. 14) A request for divine intervention, a type of meditation (centering prayer), or a form of intentionality useful in healing.

preconventional level (Ch. 20) The level of moral judgment that depends on punishment and obedience, individualism, instrumental purpose, and exchange.

preferred provider organizations (Ch. 3) A network of providers who agree to deliver services for a discounted fee. The provider generally incurs no financial risk; the financial burden is on the client rather than the provider.

preoperational stage (Ch. 18, 19) The preconceptual substage that includes the ability to function symbolically using language.

presbycusis (Ch. 23) Impaired auditory acuity.

presbyopia (Ch. 23) Farsightedness.

Preschool Readiness Experimental Screening Scale (Ch. 19) A screening tool used to detect developmental lags or abnormalities that would interfere with a child's ability to succeed in the academic and social world of school.

presence (Ch. 14) The act of being available in a situation with the wholeness of one's individual being; of "being with" rather than "doing to."

primary appraisal (Ch. 13) An appraisal of coping that includes descriptions of perceived actual and potential positive and negative outcomes.

primary care (Ch. 3) Basic health care that emphasizes general health needs rather than specialized care. It involves continual and comprehensive care that includes efforts to keep people as healthy as possible and to prevent disease. Ideally it is delivered in settings close to where people live and work.

primary care providers (Ch. 3) Health care providers who provide care in the managed care arena. They can be physicians or midlevel practitioners (physicians' assistants, nurse practitioners, or nurse midwives) who provide basic health care services.

primary sexual characteristics (Ch. 21) The physical organs necessary for reproduction.

probable signs of pregnancy (Ch. 16) Objective changes that carry a high degree of probability of pregnancy.

professional care system (Ch. 2) A system for provision of health care, characterized by specialized education and knowledge, and responsibility for care and expectation of remuneration for services rendered by the health care provider.

progesterone (Ch. 16) The hormone that prepares the uterus for reception of the fertilized ovum.

puberty (Ch. 20, 21) The period that involves the development and maturation of the reproductive, endocrine, and structural systems.

Public Law 94-142 (Ch. 20) The law stating that all disabled children must receive appropriate public education. Each child with special needs has the right to an evaluation by school or health professionals, who then develop an individualized educational plan for that child.

punishment (Ch. 20) Negative reinforcement of problem behavior.

Qi gong (Ch. 14) A part of traditional Chinese medicine that combines relaxed movements with a meditative aspect and controlled breathing to move qi energy through the energy channels. The goal of this technique is to balance, smooth, and strengthen the individual's qi energy.

qualitative studies (Ch. 1) Research studies that describe phenomena or define the historical nature, cultural relevance, or philosophical basis of aspects of nursing care.

quality of life (Ch. 1) Characteristics, conditions, and situations of life that compose the whole of a person's living. People strive for a positive quality of life. Illness or disease can diminish one's quality of life.

quantitative studies (Ch. 1) Research studies that describe situations, correlate different variables related to care, and test causal relationships between variables related to nursing care.

quickening (Ch. 16) The stage of gestation at which fetal motion is first felt by the mother.

race (Ch. 2) A biological term that refers to a grouping of individuals with distinct physical characteristics, such as skin color, hair texture, or facial features.

receptive language (Ch. 19) Language that retains information. Children can comprehend the meaning of words and phrases that are not a part of their expressive vocabulary and can make associations between concepts although they are unable to explain these concepts.

reflection (Ch. 4) A thinking process that involves bouncing back one's own thoughts and recollections of events to understand them and to take needed corrective action.

reflex (Ch. 17) A response that normally is exhibited automatically after a particular type of stimulation.

reflexology (Ch. 14) A method of moving energy by applying hand pressure to mapped points on the feet and hands.

refractive errors (Ch. 19) Defects in the ability of the lens of the eye to focus an image accurately, as occurs in nearsightedness and farsightedness.

regulations (Ch. 3) Rules or orders issued by an executive authority, agency, or department; used to implement laws.

rehearsal (Ch. 20) Repetition of an item to be learned to help with memorization.

Reiki (Ch. 14) A Japanese holistic therapy that requires training by a Reiki master. The Reiki master teaches hand placements and symbolic gestures and attunes the student. Attunement, opening the energy channel, enables the student to bring universal energy through the body and to the recipient.

relationship stages (Ch. 4) Sequential phases in a therapeutic relationship. They may overlap, vary in length, or involve issues that appear in other than a set sequence. Orientation (introductory), working, and termination phases have been identified by researchers and clinicians.

relaxation response (Ch. 12, 13) An inborn set of physiological changes that offset those of the fight-or-flight (stress) response.

reliability (Ch. 9) An assessment of the reproducibility of a test's results when the test is performed by different individuals with the same level of skill during different periods and under different conditions.

resistance training (Ch. 12) Exercise designed primarily to increase strength.

retinoblastoma (Ch. 19) A malignant tumor of the retina that develops during childhood.

risk factors (Ch. 6) Circumstances or conditions that increase the risk of health problems.

risk factor theory (Ch. 7, 8) The theory that a risk estimate can be obtained by comparing the frequency of deaths, illnesses, or injuries from a specific cause in a group that has some specific trait or risk factor with the frequency in another group that does not have this trait or in the population as a whole. The identification of human characteristics and behaviors that increase the likelihood of the manifestation of health problems.

risk-taking behavior (Ch. 21) Behaviors that bring with them an element of risk of harmful health care choices and outcomes.

ritual (Ch. 18) Routine action.

rubella (Ch. 16, 22) German measles.

S

scoliosis (Ch. 21) A lateral S-shaped curvature of the spine.

second stage of labor (Ch. 16) The stage in which the baby descends into the birth canal.

secondary appraisal (Ch. 13) An appraisal that includes the individual's identification of choices to cope with the actual or potential harm, threat, or challenge.

secondary sexual characteristics (Ch. 21) An external feature that differentiates male from female but is not essential for reproduction.

self-concept (Ch. 4) A mental picture of oneself; a composite view of personal characteristics, abilities, limitations, and aspirations.

self-disclosure (Ch. 4) Sharing aspects of the self.

self-esteem (Ch. 4, 20) The extent to which an individual believes oneself to be capable, significant, successful, and worthy.

self-insurance (Ch. 3) The instance in which an employer (or union) assumes the claims risk of its insured employees.

semantics (Ch. 20) Meaning of language.

sensitivity (Ch. 9) A measurement of the proportion of persons with a condition who correctly test positive when screened.

sensorimotor stage (Ch. 17, 18) The period (up to age 18 months) describing the infant's involvement in mastering simple coordination activities to interact with the environment.

serving size (Ch. 11) The recommended amount of food for one serving.

severe acute respiratory syndrome (SARS) (Ch. 25) A respiratory illness caused by the SARS-associated coronavirus (SARS-CoV). SARS was first reported in Asia in February 2003. Over the next few months the illness spread to more than two dozen countries in North America, South America, Europe, and Asia.

sexual abuse (Ch. 20) Use of a child for sexual, exploitative purposes. It includes any sexual contact with a child.

sexually transmitted disease (Ch. 16, 21) A contagious disease usually acquired by sexual intercourse or genital contact.

skid row (Ch. 2) A general term for an impoverished urban area where cheap housing, day labor, and marginal businesses can be found.

sleep hygiene (Ch. 13) Science and practice related to sleep and rest.

sleep talking (Ch. 20) Talking in one's sleep without awareness of doing so. Words tend to be simple, but difficult to understand.

sleepwalking (Ch. 20) Complex motor activity during sleep, usually culminating in leaving the bed and walking about. The person has no recall of the incident upon awakening.

Snellen E chart (Ch. 19) A tool that can provide a reliable estimate of the actual visual acuity of a child.

social cognitive theory (Ch. 10) A model developed by Bandera that emphasizes the influence of efficacy beliefs and outcome expectations on health behavior. Formerly known as *social learning theory.*

social learning theory (Ch. 10) The old name for social cognitive theory.

social marketing (Ch. 10) The application of commercial marketing technologies to the analysis, planning, execution, and evaluation of programs designed to influence the voluntary behavior of target audiences to improve their personal welfare and that of their society.

social support (Ch. 13) A network of close family, friends, co-workers, and professionals.

socialization (Ch. 20) The process in which a child is exposed to a variety of social roles and interactions.

socioecological model (Ch. 25) A model that describes health as a product of the interdependence among individuals and the subsystems of ecosystems, that assumes a connectedness among human beings, their physical and social environment, and their health.

somatization (Ch. 20) The transfer of feelings to a physical problem.

specificity (Ch. 9) A measurement of a test's ability to recognize negative reactions or nondiseased individuals.

spiritual practice (Ch. 13) Activities that help people find meaning, purpose, and connection for their lives.

spontaneous abortion (Ch. 16) Natural loss of conceptive products.

stagnation (Ch. 23) The result of a lack of accomplishment during developmental tasks in middle age.

Stanford-Binet test (Ch. 20) An intelligence test with a heavy emphasis on abstract thinking.

station (Ch. 16) The degree of descent of the presenting part of the fetus through the maternal pelvis, as measured in relation to the ischial spines of the maternal pelvis.

strabismus (Ch. 18, 19) A deviation of the line of vision from the midline because of extraocular muscle weakness or imbalance.

stress (Ch. 13, 22) The negative physical, psychological, social, or spiritual effects of life's pressures and events.

stress incontinence (Ch. 24) Urinary incontinence occurring during exercise, laughing, coughing, or sneezing.

stress management (Ch. 13) The process of improving the quality of life by increasing healthy, effective coping, thereby reducing the unhealthy consequences of stress.

stress warning signs (Ch. 13) The physical or emotional reactions/behaviors to a stressful experience, indicating the need to utilize more effective coping strategies to prevent illness.

stressor (Ch. 13) Any experience that disrupts homeostasis, thereby requiring change or adaptation. It can be of a physical, psychological, social, spiritual, or environmental nature.

striae gravidarum (Ch. 16) Stretch marks related to stretching of abdominal and breast skin with pregnancy.

stroke (Ch. 11) An abnormal condition of the brain characterized by occlusion by an embolus, thrombus, or cerebrovascular hemorrhage, resulting in ischemia of the brain tissues normally perfused by the damaged vessels.

structure of a community (Ch. 8) A community system or subsystem that can be seen as the formal or informal arrangement of its parts at any given time, including animate and inanimate properties.

subtle energy (Ch. 14) The energy that flows through the body, nourishing organs and promoting optimal functioning.

sudden infant death syndrome (Ch. 17) The sudden and unexpected death of an infant who has been healthy, for whom the cause of death is unexplained after a thorough postmortem examination.

sugar (Ch. 11) Any of several water-soluble carbohydrates. It supplies calories but is limited in nutrients.

syntax (Ch. 20) The part of grammar that deals with the way in which words are put together to form phrases or clauses.

syphilis (Ch. 16) A sexually transmitted disease caused by the spirochete *Treponema pallidum*.

systems theory (Ch. 7, 8) A theory that provides an overall framework in which otherwise unconnected parts can be integrated. A system is an entity composed of interrelated, interacting parts or components within a boundary that filters both the type and the rate of input and output.

T

tachycardia (Ch. 16) Fetal heart rate above 160 beats per minute or adult heart rate above 100 beats per minute.

tai chi (Ch. 14) A dancelike sequence of poses based on the movements of animals combining physical movement, breath control, and meditation. A holistic therapy that began as a Chinese martial art. The slowness of movement and focus on breathing brings an awareness of the moment-to-moment state of the body and can produce a meditative state.

Taoism (Ch. 2) The philosophical and theoretical foundation of Chinese medicine. A doctrine that states that humans are microcosms within the universe, and achieving harmony between the two is essential because the energies of both intertwine.

telehealth (Ch. 4) The use of telecommunications and data technologies to deliver health care services including diagnostic services, treatment, consultation, and health information.

teratogen (Ch. 16) A drug or other agent that causes abnormal prenatal development.

testicular self-examination (Ch. 22) A procedure recommended for detecting tumors or other abnormalities in the testes.

thalidomide (Ch. 16) A sedative-hypnotic drug that was withdrawn from general use, because it had potential to cause and did cause birth defects when taken during pregnancy.

therapeutic touch (Ch. 14) A touch therapy based on the idea that the ability to transmit universal energy is a natural ability of all humans. Therapeutic touch comprises three essential elements of practice: (1) centering, (2) assessment, and (3) treatment.

therapeutic use of self (Ch. 4) The application of cognitions, perceptions, and behaviors to create interpersonal encounters that promote health in another person, family, group, or community.

third stage of labor (Ch. 16) The stage that begins after the birth and lasts until placental expulsion.

toilet training (Ch. 18) Bowel and bladder training.

toxoplasmosis (Ch. 16) An infection resulting from the intracellular protozoan parasite *Toxoplasma gondii* that infects people through undercooked meat and the handling of cat feces. Although this infection is rare, if a pregnant woman is infected, the results to an infant can be severe.

transductive reasoning (Ch. 19) Moving only from particular to particular in making associations and solving problems.

trimester (Ch. 16) One of three equal time measurements.

Turner syndrome (Ch. 21) This is a female disorder in which only one X chromosome is present instead of two (XO).

tympanogram (Ch. 20) Test used to measure the sensitivity of the tympanic membrane to vibrations induced by pressure and sound waves.

type 2 diabetes (Ch. 11) Non–insulin-dependent diabetes mellitus; also known as adult-onset diabetes.

U

ultrasound (Ch. 16) High-frequency sound waves that bounce off the fetus and are interpreted by a computer. It allows defined visualization of the fetus and gestational structures throughout pregnancy.

underweight (Ch. 11) Body mass index of less than 18.5.

urge incontinence (Ch. 24) The inability to delay voiding once the bladder is full.

urinary incontinence (Ch. 24) Inability to control urination.

V

validity (Ch. 9) A measurement of a test's ability to distinguish correctly between diseased and nondiseased persons.

value orientation (Ch. 2) Orientation that is learned and shared through the socialization process, reflecting the personality type of a particular society. The dominant value orientations are shared by most of the group. Kluckhohn's model of value orientations incorporates themes regarding basic human nature, the relationship of human beings to nature, human beings' time orientation, valued personality type, and relationships between human beings.

value theory (Ch. 5) A theory that emerges as a result of philosophical inquiry about a good action. This type of theory is so named because it is concerned either with discovering what humans seem to value (descriptive theory) or proposing what they ought to value (normative theory) given some presupposed philosophy about the nature, or purpose of being human, or in order to achieve predetermined goals.

values (Ch. 2) Beliefs about the worth of something that serve as standards that influence behavior and thinking.

values clarification (Ch. 4, 13) A method whereby a person purposely seeks to discover what his or her values are and what importance these values have.

verbal communication (Ch. 4) Transmission of messages using spoken or written words.

Vineland social maturity scale (Ch. 19) A test that provides an objective, standardized estimate of social maturity.

voluntary migration (Ch. 2) Large-scale immigration generally motivated by the quest of the individual or group for one or more goals.

vulnerable population (Ch. 25) A population group that experiences factors that can cause or exacerbate health problems. Such factors may include poverty, lack of education, unstable or dangerous physical environments, isolation, and the lack of adequate and available health services.

W

warm-up period (Ch. 12) Physical activity that prepares both the musculoskeletal and cardiorespiratory systems for the transition from rest to exercise by increasing the blood flow, respiration, and body temperature and improving muscle flexibility.

weaning (Ch. 17) A gradual process that introduces the infant to a cup to replace the bottle or breast.

Wechsler series (Ch. 20) A series of intelligence tests that emphasize aggregate, or global, knowledge.

well-being (Ch. 1) State of being well. The status of one's condition of living. The definition of health is related to one's state of complete physical, mental, and social well-being.

wellness (Ch. 1) A state involving progression toward a higher level of functioning, an open-ended and ever-expanding future, with its challenge of fuller potential and the integration of the whole being.

wellness–illness continuum (Ch. 1) A paradigm that is a bipolar, interactive portrayal of health and illness in myriad configurations, ranging from high-level wellness to depletion of health (death).

Wilms tumor (Ch. 19) Cancer of the kidney that occurs in young children.

windshield survey (Ch. 8) Method of obtaining data about a community through direct observation involving all of the senses.

World Health Organization (Ch. 25) An international agency founded after World War II to promote health around the world.

Y

yoga (Ch. 12, 14) A form of spiritual practice involving mindful physical stretching that has Hindu origins. Awareness is focused on feeling the body as it moves.

Z

zygote (Ch. 16) The beginning of a human being, resulting from the successful penetration of a sperm cell into an egg, usually in the fallopian tube. Additional division of zygotic cells results in more differentiated structures that eventually produce an embryo and a fetus.

15-minute interview (Ch. 4) A brief interaction with a family structured by a few key questions to achieve a concise yet meaningful assessment of the family situation.

Index

A

Abuse; *See also* alcohol abuse; drug abuse
  child, 37, 395-396, 428-429, 428t, 451, 483
  of infants, 395-396
  during pregnancy, 361
  of women, 155, 535, 536
Accessibility
  in Canadian Health Act, 71, 72b
Accidents; *See also* motor vehicle accidents
  and alcohol excess, 235, 543-544
  bicycle, 455b, 457, 487-488, 490
  injuring older adults, 586-587
  injuring young adults, 532, 542
  during preschool years, 455-456
  prevention of
    in infants, 399-400
    in school-age children, 486-488, 489b, 490
  during toddler years, 430-431
Accountability
  and ethics, 106-108
Acculturation
  and diabetes, 28
  stresses in Asian American-Pacific Islanders, 29
Achievement stress, 540
Achievement tests, 479
Acne, 504-505
Acquired immunodeficiency syndrome (AIDS)
  African American youths "choosing," 521
  diet interventions for, 258
  education of school-age children concerning, 490-491
  Healthy People 2010 goals regarding, 42
  history of, 53-54
  importance of early detection, 41
  prevention and management of, 40-42
  REACH goals for, 51
  at risk infants, 401-402
  risks of
    in homeless population, 38
  screening programs for, 208t, 214
  statistics concerning people living with, 39-40
  summary of, 539t
  zidovudine (AZT) protocols, 366
Acquired lactase deficiency, 437
Active immunizations, 402
Active values, 78

Activities of daily living (ADLs)
  and exercise, 279
  of individuals, 137
  in older adulthood, 581-582
Activity-exercise patterns
  during adolescence, 510
  within communities, 183
  of families, 160
  of individuals, 136-138
  during infancy, 389-390
  during middle-age years, 555-556
  during older adult years, 577-579
  during prenatal period, 355b, 357-358
  during preschool years, 442-443
  during school years, 475-476
  during toddler years, 421-423
  during young adulthood, 531-533
Acupressure, 313-314
Acupuncture
  in Asian health culture, 30
  description of, 313
  questions to ask concerning, 3-4
  for stress management, 298-299
  for substance abuse, 313
Adaptation
  concept of, 5
Adaptive model
  of health, 5
Addiction
  in newborns, 368-369
Adipose tissue
  flowchart of life cycle growth changes in, 332t-333t
Adolescence
  definition of, 503
Adolescents, 502-521
  age and characteristics of, 330t
  age and physical changes in, 503-506
  autonomy issues with, 113
  and confidentiality, 116
  eating disorders and obesity in, 508-509
  Erikson's theory of psychosocial development, 341t
  families with, 157t-158t, 169-170, 175t
  flowchart of growth changes with time, 331t-336t
  functional health patterns, 506-516
  Healthy People 2010 goals for, 7, 8f
  homelessness among, 37, 38
  importance of peer groups to, 512-513
  pathological processes in, 516-519
  pregnancy rates among, 185, 190, 510, 513-515

Adolescents (*Continued*)
  recommended health examinations for, 507b
  risky behaviors by, 502, 510-511, 513, 516-519
  sexual activity and growth, 503t, 504-506, 513-515
  social processes affecting, 519-521
  suicide by, 502, 515-516, 521
  violence among, 517
Adrenals
  flowchart of life cycle growth changes in, 336t
Adult Treatment Panel (ATP) III, 246
Adults
  middle-age (*See* middle-age adults)
  older (*See* older adults)
  young (*See* young adults)
Advance directives
  definition of, 563-564
  and preventative ethics, 109-110, 111b
  types of, 111b
Advanced practice nurses (APNs)
  origins of, 56
Advocacy
  in nursing, 108-109
Advocates
  community nursing
    Racial and Ethnic Approaches to Community Health (REACH), 42, 51
  in global nursing, 603
  important role of nurses, 72-73
  nurses as, 18, 108-109, 603
Aerobic exercise
  definition of, 262, 531
  importance during young adulthood, 531-533
  and mental health, 272
  time and intensity recommendations, 273-275
Affective skills
  developed with play
    during preschool years, 445b, 446b
Affirmations
  and stress management, 301-302
Affluence, 496
Age
  as communication barrier, 92
  and exercise, 282-283
  as major coronary risk factor, 265t
Age-developmental focus
  of functional health patterns, 132
Agency for Health Care Research and Quality (AHRQ)
  research goals of, 7-8

Aggressive behaviors
and television habits, 166
Aging; *See also* older adults
and drug use, 588-589
effects of exercise on process of, 9,
264-265
and future health, 20
and glaucoma screening, 207t, 208t,
213-214
and health, 4
loss of function with, 6
and nutrition, 244-245
respect of
in Asian, Hispanic and Native
American cultures, 28-30, 32,
35, 36, 572
and rising health care costs, 61-64
and sexuality, 145, 584-585
theories of, 574, 575b
Aging population
and rising health care costs, 61,
62t
AIDS; *See* acquired immunodeficiency
syndrome (AIDS)
Alaskan natives
health issues in, 35
history of, 34
as race category, 25
REACH goals for, 51
Alcohol
assessing consumption of, 129-130
and cancer, 250-251
and cirrhosis, 233t
causing congenital defects, 367-368
Dietary Guidelines for Americans
2005, 234, 236, 238b
and falls by older adults, 586-588
and fetal alcohol syndrome, 368
fetal exposure to, 355
during middle-age years, 550, 552
among Native Americans, 34-35
in older adults, 589-590
statistics among men and women,
554-555
and stress, 290, 293
Alcohol abuse
during adolescence, 510, 516-517,
518b
and family risks, 156
and fetal alchohol syndrome, 368
as growing health concern, 20
Healthy People 2010 goals for, 7, 8b,
9b
and HIV and AIDS, 39-41
and homelessness, 36-38
during middle-age years, 554-555
among Native Americans, 34-35
during school years, 491-492
by seniors, 589
and sex, 523-524, 538
and stress, 290, 293
and teen drinking and driving, 178,
192t, 516-517
and violence, 535
by young adults, 543-544

Alcoholism
and cirrhosis, 233t
family risks of, 156
Alternative Co-Therapies Project, 42
Alternative medicine
questions to ask concerning, 3-4
and stress management, 298-299
used by black/African Americans, 33
Alzheimer's disease
care plan for family member with,
173
in older adults, 579-580
Ambient
definition of, 187
Amblyopia, 425, 446
Ambulatory settings
categories of, 56
American Cancer Society; *See also*
smoking
efforts on smoking awareness, 61
American Heart Association (AHA),
66
American Holistic Nurses Association,
312
American Indian/Alaska Native
as race category, 25
American Nurses Association (ANA)
agenda for the future, 73b, 74
Code of Ethics, 43, 101, 107b
defining nursing, 130
role in health care reform, 59
social policy statement, 130
Amma therapy, 314
Amniocentesis, 354
Amniotic membranes, 346
Anabolic steroids, 543
Anaerobic exercises
definition of, 262
ANA's Nurses Strategic Action Team
(N-STAT), 73
Anemia
in black/African Americans, 33
and iron deficiency, 232, 233t
related to poor nutrition, 233t
Anger
and aerobic exercise, 272
and stress, 292-293
Anorexia nervosa, 508b, 509
Anthrax, 54
Antibiotics
history of, 53
Anticipatory guidance, 340, 388, 462b
Anticonvulsants
effects on fetus, 368
Antiretroviral chemotherapy
(HAART), 40
Antisepsis, 53
Anxiety
and aerobic exercise, 272
among Asian Americans, 29
as communication barrier, 91
dreams, 444
and stress, 292-293
Apgar scoring, 353
Applied ethics, 101-102

Applied research
definition of, 20
Arab Americans
cultural values
affecting infants, 408-409
concerning pregnancy and birth,
350t
description of, 27
difficulties with researching, 24
health care issues of, 27-28
valuing family and culture, 28
Aromatherapy, 298-299, 321-322
Arteriosclerosis
during middle-age years, 550, 552
Arthritis
associated with middle-age obesity,
552-553
benefits of exercise for, 270
Healthy People 2010 goals for, 7, 8b
Asian American-Pacific Islanders
(AAPIs)
categories of, 28
culture of respect for older adults,
572
health care and cultural issues of, 28-
29
HIV and AIDS among, 40
as race category, 25
REACH goals for, 51
statistics and immigration history, 28
Asian Indians
cultural and heath issues of, 28-30
Aspiration, 455b
Assertive communication
and stress management, 302-303
Assessments; *See also* nursing
assessments
aspects of, 131t
of community functional health
patterns, 179, 183-185
definition of, 147
of families, 153-154, 156, 157t, 158-
167
of family self-worth, 161
of the individual
activity-exercise pattern, 136-138
characteristics of, 132-133
cognitive-perceptual pattern, 139-
140
coping–stress tolerance pattern,
145-146
definition of, 132
elimination pattern, 135-136
framework, 131-132
health perception/management
pattern, 134
nutritional-metabolic pattern, 134-
135
rationale for use, 133
roles-relationships pattern, 141,
142t, 143-144
self-perception-self-concept
pattern, 140-141
sexuality-reproductive pattern,
144-145

Assessments (*Continued*)
    sleep-rest pattern, 138-139
    values-beliefs pattern, 146-147
  of needs
    through communication, 93
  of nursing process, 154
  of older adults, 576
  parameters of, 134
  questions to ask
    of families, 159
  of screening target communities,
    202-203
  services in care management, 65b
Assisted living facilities, 581, 592t-
  593t, 594
Assisted suicide, 123, 124
Assurance
  versus insurance, 67
Asthma
  in homeless people, 38
  in preschoolers, 460
Astigmatism, 477
Attachment, 394-395
Attending, 82
Attention-deficit/hyperactivity disorder
  (ADHD), 479-480
Attitudes
  as communication barrier, 92
Autonomy
  and adolescents, 113
  versus beneficence, 117-120
  as civil liberty, 110, 112
  and confidentiality, 114-115
  limits on, 114
  nonmaleficence and beneficence,
    117-120
  during preschool years, 449
  as self-determination, 112-113
  in toddlers, 426-427
  and veracity, 116-117
Autosomal dominant diseases, 383

B

Baby boomers, 20
Back conditions
  Healthy People 2010 goals for, 7,
    8b
Bacterial infections
  affecting preschoolers, 457-458
  history of, 53
Bacterial vaginosis, 539t
Balance
  and Native American health
    philosophy, 35-36
Balanced Budget Act (BBA) of 1997,
  59, 70-71
Bandura's social cognitive theory, 283,
  284f
Basal metabolic rate, 529-530
Beans
  MyPyramid guidelines concerning,
    236, 240f
Bedtime rituals, 423, 443-444
Beers criteria, 589

Behaviors
  during adolescence
    substance abuse, 515-516, 518
  aggressive
    and television habits, 166
  changing, 186t, 191-192, 218-219,
    222-223
  health
    definition of, 4, 222
    models for change, 186t, 191-192
  and health history
    of young adults, 525-526, 527f,
      528
  moral
    in school-age children, 486
  in preschoolers, 439t
  risky adolescent, 502, 510-511, 513,
    516-519
  and stress, 290, 292-293
  young adult questionnaire
    concerning, 527f
Beliefs
  and healing, 27
  and nursing ethics, 121
  in toddlers, 430
Beneficence, 117-120
Beriberi, 232, 233t
Bicycles
  accidents, 455b, 472, 487-488, 490
  safety, 455b, 472, 487
Binge drinking, 523-524, 525, 543-544
Biological agents
  during adolescence, 518
  affecting fetus and mother
    during prenatal period, 365-367
  affecting infants, 401-403
  affecting middle-age adults, 565
  affecting preschoolers, 457-458
  affecting school-age children, 490-
    491
  danger to toddlers, 432
Bioterrorism, 54, 432
Birth defects, 346, 353, 364, 383-384,
  410, 540-541
Birthing centers, 56
Bisexuals
  homelessness among adolescent,
    37
  living with HIV and AIDS, 39-42
Black/African Americans (BAAs)
  and cancer, 250
  cultural values
    affecting infants, 408-409
    concerning pregnancy and birth,
      350t, 353
    and health care, 33-34
    and respect for older adults, 572
  demographics of, 32
  expectations of children, 494
  health care issues of, 32-34
  health disparities in, 10
  HIV and AIDS among, 39-41, 214,
    521
  as large uninsured population, 70-71
  pica, 357

Black/African Americans (BAAs)
    (*Continued*)
  as race category, 25, 383
  REACH goals for, 51
  reluctance of
    to participate in research, 24
  and sedentary lifestyles, 264b
  stroke statistics in, 550
  young adult health issues in, 526,
    528
Bladder
  elimination patterns
    of communities, 183
    of families, 160
    of individuals, 135-136
Blood pressure
  and diet, 247-250
  dietary and cultural aspects of, 247-
    248
  high
    associated with middle age obesity,
      552-553
    among black/African Americans,
      33
    as major coronary risk factor,
      265t
  screening programs, 207t, 208t,
    213
Bloom theory, 556-557
Body
  changes in proportion over time,
    338f
  curiosity about
    during preschool years, 452
Body image
  and self-esteem, 511-512
Body mass index (BMI)
  in CDC growth charts, 338, 382
  children's growth charts and, 254-
    255
  definition and formula of, 254
  and obesity in middle-age, 552-553
Body piercing, 511
Body work
  Bowenwork, 321
  craniosacral therapy, 321
  massage, 320-321
  Trager therapy, 321
Bonding, 394-395
Bones
  development of
    during adolescence, 505-506
  flowchart of life cycle growth
    changes in, 334t
  ossification, 469
  strength
    and exercise, 264-265, 269-270,
      577-579
    and osteoporosis, 251-253, 269-
      270
Borg Scale, 274, 275f
Boston College Health Fair, 507
Bowels
  development in toddlers, 417
  elimination patterns

Bowels (*Continued*)
of communities, 183
of families, 160
of individuals, 135-136
infant, 389
of older adults, 576-577
Bowenwork, 321
Bradycardia, 352
Brain
flowchart of life cycle growth
changes in, 335t
tumors, 460b
Breast cancer
among Asian American-Pacific
Islanders, 28-29
associated with middle age obesity,
552-553
among black/African Americans,
33
among Mexican American women,
210
in middle-age adults, 549-550
in older adults, 590
screening
description and purpose of, 204,
207t, 212
REACH goals for, 51
with self-examination, 514, 526
and stress, 290
Breast-feeding
advantages and disadvantages of,
386b
Healthy People 2010 goals to promote,
377
illustration of methods, 387
and pacifiers, 385
promotion of, 385-388
Breasts
self-examination, 514, 526
Breath meditation, 319
Breathing
disturbances
associated with middle age obesity,
552-553
exercises, 138, 278-279, 296-298,
317-319
Bubonic plague, 53, 112
Buddhism
culture and health aspects of, 28-
30
and food, 237
Bulimia nervosa, 508b, 509
Burns
prevention of
in infants, 400b
safety measures to prevent
in preschoolers, 455b, 456
during school years, 487, 488
in toddlers, 431
Business
inequities for black/African
Americans, 32
and special interest groups
affecting quality and access to
health care, 51

C
Caffeine
causing congenital defects, 367, 368-
369
positives and negatives of, 554
CAGE test, 129-130
Calcium
content in foods, 253t
needed during middle age, 554
during pregnancy, 356-357
during preschool years, 440-442
preventing osteoporosis, 252
Cambodians
cultural and heath issues of, 28-30
Canada
expenditures per capita and %GDP,
62t
universal health insurance coverage
in, 71-72
Canada Health Act
five principles of, 72b
Cancer
in adolescents, 519
among black/African Americans, 32-
33
caused by poor nutrition, 232, 233t,
250-251
diet and, 250-251
environmental carcinogens, 544,
565
Healthy People 2010 goals regarding,
7, 8b, 42-43
during infancy, 407
in Latino/Hispanic Americans, 30
leading types of
in older adults, 590t
as major cause of death, 20
in middle-age adults, 550
in preschoolers, 458-460
related to poor nutrition, 233t
in school-age children, 492
screening programs for, 207t, 208t,
212-213
warning signs of childhood, 460b
Candida albicans, 366
Capitation
definition of, 57b
system
payment mechanism of, 64-65
Car safety seats
for infants, 376-377, 406
Carbohydrates
Dietary Guidelines for Americans
2005, 234, 236, 238b
needed by infants, 384-388
during pregnancy, 356-357
Carcinogens, 544, 565
Cardiac output
changes with middle-age, 549
Cardiopulmonary diseases
signs and symptoms of, 280b
Cardiorespiratory fitness; *See also*
exercise
definition of, 262
statistics on, 262, 264f, 280-281

Cardiovascular system
changes with middle-age, 549
diseases
caused by poor nutrition, 232, 245
in Latino/Hispanic Americans, 30
REACH goals for, 51
Care
definition of, 105, 564
ethics of, 105-106
nursing models of, 105-106
Care management
definition of, 57b
description of, 65
nurses in, 18
services of, 65b
Care monitoring
services in care management, 65b
Care planning
services in care management, 65b
Caries, 38, 233t, 441-442, 469, 472,
497t
Case studies
on adolescent pregnancy rates, 185,
190
on elderly immigrant woman, 43
on ethics, 122-124
on exercise, 284-285
on family structure, 162
on health promotion and
communication, 96-97
on health promotion and prevention,
10-13
on holistic healing, 315
on homeless infants, 397.398
on middle-age cancer, 563
on obesity, 10-13, 253, 254
on possible genetic defects, 364
on prostate screening, 209
on spiritual distress, 143, 144
on stress, 295, 296
on toddlers, 431
Catastrophic chronic illnesses, 68-69
Cavities, 38, 233t, 441-442, 469, 472,
497t
Centering, 314, 445
Centers for Disease Control and
Prevention (CDC)
on body mass indexes in growth
charts, 254-255, 382
growth charts of, 338-339, 382, 417
on HIV and AIDS, 366
Racial and Ethnic Approaches to
Community Health (REACH),
42, 51
on tuberculosis, 588
Cerebrovascular accidents
in black/African Americans, 550
dietary interventions for prevention
of, 248-249
effect of exercise on, 9
Healthy People 2010 goals regarding,
7, 8b, 42-43
as major cause of death, 20
rehabilitation following, 18
screening programs, 207t, 208t, 213

Cerebrovascular disease
in middle-age adults, 549-550
Certified nurse midwives (CNMs), 56
Cervical cancer
screening programs, 204, 207t, 212
Cervical dysplasia, 544
Cervix
during prenatal period, 347b, 348
screening for cancer
REACH goals for, 51
Chadwick, Edwin, 53
Changes
goals for health behavior, 220
in lifestyle
to lower cholesterol, 247
planning within communities, 191-192
sources of resistance to, 193t
stages of, 186t
Chemical agents
during adolescence, 518-519
affecting middle-age adults, 565-566
affecting preschoolers, 458
affecting school-age children, 491-492
dangers during prenatal period, 367-370
dangers to infants, 403-406
public threats of, 54
Chemotherapy
history of, 53
Cherokees, 34-36
Chi, 312
Child abuse
cultural and legal issues, 428
and homelessness, 37
of infants, 395-396
of preschoolers, 451
of school-age children, 483
warning signs
in toddlers, 428t
Child bearing families, 157t-158t, 168-169, 175t
Child care, 407-408, 433, 450b
Childproofing, 401, 402b
Children
diabetes in, 256-258
growth charts with body mass index, 254-255
Healthy People 2010 goals for, 7, 8f
new siblings, 362b
promoting exercise in, 285
Chinese
Americans
expectations of children, 494
cultural and heath issues of, 28-30
folk medicine, 30
food culture of, 237
Chiropractic therapies
questions to ask concerning, 3-4
for stress, 298-299
Chlamydia
common in adolescents, 518
during prenatal period, 366
summary of, 539t

Chloasma, 347
Chloroma, 459
Choking, 401b
Cholera, 53
Cholesterol levels
and diet, 246-247
diseases related to high, 233-234
effect of exercise on, 9, 265-266
screening programs, 207t, 208t, 213
Chorionic membranes, 346
Chorionic villi, 3436
Christianity, 27
Chronic illnesses
benefits of exercise in coping with, 279
and families, 156
and nursing research, 19
in older men and women, 573t
and physician-assisted suicide, 585-586
Chronic obstructive pulmonary disease (COPD), 571-572
Chronic serous otitis media, 477
Cigarettes; *See* smoking
Circulatory system
adaptive changes during pregnancy, 347
development in toddlers, 418
Cirrhosis
and alcohol excess, 235
among Native Americans, 34
related to poor nutrition, 233t
Classification systems
diagnostic, 147
Clinical models
of health, 5
Clinical services
percentage of personal expenditures for, 62t
Clinics
free, 26-27
in schools, 520-521
Code of ethics
American Nurses Association (ANA), 43, 101, 107b
nursing, 107-108
Cognitive mastery, 515b
Cognitive restructuring
definition of, 300-301
four-step approach to, 301b
and stress management, 300-301
Cognitive skills
development of
during preschool years, 444-447, 445b, 446b, 448t, 449
in toddlers, 423, 424t, 425-426
in families, 161
during middle-age, 556-557
Cognitive theories
Bandura's social, 283, 284f
Cognitive values, 78
Cognitive-behavioral therapy (CBT), 299

Cognitive-perceptual patterns
during adolescence, 510-511
of communities, 184
of families, 161
of individuals, 139-140
during infancy, 392-393
during middle-age years, 556-557
during older adult years, 579-582
during prenatal period, 355b, 358-360
during preschool years, 444-447, 448t, 449
during school years, 476-480
during toddler years, 423, 424t, 425-426
during young adulthood, 532-533
Coining, 428
Collaborative partnerships
example of, 204
model of
for screening programs, 203
Collectivism
in community health, 50-51
versus individualism
in Asian Americans, 29
in Latino/Hispanic Americans, 31
Colon cancer
associated with middle age obesity, 552-553
Colorectal cancer
in middle-age adults, 550
screening programs, 207t, 208t, 212
Colostrum, 347
Columbus, Christopher, 32, 34
Communicable diseases
global efforts to prevent, 601-607
history of, 52-54
Communication
assertive, 302-303
barriers to effective, 91-93
characteristics of effective, 84-87
definition of, 81
ethical, 89
exploration of nurses', 82
within families, 154
as focus area of *Healthy People 2010*, 78
function of, 82-83
importance in nursing, 81-87
lack of, 82
patient-centered, 82b
process of, 81-87
purposeful, 88
settings for good, 93-94
steps to functional, 84-85
as topic on nursing national agenda, 73b, 74
types of, 83-84
zones of space, 87b, 88f
Communities
addressing alcohol abuse, 178, 192b, 192t
definition of, 179
examples of strengths and concerns in, 187t

Communities (*Continued*)
exercise in, 285
health promotion in
analysis and diagnoses within, 185-188
data collection and information, 180-181
developmental perspective, 182
evaluation phase, 193-194
functional health patterns, 183-185
implementation phase, 193
nurse's role, 179-180
nursing process, 179
planning phase, 188, 191-192
risk factor perspective, 182-183
system's perspective, 181-182
Healthy People 2010 education objectives in, 218, 219
hierarchical nature of, 181f
nursing process in, 179-194
retirement, 592t-593t
screening programs for, 202-203, 204
structure of, 181
systems theory of, 181
using nursing process in, 187-188, 191-194
Community diagnoses
components of, 188
Community health nursing
components of, 180
goals of, 51-52
and health promotion, 50-51
and homelessness, 38-39
Racial and Ethnic Approaches to Community Health (REACH), 42
Community lodges
for homeless people, 38
Community nursing centers, 56, 57
Community nursing interventions, 191
Community patterns, 186-187
Community risk factors, 188
Community-based care
description of, 18
residence programs
for homeless people, 38
Complementary medicine; *See also* alternative medicine
questions to ask concerning, 3-4
Comprehensiveness
in Canadian Health Act, 71, 72b
Computer games, 494
Concrete operations, 476
Condoms, 527t, 538
Confidentiality
and adolescents, 116
and autonomy, 114-115
Conformity, 515b
Congenital defects, 346, 353, 364, 540-541
Congestive heart failure
screening programs, 207t, 208t, 213
Consequentialism, 102

Conservation
concept of, 477
Consolidated Omnibus Budget Reconciliation Act (COBRA), 71
Constipation
changes with middle-age, 549
during middle-age years, 555
in older adults, 576-577
during pregnancy, 349t
related to poor nutrition, 233t
Constructive confrontation, 90
Consultants
nurses as, 18
Continuing care retirement communities (CCRCs), 594
Contraception, 536, 537t
Contract workers, 25
Control
behaviors in adolescents, 515b
sense of, 481
Conventional levels, 486
Cool-downs, 275-276
Coping skills
during adolescence, 515b, 516
case study involving, 10-13
and exercise, 261-262, 272, 280-281
in families, 166
and homelessness, 37-39
and humor, 86, 146, 305-306, 307b
during labor and delivery, 352
of preschoolers, 452-453
in school-age children, 484, 485t
and stress, 294-295, 306-307
during toddler years, 430
in young adults, 542-544
Coping strategies; *see also* coping skills
Coping–stress tolerance patterns
addressing alcohol abuse, 192b
during adolescence, 515-516
of communities, 185
of families, 166
of individuals, 145-146
during infancy, 397-399
during middle-age years, 562-564
during older adult years, 585-586
during prenatal period, 355b, 363
during preschool years, 452-453
during school years, 484-485
during toddler years, 429
during young adulthood, 538, 540
Coronary artery disease (CAD)
in young adults, 526
Coronary heart diseases (CHDs)
in Arab Americans, 27-28
benefits of exercise for, 265-268, 280
and diet, 232, 235, 245
Healthy People 2010 goals regarding, 42-43
screening programs, 207t, 208t, 213
Cost-benefit ratio analysis
of screening programs, 206
Cost-effectiveness analysis
of preventative health care, 608-609
of screening programs, 206

Cost-efficiency analysis
of screening programs, 206
Costs
breakdown of nation's health dollar, 63f
containment of, 65
factors driving, 61
of managed care, 57
and other financial factors
aging population, 61
cost containment, 65
managed care issues, 65-66
national and international expenditures, 61, 62t
payment mechanisms, 64-65
private insurance, 66-68
public insurance, 68-70
sources, 63-64
prescription drug, 61-62
reasons for inflated, 61-62
of screening programs, 205-206
total personal expenditures
for different services, 62t
in United States
inflated *versus* other countries, 56-72, 62t
Council for Nursing Centers, 56
Counseling
of adolescents, 507b
for Arab Americans, 28
Countertransference, 93
Couple families, 157t-158t, 167-168, 175t
Covered entities
in privacy rule, 115
Crack cocaine, 38
Craniosacral therapy, 321
Cretinism, 232, 233t
Creutzfeldt-Jakob disease, 241
Crisis
bonding of diverse groups during, 24
and ethnic culture, 25-26
Cubans, 30-31
Cultural competence
definition of, 8
and functional health patterns
in the individual, 133
when analyzing families, 172
Cultural diversity
changes in older population, 594
nursing journals addressing, 43
Cultural focus
of functional health patterns, 133
Cultural sensitivity; *See* multicultural awareness
Cultures; *See also* multicultural awareness
Asian American-Pacific Islanders, 29
awareness and education, 45
black/African American, 32-34
blending Western medicine with practices of, 3
changes and health improvements, 20
and child abuse, 428

Cultures (*Continued*)
  and child behavior expectations, 494
  considerations
      in health teaching, 223-224
  definition of, 26
  and fetal health, 353
  and food
      multicultural awareness of, 237
  and healing, 27
  influence on adolescents, 519-520
  influence on infants, 408-409
  influence on preschoolers, 460-461
  influence on school-age children,
      493-494
  influence on young adults, 545
  Latino/Hispanic American, 30-31
  during middle-age years, 566-567
  Native American, 34-36
  nursing awareness of transcultural
      values, 55 (*See also* multicultural
      awareness)
  passivity *versus* assertiveness, 28-29
  and pregnancy, 350t, 372
  and respect for older adults, 572
  role of
      in HIV and AIDS, 41
  of slavery, 32
  as topic on nursing national agenda,
      73b, 74
  and values, 26-27
Cupping, 428
Curative measures
  versus preventative, 54-55
Custodial care
  not provided for
      by Medicare, 68
Customs
  and ethnicity, 25
Cytomegalovirus (CMV), 365

D
Dairy products
  MyPyramid guidelines concerning,
      236, 240f
  sodium contents in, 248t
Data
  organization of, 185-186
Data analysis
  guidelines for community, 186-187
Data collection
  concerning families, 167
  methods of
      in community assessments, 180
  in nursing process, 147
Date rape, 507b, 513
Day care, 407-408, 433
Death
  among black/African Americans, 32-
      33, 535
  concept of
      in preschoolers, 454
  and firearms, 528-529, 535
  Healthy People 2010 goals regarding,
      42-43

Death (*Continued*)
  history of, 52-53
  homicide and suicide
      during young adulthood, 528-529,
          535
  leading causes of, 52, 550b
      among Native Americans, 34
  rates
      Healthy People 2010 goals
          regarding, 42-43
      statistics on, 552f
  of spouses, 561, 584
  sudden infant death syndrome
      (SIDS), 390-392
Decidua, 345
Decision making
  ethical considerations, 121-122
  proxy, 112b, 114
  and risk taking
      during young adulthood, 528-529
  steps in, 122
  strategies for ethical, 121-122
Decubitus ulcer, 582
Degenerative joint disease, 549
Deliverer of services
  nurses as, 18
Delivery; *See* health care delivery
      system
Dementia, 579
  herbal remedies
      used by older adults, 586
Demographics; *See also* populations;
      Web Site Resources
  on black/African Americans, 32
  changes in older population, 594
  concerning Asian American-Pacific
      Islanders (AAPIs), 28
  concerning older adults, 179
  of Latino/Hispanic Americans, 28-
      30
  on Native Americans-Alaska
      Natives, 34
  poverty rates
      by race and ethnic group, 188
  shifting United States, 3
Demography
  definition of, 181
Dental caries
  in homeless people, 38
  in preschoolers, 441-442
  related to poor nutrition, 233t
  during school years, 469, 472, 497t
Dental health
  during adolescence, 507b
  anticipatory guidance for, 462b
  education in school-age children,
      469b
  Healthy People 2010 goals for, 7, 8b
  among Native Americans, 35
  not provided for
      by Medicare, 68
  percentage of personal expenditures
      for, 62t
  teaching to toddlers, 418b

Dentures
  not provided for
      by Medicare, 68
Denver Developmental Screening Test
      (DDST), 339, 382
Denver Eye Screening Test, 446
Department of Defense (DOD), 60
Department of Homeland Security, 52
Depression
  during adolescence, 515-516, 521
  and aerobic exercise, 272
  among Asian Americans, 29
  herbal remedies for
      used by older adults, 586
  and obesity, 509
  in older adults, 585-586
  during school years, 485-486
  and stress, 292-293
Development
  concept of, 339
  flowchart of changes through life
      cycle, 331t-336t
  and growth (*See also* growth)
      overview of, 320-343
  milestones in preschoolers, 439t
  patterns of, 339-340
  theories of
      Erikson's theory of psychosocial
          development, 340
      Gilligan's theory of moral
          development, 341, 342t
      Kohlberg's theory of moral
          development, 341, 342t
      Piaget's theory of cognitive
          development, 340-341
Developmental approaches
  for analyzing community data, 186-
      187
  to testing, 447, 449
Developmental crises, 398
Developmental tasks
  accomplished during infancy, 378,
      381t
  of middle-age, 556b
Developmental theories
  of families, 167-172
  within nursing process
      and families, 153
Diabetes
  among Alaskan Natives, 35
  among Arab Americans, 27-28
  associated with middle age obesity,
      552-553
  benefits of exercise for, 281-282
  among black/African Americans, 33
  caused by poor nutrition, 232-236,
      233t, 255-258
  Healthy People 2010 goals regarding,
      7, 8b, 42-43
  in Latino/Hispanic Americans, 30
  during middle-age years, 550, 552
  among Native Americans, 34
  and pregnancy, 367
  prevalence and prevention of, 255-
      258

Diabetes (Continued)
REACH screening goals for, 51
risk factors for, 28
in young adults, 526, 528
Diabetes mellitus
as major coronary risk factor, 265t
screening programs for, 214-215
Diagnoses
classification systems, 147
definition of nursing, 131
early with secondary prevention, 13, 14f, 15-18
within families, 167-172
functional versus structural, 188
purpose of writing family, 171-172
variables, 148
Diagnosis-related group categories, 65
Diastolic blood pressure
changes during middle-age, 562-563
and diet, 249
screening programs for, 207t, 208t, 213
Dietary Guidelines for Americans 2005, 234, 236, 238b
Dietary Reference Intake (DRI), 234, 235b
Dietary supplements
and herbal medicines, 236-237, 239
Diets
during adolescence, 507b
for Arab Americans, 28
case study involving, 10-13
in different cultures, 237
and ethnicity, 25
fad, 257
and family risks, 156
habits of families, 156, 159-160
healthy
as stress management tool, 299
in Latino/Hispanic American communities, 30
among Native Americans, 34-35
and obesity
in young adults, 529, 530f
during pregnancy, 356-357
in Taoism, 30
Digestive system
flowchart of life cycle growth changes in, 332t
Dilantin, 368
Dilation, 348
Dilemmas
definition of, 109
Direct-to-consumer marketing (DTCM), 119
Disabilities
and exercise, 9
and health, 4
health disparities due to, 54
Healthy People 2010 goals for, 7, 8b
Public Law 94-142, 495
and rising health care costs, 61-64
risks with sedentary lifestyle, 262-263
and tertiary prevention, 18

Discipline, 482b, 483, 494
Discrimination
against Latino/Hispanic Americans, 30
Diseases; See also immunizations
brought to Native Americans, 34
definition of, 6-7
detection, instruments and resources, 201-203
diagnostic criteria, 201
Healthy People 2010 goals regarding, 42-43
history of, 52-53
in homeless people, 38
as leading cause of death in US, 52
and nursing research, 19
prevention of
in families, 152-176
and health education, 218-224
selection of screenable, 201-205
specific protection from, 17
and tertiary prevention, 18
Distant healing, 319-320
Distress, 291
Diurnal enuresis, 474-475
Divergent family structures, 161
Diversity
within Asian American-Pacific Islanders, 28-29
within Latino/Hispanic American cultures, 31
nursing journals addressing, 43
as topic on nursing national agenda, 73b, 74
in United States, 24
Divorce, 451, 485, 533-534, 561
Dolls, 452
Domestic violence
battered women's resilience, 163
educating women about, 155
during pregnancy, 361
during young adulthood, 535, 536
Down syndrome, 66, 353
Draw-a-Person and Draw-a-Family tests, 449
DRE screenings, 208t, 213
Dress
and ethnicity, 25
Drinking and driving; See alcohol abuse
Drowning
during preschool years, 455b, 456
during school years, 487, 488
toddlers, 431
Drug abuse
during adolescence, 510
and drug-resistant tuberculosis, 54
as growing health concern, 20
Healthy People 2010 goals for, 7, 8b, 9b
and Hepatitis C, 529
and HIV and AIDS, 39-42
and homelessness, 36-38
during middle-age years, 554-555
among Native Americans, 34-35
possible in older adults, 588-589

Drug abuse (Continued)
during pregnancy, 367, 368
risks for young adults, 542-543
during school years, 491-492
and stress, 290
through injections
and HIV/AIDS, 39-40
and violence, 535
Drugs
causing congenital defects, 367-368
dangers to infants, 403
Durable medical equipment
percentage of personal expenditures for, 62t
Durable power of attorney, 563-564
Duty-based theories, 102
Dysfunctional
as status of family health, 153
Dyslexia, 479

E
Early and Periodic Screening, Diagnosis, and Treatment (EPSDT), 70, 461
Eating disorders
diagnostic criteria for, 508-509
Ecology
and health, 6
Ecomaps, 163, 165
Economic ethics
and screening, 205-206
Economics
and adolescents, 520
and drug affordability
in older adult population, 589
effect of toddlers on, 434
factors
and concept of health, 4-5
influencing health care delivery system, 54
as topic on nursing national agenda, 73b, 74
of having a baby, 372
and infants, 411, 412b
and preschoolers, 461
and school-age children, 495-496
and young adults, 545-546
Education; See also health teachings; Web Site Resources
challenges of, 217-218, 612-613
concerning HIV and AIDS, 39-42
disparities
in black/African American community, 32
and screening programs, 209-210
about exercise benefits, 283-285
facilitating transcultural, 45
health
definition of, 219
goals of, 220-221
Internet as tool for, 229
key factors in, 51
health disparities due to poor, 54
and homelessness, 37-38

Education (*Continued*)
  importance of
    to Asian American-Pacific
      Islanders (AAPIs), 28
    and Latino/Hispanic Americans,
      30
    among major ethnic groups, 28
    among Native Americans, 34
  nurse's role in health
    behavior changes, 222
    cultural considerations, 223-224
    defining goals, 220-221
    defining health education, 219
    ethics, 223
    facilitating learning, 221
    family health, 221-222
    social cognitive theory, 222-223
  opportunities with higher, 24
  and promotion, 16
  and school nurse, 498-499
  and sedentary lifestyles, 264b
  social marketing, 224
  teaching and organizing skills, 228-
    229
  teaching plans, 224-228
  as topic on nursing national agenda,
    73b, 74
Educators
  nurses as, 18-19
Effacement, 348
Egocentrism
  in preschoolers, 445
  in toddlers, 423
Egyptians, 27
Ehrlich, Paul, 53
Elderly; *See* older adults
Elimination patterns
  during adolescence, 509
  within communities, 183
  within families, 160
  of individuals, 135-136
  during infancy, 388-389
  during middle-age years, 555
  during older adult years, 576-577
  during prenatal period, 355b, 357
  during preschool years, 442
  during school years, 474-475
  during toddler years, 421
  during young adulthood, 531
Elizabethan poor laws, 53
Emancipated minors, 520
Embryos, 345
Emerging populations
  rural and urban, 36-42
  in the United States, 24-34
Emotions
  changes during pregnancy, 359
Empathy
  in nursing
    definition of, 8, 82
  and stress management, 303-304
  in therapeutic relationships
    definition of, 88-89
Employee Retirement and Income
  Security Act (ERISA), 68

Employer-based health insurance, 65-66
Empty nests, 170
Encopresis, 475
Endocrine system
  adaptive changes during pregnancy,
    347
  flowchart of life cycle growth
    changes in, 336t
End-of-life issues
  and nursing research, 19
  and terminal illness, 548
Endometrial cancer, 552-553
Endometrium, 345
Energy
  definition of, 312
  feeling one's own, 312b
Engrossment, 395
Enuresis, 474-475
Environmental quality
  Healthy People 2010 goals for, 7, 8b,
    9b, 78
  pollution and hazardous waste issues,
    20, 21, 406t, 492, 531
Environments
  assessment of home family, 159
  carcinogens, 544, 565
  chemicals in
    affecting fetal development, 369
  creating safe
    for preschoolers, 455b
  and death in US, 52
  and energy work, 312-316
  and eudaimonistic model of health,
    5
  factors and screening, 210-211
  factors during middle-age years, 565
  nursing work, 52
  teaching preschoolers about
    protecting, 450
  as topic on nursing national agenda,
    73b, 74
  toxin risks to infants, 405-406
Enzyme immunoassay (EIA)
  for HIV screening, 208t, 214
Epidemics, 53
Epidemiology, 156
  definition of, 4
Episiotomy, 351
Epstein-Barr virus, 518
Erikson's eight life stages, 141, 142t-
  143t
Erikson's theory of psychosocial
  development
  and adolescents, 510-511
  description of, 340
  eight stages of human, 341t
  and infant development, 378, 396
  and middle-age adults, 557-558
  and older adulthood, 583
  and preschoolers, 449
  and school-age children, 480-481
  during young adulthood, 532
Escherichia coli, 529
Estrogen, 347, 503-504, 549, 558
Ethic of care, 105-106

Ethics
  in communication, 89
  definition of, 101
  economic
    and screening, 205-206
  health care
    accountability, 106-108
    and adolescents, 113, 116
    advance directives, 113
    advocacy, 108-109
    autonomy, 110-114
    case studies, 122-124
    confidentiality and privacy, 114-
      115
    decision-making, 112b, 114, 121-
      122
    ethic of care, 105-106
    feminist, 104-105
    informed consent, 113
    justice, 120
    moral theory, 101, 102-104
    nonmaleficence and beneficence,
      117-120
    origins of, 101-102
    problem solving, 109-110
    and screening, 205
    types of, 102
    veracity, 116-117
  and health education, 223
  in health promotion
    case studies, 122-124
    decision-making strategies, 121-
      122
    health care ethics, 101-106
    principles of, 110, 112-120
    professional responsibility, 106-
      110, 111b
  recognizing barriers, 107
  in screening, 200-201
  types of
    descriptive value theories, 102
    moral theories, 101, 102-104
    normative theories, 102
Ethnic diversity
  advantages and disadvantages of,
    25
Ethnic groups
  Asian American-Pacific Islanders,
    28-30
  black/African Americans, 32-34
  blending Western medicine with
    practices of, 3
  death rate statistics by, 552f
  and health, 4
  influences on school-age children,
    493-494
  Latino/Hispanic Americans, 30-
    32
  migration factors, 24-25
  nursing journals addressing, 43-44
  researching and working with, 24
  screening programs for different, 208-
    210
  statistics on HIV and AIDS in, 39-
    41

Ethnicity
  and adolescents, 519-520
  classification of, 25
  as communication barrier, 92
  definition of, 25, 26
  health disparities due to, 54
  and infants, 408-409
  during middle-age years, 566-567
  and pregnancy, 350t, 372
  and school-age children, 493-494
  shaping of
    during preschool years, 460-461
  and young adults, 545
Ethnocentric perspective
  nursing avoidance of, 27
Ethnocentrism
  definition of, 8
Eudaimonistic model
  of health, 5
Eustress, 291
Euthanasia, 585-586
Evaluations
  community, 188, 191-192
  phases, 193-194
Evidence-based practices
  description of, 18-20
  development and standards of, 51
Exercise
  activity level goals, 272-273
  adherence and compliance with
    program of, 282-284
  during adolescence, 507b
  and aging, 264-265, 577-579
  anticipatory guidance for, 462b
  benefits of
    for coronary heart disease, 265-
      268, 280
    for diabetes, 281-282
    for immune function, 271-272
    for low back pain, 270-271
    for mental health, 272
    for obesity, 268-269
    in older adults, 577-579
    for osteoporosis, 269-270, 577-579
  case study involving, 10-13, 284-285
  climate that encourages, 284-285
  creating program for, 283-285
  definition of, 262
  Dietary Guidelines for Americans
    2005, 234, 236, 238b
  and family risks, 156
  as functional health pattern
    of communities, 183
    of families, 160
    of individuals, 136-138
  Healthy People 2010 goals for, 262-
    264
  hydration during, 279-280
  importance of
    during middle-age years, 555-556
    during young adulthood, 531-533
  knowing *versus* doing, 261
  MyPyramid guidelines concerning,
    236, 240f
  by older adults, 577-579

Exercise (*Continued*)
  parameters of, 137
  physical activity pyramid, 274f
  precautions concerning, 279-280
  during pregnancy, 357-358
  relaxation response, 278-279
  risks of, 280-282
  and stress management, 299-300
  types of
    aerobic, 273-275
    flexibility, 276
    resistance training, 276, 277b,
      278b
    warm-ups and cool-downs, 275-
      276
Expenditures
  national health, 61, 62t
  US *versus* other countries, 62t, 71-72
Expressive language
  during adolescence, 511
  definition of, 447
  during preschool years, 447, 448t
  during toddler years, 424t
External locus of control, 481
Eye Patch Club, 426
Eyes
  changes in older adulthood, 581-582
  development in toddlers, 425-426
  development of preschoolers, 445-
    446
  flowchart of life cycle growth
    changes in, 332t
  problems during middle age, 557
  retinoblastoma, 459
  and vision in school-age children,
    477

F
Faith
  communities
    importance to health, 9, 12
  in elderly Native Americans, 35-36
Falls
  infant, 400
  in older adults, 587-588
False-negative test results, 202
False-positive test results, 202
Family developmental tasks, 155
Family history
  and diabetes screening, 207t, 208t,
    214-215
  and ethnicity, 25-26
  as major coronary risk factor, 265t
Family (ies)
  definition of, 154
  exercise in, 285
  genograms and ecomaps, 163, 164f,
    165
  health promotion of
    analysis and nursing diagnoses,
      167-172
    assessment of, 153, 156, 157t, 158
    care planning, 172
    caring for older adults, 152

Family (ies) (*Continued*)
  developmental perspective, 155-
    156
  evaluations, 175-176
  functional health patterns, 156,
    158-167
  implementation, 172-175
  nursing process and, 153-154
  risk-factor perspective, 156, 157t-
    158t
  systems perspective, 154-155
  health status
    description of, 153
  importance of
    among Asian American-Pacific
      Islanders, 29
    among black/African Americans,
      33
    in health promotion, 153
    to Latino/Hispanic Americans, 30-
      32
    among Native Americans, 35-36
  intervention effectiveness measures,
    176
  in Latino/Hispanic American
    culture, 30
  resilience, 162
  six characteristics of healthy, 158
  strengths, 174
  structures and functions of, 154-155,
    161, 162t
  tasks for survival and continuity,
    155t
  types of
    child bearing family, 157t-158t,
      168-169, 175t
    couple family, 157t-158t, 167-168,
      175t
    family with adolescents, 157t-158t,
      169-170, 175t
    family with middle-aged adults,
      157t-158t, 170-171, 175t
    family with older adults, 157t-
      158t, 171, 175t
    family with school-aged children,
      157t-158t, 169, 175t
    family with young adults, 157t-
      158t, 170, 175t
    with young, middle-aged and older
      adults, 157t-158t, 170-171,
      175t
  young adults starting, 533-534
Family nursing diagnoses
  purpose of writing, 171-172
Family of choice, 161
Farsightedness, 477, 557
Fat (s); See also obesity
  and cancer, 250-251
  changes with middle-age, 549
  Dietary Guidelines for Americans
    2005, 234, 236, 238b
  Healthy People 2010 goals for, 7, 8f
  and metabolic rates, 268-269
  MyPyramid guidelines concerning,
    236, 240f

Fat (s) (*Continued*)
   needed by infants, 384-388
   during pregnancy, 356-357
   during preschool years, 440-442
Fatalism
   definition of, 41
Federal Food Assistance Programs, 242,
   243t
Federal government
   health care responsibilities of, 60-61
   health policies of, 72-74
   role in health care, 58
Feedback
   within communication system, 83f,
     85
   importance to self awareness, 81
Fee-for-service
   in Canada, 62t, 71-72
   definition of, 56
   plans, 67
Feelings
   and families, 161
Feminist ethics, 104-105
Fertilization, 345
Fetal alchohol syndrome, 368
Fetal heart monitors, 351
Fetal hydantoin syndrome, 368
Fetuses
   cognitive-perceptual patterns of, 358-
     359
   definition of, 345
   early activity by, 357-358
   effects of biological agents on, 365-
     367
   effects of chemical agents on, 367-
     370
   elimination patterns, 355b, 357
   illustration of, 346f
   low-birth-weight, 410b
   physical changes in, 345-348
   sleep-rest patterns of, 358
   transition to newborn, 352-354
Fiber, 250-251
Fight-or-flight response, 278, 291
Filipinos
   cultural values
     concerning pregnancy and birth,
       350t
     and health issues of, 28-30
   expectations of children, 494
   folk medicine, 30
Financial factors; *See also* economics
   aging population, 61
   cost containment, 65
   costs (*See* costs)
   managed care issues, 65-66
   national and international
     expenditures, 61, 62t
   payment mechanisms, 64-65
   private insurance, 66-68
   public insurance, 68-70
   sources, 63-64
Firearms
   access to
     during young adulthood, 528-529

Firearms (*Continued*)
   death rates in black men from, 535
   safety, 535
   during school years, 487, 488
First stage of labor, 348
Fitness; *See* physical fitness
Flexibility
   definition of human, 262
   in exercise, 276, 277b-278b
   in functional communication, 86
Fluids; *See also* water
   hydration during exercise, 279-280
Fluoride, 385, 418
Folic acid
   during pregnancy, 356-357
Folk medicine
   in Asian American-Pacific Islanders,
     30
   description of healing, 27
   among Latino/Hispanic Americans,
     31-32
   and pregnancy, 359-360
   used by black/African Americans,
     33-34
Follicle-stimulating hormones, 503-
   504
Food Guide Pyramid, 236
Food safety
   causes of food-borne illnesses, 241
   Dietary Guidelines for Americans
     2005, 234, 236, 238b
   Mad Cow disease, 241
   practices to enhance, 241-242
Food Stamp Program, 242-243, 397
Food(s)
   additives, 404-405, 554
   and cancer, 250-251
   Dietary Guidelines for Americans
     2005, 234, 236, 238b
   family habits regarding, 156, 159-
     160
   Healthy People 2010 goals for, 7, 8f
   multicultural awareness of, 237
   during pregnancy, 356-357
   during preschool years, 440-442
   recommendations concerning, 234,
     235b, 236
   solid for infants, 386, 388
   during toddler years, 419-421
Formal operations, 510
Foster family care
   for homeless people, 38
Fourth stage of labor, 351
Free-market approach
   to health care in US, 61-62
Friends; *See* peer groups
Fruits
   Healthy People 2010 goals for, 7, 8f
   MyPyramid guidelines concerning,
     236, 240f
   during preschool years, 440-442
   recommendations for school-age
     children, 473, 474f
   safety guideline, 241-242
   sodium contents in, 248t

Functional
   focus
     of health patterns, 133
   as status of family health, 153
Functional health patterns
   activity-exercise pattern
     during adolescence, 510
     of communities, 183
     of families, 160
     of individuals, 136-138
     during infancy, 389-390
     during middle-age years, 555-556
     during older adult years, 577-579
     during prenatal period, 355b, 357-
       358
     during preschool years, 442-443
     during school years, 475-476
     during toddler years, 421-423
     during young adulthood, 531-533
   characteristics
     of communities, 179-182
     of families, 179-185
     of individuals, 132-133
   cognitive-perceptual pattern
     during adolescence, 510-511
     of communities, 184
     of families, 161
     of individuals, 139-140
     during infancy, 392-393
     during middle-age years, 556-557
     during older adult years, 579-582
     during prenatal period, 355b, 358-
       360
     during preschool years, 444-447,
       448t, 449
     during school years, 476-480
     during toddler years, 423, 424t,
       425-426
     during young adulthood, 532-533
   coping–stress tolerance pattern
     during adolescence, 515-516
     of communities, 185
     of families, 166
     of individuals, 145-146
     during infancy, 397-399
     during middle-age years, 562-564
     during older adult years, 585-586
     during prenatal period, 355b, 363
     during preschool years, 452-453
     during school years, 484-485
     during toddler years, 429
     during young adulthood, 538,
       540
   definition of, 132
   elimination pattern
     during adolescence, 509
     of communities, 183
     of families, 160
     of individuals, 135-136
     during infancy, 388-389
     during middle-age years, 555
     during older adult years, 576-577
     during prenatal period, 355b, 357
     during preschool years, 442
     during school years, 474-475

Functional health patterns (*Continued*)
 during toddler years, 421
 during young adulthood, 531
 framework, 131-132
 health perception/management
  pattern
  during adolescence, 506, 507b, 508
  of communities, 183
  of families, 158-159
  of individuals, 134
  during infancy, 384
  during middle-age years, 552
  during older adult years, 575
  during prenatal period, 354-356,
   355b
  during preschool years, 440
  during school years, 471-473
  during toddler years, 419
  during young adulthood, 525-526,
   527f, 528-529
 nutritional-metabolic pattern
  during adolescence, 508-509
  of communities, 183
  of families, 159-160
  of individuals, 134-135
  during infancy, 384-388
  during middle-age years, 552-555
  during older adult years, 575-576
  during prenatal period, 355b, 356-
   357
  during preschool years, 440-442
  during school years, 473-474
  during toddler years, 419-421
  during young adulthood, 529-531
 during pregnancy, 355b, 356-364
 rationale for use
  of individuals, 133
 roles-relationships pattern
  during adolescence, 512-513
  of communities, 184
  of families, 161-163
  of individuals, 141, 142t, 143-144
  during infancy, 394-397
  during middle-age years, 558-561
  during older adult years, 583-584
  during prenatal period, 355b, 361-
   363
  during preschool years, 449-451
  during school years, 482-483
  during toddler years, 427-429
  during young adulthood, 533-535
 self-perception-self-concept pattern
  during adolescence, 511-512
  of communities, 184
  of families, 161
  of individuals, 140-141
  during infancy, 393-394
  during middle-age years, 557-558
  during older adult years, 582-583
  during prenatal period, 355b, 360-
   361
  during preschool years, 449
  during school years, 480-481
  during toddler years, 426-427
  during young adulthood, 533

Functional health patterns (*Continued*)
 sexuality-reproductive pattern
  during adolescence, 513-515
  of communities, 184-185
  of families, 165-166
  of individuals, 144-145
  during infancy, 397
  during middle-age years, 561-562
  during older adult years, 584-585
  during prenatal period, 355b, 363
  during preschool years, 451-452
  during school years, 483-484
  during toddler years, 429
  during young adulthood, 535-538
 sleep-rest pattern
  during adolescence, 510
  of communities, 183-184
  of families, 160-161
  of individuals, 138-139
  during infancy, 390-392
  during middle-age years, 556
  during older adult years, 579
  during prenatal period, 355b, 358
  during preschool years, 443-444
  during school years, 476
  during toddler years, 423
  during young adulthood, 532
 values-beliefs pattern
  during adolescence, 516
  of communities, 185
  of families, 166-167
  of individuals, 146-147
  during infancy, 399
  during middle-age years, 564-565
  during older adult years, 586
  during prenatal period, 355b, 363-
   364
  during preschool years, 453-454
  during school years, 486
  during toddler years, 429-430
  during young adulthood, 540-542
Functioning
 in life, 6
Fundus, 347

G

Gallbladder disease
 associated with middle age obesity,
  552-553
Garden plants, 404t, 405b
Gastrointestinal system
 changes with middle-age, 549
 development in toddlers, 417
 flowchart of life cycle growth
  changes in, 332t
Gatekeepers
 definition of, 57b
Gays
 and alternative lifestyle stress, 546
 effected by HIV and AIDS, 39-42
 wellness series, 533, 534
Gender
 all effected by HIV and AIDS, 39-42
 and cancer rates, 590

Gender (*Continued*)
 and chronic illnesses
  in older men and women, 573t
 as communication barrier, 92
 and exercise, 282-283
 expectations and roles
  during preschool years, 449-450,
   451-452
 and fetal growth, 353
 and health, 4
 health disparities due to, 54
 issues
  during adolescence, 505-506
  during preschool years, 438
  in school-age children, 469-470,
   484
 and mortality rates, 550
 screening programs for different,
  207t, 208t
 and self-esteem, 343
 significance in infants, 382-383
Generativity, 557
Genetic counseling, 104b, 119, 383-
 384
Genetic defects, 346, 353, 364
Genetic impairments, 66, 540-541
Genetic testing
 ethical considerations concerning,
  119
Genetics
 defects, 346, 353-354, 364
 disorders during adolescence, 506
 effects on school-age children, 470-
  471
 and infants, 383-384
 during middle-age years, 550, 552
 research, 364
  and privacy rule, 115-116
Genital herpes virus, 529
 summary of, 539t
Genital warts, 539t
Genitourinary system
 health during pregnancy, 357
Genograms, 163, 164f
Genome Project, 364
Gentrification
 causing homelessness, 37
Geographical locations
 health disparities due to, 54
Geriatrics; *See* older adults
Germ theory, 53
Germany
 expenditures per capita and %GDP,
  62t
 universal health insurance coverage
  in, 72
Gestation
 illustrations of, 346f, 347f
 and low-birth-weight, 410b
Gilligan's theory of moral development
 description of, 341, 342t
Glaucoma
 in older adults, 557
 screening programs for, 207t, 208t,
  213-214

Global health
  challenges for 21st century, 600-615
  Health for All, 603-608, 605b
Goal setting
  and stress management, 305
Goals; *See also Healthy People 2010*
  direction in helping relationships, 89
  of families, 172
  learning, 225-226
Goiter, 232, 233t
Gonadotropin hormones (GnRF), 503-504
Gonococcus (GC), 366
Gonorrhea
  common in adolescents, 518
  summary of, 539t
Good health practices
  definition of, 4
Goodell sign, 347b
Gordon's functional health patterns;
  See functional health patterns
Gout
  during middle-age years, 550, 552
Government
  legislation concerning childbearing, 372-373
  official agencies of, 60-61
  role in health care reform, 56-61
  and special interest groups
    affecting quality and access to health care, 51
Grains
  Healthy People 2010 goals for, 7, 8f
  MyPyramid guidelines concerning, 236, 240f
  needed by infants, 384-388
  during preschool years, 440-442
  recommendations for school-age children, 473, 474f
  sodium contents in, 248t
Grieving process, 454
  for sudden infant death syndrome (SIDS), 391b
Gross domestic product (GDP)
  and per capita expenditures
    in US *versus* other countries, 62t
  percentage of health care in, 61, 62t
Group B *Streptococcus*, 366
Group processes, 84
Group screening, 200
Growth
  during adolescence, 503-506
  CDC charts with body mass index, 254-255, 338-339
  concept of, 330
  and development
    during infancy, 378, 379b-380b, 380t, 381-384
    overview of, 320-343
  developmental periods, 330t
  failure
    related to poor nutrition, 233t
  flowchart of changes through life cycle, 331t-336t

Growth *(Continued)*
  patterns of, 337, 338f
  rates
    during prenatal period, 345-346
    during preschool years, 437-438, 439t, 440
    during school years, 467-471, 470t
    during toddler years, 417-419
Growth and Access Increase for Nursing Students (GAINS), 44
Growth charts, 337-339
  for infants, 379b-380b, 381-384
Growth index, 382
Guided imagery, 320
Gynecomastia, 505, 506f

H

Habits; *See* lifestyle
Haitian Health Foundation, 613, 614
Halfway houses
  for homeless people, 38
Handwriting, 478-479
Hantavirus pulmonary disease, 529
Harmony
  in Native American health philosophy, 35-36
Hatha yoga, 317-318
Havighurst theory, 142t-143t, 556
Hazardous waste, 20, 21
Hazards
  occupational biological, 565, 566t
  structural, 430-431
  work-related, 542
Head Start, 397
HEADSSS assessment, 521b
Healers
  nurses as, 19
  used by black/African Americans, 33-34
Healing
  energies affecting, 312-313
  practices among Native Americans, 35-36
Healing circles, 319-320
Healing systems
  components of, 27
Healing touch (HT), 314-315
Health; *See also* health promotion
  definition of, 4
    among black/African Americans, 33
  developmental perspective of, 4
  within ethnic groups, 25-26
  exploring concepts of, 4-6
  history of the concept of, 4-5
  among homeless, 36-39
  improving prospects for, 20
  leading indicators of, 78
  models of, 5-6
  as philosophy of care, 4
  planning for, 7
  two major paradigms, 4-6
  as a value, 26-27

Health behaviors
  changing, 222-223
  definition of, 4, 222
  models for change, 186t, 191-192
Health belief model, 15, 222
Health care
  challenges of twenty-first century, 600-615
  delivery system (*See* health care delivery system)
  financial factors
    aging population, 61
    cost containment, 65
    costs (*See* costs)
    managed care issues, 65-66
    national and international expenditures, 61, 62t
    payment mechanisms, 64-65
    private insurance, 66-68
    public insurance, 68-70
    sources, 63-64
  Healthy People 2010 education objectives in, 218, 219
  history of
    early influences, 52-53
    among homeless, 36-39
    moving toward solutions, 20-21
    quality and access problems
      in United States, 51
    systems
      in other countries, 62t, 71-72
Health care costs
  definition of, 4
  escalation of, 4-5
  total personal expenditures, 62t
Health care delivery system
  definition and history of, 4-5
  health maintenance organizations (HMOs), 57-58
  history of, 51-56
  managed care, 57
  for middle-age adults, 567
  options for adolescents, 520-521
  organization of, 56-61
  physical fitness programs, 51
  political and economic influences, 54
  during prenatal period, 372
  private sector, 56-58
  public sector, 58-61
  quality and access problems
    in United States, 51
  skyrocketing costs in US, 609-610
  and toddlers, 434
  as topic on nursing national agenda, 73b, 74
Health care delivery systems
  in other countries, 62t, 71-72
Health care providers
  cultural challenges to, 3-4
Health care reimbursement account, 59
Health data
  sources in community, 180

Health disparities
  agencies that address, 42
  among Asian American-Pacific
      Islanders, 28-29
  in different population segments, 54
  and ethics, 100-124
  among ethnic groups
      and screening, 208-210
  globally, 605-607
  goals for reducing, 7-8, 51-52, 54
  among Latino/Hispanic Americans,
      30-32
  and nursing research, 19
  Racial and Ethnic Approaches to
      Community Health (REACH),
      42
Health ecology
  definition of, 6
Health education; *See* education
Health for All, 603-608
Health history
  behavioral, 527f
Health insurance
  versus assurance, 67
  in Canada, the United Kingdom and
      Germany, 62t, 71-72
  companies
      within private sector, 67
  lack of
      in black/African Americans, 32-
          33
      in ethnic minorities and poor
          communities, 26
      and homelessness, 37-38
      in Latino/Hispanic American
          communities, 31
  long-term care, 595
  for older adults, 594-595
  positives and negatives of US, 51-52,
      65-67
  public health and assistance
      Medicaid, 69-70
      Medicare, 68-69
  and special interest groups
      affecting quality and access to
          health care, 51
  the uninsured, 70-71
Health Insurance Portability and
    Accountability Act (HIPPA)
  addressing un- and underinsured, 71
  privacy rule, 115-116
Health literacy, 95
Health maintenance
  definition of, 4
  in school-age children, 496, 497t
Health Maintenance Organizations
    (HMOs)
  advantages and disadvantages of, 67
  definition of, 57b
  payment mechanisms of, 64-65
  structure and success of, 57-58
Health perception/management
    patterns
  during adolescence, 506, 507b, 508
  within families, 158-159

Health perception/management
    patterns (*Continued*)
  of the individual, 134
  of individuals, 134
  during infancy, 384
  during middle-age years, 552
  during older adult years, 575
  during prenatal period, 354-356,
      355b
  during preschool years, 440
  during school years, 471-473
  during toddler years, 419
  during young adulthood, 525-526,
      527f, 528-529
Health policies
  nursing influences on, 72-74
  in the United States
      history of, 58-61
Health problems
  in black/African Americans, 33
  in families, 156, 157t
  during preschool years, 454-460
Health promotion
  aimed at older adults, 571-596
  case study involving, 10-13
  challenges of twenty-first century
      developing country challenges,
          601-603, 606-607, 610
      global strategies, 602-603, 604-615
      HIV and AIDS, 602-603
      nursing education implications,
          612-613
      nursing implications and
          challenges, 612-615
      socioecological model, 606
      target populations, 606-507, 610
  in communities
      analysis and diagnoses within, 185-
          188
      data collection and information,
          180-181
      developmental perspective, 182
      evaluation phase, 193-194
      functional health patterns, 183-
          185
      implementation phase, 193
      nurse's role, 179-180
      nursing process, 179
      planning phase, 188, 191-192
      risk factor perspective, 182-183
      system's perspective, 181-182
  community health efforts
      concerning, 50-52
  definition of, 4, 15-16, 17b
  and education, 227
  ethics in
      case studies, 122-124
      decision-making strategies, 121-
          122
      health care ethics, 101-106
      principles of, 110, 112-120
      professional responsibility, 106-
          110, 111b
  and exercise, 261-286
  and the family

Health promotion (*Continued*)
  analysis and nursing diagnoses,
      167-172
  assessment of, 153, 156, 157t, 158
  care planning, 172
  caring for older adults, 152
  child bearing family, 157t-158t,
      168-169, 175t
  couple family, 157t-158t, 167-168,
      175t
  developmental perspective, 155-
      156
  evaluations, 175-176
  family with adolescents, 157t-158t,
      169-170, 175t
  family with middle-aged adults,
      157t-158t, 170-171, 175t
  family with older adults, 157t-
      158t, 171, 175t
  family with school-aged children,
      157t-158t, 169, 175t
  family with young adults, 157t-
      158t, 170, 175t
  functional health patterns, 156,
      158-167
  implementation, 172-175
  nursing process and, 153-154
  risk-factor perspective, 156, 157t-
      158t
  systems perspective, 154-155
history of, 54-56
importance of value clarification in,
    77-79
and the individual, 129-140 (*See also*
    individuals)
for individuals
  activity-exercise pattern, 136-138
  characteristics of, 132-133
  cognitive-perceptual pattern, 139-
      140
  coping–stress tolerance pattern,
      145-146
  definition of, 132
  elimination pattern, 135-136
  framework, 131-132
  health perception/management
      pattern, 134
  nutritional-metabolic pattern, 134-
      135
  rationale for use, 133
  roles-relationships pattern, 141,
      142t, 143-144
  self-perception-self-concept
      pattern, 140-141
  sexuality-reproductive pattern,
      144-145
  sleep-rest pattern, 138-139
  values-beliefs pattern, 146-147
for infants, 412, 413t
interventions
  during preschool years, 461, 462b
levels of prevention, 13, 14f, 15-17
making it real, 50-51
for older adults, 571-596
program incentives, 17

Health promotion (Continued)
  sources of resistance to programs,
    193t
  two strategies for, 16-17
  via telephone, 228
Health Promotion Center (HPC), 9
Health promotion models, 15
Health savings accounts, 59
Health teachings
  on anticipatory guidance, 340
  on assessing and treating obesity,
    15
  on awareness of genetics/test
    marketing, 119
  on breast and testicular self-
    examination, 514
  on breast-feeding
    methods of, 387
  concerning health promotion
    to preschoolers and school-aged,
      221
  on domestic violence, 155
  on effective discipline, 482, 483
  on exercise, 269
  on fad diets, 257
  for families, 221-222
  on Internet informational resources,
    66
  on Pender's health promotion model,
    210
  on problem solving
    in communication, 91
  on urinary tract infection
    prevention
    during pregnancy, 357
Healthy People 2000, 7, 51
Healthy People 2010
  28 focus areas of, 8b
  addressing health disparities, 51-52,
    54
  description and goals of, 42
  ethics goals of, 101
  focus on communities, 179
  focus on exercise, 262-264
  focus on families, 153, 156, 158
  focus on individuals, 130-131
  global goals of, 603-608
  goals and objectives of, 7, 8f, 51-52,
    54
    for adolescents, 503
    concerning education, 218, 219
    for hearing, 7, 8b
    for infants, 377
    for middle-age adults, 551
    for older adults, 573-574
    for preschoolers, 438
    for toddlers, 419-430
    for young adults, 525
  on holism, 312
  on infant mortality rates, 354
  Internet site, 8, 10
  progress made, 10, 52, 262-263
  screening objectives, 211
  ten leading health indicators, 233
Healthy pleasures, 304

Hearing
  changes in older adulthood, 581-582
  development of
    during infancy, 392-393
    in toddlers, 424t, 425
  flowchart of life cycle growth
    changes in, 332t
  Healthy People 2010 goals for, 7, 8b
  landmarks during preschool years,
    448t
  and noise pollution, 542
  during preschool years, 446
  during school years, 477-478
Hearing aids
  not provided for
    by Medicare, 68
Heart
  flowchart of life cycle growth
    changes in, 331t
Heart attacks; See heart diseases
Heart diseases
  in Arab Americans, 27-28
  associated with middle age obesity,
    552-553
  benefits of exercise for, 9, 265-268,
    265-269, 280
  caused by poor nutrition, 232, 235,
    245-247
  changes with middle-age, 549
  and diet, 232, 235, 245
  Healthy People 2010 goals regarding,
    7, 8b, 42-43
  Internet resources concerning, 66
  as major cause of death, 20
  during middle-age years, 550, 552
  and poor nutrition
    Healthy People 2010 goals
      concerning, 233-234, 235
  during pregnancy, 367
  screening programs, 207t, 208t, 213
  and stress, 562-564
  in women, 148
Heart rate (HR)
  during exercise, 274-275, 281
  in toddlers, 418
Heimlich maneuver, 401f
Helmets, 472, 541-532
Helping relationships; See therapeutic
    relationships
Hemophilia, 383
Hemorrhoids
  during pregnancy, 349t
Henry Street Settlements, 52, 56
Hepatitis B
  in adolescents, 518
  prenatal, 366
  in young adults, 529
Hepatitis C
  and drug abuse, 529
Herbal medicines
  and dietary supplements, 236-237,
    239
  questions to ask concerning, 3-4
  for stress, 298-299
  used by older adults, 586

Herbs
  used by Asian American-Pacific
    Islanders, 30
  used in black/African American
    medicine, 33-34
Heredity
  and birth defects, 383-384
  and disease, 156
Heroin, 543
Herpes simplex virus
  common in adolescents, 518
  during prenatal period, 365-366
Heterotropia, 446
High blood pressure
  associated with middle age obesity,
    552-553
  among black/African Americans, 33
  case study involving, 10-13
  caused by poor nutrition, 232, 233t,
    235, 247-250
  and diet, 247-250
  dietary and cultural aspects of, 247-
    248, 247-249
  epidemiology of, 247-248
  as major coronary risk factor, 265t
  and poor nutrition
    Healthy People 2010 goals
      concerning, 233-234, 235
  during pregnancy, 367
  during school years, 468
  screening programs for, 207t, 208t,
    213
  in young adults, 526
High-density lipoprotein (HDL)
  cholesterol, 266
High-level wellness, 5, 6f
  research on, 4
Hinduism
  and food, 237
Hispanics; See Latino/Hispanic
  Americans
HIV; See human immunodeficiency
  virus (HIV)
Hmongs
  cultural and heath issues of, 28-30
  women, 351
Holistic health strategies, 310-323
  aromatherapy, 322
  body work
    Bowenwork, 321
    craniosacral therapy, 321
    massage, 320-321
    Trager therapy, 321
  defining holism, 311-312
  energy work, 312-316
    acupressure, 313-314
    acupuncture, 313
    chi, 312-313
    healing touch, 314-315
    reflexology, 314
    Reiki, 315, 316
    therapeutic touch, 314
  guided imagery, 320
  for healing, 27
  meditation, 318-319

Holistic health strategies (Continued)
movement arts, 315-316
Qi Gong, 316-317
Tai chi, 317
yoga, 317-318
music therapy, 320
prayer and distant healing, 319-320
presence, 322
self-knowledge, 322
Holistic nursing
definition of, 130
Home
childproofing, 402b
Home health care
percentage of personal expenditures
for, 62t
Home visits
guidelines for, 153b
Homelessness
and alcohol/drug abuse, 535
as an emerging population, 24
children facing, 496
definition of, 36-37
and drug-resistant tuberculosis, 54
health care issues of, 38
during infancy, 396-397, 398
resources for, 38-39
strategies to address, 38-39
three characteristics of, 36
during young adulthood, 545-546
Homeostasis, 437
Homework, 467
Homicides
and alcohol excess, 235
confidentiality issues, 115
among Native Americans, 34
during young adulthood, 528-529,
535
Homosexuals
and alternative lifestyle stress, 546
homelessness among adolescent, 37
living with HIV and AIDS, 39-42
school-age
challenges facing, 483-484
wellness, 533, 534
Hormones
development during adolescence,
503-504
flowchart of life cycle growth
changes in, 336t
during pregnancy, 346-348
Hospitals
care
percentage of personal
expenditures for, 62t
history of, 54-55
and the uninsured, 71
Hot and cold concept of disease, 31
Human chorionic gonadotropin
(HCG), 346-347
Human immunodeficiency virus (HIV)
in adolescents, 518
and drug-resistant tuberculosis, 54
education of school-age children,
490-491

Human immunodeficiency virus (HIV)
(Continued)
Healthy People 2010 goals regarding,
7, 8b, 42
history of, 53-54
importance of early detection, 41
in Latino/Hispanic American
community, 30-31
and poor nutrition
diet interventions, 258
Healthy People 2010 goals
concerning, 233-234, 235
prevention and management of, 40-
42, 538
REACH goals for, 51
risks of
in homeless population, 38
in infants, 401-402
screening programs for, 208t, 214
statistics on people living with, 39-
40
transmission of, 538
in young adults, 529, 538, 539t
zidovudine (AZT) protocols, 366,
538
Human papilloma virus (HPV)
in adolescents, 518
in young adults, 529
Humor
aiding coping, 146
in communication, 86
and friendliness, 82
and stress management, 305-306,
307b
Humor Potential, Inc., 146
Hunchback, 549
Huntington's chorea, 383, 550
Hydantoin, 368
Hydration, 279-280
Hypercholesterolemia
as major coronary risk factor, 265t
related to poor nutrition, 233t
Hyperinsulinemia, 266, 267-268
Hyperlipidemia
case study involving, 10-13
Hyperopia, 477
Hypertension
case study involving, 10-13
caused by poor nutrition, 232, 233t,
235, 247-250
and diet, 247-250
dietary and cultural aspects of, 247-
249
epidemiology of, 247-248
as major coronary risk factor, 265t
and poor nutrition
Healthy People 2010 goals
concerning, 233-234, 235
during pregnancy, 367
during school years, 468
in young adults, 526
Hypnosis, 298-299
Hypophysis
flowchart of life cycle growth
changes in, 336t

Hypothalamus, 503, 504f
Hypothermia, 588t

I

Identity, 510-511, 512
Illiteracy, 187
Illnesses
definition of, 7
within wellness-illness continuum,
5, 6f
within ethnic groups, 25-26
Immigrants
and homelessness, 36-38
Immigration
factors influencing, 24-25
waves by Arabs, 27
Immune system
benefits of exercise for, 271-272
development in preschoolers, 438
development in toddlers, 418
Immunizations
during adolescence, 507b
in black/African Americans, 33
Healthy People 2010 goals for, 7, 8b,
9b, 78
during infancy, 377, 402-403
issues and controversies, 329
in older adults, 588
during preschool years, 457-458
REACH goals for, 51
schedules in toddlers, 418
and specific protection, 17
during young adulthood, 529
Impartialist perspective, 120
Implementation
with families, 172-173
of nursing plans, 149
phase
within communities, 193
Income
affluence, 496
disparities
and screening programs, 209-210
health disparities due to, 54
and nutrition, 242
and sedentary lifestyles, 264b, 282
Incontinence, 576-577
Indentured servitude, 25
Independent living, 592t-593t
Independent practice associations
(IPAs)
definition of, 57b, 58
Indian Health Service, 35
Indians
American (See Native Americans)
Individual-environmental focus
of functional health patterns, 132
Individualism
versus collectivism, 29, 31
versus community health, 51-52
Individuals
assessments and functional patterns
of
activity-exercise pattern, 136-138

Individuals *(Continued)*
  characteristics of, 132-133
  cognitive-perceptual pattern, 139-140
  coping–stress tolerance pattern, 145-146
  definition of, 132
  elimination pattern, 135-136
  framework, 131-132
  health perception/management pattern, 134
  nutritional-metabolic pattern, 134-135
  rationale for use, 133
  roles-relationships pattern, 141, 142t, 143-144
  self-perception-self-concept pattern, 140-141
  sexuality-reproductive pattern, 144-145
  sleep-rest pattern, 138-139
  values-beliefs pattern, 146-147
  screening programs for, 200
Inductive explanation, 453
Industry *versus* inferiority, 480
Infant mortality rates (IMRs)
  among Asian American-Pacific Islanders, 28-29
  among black/African Americans, 32-33
  Healthy People 2010 goals regarding, 42-43
  REACH goals for, 51
  risk factors contributing to, 410-411
  in United States, 353
Infants, 376-414
  accidents and injuries, 399-400
  age and physical changes in, 378, 379b-380b, 380t, 381-384
  attachment and bonding with, 394-395
  biological agents affecting, 401-403
  breast feeding, 385-388
  cancer in, 407
  car seats for, 376-377, 406
  chemical agents affecting, 403-406
  culture and ethnicity factors, 408-410, 411
  Erikson's theory of psychosocial development, 341t
  family income levels affecting, 411-412
  flowchart of growth changes with time, 331t-336t
  Gordon's functional health patterns in, 383-399
  growth and development of, 378, 379b-380b, 380t, 381-384
  homelessness, 396-397, 398
  immunizations of, 402-403
  legislation concerning, 410-411
  motor vehicle accidents injuring, 406
  nursing interventions, 411-412, 413t
  radiation, 406-407
  schedule of health care for, 413t

Infants *(Continued)*
  social processes affecting, 407-408
  sudden infant death syndrome (SIDS), 390-392
Infectious diseases
  before 1940, 4
  Healthy People 2010 goals for, 7, 8b
  history of, 52-54
  in homeless people, 38
Infertility, 536
Influenza, 53, 588
Informed consent, 113-114
Injection drug users
  and Hepatitis C, 529
  living with HIV and AIDS, 39-40
Injuries
  among black/African Americans, 33
  Healthy People 2010 goals for, 7, 8b, 9b, 78
  among Native Americans, 34
  in older adults, 587-588
  potential during exercise, 275
  during preschool years, 455-456, 462b
  risks of
    in homeless population, 38
  during toddler years, 431-434
Input
  of information, 83
Institute of Medicine (IOM), 52
Instruments
  for screening
    reliability and validity, 201-202
Insulin; *See also* diabetes
  and diabetes
    exercise benefits, 281-282, 283t
    hyperinsulinemia and exercise, 266, 267-268
Insulin-dependent diabetes mellitus (IDDM)
  and exercise, 266, 267-268, 281-282
Insurance; *See* health insurance
Integumentary system
  adaptive changes during pregnancy, 347
  changes with middle-age, 549
  flowchart of life cycle growth changes in, 336t
Intelligence
  abilities during middle-age, 556
  concept of, 479
  growth during young adulthood, 532
Intelligence quotient (IQ), 479
Intergenerational relationships
  among Asian American-Pacific Islanders, 29
Internal locus of control, 481
Internet
  as health education tool, 229
  therapeutic relationships in age of, 98
Interobserver reliability, 202
Interventions
  effectiveness measures in family, 176
  to facilitate behavior changes, 223

Interventions *(Continued)*
  and functional health patterns, 131-140
  for infant health promotion, 412, 413t
  for middle-age adults, 567-568
  nursing, 149
  for pregnant women, 372-373
  during preschool years, 461, 462b
  with school-age children, 498
  and treatment modalities and screening, 203-205
  types of family, 172-174
  via telephone, 228
Interview data, 180
Interviews
  for data collection, 180
Intraobserver reliability, 202
Intraocular pressure, 557
Intravenous drug users, 366
  and Hepatitis C, 529
Involuntary migration
  of black/African Americans, 32-34
  definition of, 25
Iodine
  diseases caused by deficiencies in, 233t
Iron
  diseases caused by deficiencies in, 233t
  during pregnancy, 356-357
  during preschool years, 440-442
Iron deficiency, 232, 233t
Irreversibility, 445
Ishihara's test, 446
Islam, 27, 237
Islets of Langerhans
  flowchart of life cycle growth changes in, 336t

J

Japanese
  cultural and heath issues of, 28-30
  folk medicine, 30
Johari windows, 79, 80f
Journal of Cultural Diversity, 43
Journal of Multicultural Nursing and Health, 43
Journal of Transcultural Nursing, 43
Journal writing
  and stress management, 299
Judaism
  and food, 237
  health and cultural aspects of, 27
Justice
  ethics of
    versus care, 105-106
  principle of
    in health care ethics, 120

K

Kant, Immanuel, 102
Kidney tumors, 460b

Kidneys
    development in toddlers, 417
    diseases
        Healthy People 2010 goals for, 7,
            8b
Klinefelter syndrome, 506
Kluckhohn's model, 26
Koch, Robert, 53
Kohlberg's theory of moral development
    description of, 341, 342t
    in school-age children, 486
    in young adults, 532-533
Koreans
    cultural and heath issues of, 28-30
    folk medicine, 30
Kwashiorkor, 232, 233t
Kyphosis, 549

L

Labor and delivery
    first pregnancy, 345
    health care options for, 372
    medications given during, 369-370
    overview of care during, 351-352
    signs of beginning of, 351t
    stages of, 348, 351
Lamaze childbirth, 348
Language
    during adolescence, 511
    barriers
        and health teaching, 223-224
    as communication barrier, 92-93
    development of
        during infancy, 393
        during preschool years, 447, 448t,
            449b
        during school years, 478
        in toddlers, 424t, 425
    and ethnicity, 25
    expressive and receptive, 424t, 447,
        448
    in families, 161
    juvenile interpreters
        ethical questions concerning, 100-
            101
    landmarks during preschool years,
        448t
    nursing sensitivity to, 410
Laotians
    cultural and heath issues of, 28-30
Latchkey children, 493b
Latino/Hispanic Americans (LHAs)
    and cancer, 550
    cultural and health issues of, 30-32
    cultural values
        affecting infants, 408-409
        and respect for older adults, 572
    employment trends, 31
    health paradox, 302
    HIV and AIDS among, 39-42
    as large uninsured population, 70-71
    as race category, 25
    REACH goals for, 51
    and sedentary lifestyles, 264b

Latino/Hispanic Americans (LHAs)
        (*Continued*)
    subgroups of, 30-32
    supernatural beliefs of, 31
Latinos; *See* Latino/Hispanic
    Americans
Lead poisoning
    in black/African Americans, 33
    in Hispanic children, 337
    risks for infants, 405
    screening programs for, 214
    in toddlers, 433
Leadership
    global challenges for nursing, 600-
        615
    as topic on nursing national agenda,
        73b, 74
Learning
    climate for, 227
    designing strategies for, 226-227
    general principles of, 221b
    levels of, 226
    during preschool years, 442-443,
        445b, 446b
    and teaching planning process
        assessments, 224-225
        evaluation, 227-228
        expected outcomes, 225b, 226
        learning strategies, 226-227
        referrals, 228
        selected content, 226
    three domains of, 226, 227
Learning disabilities, 479-480
Leavell and Clark's
    three levels of prevention, 13,
        14f
Lebanese, 27
Leg cramps
    during pregnancy, 349t
Legal issues; *See* legislation
Legislation
    aimed at adolescents, 520
    concerning childbearing, 372-373
    concerning infants, 410-411
    related to toddlers, 433-434
    for school-age children, 495
    as topic on nursing national agenda,
        73b, 74
Lesbians
    and alternative lifestyle stress,
        546
    wellness series, 533, 534
Leukemia
    in preschoolers, 459
    in school-age children, 492
Leukorrhea
    during pregnancy, 349t
Levels of prevention
    discussion of, 13, 14f, 15-18
Levinson's theory, 557
Libraries
    as information sources, 180
Lice, 490
Life
    functioning in, 6

Life cycle
    and developmental and wellness
        tasks, 142t-143t
    flowchart of growth changes through,
        331t-336t
Life expectancy
    in black/African Americans, 33
    during middle-age years, 550
    statistics for older adults, 572
Lifestyle
    case study involving, 10-13
    changes
        with health promotion, 16
        to lower cholesterol, 247
        with middle-age, 549
    creating an active, 283-285
    and exercise, 261-286
    of families, 153, 156
    health disparities due to, 54
    and HIV and AIDS, 39-42
    among Native Americans, 34-35
    and nursing research, 19
    and nutritional self-assessment, 231-
        232
    during pregnancy, 357-358
    programs to help change, 568
    responsibility for healthy, 9
    and stress, 290, 293
Limit-setting, 426, 454, 482
Listening
    importance of, 85-86
    and self awareness, 81
Lister, Joseph, 53
Liver disease
    cirrhosis, 232, 233t
    among Native Americans, 34
Living spaces
    of families, 154
Lobbying (and lobbyists), 73-74
Local government
    health policies of, 72-74
Long term care
    issues in older adults, 590-591, 592t-
        593t, 594-596
    options for housing, 592t-593t
    percentage of personal expenditures
        for, 62t
Low back pain
    benefits of exercise for, 270-271
    during pregnancy, 349t
Low-birth-weight
    risk factors, 410b
Low-density lipoprotein (LDL)
    cholesterol, 246
Low-income populations
    and exercise, 9
    health disparities in, 54
    lack of insurance in, 71
    and nutrition, 242
    screening disparities in, 209-210
    and sedentary lifestyles, 264b, 282
Lung cancer
    among black/African Americans, 33
    in middle-age adults, 549-550
    and smoking, 156

Luteinizing hormones, 503-504
Lyme disease, 529
Lymphoid tissue
  flowchart of life cycle growth
    changes in, 333t

M

Mad cow disease, 54, 241
Malaysians
  cultural and heath issues of, 28-30
Malnutrition
  in black/African Americans, 33
  maternal, 356
  from protein deficiency, 232, 233t
Managed care; *See* managed health
    care
Managed competition
  definition of, 57b, 59
Managed health care
  financial issues, 65-66
  organizations
    glossary of terms, 57b
    philosophy of, 57
Management-by-objectives, 7
Mapping, 186
Marketing
  direct-to-consumer
    of drugs and tests, 119
Mass screening, 200
Massage, 30, 320-321
Maternal mortality rates, 524
  among black/African Americans, 32-
    33
Maturation
  definition of, 340
Maximum heart rate (MHR), 274
Meals on Wheels, 244-245
Measurement data, 180
Meat
  MyPyramid guidelines concerning,
    236, 240f
  recommendations for school-age
    children, 473, 474f
  sodium contents in, 248t
Meconium, 352
Medicaid
  definition of, 69
  history of, 59
  origins of, 54
  spending, 61-64
Medical nutrition therapy (MNT), 256-
    257, 258t
Medical savings accounts (MSAs), 59,
    71
Medicare
  cost and quality concerns, 68
  and cost containment, 65
  costs of, 61-64
  description and evolution of, 68-
    69
  history of, 59
  for older adults, 594-595
  origins of, 54
  web resources, 74

Medications; *See also* prescription drugs
  causing congenital defects, 367
  given during labor and delivery, 369-
    370
Meditation, 30, 138, 278-279, 296-298,
    318-319
Memory
  development of
    during preschool years, 447
  lapses, 140
  during school years, 478-479
Men
  changes with middle-age, 549
  chronic conditions in older, 573t
  midlife crisis, 558
  role during pregnancy, 361-362
  screening guidelines for, 208t
  self-esteem *versus* women, 343
  sexual development of, 504t, 505-506
Menarche, 470-471, 497t, 504, 505,
    506f
Menopause, 549-550, 558, 562
Menstruation, 505, 506f
Mental health
  and adolescent substance abuse, 515-
    516, 518-519
  in Arab Americans, 28
  among Asian American-Pacific
    Islanders, 29
  benefits of exercise for, 261-262, 272
  among black/African Americans,
    33
  coverage in Canada, 71
  and economic status, 567
  and homelessness, 36-38
  during middle-age years, 558, 560
  among Native Americans, 35
  in older adults, 579-582, 585-586
  during pregnancy and fetal
    development, 359
  and stress, 298-300
Mental illnesses
  in Arab Americans, 28
  Healthy People 2010 goals for, 7, 8b,
    9b, 78
  in homeless people, 38
Mental retardation
  and infant genetics, 383
  and phenylketonuria screening
    programs, 207t, 208t, 211
Metabolic rates
  and exercise, 268-269
Metabolic syndrome, 247, 526-527
Metabolic system
  adaptive changes during pregnancy,
    347-348, 356
  during middle age, 552
Metacommunication, 84
Metaethics, 102-103
Mexican Americans, 30, 55, 210
  cultural values
    concerning pregnancy and birth,
      350t
  expectations of children, 494
  health paradox, 302

Middle-age adults
  age and characteristics of, 330t
  age and physical changes in, 459-
    551, 552f
  biological and chemical agents
    affecting, 565-566
  definition of, 549
  environmental factors affecting, 565-
    566
  Erikson's theory of psychosocial
    development, 341t
  families with, 157t-158t, 170-171,
    175t
  flowchart of growth changes with
    time, 331t-336t
  functional health patterns, 552-565
  Healthy People 2010 goals for, 551
  nursing interventions promoting
    health in, 567-568
  risk factors, 552-553
  sexual activity for, 561-562
  social processes affecting, 566-567
Midlife crisis, 558
Mild cognitive impairment (MCI), 579
Milk
  advantage of breast, 386b
  MyPyramid guidelines concerning,
    236, 240f
  needed by infants, 384-388
  during pregnancy, 356-357
  recommendations for school-age
    children, 473
  safety guideline, 241-242
Millennium Development Goals
  (MDGs), 605
Mind-body connection
  in Latino/Hispanic American
    culture, 30
  research during middle-age, 564
Mindfulness meditation, 318-319
Minerals
  needed by infants, 384-388
  during pregnancy, 356
Minimal wellness tasks, 142t-143t
Mini-Mental State Examination
  (MMSE), 580f
Mini-relaxations, 298, 307
Minorities
  as an emerging population, 24
  cultural issues in adolescent, 519-520
  HIV and AIDS among, 39-42
  and homelessness, 545-546
  Native Americans, 34-36
  Office of Minority Health, 43
  poor insurance coverage among, 31
  sexually transmitted diseases (STDs)
    in, 518
  in the United States, 24-34
Minority groups
  classification of, 25
  description of, 26
Minority Nurse Newsletter, 43-44
Model minority myth, 29
Monkey pox, 54
Mononucleosis, 518

Moral development
   in school-age children, 486
   during young adulthood, 532-533
Moral philosophy
   autonomy, 112-113
   definition of, 101-102
   limitations of, 102-104
Moral reasoning, 105
Moral theories
   religiously based, 102-103
Morals
   and autonomy, 112-113
   definition of, 101
Morbidity
   effect of health promotion on, 16-17
   risks with sedentary lifestyle, 262-263
   and stress, 293
Mortality rates
   disease-specific, 201
   effect of health promotion on, 16-17
   in middle-age adults, 549-550
   risks with sedentary lifestyle, 262-263
Motion
   at birth, 393
Motor development
   during school years, 470t
Motor vehicle accidents
   during adolescence, 178, 192t, 507b,
      516, 517
   and infant car seats, 406
   injuring school-age children, 489-490
   injuring toddlers, 431-432
   during pregnancy, 370
   and teen drinking and driving, 178,
      192t
Mucus
   suctioning of newborn, 352-353
Multicultural awareness
   African American youths "choosing"
      AIDS, 521
   and child behaviors, 494
   concerning lead poisoning, 337
   of cultural practices during
      pregnancy, 372-373
   culture and teaching, 223-224
   cupping and coining, 428
   facilitating transcultural education,
      45
   of foods and culture, 237
   LHA's self-assessments of health,
      134
   of Native Americans, 612
   nurse facilitation of, 409b
   personal cultural values
      affecting health care delivery, 8
   of poverty in racial and ethnic
      categories, 188
   preconception care, 168
   transcultural values and beliefs
      about health care, 55
Multiinfarct dementia, 579
Multiple test screening, 200
Muscle system
   flowchart of life cycle growth
      changes in, 334t

Muscular fitness
   definition of, 262
   and resistance training, 262, 276,
      277b-278b
Musculoskeletal system
   adaptive changes during pregnancy,
      347
   changes with middle age, 549
   effects of stress on, 291, 292f
   flowchart of life cycle growth
      changes in, 334t
   and food, 251-253
   importance of exercise for strong,
      264-265
   pain
      acupuncture to treat, 313
Music
   and ethnicity, 25
   therapy, 320, 321
Mutual storytelling, 452
Myocardial infarctions (MIs)
   case study involving, 10-13
   in women, 550
Myopic vision, 446, 477
MyPyramid, 234, 236, 240f, 440, 473

N

Nägele's rule, 345
Narcotics
   during pregnancy, 368
National Acupuncture Detoxification
   Association (NADA), 313
National Arthritis Foundation, 9
National Blueprint Project, 9
National Center for Complementary
   and Alternative Medicine, 3
National Center for Nursing Research,
   60
National Committee for Quality
   Assurance's Quality Compass, 66
National health care systems
   in other countries, 62t, 71-72
National Heart, Lung and Blood
   Institute's (NHLB)
   Obesity Education Initiative, 15
National Institute of Nursing Research
   (NINR), 19-20
National Institutes of Health (NIH), 60
National League for Nursing, 56
National School Lunch Program, 243
National Society for the Prevention of
   Blindness, 446
Nation's Health Dollar in 2002, 63f
Native Americans
   cultural values
      affecting infants, 408-409
      concerning pregnancy and birth,
         350t
      concerning respect for older adults,
         572
      and health care issues in, 34-36
   expectations of children, 494
   in harmony with nature, 35-36
   HIV and AIDS among, 40

Native Americans (Continued)
   multicultural awareness of, 612
   nutritional programs for, 244
   physical activity issues among,
      471
   REACH goals for, 51
   tribe health cultures, 36
   women
      substance abuse among, 34-35
Native Hawaiians, 28
Natural disasters, 25
Natural history
   and phenylketonuria screening
      programs, 211
Nature
   and health in Native American
      culture, 35-36
Nausea
   during pregnancy, 349t
Navajo, 34-36, 612
Nearsightedness, 477
Neighborhoods
   assessment of, 159
Nervous system
   cancer of, 459-460
   flowchart of life cycle growth
      changes in, 335t
Neuroblastoma, 459-460
New Deal, 58
New Federalism, 58
Newborns
   and phenylketonuria screening
      programs, 211
   stimulation of, 377-384
   transition from fetus to, 352-354
Nicotine
   causing congenital defects, 367-368
   use during middle-age years, 566
Night terrors, 423, 444, 476
Nightingale, Florence, 52, 130
Nightmares, 444
Nipah virus, 54
Nocturnal emissions, 505
Nocturnal enuresis, 474-475
Noise, 542
Noninsulin-dependent diabetes mellitus
   (NIDDM)
   and exercise, 266, 267-268, 281-282
Nonmaleficence, 117
Nonprofit organizations, 61
Nontraditional therapies
   complementary and alternative, 3-4
Nonverbal communication, 84
Normative theories
   of ethics, 102
North American Nursing Diagnosis
   Association (NANDA)
   defining nursing diagnosis, 131
   diagnosis classifications, 147
Nurse practitioners (NPs)
   origin of, 56
Nurses
   challenges of twenty-first century,
      600-615
   code of ethics, 107-108

Nurses (*Continued*)
　communication process for, 81-87,
　　89-93
　cultural awareness by (*See*
　　multicultural awareness)
　health promotion strategies for, 15-
　　18
　health teaching
　　on obesity and weight
　　　management, 15
　lobbying efforts for, 73-74
　pivotal roles of, 4
　policy decision making by, 73
　role of
　　in community health promotion,
　　　179-180
　　in health promotion, 18-19
　　in screening program design, 215
　social policy statement, 107b
　stress management strategy for, 304b
　transcultural role of, 55
　values of
　　versus patient's values, 77-78
　work environment of, 52
Nurses for Political Action Coalition
　(N-PAC), 73
Nursing; *See also* multicultural
　awareness
　ANA definition of, 130
　awareness by
　　of transcultural values and beliefs,
　　　55
　challenges of twenty-first century,
　　600-615
　costs of, 64
　facilitating transcultural awareness,
　　45
　health promotion by, 50-51
　history of, 51-56
　holistic strategies, 310-323
　home visits guidelines, 153b
　importance of communication in, 81-
　　87
　journals of, 43
　during labor and delivery, 351-352
　multicultural awareness (*See*
　　multicultural awareness)
　national agenda for future, 73b, 74
　Native American principles of, 36
　response of
　　to emerging populations and
　　　health, 43-44
　role in health care reform, 59
　transcultural, 26-27
　　models for, 44b
　two major paradigms of literature, 4-
　　6
Nursing assessments; *See also* functional
　health patterns
　aspects of, 131t
　of community functional health
　　patterns, 179, 183-185
　definition of, 147
　of families, 153-154, 156, 157t, 158-
　　167

Nursing assessments (*Continued*)
　of family self-worth, 161
　of the individual
　　activity-exercise pattern, 136-138
　　characteristics of, 132-133
　　cognitive-perceptual pattern, 139-
　　　140
　　coping–stress tolerance pattern,
　　　145-146
　　definition of, 132
　　elimination pattern, 135-136
　　framework, 131-132
　　health perception/management
　　　pattern, 134
　　nutritional-metabolic pattern, 134-
　　　135
　　rationale for use, 133
　　roles-relationships pattern, 141,
　　　142t, 143-144
　　self-perception-self-concept
　　　pattern, 140-141
　　sexuality-reproductive pattern,
　　　144-145
　　sleep-rest pattern, 138-139
　　values-beliefs pattern, 146-147
　of needs
　　through communication, 93
　of nursing process, 154
　of older adults, 576
　parameters of, 134
　questions to ask
　　of families, 159
　of screening target communities,
　　202-203
　services in care management, 65b
Nursing centers
　case study, 57
　function of, 56
Nursing diagnoses
　purpose of writing family, 171-172
Nursing homes
　percentage of personal expenditures
　　for, 62t
　types and functions of long-term
　　care, 592t-593t
Nursing interventions
　effectiveness measures in family, 176
　to facilitate behavior changes, 223
　to foster positive self-concept, 481b
　and functional health patterns, 131-
　　140
　for infant health promotion, 412,
　　413t
　for middle-age adults, 567-568
　for pregnant women, 373
　during preschool years, 461, 462b
　with school-age children, 498
　and treatment modalities
　　and screening, 203-205
　types of family, 172-174
　via telephone, 228
Nursing process
　and the community, 179-194
　in community health promotion,
　　187-188, 191-194

Nursing process (*Continued*)
　data collection
　　concerning individuals, 147-148
　definition of, 147
　and the family, 153-154
　planning and implementation
　　in families, 172-173
　planning care, 148-149
　role in family health promotion, 175t
Nutrition; *See also* diet; obesity
　counseling for health promotion,
　　231-259
　dietary excess and imbalance, 232
　dietary guidelines for good, 236,
　　238b-239b
　dietary reference intakes, 234, 235b
　dietary supplements and herbal
　　medicines, 236-237, 239
　diseases caused by poor
　　cancer, 232, 233t, 250-251
　　cardiovascular diseases, 232, 245
　　diabetes, 232-236, 233t, 255-258
　　heart diseases, 232, 235, 245-247
　　hypertension, 232, 233t, 235, 247-
　　　250
　　obesity, 232-236, 233t, 253-255
　　osteoporosis, 233t, 235, 251-253
　food guidelines, 234-236
　food safety issues, 241-242
　habits
　　in families, 156, 159-160
　Healthy People 2010 goals for, 7, 8f,
　　232-234, 235
　among homeless, 38
　and human immunodeficiency virus,
　　235, 258
　individual patterns of, 134-145
　MyPyramid, 236, 240f
　among Native Americans, 34-35
　and obesity in young adults, 529,
　　530f
　and poverty, 242-245
　during pregnancy, 356-357
　problems related to poor, 233t, 234,
　　235, 247-253
　programs
　　Federal Food Assistance, 242-243
　　Food Stamp Program, 242-243
　　low income women and children
　　　(WIC), 244
　　National School Lunch, 243
　　for older adults, 244-245
　　School Breakfast Program, 243-
　　　244
　requirements in infants, 384-388
　screening, 245
　self-assessment, 231-232
　during toddler years, 419-421
　vitamin toxicity, 239, 241
　vitamin-deficiency diseases, 232, 233t
Nutrition Program for the Elderly
　(NPE), 244-245
Nutritional-metabolic patterns
　during adolescence, 508-509
　within communities, 183

Nutritional-metabolic patterns
(*Continued*)
within families, 159-160
of individuals, 134-135
during infancy, 384-388
during middle-age years, 552-555
during older adult years, 575-576
during prenatal period, 355b, 356-357
during preschool years, 440-442
during school years, 473-474
during toddler years, 419-421
during young adulthood, 529-531

O

Obesity
assessing and treating, 15
benefits of exercise for, 266, 268-269
and body mass index, 254-255
case study involving, 10-13, 253, 254
childhood, 232
definition of, 552
and depression, 509
and eating disorders, 508-509
epidemiology of, 253-254
as growing health concern, 20
Healthy People 2010 goals
concerning, 7, 8b, 8f, 9b, 78, 233-234, 235
in middle-age adults, 552-553
and poor nutrition, 232-236, 233t, 253-255
during school years, 473-474
and size sensitivity, 256
statistics on, 530f
and stress, 290, 293
and television habits, 166
in young adults, 529-531
Object permanence, 423-424
Observation data, 180
Occupational health and safety; *See also* work
Healthy People 2010 goals for, 7, 8b
Occupational Safety and Health
Administration (OSHA)
employee health issues, 568
and work hazards, 542
Office of Minority Health, 43
Older adults, 571-596
age an physical changes in, 571
age and characteristics of, 330t
alcohol, drugs and tobacco use by, 588-590
assessment of, 576
biological agents affecting, 588
caring for, 152
continuum of care for, 591f
drug use among, 588-589
Erikson's theory of psychosocial
development, 341t
and exercise, 9
falls and accidents in, 586-588
families with, 157t-158t, 171, 175t

Older adults (*Continued*)
flowchart of growth changes with
time, 331t-336t
and glaucoma screening, 207t, 208t, 213-214
Gordon's functional health patterns
in, 575-586
health promotion goals for, 573-574
Healthy People 2010 goals for, 573-574
importance of exercise for, 264-265
long term care issues in, 590-591, 592t-593t, 594-596
loss of function in, 6
middle-agers caring for, 561
nutrition programs for, 244-245
pathological processes affecting, 586-587
respect of
in Asian cultures, 30-32
in different cultures, 572
in Latino/Hispanic American
cultures, 31
in Native American cultures, 35
and rising health care costs, 61-64
sex myths concerning, 145
sleep issues of, 579, 591
sleep patterns of, 139
social processes affecting, 590-591, 592t-593t, 594-596
and theories of aging, 574, 575b
US Census Bureau statistics on, 179
Omnibus Reconciliation Act of 1989, 68-69
One-test disease-specific screening, 200
Oral stage
of infant development, 378
Ossification, 460
Osteoporosis
benefits of exercise for, 264, 269-270, 577-579
and calcium, 554
caused by poor nutrition, 233t, 235, 251-253
epidemiology of, 251
and falls by older adults, 586-587
Healthy People 2010 goals for, 7, 8b
and menopause, 549
pathophysiology, 251-252
and poor nutrition
Healthy People 2010 goals
concerning, 233-234, 235
prevention of, 252-253
Otitis media, 417, 425, 437, 478
Ottawa Charter, 604, 606
Outcomes
from abuse during pregnancy, 361
community, 188, 191-192
in toddler limit-setting, 426
for weight loss, 258t
Outpatient care
definition of, 56
focus of HMOs on, 67
Output
of information, 83

Ovaries, 549
Overflow incontinence, 577
Over-the-counter drugs
using during pregnancy, 367, 368
Overweight; *See also* obesity
definition of, 253

P

Pacific Islanders; *See* Asian American-
Pacific Islanders
Papanicolaou (Pap) smear, 528t, 544
Parallel play, 422
Parathyroid
flowchart of life cycle growth
changes in, 336t
Parental divorce, 451, 485, 561
Parenting
in Asian American-Pacific Islanders, 30
breast-feeding and weaning, 385-388
consistent limit-setting, 426, 454
and divorce issues, 451, 485, 533-534
education agencies, 412b
and infant stimulation, 378-384, 389-390
during middle-age years, 558-559
tasks for infant development, 380t
values involved in, 540-542
by working parents, 493
Passive immunizations, 403
Passivity
versus assertiveness
in different cultures, 28-31
Pasteur, Louis, 53
Patient Self-Determination Act, 61
Patients
therapeutic relationships with, 77-98
Pattern focus
definition of, 132
Patterns; *See* functional health
patterns
Peabody Picture Vocabulary Test, 447, 449, 479
Pediculosis, 490
Peer groups
activity and exercise in, 475f
definition of, 473
importance to adolescents, 512-513
importance to school-age children, 492-493
and self-esteem, 481
sharing sexual information
during school-age years, 484
Pellagra, 232, 233t
Pender's health promotion model, 15, 191, 210
People with Arthritis Can Exercise
(PACE), 9
Per diem
definition of, 57b
Perceptual skills; *See* cognitive-
perceptual patterns
Periodontitis, 555

Pharmaceutical companies
  and special interest groups
    affecting quality and access to
      health care, 51
Pharmaceuticals; *See also* prescription
    drugs
  spiraling costs of, 70
Phenylketonuria
  screening programs, 207t, 208t, 211
Phonics, 478
Physical activities
  activity level goals, 272-273
  adherence and compliance with
    program of, 282-284
  during adolescence, 507b
  and aging, 264-265, 577-579
  anticipatory guidance for, 462b
  benefits of
    for coronary heart disease, 265-
      268, 280
    for diabetes, 281-282
    for immune function, 271-272
    for low back pain, 270-271
    for mental health, 272
    for obesity, 268-269
    in older adults, 577-579
    for osteoporosis, 269-270, 577-579
  case study involving, 10-13, 284-285
  climate that encourages, 284-285
  creating programs for, 283-285
  definition of, 262
  Dietary Guidelines for Americans
    2005, 234, 236, 238b
  and family risks, 156
  as functional health pattern
    of communities, 183
    of families, 160
    of individuals, 136-138
  Healthy People 2010 goals for, 262-264
  hydration during, 279-280
  importance of
    during middle-age years, 555-556
    during young adulthood, 531-533
  knowing *versus* doing, 261
  MyPyramid guidelines concerning,
    236, 240f
  by older adults, 577-579
  parameters of, 137
  physical activity pyramid, 274f
  precautions concerning, 279-280
  during pregnancy, 357-358
  relaxation response, 278-279
  risks of, 280-282
  and stress management, 299-300
  types of
    aerobic, 273-275
    flexibility, 276
    resistance training, 276, 277b,
      278b
    warm-ups and cool-downs, 275-
      276
Physical activity pyramid, 274f
Physical examinations
  not provided for
    by Medicare, 68

Physical fitness; *See also* exercise
  benefits of
    for coronary heart disease, 265-
      268, 280
    for diabetes, 281-282
    for immune function, 271-272
    for low back pain, 270-271
    for mental health, 272
    for obesity, 268-269
    in older adults, 577-579
    for osteoporosis, 269-270, 577-579
  definition of, 262
  Healthy People 2010 goals for, 7, 8b,
    9b, 78
  nursing promotion of, 51
Physician-assisted suicide, 585-586
Physicians
  Canadian, German, and the United
    Kingdom, 62t, 71-72
  percentage of personal expenditures
    for, 62t
Piaget's theory of cognitive
    development
  during adolescence, 510-511
  description of, 340-341
  and infant development, 378, 381-
    382
  during middle-age, 556
  during preschool years, 444-445
  during school years, 476-477
  stages of, 342t
  during young adulthood, 532
Pica, 357
Pituitary gland
  flowchart of life cycle growth
    changes in, 336t
Placenta
  definition of, 345
  elimination function of, 355b,
    357
Plague, 53, 54, 112
Plan for Your Young Child . . . The
    Pyramid Way, 420, 420f
Planning phase
  of nursing process
    addressing alcohol abuse, 192b,
      192t
    within communities, 188, 191-192
    with families, 172
    with individuals, 148
Planning process
  for teaching
    assessments, 224-225
    evaluation, 227-228
    expected outcomes, 225b, 226
    learning strategies, 226-227
    referrals, 228
    selected content, 226
Play
  during infancy, 389-390
  during preschool years, 442-443,
    445b, 446b, 452
  during school years, 475-476
  during toddler years, 421-423, 425
Pneumococcal infections, 588

Pneumonia
  among Native Americans, 34
Point-of-service plans (POS)
  advantages and disadvantages of, 67
  benefits of, 58
  definition of, 57b
Poisoning
  with garden plants, 404t, 405b
  lead, 337, 433
  in preschoolers, 458
  preventing in toddlers, 432-433
  safety, 455b
Polarity therapy, 316
Policies
  health
    nursing influences on, 72-74
    as topic on nursing national agenda,
      73b, 74
Policy decision making, 73
Political freedom
  opportunities and education, 24
Politics
  inequities for black/African
    Americans, 32
  influencing health care delivery
    system, 54
  and nursing, 73
Pollution, 20, 21, 492
  health effects to infants, 406t
  noise, 542
  reducing with bicycles/motorcycles,
    531
Poor laws, 53
Populations; *See also* demographics
  aging of
    and health, 20
  community concerns in different,
    187-188
  diversity of, 24
  effected by HIV and AIDS, 39-42
  emerging
    health in, 23-46
    rural and urban, 36-42
  health disparities in different, 54
  with sedentary lifestyles, 264b
  selection of screenable
    environment-dependent factors,
      210-211
    person-dependent factors, 206,
      207t, 208-210
  targeted for screening, 200
Positive reinforcement, 483
Positive signs of pregnancy, 346-347
Postconventional levels
  of moral development, 532-533
Postwesternization
  definition of, 28
Potassium
  Dietary Guidelines for Americans
    2005, 234, 236, 238b
Potentially dysfunctional
  as status of family health, 153
Poverty
  affecting black/African Americans,
    32-33

Poverty (*Continued*)
  among Asian American-Pacific
    Islanders, 29
  effect on school-age children, 495-
    496
  ethical considerations, 121, 123
  and exercise, 9
  health disparities due to, 54
  and HIV/AIDS, 40-41
  and homelessness, 36-38
    during young adulthood, 545-546
  and infant mortality rates (IMRs),
    411b
  influencing preschoolers, 461
  issues among Native Americans, 34
  in middle-age minorities, 567
  and nutrition, 242-245
  poor laws, 53
  and risks of uninsured, 71
  and sedentary lifestyles, 264b
Prana, 312, 317-318
Pranic healing, 315
Prayer
  by elderly Native Americans, 35-36
  research on effectiveness of, 319
Preconception care, 168
Preconventional levels, 486
Preferred provider organizations (PPOs)
  advantages and disadvantages of, 67
  and cost control, 58
  definition of, 57b
Pregnancy
  during adolescence, 510, 513-515
  alcohol use during, 129-130, 367,
    368
  biological infections, 365-367
  chemical agents affecting, 367-370
  cultural values related to, 350t
  duration of, 345
  emotions during, 359
  fertilization and implantation, 345
  fetal growth and development, 345-
    346
  Gordon's functional health patterns
    concerning, 354-364
  Healthy People 2010 goals, 354
  maternal changes and problems, 346-
    348, 350t, 351-352
    abuse during, 361
    body system changes, 347
    labor and delivery, 348, 351
    overview of, 351-352
    reproductive and other system
      changes, 347-348
    role development, 360
    signs of, 346-347
  mechanical forces affecting, 370
  normal discomforts during, 349t
  nursing interventions, 373
  pathological processes during, 364-
    370
  placental development and function,
    346
  probable and positive signs of, 346-
    347

Pregnancy (*Continued*)
  radiation affecting, 370
  rates
    in adolescents, 185, 190
    response to first, 362t
  social processes during, 370-372
  unintended, 536-537
Prejudice
  against minority groups, 26
  racial and slavery, 32
Premiums
  high costs of insurance
    causing high numbers of
      uninsured, 70-71
Prenatal care
  access to, 537
  teaching of, 344
Prenatal period
  biological infections during, 365-367
  and chemical agents, 367-370
  cultural values related to, 350t
  duration of, 345
  emotions during, 359
  fertilization and implantation, 345
  fetal growth and development, 345-
    346
  fetus to newborn transition, 352-354
  functional health patterns of, 354-
    364
  genetic impairments diagnosed
    during, 540-541
  Gordon's functional health patterns
    concerning, 354-364
  Healthy People 2010 goals, 354
  maternal and prenatal physical
    changes, 345-348, 349t, 350t,
    351-352
  mechanical forces affecting, 370
  normal discomforts during, 349t
  nursing interventions, 373
  pathological processes during, 364-
    370
  placental development and function,
    346
  radiation affecting, 370
  response to first pregnancies, 362t
  social processes during, 370-372
Preoperational stages, 423, 444
Presbyopia, 557
Preschool Readiness Experimental
    Screening Scale (PRESS), 447
Preschoolers, 436-462
  age and characteristics of, 330t
  biological or bacterial infections in,
    457-458
  building relationships, 451
  culture and ethnicity issues, 460-461
  development milestones in, 439t
  developmental testing in, 447, 449
  flowchart of growth changes with
    time, 331t-336t
  Gordon's functional health patterns,
    440-454
  injuries, burns and drowning, 455-
    457

Preschoolers (*Continued*)
  language development in, 447, 448t,
    449b
  pathological processes affecting, 454-
    460
  physical changes of, 437-438, 439t,
    440
  social processes of, 460-461
  teaching health promotion to, 221
Prescription drugs
  affordability of, 589
  costs of outpatient, 69
  coverage in Canada, 71
  dangers to infants, 403
  percentage of personal expenditures
    for, 62t
  plans, 69
  spiraling costs of, 61-62, 70
  used by older adults, 588-589
  using during pregnancy, 367-368
Presence, 322
Preventative ethics, 109-110, 111b
Prevention; *See also* screening
  case study involving, 10-13
  versus curative measures, 54-55
  efforts for young adults, 526
  and healthy lifestyles, 9
  importance in nursing, 130-131
  importance of screening to, 200
  key nursing role in, 50-51
  in Latino/Hispanic American
    communities, 31
  levels of, 13, 14f, 15-18
  and management of HIV/AIDS, 40
  primary
    definition and illustration of, 13,
      14f, 15-17
    and screening, 200
  versus treatment, 55
Primary appraisals, 295
Primary care
  definition of, 56, 57b
Primary care providers (PCPs)
  definition of, 57
Primary prevention
  definition and illustration of, 13, 14f,
    15-17
  and screening, 200
Primary sexual characteristics, 505, 506f
Privacy Rule, 115-116
Private health insurance, 67-68
Private sector
  of health care delivery system, 56-58
Probable signs of pregnancy, 346-347
Problem solving
  and ethical issues, 109
Professional care systems
  description of, 27
  percentage of personal expenditures
    for, 62t
Professions
  nursing as, 106
Progesterone, 345
Prospective payment system
  for Medicare, 65

Prostate cancer
associated with middle age obesity,
552-553
among black/African Americans, 33
in older adults, 590
screening
case study, 209
programs, 208t, 212-213
Proteins
diseases caused by deficiencies in,
233t
needed by infants, 384-388
during pregnancy, 356
Proxy decision making, 112b, 114
PSA screenings, 208t, 213
Psychiatric illnesses
in Arab Americans, 28
among black/African Americans,
33
Healthy People 2010 goals for, 7, 8b,
9b, 78
and stress, 298-300
Psychological health
among homeless, 38
during pregnancy and fetal
development, 359
Psychomotor skills
developed with play
during preschool years, 445b, 446b
Psychosocial development
assessment of
HEADSSS, 521b
theories of, 340, 341t
Psychotherapy
in Arab American communities, 28
Puberty, 467, 503-506
Public administration
in Canadian Health Act, 71, 72b
Public agencies
as information sources, 180
Public health
autonomy, 110, 112
Healthy People 2010 goals for, 7, 8b
history of, 52-54
new global movement, 606
nursing
goals of, 51-52
obesity issues in, 15
screening approaches, 203, 204
system
in US, 54
Public health insurance
and assistance
Medicaid, 69-70
Medicare, 68-69
Public relations
as topic on nursing national agenda,
73b, 74
Public sector
health agencies associated with, 58-
61
of health care delivery system, 58-61
Puerto Rico
cultural and health aspects of, 30
food culture of, 237

Punishment, 483
Puppet play, 452

Q

Qi, 312
Qi Gong, 315-316
Qualitative studies
in evidence-based practices, 20
Quality of life
focus of Healthy People 2010, 42-43
and health, 4-5
and health promotion, 15-18
Healthy People 2010 goals for, 7, 8f
and nursing research, 4, 19
responsibilities that go with, 9
and screening, 201
Quantitative studies
in evidence-based practices, 19-20
Quantity of life, 201
Quickening, 358

R

Race(s)
awareness development of, 438
classification of, 25
as communication barrier, 92
and culture of slavery, 32
definition of, 25
and exercise, 282-283
and fetal health, 353
and health, 4
and health disparities, 8, 54
and homelessness, 37
issues in school-age children, 470
and minority groups
hierarchy of, 26
screening programs for different, 208-
209
types of, 383
Racial and Ethnic Approaches to
Community Health (REACH), 42,
51
Racism
definition of, 8
and slavery, 32
Radiation
damage to infants, 406-407
ionizing, 565
during pregnancy, 370
and sun exposure, 531
x-ray exposure, 492
Rapid Assessment, Response, and
Evaluation (RARE), 42
Rapport, 88
Rating perceived exertion (RPE), 274,
275f
Receptive language
during adolescence, 511
definition of, 447
during preschool years, 447, 448t
during toddler years, 424t
Reciprocity
in communication, 86

Recommended Daily Allowances
(RDAs), 234, 235b
Recruitment
as topic on nursing national agenda,
73b, 74
Referrals
educational resource, 228
Reflection
communication technique of, 90
definition of, 81
and nursing ethics, 121-122
Reflexology, 298-299, 314
Refractive errors, 446
Refugees
definition of, 24-25
Regulations
health care, 73
as topic on nursing national agenda,
73b, 74
Rehabilitation
following strokes, 18
with tertiary prevention, 13, 14f, 15-
18
Rehearsals, 478-479
Reiki, 315, 316, 322
Reimbursements
definition of, 57b
Relationship stages, 94-95
Relaxation response (RR)
definition of, 278
exercise and, 278-279
and stress, 296-298
Relaxation techniques
in Asian culture, 30
exercises, 138
and stress management, 296-298
Reliability
of screening instruments, 202
Religion; See also faith communities
as communication barrier, 92
in elderly Native Americans, 35-36
and ethnicity, 25
and food culture, 237
among Latino/Hispanic Americans,
31
nursing sensitivity to, 410
and prayer
by elderly Native Americans, 35-
36
research on effectiveness of, 319
Religious freedom
opportunities and education, 24
Reproductive system
adaptive changes during pregnancy,
347-348
flowchart of life cycle growth
changes in, 335t
and infertility, 536
Research; See also research highlights
challenges of twenty-first century,
613-615
on developmental perspective of
health, 4-5
importance of, 4
and privacy rule, 115-116

Research (*Continued*)
  studies on behavioral interventions, 19
  on wellness-illness continuum, 4
  working with ethnic groups, 24
Research highlights
  on advance directives for adolescents, 113
  on behavioral interventions, 19
  on bicycle injuries and safety helmets, 182
  on domestic violence, 163
  on faith and prayer
    and health of elderly Native Americans, 35
  on health promotion via telephone, 228
  on Hispanics with chronic diseases, 60
  on music therapy, 321
  on Native Americans
    physical activity issues, 471
  on nurse cancer survivors, 293
  on nursing communication, 82
  on reducing falling in women with strength training, 270
Researchers
  nurses as, 19
Residential services
  for mentally ill homeless people, 38
Resistance
  as communication barrier, 93
Resistance training
  description of, 276
  guidelines for, 277b-278b
Respiratory system
  adaptive changes during pregnancy, 347
  diseases
    Healthy People 2010 goals for, 7, 8b
  flowchart of life cycle growth changes in, 333t
Responsibility
  acceptance of
    for healthy lifestyles, 9, 16
Rest; *See also* sleep-rest patterns
  habits in families, 160-161
Resting heart rate (RHR), 274
Restoration
  with tertiary prevention, 13, 14f, 15-18
Retinoblastoma, 459
Retirement communities, 592t-593t
Rh blood group incompatibility, 367
Ricin, 54
Rickets, 16, 385
Risk factors
  assessment of
    in families, 156, 157t
    in individuals, 148
  for cardiovascular diseases
    and Healthy Start program, 442
  for low-birth-weight, 410b
  during middle-age years, 552
  screening to identify, 199-200

Risk factors (*Continued*)
  theories
    in families, 156
    within nursing process, 153
Risks
  during adolescence, 502, 503, 506, 508, 518
  areas for older adults, 587t
  and cancer, 250-251
  and ethical dilemmas, 109
  within families, 153, 154, 156
  global populations with greatest, 611
  with sedentary lifestyle, 262-263
Risk-taking behaviors
  during adolescence, 502, 503, 506, 508, 518
Rituals, 423, 443-444
Robert Wood Johnson Foundation, 9, 70
Role performance model
  of health, 5
Roles-relationships patterns
  addressing alcohol abuse, 192b
  during adolescence, 512-513
  case study involving, 143, 144
  in communities, 184
  description of, 141, 143-144
  of families, 161-163
  of individuals, 141, 142t, 143-144
  during infancy, 394-397
  during middle-age years, 558-561
  during older adult years, 583-584
  during prenatal period, 355b, 361-363
  during preschool years, 449-451
  during school years, 482-483
  during toddler years, 427-429
  during young adulthood, 533-535
Rosenstock's model, 191
Rubella, 365, 529
Rural populations, 36-42

S

Safety
  automobile precautions, 407b
  car seats, 376-377, 406
  concerns for school-age children, 487
  firearm, 535
  issues during school years, 472, 487-492
  issues for preschoolers, 455b
  and Occupational Safety and Health Administration (OSHA), 7, 8b, 542, 568
  risk areas for older adults, 587t
  tips to prevent infant falls, 400b
  during toddler years, 433-434
Salmonella typhimurium, 54
Salt; *See also* sodium
  MyPyramid guidelines concerning, 236, 240f
  during preschool years, 440-442
Same-sex marriage, 533, 534

Same-sex partners (couples)
  and alternative lifestyle stress, 546
  legal rights of, 533
  wellness series, 534
Sanitarians, 55
Sanitary engineering, 53
Sanitation
  history of, 53
  and infectious diseases, 55
Sarin, 54
Satellite housing
  for homeless people, 38
Scabies, 490
School Breakfast Program, 243
School nurses
  treating adolescents, 520-521
  treating school-age children, 498-499
School-age children, 466-499
  age and characteristics of, 330t, 467-470
  encopresis, 475
  enuresis, 474-475
  Erikson's theory of psychosocial development, 341t
  families with, 157t-158t, 169, 175t
  flowchart of growth changes with time, 331t-336t
  gender issues in, 469-470
  Gordon's functional health patterns in, 471-486
  health maintenance of, 496b
  health perceptions of, 471-473
  homework procrastination by, 467
  moral development of, 486
  motor development of, 470t
  nutrition and obesity issues in, 473-474
  pathological processes affecting, 486-492
  physical changes with age, 467-470
  play activities of, 475-476
  race issues in, 470
  social processes affecting, 492-497
  teaching health promotion to, 221
  well-child care, 496
Schools
  clinics in, 520-521
  exercise in, 285
  Healthy People 2010 education objectives in, 218, 219
  and the nurse, 498-499, 520-521
Scoliosis, 504, 505f
Screening, 199-215; *See also* prevention
  of adolescents, 507b
  advantages and disadvantages of, 200-201
  concept of, 200
  conditions commonly chosen for, 211-215
    breast cancer, 212, 590
    cervical cancer, 212
    cholesterol, 213
    colorectal cancer, 212
    diabetes mellitus, 214-215
    glaucoma, 213-214

Screening (*Continued*)
  human immunodeficiency virus
    (HIV), 214
  hypertension, 213
  lead poisoning, 214
  phenylketonuria, 211
  prostate cancer, 212-213, 590
  ethical and financial considerations
    cost-benefit ratio, 206
    cost-effectiveness and efficiency,
      206
    economic ethics, 205-206
    health care ethics, 205
  to identify risk factors, 199-200
  instruments for
    reliability and validity, 201-202
  men's guide to recommended, 208t
  for middle-age adults, 553b
  nurse's role in, 215
  nutritional, 245
  partnerships, 203, 204
  populations selected for, 206, 207t,
    208-211
  of preschoolers, 456
  and prevention, 200
  for scoliosis, 504, 505f
  as secondary prevention, 14f, 17
  selection of diseases for, 201-205
  women's guide to recommended,
    207t
  of young adults, 528t
Scurvy, 232, 233t
Second stage of labor, 348, 351
Secondary appraisals, 295
Secondary prevention
  description and illustration of, 14f,
    17
  and screening, 200
Secondary sexual characteristics, 505,
  506f
Sedentary lifestyles
  as major coronary risk factor, 265t
  during middle age, 549
  populations at risk for, 264b
Self
  therapeutic use of
    components of, 80b
    Johari windows, 80f
Self-assessment
  of nutritional status, 231-232
Self-awareness
  description of, 79-81
  ethical, 103
  and holistic health, 322-323
  Johari windows, 79, 80f
  and stress management, 295-296,
    297f
Self-concept
  definition and evolution of, 79
  development of
    during adolescence, 511-512
    in school-age children, 480-481
  of families, 161
  fostering positive
    in school-age children, 482b

Self-disclosure, 81
Self-efficacy
  and health behaviors, 222-223
  and health promotion, 15
Self-esteem
  and body image, 511-512
  definition and evolution of, 79, 480
  development of
    during adolescence, 511-512
    during preschool years, 449,
      452
    in school-age children, 480-481
  in males *versus* females, 343
  during middle-age, 558, 560
  and obesity, 553
Self-funded plans, 67
Self-insurance
  advantages and disadvantages of, 67-
    68
  description of, 67
Self-knowledge
  and holistic health, 322
Self-perception-self-concept patterns
  during adolescence, 511-512
  affecting progress toward tasks, 142t-
    143t
  of communities, 184
  within communities, 184
  of families, 161
  of individuals, 140-141
  during infancy, 393-394
  during middle-age years, 557-558
  during older adult years, 582-583
  during prenatal period, 355b, 360-
    361
  during preschool years, 449
  during school years, 480-481
  during toddler years, 426-427
  during young adulthood, 533
Self-reflection
  description of, 80-81
  ethical, 103, 122
  with journaling, 299
Self-worth
  and families, 161
Semantics, 478
Senses
  changes in older adults, 581-582
  development during preschool years,
    446-447
  flowchart of life cycle growth
    changes in, 332t
Sensitivity
  to criticism
    during preschool years, 449
  of screening tests, 202
Sensorimotor stages, 423
Sensory barriers, 93
Sensory perception
  during older adult years, 581-582
  during preschool years, 446-447
  during school years, 478
Separation, 533-534
September 1, 2001, 24, 52
Serum lipid levels, 246t, 266

Seventh Day Adventists
  and food, 237
Severe acute respiratory syndrome
  (SARS), 529, 602, 609
Severe acute respiratory syndrome-
  associated coronavirus, 54
Sewage systems
  sanitary, 16
Sex
  behaviors
    by adolescents, 507b
    biological infections from, 365-367
  curiosity about
    during preschool years, 452
  education, 484
  goals for responsible, 78
  history
    and HIV screening, 208t, 214
  individual patterns of, 144-145
  in middle-age, 561-562
  in older adults, 584-585
  primary and secondary
    characteristics, 505, 506f
  teaching safe-sex skills, 41-42
Sexual abuse
  and homelessness, 37
  of school-age children, 483
Sexual identity
  issues during school age years, 484
  and the workforce, 533, 534
Sexual maturity ratings
  of adolescents, 502t, 505
Sexual orientation
  children struggling with, 484
  health disparities due to, 54
  wellness series, 533, 534
Sexuality
  challenges for homosexual children,
    484
  definition of, 144
  and families, 165-166
  in older adults, 145, 584-585
  and television habits, 166
Sexuality-reproductive patterns
  during adolescence, 513-515
  of communities, 184-185
  of families, 165-166
  of individuals, 144-145
  during infancy, 397
  during middle-age years, 561-562
  during older adult years, 584-585
  during prenatal period, 355b, 363
  during preschool years, 451-452
  during school years, 483-484
  during toddler years, 429
  during young adulthood, 535-538
Sexually transmitted diseases (STDs)
  common in adolescents, 518
  education
    and HIV and AIDS, 39-42
  Healthy People 2010 goals for, 7, 8b,
    9b
  in homeless people, 38
  in pregnant women, 355, 366
  and stress, 290

Sexually transmitted diseases (STDs) (*Continued*)
summary of selected, 539t
in young adults, 538, 539t
Shaman, 36
Shelters
for abused women, 155, 163
homeless, 36-38
Shiatsu, 314
Siblings
preparing for newborn, 362b
Sickle cell anemia, 156, 201, 353, 383
Silence
during communication, 86
Single-payer arrangements, 71-72
Situational crises, 398-399
Skeletal system
flowchart of life cycle growth changes in, 334t
Skid row, 36, 37
Skin
changes with middle-age, 549
elimination patterns
of communities, 183
of families, 160
of individuals, 135-136
flowchart of life cycle growth changes in, 336t
wrinkles and xerosis in middle-age, 558
Slavery
history of, 32
Sleep
creating safe environment for, 455b
disturbances
associated with middle age obesity, 552-553
during infancy, 390t
during older adulthood, 579, 591
Sleep hygiene
and stress management, 300
Sleep talking, 476
Sleep-rest patterns
during adolescence, 510
of communities, 183-184
of families, 160-161
of individuals, 138-139
during infancy, 390-392
during middle-age years, 556
during older adult years, 579
during prenatal period, 355b, 358
during preschool years, 443-444
during school years, 476
during toddler years, 423
during young adulthood, 532
Sleepwalking, 476
Smallpox, 53, 54
Smell
at birth, 393
changes in older adulthood, 582
development in toddlers, 426
Smoking
and accidents, 560
by adolescents, 518-519

Smoking (*Continued*)
American Cancer Society's efforts on, 61
anticipatory guidance for prevention of, 462b
case study involving, 10-13
cessation programs
globally, 610
for older adults, 571-572
during pregnancy, 369
causing congenital defects, 367-368
effect of health promotion on, 16-17
as growing health concern, 20
Healthy People 2010 goals for, 7, 8b, 9b, 78
as leading cause of preventable death, 544
and lung cancer
in families, 156
as major coronary risk factor, 265t
among Native Americans, 34-35
by older adults, 571-572, 589-590
during school years, 491-492
and stress, 293
by young adults, 544
Snellen E chart, 446
Social cognitive theory, 222-223
Social isolation
and alcohol/drug abuse, 535
Social justice, 120
Social learning theories, 222-223
Social marketing
definition of, 224
Social processes
affecting adolescents, 519-521
affecting young adults, 544-545
and day care for infants, 407-408
during pregnancy, 370-371
during preschool years, 460-461
in school-age children, 492-493
support
and stress management, 302
Social Security Act (SSA), 54
Socialization, 492
Socioecological model, 606
Socioeconomic factors
affecting AIDS/HIV prevention, 40
among Asian American-Pacific Islanders, 29
in black/African American communities, 33
changes and health improvements, 20
as communication barrier, 92
and health, 4
history and influence on health, 53
issues among Native Americans, 34
in Latino/Hispanic American communities, 30
Socioeconomic status
health disparities due to, 54
and minority groups, 26

Sodium
contents in foods, 248t
Dietary Guidelines for Americans 2005, 234, 236, 238b
diets high in, 554
Healthy People 2010 goals for, 7, 8f
MyPyramid guidelines concerning, 236, 240f
Somatization, 485-486
Space
between communicators, 86-87
zones of, 87b, 88f
Special interest groups, 51
Specific protection, 13, 14f, 17
Specificity, 202
Speech; *See also* language
development in toddlers, 424t, 425
landmarks during preschool years, 448t
Sperm, 345
Spiritual distress
case study involving, 143, 144
Spiritual healing
among Latino/Hispanic Americans, 31
practice of stress management with, 304-305
questions to ask concerning, 3-4
Spirituality
among black/African Americans, 33
changes during pregnancy, 363-364
and stress management, 293, 304-305
Spontaneous abortion, 364
Sports; *See also* physical activities
activities during young adulthood, 531-532
hazards to toddlers, 431
safety issues, 455b, 487, 488
Sports drinks, 279, 280t
Stages of change theories, 15
Stagnation, 557
Stanford-Binet Test, 479
Staphylococcus aureus, 54
State Children's Health Insurance Program (SCHIP), 59, 61, 71
State governments
health policies of, 72-74
and Medicaid, 69-70
role in health care, 58, 60
Station, 348
Step Up to Health, 9
Strabismus, 425, 446
Streptococcus, 366
Streptococcus pneumoniae, 54
Stress
achievement, 540
assessment of, 294-295
benefits of exercise on, 272
definition of, 290
and family risks, 156
health benefits of managing, 293-294
and heart disease, 562-564
infant, 398, 399b
management of (*See* stress management)

Stress (*Continued*)
  physiological effects of, 291-292
  during pregnancy, 358-360
  psychological effects of, 292-293
  response, 291, 292f
  sociobehavioral effects of, 293
  sources of, 290-291
  spiritual effects of, 293
  strategies for reducing, 295-306
  tolerance patterns, 145-146
  warning signs, 295-296, 297f
  Yerkes-Dodson Law, 291f
  in young adults, 538, 540
Stress incontinence, 577
Stress management, 289-307
  assessment of, 294-295
  and effective coping, 306-307
  goals of, 290
  health benefits of, 293-294
  and humor, 146
  interventions, 296-306
    affirmations, 301-302
    alternative/complementary
        therapies, 298-299
    assertive communication, 302-
        303
    cognitive restructuring, 300-301
    empathy, 303-304
    exercise, 272, 299-300
    goal setting, 305
    healthy diet, 299
    healthy pleasures, 304
    humor, 305-306, 307b
    journal writing, 299
    relaxation techniques, 296-299
    self-awareness, 296, 297f
    sleep hygiene, 300
    social support, 302
    spirituality, 304-305
    values clarification, 305
  strategy for nurses, 304b
Stressors
  categories of, 290-291
  definition of, 290
Stretching
  in exercise routine, 275-276, 277b-
      278b
Strokes
  in black/African Americans, 550
  dietary interventions for prevention
      of, 248-249
  effect of exercise on, 9
  Healthy People 2010 goals regarding,
      7, 8b, 42-43
  as major cause of death, 20
  rehabilitation following, 18
  screening programs, 207t, 208t, 213
Structural hazards, 430-431
Substance abuse; *See also* alcohol abuse;
      drug abuse
  acupuncture for, 313
  by adolescents, 507b, 518b
  Healthy People 2010 goals for, 7, 8b,
      9b, 78
  and HIV and AIDS, 39-41
  and homelessness, 36-38

Substance abuse (*Continued*)
    among Native Americans, 34-35
    warning signs in adolescents, 518b
Subtle energy, 312
Sudden infant death syndrome (SIDS)
    description and statistics, 390-392
    Healthy People 2010 goals to reduce,
        377
Sugar
    during preschool years, 440-442
Sugars
    MyPyramid guidelines concerning,
        236, 240f
Suicide
    during adolescence, 515-516, 521
    and alcohol excess, 235
    confidentiality issues, 115
    among Native Americans, 34
    in older adults, 585-586
    physician-assisted, 585-586
    risks of
        in homeless population, 38
    warning signs
        in young adulthood, 528-529, 535,
            540
Sulfonamides, 53
Sun exposure, 531
Supplemental Security Income (SSI),
    69
Swallowing
    development in toddlers, 418
    of foreign objects during infancy,
        401
Symbols
    and ethnicity, 25
Syntax, 478
Syphilis
    common in adolescents, 518
    summary of, 539t
Syrians, 27
Systems theory
    of community, 181
    within families, 154-155
    within nursing process, 153
Systolic blood pressure
    changes during middle-age, 562-
        563
    and diet, 249
    screening programs for, 207t, 208t,
        213

T

T-ACE test, 129-130
Tachycardia, 351
Tactile system
    at birth, 393
    flowchart of life cycle growth
        changes in, 332t
    as nonverbal communication, 86
Tai Chi, 272, 279, 317
Tanger Center for Health Management,
    534
Tanner stages of sexual development,
    502t, 505
Taoism, 30

Target populations; *See also Healthy
        People 2010*
    global populations with greatest risk,
        610-611
    during school years, 472
    in social marketing, 224
Tasks
    family developmental, 155
Taste
    at birth, 393
    changes in older adulthood, 581-582
    development in toddlers, 426
    lessening during middle-age, 557
Tattooing, 511
Tay-Sachs disease, 156, 383
Teaching
    health education to families, 221-222
    and organizing skills, 228-229
    planning process
        assessments, 224-225
        evaluation, 227-228
        expected outcomes, 225b, 226
        learning strategies, 226-227
        preparation of, 225
        referrals, 228
        selected content, 226
Teenagers; *See* adolescents
Teeth
    during adolescence, 504
    development in toddlers and
        preschoolers, 418, 438
    development of deciduous and their
        sequence of eruption, 486f
    development of permanent and their
        sequence of eruption, 486f
    learning basic brushing of, 418b
    of older adults, 582
Television
    effects of
        on sexuality, violence and obesity,
            166
    influence on school-age children,
        494
Temperament
    of preschoolers, 452-453
    during toddler years, 430
Temporary Assistance for Needy
        Families (TANF), 64, 69, 411b
Teratogen, 356
Terminal illnesses, 548
Terrible twos, 416, 430
Terrorists attacks, 24, 52
Tertiary prevention, 14f, 18
Testicular self-examination (TSE), 514,
    526
Testosterone, 503, 504f
Thailand
    cultural and heath issues of, 28-30
Thalidomide, 367
The Humor Potential, Inc., 146
The Wellness Community, 174
Theory of reasoned action, 15
Therapeutic relationships, 77-98
    characteristics of, 87-89
    communication barriers, 91-93
    communication process, 81-87, 89-93

Therapeutic relationships (*Continued*)
  development of, 87
  ethics in, 89
  and the Internet, 98
  settings for, 93
  stages of, 94-95
  techniques, 89-91
  values clarification in, 77-81
Therapeutic touch (TT), 30, 314
Therapeutic use of self, 79-80
Thiamine
  diseases caused by deficiencies in, 233t
Third stage of labor, 351
Thyroid gland
  flowchart of life cycle growth changes in, 336t
Tobacco use
  and accidents, 560
  by adolescents, 518-519
  American Cancer Society's efforts on, 61
  anticipatory guidance for prevention of, 462b
  case study involving, 10-13
  cessation programs
    globally, 610
    for older adults, 571-572
    during pregnancy, 369
  causing congenital defects, 367-368
  effect of health promotion on, 16-17
  as growing health concern, 20
  Healthy People 2010 goals for, 7, 8b, 9b, 78
  as leading cause of preventable death, 544
  and lung cancer
    in families, 156
  as major coronary risk factor, 265t
  among Native Americans, 34-35
  by older adults, 571-572, 589-590
  during school years, 491-492
  and stress, 293
  in young adults, 544
Toddlers
  accidents, 430-432
  age and characteristics of, 330t
  biological agents affecting, 432
  culture and ethnicity influences on, 433
  Erikson's theory of psychosocial development, 341t
  flowchart of growth changes with time, 331t-336t
  functional health patterns in, 419-430
  physical growth in, 417-419
  poisoning of, 432-433
  social processes, 433-434
  speech, language and hearing landmarks in, 424t
  terrible twos, 416
  toilet training, 421, 422, 429
Toilet training
  in preschoolers, 442
  in toddlers, 421, 422, 429

Toileting; *See* elimination patterns; toilet training
Touch
  at birth, 393
  flowchart of life cycle growth changes in, 332t
  as nonverbal communication, 86
Touch therapies, 314
Toxins
  risks for infants, 405-406
Toxoplasmosis, 365
Toys
  hazards to toddlers, 431
Traditional medicine
  in Native American culture, 36
Trager therapy, 321
Trance surgery, 316, 317
Transcendental Meditation (TM), 318
Transcultural nursing; *See also* multicultural awareness
  definition of, 26-27
  models for, 44b
Transcultural values
  and beliefs
    nursing awareness of, 55
Transductive reasoning, 445
Transference, 93
Trauma
  during pregnancy, 370
Treatment
  with secondary prevention, 13, 14f, 15-18
Trichomoniasis
  common in adolescents, 518
  summary of, 539t
Trimesters, 345, 346-347, 362t, 363
Trust
  and accountability, 106-107
  and confidentiality, 115
  in therapeutic relationships, 88
Tuberculosis
  among Asian American-Pacific Islanders, 28-29
  drug-resistant, 54
  history of, 53
  in minority young adults, 529
  in older adults, 588
  risks of
    in homeless population, 38, 54
Turner syndrome, 506
Tuskegee Syphilis Study, 24, 41
Twins, 353, 410b
Tympanograms, 478
Type 2 diabetes
  prevalence and prevention of, 255-258
  related to poor nutrition, 233t
Typhoid, 53

U

Ulcers
  in homeless people, 38
Ultrasonography, 346-347
Uninsured persons, 70-71

United Kingdom
  expenditures per capita and %GDP, 62t
  health care in, 72
  universal health insurance coverage in, 72
United Nations Children's Fund (UNICEF)
  on breast-feeding promotion, 385-386
United States
  expenditures *versus* other countries, 62t, 71-72
  food culture of, 237
  inflated health care costs in, 56-71
Universal health care
  in other countries, 62t, 71-72
Universality
  in Canadian Health Act, 71, 72b
Upper respiratory tract infections (URTIs), 271f, 490
Urge incontinence, 577
Urinary frequency
  during older adult years, 577b
  during pregnancy, 349t
Urinary incontinence, 577
Urinary system
  adaptive changes during pregnancy, 347
  changes in older adults, 576-579, 577b
  flowchart of life cycle growth changes in, 331t
US Census Bureau
  defining race and ethnic groups, 25
  statistics on older adults, 179
  statistics on young adult workforce, 533
US Department of Health and Human Services (USDHHS)
  description of, 4
  Healthy People 2010 (*See Healthy People 2010*)
  on infant health care, 405, 412b
  Web site resources, 74
US Office of Management and Budget
  on race classification, 25
Uterus
  illustrations of, 346f, 347f
  trauma during pregnancy, 370
Utilization reviews
  definition of, 57b

V

Vaccines; *See* immunizations
Vaginal cytology, 55
Validity
  of screening instruments, 202
Value orientation
  definition of, 26
Value systems
  assessment of, 146-147
Value theories, 102

Values
of Asian Americans, 29
clarification of, 78-79
and culture, 26-27
definition of, 26, 78
ethical theories concerning, 102
and ethnicity, 25
within families, 154
and healing, 27
nurse's *versus* patient's, 77-78
and nursing ethics, 121
process of determining one's, 79b
in toddlers, 430
Values clarification
definition of, 78-79
and nursing ethics, 121
and self, 79-81
and stress management, 305
Values-beliefs patterns
during adolescence, 516
of communities, 185
of families, 166-167
of individuals, 146-147
during infancy, 399
during middle-age years, 564-565
during older adult years, 586
during prenatal period, 355b, 363-364
during preschool years, 453-454
during school years, 486
during toddler years, 429-430
during young adulthood, 540-542
Varicosities
during pregnancy, 349t
Vegetables
Healthy People 2010 goals for, 7, 8f
MyPyramid guidelines concerning, 236, 240f
during preschool years, 440-442
recommendations for school-age children, 473, 474f
safety guideline, 241-242
sodium contents in, 248t
Vegetarianism, 237
Veracity, 116-117
Verbal communication, 83
Veterans
homeless, 38
Veterans Administration, 60
Video games, 494
Vietnamese
cultural values
affecting infants, 408-409
concerning pregnancy and birth, 350t
and heath issues of, 28-30
Vineland Social Maturity Scale, 451
Violence
anticipatory guidance for prevention of, 462b
among black/African Americans, 33, 535
confidentiality issues, 115
counseling during adolescence, 507b

Violence *(Continued)*
domestic, 155, 163, 361, 535, 536
factors contributing to
during adolescence, 517f
and firearms, 487, 488, 528-529, 535
Healthy People 2010 goals for, 7, 8b, 9b
influence on school-age children, 494-495
male and female risk of, 535
against women, 155, 163, 535, 536
during pregnancy, 361
workplace, 189, 560
Vision
and accidents by older adults, 586-588
changes in older adulthood, 581-582
development of
during infancy, 392t
in preschoolers, 445-446
during toddler years, 425-426
difficulties
among homeless people, 38
during middle age, 557
among older adults, 581-582, 586-588
flowchart of life cycle growth changes in, 332t
Healthy People 2010 goals for, 7, 8b
and retinoblastoma, 459
during school years, 477
Vision care
not provided for
by Medicare, 68
Visual acuity, 445
Vitamin A
diseases caused by deficiencies in, 233t
Vitamin C, 233t
Vitamin D, 16
Vitamins
classic deficiency diseases, 232, 233t
needed by infants, 384-388
during pregnancy, 356
during preschool years, 440-442
toxicity, 239, 241
Voluntary health agencies, 61
Voluntary migration
description of, 24-25
Vomiting
during pregnancy, 349t
Voodoo, 34
Vulnerable populations, 610, 611
Vulvovaginal candidiasis, 539t

W

Wald, Lillian, 52, 56
Walking
importance of, 275
by older adults, 577-579
Walking meditation, 319
Warm-ups and cool-downs, 275-276

Warning signs
of child abuse
in preschoolers, 428
in school-age children, 484b
of stress, 295-296, 297f
of substance abuse
in adolescents, 518b
of suicide
risk in adolescents, 516b
risk in young adulthood, 540
of workplace violence, 189
Water
hydration during exercise, 279-280
maintaining clean, 16
needed by infants, 384-388
safety, 455b, 487
Water aerobics, 275, 578
Weaning, 386, 388
Web sites; *See* last page of individual chapters
Wechsler Series, 479
Weight; *See also* obesity
assessing and treating excess, 15
Healthy People 2010 goals for, 7, 8f, 78
management
process of, 15
obesity statistics, 530f
Weight training; *See* resistance training
Welfare, 69
Well child care, 496, 497t
Well-being
research on patient, 4
Wellness
definition of
within wellness-illness continuum, 5, 6f
and self-knowledge, 322
tasks, 142t-143t
Wellness Community, 174
Wellness-illness continuum
description and illustration of, 5, 6f
description of, 4
White
as race category, 25
WIC program; *See* Women, Infant, Children (WIC) program
Wilms tumor, 459
Windshield surveys, 180
Women
alcoholism in, 554-555
assessing drinking in pregnant, 129-130
breast cancer
among Asian American-Pacific Islanders, 28-29
among black/African Americans, 33
in older adults, 590
changes with middle-age, 549
chronic conditions in older, 573t
disparities for
in Arab American culture, 27-28
domestic violence against, 155, 163
and exercise, 9

Women (*Continued*)
Gilligan's stages of moral development
 for, 341, 342t
 heart disease in, 148
 HIV and AIDS prevention in, 40-42
 Latinas
  HIV and AIDS issues in, 39-40, 42
 menopause, 549, 558
 middle-age challenges, 558, 561-564
 Native American, 34-35
 pregnancy (*See* pregnancy)
 reducing falls in
  with strength training, 270
 in rural areas, 551
 screening guidelines for, 207t
 and sedentary lifestyles, 264b
 self-esteem *versus* men, 343
 sexual development of, 504t, 505-
  506
 sexuality in older, 145
 Women, Infant, Children (WIC)
  program, 243t, 244
Women, Infant, Children (WIC)
 program, 243t, 244, 397, 411b
Work
 dual careers, 546, 560
 Healthy People 2010 education
  objectives in, 218, 219
 during middle-age years, 559-560

Work (*Continued*)
 occupational health and safety
  Healthy People 2010 goals for, 7, 8b
 statistics on women who, 533, 560
 violence in place of, 560
Workforce
 sexual identity and, 534
 women in, 533, 560
Working parents, 493
Workplace violence
 actions to prevent, 189
 plan for, 560
World Health Organization (WHO)
 on breast-feeding promotion, 385-
  386
 defining community, 179
 defining health, 6
 functions of, 61
 global health challenges facing, 602-
  608
 on global health promotion, 51
 on HIV/AIDS, 602
World Trade Center bombing, 24, 52
Wounded Knee, 34
Wrinkles, 558

X

Xerosis, 558

Y

Yerkes-Dodson law, 291f
Yoga, 138, 279, 317-318
Young adults, 523-546
 age and characteristics of, 330t
 age and physical changes in, 524-525
 college drinking behavior, 523-524
 communicable diseases, 529
 Erikson's theory of psychosocial
  development, 341t
 families with, 157t-158t, 170, 175t
 flowchart of growth changes with
  time, 331t-336t
 functional health patterns, 525-542
 gay and lesbian wellness, 533, 534
 health screening for, 528t
 Healthy People 2010 goals for, 525
 sexual behaviors and diseases, 535-
  538, 539t
 stress issues for, 539-540

Z

Zidovudine (AZT) protocols, 366, 538,
 602
Zygote, 345

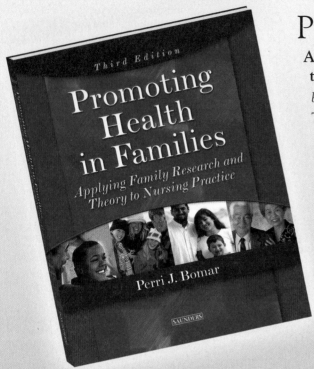
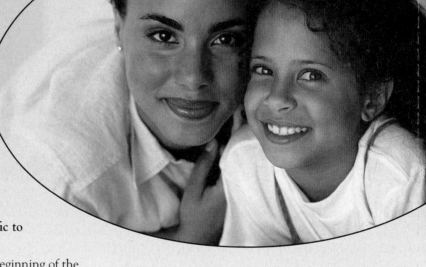

Study Questions

DARLENE NEBEL CANTU

CHAPTER 1

1-1. The client who would be least likely to participate in health teaching activities would choose which model?
1. Clinical model
2. Adaptive model
3. Role performance model
4. Eudaimonistic model

1-2. The nurse is teaching about primary prevention and includes which educational statement in the instructions?
1. Everyone should participate in colorectal cancer screening.
2. Health teaching about the risk factors of heart disease should be performed.
3. Limiting disability is a vital role of nursing, because preventive measures are therapeutic.
4. The nurse is involved in minimizing the effects of disease and disability by surveillance and maintenance.

Innovative Item

1-3. The nurse assesses a community for evidence of health-promotion strategies. Identify all of the health-promotion strategies.
1. Seeking primary care in the acute care hospital
2. Self-care for minor illness
3. Entry into acute care facilities to manage chronic illness
4. Environmental changes to enhance clean air
5. Supporting Habitat for Humanity house construction

1-4. Public health nurses are involved in supporting active health-promotion strategies such as:
1. Supporting clean water
2. Advocating for vitamin D in all milk
3. Supporting sanitary sewage systems
4. Participating in an individual daily exercise program

1-5. Identify the National Institute of Nursing Research theme that focuses the least on health promotion.
1. Changing lifestyle behaviors for better health
2. Managing the effects of chronic illness to improve health and quality of life
3. Identifying effective strategies to reduce health disparities
4. Enhancing the end-of-life experience for individuals and their families

CHAPTER 2

2-1. Which situation supports voluntary as opposed to involuntary immigration?
1. Volcanic eruptions
2. Economic benefits
3. Indentured servitude
4. Fleeing a hostile army

2-2. The nurse recognizes that a minority group is perceived as:
1. Capturing biological variations within human populations
2. People who receive less than their share of wealth, power, or social status
3. People set apart on the basis of cultural or national origin characteristics
4. Socially organized groups with salient differences with respect to other groups in society

2-3. The focus on health promotion in Arab Americans should be based upon their most prevalent health care problem which is:
1. Colon cancer
2. Coronary artery disease
3. Adult-onset diabetes
4. End-stage renal disease

2-4. Priority nursing assessments of Asian Americans/Pacific Islanders should be on which disease process, because these groups have the highest rates of:
1. Tuberculosis
2. Hypertension
3. Diabetes mellitus
4. Breast cancer

2-5. Priority nursing assessments of the Latino/Hispanic Americans should focus on what disease process due to its higher incidence in this population?
1. Cancer
2. Stroke
3. Diabetes
4. Cardiovascular disease

Innovative Item

2-6. Rank from the highest to the lowest the following ethnic populations according to their incidence of human immunodeficiency virus (HIV) and acquired immunodeficiency syndrome (AIDS).

1. White Americans
2. Latino/Hispanic Americans
3. Asian Americans/Pacific Islanders
4. Black Americans
5. Native Americans

CHAPTER 3

3-1. A major public health concern requiring involvement by the nurse in health promotion and teaching focuses on elimination of:
   1. Terrorist attacks
   2. Chronic diseases
   3. Medical errors
   4. Infant mortality

Innovative Item
3-2. The Patient Self-Determination Act requires health care facilities to have (select all that apply):
   1. Policies and procedures for advance directives
   2. Documentation of individual decision about life-sustaining treatment
   3. Documentation of health care coverage
   4. Education about advance directives
   5. Written prohibition of employment discrimination
   6. Guidelines for provision of services to people with disabilities

3-3. Preventive services in the health care facility promote safety for nurses. The governmental agency responsible for preventive services is:
   1. Centers for Disease Control and Prevention (CDC)
   2. National Institutes of Health
   3. Occupational Safety and Health Administration
   4. Health Resources and Services Administration

3-4. In the private sector, which organization provides health care insurance that includes independent prepayment plans?
   1. Self-insurance
   2. Health maintenance organization
   3. Preferred provider organization
   4. Point-of-service plans

3-5. The most positive influence of managed care on both nurses and the people in their care is the:
   1. Delivery and financing of illness care
   2. Curative aspects of episodic acute diseases
   3. Emphasis on and access to preventive care
   4. Short-term cost containment

CHAPTER 4

4-1. One concern that nurses have when using self-disclosure during therapeutic interactions is that:
   1. Revealing oneself assists in developing a helping relationship.
   2. It may cross a boundary from a professional to a personal relationship.
   3. People value nurses who engage in interactions as real people.
   4. It creates reciprocity involving a mutual exchange between the nurse and individual.

4-2. An individual is scheduled for ambulation in the early morning of the first day after undergoing abdominal hysterectomy. The nurse uses consensual validation of the individual's understanding of the plan of care by stating:
   1. "I will be back at 9:00 AM to take you for a walk."
   2. "The doctor wants you to walk 1 time this morning."
   3. "Tell me your thoughts of how you would like to walk this morning."
   4. "Walking soon after a surgical procedure prevents complications."

4-3. The nurse demonstrates empathy toward a crying woman whose baby was stillborn by stating:
   1. "I know exactly how you feel; that happened to me once."
   2. "You are young and will be able to have another baby."
   3. "It was God's will that your baby was taken to heaven with him."
   4. "Loss of a baby is truly a sad occurrence."

4-4. Which question best assists the nurse who is helping a person to formulate the problem as a step in the problem-solving process?
   1. "What pattern is there?"
   2. "What do you want to see changed?"
   3. "What would you do the next time?"
   4. "What meaning does this have for you?"

Innovative Item
4-5. The nurse uses strategies associated with client-centered communication by (select all that apply):
   1. Not being too busy to talk
   2. Focusing on the nurse's views
   3. Developing mutual understanding
   4. Emphasizing the technical aspects of care
   5. Using a conversational interviewing style
   6. Tuning in to the client's preferences and style

CHAPTER 5

5-1. Which nursing intervention would be based upon utilitarian theory?
1. Initiating resuscitation of a newborn at 20 weeks' gestation
2. Preparing a 52-year-old woman with uterine cancer for a hysterectomy
3. Placing a 92-year-old person with terminal congestive heart failure on a ventilator
4. Administering chemotherapy to a 17-year-old with leukemia who states that he wants everything terminated

Innovative Item
5-2. The nurse participates in the process of ethical inquiry in health promotion to (select all that apply):
1. Facilitate in-depth data gathering
2. Resolve all ethical problems related to health promotion
3. Understand what is expected of the health-promotion agent viewed as a moral agent
4. Gain clarity on actual or potential issues regarding health-promotion endeavors
5. Foresee all possible consequences of ethical issues related to health promotion
6. Permit the uncovering of hidden agendas and interests
7. Focus on salient aspects of problems, thus enhancing professional judgment

5-3. The nurse recognizes that the American Nurses Association Code of Ethics identifies expectations of ethical behavior through statements regarding:
1. The primary goals, values, and obligations of the profession
2. Specific standards of care for selected populations
3. Disciplinary actions for incompetent nursing practice
4. Legal standards of practice

5-4. Which statement supports the principle of beneficence that overrides a person's autonomy?
1. The nurse presses the button to administer pain medication through a client-controlled analgesia infusion.
2. The nurse maintains confidentiality to an HIV-positive husband who does not want his wife informed of his HIV status.
3. The nurse instructs parents that their newborn must be placed in a car seat that faces the back of the seat in the back seat of the car.
4. The nurse counsels a 21-year-old woman delivering her third child that she should request a tubal ligation.

5-5. Identify the statement that best supports the ethical principle of justice.
1. Access to health care should be provided for all people.
2. Dialysis should be available for persons who adhere to their prescribed dietary regimen.
3. Transplant organs should be allocated based upon ability to pay for hospital costs.
4. Health-promotion interventions should be provided to those who agree to pay more for health services.

CHAPTER 6

6-1. The nurse is performing an initial antepartum assessment on a client who has missed two periods. Assessment of this woman for alcohol consumption is best determined by the:
1. CAGE test
2. T-ACE test
3. Nonstress test
4. Protein dipstick test

6-2. The nurse, teaching a class on primary prevention at a women's health club, emphasizes participation in:
1. Physician visits during illness
2. Recommended immunization schedules
3. Taking antibiotics at the first sign of symptoms
4. Water aerobics to develop muscle building

Innovative Item
6-3. Major goals in assessing each person's functional pattern are to determine (select all that apply):
1. Ability to manage health-promoting activities
2. Herbal medications that promote health
3. Knowledge of health promotion
4. Need for physician referral for illness care
5. Value that the individual ascribes to health promotion

6-4. The individual's perceived health and well-being and how health is managed describes:
1. Cognitive-perceptual pattern
2. Coping–stress tolerance pattern
3. Health perception–health management pattern
4. Self-perception–self-concept pattern

6-5. In assessing the nutritional-metabolic pattern, the nurse performs an examination of:
1. Attention span
2. Blood pressure
3. Mucous membranes
4. Urine color

6-6. When teaching about proper nutrition to a person with congestive heart failure, which affective

component should be included in the educational plan?
1. Eating with someone
2. Food preparation techniques
3. Knowledge of dietary restrictions
4. Values of adhering to the diet

6-7. The nurse is preparing education on prevention of urinary tract infections. A principle emphasized in the teaching plan would be:
1. Decreasing oral intake facilitates urinary dilution.
2. Empty the bladder at the first sensation of fullness.
3. Frequency is a common symptom that can be ignored.
4. Increasing time between urinations decreases the risk of infections.

6-8. A person reports his exercise pattern is 1 golf game per week. The nurse evaluates this pattern and teaches the individual that:
1. Exercise should include jogging.
2. Exercises should be repetitive.
3. Golfing 1 time per week is adequate.
4. Weekly workouts at the gym should be included.

6-9. When assessing the older adult for sleep quality, the nurse expects to find that the person will state:
1. "I continue to be a night owl."
2. "I experience difficulty returning to sleep."
3. "I experience a night of deep sleep."
4. "I rarely wake up during the night."

6-10. The nurse is preparing a class on wellness and health promotion for a group of middle school students. Developmental tasks of early adolescence include a learning focus emphasis on:
1. Coping with life events and problems
2. Economic responsibility
3. Risk taking and its consequences
4. Social responsibility for self and others

CHAPTER 7

Innovative Item
7-1. Improvement of which five of the following habits would substantially reduce mortality rates?
1. Smoking
2. Stress
3. Poor diet
4. Alcohol abuse
5. Medication use
6. Lack of exercise
7. Emergency room visits

7-2. The cognitive-perceptual pattern assessment includes:
1. Who decides when children go to sleep
2. What types of daily activities include physical exercise
3. What kinds of feelings family members have for each other
4. How the family makes decisions about health promotion and disease prevention

7-3. The nurse assesses a family's coping–stress tolerance pattern by exploring their:
1. Cultural beliefs
2. Traditions and practices
3. Dysfunctional adaptive strategies
4. Expectations of marriage and parenthood

7-4. The nurse uses developmental theory by evaluating the family's:
1. Analysis of baseline data
2. Rigid and permeable boundaries
3. Structural and functional components
4. Prospective tasks and progression through cycles

7-5. The nurse teaches parents that the most important factor in the child's physical, emotional, and cognitive development is:
1. Parental maturity
2. Parental influence
3. Experiences with children
4. How they were nurtured as children

7-6. The nurse uses client teaching as an intervention to prevent family violence by:
1. Assisting the woman to develop an escape plan
2. Advising the woman to try to identify reasons for the violence
3. Encouraging the woman to have an intrauterine device inserted to prevent pregnancy
4. Explaining that her situation is unique and requires psychiatric intervention

7-7. The nurse's educational role reflecting health promotion and disease prevention during the couple stage of family development is:
1. Teacher of risk factors to health
2. Coordinator with pediatric services
3. Teacher of first aid and emergency measures
4. Coordinator for genetic counseling

7-8. The nurse evaluates the home environment of a family with school-age children. Which observation is considered a risk factor related to heath maintenance?
1. Both parents working with children in child care after school

2. Children watching television at least 6 to 8 hours per day
3. Three children ages 6, 8, and 10 living with two parents
4. All children participating in school volleyball teams

7-9. During the critical stage in the natural history of chronic diseases, the nurse teaches the individual that the disease process:
1. Cannot be reversed
2. Is underway, but there are probably no noticeable signs
3. Is advanced with acute symptoms
4. Will have a significant effect on future heath

7-10. The nurse's role with the family with older adults includes serving as a counselor of:
1. Bereavement
2. Menopause
3. Family planning
4. Sexually transmittable diseases

CHAPTER 8

8-1. The health care strategy identified as the major improvement intervention for the population's health is:
1. Increased use of technological interventions
2. Hospital admission for the control of chronic disease
3. Self-care based on heath promotion activities
4. Medical treatment through outpatient clinics

8-2. Collaboration with community members and the interdisciplinary teamwork describes the nursing function as:
1. Independent
2. Interdependent
3. Dependent
4. Multidisciplinary

8-3. Measurement, as a community data collection method, would include:
1. Epidemiological data
2. Verbal statements from key community officials
3. The type and state of residential dwellings
4. The use of senses to determine community appearances

Innovative Item
8-4. Rank order the steps in the Rosenstock model that individuals and groups demonstrate when undergoing a change in health behavior.
1. Taking action to adopt preventive health practices

2. Believing the behavior is a threat to health
3. Reinforcing the new behavior
4. Perceiving the behavior as a threat in terms of susceptibility and seriousness

8-5. The nurse employs the observation data collection method in assessing the community's nutritional-metabolic pattern by asking:
1. What shopping facilities are visible?
2. What is the water quality in the community?
3. What nutritional services are available to community residents?
4. What percentage of community housing has no or inadequate kitchen and plumbing facilities?

CHAPTER 9

9-1. Identify a *Healthy People 2010* goal related to the screening of infants and children.
1. Increase the proportion of newborns screened for chlamydia infections at birth.
2. Increase the proportion of school-age children ages 6 to 10 who receive vision screening.
3. Increase the proportion of infants who receive an audiologic evaluation by 3 months of age.
4. Increase the proportion of newborns who are screened for hearing loss by 1 week of age.

9-2. Disease screening instruments provide accurate measurement outcomes of sensitivity when they:
1. Identify the person whose test results indicate infection with the disease.
2. Reproduce the test results when different individuals perform the test.
3. Correctly distinguish between individuals with and without disease.
4. Measure the test's ability to recognize negative reactions or individuals without disease.

Innovative Item
9-3. Screening processes are performed on apparently well individuals to determine their disease risk. These screening programs cause ethical issues to occur, such as (select all that apply):
1. Maintaining a high cutoff point for screening a disease that is potentially life threatening
2. Lack of resources of individuals identified with risk factors to seek referral and follow-up
3. Determining the screening cutoff points for the screening instrument and borderline results
4. Individual misinterpretation of screening results as diagnostic of a disease state
5. Provision of information to individuals at risk who may need further follow-up or evaluation
6. Evaluating whether the benefits received by those correctly screened are worth the problems experienced by those incorrectly screened

9-4. The nurse is presenting a class for women on Papanicolaou (Pap) smears. The nurse recommends that screening should be performed on women who:
1. Have a history of multiple sex partners
2. Are age 65 and older whose recent Pap smear result was normal
3. Have a history of total hysterectomy as a result of benign disease
4. Are in a monogamous relationship and age is between 18 and 20 years

9-5. The nursing role when incorporating multicultural awareness into the screening process initially begins with:
1. Evaluating the screening program that targets a specific population
2. Identifying factors influencing the population's access to health care
3. Planning for population characteristics such as lifestyle, socioeconomic status, and religious and cultural beliefs
4. Partnering with individuals and organizations in the community to facilitate success in implementing the screening program

CHAPTER 10

10-1. Which client characteristic represents the most controllable area of influence over the future health forecast?
1. Heredity
2. Educational level
3. Behavior patterns
4. Economic status

Innovative Item
10-2. Nurses provide health education to clients to assist them in achieving a goal of (select all that apply):
1. Enhanced wellness
2. Physician-directed care
3. Management of a chronic condition
4. Admission to tertiary care facilities
5. Wisely handling daily health care decisions
6. Fostering successful changes in health behaviors

10-3. The nurse incorporates cultural considerations into the health teaching plan by:
1. Assessing a person's beliefs
2. Using medical terminology
3. Presenting evidence-based information
4. Explaining that universal health practices are the best

10-4. Which assessment technique will elicit the best information on the quality of life from individuals and families in a target population?

1. Collect information on infant mortality
2. Involve the people in a self-study
3. Analyze health care coverage statistics
4. Review the epidemiological data of the people

10-5. Which methodology would the nurse use for teaching psychomotor skills?
1. Field experiences
2. Programmed instruction
3. Drill and practice
4. Computer-assisted programs

CHAPTER 11

11-1. The nurse, presenting a nutrition class to high school students, emphasizes that the leading cause of death associated with diet is:
1. Anemia
2. Infection
3. Cirrhosis of the liver
4. Coronary heart disease

11-2. The client asks the nurse, "Should I take a nutrient supplement?" The nurse explains that nutrient supplementation is indicated in situations such as:
1. Folic acid prior to pregnancy
2. Vitamin A during the first trimester of pregnancy
3. Vitamin E during anticoagulation therapy
4. Calcium in iron-deficiency anemia

11-3. Which statement requires further teaching related to food safety practices?
1. Always drink pasteurized juices.
2. Wash fresh fruits and vegetables thoroughly.
3. When shopping, buy perishable foods last and take them straight home.
4. Cooked meat, poultry, and eggs may be left out at room temperature for up to 3 hours.

11-4. Which woman has the highest priority for being served by the Women, Infants, and Children (WIC) program?
1. Non–breast-feeding postpartum women with any nutritional risk
2. Individuals at nutritional risk only because they are homeless
3. Children (up to age 5) at nutritional risk from serious medical problems
4. Infants determined to be at nutritional risk from serious medical problems

11-5. When assessing elderly adults, the nurse determines that malnutrition may be present in the person with:
1. Serum albumin level of 5 g/dl
2. Midarm muscle circumference at the 25th percentile

3. Triceps skin fold thickness at the 20th percentile
4. Involuntary decrease of weight of more than 10 pounds during the last 6 months

11-6. The nurse, teaching a class on reducing the incidence of heart disease, emphasizes the major risk factors for heart disease are:
1. Peripheral arterial disease
2. High-density lipoprotein (HDL) level higher than 40 mg/dl
3. Age between 45 and 55
4. Fasting blood glucose between 90 and 100 mg/dl

Innovative Item
11-7. Identify all of the *Healthy People 2010* objectives for heart disease (select all that apply):
1. Reduce the mean total blood cholesterol levels among adults from 206 mg/dl to 199 mg/dl.
2. Decrease the number of people requiring open heart surgery.
3. Increase the proportion of people aged 2 years and older who receive less than 10% of calories from saturated fat.
4. Reduce the proportion of adults with high total blood cholesterol levels.
5. Increase the proportion of people aged 2 years and older who receive no more than 30% of calories from fat.
6. Increase the number of people with heart disease who receive an aspirin at discharge.

CHAPTER 12

12-1. The nurse is presenting information on the effects of exercise on lipid metabolism. The nurse emphasizes that:
1. Increase in HDL level lowers the total cholesterol-to-HDL ratio.
2. Longer periods of exercise produce smaller increases in HDL levels.
3. The effect of exercise on lipid metabolism is related to the intensity of the exercise.
4. Exercise has little influence on plasma levels of HDL and triglyceride levels.

12-2. The nurse is teaching a class to nursing students on the relationship between exercise and immune system function. Content should include:
1. High-intensity exercise decreases the incidence of upper respiratory infections.
2. Moderate exercise decreases the release of immunostimulatory hormones.
3. Intense exercise is associated with a decrease in catecholamine and corticosteroid levels.
4. Moderate exercise is associated with a prolonged improvement in the killing capacity of neutrophils.

12-3. The nurse is developing a physical activity program for populations with low rates of physical activity. This program should focus on individuals with:
1. Lower incomes
2. Higher education levels
3. No disabilities
4. Age less than 50 years

Innovative Item
12-4. Recommendations and precautions for people with diabetes who are interested in regular physical activity and exercise include (select all that apply):
1. Monitor blood glucose levels before and 20 to 30 minutes after exercise.
2. Exercise at the peak time of the insulin effect.
3. Inject the insulin into a muscle area that will be active during exercise.
4. Exercise approximately 1 hour before meals.
5. Avoid high-impact activity when prone to neuropathy in the legs and feet.
6. Carry a concentrated form of carbohydrate when exercising.

12-5. In an attempt to encourage increased participation in physical activity, the CDC and the American College of Sports Medicine recommend that:
1. Activity needs to be continuous for 30 to 60 minutes per day.
2. Lower intensity activities should be performed more often, or for longer periods, or both.
3. Only activities such as running, bicycling, swimming should be counted as exercise.
4. Adults should accumulate 30 minutes or more of vigorous intensity physical activity on all days of the week.

CHAPTER 13

13-1. Physiological effects of stress includes:
1. Decreasing the antiinflammatory response
2. Decreasing musculoskeletal tension and tone
3. Increasing the heart rate, blood pressure, and respiratory rate
4. Shifting of blood for the large muscle groups to the visceral organs

13-2. Research has demonstrated the role of stress-hardy characteristics of individuals in promoting better health. These characteristics of stress hardiness include:
1. Viewing stress as a challenge rather that a threat
2. Feeling as though one does not have internal control over stressful situations
3. Having to focus commitment on primarily one component (home or work) in life

4. Reporting more physical symptoms related to the degree of stress

13-3. The nurse is discussing strong evidence on effectiveness of alternative and complementary therapies in reducing harmful effects of stress. Emphasis is placed on the effectiveness of:
1. Aromatherapy
2. Acupuncture
3. Chiropractic therapy
4. Herbal therapy

13-4. The nurse is implementing cognitive restructuring as a stress management intervention with a group of pregnant teens. The nurse explains that cognitive restructuring reduces stress by:
1. Glossing over misfortune, suffering, or negative feelings
2. Helping people identify who is responsible for their stress
3. Recognizing that negative thinking often causes emotional distress
4. Assisting people to focus on a narrow range of feelings causing their stress

Innovative Item
13-5. The nurse is providing suggestions to individuals with sleep disturbances resulting from stress-related issues. The nurse recommends (select all that apply):
1. Have a glass of wine right before bedtime.
2. Establish a regular sleep-wake schedule, even on weekends.
3. Limit naps during the day to 45 minutes.
4. Exercise within 1 hour of bedtime.
5. Take a hot bath 2 hours before bedtime.
6. Sleep in a warm room.

CHAPTER 14

14-1. The nurse understands that holistic health care practice:
1. Has no scientific basis
2. Is not covered by health care insurance
3. Treats the symptoms that the client demonstrates
4. Considers that people have emotions, spirits, and relationships that combine with the physical body

14-2. The nurse explains that the philosophical base for energy medicine involves:
1. Reading auras
2. Rebalancing life energy
3. Placing the hands and making symbolic gestures
4. Inserting fine needles into precisely mapped points on the skin surface

14-3. The nurse advocates that acupuncture is useful in management of:
1. Hypertension
2. Osteoporosis
3. Substance abuse
4. Gastrointestinal bleeding

Innovative Item
14-4. Music therapy has been used to produce desired outcomes in which of the following conditions (select all that apply):
1. Postoperative pain
2. Postpartum depression
3. Acute myocardial infarction
4. Pain associated with labor
5. Osteoarthritis pain
6. Nausea and vomiting induced by chemotherapy

14-5. The nurse is asked how essential oils may be used as part of aromatherapy. The nurse responds:
1. "They may be mixed with carrier oils and used during massage."
2. "They may be swallowed in small amounts for stomach distress."
3. "They may be applied during pregnancy to prevent stretch marks."
4. "They may be placed on herpes lesions on the eye."

CHAPTER 15

15-1. The nurse is teaching a class to students of pediatric nursing on comparing the concepts of growth and development. Which statement most accurately represents these concepts?
1. Growth patterns are qualitative changes.
2. Growth proceeds from the head to toe (cephalocaudal progression).
3. Development reflects an increase in the number and size of cells.
4. Development is a gradual change that includes advances in skills.

15-2. During health screening of Hispanic children for lead poisoning, the initial question the nurse should ask is:
1. "How old is the house you are living in?"
2. "Do you eat canned foods from the U.S. only?"
3. "Are there any areas in your home where paint is chipping off?"
4. "Do you use ceramic containers made outside the United States for cooking?"

15-3. Erikson's theory of psychosocial development identifies the toddler stage as:
1. Trust versus mistrust

2. Initiative versus guilt

3. Industry versus inferiority

4. Autonomy versus shame and doubt

15-4. Piaget's theory of cognitive development states that characteristics of the sensorimotor stage include:
1. Development of egocentric animistic and magical thinking
2. Development of the concept of object permanence
3. Consideration of others' point of view
4. Thought dominated by senses

Innovative Item

15-5. Identify the goals of Gilligan's stages of moral development for women in the postconventional stage (select all that apply):
1. Agree upon rights
2. Principle of nonviolence
3. Justice
4. Personal moral standards
5. Do not hurt self or others

CHAPTER 16

16-1. The goal for the couple that attends childbirth education classes is to:
1. Have a medication-free birth
2. Prepare for an early discharge
3. Increase knowledge of labor and delivery
4. Obtain information about hospital policies

16-2. The nurse performs assessments of the mother and her fetus throughout the labor process. Which finding indicates a complication?
1. Clear amniotic fluid
2. Active fetal movement
3. Fetal heart rate below 100 beats per minute
4. Contractions every 3 minutes, lasting 60 seconds

16-3. The nurse prevents cold stress in the newborn in the delivery room by:
1. Maintaining the delivery room temperature at 73° F
2. Drying the baby with warm blankets
3. Bathing the baby immediately after delivery
4. Placing the baby in an open warmer on manual control

16-4. Which maternal action demonstrates a mother's ability to ensure safe passage for her fetus?
1. Fantasizes about the gender of her baby
2. Seeks prenatal care from a health care provider
3. Integrates the fetus as an integral part of her
4. Examines what she will gain and lose by becoming a mother

16-5. The nurse teaches the expectant woman about interventions that decrease sibling rivalry after birth. These instructions would include:
1. Encouraging the sibling to participate in decisions such as selecting toys for the newborn
2. Disciplining the sibling when negative comments are made about the baby
3. Instructing the sibling to "be careful" and "be quiet" around the newborn
4. Requesting the grandparents to care for the sibling during prenatal visits

16-6. Which mother is a candidate for the administration of Rho(D) immune globulin (RhoGAM)?
1. An Rh-negative mother with an Rh-negative newborn
2. An Rh-positive mother with an Rh-negative newborn
3. A mother demonstrating the presence of Rh antibodies
4. A pregnant Rh-negative mother who experiences a spontaneous abortion

Innovative Item

16-7. Identify all nursing interventions that would facilitate resolution of an individual's ineffective coping related to active labor.
1. Assess labor discomfort every 20 to 30 minutes.
2. Implement nursing interventions to improve coping with labor discomfort as needed.
3. Prepare the individual for epidural anesthesia.
4. Assess cultural beliefs during labor and delivery management.
5. Provide teaching about the labor and delivery process.
6. Monitor the fetal response to maternal systemic analgesia.

16-8. The nurse assesses the woman for positive signs of pregnancy, which include:
1. Enlargement of the uterus
2. Bluish color of the cervix and upper vagina
3. Detection of fetal heart tones by Doppler auscultation
4. Positive test results for human chorionic gonadotropin

16-9. The nurse assesses the newborn 1 minute after delivery and documents the following data:
- Body pink, extremities blue
- Heart rate 120 beats per minute
- Weak cry, hypoventilation
- Some flexion of extremities
- Grimace

The nurse documents the 1 minute Apgar score as:
1. 6
2. 8

3. 9
4. 10

CHAPTER 17

17-1. The nurse suggests stimulating experiences for development of their infant to the parents of a 6-month-old. These experiences would include:
1. Singing lullabies to the baby
2. Inviting another infant over to play
3. Keeping the top of the crib free of hanging mobiles
4. Providing a toy that emits animal sounds when the buttons are pushed

Innovative Item
17-2. The nurse, teaching a class to primiparas about risk factors associated with sudden infant death syndrome (SIDS), explains that prevention strategies include (select all that apply):
1. Prone sleeping position
2. Supine sleeping position
3. Postnatal smoking
4. Sleeping on soft surfaces
5. Sleeping on hard surfaces
6. Over-wrapping the baby
7. Allowing the baby to sleep with the parents
8. Breast-feeding the baby

17-3. During the 1-month well-baby visit, a pediatric nurse explains to the mother that she should expect to hear babbling in her infant by:
1. 2 months
2. 4 months
3. 6 months
4. 9 months

17-4. The nurse is teaching prenatal couples about the critical principles of attachment. These principles include:
1. Parents of sick infants become attached as quickly as those of healthy infants.
2. The mother and father should have close contact with their infant within minutes after birth.
3. It is mandatory for the father to witness the birth process so that bonding and attachment will occur.
4. Parents take on the active role when interacting with their infant, realizing that their infant will be unresponsive.

17-5. The nurse teaches new mothers about research on pacifiers and breast-feeding. Which statement by a mother indicates an understanding of the instruction?

1. "I have no problem giving a pacifier to a breast-feeding baby."
2. "I offer a pacifier after each feeding to satisfy my baby's sucking needs."
3. "There is significant research that indicates harm is associated with occasional pacifier use."
4. "I do not give my baby a pacifier, because I know it is associated with shorter breast-feeding duration."

17-6. A new mother asks the nurse when the baby's anterior fontanel will close. The nurse explains that it will close at:
1. 2 months
2. 6 months
3. 12 months
4. 18 months

17-7. The nurse in the well-baby clinic informs the mother of a 6 month old about introducing solid foods by instructing her to:
1. Feed the baby solids before the milk.
2. Make the baby's solid foods smooth and runny.
3. Introduce solid food by adding it to the baby's formula bottle.
4. Mix a little honey in the fruit to stimulate the infant's taste buds.

CHAPTER 18

18-1. Which physical growth and development change in toddlers places them at risk for airway obstruction?
1. The diameter of the upper respiratory tract is small.
2. The respiratory rate decreases to 25 breaths per minute.
3. All 20 primary or deciduous teeth erupt by the end of toddlerhood.
4. The swallowing pattern using the tongue is fully developed.

Innovative Item
18-2. The nurse offers interventions to parents to enhance toddler's nutritional pattern by telling the parents to (select all that apply):
1. Avoid foods that may cause choking.
2. Serve the toddler's favorite foods when the child refuses to eat.
3. Send the toddler to bed if the child does not want to eat.
4. Not use food to bribe, reward, or punish the toddler.
5. Serve small portions and let the toddler ask for more.
6. Serve mixtures of foods.

18-3. The nurse is teaching a group of mothers about toddlers and their play activities by explaining that toddlers:
1. Participate in parallel play
2. Demonstrate skill in sharing and cooperative play
3. Enjoy playing together with a group of toddlers
4. Learn best with intensive drill during play

18-4. The nurse, presenting a class on strategies to prevent drowning in toddlers, instructs parents to:
1. Teach your toddler how to swim.
2. Place the toddler in the tub with 1 or 2 inches of water.
3. Make sure pails of water are less than one half full.
4. Be sure the toddler wears a personal flotation device when boating.

18-5. Which statement, if made by a parent after attending a teaching session on initiating a toilet training program for toddlers, indicates a need for further teaching?
1. "I take my child to the potty after a meal."
2. "I offer praise when my child uses the potty."
3. "I require my child to sit on the potty until she goes."
4. "I have given my child underpants as a reward for using the potty."

18-6. When the nurse is assessing a toddler for signs of child abuse, observations of parental behavior may include:
1. Difficulty leaving the child
2. Parental delays in seeking help
3. Spontaneous reporting of the details of the injury
4. Parental questions about progress and discharge

18-7. The nurse assessing a 24-month-old toddler expects expressive language to include:
1. Repeats two digits from memory
2. Jargon and echolalia are used predominately
3. Talks in phrases and two to three word sentences
4. Average sentence length is approximately two and a half words.

CHAPTER 19

19-1. The school nurse assesses preschoolers for genetic conditions such as:
1. Down syndrome
2. Congenital hypothyroidism
3. Sickle cell disease
4. Duchenne muscular dystrophy

19-2. When evaluating the health perception of a preschooler, the nurse understands that this age group views pain or illness as:
1. Punishment
2. Separation anxiety
3. A result of their actions
4. Painful regardless of the intervention

19-3. Which activity would the nurse plan for a 4-year-old girl 2 days after undergoing an appendectomy?
1. Play a game of Monopoly
2. Dress up in a Cinderella gown
3. Participate in a game of hopscotch
4. Draw pictures of her mother and father

Innovative Item
19-4. The nurse is teaching parents about typical sleep disturbances of the preschooler. Which recommendation would the nurse make to the parents?
1. Bedtime rituals of 1 hour or more should decrease sleep disturbances.
2. Frightening television shows and stories should be banned before bedtime.
3. Parents should help the child differentiate between pretend and real occurrences.
4. When the child has night wakening events, reassurance is given by taking the child to the parents' bed.

19-5. Cognitive development of the preschooler includes:
1. Transductive reasoning
2. The trait of irreversibility
3. Understanding the perspectives of others
4. An ability to consider more than one factor when solving simple problems

19-6. The nurse assesses the preschooler's coping mechanisms as being developmentally appropriate through observation of:
1. Temper tantrums
2. Fantasy play
3. Separation anxiety
4. Flexible bedtime rituals

Innovative Item
19-7. The nurse is teaching parents about strategies to help reduce preschooler unintentional poisonings in the home. Instructions would include (select all that apply):
1. Post the poison control number near every telephone.
2. Administer syrup of ipecac immediately to the child suspected of swallowing poison.
3. Transfer cleaning supplies to old unattractive canisters.
4. Teach the child about poisons at an early age.

5. Use safety latches for drawers and cabinet doors.
6. Store products in their original containers.

CHAPTER 20

20-1. The nurse assessing conventional level moral development in a 12-year-old child would expect to see which behaviors?
1. The child looks to others for approval.
2. The child views behavior as completely right or wrong.
3. The child behaves because there is a fear of punishment.
4. The child's moral development is characterized by self-interest.

20-2. The most common childhood school-age cancer is:
1. Retinoblastoma
2. Neuroblastoma
3. Wilms tumor
4. Acute lymphocytic leukemia

Innovative Item
20-3. The nurse discusses discipline for school-age children with a group of parents at a parent-teacher association meeting. Principles include (select all that apply):
1. Focusing on the misbehavior in an attempt to eliminate it
2. Using distraction or substitution to avoid a problem situation
3. Ignoring the child's whining after a decision has been made
4. Using humor to decrease the intensity of the situation
5. Modeling appropriate behavior
6. Setting age-relevant limits

20-4. The school nurse is developing an information pamphlet on prevention of obesity in school-age children. Interventions stated on the pamphlet would include:
1. Provide foods high in vitamin A and C, fruits, and vegetables for after-school snacks.
2. Eating may occur in front of the television as long as the program is news related.
3. Make different meals for children based on their likes and dislikes.
4. Reward the child with food for school achievement.

20-5. Parents of a 7-year-old boy request a discussion with the school nurse on how they can resolve the child's nighttime enuresis. The nurse advises that nighttime enuresis:

1. Is an intentional act with a psychological basis
2. Should have consequences to eliminate the behavior
3. Has no serious physical problems and should be ignored
4. Requires a family plan to deal with the wet bed to decrease family arguments

20-6. Nursing interventions to help a child develop a positive self-concept during the school-age period would include:
1. Giving positive feedback to the child for accomplishments
2. Waiting to discuss sexual changes until the child asks questions
3. Making decisions for the child so that positive consequences will be experienced
4. Counseling the child that time spent with peers should be greater than time spent with the family

20-7. The nurse is teaching 8 and 9 year olds about safe bicycling. The nurse emphasizes the principles of transportation safety including:
1. Riding on the side of the road traveling opposite to the traffic
2. Riding the bike through the crosswalks after checking for traffic
3. Wearing an approved, properly fitting helmet when bicycling
4. Using a backpack to carry objects instead of the back basket

CHAPTER 21

21-1. The nurse provides educational information to the female adolescent on decreasing the incidence of acne, which includes:
1. "Decrease chocolate intake in your diet."
2. "Expose your face to sunlight for at least 2 hours per day."
3. "Remove all pustules and papules with special instruments."
4. "Wash your face with soap and water 2 to 3 times per day."

Innovative Item
21-2. The nurse is assessing a 12-year-old female with an admission diagnosis of anorexia nervosa. The data collected that support this diagnosis should include (select all that apply):
1. Binge eating followed by purging
2. Compulsive physical activity
3. Eating an amount of food that is definitely larger than most people would eat

4. Preoccupation with food

5. Self-starvation with significant weight loss

21-3. Research has documented what symptom as the strongest predictor of adolescent obesity?

1. Depression

2. Excessive television watching

3. Lack of physical activity

4. Meal skipping

21-4. The nurse assesses the cognitive abilities of the adolescent according to Piaget's stage of formal operations as:

1. Accepting family beliefs and values

2. Developing extrovert behaviors

3. Having an intolerance of things as they are

4. Recognizing the importance of putting others' needs ahead of their own

21-5. The nurse facilitates the adolescent's self-perception–self-concept development by:

1. Complimenting the adolescent for what is accomplished

2. Developing a plan for the adolescent's future growth

3. Encouraging the adolescent to join in group activities

4. Giving praise for who the adolescent is

21-6. The nurse is preparing an educational activity for adolescents. The primary reason that emphasis is placed on teaching testicular self-examination is because:

1. Adolescents are naturally interested in their developing bodies.

2. Baseline assessment data are necessary for future comparison.

3. Rapid anatomical changes are occurring in the testes.

4. Testicular cancer is the number 1 cancer in the adolescent male.

21-7. The nurse is reviewing the immunization record of a sexually active adolescent. The adolescent should receive:

1. Hepatitis B vaccine

2. *Haemophilus influenza* vaccine

3. Measles, mumps, and rubella vaccine

4. Meningococcal meningitis vaccine

21-8. To facilitate the adolescent's need for controlling behaviors, the nurse implements the intervention that:

1. Asks how the adolescent would like to handle the situation

2. Consults with the parents regarding the adolescent's health care needs

3. Gives specific, detailed instructions in writing

4. Partners with the adolescent to develop a plan

Innovative Item

21-9. The nurse emphasizes warning signs of suicide risk in adolescents during a health education class. These signs include (select all that apply):

1. Difficulty concentrating

2. Increased accidents

3. Hyperactivity

4. Lethargy

5. Sleep disorders

21-10. The school nurse is performing scoliosis screening on 14-year-old girls. Signs indicative of scoliosis include:

1. Alignment of the spinous processes

2. Lower scapula height on the side of thoracic convexity

3. Thoracic convexity with lateral spine curvature

4. Waist and leg symmetry

21-11. Assessment of an 11-year-old girl demonstrates the following findings:

- Sparse growth of long straight, downy hair along the labia
- Enlargement of the areolar diameter
- Beginning breast bud

The nurse determines that the girl's Tanner stage is:

1. 1

2. 2

3. 3

4. 4

CHAPTER 22

22-1. *Healthy People 2010* documents that death rates related to traffic and motor vehicle injuries are highest in which age group?

1. 5 to 14 years

2. 15 to 24 years

3. 25 to 34 years

4. 35 to 44 years

22-2. Emphasis on disease prevention for the young adult, after age 25, is on modifying risk factors related to:

1. Coronary artery disease

2. Cirrhosis of the liver

3. Cervical cancer

4. Colon cancer

22-3. A new target goal of *Healthy People 2010* is to reduce the incidence of hepatitis C. The nurse focuses on individuals most at risk, which includes persons with:

1. Hepatitis A
2. Epstein-Barr virus
3. Human papilloma virus
4. Chronic renal disease on hemodialysis

22-4. According to Piaget's theory of cognitive development, the young adult is in the stage of formal operational thought and demonstrates abilities to:
1. Analyze concepts
2. Manipulate concrete objects
3. Participate in cooperative interactions
4. Perceive specific examples

Innovative Item
22-5. The nurse is preparing a class on young adult risk factors for violence. The nurse includes content on (select all that apply):
1. Homicide is the second leading cause of death in young adults.
2. Violence is becoming less prevalent globally.
3. Homicide is the leading cause of death for black young men.
4. Firearms are involved in less that 50% of homicides.
5. More women than men are at risk for death from a firearm.
6. The presence of firearms in the home is associated with the increased risk of firearm-associated injury to children.

22-6. Young adults are screened for cervical cancer through assessment of known risk factors that include:
1. Obesity
2. Smoking
3. Hypertension
4. Alcohol use

22-7. The nurse incorporates epidemiological findings in assessing for risks associated with intimate partner violence, which include:
1. Adequate economic resources
2. Equal job position of the partners
3. Both partners having achieved college graduation
4. Differences in prestige associated with the partners' careers

CHAPTER 23

23-1. During middle adulthood, physiological changes affect most bodily systems. These changes include:
1. Increased cardiac output
2. Increased glomerular filtration rates
3. Thinning of the intervertebral disks
4. Increased bone density and mass

23-2. The leading causes of death in middle adulthood, in both white and black populations, are the same and include:
1. Heart disease
2. Kidney disease
3. Respiratory disease
4. Gastrointestinal disease

23-3. The nurse initiates an exercise program with middle-age adults by:
1. Planning physical activity for a minimum of 45 minutes
2. Considering activities that have the least potential for injury
3. Counseling the adult that exercise should be rigorous to produce results
4. Advising that the heart rate should double during exercise to achieve cardiovascular benefit

23-4. Bloom has developed a hierarchy of cognitive levels in the adult learner. The analysis cognitive level for the adult learner would be:
1. Recall of specific facts
2. Grasping the meaning of the communicated message
3. Breaking down material into its constituent parts while noting their relationships
4. Application of knowledge in the form of abstractions and ideas to concrete situations

23-5. The nurse, teaching a class on smoking cessation to a group of middle-age adults, presents the adverse effects of smoking, which include:
1. Nicotine stimulates the heart.
2. Nicotine calms the central nervous system.
3. Nicotine assists in decreasing blood pressure.
4. Nicotine causes a decrease in carbon monoxide.

Innovative Item
23-6. The nurse provides anticipatory guidance to people during middle age to meet developmental tasks of (select all that apply):
1. Helping children become responsible, happy adults
2. Rediscovering new satisfaction in the relationship with one's spouse
3. Developing an affectionate, but independent, relationship with aging parents
4. Reaching the peak in one's career
5. Passing on traditions and skills to grandchildren
6. Developing leisure-time activities

CHAPTER 24

24-1. Characteristic behaviors of older adults who have successfully met Erikson's ego integrity versus despair developmental task include:

1. Fear of death
2. Feelings that life has been lived in vain
3. Identity related to career and work only
4. Honest acceptance of the life that has passed

24-2. During an initial home health visit, the nurse evaluates safety in the kitchen of an elderly woman. Which finding indicates a potential for accidental injury?
1. One nonskid rug at the sink
2. Gas oven door opened to warm the house
3. Two electrical appliances plugged into the same socket
4. Cleaning products below the sink in their original containers

24-3. The geriatric nurse practitioner is making arrangements for a geriatric assessment community service. Which individual would most benefit from this service?
1. One who is under age 70
2. One who walks with a cane
3. One with extended family in the community
4. One who is depressed because of loss of a spouse

Innovative Item
24-4. Rank the listed chronic conditions, in order from most to least frequent, in the older adult woman.
1. Arthritis
2. Heart disease
3. Hearing impairment
4. High blood pressure
5. Orthopedic impairment
6. Cataracts

24-5. The nurse is explaining services provided in assisted living to a couple considering a move to long-term housing for older adults. The nurse explains that assisted living includes:
1. Twenty-four hour protective oversight
2. Medications administered by staff personnel
3. Individual responsibility for preparation of own medications
4. Expectations that persons are independent in all care areas

CHAPTER 25

25-1. The biggest factor influencing life expectancy in developing African countries is:
1. Hepatitis
2. Tuberculosis
3. Diabetes mellitus
4. HIV

Innovative Item
25-2. Rank the categories of homeless groups from highest to lowest prevalence.
1. Families with children
2. Single men
3. Single women
4. Adolescents

25-3. One of the health targets for the twenty-first century is to reverse global trends of five major pandemics. One of the five pandemic diseases is:
1. Cancer
2. Hepatitis
3. Hypertension
4. Diabetes mellitus

25-4. The nurse is preparing a class on severe acute respiratory syndrome (SARS). Which content is essential?
1. Respiratory droplets spread SARS.
2. Initial symptoms include a dry cough.
3. SARS can be contracted while sitting in a waiting room.
4. Approximately 1 week after infection with SARS virus, symptoms of high fever, headache, and malaise develop.

25-5. Smoking rates in developing countries are rising at alarming rates, with teenage male smoking rates of:
1. 5% to 9%
2. 10% to 20%
3. 21% to 29%
4. 30% to 40%

CHAPTER 1

1-1. **Answer: 1**
Text page: 5
Rationale: The absence of signs and symptoms of disease as indicative of health would fit the clinical model of health. People who use this model to guide their use of health care services may not seek preventive services, or they may wait until they are very ill to seek care. Personal responsibility for health may not be a motivating factor for this individual, because the provider is responsible for dealing with the health problem and returning the person to a state of health. Attempts to provide health-promoting activities may not be effective. In the role performance model, social role performance is indicative of health. This model is the basis for work and school physical examinations and physician-excused absences. In the adaptive model of health, the ability to adapt positively to social, mental, and physiological change is indicative of health. In the eudaimonistic model of health, exuberant well-being is indicative of health. This model is also more congruent with integrative modes of therapy.

1-2. **Answer: 2**
Text page: 13
Rationale: Primary prevention precedes disease or dysfunction. Primary prevention intervention includes health promotion, such as health teaching about risk factors for heart disease, and specific protection, such as immunization against hepatitis B. Its purpose is to decrease the vulnerability of the individual or population to disease or dysfunction. People are taught to use appropriate primary preventive measures. Screening is secondary prevention, because the principal goal is to identify individuals in an early, detectable stage of the disease process. Delayed recognition of disease results in the need to limit future disability in late secondary prevention. Tertiary prevention occurs when a defect or disability is permanent and irreversible. The process is minimizing the effects of disease and disability by surveillance and mainte-nance activities aimed at preventing complications and deterioration.

1-3. **Answers: 2, 4, 5**
Text page: 15
Rationale: Health promotion goes beyond providing information. It is proactive decision making at all levels of society. Strategies identified within this decision-making process are screening, self-care for minor illness, readiness for emergencies, successful management of chronic illness, environmental changes to enhance positive behaviors, and health-enhancing policies within an organizational setting. Health-promotion efforts focus on maintaining or improving the general health of individuals, families, and communities through support of housing at the public and community levels, and at the personal level by voting and volunteering for improved low-income housing.

1-4. **Answer: 4**
Text page: 16
Rationale: Health-promotion strategies are either active or passive. Passive strategies involve the individual as an inactive participant or recipient. Examples of passive strategies include public health efforts to maintain clean water and sanitary sewage systems and efforts to introduce vitamin D into all milk to ensure that children will not be at risk for rickets when they are exposed to little sunlight. Active strategies depend on the individual becoming personally involved in adopting a program of health promotion. Examples of lifestyle changes are daily exercise as part of a physical fitness plan and a stress-management program as part of daily living.

1-5. **Answer: 4**
Text page: 19
Rationale: The four optional answers are four of the five themes of the National Institute of Nursing Research. Enhancing the end-of-life experience for clients and families does not focus on health promotion. This theme focuses on the creation of an experience that includes death with dignity based upon the individual's desires.

CHAPTER 2

2-1. *Answer: 2*
Text page: 24
Rationale: Voluntary immigrations are generally motivated by the quest of the individual or group for one or more of goals including:
- Educational opportunities
- Economic benefits
- Social improvements
- Political or religious freedom

Involuntary immigration involves movement based on forced reasons and occurs when individuals or groups are fleeing a hostile army, civil war, and political anarchy. Natural disasters such as floods, famines, earthquakes, and volcanic eruptions cause people to search for safer places to live. Today individuals are lured by attractive job opportunities in other countries, which may lead to indentured servitude when they find themselves trapped in low-paying jobs or prostitution.

2-2. *Answer: 2*
Text page: 26
Rationale: A minority group may be perceived as consisting of people who receive less than their share of the wealth, power, or social status. Race has been viewed as biological variations within human populations. It emphasizes physical and biological heredity. An ethnic group is one that is set apart by insiders or outsiders, primarily on the basis of cultural or national origin characteristics subjectively selected. Ethnic groups are socially organized with salient differences compared with other groups in society.

2-3. *Answer: 3*
Text pages: 27-28
Rationale: Their most relevant health problem is adult-onset diabetes. A study on the prevalence of diabetes was done on 542 participants, with prevalence rates among women at 15.5% and in men at 20.1%. There continues to be a rise in coronary artery disease in the Arab American population.

2-4. *Answer: 1*
Text page: 29
Rationale: Asian Americans/Pacific Islanders have the highest rates of tuberculosis, 36.6 cases per 100,000 people. Heart disease, cancers, and cerebrovascular problems are the leading causes of death. The women are less likely to die of breast cancer, and infant mortality rates are lower than in other ethnic groups. Their healthy diet decreases their incidence of diabetes mellitus.

2-5. *Answer: 4*
Text page: 30
Rationale: Cardiovascular disease is the number 1 cause of morbidity and mortality among Latino/Hispanic Americans. Cancer is the second most prevalent cause of morbidity and mortality. Diabetes is twice as prevalent in Latino/Hispanics as in non-Latino white Americans.

2-6. *Answer: 4, 2, 1, 3, 5*
Text page: 40
Rationale: Currently HIV/AIDS has affected people of all ages, both genders, and different populations in the United States. Through December 2001 the following incidence statistics were recorded:
- Black Americans—35%
- Latino/Hispanic Americans—22.5%
- White Americans—6.6%
- Asian Americans/Pacific Islanders—less than 1%
- Native Americans—less than 1%

CHAPTER 3

3-1. *Answer: 2*
Text page: 52
Rationale: The public health system and the nurse focus on chronic disease is most important, because it is the leading cause of death and disability in the United States. The link between the environment and the health needs of the population must be kept in the forefront when building an effective public health system. A strengthened public health system should complement both goals of *Healthy People 2010*. The Department of Homeland Security, established in April 2003, is in charge of preventing terrorist attacks. Medical errors are being studied by accrediting organizations, and institutional requirements have been established requiring client safety and an acceptable work environment for nurses. The public health departments follow infant mortality, although a major focus remains on chronic diseases.

3-2. *Answers: 1, 2, 4*
Text page: 61
Rationale: As a condition of Medicare and Medicaid payment, the Patient Self-Determination Act requires health care facilities to have the following:
- Policies and procedures for advance directives
- Individual choice in the medical record
- Individual facility policies and procedures
- Facility staff and community education about advance directives

Sections of the Americans With Disabilities Act that apply most directly to health care providers are the prohibition of employment discrimination and the requirement for provision of services to people with disabilities. Documentation of health care coverage is obtained by the hospital from the client after admission.

3-3. **Answer: 3**
Text page: 60
Rationale: The Occupational Safety and Health Administration provides and monitors preventive services in the workplace. National Institutes of Health funds and conducts research. The Health Resources and Services Administration conducts health resources planning, funds education of health personnel, and administers the Indian Health Service, the Federal Bureau of Prisons, and the Bureau of Health Professionals. The CDC investigates causes of disease, establishes policies and standards for the prevention, diagnosis, and treatment of health conditions, and provides information on diseases for all health care personnel.

3-4. **Answer: 2**
Text page: 67
Rationale: Health maintenance organizations are independent prepayment plans. Preferred provider organizations act as "brokers" between insurers and health care providers. Point-of-service plans combine classic health maintenance organizations with client choice characteristics of preferred provider organizations. Self-insurance and self-funded plans are those in which either the employer takes on the role of insurer or the enrollee sets up a trust account with tax savings.

3-5. **Answer: 3**
Text page: 66
Rationale: The most positive influence of managed care on both nurses and the people they care for is the emphasis on and access to preventive services, which has always been an important focus for nurses. The emphasis on short-term cost containment is sometimes at the expense of quality and long-term outcomes. Sick people can face obstacles receiving treatment from managed care plans.

CHAPTER 4

4-1. **Answer: 2**
Text page: 81
Rationale: Self-disclosure involves sharing experiences that the nurse has had with a client who has had a similar experience, to assist the client to recognize that the nurse demonstrates understanding of the client's need. Self-disclosure is an indicator of a healthy personality and a strategy for developing a healthy relationship with a client. Therapeutic interactions characterized by reciprocity involve a mutual exchange between the nurse and the client. Traditionally nurses have been wary of self-disclosure, because it may cross a boundary from a professional to a personal relationship. The nurse must recognize when self-disclosure is inappropriate and when it is needed in a therapeutic relationship. Literature documents that self-disclosure is an effective clinical strategy when developing a helping relationship. Clients value nurses who engage in interactions as real people and who are willing to share information about themselves.

4-2. **Answer: 3**
Text page: 85
Rationale: Consensual validation is a confirmation that both the sender and receiver understand the same information. The nurse should ask the person to explain her sense of the message and how to ask the nurse for further information. Consensual validation in communication is essential when providing health-promotion interventions. Without validating that the individual understands the information and its importance and that the individual had a behavioral plan to follow, health-promotion efforts are likely to fail. Option 3 is the only response that asks the person for her input regarding her understanding of the plan of care. The other options stated by the nurse contain information given to the person.

4-3. **Answer: 4**
Text pages: 88-89
Rationale: Empathy involves the ability to understand another's feelings without losing personal identity and perspective. It is the critical element creating the caring climate through therapeutic use of self. Empathy decreases client distress. When the nurse acknowledges the content of the person's communication she transmits empathy. It is important that the nurse remain with the individuals, spending time listening and assisting them to discuss problems, fears, and anxieties. Nurses do not empathize by switching the focus of the interaction to themselves, as in response number 1, or by sympathizing. The only statement that demonstrates empathy is number 4, which states an observation reflective of the woman's crying. Response number 2 does not focus on the loss of this baby, which is important for the grieving process. Response number 3 does not take the person's beliefs into consideration.

4-4. **Answer: 2**
Text page: 91, Health Teaching box
Rationale: Option 2 assists the person to focus on formulating the problem, but having the person state what he wants to see changed to resolve the problem. Options 1 and 4 both assist the person to analyze the parts of the experience and see relationships to other events. Option 3 assists the person to identify how another similar problem could be resolved.

4-5. **Answers: 1, 3, 5, 6**
Text page: 82, Box 4-4
Rationale: Strategies associated with client-centered communication include options 1, 3, 5, and 6. All of those responses focus attention on the individual. Options 2 and 4 focus on the nurse, and emphasizing the technical aspects of care is for information giving, again with the major focus on the nurse.

CHAPTER 5

5-1. **Answer: 2**
Text page: 102
Rationale: Utilitarian theory proposes that actions are good insofar as they are aimed at yielding the greatest amount of happiness or pleasure or cause the least amount of harm or pain to people and overall within the society. Any decision making must take into account the consequences. The professional involved in the decision making must also possess the appropriate skills and knowledge to undertake actions that will promote a "good" for people. The situations stated above require the nurse to determine which situation has the greatest amount of good for society and which causes the least amount of pain. The woman with the uterine cancer diagnosis preparing for surgery has the most promising outcome and therefore should be selected as the priority intervention based upon utilitarian theory. The newborn of 20 weeks' gestation has almost no chance of surviving outside of the mother's womb. The adolescent with leukemia who has stated that he does not want the chemotherapy should be respected, even though his parents will make the final decision. Being placed on the ventilator will not cure the 92-year-old person with terminal congestive heart failure. Even with extraordinary interventions, the individual with a terminal disease prognosis is one who will not be cured of that disease.

5-2. **Answers: 1, 3, 4, 6, 7**
Text page: 106
Rationale: The purpose of ethical inquiry in health promotion is to gain clarity on actual or potential moral issues arising in the context of health-promotion endeavors and to understand what is expected of the health-promotion agent viewed as a moral agent. Ethical inquiry will not permit the resolution of all problems, mainly because the environments in which health-promotion efforts are conceptualized are incredibly complex. It is impossible to foresee all possible consequences of an action. Ethical reasoning can facilitate appropriate and in-depth data gathering, permit the uncovering of hidden agendas and interests, and focus on salient aspects of a particular problem, thus enhancing professional judgment.

5-3. **Answer: 1**
Text page: 107
Rationale: The American Nurses Association Code of Ethics identifies the primary goals, values, and obligations of the profession of nursing. The specific standards of care and practice are developed by professional organizations and the nursing practice acts of each state based upon evidence-based practice. The board of nurse examiners for each state has been charged with the disciplinary actions for incompetent nurse in the respective state.

5-4. **Answer: 3**
Text pages: 117-119
Rationale: Beneficence means to do good. As a moral principle, beneficence presents us with the duty to maximize the benefits of actions while minimizing harm. When society formulates rules that are designed to protect people against the negative effects of their own actions, these rules are considered beneficent, yet they override a person's autonomy. One example of this is the use of safety restraints—car seats for children and seat belts for adults—when driving or riding in an automobile. It is inappropriate to consider beneficence as a moral principle when holding confidential information that may harm another, as in the case of the husband with HIV. The client must control the client-controlled analgesia infusion and choose when to administer additional pain medication. If the nurse presses the button to administer additional medication, the client may suffer adverse effects related to receiving too much medication, because the client is not determining pain medication needs. Counseling a person regarding when to request a tubal ligation is inappropriate based upon the nurses' cultural values. The person should be given information on the advantages and disadvantages of the surgical procedure and its consequences, and the person has the autonomy to make her decision.

5-5. **Answer: 1**
Text page: 120

Rationale: Justice is an ethical principle of major importance in health-promotion settings. Justice is involved with the fair distribution of goods such as health, education, food, and shelter. Justice is the equalizing of benefits across society regardless of merit. Evaluating the four options given, it is apparent that the first statement supports justice related to provision of health care to all people, without regard to ability for payment. The other options place conditions on receiving care and interventions based upon ability to pay or maintain medical regimens, which are not consistent with the concept of justice.

CHAPTER 6

6-1.   **Answer: 2**
        Text page: 129
        Rationale: The T-ACE test provides a much more sensitive measure of alcohol intake patterns than that derived from the CAGE test. The T-ACE test comprises the following assessment criteria:
        - How many drinks does it **T**ake to make you feel high?
        - Have you ever been **A**nnoyed by people criticizing your drinking?
        - Have you ever felt you ought to **C**ut down your drinking?
        - Have you ever had a drink first thing in the morning (**E**ye opener) to steady your nerves or get rid of a hangover?

        The CAGE test considers data collected from the client on **C**utting down on drinking, been **A**nnoyed by criticism of drinking, feeling **G**uilty about drinking, and using alcohol as an **E**ye opener.

        The nonstress test evaluates the fetal heart rate response to fetal movement, which is assessed after the fetus is 20 weeks or older. The protein dipstick test is performed at each prenatal visit and measures the amount of protein in the client's urine. Proteinuria is a symptom seen with preeclampsia.

6-2.   **Answer: 2**
        Text page: 130
        Rationale: Primary prevention is a concept central to nursing and includes generalized health promotion and specific protection from disease. Health promotion connotes an active process involving specific protections, including immunizations, occupational safety, and environmental control, along with a set of behaviors that enhances health. Physician visits that promote health promotion focus on screening and wellness visits that include teaching on preventive health practices. Antibiotics should be taken only when there is evidence of an infec-

tion. Water aerobics focuses on flexibility, not muscle building.

6-3.   **Answers: 1, 3, 5**
        Text page: 134
        Rationale: A major goal in assessing each pattern is to determine the individual's knowledge of health promotion, the ability to manage health-promoting activities, and the value that the individual ascribes to health promotion. Assessment of herbal medication use is important to determine potential for interactions with other prescribed medications and adverse effects produced by the herbal medications. Referral to the physician for illness care would not be part of the assessment of functional health patterns.

6-4.   **Answer: 3**
        Text page: 134
        Rationale: The health perception–health management pattern provides an overview of the individual's health status and the health practices that are used to reach the current level of health or wellness. The focus is on perceived health status and the meaning of health, along with the individual's level of commitment to maintaining health. The cognitive-perceptual pattern focuses on sensory, perceptual, and cognitive patterns. The coping–stress tolerance pattern identifies the general coping pattern and effectiveness on stress tolerance. The self-perception–self-concept pattern describes the individual's perception of self to include body comfort, body image, and feeling state, as well as self-concept and self-esteem.

6-5.   **Answer: 3**
        Text page: 134
        Rationale: Assessment of the mucous membranes determines hydration status, which is part of the nutritional-metabolic pattern. Other assessment findings for this pattern may point to an individual who is overweight, underweight, overly hydrated, dehydrated, or experiencing difficulties in skin integrity, such as skin breakdown or delayed healing. The attention span is part of the self perception–self-concept pattern. Measurement of blood pressure is part of the activity-exercise pattern. Urine color is part of the elimination pattern.

6-6.   **Answer: 4**
        Text page: 135
        Rationale: The affective component of education addresses the attitudes and values of the individual regarding the education and how it will affect life beliefs. If education is valued, the person will be more likely to comply, opposite to what occurs when the education is not congruent with the person's

values. Even when the individual possesses the knowledge base, assessment of whether the individual also values the importance of adhering to the modifications in lifestyle is vital.

6-7. **Answer: 2**
Text page: 136
Rationale: The nurse uses evidence to guide practice. Emptying the bladder as soon as the sensation of fullness occurs is a practice that decreases the time the urine remains in the bladder, thus decreasing the chance for bacterial growth to occur. Decreasing oral intake will cause the urine to become concentrated. Urinary frequency is a symptom seen with urinary tract infection. Research indicates that delayed time between urinations is associated with increased incidence of urinary tract infection.

6-8. **Answer: 2**
Text pages: 136-137
Rationale: Exercise is a type of physical activity that is planned, structured, and repetitive and performed to improve or maintain physical fitness. Active social activities, such as backyard softball or golf, would be considered physical activity. Jogging, walking, or a gym workout would be considered exercise. Sedentary social activities such as bingo, reading, knitting, stamp collection, cards, or discussion groups would not be considered physical activity.

6-9. **Answer: 2**
Text page: 139
Rationale: Most difficulties associated with sleep are amenable to nursing therapies. Frequent awakenings do not necessarily imply sleep interruption. Many individuals awaken numerous times during the night but return to sleep within seconds. This may be especially true of older adults who generally spend most of the night in stages of light sleep. Their normal developmental pattern does not include deep sleep; therefore, awakenings may not affect the sleep cycles and resultant feelings in the morning. More commonly the older adult experiences difficulty returning to sleep because of discomfort, fears, or other variables.

6-10. **Answer: 3**
Text page: 142
Rationale: Early adolescence developmental focus is on industry verses inferiority, as identified by Erikson. The wellness tasks identified include:
- Learning that health is an important value
- Learning self-regulation of physiological needs— sleep, rest, food, drink, and exercise

- Learning risk taking and its consequences (injury prevention)

The three other options define adolescent (identity verses role confusion) wellness developmental tasks, which include learning to cope with life events and problems, learning economic responsibility, and learning social responsibility for self and others.

CHAPTER 7

7-1. **Answers: 1, 2, 3, 4, 6**
Text page: 156
Rationale: At least 7 of the 10 leading causes of death listed in the *Healthy People 2010* report might be reduced substantially by improving only five habits: poor diet, smoking, lack of exercise, alcohol abuse, and stress.

7-2. **Answer: 4**
Text page: 161
Rationale: How the family makes decisions about health promotion and disease prevention is part of the cognitive-perceptual pattern. Option 1 is an assessment included in the sleep-rest pattern. Option 2 falls within the realm of the activity-exercise pattern. Option 3 is included in the self-perception–self-concept pattern.

7-3. **Answer: 3**
Text page: 166
Rationale: The coping–stress tolerance pattern helps to depict the family's adaptation to both internal and external pressures. Assessments include the kinds of dysfunctional adaptive strategies that are used. The remaining options are assessments for the values-beliefs pattern.

7-4. **Answer: 4**
Text page: 167
Rationale: Developmental theory approaches families from the perspective of tasks and progression through cycles. The nurse analyzes data for cues to identify the stages of the family life cycle and tasks to accomplish for successful family function. The systems approach determines both the structural and functional components of the family as a system. The stages of family development guide the analysis of the baseline data.

7-5. **Answer: 2**
Text page: 168
Rationale: Couples who find satisfaction in parenthood seem to realize that parental influence begins at birth and is the single most important factor in the child's physical, emotional, and cognitive devel-

opment. The parents' ability to assume responsibility depends on a complex array of factors, some of which are their own maturity, how they were nurtured as children, their values and philosophy of life, their conceptions about self, culture, social class, and religion, and their perceptions of and experiences with children and other adults.

7-6. **Answer: 1**
Text page: 155
Rationale: The nurse intervenes in a situation of suspected domestic violence by helping the woman develop an escape plan. The abused woman should not attempt to identify the reasons for the abuse, because it is not based upon identifiable reasons. She should be encouraged to control her fertility through contraceptive methods, although the type of contraception used should be based upon the woman's reproductive history and choice. The abuse situation should be discussed with the nurse, and the individual should be assured that she is not alone. A psychiatric intervention is usually not the first intervention.

7-7. **Answer: 4**
Text pages: 167-168
Rationale: The coordinator for genetic counseling is identified as a possible nursing role for the couple stage. The coordinator with pediatric services is part of the nurse's role for the childbearing family. The teacher of first aid and emergency measures is addressed in the family with preschool or school-age children. The teacher of risk factors to health is part of the role with the family with adolescents.

7-8. **Answer: 2**
Text page: 169
Rationale: Some of the risk factors for a family with school-age children include an unstimulating home environment, working parents with inappropriate use of resources for child care, multiple, closely spaced children, and abuse or neglect of the children.

7-9. **Answer: 2**
Text page: 156
Rationale: During the critical stage, signs are present but are probably not noticeable to the individual. The stage is the transition from wellness to illness. If the risks had been eliminated before this stage, then the disease process might have been reversed or significantly decelerated. The individual is likely unaware that a disease process is underway. Arresting or reducing the seriousness of the disease and enhancing longevity are still possible.

7-10. **Answer: 1**
Text page: 168
Rationale: The nurse's role in the family with older adults includes the counselor of bereavement. The counselor of menopause would be part of the nurse's role with the family with young or middle-aged adults. The nurse's role with the family with adolescents would be the counselor of family planning and sexually transmitted diseases.

CHAPTER 8

8-1. **Answer: 3**
Text page: 179
Rationale: The health care literature proposes that the major improvements in the population's health will be derived from self-care and strategies of health promotion and disease prevention, not from medical technology and services. The goal for maintaining health in the population focuses on the active involvement of individuals in caring for their health through use of health-promotion strategies. Hospital admissions and interventions provided at clinics are to be used when self-care activities are not successful in maintaining health.

8-2. **Answer: 2**
Text page: 180
Rationale: Interdependent nursing functions include collaboration with community members and interdisciplinary teamwork functions that are crucial to effective community health. Independent nursing functions include assessing, analyzing, diagnosing, planning, implementing, and evaluating nursing activities such as health promotion and health education. Dependent nursing functions include implementing the therapeutic plans of team members. Multidisciplinary functions involve many members of the entire health care team, not solely nursing.

8-3. **Answer: 1**
Text page: 180
Rationale: Measurement uses instruments to quantify data in information collection. Measurement data include population statistics, pollution indexes, morbidity and mortality rates, census statistics, and epidemiological data. The interview is a method for collecting data from people. Interview data include verbal statements from community residents, key community officials, health care personnel, and various community agency staff. This method of data collection is an excellent way to determine how members perceive their community. The "windshield survey" approach to data collection includes the use of the senses to determine commu-

nity appearances. These appearances include the type and state of residential dwellings, the people, and the physical and biological characteristics.

8-4.   ***Answer: 4, 2, 1, 3***
Text page: 191
Rationale: The Rosenstock model identifies four steps, which sequence how individuals undergo a change in health behavior. These steps are:
- Perceiving the behavior as a threat in terms of susceptibility and seriousness
- Believing the behavior is a threat to health
- Taking action to adopt preventive health
- Reinforcing the new behavior

In this model the consumer first takes on a passive role, progressing from passive to active in steps 2 and 3. The consumer then, in step 4, is actively involved in reinforcing the new behavior.

8-5.   ***Answer: 1***
Text page: 183
Rationale: Observation data collection is a visual assessment of the community related to the nutritional-metabolic pattern. The shopping facilities are visible to the data collector. The water quality is a measurement derived from statistics. The percentage of the community housing that possesses inadequate kitchen and plumbing facilities is also a measurement expressed as a percentage. The nutritional services available in the community would be collected through the interview process.

CHAPTER 9

9-1.   ***Answer: 3***
Text page: 211
Rationale: The *Healthy People 2010* goals related to infant and children screening include:
- Ensure appropriate newborn bloodspot screening, follow-up testing, and referral to services.
- Increase the proportion of newborns who are screened for hearing loss by age 1 month, have audiologic evaluation by age 3 months, and are enrolled in appropriate intervention services by age 6 months.
- Increase the proportion of preschool children aged 5 years and under who receive vision screening.

There is not a goal that speaks to the screening of newborns for chlamydia infections. The mother at risk for sexually transmitted diseases is screened for chlamydia infection during pregnancy.

9-2.   ***Answer: 1***
Text pages: 201-202

Rationale: Sensitivity measures the proportion of people with a condition who correctly test positive when screened. Reliability is an assessment of the reproducibility of the test's results when different individuals with the same level of skill perform the test during different periods and under different conditions. Validity measures the test's ability to distinguish correctly between diseased and nondiseased individuals and is an indicator of the accuracy of the test. Specificity measures the test's ability to recognize negative reactions or nondiseased individuals.

9-3.   ***Answers: 2, 3, 4, 6***
Text page: 205
Rationale: People who submit to screening tests may assume that the results they receive are diagnostic and classify them as disease free or disease laden. This is untrue, because the screening goal is only identification and referral of individuals at risk or who may need follow-up or further evaluation. Participants need to be informed of the limitations of the screening and the results. Because sensitivity and specificity are not 100% accurate, false-positive and false-negative results occur. It becomes difficult as an ethical issue to evaluate whether the benefits received by those correctly screened are worth the problems experienced by those incorrectly screened. Additional issues that confound the medical ethics of screening are cutoff points for the screening instrument and borderline cases. If the disease were potentially life threatening, an increase in false-positive results (lower cutoff point) would be preferred to missing individuals who may have the disease. A problem closely related to the cutoff point is defining a policy for borderline results.

9-4.   ***Answer: 1***
Text page: 212
Rationale: Although all sexually active women are at risk for cervical cancer, the disease is more common among women of low socioeconomic status, women with a history of multiple sex partners, women with an early first sexual intercourse, smokers, and women infected with certain types of human papilloma virus and HIV.

The official guidelines for Pap smear testing include the following:
- Screening should be performed on all women aged 21 years and older or within 3 years of the onset of sexual activity and at least 3 years thereafter.
- Routine screening is not recommended for women who are not at high risk, aged 65 and older, whose recent Pap smear results have been normal.

- Screening is not recommended for women with a history of total hysterectomy for benign disease.
- There is insufficient evidence to recommend for or against the use of the new technologies for routine screening.

9-5. **Answer: 2**
Text page: 209
Rationale: Racial and ethnic health disparities and factors such as access to care need to be taken into consideration when planning screening programs. In order to plan, implement, and evaluate a screening program that targets a specific population, the provider must have an awareness of that particular population's characteristics. The components of awareness include lifestyle, socioeconomic characteristics, education, heredity and environmental factors, values, and religious and cultural beliefs. Partnering with the community through the entire process is also necessary if the program is to be successful.

CHAPTER 10

10-1. **Answer: 3**
Text page: 218
Rationale: McGinnis (2003) states that behavior patterns currently account for 40% to 50% of early deaths among Americans and represent the single most controllable area of influence over the future health forecast. Heredity is not controllable, and inheritance does influence one's future health. Educational level enhances knowledge of information that should be used to incorporate health practices into one's lifestyle. Economic status allows a person the ability to purchase healthy food and access to health promotion through primary care interventions.

10-2. **Answers: 1, 3, 5, 6**
Text page: 220
Rationale: The goal of health education is to assist individuals, families, and communities to achieve, through their own actions and initiative, optimal states of health, therefore enhanced wellness. Other goals of health education are for the detection of illness, treatment, rehabilitation, and long-term care. Health education encourages positive, informed changes in lifestyle behaviors that prevent acute and chronic disease, decrease disability, and enhance wellness. Health education fosters successful changes in health behavior, which then empowers the client. People who believe that their behaviors will make a difference in their health and who are involved in the decision making are more likely to make changes. Health education enables the individual to wisely handle daily decisions and to manage a chronic illness.

10-3. **Answer: 1**
Text pages: 226-227
Rationale: The health professional must take the time to assess cultural beliefs that influence social and health practices and must make every effort to analyze educational interventions that are acceptable and satisfying to the individual. Nurses should recognize that a person's or group's background, beliefs, and knowledge may differ significantly from their own and seek to understand and show respect for these differences. Nurses should endeavor to provide culturally sensitive education to the individual. Medical terminology may be confusing and interpreted in different ways and therefore should be used only when the meaning can be made clear. Nurses should present evidence-based information to all persons regardless of cultural background. Universal health practices, which are based upon research, should be presented regardless of cultural background.

10-4. **Answer: 2**
Text page: 227
Rationale: The nurse evaluates the quality of life in a population by analyzing social, economic, communication, or spiritual patterns, concerns, and problems. Involving the people in a self-study of their needs and aspirations is the best way to accomplish this task. Relating a health problem to social problems helps the nurse and the individuals expand the rationale or justification of the health education project. The nurse collects data by analyzing infant mortality rates, health care coverage, and the population's demographic information. These are assessment techniques used to formulate the intervention plans for the population. Active involvement in a self-study secures participation in the interventions leading to positive outcomes.

10-5. **Answer: 3**
Text page: 227
Rationale: Drill and practice would be an appropriate methodology used to teach psychomotor skills. Other teaching methods for psychomotor skill acquisition would include performing procedures through demonstrations, games, role-playing exercises, and peer teaching. Cognitive teaching is best accomplished through programmed instruction, lecture, simulations, games, and computer-assisted programs. Teaching in the affective domain involves a change in attitudes or emotions that will affect behaviors. Suggested teaching strategies include discussion, simulations, role playing, and field experiences.

CHAPTER 11

11-1. *Answer: 4*
Text page: 232
Rationale: The four leading causes of death directly associated with diet are coronary heart disease, some types of cancer, stroke, and diabetes mellitus. Anemia may be due to inadequate iron and folate intake. Risk for infection is increased if a person is malnourished. Cirrhosis of the liver is caused by alcohol abuse.

11-2. *Answer: 1*
Text pages: 239, 241
Rationale: Supplements are sometimes necessary for specific populations to obtain desirable amounts of particular nutrients. These include:
- Folic acid for females who could be pregnant to help prevent neural tube defects
- Iron during pregnancy
- Calcium for individuals who do not meet the recommended intake of calcium
- Vitamin D for elderly people who do not drink generous quantities of fortified milk or who do not manufacture vitamin D from sunlight
Large doses of vitamin A may be teratogenic, and supplementation should be avoided during the first trimester of pregnancy unless there is a specific deficiency. Calcium supplements interfere with iron absorption. High doses of vitamin E can interfere with vitamin K action and enhance the effect of some anticoagulant drugs (e.g., coumadin).

11-3. *Answer: 4*
Text pages: 241–242
Rationale: Hand washing is one of the most important practices in the prevention of food-borne illness. Raw, cooked, and ready-to-eat foods should be separated while shopping, preparing, or storing foods. Additional preventive safety measures include:
- Wash fresh fruits and vegetables thoroughly.
- Drink pasteurized juices.
- Do not consume raw (unpasteurized) milk or cheeses made from raw milk.
- Eat food that has been chilled and refrigerated properly.
- When eating out, make sure that food has been chilled and refrigerated properly.
- When shopping, buy perishable foods last and take them straight home.
- Whether raw or cooked, never leave meat, poultry, eggs, fish, or shellfish out at room temperature for more then 2 hours. Be sure to chill leftovers as soon as you are finished eating.

11-4. *Answer: 4*
Text page: 244
Rationale: When the local WIC agency has reached its maximal caseload, vacancies generally are filled in the order of the following priority levels:
- Pregnant women, breast-feeding women, and infants determined to be at nutritional risk from serious medical problems
- Infants up to 6 months of age whose mothers participate in WIC or are eligible to participate and have serious medical problems
- Children (up to age 5) at nutritional risk from serious medical problems
- Pregnant or breast-feeding women and infants who are at nutritional risk from dietary problems
- Children (up to age 5) at nutritional risk for dietary problems
- Non–breast-feeding postpartum women with any nutritional risk
- Individuals at nutritional risk only because they are homeless or migrants and current participants who would likely continue to have medical or dietary problems without WIC assistance

11-5. *Answer: 4*
Text page: 245
Rationale: The single largest group at risk for malnutrition is composed of elderly adults. The health care professional should refer the individual to a physician when there has been an involuntary weight loss of 10 pounds or more within a 6-month period. Additional anthropometric measurements suggesting malnutrition include:
- Triceps skin fold thickness less than 10th percentile
- Midarm muscle circumference less than 10th percentile
- Serum albumin level less than 3.5 mg/dl
- Evidence of osteoporosis or mineral deficiency (indicated by a history of bone pain or fractures, particularly in older women)
- Evidence of vitamin deficiency (indicated by inadequate intake of fruits and vegetables; angular stomatitis, glossitis, or bleeding gums; pressure ulcers in bedridden individuals)

11-6. *Answer: 1*
Text page: 247
Rationale: Major risk factors for heart disease include:
- HDL level less than 40 mg/dl
- Clinical forms of atherosclerotic disease (peripheral arterial disease, abdominal aortic aneurysm, and symptomatic carotid artery disease)
- Age 55 for men and 65 for women
- Cigarette smoking

- Hypertension (BP 140/90 mm Hg or higher, or on antihypertensive medication)
- Diabetes (fasting blood glucose 110 mg/dl or higher)
- Family history of premature heart disease (heart disease in a first-degree relative at age 55 or younger for men or age 65 or younger for women)

11-7. *Answers: 1, 3, 4, 5*
Text page: 235, Healthy People 2010 box
Rationale: Options 1, 3, 4, and 5 are stated as the objectives for heart disease in the *Healthy People 2010*. Option 2 is not part of that document. Option 6 is part of the core measure requirements at discharge for a person who has been hospitalized for an acute myocardial infarction.

CHAPTER 12

12-1. *Answer: 1*
Text page: 266
Rationale: Exercise has a major influence on lipoprotein metabolism, primarily on the levels of HDL and triglycerides (TRG). Increases in HDL lower the total cholesterol-to-HDL ratio. Exercise has a potent lowering effect on levels of plasma TRG that is evident within hours after a bout of exercise. TRG levels are lower and HDL levels are higher in physically active people than in the sedentary population. The effect of exercise on lipid metabolism may be related more to the volume (duration and frequency) rather than to the intensity of the exercise. Short periods of exercise training result in modest increases in HDL, but longer periods of training produce larger increases in HDL. Exercise's lowering effect on TRG is cumulative; therefore, frequent bouts of exercise result in a progressive decrease in TRG.

12-2. *Answer: 4*
Text page: 271
Rationale: Changes in immune markers, such as CD4 and CD8 cell counts and the number and activity of natural killer cells, indicate that moderate exercise may help bolster an impaired immune system. Evidence indicates that moderate exercise stimulates the neuroendocrine system, which causes changes in the function and numbers of various immune system cells. Evidence also indicates that moderate exercise is associated with a prolonged improvement in the killing capacity of neutrophils. Moderate exercise may decrease the risk of upper respiratory tract infection. High-intensity marathoner runners have a significantly higher incidence of upper respiratory tract infections. Intense exercise is associated with a decrease in catecholamine and corticosteroid levels. Moderate exercise increases the release of immunostimulatory hormones.

12-3. *Answer: 1*
Text page: 264, Box 12-2
Rationale: Populations with low rates of physical activity:
- Women generally are less active than men are at all ages.
- People with lower incomes and less education typically are not as physically active as those with higher incomes and more education.
- African American and Hispanic people are generally less physically active than whites.
- Adults in northeastern and southern states tend to be less active that adults in north central and western states.
- People with disabilities are less physically active than people without disabilities.
- By age 75, one in three men and one in two women engage in no regular physical activity.

12-4. *Answers: 1, 5, 6*
Text page: 282, Box 12-5
Rationale: Recommendations and precautions for people with diabetes who are interested in physical activity and exercise include:
- Monitor blood glucose levels before and 20 to 30 minutes after exercise to determine the response to exercise.
- Exercise approximately 1 hour after meals when blood glucose level is the highest.
- Know the action and peak times of insulin effect and avoid exercising at peak times.
- Avoid injecting insulin into a muscle area that will be active during exercise: the pumping action of the muscle may speed up absorption of the insulin and cause a rapid decrease of blood glucose.
- Carry a concentrated form of carbohydrate when exercising to be used if signs of hypoglycemia are felt.

12-5. *Answer: 2*
Text page: 273, Hot Topics box
Rationale: Recommendations from the CDC and the American College of Sports Medicine are:
- Adults should accumulate 30 minutes or more of moderate intensity physical activity on most (or all) days of the week, for a weekly total of 3 to 4 hours.
- The activity need not be continuous; benefits can be realized with short bouts of activity (a minimum of 10 minutes) over the course of the day.

- This activity will expend about 150 to 200 calories per day or 1000 to 1400 calories per week.
- All types of activity can be applied to the daily total exercise for the day.

CHAPTER 13

13-1. **Answer: 3**
Text page: 291
Rationale: Stress causes physiological arousal along three pathways: the musculoskeletal system, the autonomic nervous system, and the psychoneuroendocrine system. The musculoskeletal system responds to stress by increasing tension and tone. The autonomic nervous system causes an increase in heart rate, blood pressure, and respiratory rate. Heightened awareness of the environment is triggered, and the blood shifts from the visceral organs to the large muscles. The psychoneuroendocrine system stimulates the secretion of corticosteroids and other neuroendocrine substances into the systemic circulation, which increases glucose levels and the antiinflammatory response.

13-2. **Answer: 1**
Text page: 294
Rationale: Individuals who possess characteristics of stress hardiness are shown to be less vulnerable to stress-related symptoms and disease. The characteristics of stress hardiness are control, challenge, and commitment. For stress-hardy individuals, stress is viewed as a challenge rather than a threat; they feel in control of situations in their lives, and they are committed to rather than alienated from work, home, and family.

13-3. **Answer: 2**
Text page: 298
Rationale: A variety of alternative and complementary therapies are available as techniques to prevent and reduce harmful effects of stress. Common therapies include acupuncture, hypnosis, aromatherapy, reflexology, chiropractic therapy, and herbal therapies. People are increasingly using alternative therapies as self-help measures, and research to study their effects has grown enormously in recent years. Nurses can assist individuals to base their use on evidence of safety and efficacy. Among the variety of alternative therapies available, acupuncture and hypnosis have strong evidence of effectiveness. Herbal remedies require caution, because they can have harmful as well as beneficial effects and may interfere with other treatments.

13-4. **Answer: 3**
Text pages: 300–301

Rationale: Cognitive therapy is a conceptual model for short-term intervention to modify thinking and reduce stress. In the context of cognitive therapy, cognitive restructuring is a technique or series of strategies that help people evaluate their thoughts, challenge them, and replace them with responses that are more rational. Cognitive restructuring:
- Teaches people to recognize that negative thinking often causes emotional distress
- Does not gloss over or deny misfortune, suffering, or negative feelings
- Assists people to become "unstuck" from negative moods so that they can experience a broader range of feelings

13-5. **Answers: 2, 3, 5**
Text page: 301, Box 13-2
Rationale: The nurse can provide suggestions to the client with stress-related sleep disturbances using the following strategies:
- Keep a sleep diary, which helps determine sleep patterns.
- Reduce consumption of alcohol and caffeine.
- Have a regular sleep-wake schedule, even on weekends.
- If unable to fall asleep within 20 to 30 minutes or if waking up and unable to fall back to sleep within that time, get out of bed and do something until groggy and sleepy again.
- Use a relaxation tape or practice diaphragmatic breathing to help release tension and calm down.
- Limit naps during the day to 45 minutes.
- Exercise within 3 to 6 hours of bedtime.
- Take a hot bath 2 hours before bedtime.
- Sleep in a cool room.

CHAPTER 14

14-1. **Answer: 4**
Text page: 311
Rationale: Holistic health practices are used to promote wellness. They are used to treat illness and reduce pain. Holism is the understanding that people are not just physical bodies; people have emotions, spirits, and relationships that combine with the physical body to make a whole person. The holistic movement in the healing arts reflects the theory of holism and recognizes that all these aspects of the person must be considered when planning and delivering care. The entire person is treated, not only symptoms. It is important to identify the cause of the symptom and treat the cause. Many of the interventions used in holistic health practices are backed by centuries of tradition, and

today research is being carried out to document their scientific merit. These holistic practices often are considered alternative practices, some of which are covered by health insurance.

14-2. **Answer: 2**
Text page: 313
Rationale: The basic premise behind energy work is releasing blockages to energy flow, stimulating deficient life energy, and rebalancing life energy. Acupuncture is the insertion of fine needles into precisely mapped points on the skin surface. Reading auras is the extension of the energy field beyond the physical body. Reiki is placing the hands and making symbolic gestures that create attunement or the opening of the energy channel.

14-3. **Answer: 3**
Text page: 313
Rationale: Acupuncture is a useful treatment for substance abuse. It has also been found to be effective in postoperative pain, nausea and vomiting from chemotherapy, other pain syndromes, stroke rehabilitation, and asthma.

14-4. **Answers: 1, 3, 4, 5, 6**
Text page: 320
Rationale: Music therapy influences the area of the brain involved with emotions and feelings, the limbic system. Music therapy has been documented as decreasing anxiety and increasing pain thresholds in postoperative individuals. It has had a significant effect on pain and distress in laboring mothers. Others have found music therapy useful for people with osteoarthritis pain. Classical music used with persons with acute myocardial infarction was associated with a significant decrease in heart rate, respiratory rate, and oxygen demand after these individuals listened to 20 minutes of music. Music therapy has produced a significant decrease in nausea and vomiting associated with administration of chemotherapy.

14-5. **Answer: 1**
Text pages: 321–322
Rationale: Essential oils may be used in the following ways:
• They may be added to the bath or used in a douche.
• They may be mixed with carrier oils and used during massage.
• They may be applied directly to minor injuries to speed healing.
• They may be placed on cloth and applied as a compress.
• They may be inhaled after vaporization.
Precautions that should be considered when using essential oils include:

• They are for external use only.
• The oils should be diluted in carrier oil before direct application to the skin.
• Avoid application to the eyes and mucous membranes.
• Many of the oils are contraindicated for use during pregnancy.
• Essential oils should be used with caution in people with epilepsy, hypertension, and estrogen-dependent tumors.

CHAPTER 15

15-1. **Answer: 4**
Text pages: 330, 339
Rationale: Growth refers to changes in the structure, reflects an increase in the number and size of cells, and results in an increase in the size and weight of the whole or any of its parts. During childhood, physical changes in head circumference, weight, height, and overall body proportion are part of growth. Growth also refers to increases or decreases, as in old age, in the size of organs and systems.

Development refers to gradual change and expansion of ability and advance in skill from lower to more advanced complexity. In contrast to growth, which is a quantitative or precisely measurable change, development is a qualitative change. Development has best been conceptualized as a process that follows certain pattern sequences, although the timing of the advancements is individual.

15-2. **Answer: 4**
Text pages: 337, Multicultural Awareness box
Rationale: Questions addressing the age of a house, where lead paint was used, targets only children whose exposure to lead is through lead-based paint. During the past 2 decades, assessment of children from homes with lead-based paint has resulted in a 90% decline in the overall number of children affected; however the risk for Hispanic children has remained steady. Lead-based paint is not the primary source of lead poisoning for these children. Food and culturally defined health practices bring additional unscreened risk to this population. Foods packaged or canned outside the United States or foods prepared in ceramic containers or pottery made outside the United States and wrapped Mexican candies all increase lead exposure of these children.

15-3. **Answer: 4**
Text page: 341, Table 15-3

Rationale: Erikson identifies eight stages of psychosocial development across the lifespan. These are:

- Infancy: trust versus mistrust
- Toddler: autonomy versus shame and doubt
- Preschool: initiative versus guilt
- School age: industry versus inferiority
- Adolescence: identity versus role confusion
- Young adulthood: intimacy versus isolation
- Middle adulthood: generativity versus stagnation
- Older adulthood: ego integrity versus despair

15-4.   *Answer: 2*
   Text page: 342, Table 15-4
   Rationale: Development of the concept of object permanence occurs from birth to 2 years old and is in the sensorimotor stage. Development of egocentric animistic and magical thinking occurs in children 2 to 7 years old in the preoperational stage, as does thought dominated by senses. Consideration of others' point of view is in the concrete operations stage, which is from 7 to 11 years of age.

15-5.   *Answers: 2, 5*
   Text page: 342, Table 15-6
   Rationale: Gilligan identifies the goals for women in the postconventional stage as principle of nonviolence and do not hurt self or others. Kohlberg's postconventional stage identifies the goals as agree upon rights, personal moral standards, and justice.

CHAPTER 16

16-1.   *Answer: 3*
   Text page: 348
   Rationale: The nurse refers couples to early pregnancy and Lamaze childbirth preparation classes to increase their social support and help them increase their knowledge about labor and delivery. Couples make many of their decisions regarding pain relief for labor and birth based upon information provided in the childbirth classes. Information provided during childbirth classes does facilitate a smooth transition to an early discharge, but that is not the goal of the education. Childbirth education may be provided to couples who are planning to deliver at different health care settings. The focus is not on sharing the policies of each of these facilities.

16-2.   *Answer: 3*
   Text pages: 351-352
   Rationale: Events that may signal difficulties with the progression of labor or development of a complication include unusual fetal or uterine activity, presence of meconium in the amniotic fluid, fetal tachycardia (heart rate above 160 beats per minute), fetal bradycardia (heart rate below 120 beats per minute) in a full-term infant, and fetal heart rate decreases with uterine activity (late deceleration) during labor. Clear amniotic fluid is a normal finding during labor. The presence of fetal activity during labor is considered a good finding. Contractions with a frequency of 3 minutes and duration of 60 seconds indicates an acceptable pattern.

16-3.   *Answer: 2*
   Text page: 352
   Rationale: Cold stress should be avoided by keeping the newborn dry, warmly wrapped, and avoiding environments that cause heat loss. The labor and delivery room temperature should be increased to at least 78° F at the time of delivery. The infant should not be bathed immediately after birth, because heat loss will occur as the water evaporates from the skin. The baby should be placed in an open warmer with servo control so that the heat output is regulated according to the newborn's skin temperature.

16-4.   *Answer: 2*
   Text pages: 359-360
   Rationale: The woman attempts to ensure safe passage for herself and her infant by seeking health care from a doctor, midwife, or cultural health practitioner, by gaining support and information from family and friends, and by reading and watching videotapes. Fantasizing about the gender of her baby is a behavior seen in the mother as she attempts to ensure acceptance of her child. Integrating the fetus as an integral part of her is seen in the pregnant woman as she binds into her unknown child. The woman is learning to give of herself by examining what she will gain and lose by becoming a mother.

16-5.   *Answer: 1*
   Text page: 362, Box 16-4
   Rationale: The older sibling must be involved in the pregnancy and birth experience according to the child's growth and development. After delivery, involving the sibling in choosing toys and clothes for the new baby will decrease sibling rivalry. The sibling may make negative comments, because now time with the parents must be shared with the baby. Explanations and planning separate time for the sibling, not discipline, should be the intervention. If the sibling is admonished to "be careful" and "be quiet" he or she may not accept the baby with open arms. Involving the sibling during prenatal visits helps set the stage for the arrival of the new baby. It provides an extended time for the sibling to begin to understand the addition to the family.

16-6. *Answer: 4*
Text page: 367
Rationale: The Rh-negative pregnant woman should be given RhoGAM after delivery of an Rh-positive infant within 72 hours of delivery, between 24 and 28 weeks of gestation, or after a miscarriage or therapeutic abortion, even if the fetal blood type is unknown. The RhoGAM prevents the mother's sensitization to fetal Rh-positive cells by inactivating fetal red blood cells in the mother before the mother can develop an antibody response. RhoGAM must be given to the Rh-negative woman after each delivery of an Rh-positive baby.

16-7. *Answers: 1, 2, 4, 5*
Text page: 352, Care Plan
Rationale: Options 1, 2, 4, and 5 are all interventions that will assist the labor client to cope with her contractions. Preparing the client for epidural anesthesia will eliminate the pain of contractions, but is not the priority nursing intervention for ineffective coping during active labor. Systemic analgesia administration and monitoring are important during labor but do not directly address the client need of ineffective coping.

16-8. *Answer: 3*
Text page: 347, Box 16-1
Rationale: Positive signs of pregnancy are those that document the existence of the fetus. The presence of fetal heart tones is a positive sign of pregnancy. Others include the detection of fetal parts through Leopold's maneuvers, objective detection of fetal movements, and radiological or ultrasonographic demonstration of fetal parts. Options 1, 2, and 4 are all probable signs of pregnancy. They indicate that a pregnancy is likely, but they do not confirm it.

16-9. *Answer: 1*
Text page: 353, Table 16-3
Rationale: The nurse determines the Apgar score at 1 and 5 minutes after birth. It is based on five signs noted in the newborn. The nurse evaluates the newborn for these five signs and then adds the numbers for the total score. The score is from 0 to 10. The higher the score, the better the newborn is adapting to the extrauterine environment. The actual Apgar scoring tool is below.

Sign	0	1	2
Heart rate	Absent	Slow (under 100)	Over 100
Respiratory effort	Absent	Weak cry, hypoventilation	Good strong cry
Muscle tone	Flaccid, limp	Some flexion of extremities	Active motion, extremities well flexed
Reflex irritability	No response	Grimace	Cry
Color	Blue, pale	Body pink, extremities blue	Completely pink

CHAPTER 17

17-1. *Answer: 1*
Text page: 389
Rationale: The infant's first play is an exercise of the senses, and the toys are visual in nature. The infant needs experiences that involve sight, sound, and touch. Singing to the infant will stimulate hearing. The parents should hang a mobile over the crib to stimulate the infant's sight. During infancy, the baby's play is solitary and repetitive. The 6-month-old infant does not possess the fine motor skills to push a button on a toy.

17-2. *Answers: 2, 5, 8*
Text page: 390
Rationale: Observational studies have found an association between SIDS and several risk factors, including prone sleeping position, prenatal or postnatal exposure to tobacco smoke, soft sleeping surfaces, hyperthermia or over-wrapping, bed sharing, and lack of breast-feeding. The American Academy of Pediatrics Task Force on SIDS recommends that those risk situations be eliminated as preventive strategies.

17-3. *Answer: 3*
Text page: 393
Rationale: During the first 2 months, most of the infant's sounds are vowels and are made primarily in the front part of the mouth. Cooing sounds are heard at approximately 2 to 3 months, usually in response to an adult's voice. By 6 months babbling sounds are heard, and by 9 to 10 months the infant forms two-syllable sounds.

17-4. *Answer: 2*
Text page: 394
Rationale: In early studies on attachment, Klaus, Kennell, and Klaus have formulated seven critical principles in the process of attachment. These include:
- A sensitive period appears to exist during the first minutes and hours after birth, when it seems necessary for the mother and father to have close contact with their infant for later development to be optimal.
- Species-specific responses to the infant appear to exist in the human mother and father when the infant is first given to them.
- The attachment process seems to be structured such that the parents become attached to only one infant at a time.
- For attachment to occur appropriately, the infant must respond to the mother and father by some signal, such as body or eye movements.
- Individuals who witness the birth process become strongly attached to the infant.
- Some adults find it difficult to go through the processes of attachment and detachment simultaneously. Becoming attached to an infant while mourning the loss or threatened loss of another person is difficult for parents.
- Some early events may have long-lasting effects.

17-5. *Answer: 4*
Text page: 385, *Research Highlights box*
Rationale: Research on breast-feeding and pacifiers includes the following findings:
- Shorter breast-feeding duration has been associated with pacifier use.
- Weight of evidence does suggest that pacifier use may cause a reduction in long-term breast-feeding.
- There is little harm associated with occasional pacifier use. Offering a pacifier after each feeding is not recommended. The mother should encourage the baby to satisfy sucking needs on her breasts.

17-6. *Answer: 4*
Text page: 380, *Box 17-1*
Rationale: At 2 months the posterior fontanel closes, and at 18 months the anterior fontanel closes.

17-7. *Answer: 2*
Text pages: 386, 388, *Box 17-6*
Rationale: Tips for introducing solid foods to infants:
- The infant's first solid foods should be smooth and runny.
- Puréed foods are used until the infant has teeth; chopped foods are used when the infant can chew.
- Introduce only one food at a time and in small amounts.
- Do not mix solid foods together; the infant should learn to appreciate different tastes and textures.
- Do not add solid foods to the infant's bottle.
- Do not start to reduce the milk supply until the infant is taking food successfully from the spoon.
- Until 1 year of age, feed the baby milk before solid foods.
- Do not give honey to infants less than 12 months of age. Honey is a known source of bacterial spores that produce a toxin, which can cause infant botulism.

CHAPTER 18

18-1. *Answer: 1*
Text pages: 417, 418
Rationale: No difference exists in lung topography or function after infancy. As the toddler grows the respiratory rate decreases, for a mean of 30 breaths per minute at 1 year of age to 25 breaths per minute at 3 years of age. The diameter of the toddler's upper respiratory tract is small when compared with that of an older child. This small diameter, coupled with the toddler's exploratory nature and lack of judgment in deciding what to place in the mouth, can result in airway obstruction. All 20 primary teeth erupt by the end of toddlerhood, but it is extremely rare that one of these teeth becomes loose. A mature swallowing pattern, using the tongue rather than the cheeks, has not yet developed, and toddlers continue to be at risk for choking.

18-2. *Answers: 1, 4, 5*
Text page: 421
Rationale: Nursing interventions to assist parents to meet nutritional needs of toddlers.
- Offer simple, single foods, because mixtures of foods are often rejected.
- Serve the toddler's favorite foods along with the new ones. It may take several introductions before the toddler accepts a new food.
- Encourage the use of utensils, but accept that toddlers still often need to use their fingers.
- Routines are important to toddlers. Serve scheduled meals and snacks.
- Mealtime should be a relaxed and pleasant time, free of distractions.
- Do not use food to bribe, reward, or punish the toddler.

- Schedule meals and sleep periods such that the child is awake and alert during mealtime.
- Serve small portions and let the toddler ask for more.
- Avoid foods that may cause choking.
- Drinking more than 2 cups of milk per day can reduce the child's appetite for other healthy foods.

18-3. **Answer: 1**
Text page: 422
Rationale: Most toddlers are interested in other children. However, this interest is limited, because toddlers, although ready to be with other children, are not ready to share. Successful social encounters with toddlers are best described as parallel play, where children play side by side, doing similar things with similar toys, but each working independently; sharing and cooperative play will not develop until well into the preschool years.

18-4. **Answer: 4**
Text page: 431
Rationale: Children between the ages of 1 and 3 years old are at the highest risk for drowning, because most do not know how to swim and do not have the skills to keep their heads above water or to get out of the water. Toddlers can drown in water just deep enough to cover their noses and mouths. Although swimming pools and natural bodies of water are a big part of the problem, even pails of water, toilets, bathtubs, and wading pools are dangerous. When a toddler falls into a pail of water or a toilet, it is hard for the child to straighten up because the entire weight is forward. Toddlers should never be left unattended—even for a few seconds—near the bathtub, hot tub, wading or swimming pool, toilet, or pail of water. All swimming pools should be fenced and have self-closing gates and latches. Toddlers must be supervised constantly and competently whenever they are near water and fitted properly with personal flotation devices whenever they are on a boat.

18-5. **Answer: 3**
Text page: 421, Health Teaching box
Rationale: Before beginning toilet training, parents should begin to check their toddlers for the prerequisite skills for toileting, which include being able to walk well, stoop and recover, stay dry for at least 2 hours during the day, communicate sensations before elimination, as well as the discomfort of wet or messy pants and the need for assistance. First, introduce the child to the potty seat or chair. The potty should provide secure seating with the child's feet touching the floor.

Because of the gastrocolic reflex, bowel elimination is more likely to occur after a meal; this is a good time to place the toddler on the potty. Encourage the toddler to stay on the chair for 2 to 3 minutes and always explain what to do ("Go potty") rather than what not to do ("Don't wet your pants"). Do not refer to elimination as *dirty* or *yucky*. Remember that this is your child's first creation.

Praise the child for the desired behavior. Introduce underwear as a badge of success. Ignore undesired behavior and never punish the child by scolding, spanking, or other punitive measures.

18-6. **Answer: 2**
Text page: 428, Box 18-2
Rationale: Indicators of child abuse that are observed by the nurse during an admission assessment of a toddler include:
- Parental delays in seeking help
- Inconsistencies in the history of how the injury occurred
- Injury inconsistent with the history or child's developmental capacity
- Radiographs showing old, unexplained fractures
- Bruises confined to back surface of the body—neck to knees
- Bare spots and broken hair
- Pattern to injury or bruising descriptive of object used to inflict injury
- Burns with sharply demarcated edges or circumferential patterns
- Perineal injuries of any kind

18-7. **Answer: 3**
Text page: 424, Table 18-1
Rationale: The 18 month old uses jargon and echolalia. The 24 month old talks in phrases and two to three word sentences. The 30-month-old toddler repeats two digits from memory, and the average sentence length is approximately two and a half words.

CHAPTER 19

19-1. **Answer: 4**
Text page: 440
Rationale: During the preschool years the genetic conditions that are most likely to appear are cystic fibrosis, Duchenne muscular dystrophy, fragile X syndrome, and Williams syndrome. Down syndrome usually is diagnosed soon after birth, because the infant exhibits physical characteristics that warrant evaluation for the chromosome karyotype. Congenital hypothyroidism and sickle cell disease are determined during the neonatal period through the newborn screening test.

19-2. *Answer: 1*
Text page: 440
Rationale: By age 4 or 5 children possess their own beliefs about health. They begin to understand that they play a role in their own health. The preschooler often becomes upset over minor injuries. Pain or illness frequently is viewed as punishment. The infant and toddler from 6 to 30 months will demonstrate signs of separation anxiety. The school-age child views illness as being related to failure to follow parents' instructions for wearing warm clothes, eating nutritious meals, and getting enough rest. The toddler responds to all interventions as if they will be painful, because pain is viewed concretely.

19-3. *Answer: 4*
Text pages: 442-443
Rationale: Most 4-year-old children play simple interactive games, dress themselves, copy a number of basic geometric figures well, and draw recognizable people. Preschoolers enjoy using language skills in telling stories and asking questions, and they can balance on one foot, jump, and run well. Because the child had an appendectomy 2 days earlier, the activity selected would have to be one that is appropriate for her condition and stage of recovery. Dressing up in fairy tale clothing would be an activity of a healthy 4-year-old, but not one who is recovering from surgery. Hopscotch is too vigorous. A game of Monopoly is at a higher level than her intellectual development. Drawing pictures of her family would be the best choice for a play activity.

19-4. *Answer: 2 and 3*
Text pages: 443-444
Rationale: Parents of preschoolers can benefit from the following recommendations:
* Bedtime rituals of 30 to 45 minutes are common.
* Night wakening events are common in the preschool years. Children who wake up at night should be reassured and encouraged to return to their own beds.
* Restricting frightening television shows and stories and discussing real versus pretend ideas and stories can help lessen the incidence of nightmares.

19-5. *Answer: 1*
Text pages: 444-445
Rationale: Piaget describes the preoperational stage of thinking as transductive reasoning. The child moves only from particular to particular in making associations and solving problems. The preschooler exhibits the concept of concrete thinking. At this stage, children concentrate on only their own per- spective. These children focus on one part of an object without shifting. The child does not possess the ability to consider more than one factor at a time when solving simple problems. The preschooler is not able to demonstrate the concept of irreversibility, being unable to connect the reverse operation to reach a logical conclusion.

19-6. *Answer: 2*
Text page: 452
Rationale: Preschoolers use many of the coping mechanisms developed during their toddler years, however, the preschooler generally shows greater ability to verbalize frustration, fewer temper tantrums, and more patience in experimentation to resolve difficulty than the typical toddler. Preschoolers refine their problem-solving skills. Through fantasy play, preschoolers investigate solutions or responses to stressful events and find inner control for challenging situations. Strict adherence to rituals or game rules controls situations for the preschooler. The preschooler has longer and more rigid bedtime rituals than the toddler.

19-7. *Answers: 1, 4, 5, 6*
Text page: 458
Rationale: There are many strategies that the nurse should recommend to parents to reduce or eliminate unintentional poisonings. Option 1 supports the ease of having the poison control number readily available in case of an emergency. Option 2 is incorrect, because syrup of ipecac is not administered for all swallowed poisons. Some poisons will cause more harm if vomiting is induced. Making the environment safe by keeping the products in their original containers and placing safety latches on drawers and cabinets that contain these chemicals help to prevent poisonings, because the child will not be able to get at the poison. Teaching the child about poisons is an important task so that the child will recognize when something is "bad." Never transfer products out of their original containers, because then it will be difficult to determine exactly what the chemical is and what the components of the product are.

CHAPTER 20

20-1. *Answer: 1*
Text page: 486
Rationale: Kohlberg describes the younger school-age child at the preconventional level of moral development, characterized by self-interest. This child behaves because there is a fear of punishment. The young child, approximately 6 or 7 years of age, views behavior as completely right or wrong. The

school-age child in the conventional level of moral development looks to others for approval.

20-2. **Answer: 4**
Text page: 492
Rationale: Acute lymphocytic leukemia is the most common form of cancer in the school-age population. Retinoblastoma, a tumor involving the retina of the eye, usually is diagnosed before the child is 2 years of age. Wilms tumor, affecting one or both kidneys, usually is diagnosed at approximately 2 years old. Neuroblastoma is a solid cancerous tumor that begins in the nerve tissue in the neck, chest, abdomen, or pelvis. It is primarily a disease of infancy and early childhood. More than 80% are recognized by 5 years of age.

20-3. **Answers: 2, 4, 5, 6**
Text page: 482, Health Teaching box
Rationale: The goal of discipline is to encourage and reinforce positive child behaviors, improve parent-child communication, meet parental needs, and eliminate inappropriate child behaviors. The specifics of discipline include:
- Using distraction or substitution to avoid a problem situation
- Using humor to decrease the intensity of the situation
- Modeling appropriate behavior
- Setting age-relevant limits
- Ignoring the misbehavior and acknowledging the appropriate behavior
- Offering choices to prevent inappropriate behavior such as whining or an emotional outburst
- Giving specific and clear commands for behavior appropriate to the child's age
- Talking calmly, being a good listener, and encouraging negotiation, perhaps in a family meeting, to allow problem resolution
- Setting clear and consistent consequences for misbehavior
- Providing one-to-one time, focusing on positive attention

20-4. **Answer: 1**
Text page: 474, Box 20-2
Rationale: Nursing interventions to prevent obesity during the school-age years include:
- Encourage the parents to evaluate their own nutritional values, patterns, and choices.
- Explain to parents that there is a relationship between eating in front of the television and obesity.
- Encourage the parents to assess snacking habits. Help parents choose healthy snacks such as fruits and vegetables.
- Help the child assess personal nutrition and make reasonable choices for diet improvement.

- Encourage the family to assess "fast food" eating habits and ways to change these habits.
- Encourage the child to occasionally prepare meals of his choosing that meet requirements of the food pyramid.

20-5. **Answer: 4**
Text pages: 474-475
Rationale: Helpful information for parents about nighttime enuresis includes:
- Usually no serious physical problems exist, although the parents should be told that it is uncommon after age 8.
- Enuresis is often inherited. With time and patience, the child will be cured.
- The child does not wet the bed intentionally; it is not a conscious act.
- The parents are not at fault for creating the problem in most cases.
- The child should be responsible for dealing with both the problem and the proposed treatment.
- Delivery of consequences to the child when wet should be replaced with praise when the child is dry.
- Parents might wake the child to urinate before they go to bed as one form of management.
- A family plan to deal with the wet bed may decrease family arguments.

20-6. **Answer: 1**
Text page: 481, Box 20-4
Rationale: Nursing interventions to help a child develop a positive self-concept during the school-age period include:
- Remind people that a sense of success is important for all children. They are mastering Erikson's stage of industry versus inferiority. All children must believe that they are good at something.
- Parents should learn the importance of giving positive feedback to their children, of setting realistic goals, of spending quality time with their children, and of helping them to attempt realistic tasks.
- School-age children should be encouraged to make choices to develop their sense of control and decision-making skills and to experience consequences of their choices.
- Questions of school-age children about bodily changes should be acknowledged and discussed sensitively.
- Discuss with the parents and the child that it is important for the school-age child to spend time with peers for social development.

20-7. **Answer: 3**
Text page: 487, Hot Topics box

Rationale: Suggestions for safe bicycling include (see also Web Site Resource 20E):

- Parents should discuss and enforce safe and permitted locations for a child's bike riding.
- Families should agree on some general rules for safe riding, such as not riding in the dark, while barefoot, with someone else on the bicycle, in bad weather, on poorly constructed surfaces, or with loose clothing that may get tangled in the wheels.
- Children on bicycles should wear properly fitting American National Standards Institute–approved helmets.
- Bicyclists must follow all traffic signs and signals.
- A front basket or back basket should be used for carrying objects, not a backpack.
- Children should ride on the side of the road traveling with traffic, keeping close to the side of the road.
- Children should approach intersections with caution and walk bikes in crosswalks.
- Children should not wear large hats or listen to music, because vision and hearing may be blocked.

CHAPTER 21

21-1. ***Answer: 4***
Text page: 505
Rationale: Washing with soap and water 2 or 3 times a day is the best way to remove dirt and oil. The adolescent should not attempt to remove the pustules and papules that form. Squeezing the lesions can result in further irritation of the glands and permanent injury to the tissue. Sunlight can have a beneficial effect on acne; however, prolonged exposure should be avoided. The effect of diet on acne is a highly controversial issue. Evidence indicates that dietary restrictions specific to acne are unnecessary.

21-2. ***Answers: 2, 4, 5***
Text pages: 508-509, Box 21-2
Rationale: Symptoms of anorexia nervosa include self-starvation with significant weight loss, amenorrhea, compulsive physical activity, preoccupation with food, and a distorted body image. Another eating disorder is bulimia nervosa, which involves a pattern of binge eating followed by purging by induced vomiting or use of laxatives. This person eats an increased amount of food in a discrete period.

21-3. ***Answer: 1***
Text page: 509, Research Highlights box
Rationale: The obese adolescent consumes too many calories for the amount of energy expended.

Studies have shown a strong correlation between inactivity, such as viewing television, and the tendency to be overweight. Teens who watch more than 5 hours of television each day are more than 4 times more likely to be obese than those who spend 2 hours or less in front the of the television. Depression is the strongest predictor of adolescent obesity.

21-4. ***Answer: 3***
Text page: 510
Rationale: Adolescence is characterized by a shift in cognitive abilities to Piaget's stage of formal operations. A behavioral manifestation of an adolescent's formal operations is intolerance of things as they are. They constantly challenge the way things are and challenge themselves to consider the way things can or should be. Adolescents begin to "think about their thinking." This causes them to become highly introspective. Introspection also combines with a reemergence of egocentrism leading to adolescents' sense of being the primary focus—special, unique, and exceptional. Teens can be vehement in trying to convince others of their viewpoints. Their idealism can lead to a rejection of family values, religion, or social causes.

21-5. ***Answer: 4***
Text page: 512
Rationale: Assessment, anticipatory guidance, education, and counseling are strategies the nurse can use to guide the adolescent in developing a healthy self-perception that incorporates a healthy body image. It is important for nurses to remember to praise adolescents for who they are rather than for what they do, value each of them as unique, demonstrate belief in their abilities to grow and develop, and delight in their discoveries of themselves and their unique means of expressing it.

21-6. ***Answer: 4***
Text page: 519
Rationale: Testicular cancer is the number 1 cancer in adolescent and young adult males. Adolescent males should learn to do a testicular self-examination and continue this practice monthly. Nurses should introduce and teach methods of self-examination to adolescents, who are naturally interested in their developing bodies. Even though the adolescent's body is undergoing anatomical changes, the primary reason for testicular self-examination is preventive for early identification of cancer. Baseline data collected during adolescence for future comparison is not a priority.

21-7. ***Answer: 1***
Text page: 518
Rationale: Because hepatitis B is sexually transmitted, this vaccine should be given to the sexually

active adolescent who has not received it. Data do not support administration of the measles, mumps, and rubella vaccine. Data should be collected from immunization records or from history of exposure to those communicable diseases. The influenza vaccine is given to adolescents who have chronic illness. The meningococcal meningitis vaccine is administered to college students residing in a dormitory.

21-8. **Answer: 4**
Text page: 515, Box 21-4
Rationale: Adolescents must be in charge of some aspects of life and can no longer accept family and school rules without question as they did in the past. This need to control extends to health care. The nurse cannot simply give directions or instructions but rather should present the options and partner with the adolescent to work out an acceptable plan. The primary discussion needs to be performed with the adolescent, instead of with the parents.

21-9. **Answers: 1, 2, 5**
Text page: 516, Box 21-5
Rationale: Typical warning signs of suicidal risk in adolescents include: behavior changes, increased risk taking, increased accidents, substance use or abuse, physical violence to self, others, or animals, decreased appetite, alienation from family or peer group, giving away personal items, writing letter or notes, essays, and poems with suicidal content, cognitive and mood changes, expression of hopelessness, increasing rage or anger, dramatic swings in affect, sleep disorders, preoccupation with death, difficulty concentrating, hearing voices or seeing things or people, and newfound interest in religion or a cult.

21-10. **Answer: 3**
Text pages: 504, 505, Figure 21-2
Rationale: Scoliosis screening begins during early adolescence. So that the entire back can be seen, the adolescent should remove all clothing from the upper body. While the adolescent stands up straight, check for asymmetry; observe and palpate for differences in shoulder or scapular height, a prominence of either scapula or hip, waist asymmetry, and misalignment of the spinous processes. Lateral curvature and thoracic convexity of the spine indicate scoliosis. With the feet together, legs straight, and arms hanging freely, the adolescent bends forward until the back is parallel with the floor. The adolescent is assessed for prominence of the ribs, or rib hump, on one side only and hip and leg asymmetry. With scoliosis, the chest wall on the side of convexity is prominent, and the scapula on the side of convexity is elevated.

21-11. **Answer: 2**
Text page: 503, Table 21-1
Rationale: Sexual maturity rating based on the Tanner scale for stage 2 female development includes: sparse growth of long, straight, downy hair along the labia; enlargement of areolar diameter, with a small area of elevation around papillae; and beginning breast bud.

CHAPTER 22

22-1. **Answer: 2**
Text page: 524
Rationale: *Healthy People 2010* documents that death rates related to traffic and motor vehicle injuries are highest in the age group of 15 to 24 years.

22-2. **Answer: 1**
Text page: 526
Rationale: After age 25 the emphasis is on modifying coronary risk factors. Recommendations for screening young adults are undergoing revision as more information becomes available about the interactive risks of high cholesterol levels, familial high lipid levels, diabetes mellitus, and smoking.

22-3. **Answer: 4**
Text page: 529
Rationale: Individuals most at risk for hepatitis C are those who have injected illicit drugs, received clotting factors before 1987, are on hemodialysis, are infected with HIV, or have elevated liver function values. The other diseases listed do not have a positive correlation to hepatitis C.

22-4. **Answer: 1**
Text page: 532
Rationale: Piaget's stage of formal operational thought evolves from concrete operational thought in adolescence and extends through the reasoning process of young adults. Achievement of formal operational thinking allows a person to analyze all combinations of possibilities and construct hypotheses that can being tested. Young adult thought becomes more perceptive and insightful; issues can therefore be evaluated realistically and objectively. The person in the concrete operational thought stage is able to manipulate concrete objects, participate in cooperative interactions, and perceive specific examples.

22-5. **Answers: 1, 3, 6**
Text page: 535
Rationale: Homicide is the second leading cause of death in those 15 to 24 years old and the leading

cause of death for black men in the same age category. Firearms are involved in approximately two thirds of these deaths, and men have twice the risk of dying than women. The presence of firearms in the home is associated with the increased risk of unintentional and intentional firearm injury to children. Violence is becoming more prevalent globally related to organized terrorism.

22-6. **Answer: 2**
Text page: 544
Rationale: Known risk factors for cervical cancer include smoking, early age of first intercourse, increasing number of sexual partners, and infection with human papilloma virus.

22-7. **Answer: 4**
Text page: 536, Hot Topics box
Rationale: Epidemiological studies have attempted to determine the risks for intimate partner violence. Poverty and associated stress stemming from lack of economic resources appear to contribute to abuse against women. The unequal position of women in a relationship and the manner in which conflict is managed, as well as differences in education and prestige associated with the partner's occupations, are related to risk of violence.

CHAPTER 23

23-1. **Answer: 3**
Text page: 549
Rationale: Physiological changes that occur during middle adulthood include:
- Hair of the adult begins to thin and turn gray.
- The skin's moisture and turgor decrease and with the loss of subcutaneous tissue, wrinkles appear.
- Fat deposits increase during these years with increases in weight gain.
- Cardiac output decreases.
- Bone density and mass progressively decrease.
- Thinning of the intervertebral disks accounts for approximately a loss of 1 inch in height.
- Acid indigestion and belching increase due to decreased gastrointestinal motility.
- Stools become harder and dry due to deceased gastrointestinal motility.
- As blood supply to the kidneys decreases, the glomerular filtration rate is decreased.
- Blood vessels lose elasticity and become thicker.

23-2. **Answer: 1**
Text pages: 549-550
Rationale: The three leading causes of death in both white and black populations are the same: heart disease, cancer, and cerebrovascular accident.

23-3. **Answer: 2**
Text pages: 555-556
Rationale: Moderation is the key, along with increased caution as the adult approaches age 65. The exercise program should be realistic and the activities selected should be ones that the individual enjoyed in the past. Activities should be selected with consideration of the potential for injury. Physical exercise should involve as many muscles as is possible, performed on a regular basis, preferably 3 to 4 times a week, for a minimum of 30 minutes each time. The appropriate level of performance for aerobic exercise is determined by achieving a pulse rate that is established for each individual: taking the number 220, subtracting the person's age, and then computing 75% of that number.

23-4. **Answer: 3**
Text page: 557
Rationale: Bloom (1984) developed a hierarchy of cognitive levels in the adult learner. The first level is knowledge, which is the recall of specifics. The second level is comprehension. The learner grasps the meaning of communicated messages and relates it to other material. The third level is application. The learner applies knowledge in the form of abstractions and ideas to concrete situations. Analysis is the fourth level, in which the adult breaks down the material into its constituent parts while noting their relationships. The final and fifth level is synthesis, in which the person is able to combine various elements to form a plan and then judge the extent to which the ideas and materials satisfy the established criteria.

23-5. **Answer: 1**
Text page: 566
Rationale: Nicotine acts on the two divisions of the nervous system: central the (brain and spinal cord) and peripheral (autonomic nervous system and motor and sensory fibers to the arms and legs). Nicotine stimulates the heart, leading to increased pulse and elevated blood pressure. Although smokers frequently believe that cigarettes have a calming effect, this notion is misleading. Nicotine stimulates the body, whereas increasing levels of carbon monoxide cause lethargy. Smokers may feel calm, although they are actually having their sensations dulled by the elevated level of carbon monoxide.

23-6 **Answers: 1, 2, 3, 4, 6**
Text page: 556, Box 23-3
Rationale: The developmental tasks of middle age include:
- Helping children become responsible, happy adults

- Rediscovering new satisfaction in the relationship with one's spouse
- Developing an affectionate, but independent, relationship with aging parents
- Reaching the peak in one's career
- Developing leisure-time activities
- Achieving mature social and civic responsibility
- Accepting and adapting to biological changes
- Maintaining or developing friendships

CHAPTER 24

24-1. **Answer: 4**
Text page: 583
Rationale: Ego integrity versus despair is the developmental stage of older adults. The quality associated with successful passage of this stage is integrity, defined as an honest acceptance of the life that has passed and the stage of life that is currently being lived. Individuals who have reached this stage are said to be at peace with themselves. The inability to reach this stage leads to fear of death and despair that life has been lived in vain. Ego differentiation, which is a part of the developmental stage of ego integrity, involves achieving an identity apart from work.

24-2. **Answer: 2**
Text page: 587, Table 24-2
Rationale: Nurses in the home care environment are in an ideal position to assess risks and prevent injuries in the older adult population. During the initial and subsequent assessments, the nurse can evaluate individuals' homes for factors common to poisoning, fires, and falls. Determining the causes of potential injuries in homes, such as frayed wires on electrical appliances that can produce sparks and start fires or improperly labeled cleaning products that can be accidentally ingested, allows the nurse to intervene at an early point to prevent injuries. Any rugs used in the kitchen must be the nonskid types. The person should also make sure that the floor has not been waxed, which would make it slippery. Most electrical outlets have two receptacles, so having two appliances plugged in would be acceptable.

24-3. **Answer: 4**
Text page: 576, Innovative Practice box
Rationale: A person who might benefit from geriatric assessment would be:
- Over age 80
- Falling frequently
- Losing weight because of poor nutrition
- Depressed because of loss of spouse and friends
- Experiencing mild memory loss
- Hospitalized 3 times in 2 months

- Taking more than 5 medications regularly and frequently getting them confused
- Without close family in the community
- In need of health teaching

24-4. **Answer: 1, 4, 2, 3, 6, 5**
Text page: 573, Table 24-1
Rationale: The ranking is determined by the number of chronic conditions by gender (female) per 1000 population.

24-5. **Answer: 1**
Text page: 592, Table 24-5
Rationale: Assisted living includes 24-hour oversight for people. The person must be mobile but may require some assistance. All meals and snacks are provided. Persons may request assistance with bathing and hygiene. Housekeeping and laundry services are provided. Individuals may require occasional assistance with dressing. The person should self-administer medications, or personnel may monitor medication administration. Option 2 describes the care rendered in a nursing facility. Options 3 is found in a retirement community. Option 4 is the expectation of clients in an independent living community.

CHAPTER 25

25-1. **Answer: 4**
Text page: 604
Rationale: Infectious diseases are the major disease conditions found in developing African countries. The number 1 cause of mortality is HIV leading to AIDS.

25-2. **Answer: 2, 1, 3, 4**
Text page: 611
Rationale: Data compilation of the homeless population states that families with children account for 36.5%, single men for 46%, single women for 14%, and adolescents for 3.5%.

25-3. **Answer: 2**
Text page: 605, Box 25-1
Rationale: The five major pandemics are malaria, AIDS, tuberculosis, hepatitis, and influenza.

25-4. **Answer: 1**
Text page: 609, Hot Topics box
Rationale: It is believed that SARS is spread by close person-to-person contact, especially by respiratory droplets. Examples of close contact include kissing or hugging, sharing eating or drinking utensils, talking to someone within 3 feet, and touching

someone directly. Close contact does not include activities such as walking by a person or briefly sitting across a waiting room or office. The virus can be deposited on the mucous membranes of the mouth, nose, or eyes of a person who is within a 3-foot distance when an infected person coughs or sneezes. The early symptoms include high fever, headache, malaise and body aches, diarrhea, and mild respiratory symptoms. Two to seven days later, dry cough develops.

25-5. **Answer: 4**
Text page: 610, Health Teaching box
Rationale: In China and Malaysia 30% of male teenagers smoke. In the Philippines the number is higher, at 40%.